Biodiversity of Malaria in the World

ISBN 978-2-7420-0616-8

Éditions John Libbey Eurotext
127, avenue de la République, 92120 Montrouge, France
Tél : 01 46 73 06 60
E-mail : contact@jle.com
Site internet : http://www.jle.com

John Libbey Eurotext Limited
42-46 High Street
Esther, Surrey, KT 10 9QY
United Kingdom

© 2008, John Libbey Eurotext, Paris

It is prohibited to reproduce this work or any part of it without autorisation of the publisher or of the Centre Français d'Exploitation du Droit de Copie, 20, rue des Grands-Augustins, 75006 Paris, France.

Biodiversity of Malaria in the World

English version completely updated

Coordinated by: Sylvie Manguin, Pierre Carnevale
and Jean Mouchet

Marc Coosemans
Jean Julvez †
Dominique Richard-Lenoble
Jacques Sircoulon

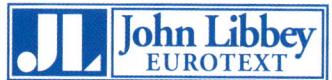

Carnevale Pierre, PhD, Research Director, Institute of Research for Development (IRD), Montpellier, France.

Coosemans Marc, PhD, Professor, Prince Leopold Institute of Tropical Medicine (ITM), Antwerp and Faculty of Biomedical Sciences, University of Antwerp, Belgium.

Julvez Jean (†), MD, PhD, Inspector-General of Health.

Manguin Sylvie, PhD, Research Director, Institute of Research for Development (IRD), Montpellier, France.

Mouchet Jean, Pharmacist, Honorary Inspector-General, Institute of Research for Development (IRD), Paris, France.

Richard-Lenoble Dominique, MD, Professor, Department of Parasitology and Tropical Medicine, Medical University of Tours, France.

Sircoulon Jacques, PhD, Hydrology Engineer, Institute of Research for Development (IRD), Saint-Germain-en-Laye, France.

Foreword

"Intermittent fevers" were described by Hippocrates in the 5th century BC, and later, by Celsus in the 1st century AD. In the 17th century, Europeans discovered from Amerindian traditional medicine that cinchona bark had curative effect against malaria fevers. Then it is only in 1880 that the mystery of malaria began to be lifted with the identification of the pathogen, *Plasmodium*, by Alphonse Laveran in Constantine (Algeria). In the following decade, the parasite's life cycle with *Anopheles* as biological vector was elucidated by Ross in India and by Grassi *et al.* in Italy. This revealed the tight, *Anopheles*-dependent links between the disease and environmental conditions.

In the Age of Discovery, it emerged that such fevers were not the prerogative of Europe and the Mediterranean Basin but ravaged throughout most of the Tropics. Until the 19th century, Africa was known as the land of fevers, the "White Man's Grave", where just a few merchants, adventurers, explorers and missionaries dared to set foot. Quinine later opened the continent up for soldiers and colonial administrators. In Asia, danger spots—the mountainous jungles—rose from the healthy, densely populated, plains. Soon after the discovery of the Americas, the New World was being ravaged by malaria, introduced by slaves from Africa.

As of 1880, knowledge about the biology of parasites and vectors as well as about the epidemiology and distribution of the disease expanded at a great rate. In 1930, Hackett estimated that malaria had reached its epitome: the disease had spread to all parts of the world where conditions were propitious for the parasite's development.

By the end of the 18th century in Europe and North America, better standards of living coupled with improved environmental conditions (notably the removal of livestock from living quarters) was leading to regression of the incidence of malaria, although the disease remained a scourge around the Mediterranean peninsulas and islands—Italy, the Balkans, Corsica, Sardinia, Sicily and Cyprus. Measures to control malaria were designed on the basis of the knowledge at that time: prevention and treatment using quinine, zooprophylaxis, and vector control by the drainage and/or chemical treatment of potential larval habitats. In many places, such measures were highly effective: in Italy, the incidence of malaria had been reduced by 80% by 1940 and similar successes were achieved in other parts of Southern Europe, the Netherlands, North Africa and the United States; however, the results of trials in sub-Saharan Africa and in the Tropics in general were far less promising.

In 1945 at the end of the Second World War, malaria control strategies were revolutionised by the development of synthetic insecticides, notably DDT. In 1955 began the euphoric era of eradication in which control programmes were instigated in most countries on all the continents, apart from tropical Africa. Malaria was completely eradicated in many countries but, more importantly, the geographical territory of the disease and its incidence in affected zones were brought down by over 70%. By 1962 in pilot zones in West Africa, it was beginning to become apparent that the currently available means would never be able to block the transmission of malaria (Cavalié & Mouchet, 1962). Since Africa had never been included in the Global Eradication Programme, these observations raised little interest at the relevant international institutions at the time but, in subsequent years, difficulties were encountered in eradication programmes in many countries, leading to the repeated postponement of targets.

At the 1966 International Congress on Tropical Medicine and Malaria in Tehran, Gabaldon, one of the godfathers of eradication, reported that the ultimate goal was unachievable even in his own country, Venezuela. His announcement was no surprise to anyone who had worked in Africa but its effect was like that of a bombshell. In 1970, WHO decided to abandon a strategy aimed at eradication in favour of one of "control", although complete eradication was nevertheless preserved as the ultimate goal.

Beginning in 1970 and at a faster pace as of 1975, eradication programmes were abandoned one by one and replaced with poorly defined control programmes. Over the twenty subsequent years of prevarication, the number of cases of malaria steadily rose, reaching several million per annum outside of Africa.

A Global Malaria Control Programme was finally proposed at the 1992 Amsterdam Conference, to be based on strategies conceived in the light of epidemiological and ecological realities as well as the socio-economic capacities of different countries. Control would be based on diagnosing and treating patients, selective prophylaxis in high-risk groups, individual protection measures, and vector control. In addition, measures—notably training programmes—would be implemented to prevent and control epidemics of the disease.

In 1999, WHO launched the Roll-Back Malaria programme (RBM), the main goal of which is to reduce or abolish malaria mortality through concerted implementation of the Global Malaria Control Programme.

It is as yet too early to evaluate the outcome of this strategy which has proved difficult to implement in many places for economic reasons (a perennial obstacle) and because of the lack of trained and—even more important—motivated operatives. Lukewarm political responses—in which control is more often addressed with words than with concrete actions—has also slowed things down. *Plasmodium vivax* has even returned to places from which it had supposedly been eradicated (following the collapse of the Soviet Union but also in the Koreas, especially the North), as a result of health system breakdown.

The goal of this book is to detail the variable epidemiology of malaria across the planet. Countries and regions are home to different vectors according to local ecological conditions which dictate both their seasonality and geographical distribution. And it is the density and most importantly the longevity of the vectors coupled with their differential capacities to transmit the parasites which govern the incidence of malaria. We use the word "biodiversity" because it is the profile of anopheline species or taxonomic forms present which is the key determinant of the local intensity of the disease, the clinical cases of which ultimately represent only the tip of the iceberg. We have introduced the terms "facies" and epidemiological "stratum" to unite distinct geographical regions in which the same vectors cause similarly endemic disease with comparable morbidity and mortality rates. This classification system has been used for sub-Saharan Africa but it cannot be extended to the rest of the world because of the skewing effects of indoor insecticide spraying operations which have, in many places and/or at certain times, considerably reduced the prevalence and incidence of malaria thereby giving birth to "secondary facies" in which the disease rises and ebbs according to the efficacy of local treatment programmes.

We hope that this snapshot of the situation in 2002-2006 can be used as a basis to follow the fluctuations of malaria in coming years, even though the data that we have tried to gather is no doubt incomplete, despite our best efforts.

We address all the factors that could conceivably have an impact on malaria in both the short and medium terms: from natural climatic (global warming, El Niño, drought, floods) through man-made environmental modifications (deforestation, land clearance, surface water management, migration, urbanisation, transport), socio-economic (development) and even political (war, the break-up of states) phenomena. We end by reviewing current control methods, including the available drugs and patient care options, chemoprophylaxis, vector control, individual protection, the prevention and control of epidemics, and some perspectives for drug development and the future of immunisation.

Since 1975, WHO has been asking scientists (including those involved in basic research) to bring their expertise to the development of new ways of controlling malaria. After thirty years, it has to be said that the fruits have been few and far between. Only research in the pharmaceutical sector has yielded results with medicinal products available and the development of the artemisinin derivatives (natural products made from the plant *Artemisia annua* which has been in the traditional Chinese apothecary for over 3,000 years).

Despite optimism in the 1980's when it was predicted that an effective vaccine would be available within five years, there is no effective way of immunising against malaria. Current research is focusing on a vaccine aimed at a combination of three different targets, namely sporozoites and hepatic stages, erythrocytic stages, and vector stages (which would block development in *Anopheles*). However, none so far have proved either sufficiently immunogenic or long-acting to have a place in a rational immunisation strategy. And no one is in a position now to say when an effective vaccine might become available.

Apparently unfettered progress in molecular biology has yielded sequences for the genomes of the human host, one of the malarial parasites (*Plasmodium falciparum*) and a vector strain (*Anopheles gambiae* mixture of S and M forms). We are waiting to see what this new knowledge will contribute to malaria control in practical terms. Similarly, we are waiting to see whether and what the capability of generating transgenic *Anopheles* that cannot carry *Plasmodium* will bring; can they be used to compete out competent vectors? In any case, this possibility is probably not on the immediate horizon.

While we wait for the miracles of high technology, malaria is still a massive killer in the poorest countries of the world. Malaria control cannot be allowed to stagnate on the pretext that science will be providing new, more effective tools in the near future. The most has to be made of the tools at our disposal, and at the same time we must be ready to integrate any new drugs or vector control methods that emerge in as quickly as possible. It seems barely credible that a disease

Foreword

which is easy to cure at a very low cost is still killing a million people every year, mostly children. The response to AIDS should set an example in the fight against malaria.

This book represents the fruit of fifty years of experience and reflection about controlling malaria on the part of the authors—fifty years in which successive periods of euphoria and disappointment have never undermined our confidence that this scourge can one day be eliminated. Its writing has been a collective enterprise, based not only on our combined knowledge and expertise but also on friendship. Jean Mouchet has been the overall coordinator and has been involved in almost all the chapters. Jean Julvez who was one of the originators of the idea underlying the book died before his time. Marc Coosemans reread many of the chapters on Africa and Asia, and wrote much of the part on malaria control. Pierre Carnevale focused on the general sections and Africa, which he has rarely left in over twenty-five years. Sylvie Manguin has been an unpitying editor of almost the whole book, and wrote much of the chapter on the Americas. Dominique Richard-Lenoble wrote the part about treatment, drugs and chemoprophylaxis. Jacques Sircoulon put all his vast knowledge of climate and water systems at our disposal. Michèle Guillet compiled the reference section and the indices. Valérie Delplanque has been a dedicated secretary, forever available and attentive. All the authors have enthusiastically taken part in this collective effort.

Before concluding this foreword, it is a pleasurable duty to address—on behalf of all the authors—all those who have helped in the writing of this book as well as all our colleagues who welcomed us in the field and provided us with up-to-date information.

We would also like to thank Sanofi Aventis, especially its Impact Malaria Programme which is the embodiment of the company's commitment to helping developing countries control this formidable scourge. It is a concrete, long-term programme which aims to provide the poorest victims who are the most affected by the disease with effective ways of fighting it. The goals of Impact Malaria are to foster research to identify new drugs, to develop novel treatment strategies, to design training and education programmes to raise consciousness about the disease and how it can be treated, and to make every effort to ensure that people living in affected areas can get access to the drugs they so badly need.

We owe a great deal to Impact Malaria for distributing the book in poor countries. A special thank to Dr Jean-Marc Bouchez who has been responsible for the publication of this work.

We thank Dr. JE Najera, the former Director of the WHO Malaria Division for his encyclopaedic knowledge of the history of malaria control and the epidemiology of the disease which has been so precious to us. We also thank Dr. Umberto d'Alessandro of the Antwerp Institute of Tropical Medicine for writing the chapter on prophylaxis in pregnant women.

Dr. Pierre Guillet of WHO and his wife Michèle have always generously made themselves available to provide the Organisation's documents as well as those archived in the rich library in Geneva.

Dr. Anatoli Kondrashin has helped us with his extensive knowledge of malaria in the Russian-speaking parts of Europe and Asia.

Dr. Charles Delacollette and Dr. Morteza Zaim from Roll Back Malaria provided us with up-to-date information.

I cannot forget the archivist for the Malaria Division, Mireille Deplombain, for her search of particularly difficult to find literature which were often indispensable.

Our friend, Dr. Charles Ravaonjanahary, liaised with the African Regional Office and facilitated our access to a great deal of information on eastern and southern African countries.

Our friends, Dr. Sixte Blanchy and Dr. Ahmed Ouledi, who welcomed us in Madagascar and the Comoros Islands.

Dr. Jean-François Molez of IRD was a very dedicated collaborator in our work on the Congo, Senegal and Burkina Faso.

Professor Yeya Touré and Dr. Ogobara made us welcome in Mali and provided a great deal of pertinent information on malaria in that country.

Professor Jean Roux welcomed us at the Pasteur Institute of Antananarivo where we could develop (together with Drs. Stephane Laventure and Laurence Marrama) our surveys of mainland Madagascar. Special mention should be made of Sister Rosela who, despite many problems, kept the Analaora Dispensary open so that we could find all the information we needed about the epidemic of 1985-1987 in Madagascar.

Our collaboration with Dr. Ousmane Faye of the University of Dakar shed much light on the changes in vector ecology and malaria epidemiology seen during the drought in the Sahel.

Ambrose W. Onapa was involved in all the work on highland malaria in south-western Uganda.

The Muraz Centre at Bobo-Dioulasso in Burkina Faso has been a stopping point and reception centre for all the entomologists and many French-speaking and English-speaking parasitologists. Thank you to all the generations of staff, in particular Professor Robert Guigemdé, one of the few "survivors" of the storm that tore the OCCGE apart.

We were particularly warmly welcomed by Drs. Maureen Coetzee and Richard Hunt at the National Institute for Communicable Diseases in Johannesburg where we had very useful exchanges and were able to see research into malaria conducted between the World Wars. We regret the passing of our friend, Botha de Meillon, the former Director of the Institute, although he reached 98.

Thanks to Drs. P. K. Rajagopalan, then P. K. Das, the Directors of the Vector Control Research Institute at Pondicherry where we were able to get insight into the malaria situation in India, especially in Orissa and the south.

In Vietnam, we benefited from the experience of Professor Nguyen Tang Am, the author of the authoritative Treatise on Parasitology, Dr. Nguyen Tho Vien, a longstanding stalwart of malaria control, Dr. Ho Dinh Trung, our precious and knowledgeable collaborator on malaria vectors for more than 10 years, as well as Drs. Tho Sochantha from Cambodia and Kalounna Keokenchanh from Laos. Our current collaborations with the Institutes of Malariology, Parasitology and Entomology of Vietnam (Profs. Le Dinh Cong and Le Khanh Thuan), Laos (Dr. Samlane Phompida) and Cambodia (Dr. Doung Socheat), along with Mahidol and Kasetsart Universities of Thailand, respectively Dr. Visut Baimai and Dr. Theeraphap Chareonviriyaphap, represent a highly productive source of information and scientific exchange. We also thank Dr. Indra Vythilingam from the Institute for Medical Research, Kuala Lumpur, Malaysia for her knowledge on malaria vectors in Southeast Asia and her warm welcome in Malaysia.

Professors Neila Salazar and Dorina Bustos received us warmly in Manila and gave us a valuable, up-to-date picture of malaria in the Philippines.

At the South Pacific Commission in Nouméa, Dr. Sweeney gave us current literature on Australasia. At Namru 2 in Jakarta, Dr. Church told us about his most recent results from Western New Guinea and Dr. Mike Bangs contributed with us to the advances on the Sundaicus Complex.

Dr. Ralph E. Harbach of the Natural History Museum in London, Dr. Bruce Harrison from the Division of Environmental Health Services, Winston-Salem, North Carolina, USA and the late E. L. Peyton of the Walter Reed Biosystematics Unit in Suitland, Maryland, USA made their contributions by virtue of their understanding of malaria in Asia and in the Americas.

In Latin America, great thanks for welcoming us and for endless discussions on mosquitoes go to Dr. Yasmin Rubio-Palis from the Escuela de Malariologia y Saneamiento ambiantal, Maracay, Venezuela, and in Mexico, to Drs. Ildefonso Fernandez-Salas and Juan Arredondo-Jimenez from respectively the University of Nuevo Leon, Monterrey and Centro de Investigacion de Paludismo, Tapachula.

Our secretariat was helped by Yvonne Lafitte (IRD), Marinette Teppaz (ex-IRD), Sylvie Hart (IRD) and Suzanne Balthazar-Gajeski (Société de Pathologie Exotique).

I give my sincere thanks to all at Editions John Libbey Eurotext, in particular Mrs. Catherine Cahn and Mrs. Valérie Parroco.

Finally, it is a very pleasurable duty to be able to thank Professor Marc Gentilini who has agreed to write a preface to the book. A longstanding friend, Emeritus professor, member of National Academy of Medicine, former President of the French Red Cross (1997-2004), he has never ceased fighting on behalf of the most underprivileged. His work on behalf of Africa where malaria is such a major cause of mortality makes him ideal to introduce this work. At last but not least, we are extremely grateful to Dr. Donald R. Roberts of USUHS in Bethesda, Maryland, USA, internationally recognized as malaria expert and researcher particularly involved in the need for DDT to control malaria, for prefacing the English version of the book. He was one of our information sources on the Americas; his friendship and knowledge have substantially enriched this book.

Jean Mouchet

Preface

By virtue of its impact on humanity, malaria has long been considered as the most important of all transmissible, infectious diseases. It was the disease most dreaded by explorers who were reluctant to penetrate deep into the African continent until ways of protecting and treating it became available.

It is difficult to be sure about what exactly was meant by the word "fever" before the end of the 19th century, until which time malaria was regularly confused with other fevers of diverse etiologies, notably typhoid and yellow fever.

In the Tropics, the absence of the possibility of microscopic diagnosis in 90% of cases—at least in Africa—coupled with the failure of the health authorities to submit figures, undermine the reliability of the official WHO statistics.

In recent years, efforts have been made to produce more accurate mortality figures, resulting in an estimate of the annual number of deaths at 800,000-900,000 in Africa. This figure is probably closer to the truth than the estimate of between 1 and 2.7 million deaths annually published by WHO.

No recent surveys of morbidity have been conducted. The number of cases per annum in Africa is estimated at 200 to 300 million, while an estimated 430 million people are carrying the parasite.

The African situation is by far the worst. The main reason is the widespread presence of *Plasmodium falciparum* (the species which accounts for almost all malaria mortality). After a nadir in malaria incidence in 1970, the number of cases has steadily risen since 1975 because of the abandonment of indoor insecticide spraying operations when the establishment of primary health care systems was prioritised following the Alma Ata Declaration (1978).

Today, the biodiversity situation is still changing with the distribution and ecology of vectors evolving in an ever-changing man-made and climatic environment. This biodiversity is governed by a number of key determinants:
- biogeographical factors: the distribution of anopheline species and taxa;
- ecological factors: the ability of vectors to reproduce;
- biological factors: vector capacity (the ability to transmit *Plasmodium*) and the physiology of the various plasmodial species;
- environmental factors: short- and longer-term climatic variations (temperature, rainfall), the consequences of global warming, climatic phenomena (El Niño and the Sahelian drought).

Biodiversity also depends on man-dependent factors: deforestation, surface water management, urbanisation (which tends to reduce the incidence of the disease), rapid transport (imported and airport malaria) and economic changes—be they positive or negative.

Another key determinant is malaria control. The development of drug resistance has necessitated the substitution of monotherapy with combinations of drugs. Chemoprophylaxis is mainly targeted at pregnant women, tourists or emigrants returning home after spells abroad. Vector control—still as effective as ever wherever it is feasible—is based on indoor insecticide spraying and the use of treated mosquito nets although the efficacy of these measures is spatially restricted and mitigated by limited participation on the part of communities. In contrast, antilarval measures have only proven effective in a few very special cases.

What about research?

To combat the emergence and spread of resistance to chloroquine and other antimalaria drugs, few new drugs have been added to the therapeutic and prophylactic arsenals, although mefloquine and halofantrine have proven very valuable. More recently, artemisinin derivatives have raised hopes although these hopes remain fragile.

Apart from these advances, better, simpler diagnostic methods have been developed as has the use of insecticide-treated mosquito nets, although the overall picture is still less than satisfactory.

Certainly, we know more about *Plasmodium*, especially *Plasmodium falciparum* and its polymorphism but this has as yet had little practical impact on malaria control. Nor has elucidation of the mechanisms underlying resistance to drugs and insecticides yielded any concrete progress in the fight against the disease.

The regular announcements of imminent progress in the field of immunisation are all the more frustrating in the absence of any actual vaccine. Is it not paradoxical to propose a vaccine aimed at three targets when none at all have yet been developed, when no candidate has yet been shown to be immunogenic, and when how long any vaccine is likely to remain active is unknown? Is it really worth expending such great effort on preparing for vaccine trials when no vaccine is available?

This illusory hope is compromising practical control operations based on means that we actually have at our disposal—which are considerable. While it is true that political will is often lacking and civil unrest (especially in Africa) undermines such operations which require sustained effort, it is nevertheless unacceptable that this disease is still killing a million people every year. The WHO Roll Back Malaria programme must be supported to the hilt, but for this to happen, consciousness of the gravity of the problem will have to be raised and motivated, responsible operators ready to commit themselves will have to be engaged.

Jean Mouchet belongs to this band. He is an assiduous scientist, forever attentive, a sometimes pointed critic but always right, erudite but modest. Never one to shy away from knocking down a baseless theory, an incorrect assumption or an unrealistic speculation.

Dedicated for many years to vector control, to paying sufficient attention to environmental factors, and to analysing patients' clinical histories. In this book, Jean Mouchet (together with his collaborators) sheds new light on the epidemiological biodiversity of malaria throughout the world, based on years of experience and reflection over a long, distinguished career of service in the field of malaria control.

Professor Marc Gentilini

Preface to the English Version

The French version of this encyclopedic work was first published in 2004. After seeing the French text I expressed hope to co-author Sylvie Manguin that an English version would soon be available. That hope has now become reality, and I am greatly honored to write a preface to this long-awaited text.

In 2000 I attended an international conference on malaria in Lausanne, Switzerland. Jean Mouchet was there, and I enjoyed the brief times we had to discuss the environmental determinants of malaria and the burgeoning issues of malaria control. I valued his thoughts and views so much because he spoke from the perspective of one who has researched and worked with malaria for many years in numerous countries, especially those in Africa.

Jean Mouchet took prodigious notes during the Lausanne conference. I recall wondering how he could possibly use notes on such diverse topics as demography, climatology, and status and determinants of malaria in different regions around the world. A brief examination of topics covered in this book shows how those notes relate to Jean Mouchet's scholarly vocation. I now know that the note taking was Jean Mouchet, malaria expert and scholar, hard at work collecting data, synthesizing information, and documenting findings.

Jean Mouchet and his illustrative co-authors have produced an authoritative and invaluable referenced text. The authors have carefully documented a wealth of important facts. However, and perhaps more important than the facts themselves, is their careful interpretation of those facts in a global context of malaria diversity in the many countries, cultures and climates around the world. The authors engage controversial issues and contribute to those controversies by presenting facts and figures that are simply not available in any other malaria textbook. Not the least of those controversies is the role of climate change on the re-emergence of malaria and ongoing extensions of endemic malaria into regions that had been freed of malaria during the eradication era. The authors raise the issue of DDT and the unique chemical actions of DDT on vector behaviour and describe how those actions function to protect people from indoor transmission of malaria. They describe how DDT spraying can, in some environments, continue to control disease even when vectors are resistant to DDT toxicity. They engage the issues of malaria treatment, insecticide resistance, and changes in malaria control policies that have, directly or indirectly, contributed to the re-emergence of malaria. There is much in this book that has bearing on the modern public debate of how best to use new resources in the fight to reduce the burdens of malaria in Africa.

I am confident this comprehensive work will become the premier textbook on malaria. It should be required reading for any malaria worker or serious student of malaria. It covers a broad spectrum of current topics, to include the history and diversity of malaria and its vectors, malaria therapy, malaria epidemiology, vector control, the various facets of climatic and anthropogenic change, and distribution of malaria across the landscape. Many of these topics formed the centerpiece of research funded in the 1980s and 1990s by the U.S. National Aeronautics and Space Administration (NASA) to use remote sensing and geographic information systems to study environmental determinants of malaria in the Americas. Those technologies are increasingly a valuable part of malaria research and malaria control operations. Now, with renewed attention on the battle to control this ancient scourge of mankind, we owe a great debt of gratitude to Jean Mouchet and co-authors for this new and exciting textbook.

Donald R. Roberts, PhD, Professor

Malaria, a Vector-Borne Parasitic Disease

Increase Knowledge about Malaria and Development of Control Measures
Parasites and Vectors
Plasmodium Life Cycles in Humans and Anopheline Vectors
Epidemiological Basis
Man Facing Malaria
Year 2000: Time to Take Stock

Epidemiological Biogeography of Malaria

Malaria in the Main Biogeographical Regions
Afrotropical Region
Australasian Region
Oriental Region
Palaearctic Region
American Regions

Spatiotemporal Dynamics of Malaria

Climate and Malaria
Anthropogenic Changes of the Environment and Malaria
Habitat, Urbanisation and Professional Activities
The Role of Humans in the Dispersal of Malaria and its Vectors

Malaria Control

History of Control Policies
Patient Care and Malaria Diagnosis
Drug and Treatment Policies
Chemoprophylaxis
Prevention by Means of Control Vector
Detection, Control and Prevention of Epidemics
Vaccination

Contents

Malaria, a Vector-Borne Parasitic Disease

Increase Knowledge about Malaria and Development of Control Measures

Empirical period 3
Naturalist period 4
    Elucidation of *Plasmodium* life cycles 4
    Vector ecology and malarial control 5
Chemical phase: the dream of eradication 7
    Theory of eradication 7
    Failures and successes 9
    Drug development 9
Current questions: public health and research priorities 10

Parasites and Vectors

Early ancestors of *Plasmodium* and its vectors 12
Malaria parasites 12
    Plasmodium taxonomy 12
    Phylogeny 13
Malaria vectors 15
    Anopheles taxonomy 15
    Complexes of species 15
    Plasmodium "capture" by anophelines 16
    Vector species 17
    Anopheline biology 17
    Anopheline ecology and behaviour 20
        • Larval ecology 20
        • Ecology and behaviour of adults 20

Plasmodium Life Cycles in Humans and Anopheline Vectors

Pathogenic malaria complex 22
Plasmodium cycles 23
    Asexual phase in the human host 23
        • *Plasmodium falciparum* 23

Biodiversity of Malaria in the World

• *Plasmodium malariae*	23
• *Plasmodium vivax* and *Plasmodium ovale*	24
Sexual phase in *Anopheles*	25
Polymorphism in *Plasmodium falciparum*	26

Epidemiological Basis

Requisites for autochthonous malaria	27
Malaria indicators	27
Diagnosing plasmodial infection	27
Parasitological indicators	29
• Prevalence	29
• Parasite load and pyrogenic threshold	30
• Incidence	31
• Gametocyte Rate	31
Serological indicators	31
• Theoretical aspects and technical solutions	31
• Interpreting results	32
Measuring transmission and estimating infection levels in populations	32
Sporozoite Rate	32
Entomological Inoculation Rate and Parasite Inoculation Rate	33
Stable and unstable malaria	34
Vectorial Capacity	35
Parasite Propagation Rate	35
Classifying malaria endemicity	35
Epidemiological facies and strata	36
Epidemics	36
Man, carrier of malaria	37

Man Facing Malaria

Pathogenicity	38
The human victim	39
Difficulties in diagnosing and defining malaria disease	39
Simple primary paroxysms, relapses and recrudescence	39
Severe *Plasmodium falciparum* malaria	40
Very low parasitaemia	40
Human resistance to malaria parasites	40
Resistance of Melano-Africans to *Plasmodium vivax*	40
Development of immunity	41
Genetics and the host-parasite relationship	41
Haemoglobinopathies	42
Malaria mortality	43
Measuring mortality	43
• Direct method	43
- Official State figures	43

- Autopsies	43
- Verbal autopsies	43
• Indirect methods	44
Variable mortality rates	44
Epidemics and mortality	45
Medium-term consequences of vector control on malaria mortality: a controversial subject	46

Malaria morbidity ... 46
Measuring morbidity ... 46
Malaria morbidity on the different continents ... 46

Year 2000: Time to Take Stock

Malaria and malaria control over the last two centuries ... 48
An overview of malaria 2000 ... 48
Health figures ... 49
• How many people die of malaria every year? ... 49
• Malaria morbidity on the different continents ... 49
Towards a new geography of malaria ... 50
• Maps ... 50
- National and regional maps ... 50
- Global maps ... 50
• Epidemiological classification of malaria regions ... 51
- Areas of high endemicity ... 51
Afrotropical area ... 51
Australasian expanse ... 52
- Foci ... 52
Southeast Asian forest ... 52
Historical epidemic foci ... 52
Afghanistan and Tajikistan ... 52
Turkey ... 52
Meso-American foci ... 52
Guyana and its neighbours ... 52
The Amazon ... 52
North-western Andes ... 53
- Regions with very low-level disease ... 53
- "Re-emergent" malaria ... 53
The socio-economic impact of malaria ... 53
• Malaria and poverty ... 53
• Cost of prevention and treatment ... 54
- Personal medical costs ... 54
- Medical costs for health care services ... 54
• Infant mortality and birth rates ... 54
• Productivity ... 54
• Financial needs in the next decade ... 54

Epidemiological Biogeography of Malaria

Malaria in the Main Biogeographical Regions

Factors which affect the distribution of malaria 59
Major malaria biogeographical regions 59
    Afrotropical (or Ethiopian) Region 60
    Australasian (or Oceanian) Region 60
    Oriental Region 61
    Palaearctic Region 62
    American Regions 63
Classification of regions 63

Afrotropical Region

Main characteristics of malaria in the Afrotropical Region 64
    Peoples and countries 64
    Geography, elevation, climate, flora and fauna 64
    Malaria vectors 66
        • *Anopheles gambiae* Complex 66
            - *Anopheles gambiae s.s.* Giles 1902 68
            - *Anopheles arabiensis* Patton 1905 70
            - *Anopheles merus* Dönitz 1902 and *Anopheles melas* Theobald 1903 71
            - Zoophilic species of the *Anopheles gambiae* Complex 72
        • *Anopheles funestus* Group 72
        • *Anopheles nili* Theobald 1904 Group 74
        • *Anopheles moucheti* Evans 1925 Complex 74
        • Localised species and secondary vectors 75
    Parasites 76
        • *Plasmodium falciparum* 76
        • *Plasmodium vivax* 76
        • *Plasmodium malariae* 76
        • *Plasmodium ovale* 76
        • Haemoglobinopathies 76
    Epidemiological strata 77
        • Epidemiological facies and strata 77
        • Equatorial stratum 78
        • Tropical stratum 79
        • Sahelian and Sub-desert strata 79
        • Southern stratum 80
        • Mountainous strata 81
    Local and anthropogenic facies 82
        • Relief 82
        • Soil 83
        • Water systems 83
            - Rivers and streams 83
            - Lakes and lagoons 83

• Anthropogenic modifications of the environnement	83
Stability of malaria, Sporozoite Rates and Inoculation Rates	84

Malaria in the different countries of the Afrotropical Region — 84

West Africa	85
• Countries on the Atlantic coast	85
- Republic of Cape Verde	86
- Mauritania	86
- Senegal and Gambia	87
Senegal River Valley	88
Sahel	89
Coastal Sahel: the Niayes	89
Sudanese zone	90
Casamance	91
Mangrove of the southern rivers	91
Urban malaria	91
- Guinea-Bissau	92
- Guinea	93
- Sierra-Leone	93
Malaria in the estuary of Freetown	93
Transmission in rural zones	94
Epidemiology	94
- Liberia	94
• Nations of the northern coastline of the Gulf of Guinea	95
- Ivory Coast	96
Description	96
A long epidemiological history	97
Malaria in the southern forest region	97
Malaria in the wet savannah	98
Bouaké	98
Impact of rice farming	98
Anopheles gambiae resistance to pyrethroids	98
Drug resistance	99
Malaria mortality and morbidity	99
- Ghana	99
Malaria in the Accra Region	99
Malaria in rural areas	99
Lake Volta and the Volta Region	100
Diagnosis and clinical incidence	101
Control measures	101
- Togo	101
Malaria	102
Malaria and nutrition	102
- Benin	102
Vectors and transmission	102
Epidemiology	103
- Nigeria	103
Demographics	104
Vectors and general characteristics of malaria	104
Southern Nigeria	104
Northern savannahs	105
Clinical research	106
• Sahelian States	106
- General characteristics of the Sahelian States	106
- Mali	107
Epidemiology of malaria	107

Vectors	107
Haemoglobinopathies	109
- Burkina Faso	109
Epidemiology of malaria in the Sudanese zone	109
Epidemiolgy of malaria in the Sahelian zone	110
Urban malaria	110
Entomological research in Burkina Faso	111
Human genetics	111
- Niger	111
Epidemiology of malaria	112
- Chad	113
Epidemiology and entomology	113
Central Africa	114
• Geographical boundaries and general characteristics	114
• Cameroon	114
Epidemiology	114
Entomology	115
Morbidity	116
Mothers and children	117
Genetics	117
Gametocytes in the blood	117
• Central African Republic	117
Epidemiology	117
Entomology	117
Rodent *Plasmodium*	117
• Equatorial Guinea	118
• The Republic of São Tomé and Principe	118
• Gabon	118
Epidemiology	118
Entomology	119
• The Republic of Congo	120
Epidemiology	120
Morbidity and mortality	122
Entomology	123
• The Democratic Republic of Congo	123
History	124
Epidemiology	124
Entomology	125
Malaria morbidity and mortality	126
• Rwanda and Burundi	126
Epidemiology	127
- Rwanda	128
- Burundi	130
Endemic disease and epidemics	130
Entomology	132
East Africa	132
• Geographical boundaries and general characteristics	132
• Sudan	132
Epidemiology	133
Entomology	135
Epidemiology of unstable malaria	135
• The Horn of Africa	136
- Ethiopia	137
Epidemiology	137

Entomology	138
Problems of displaced populations	139
- Eritrea	139
- Republic of Djibouti	140
- Somalia	141
• The Plateaux of East Africa	142
- Geographical, climatic and ethnic characteristics	142
- Kenya	142
Epidemiology	142
Hyperendemic plateaux	142
Coastal regions	143
Mountain epidemics	143
Epidemics of the semi-dry regions and the effects of El Niño	145
Entomology, taxonomy, and ecology	145
Transmission	146
Mapping malaria and predicting epidemics	146
- Uganda	147
Natural regions and endemicity	147
Vectors	148
Regional epidemiology	148
Occupational malaria	151
Refugee camps	151
- Tanzania	151
Epidemiology	151
Research on transmission	152
Entomology	152
Malaria control programmes	153
Plasmodial biology	153
Southern Africa	154
• Boundaries and characteristics of Southern Africa	154
• Angola	154
• Zambia	156
Epidemiology	156
Entomology	158
• Malawi	158
• Mozambique	159
Epidemiology	159
Entomology	161
• Zimbabwe	161
Epidemiology	161
Entomology	163
• Swaziland	163
Epidemiology	163
Entomology	164
• Botswana	164
• Namibia	164
• South Africa	165
History of malaria and the malaria control programme	165
Epidemiology	166
Entomology	167
South-western islands of the Indian Ocean	167
• Geographical and historical outline	167
• Madagascar	168
Geography	168

Biodiversity of Malaria in the World

    History 168
    History of epidemics and the malaria control programme 169
    Epidemiological coverage and stratification 170
    Entomology 173
  • Comoros Islands 174
    History of malaria 175
    Stratification and diversity of malaria on the four islands 175
    Malaria vectors in the Comoros 177
  • Mascarene Islands 177
   - Epidemics and how malaria became endemic in Mauritius 177
    Eradication and re-introduction 178
    Why malaria became established in Mauritius 178
   - Epidemics and how malaria became endemic in La Réunion 178
  • Seychelles 179

Australasian Region

Geography and malaria prevalence 180
Anopheline vectors 181
  Taxonomy and distribution 181
  Larval ecology 181
  Adult ecology and behavioural changes 183
  Vectorial capacity and vector longevity 183
  Parasites and immunity 183
The malaria situation in the islands groups 184
  The Molucas or Maluku 184
  Western New Guinea and Papua New Guinea 184
  Solomon Islands 186
  Vanuatu 186
  Australia 187
Conclusion 187

Oriental Region

Limits and subdivisions of the Oriental Region 188
Populations and ethnic minorities 189
Forest malaria and migration 191
  Traditional jungle exploitation 192
  Industrial exploitation of jungle resources 192
  Permanent settlements within the jungle 193
  Degradation of the jungle 193
  Occupational malaria. Temporary labour 193
  Population displacements and migration 193
Parasites 194
  Plasmodial species 194
  Asymptomatic malaria 195

Biodiversity of Malaria in the World

The eradication period	270
Implementation of the Global Control Strategy	272
Current malaria situation	272
Ecological zones	**272**
Coastal	273
Wooded lowlands	274
Savannah	274
Foothills	274
• East of the Andes	274
• West of the Andes	274
• Mexico, Central America and the Caribbean islands	275
High valleys	275
North America	275
Anopheline vectors	**275**
Regional vectors	275
• *Anopheles darlingi*	275
• *Anopheles albimanus*	276
• *Anopheles aquasalis*	278
• *Anopheles nuneztovari*	278
• *Anopheles pseudopunctipennis*	278
• *Anopheles vestitipennis*	279
• Maculipennis Group	279
Local vecctors	280
Parasites	**280**
Epidemiology	**280**
Country by country	**282**
North America	282
• United States	282
• Canada	282
• Mexico	282
Central America	282
• Guatemala	283
• Belize	283
• Honduras	283
• El Salvador	284
• Nicaragua	284
• Costa Rica	284
• Panama	284
Caribbean islands	285
• Haiti and the Dominican Republic	285
• Cuba, Jamaica, Puerto Rico, the Lesser Antilles, Grenada, Trinidad and Tobago	285
South America	286
• The Andes	286
- Venezuela	286
- Colombia	287
- Ecuador	288
- Peru	288
- Bolivia	289
• The Southern Cone	290
- Chile	290

Mediterranean Subregion 246
Climate and the history of malaria 246
The disease today and control measures 246
The Maghreb 247
- Characteristics 247
- Morocco 247
- Algeria 248
- Tunisia 248
Libya and Egypt 249
Eastern Mediterranean countries 250
Turkey 251

Arabo-Persian Subregion 252
Limits and characteristics 252
Geography 252
Arabian Peninsular 253
Mesopotamian plain and the plateaux of Iran and Afghanistan 256
- Iraq 256
- Iran 257
- Afghanistan 259
Central Asia 259

Chinese Subregion 260
Borders 260
General characteristics 261
China 261
- Stratification 261
- Changes in the malaria situation 262
Korea 263
Japan 263
Far-eastern Russia 263

American Regions

Introduction of malaria into the Americas 265
History, development and distribution of malaria 265
From Colombus to DTT 266
- North America and Mexico 266
  - Canada 266
  - United Sates 266
  - Mexico 266
- Central America and the Caribbean 267
  - Central America 267
  - The Caribbean 267
- South America 267
  - The south-west: Argentina, Bolivia, Chile, Paraguay, Peru 269
  - The northern Andes: Colombia, Ecuador, Venezuela 269
  - Guyana and its neighbours 269
  - Brazil 270

Biodiversity of Malaria in the World

Tribal malaria	220
Urban malaria	221
Malaria in different countries	221
• India	221
• Pakistan	223
• Afghanistan	224
• Sri Lanka	224
• Maldives	225

Palaearctic Region

Borders and subdivisions	226
General characteristics	227
Diverse climates and flora	227
Highly variable population densities and levels of economic growth	227
Propitious conditions for malaria control	228
What does the future hold for Eurasian malaria?	229
Parasites	229
Frequency of the various parasite species	229
Plasmodium vivax "hibernation"	230
• *Plasmodium vivax* hibernation in the northern regions	230
• Gonotrophic dissociation in winter	230
Haemoglobinopathies	231
Vectors	231
Maculipennis Subgroup	231
• *Anopheles sacharovi* and *Anopheles martinius*	232
• *Anopheles labranchiae* and *Anopheles sicaulti*	232
• *Anopheles atroparvus*	233
• *Anopheles maculipennis*	234
• *Anopheles messae* and *Anopheles beklemishevi*	234
• *Anopheles melanoon*	235
• *Anopheles daciae* and *Anopheles persiensis*	235
• Compatibility of different plasmodia with the various members of the Maculipennis Subgroup	235
Anopheles sergentii (Theobald 1907)	235
Anopheles superpictus (Grassi 1899)	236
Hyrcanus Group	236
• *Anopheles hyrcanus*	236
• *Anopheles sinensis* and *Anopheles lesteri*	236
Secondary and localised vectors	237
Oriental and Afrotropical vectors in the Palaearctic Region	238
Euro-Siberian Subregion	238
Climatic changes and the history of malaria	238
Control and eradication of malaria	239
Mediterranean peninsulas and islands	240
Western, Central and Northern Europe	242
Eastern Europe and Siberia	243
Caucasian Republics	244

Vectors	195
General information about the anopheline fauna of the Oriental Region	195
Minimus Complex	195
Leucosphyrus Group	198
• Dirus Complex	198
• Leucosphyrus Complex	200
- *Anopheles balabacensis*	200
- *Anopheles latens*	200
- *Anopheles leucosphyrus*	200
Maculatus Group	200
Sundaicus Complex	201
Vectors of Malaysia, Indonesia and the Philippines	202
Anopheles fluviatilis James 1902	204
Anopheles culicifacies Giles 1901	205
Anopheles stephensi Liston 1901	206
Palaeartic species that overflow into the Oriental Region	207
• "Chinese" species	207
• Palaearctic species	207
Vectors of limited significance	207
The epidemiology of malaria in the Indo-Chinese Subregion	208
General characteristics and stratification	208
Country by country	209
• Nepal	209
• Bhutan	210
• Northeast India	210
• Bangladesh	210
• Myanmar	211
• Thailand	211
• Cambodia	211
• Laos	213
• Vietnam	213
• Southern China	214
• Taiwan	214
• Japan	214
The epidemiology of malaria in the Malayo-Indonesian Subregion	215
General characteristics	215
Country by country	216
• Malaysia	216
• Indonesia	216
- Java and Bali	216
- Sumatra	217
- Kalimantan	217
- Sulawesi	217
- Lombok, Soembava, Soemba, Flores, West Timor	217
• East Timor	217
• Philippines	217
The epidemiology of malaria in the Indo-Pakistani Subregion	218
General characteristics of the subregion	218
The balance between *P. vivax* and *P. falciparum* and haemoglobinopathies	219
Epidemic malaria	219

- Argentina	290
- Paraguay	290
- Uruguay	291
• Guyana and its neighbours	291
- Guyana	291
- Suriname	292
- French Guiana	292
• Brazil - Amazonia	293
- Migrations and recent epidemiological changes	294
- Malaria and the Amerindians	294
- Primate malaria	294
- Regional epidemiology	295
Conclusions on malaria in the Americas	298

Spatiotemporal Dynamics of Malaria

Climate, humans and malaria from a global point of view	301
Malaria determinants	302

Climate and Malaria

Direct impact of temperature and rainfall on malaria	303
Malaria since the Quaternary Period	303
Appearance of humans and of the pathogenic malaria complex	303
Glaciation events and post-glacial periods in Holarctic Regions	304
Recent climatic changes in the Palaearctic Region	305
Recent climatic changes in the tropics	306
Global warming	308
El Niño, La Niña and the ENSO	309
• Global climatic effects of the El Niño (a hot episode)	310
• Regional effects: the Sahel	311
• Regional effects: southern Africa	311
• The exceptional El Niño of 1997-1998	311
Climate and other factors that affect malaria	311

Anthropogenic Changes of the Environment and Malaria

Different stages of demographic and technological development	312
Changes in vegetation	313
Deforestation	313
• Forests and forest-dwellers	313
• Exploitation of forest	313

• Destruction of the forest	314
Damaged herbaceous strata	314
• Over-grazing of dry pastureland	314
• Draining wetlands	314

Interference with surface water — 315

Bore holes	315
Cisterns and wells	315
Dams and watering basins	315
Irrigation ditches and irrigated land	316
Rice paddies	316

Cultivation and animal husbandry — 317

Arable farming	317
Livestock raising	318

Habitat, Urbanisation and Professional Activities

Habitat — 320

Habitat and dwellings	320
Building houses	321

Urbanisation — 321

Urban malaria	321
Urbanised malaria	322
Malaria-free towns	322

Excavation work — 322

The Role of Humans in the Dispersal of Malaria and its Vectors

Spread of the parasites and the disease — 324

Great historical migration events	324
• Population displacements at the dawn of humanity	324
• Migrations in the Afrotropical Region	324
• Migrations in Southeast Asia	325
• Arrival of Europeans and the slaves in the Americas	325
Recent and ongoing migration events	326
• Reasons for population shifts	326
• Rural exodus	326
• Quest for arable land	326
• Refugees and people who have been displaced within their own country of birth	326
• Temporary, seasonal and long-term migrants	327
• Travellers	327
Risks associated with migration	327
• Risks to the migrants	327
- For those from malaria-free places	327
- For those from malaria-endemic places	328
• Malaria in refugees	328
• Epidemiological dangers for the host country	328
Imported malaria	329

- • Backgroud 329
- • Impact on public health 329
- • Marginal cases 329
- • Seriousness of imported malaria 331

Anthropogenic vector spread 331
Introduction of *Anopheles* 331
- • Active spread 331
- • Passive spread 332
Vector acclimatisation and establishment 332
Epidemiological consequences of vector importation 333

Airport malaria 333
Earliest cases 333
Scale of the problem 334
Infection pathways 334
- • Inside airplanes 334
- • Inside the airport and associated buildings 334
- • Infection of those living near the airport 334
- • Infection further away 334
- • Baggage handling 335
Sources of infection 335
Distribution of cases 335
Uncertainties of airport malaria 336

Malaria Control

History of Control Policies

Control measures before the Second World War 339
- Italian strategy 339
- Larval control in the Americas 340
- Adult control by indoor pyrethrin spraying 340
- Return to drugs 340
- Disappearance of malaria from Europe 341

World Eradication Programme 341
- DDT and the hope of eradication 341
- Launch of the Eradication Programme 341
- Eradication problems 342
- End of the programme: lessons learned 342

Revision of the Global Malaria Control Strategy in 1992 342
- Problems with the switch from eradication to control 342
- Amsterdam Conference (1992) and the Revised Global Malaria Control Strategy ... 342

Conclusion 343

Patient Care and Malaria Diagnosis

Clinical diagnosis 345
    Attitudes of mothers and family members 345
    Attitudes of local health care workers 346
Parasitological diagnosis 346
Modern diagnostic methods 346
    Simple attacks 346
    Severe paroxysms 346

Drug and Treatment Policies

National drug policies 349
    Choice of drugs 349
    Changing national policies: monotherapy or multiple drugs? 349
Therapeutic arsenal 351
    Drugs used in monotherapy 351
    Combination therapy 352
    New drugs in development 353
    Counterfeit drugs and inappropriate products 354
Resistance to malaria drugs 354
    What induces resistance 354
    Monitoring resistance 354
        • *In vivo* tests 354
        • *In vitro* tests 355
        • Molecular methods 355
    Distribution of resistance 355
Treatment 355

Chemoprophylaxis

Definition and mass trials 357
Prophylaxis for pregnant women 357
    Rationale 357
    Intermittent Preventive Treatment (IPT) 358
    Insecticide-treated mosquito nets in the protection of pregnant women 358
    Conclusions: the future 359
Prophylaxis for travellers 359
    Destination 359
    Other factors which determine prophylactic strategy 359
    Prophylaxis 359
Prophylaxis for non-immune inhabitants 360

Prevention by Means of Vector Control

Objectives 361
Targets 361
Personal measures 363
   Treated mosquito nets and protective screens 363
   Treated curtains 365
   Protecting living quarters 365
   Domestic spraying of insecticide and repellents 365
      • Repellent products 365
      • Domestic insecticide products 366
   Clearance of larval habitats around the house 367
Community-based preventive measures 367
   Methods 367
   Indoor spraying with long-acting insecticides 367
      • Vector behaviour in response to indoor spraying 367
      • Insecticide toxicity and excito-repellent effects 368
      • Current trends 368
      • Insecticide: choice, safety, poisoning 369
      • Application 370
         - Logistics 370
         - Formulations, specifications, dosages, cycles 370
         - Method of application and auxiliary equipment 371
      • Treating the tents of nomads and refugees 372
      • Indoor low volume insecticide spraying 373
   Community-based protection using treated nets 373
      • Mass effect 373
      • Efficacy 373
         - Fewer bites 374
         - Curtailed transmission 374
         - Lower incidence 374
         - Reduced mortality 374
         - Curtains 374
      • Problems associated with treated nets 375
   Antilarval and environmental measures 376
Resistance to insecticides 377
   Main resistance mechanisms 378
   Resistance and control measures 378
   What to do about resistance 379

Detection, Control and Prevention of Epidemics

Control of epidemics 381
   Detection 381
   Combating epidemics 381
Prevention 382
   Predicting epidemics? 382
   What strategy to adopt? 383

Biodiversity of Malaria in the World

Temporal and spatial targeting 383
  • Targeting in time 383
  • Targeting in space 383
Reflections on different vector control methods 383

Vaccination

Vaccines and fundamental problems associated with the physiology of *Plasmodium* 384
Candidate antigens 385
Vaccine trials 385
Until a vaccine is developed 385

Bibliography 387
Species Index 425

Malaria, a Vector-Borne Parasitic Disease

Increase Knowledge about Malaria and Development of Control Measures

The history of the growth in our knowledge about malaria and the development of disease control can be divided into four phases of highly disparate duration: a first or empirical phase, followed by a naturalistic phase, then a chemical phase and finally the current phase in which, despite enormous progress in the fundamental sciences, malaria still represents a massive public health problem. The second and third phases were characterised by massive expansion of anti-malarial measures and operations which resulted in substantial reductions in the prevalence of the disease throughout the world. As of the mid-1960's, the failure to eradicate malaria or even further reduce its prevalence led to profound disillusion. This resulted in repeated shifts in the strategies used to combat the disease from the 1970's on until, in 1992, all governments came together to adopt a global strategy.

Empirical period

This period spans from the dawn of humanity up until 1880 when Laveran, working at Constantine in Algeria, identified the parasite that causes malaria.

In the absence of fossil evidence—either direct (i.e. fossils of the parasite itself) or indirect (traces of the disease in fossilised human bones)—the earliest trace of malaria is *Plasmodium falciparum* DNA found in mummies dating from 3,200 BC (Miller *et al.*, 1994). If we want to learn about malaria before then, our only option therefore is to retrace the history of the disease in written texts—and it is believed that modern humans have been infected ever since they first appeared on Earth (Bruce-Chwatt, 1980). The palaeogenesis of *Plasmodium* species and their spread in early humans are addressed in the Chapter entitled "*Plasmodium* Life Cycles in Humans and Anopheline Vectors".

Intermittent fevers—possibly malaria— are mentioned in texts from Mesopotamia, India, China and Europe (in Greece, in Homer's Iliad which was written around 800 BC). Mosquito nets were in use in Ancient Egypt but this may have been as much a measure against the simple inconvenience of bites as against disease.

In the 5th century BC, Hippocrates was the first to describe benign tertian and quartan fevers. He recorded that these fevers were seasonal and were associated with splenomegaly. He also noted a relationship with stagnant water in marshlands—so already in antiquity, malaria was perceived as a disease related to the environment (as evidenced by the etymology of the word which is derived from the Italian for "bad air"). The Roman authors Celsus (25 BC to 54 AD) and Galen (130-200 AD) described intermittent forms of fever (*in* Grmek, 1994) and singled out malignant tertian fever (due to *P. falciparum*), although it was not until the end of the 19th century that these different forms were attributed to *P. vivax, P. malariae* and *P. falciparum*.

The spread of malaria as of the 4th century BC and through the Graeco-Roman era probably followed the introduction of *P. falciparum* and has been attributed to the presence or importation of two anopheline species, *Anopheles sacharovi* in Greece and *An. labranchiae* in southern Italy, both highly efficient vectors. However, there is no concrete evidence that new vectors appeared at this time and the historical evidence about malaria during the Graeco-Roman era remains largely conjectural.

For nearly five centuries, malaria ravaged southern Europe. Rome, the centre of Christianity, was famously unhealthy and several Popes apparently died of malaria. In the Middle Ages, fevers were killing people through a large part of Europe: in the Thames estuary in England where the disease was called ague; in Flanders and the Netherlands; in France: in the Camargue delta near the Mediterranean Sea, in the Dombes Region in the South-West, and in Sologne near Paris; in Spain, irrigated rice cultivation was proscribed by the Catholic Kings as a measure against fever.

Based on ideas inherited from the Ancients, only two ways of protecting against infection were recognised, namely avoiding insalubrious areas and draining deposits of stagnant water. No curative modalities are described in either the European Pharmacopoeias of the Middle Ages or those of the Arab world. It is only recently that it was realised that *Artemisia annua* had been in use for 2,000 years against fever in China.

The first decisive advance in malaria control came from South America, ironically since the disease was most likely absent during the Pre-Columbian era. The curative properties of the bark of *Cinchona* trees were described in a series of works which reported various different—and sometimes contradictory—effects and anecdotes. The importance of the cure of the beautiful Countess of Chinchon in the spread of the news around Europe depends on the source. Bovay (1972) gives a well-referenced summary of the "*History of Quinquina*". The first documented cure using *Cinchona* powder seems to have been that of a Jesuit priest called Juan Lopez in around 1600, who was treated by a traditional Indian healer, Pedro Liva, at Loja in Ecuador (at an altitude of 2,300 metres). When the town's corregidor (a local magistrate in the Spanish colonies) learned of this event, he broadcast the news; eventually, Cardinal Juan de Lugo told the Pope who commissioned his personal physician, Gabriel Fonseca, to test the material at the Santo-Spirito hospital in Rome. In 1649, Jesuits started using *Cinchona* bark at their missions but the new drug was very expensive. The Spanish initially had a monopoly on it and this was later transferred to the newly independent Latin American States.

In the 17th century, Morton and Sydenham were already studying how *Cinchona* bark works (reviewed *in* Najera, 2001) and at the end of the century, Talbot used the powder to treat the Dauphin of France. In Italy in 1712, Torti distinguished between those forms of fever that responded to quinine and those that did not (*in* Najera, 2001).

Quinine was not synthesised until much later so the drug had to be extracted from *Cinchona* bark. As described by La Condamine and classified by Linnaeus, twenty-odd *Cinchona* species are found on the eastern side of the Andes Mountains, with alkaloid contents varying from 15% to 39%. After numerous attempts at transplantation, in 1865 Ledger sent back to England some seeds which his agent had found at Chulumani in Bolivia. This alkaloid-rich species, *Cinchona ledgeriana*, was ultimately used for all the plantations in Java which, by 1941, were yielding 20 million pounds of bark per annum (Bovay, 1972).

By 1820, Pelletier and Caventou had isolated quinine and quinidine. In 1822, quinine was already being used by the French in Senegal and, in 1844, it was being administered prophylactically to railroad workers in the United States of America. The availability of a convenient, effective drug against malaria meant that no part of the planet was off limits. This was probably a key factor in colonial expansion, especially through Africa.

Intercontinental travel leading to exploration of the entire world led to a realisation of the scale of the malaria problem. Tropical Africa was justifiably seen as a high-risk environment for potential travellers and invaders—the White Man's Grave. Fever was no longer seen as a peculiarity of the Mediterranean rim—it was prevalent in most tropical and sub-tropical regions of the world. In America, *P. vivax* and/or *P. malariae* may have been infecting Amerindians in Pre-Columbian times but *P. falciparum* seems to have been introduced with slaves from Africa.

Naturalist period

This period lasted from 1880 to the Second World War.

Elucidation of Plasmodium *life cycles*

The last quarter of the 19th century and the beginning of the 20th were a golden age for discoveries in the natural and medical sciences, not least when it comes to parasites and their vectors. Only a little more than fifty years passed between the discovery of the guinea worm cycle in *Cyclops* crustaceans (by Fedschenko in Ukraine in 1869) and full descriptions of the cycles of the most important, arthropod-transmitted pathological parasites (filaria, trypanosomes and plasmodium) and bacteria (*Yersinia pestis* which causes bubonic plague).

In 1880*, at Constantine, Alphonse Laveran described the agent which causes malaria and named it *Oscillarium malariae*. In the United States, Laveran's discovery was confirmed by Osler (1882), Abbott (1885) and Sternberg (1886). In Italy, Marchiafava described *Plasmodium* in 1885 (although he initially resisted the idea that it was a parasitic organism) and in 1886, Golgi made a distinction between *P. vivax* and *P. malariae*. Soon after in 1889, Celli and Marchiafava described *P. falciparum*. In the United States in 1897, MacCallum observed exflagellation of male *P. falciparum* gametocytes and their penetration into the female gametocyte.

The development of eosin-methylene blue staining for blood-borne parasites by Romanovsky in 1891 greatly enhanced microscopic parasite identification.

P. ovale, the fourth plasmodial species that can infect humans, was not identified until 1922 by Stephens.

Already in 1717, Lancisi in Italy had proposed that mosquitoes may be involved in the transmission of malaria, a hypothesis based on the abundance of these insects in wetlands. A role for mosquitoes was also suspected in Mobile, Alabama in the United States (1848) and in Caracas, Venezuela by Beauperthuy (1854).

---

* The chronology of discoveries in malaria research between 1847 and 1978 is reviewed in Bruce-Chwatt, 1980: 5-9.

The discovery by Manson in China that filariae are transmitted by *Culex* mosquitoes (1877) supported the idea that malaria might be transmitted by mosquitoes. In 1895, Ross detected oocysts in the stomachs of anopheline mosquitoes and, in 1898, he documented the transmission of avian malaria by *Culex*.

In 1899, Grassi, Bastianelli & Bignami elucidated the entire developmental cycle (sporogony) of *P. falciparum*, *P. vivax* and *P. malariae* in *Anopheles claviger*.

In 1898, Grassi & Bignami infected a volunteer with *P. falciparum* using *Anopheles* collected in the highly endemic rural surroundings of Rome. In 1899, three similarly successful experiments were carried out by Bastianelli, Grassi & Bignami, who also published details of the *Plasmodium* cycle in *Anopheles*. In 1900, Manson confirmed the cycle of transmission in volunteers in the countryside around both Rome and London.

In 1901, Grassi had hypothesised that the parasite cycle includes a third phase and in 1937, James and Tate saw the schizogonic form of *P. gallinaceum* in the brains of infected chickens ("blue bodies"). Shortt & Garnham first described pre-erythrocytic forms of *P. cynomolgi* in the livers of macaque monkeys and later, analogous forms of *P. vivax* (1948), *P. falciparum* (1949) and *P. ovale* (1953) in human livers. The existence of *P. vivax* hypnozoites was not reported until 1972 (*see the Chapter on "*Plasmodium* Life Cycles in Humans and Anopheline Vectors"*) although Krotoski had actually observed them as early as 1940.

Thus, all the phases in the developmental cycle of plasmodia were eventually elucidated.

Vector ecology and malaria control

As soon as it was recognised that malaria was transmitted by anopheline mosquitoes, killing the vectors became the goal of all experts because it was believed that the disease could thereby be eradicated. In parallel with widespread quinine treatment, vector destruction became the spearhead of malaria control. The main targets for destruction were larval habitats (mainly by draining) and the larvae themselves (using mineral oil or copper acetoarsenite [Paris Green]). This was coupled with measures aimed at personal protection, mainly equipping homes with anti-mosquito screens.

Ross instigated malaria control measures at Freetown in Sierra Leone in 1899, then at Ismailia in Egypt in 1901. Gorgas and Le Prince implemented all-out attacks on mosquito larvae in Cuba (1899) and Panama (1904), specifically aimed at *Aedes aegypti*. Although the results of Ross were generally ignored, those of Gorgas and Le Prince were widely publicised and have been used as a reference for malaria control on the American continent—and not always happily.

In Italy, France, Albania, Algeria and the United States, drainage and environmental management (with reclamation of the recovered land) and other environmental measures together with comprehensive quinine treatment of local people resulted in a marked drop in the prevalence of malaria, with complete disappearance in certain places. Whereas the Americans continued with total larval control (suitable to the local conditions, it must be said), as of 1920, Europeans (e.g. Swellengrebel) recommended rigorous assessment of local conditions before deciding which strategy to pursue (reviewed *in* Najera, 2001). This led, by 1935, to campaigns in South Africa based on killing adult mosquitoes by weekly spraying with a pyrethrin-based insecticide (Park Ross, 1936; Swellengrebel *et al.*, 1939). Dichloro-diphenyl-trichloroethane (DDT), which had been discovered in 1938 (Müller, 1955) was first used in 1943 in the United States.

Malaria had spontaneously begun to disappear in Europe in the 18th century, and in North America by the middle of the 19th century. By the end of the 19th century, it had completely disappeared from England and was rare in France and many other European countries. However, in Italy, Corsica (France), Greece, the Balkans, The Netherlands and Germany as well as the United States, it persisted until 1945, and in the Soviet Union until 1959. Throughout this period, the disease remained endemic and highly prevalent throughout almost all tropical and sub-tropical regions.

During the First World War, deadly epidemics swept through the ravaged Balkans. Beginning in 1920—against a background of the governmental, economic and social repercussions of the Russian Revolution—a pandemic ravaged the Soviet Union lasting until 1935, causing 9 million cases per annum and reaching as far north as Arkhangelsk, a port on the White Sea beyond the Arctic Circle (Lysenko & Kondrashin, 1999).

The spontaneous regression of malaria has been attributed to economic development linked with improvements in living conditions, notably the separation of human living quarters from those of livestock; however, during the pandemic of 1921-1935 in the USSR, it seems that the disappearance of livestock played an important exacerbatory role because zoophilic *Anopheles* species (especially *An. messae*) found themselves obliged to feed on humans.

Many experts, including Roubaud (1937), advocated zooprophylaxis, i.e. introducing animals between larval breeding sites and human habitations in order to divert the mosquitoes, a practice which was widespread in eastern Europe.

The highly variable distribution of malaria in Europe despite the quasi-omnipresence of *Anopheles* mosquitoes—notably of *An. maculipennis s.l.*—led to Roubaud's concept of "anophelism without malaria" (Roubaud, 1925) which resulted from the weakness of taxonomic classification systems at that time. In fact, the maculipennis name included several species which can only be differentiated on the basis of egg morphology (Hackett, 1934; Missiroli *et al.*, 1933). Some of these species were efficient vectors, such as *An. labranchiae* in Italy, France (Corsica) and North Africa, and *An. sacharovi* in Corsica, Italy, Greece,

Biodiversity of Malaria in the World

		Chronology of discoveries relevant to malaria	
Year/period	**Discoverer**	**Country**	**Discovery**
5th century BC.	Hippocrates	Greece	Description of benign tertian and quartan fevers
1st millenium BC.	Anonymous	China	Antimalaria activity of *Artemisia annua* (Quinghaosu)
Beginning of christianity	Celsus	Rome	Description of malignant tertian fever
1600	Juan Lopez	Ecuador	Use of quinquina bark to treat "fever"
1820	Pelletier & Caventou	France	Isolation of quinine and quinidine
1822	Anonymous	Senegal	First use of quinine as a drug
1869	Fedschenko	Ukraine	Elucidation of the first cycle of a parasite in an invertebrate— that of dracunculus in *Cyclops*
1877	Manson	China	Vector role of *Culex quinquefasciatus* in lymphatic filariasis transmission
1880	Laveran	Algeria	Observation and description of the malaria parasite in human blood
1886	Golgi	Italy	Description of *P. vivax* and *P. malariae*
1889-1890	Celli & Marchiafava	Italy	Description of *P. falciparum*
1891	Romanovsky	Russia	Development of staining systems for *Plasmodium*
1897	Manson	United Kingdom	Hypothesis that malaria is transmitted by a vector
1897	Ross	Italy	Discovery of oocysts on the stomach wall of an *Anopheles* mosquito
1897	MacCallum	United States	Exflagellation of *P. falciparum*
1898	Grassi, Bignami & Bastianelli	Italy	Parasite cycle in *Anopheles*
1900	Manson	Italy and United Kingdom	Confirmation of the transmission mechanism in volunteers
1901	Grassi	Italy	Hypothesis that the cycle includes a third phase in the liver
1922	Stephens	United States	Description of *P. ovale*
1934	Anonymous	Germany	Discovery of chloroquine
1935-1939	de Meillon	South Africa	Use of pyrethrin in indoor spraying operations
1936-1939	Muller	Switzerland	Discovery of the insecticidal activity of DDT
1943	Gahan	United States	Indoor spraying with DDT
1946-1951	Anonymous		Mass DDT spraying campaigns in Cyprus, Italy, Greece, Corsica, Venezuela and Guyana
1948	Shortt *et al.*	United Kingdom	Description of pre-erythrocytic forms of *P. vivax*
1948	Rodhain	Congo	Discovery of *P. malariae* in chimpanzees
1949	Shortt *et al.*	United Kingd. and Kenya	Discovery of pre-erythrocytic forms of *P. falciparum*
1952	Elderfield	United States	Discovery of primaquine
1952	Hichings	United States	Discovery of pyrimethamine
1953	Belios & Livadas	Greece	Anopheline insecticide resistance
1955	Anonymous WHO		Launch of the Global Eradication Programme
1957	Macdonald	United Kingdom	Mathematical models for malaria epidemiology

Increase Knowledge about Malaria and Development of Control Measures

Chronology of discoveries relevant to malaria

Year/period	Discoverer	Country	Discovery
1960-1966	Hichings	United States	Development of sulfadoxine-pyrimethamine (Fansidar®)
1961	Anonymous		Appearance of drug resistance
1967-1974	Anonymous	United States	Development of mefloquine
1967-1974	Anonymous	United States	Development of halofanthrine
1969	OMS		Review of malaria control strategies, the situation having been unclear for nearly thirty years
1975			As of 1975, abandonment of indoor spraying in favour of primary health care development
1980			Recrudescence and re-emergence of malaria on the abandonment of eradication operations
1984	Darriet *et al.*		Use of mosquito nets treated with permethrin in Burkina Faso
1985		China	Development of artemisinin derivatives
1992	Conference	The Netherlands	Global Malaria Control Strategy
1998	WHO		Roll-Back Malaria Programme

the Balkans and the Middle East. In contrast, *An. atroparvus*, a vector which is found in coastal regions, is relatively zoophilic, and both *An. messae* and *An. maculipennis* are highly zoophilic and rarely transmit malaria to humans. Since that time, the idea of species complexes—largely supported by the techniques of cytogenetics and molecular biology—has been extended to other groups, including *An. gambiae* in Africa, *An. leucosphyrus* in Southeast Asia, *An. culicifacies* on the Indian sub-continent, and *An. farauti* in Australasia. Now, complexes are the basis of anopheline taxonomy and, in the final analysis, there are not many species which are not in fact members of some complex (*An. darlingi* in South America and *An. stephensi* in India seem to constitute exceptions).

In tropical Africa, Southeast Asia, Australia and South America, anti-malarial measures were generally limited to the distribution of quinine to European colonists and the better-off inhabitants, less often to the indigenous population as a whole. In consequence, the disease remained endemic in these tropical regions without any significant changes in prevalence prior to 1945.

Above and beyond these limited successes, it is important to point to, on the one hand, the uniquely successful operations in South Africa where the novel strategy of killing adult mosquitoes when they are resting in houses using pyrethrin-based insecticides was pioneered (de Meillon, 1936), and, on the other hand, the effective eradication of *An. gambiae s.l.* in Brazil (Soper & Wilson, 1943) and Egypt (Shousha, 1948). This afrotropical *Anopheles*—probably *An. arabiensis*—had invaded northeastern Brazil and it took ten years to dislodge it; in Egypt, it persisted in the Middle Nile Valley through three winters.

Chemical phase: the dream of eradication

Theory of eradication

During the Second World War, malaria control was revolutionised by the development on the one hand of synthetic, long-acting insecticides, and on the other, of new antimalarial drugs which were both effective and easy to administer.

Insecticides which kill adult mosquitoes, notably the pyrethrins which can be used for indoor spraying, had been shown to be effective in South Africa, The Netherlands, Brazil, Egypt and India by the end of the 1930's. But the practicality of this anti-vector strategy was limited by the necessity of weekly treatment and the high cost of the products used. The arrival of DDT, which was both cheap and persistent (more than six months), led to more widespread implementation of strategies directed against adult insects.

Although DDT was synthesised by Zeidler in 1874 in Germany, it was not until 1939 that its insecticide activity was discovered by Müller in Basel (1946; 1955) (Geigy). The compound was tested in the United States and, in 1943, Gahan & Lindquist (1945) showed that it remained active for a long time after indoor spraying. In 1944, field tests around Voltunero in Italy and in the United States, Africa and Asia convincingly demonstrated the efficacy of such treatment. In 1945, Gabaldon working in Venezuela was the first to apply the principle of total coverage of an entire country by DDT spraying (reviewed *in* Boyd, 1949). He concluded that such a strategy effectively increased the size of a country since arable land could be recovered—without even the need for war.

The practice of indoor spraying spread with successful results. In 1949, campaigns were launched in Madagascar, Mauritius and La Réunion, and by 1954, it had become clear that malaria had been eradicated in the United States, Venezuela, British Guiana, Italy, Greece, and Corsica, among others.

Given this success, the Pan-American Sanitary Bureau (PASB/WHO) drew up a plan for the eradication of malaria from the Americas in 1954 (reviewed in WHO, 1957).

In many other countries, malaria indices and mortality fell dramatically. Based on experiments conducted in Greece, Livadas (1952) proposed stopping spraying once the "parasite reservoir" had been eliminated—an idea which subsequently underpinned eradication theory.

In 1951, evidence of resistance to DDT was first documented in Greece in the species *An. sacharovi* (Livadas and Georgiopoulos, 1953). This Damocles' sword spurred international institutions to step up operations so that malaria would be eradicated before resistance had the time to become established. This was one of the arguments—albeit a somewhat naive one—that led to the adoption of a **Global Malaria Eradication Programme** by the 8th World Health Assembly in Mexico City in 1955; the dream of Soper and many American experts was finally going to be made reality. The underlying principle was interrupting transmission with time-limited spraying campaigns. The following year, a committee of experts formulated a strategy of spraying homes with DDT. Across-the-board strategies were implemented in many countries, often without any epidemiological insight into the problem and in many cases without the necessary administrative back-up (Najera, 1989).

The resolution was not adopted with universal enthusiasm and the 6th Expert Committee on Malaria (WHO, 1957) decided that Africa would not be included in the programme for the time being because of particular properties of the vectors there, the lack of knowledge about interrupting transmission, and the local lack of resources and qualified personnel. Pilot areas were designated in Burkina Faso, Nigeria, Liberia, Cameroon, Benin, Tanganyika and Uganda to investigate the possibilities of eradication in Africa. The results of these experiments were going to justify the Assembly's reticence. Without Africa—the continent in which the prevalence of malaria was highest—the Global Malaria Eradication Programme was no longer global, and doubt was cast on the possibility of sustained eradication given the vast reservoir of parasites that Africa represented. The etymology of the word—*ex-radicis* meaning literally "to destroy the roots"—was betrayed, and was it even justified to describe this geographically restricted programme as one of elimination—*ex-liminis* meaning without limits?

Moreover, resurgence of the disease remained a major preoccupation in countries in which malaria had already been eradicated or which were on the way to eradication. This really began to be observed as of 1975 when the regularity of treatment started to drop off.

The 6th Expert Committee (WHO, 1957) defined eradication as the arrest of transmission and a reduction in the size of the infectious reservoir, achieved through a time-limited campaign and conducted such that the disease would not ultimately re-emerge.

Operations proceeded in four phases:
- a preparatory phase lasting twelve to eighteen months, in which endemic zones were mapped and it was confirmed that the country possessed the infrastructure necessary to undertake eradication. Pampana (1969) emphasised that, before beginning a campaign, it was crucial to ensure that stopping transmission was an achievable goal, a recommendation that many programmes fatally failed to take on;
- an attack phase involving total coverage of all houses in the country's endemic zones with DDT sprayed to a concentration of 2 g/m². This phase was to last for three or four years, or longer if necessary to eliminate the parasite reservoir—an interval estimated as being three years after the last documented local transmission event, meaning that a malaria detection system had to be set up. Hexachlorocyclohexane (HCH), the action of which is relatively short-lived, was soon abandoned as was dieldrin, an excellent compound but one to which most *Anopheles* species rapidly developed resistance. Malathion, propoxur and fenitrothion were used against resistant mosquitoes;
- a consolidation phase after the end of the spraying campaign. In this phase, residual cases and "foci of infection" were identified and then eliminated by targeted (although relatively comprehensive) treatment. Thus was created an "epidemiology of malaria on the way to eradication": any new transmission was considered as an epidemic—even if there were only a handful of cases (e.g. just eight!)—and classified as a focus of infection which must be treated, if necessary in the same way as during the attack phase;
- a maintenance phase intended to sustain the new *status quo* and prevent malaria from becoming re-established. This phase was to last as long as there remained any parasites anywhere in the world.

The "theory of eradication" was in vogue from 1956 onwards. Within each affected country's health authority, the malaria eradication division was made autonomous and given its own budget. In 1962, the World Health Assembly recognised that wherever health authorities were insufficiently developed (especially in Africa), eradication could not be embarked upon. Instead, a pre-eradication programme would be implemented, on the one hand to develop basic health services in all the countries in which malaria was still endemic, and on the other hand to study local epidemiology.

New indices were devised to replace the classic ones: the Annual Parasite Incidence (API) which describes the number of new cases per 1,000 people in a given year became one of the basic ways of evaluating the outcome of operations. As soon as the API dropped below 0.1, spraying could be discontinued (Pampana, 1969). The number of new cases was evaluated using the Annual Blood Examination Rate (ABER) which had to be at least 10% of the population. This entailed the analysis of very large numbers of smears, so the microscopists were often overworked and did not always perform the examinations with the necessary rigour.

Failures and successes

Resistance to DDT appeared in Greece in 1951 (Livadas & Georgiopoulos, 1953). This phenomenon was considered as a major obstacle on the road towards eradication although in practice, its consequences were less marked. In some countries, DDT still proved useful although in others, a switch had to be made to malathion (Pakistan, Sudan and Burundi).

Drug resistance, in particular to chloroquine, began to emerge as a problem in 1960 in the border regions between Colombia and Venezuela, and between Thailand and Cambodia. From 1980 onwards, this problem spread throughout the world.

Vectors leaving the house after feeding (exophilic behaviour) were considered as a special problem, notably *An. dirus* in Southeast Asia, *An. fluviatilis* in Iran and *An. nuneztovari* in Venezuela. Even more of a problem in the pilot zones of the African savannah, it was shown that transmission could not be stopped using DDT (Cavalié & Mouchet, 1961; Choumara *et al.*, 1959); undoubtedly, the effect of DDT driving the vectors outside of houses was involved, but other factors have to be considered.

In 1968, there was a recrudescence of malaria in Sri Lanka where the disease was believed to be close to eradication (Bruce-Chwatt, 1974).

In Mexico City in 1962, it was recognised that "problem areas" existed and the World Health Assembly adopted a resolution in 1967.

At the 1968 International Congress on Tropical Medicine and Malaria in Tehran, Gabaldon*—one of the godfathers of eradication—recognised that it might not be possible to eradicate malaria throughout the world. This was based not only on the results from Venezuela, but also on data from many countries in Africa and Asia. No global strategy could be implemented in a uniform fashion without operational rural support services, so the Congress asked WHO to adapt its policy on eradication.

In 1969, the 22nd World Health Assembly acknowledged this failure but eradication remained the ultimate goal until an entirely new strategy was adopted in 1972.

At Brazzaville in 1972, a meeting was held between countries which could not support an eradication programme, mostly African countries but also some from the Pacific Region (Papua New Guinea). One by one, a whole series of countries abandoned eradication programmes in favour of more flexible, less onerous control programmes.

Despite its ultimate failure, the Global Malaria Eradication Programme had positive aspects. It is certainly the biggest health-related operation ever implemented:
- it brought about a massive reduction in the level of malaria in the world, in terms of both the total surface area across which the disease is endemic and the overall prevalence of the disease. Outside of Africa (which currently accounts for 80-90% of cases), holoendemicity is now rare;
- it led to a substantial reduction in mortality due to malaria, reductions of 71% to 100% depending on country. By way of example, some figures: in Central America and the Philippines, malaria mortality fell from 15.6‰ to 2.9‰, and in Thailand from 63‰ to 14‰. The Programme therefore fulfilled ethical public health principles (Gramiccia & Hempel, 1972) and it was the first with universal, democratic ambitions, aiming to cover populations as a whole. It brought public health to the most isolated spots, often with training of local volunteers.

In the end, the Global Malaria Eradication Programme had a huge beneficial effect on human health even if the exact proportion of the reduction in mortality (which has occurred throughout the world) that is due to anti-malarial initiatives alone may be questioned in some countries. Some have even attributed the population growth seen since the 1950's to the success of malaria control, a claim which is obviously overblown since a similar explosion has been observed in many African countries where no eradication programme was ever implemented, e.g. Nigeria and Niger.

Drug development

In this historical review, it is impossible to ignore the considerable progress over the last sixty years in the availability of effective drugs against malaria. Here, we will not give an exhaustive list of all the compounds and how they are used which can be found in Bryskier & Labro (1988) and Danis & Mouchet (1991), and is reviewed in the Chapter on "Drug and Treatment Policies".

Initially, *Cinchona* bark and later quinine were practically the only drugs ever prescribed for "fever" before the Second World War. Beginning in 1936 but more generally from 1940 on when the sources of quinine in Indonesia came under threat, research into synthetic alternatives really took off. Nevertheless, even today quinine remains a valued compound, especially in severe cases.

---

* Inaugural Conference (unpublished).

The amino-4-quinolines—chloroquine and amodiaquine—were discovered between 1939 and 1941. These compounds which are only active against the schizont are extremely effective, relatively non-toxic, cheap and easy to use. They were widely used for both treatment and prophylaxis throughout the world for over fifty years although, as of 1975, amiodaquine was no longer recommended for prophylaxis because of the risk of liver damage (rare but, in some cases severe). Similarly, the spread of resistance to chloroquine has considerably compromised its efficacy. To date, no compounds have fully replaced them as prophylactic agents and their loss has created a major gap in the therapeutic arsenal.

The first amino-8-quinoline (pamaquine) was discovered in 1925; currently, only one member of this family is used as a drug, namely primaquine which is the only compound which kills gametocytes as well as the only one which is active against the hypnozoites of *P. vivax* and *P. ovale*; it is an effective drug but is contraindicated in people with glucose-6-phosphate dehydrogenase deficiency.

The aryl-amino alcohols—mefloquine (Lariam®) and halofantrine (Halfan®)—are very active against the shizont. The first has a synergistic effect with artemisinin derivatives and is often prescribed in combination therapy, although it is associated with a high incidence of side effects. Halofantrine causes heart problems in one case out of 10,000 and is no longer recommended for prophylaxis.

Pyronaridine was reported as being effective by Zhang *et al.* in 1982 (reviewed *in* Bryskier & Labro, 1988) but to date, it has only been marketed in China (Lonaiding®).

Sulfadoxine-pyrimethamine (Fansidar®) is a fast-acting, potent anti-malarial which has been in use since the 1960's. It used to be prescribed for first-line treatment in Africa in areas where the incidence of chloroquine resistance is high, although these days, more and more strains of *P. falciparum* are also resistant to the newer drug.

The antibiotics doxycycline (Vibramycin®) and clindamycine (Dalacine®) are often combined with quinine in places where there is doubt about sensitivity to the latter drug.

Proguanil, in combination with chloroquine (Savarine®) or atovaquone (Malarone®), is used for prophylaxis, as is Dapsone®, combined with either pyrimethamine (Maloprim®) or chlorproguanil (Lap-Dap®).

From a completely different source, Qinghaosu has been used in traditional Chinese medicine for 2,000 years. It is an extract of *Artemisia annua*, the only member of its genus with anti-malarial activity. The structure of Qinghaosu was elucidated in 1973 and it was first synthesised in 1984. It is a lactone with an endoperoxide chain which is responsible for the anti-malarial activity.

Artemisinin and its derivatives artemeter (Paluther®) and artesunate (Arsumax®) are fast-acting and potent substances which are ideal for treating cases of severe malaria. However, they are cleared rapidly and sometimes it is necessary to extend their action by combining with mefloquine with which they act synergistically. Combinations of lumefantrine and artemisinin (Coartem®, Riamet®) are marketed in Africa.

Traditional medicine offers many and various compounds, the antimalarial activity of which warrants serious evaluation. However, quassia and simarouba from South America are toxic, and "Neem" from Africa has not lived up to local hopes. There are many candidate drugs but none have yet been singled out for large-scale development.

At the beginning of the new millennium, plasmodial resistance to drugs is one of the main problems encountered when treating malaria (*see the Chapter on* "Drug and Treatment Policies").

Chloroquine-resistant *P. falciparum* appeared independently at two different places in Colombia in 1959, then in Thailand in 1959-1960, and in Vietnam in 1964. It subsequently spread throughout Asia and South America. In Africa, it reached Kenya in 1978 and then slowly spread, reaching the centre of the continent and South Africa between 1982 and 1985, and finally West Africa in 1986 since when, its spread seems to have been stabilised.

P. falciparum resistance to chloroquine and later to sulfadoxine-pyrimethamine is changing how patients are cared for and increasing the cost of treatment.

The shrinking therapeutic arsenal constitutes a serious problem in malaria control and preserving the usefulness of the currently available compounds is vital. The only existing strategic option is to replace regimens based on a single drug with compounds, to avoid resistance as well as improve efficacy and safety. However, the cost of combination therapy is far higher—sometimes ten times more expensive than simple treatment with chloroquine or sulfadoxine-pyrimethamine.

This question is addressed in the Chapter on "Patient Care and Malaria Diagnosis".

Current questions: public health and research priorities

The gradual substitution of a strategy of eradication with one of control was very disruptive for public health institutions which found it difficult to define objectives and targets.

The control strategy was ratified by the 31st World Health Assembly in 1978 which put an end to the confusion which had reigned since 1969, during which time certain States had been obliged to switch from eradication to control without adequate technical back-up.

In 1992, the Amsterdam Ministerial Conference defined a Global Strategy based on four foundation stones: early diagnosis and rapid treatment of new cases; prevention (including measures against vectors); the prevention and containment of epidemics; and the consolidation of national capacities. These measures were to be implemented in a framework of epidemiological and socio-economic stratification. This was a long-term strategy dependent on the development of solid public health institutions. The results would be proportional to the scope of the initiatives launched, and it would not be possible to judge them in the short term.

Deadly epidemics in Sri Lanka, India, Pakistan and Madagascar retrospectively proved that eradication was not sustainable, as has also been shown by the recent re-emergence of malaria in Korea and some States of the former Soviet Union (Armenia, Azerbaijan and Tajikistan).

Indoor spraying—possibly with DDT (Roberts *et al.*, 2002b)—has again been proposed by many experts although only as a temporary, local measure to remedy "problem" situations rather than as a general, country-wide measure.

While malaria control has to face massive technical, administrative and financial difficulties, certain lines of research seem to be particularly promising although no solutions to any of the central problems have as yet resulted. Three types of vaccine are being investigated: directed against sporozoites and liver forms; against blood-borne forms; and against sexual stages. However, no effective vaccine is yet available. The possibility of combined vaccines is also being contemplated but again, none as yet exist.

Our understanding of resistance mechanisms, both of *Plasmodium* to drugs and *Anopheles* mosquitoes to insecticides, is increasing steadily but this has not had any great practical consequences in terms of the impact of these phenomena.

Genetic and cladistic analysis of complexes of *Anopheles* species has led to the classification of each taxon in its correct place in the transmission of malaria which in turn should make it possible to target measures against vectors in a more effective way; however, this pre-supposes enhancing the specificity of such measures which is not yet happening.

The development of transgenic mosquitoes which are resistant to *Plasmodium* would open long-term possibilities if we could devise ways of introducing them in such a way that they compete with wild-populations of vectors.

When it comes to identifying possible targets for drugs and/or insecticides, great hopes are being pinned on DNA sequencing, of both the human genome and the genomes of *P. falciparum* and *An. gambiae*. Attitudes to the possibility of genetically modifying vectors to be refractory to parasites are more reserved.

In contrast, new simple and fast diagnostic tools have been developed for *Plasmodium* (e.g. the dipstick method) and will soon be in use in the field (in Cambodia and Guyana); however, these methods are expensive and give a high proportion (10-20%) of false negative results.

Finally, no progress at all is being made when it comes to developing either new insecticides or biological agents to control the vectors.

Parasites and Vectors

In this Chapter, we will first address the taxonomic status of the parasites in the context of their evolution. Later, the various species will be described together with their life cycles. Vector taxonomy, biology and ecology will also be reviewed to establish the basic ideas which will be essential to understanding the parasites' life cycles (*see the Chapter on "Plasmodium Life Cycles in Humans and Anopheline Vectors"*) and the epidemiology of malaria (*see the Chapter on "Epidemiological Basis"*).

Early ancestors of *Plasmodium* and its vectors

In the absence of physical evidence in the form of fossils, the phylogeny of the early ancestors of *Plasmodium* and its vectors remains highly speculative. It is accepted that precursors of today's human plasmodia existed before or emerged at the same time as the first insects. In reptiles, intestinal coccidian parasites have been observed to be able to adapt to a blood habitat, in the course of which evolutionary process, a new host may be acquired, e.g. the *Haemosporidae* which gave rise to the genera *Haemoproteus* (plasmodia found in amphibians, reptiles and birds) and, more recently, *Hepatocystis* which includes mammalian plasmodia (*Table I*).

A rich insect fauna appeared in the Carboniferous Period (in the Palaeozoic Era, some 290 million years ago) and protodiptera first emerged in the Permian Period (towards the end of the Palaeozoic, about 260 million years ago) although the oldest dipteran fossils date from only the Jurassic Period (in the Mesozoic Era about 172 million years ago). Fossilised Culicidae appear in the Eocene but the family really expanded in the Oligocene (in the Tertiary Period 38 million years ago). Recently, a fossil of *An. (Nyssorhynchus) dominicanus* sp.n. has been found from Dominican Amber (Zavortink & Poinar, 2000). In the course of their evolution towards haematophagia, these insects may have preyed upon other insects before switching to amphibians. Some Culicidae species still prefer to feed on amphibians.

Tight dependence of one group of parasites on one group of insects reflects mutual adaptation—and therefore long-standing co-evolution. Overlap between the ecological niches of apes and those of early hominids in Africa may explain why the parasite could transfer horizontally within the same zoological group.

In any event, haematophagous anophelines were present before hominids in areas in which the parasite had become established.

Malaria parasites

Plasmodium *taxonomy*

The agents responsible for malaria are protozoa belonging to the Class Sporozoa, genus *Plasmodium*.

At the end of the 19th century, Mesnil (1899) and Schaudlin observed that Plasmodium was related to Coccidium, both of which were classified together with the gregarines (insect parasites) in the order *Coccidiomorpha* which was divided into three sub-orders (Garnham, 1966), namely *Eimeriidae* (which includes Coccidium, parasites of the vertebrate digestive tract), the *Adeleidae* (gregarine parasites of insects) and the *Haemosporidae* (*Table I*). The latter have a biphasic life cycle alternating between vertebrate blood and arthropod tissues.

The sub-order *Haemosporidae* (*Table I*) contains three families:
- *Plasmodidae* including the genus *Plasmodium* which contains 66-80 species (according to the source), almost all of which are transmitted by *Culicinae* and *Anophelinae*;
- *Haemoproteidae* including some ten genera of parasites of higher vertebrates transmitted by *Culicoides, Stomoxys* and *Hippoboscidae*;
- *Leucocytozoonidae* which parasitise the white blood cells of birds and are transmitted by flies of the genus *Simulium*.

Parasites and Vectors

Table I. From coccidia to human *Plasmodium*.

Classifications of coccidiomorphic sporozoans

Sub-order Haemosporidae	Sub-order Eimeriidae	Sub-order Adeleida
Vertebrate blood parasites	Vertebrate digestive tract parasites	Gregarines, insect parasites

Classification of *Haemosporidae*

Plasmodidae family	Haemoproteidae family	Leucocytozoonidae family
Plasmodium transmitted by *Culicinae* and *Anophelinae*	Many genera: *Hepatocystis, Haemoproteus, Nycteribia, Polychromophilus* transmitted by *Culicoides* and also *Hippoboscidae, Stomoxys*, etc.	Bird leukocyte parasites tranmsitted by Simulium

Classification of *Plasmodidae*

Mammals	Sg. Laverania	2*	Primates	Vectors: *Anopheles*
	Sg. Plasmodium	20 or 22		
	Sg. Vinckeia	14	Rodents, ungulates, cheiroptera	
Birds	Sg. Haemamoeba	7	Birds	Vectors: *Culicidae* (*Culex, Aedes, Mansonia*)
	Sg. Giovannolaia	10		
	Sg. Novyella	5		
	Sg. Huffia	2		
Reptiles	Sg. Sauromoeba	14	Lizards	Vectors: mostly unknown. Phlebotomine sandflies for *P(S) mexicanum*
	Sg. Carinia	8		
	Sg. Ophidiella	1	Snakes	

Plasmodial parasites of humans and African apes—adapted to American and Asian monkeys

Sub-genus	**Human**	Chimpanzee	Gorilla	American and Asian monkeys
Plasmodium	P. malariae P. vivax P. vivax-like P. ovale	P. malariae P. schwetzi	P. schwetzi	P. brasilianum = P. malariae P. simium = P. vivax P. simiovale = P. vivax-like
Laverania	P. (L.) falciparum	P.(L.) reichenowi		

* Number of species in the subgroup

The *Plasmodidae* (*Table I*) family which is only represented by the genus *Plasmodium* has been divided into ten sub-genera. Three of these are parasites of mammals, four of birds and three of reptiles. All the mammalian parasites are transmitted by *Anopheles*, those of birds by *Culicinae*, and those of reptiles by Culicinae or *Phlebotomus*.

Phylogeny

"Malaria" is very common in the animal kingdom—occurring in reptiles, birds, rodents and primates—although its pathogenicity varies. The inventory of the various species has yet to be completed. All the parasites of primates belong to the sub-genus *Plasmodium* which evolved from parasites of reptiles.

The first pro-simian primate (a lemur) appeared in the Eocene (Tertiary Period, 55 million years ago) at the same time as *Hepatocystis* and also, perhaps, contemporaneously with the species of *Plasmodium* that are responsible for quartan fevers (*P. malariae* and *P. inui*). Monkeys appeared in the New World (South America) towards the end of the Eocene, and in the Old World at the beginning of the

Biodiversity of Malaria in the World

Oligocene (about 35 million years ago). As the main simian species diverged during this Period, plasmodia that cause tertian fever emerged, i.e. *P. vivax, P. ovale, P. cynomolgi, P. schwetzi* and *P. simium* which were soon followed by *P. knowlesi*. It was not until the Pliocene (15 million years ago) or the beginning of the Pleistocene (8 million years), not long before the divergence of humans from the apes, that the sub-genus *Laverania* (*P. falciparum, P. reichenowi*) first emerged (Garnham, 1966).

Long co-evolution of plasmodia and their hosts means that relationships are as a general rule highly specific, apart from in certain higher primates (Bruce-Chwatt, 1965). *P. malariae* (described as *P. rodhaini*) is the only parasite found in both humans and chimpanzees (the animal species which is genetically closest to Man). Two simian species are morphologically indistinguishable from their human homologues: *P. reichenowi* which is found in chimpanzees is homologous to *P. falciparum*, and *P. schwetzi* which infects chimpanzees and gorillas is homologous to *P. vivax*. The sub-genus *Laverania* was created for the human *P. falciparum* and the chimpanzee *P. reichenowi*. The sub-genus *Plasmodium s.s.* brings together the other three species which parasitise humans.

Based on the genealogy of primates (*Figure 1*), Garnham (1966) has estimated the age of different members of the sub-genera *Plasmodium* and *Laverania*.

P. ovale is only found in humans and has not yet been shown to have had any homologue in African apes. The morphologically similar *P. simiovale* has been reported infecting macaques in Sri Lanka (Dissanaike *et al.*, 1965), Papua New Guinea and Brazil; in the latter country, it is believed that *P. simiovale* is the same as a human *P. vivax-like* parasite which might therefore represent a fifth plasmodial species that can parasitise humans (Qari *et al.*, 1993a et 1993b). The taxonomy of the *P. vivax* Group is still a highly controversial topic.

P. falciparum and *P. reichenowi* on the one hand, and *P. vivax* and *P. schwetzi* on the other, descend from two common trunks according to Garnham (1966). It was not until the Pliocene, i.e. relatively recently, that gorillas diverged from the hominids, followed by the chimpanzees. This might account for why the morphology of the human parasites is so similar to that of those which infect apes, further support for the idea that higher primates arose in Africa (Bruce-Chwatt, 1965).

In New World monkeys, *P. brasilianum* and *P. simium* are morphologically indistinguishable from *P. malariae* and *P. vivax* respectively, and constitute a zoonosis which can be transmitted to humans (Dean *et al.*, 1966).

Human parasites can infect two South American monkeys, namely *Aotus trivirgatus* which is susceptible to

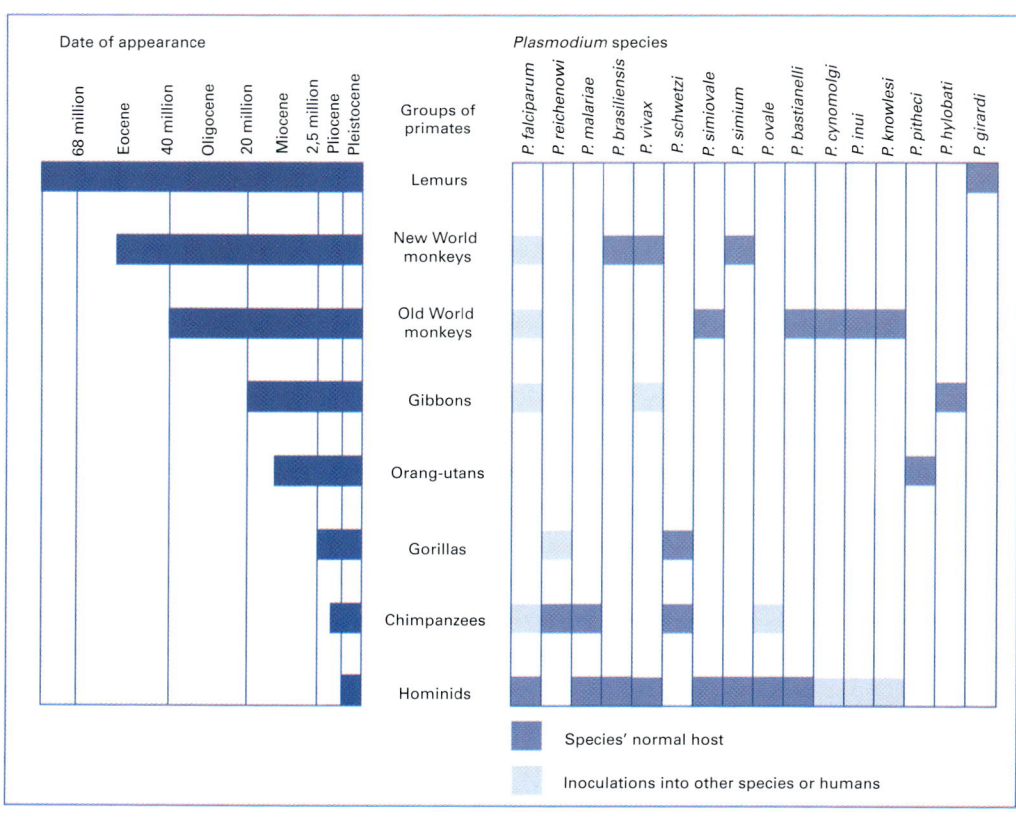

Figure 1. Plasmodium *species associated with various groups of primates.*

P. falciparum, and *Saimiri sciureus* which is susceptible to *P. vivax* as well as some strains of *P. falciparum*.

Several species—*P. inui, P. cynomolgi, P. knowlesi* and *P. bastianelli*—which infect Asian monkeys, mainly macaques, can be productively inoculated into humans (Chin *et al.*, 1965). *P. bastianelli* has been reported to have naturally infected human subjects in Malaysia and it was even worried that this species could represent a zoonosis which might spread following the eradication of the classic human parasites. In the 1970's, studies of *Plasmodium* in monkeys was a research priority in Malaysia and the United States (Coatney *et al.*, 1971; Sandosham *et al.*, 1970) but in fact, this phenomenon never amounted to more than a parasitological curiosity.

Gibbons appeared during the Oligocene and orang-utans in the Miocene. The parasites that infect these animals (*P. hylobati, P. yangi, P. eylesi, P. jeffreyei* and *P. pitheci*) are unrelated to those of African apes (Garnham, 1966).

Treatises on malaria (Boyd, 1949; Russel *et al.*, 1963) only provide descriptions of human parasites, ignoring those that infect other mammals. For detailed descriptions of other mammalian plasmodia and *Hepatocystis*, it is necessary to refer to the writings of specialists in protozoology, notably Garnham's excellent monograph (1966).

Malaria vectors

Anopheles *taxonomy*

All vectors of mammalian *Plasmodium* belong to the *Culicidae* family, more specifically to the sub-family of *Anophelinae*. Detailed descriptions of the morphology, biology and ecology of anopheline mosquitoes are provided in most treatises on malaria (Boyd, 1949; Bruce-Chwatt, 1980; Gillies & de Meillon, 1968; Russel *et al.*, 1963) and parasitology (Brumpt, 1949; Wernsdorfer & McGregor, 1988). Three genera are recognised in the *Anophelinae* family: species belonging to the genera of *Bironella* (found in New Guinea) and *Chagasia* (South America) are not vectors, but members of the genus *Anopheles* are. This genus contains 484 species (including all the vectors of human malaria) which are found across the entire planet apart from the Antarctic, central and eastern Polynesia, and a few islands, notably Greenland and Iceland. A list of Culicidae (which includes *Anopheles*) in the world was compiled by Knight & Stones in 1977 and updated by Knight in 1978, then again by Ward in 1984 and 1992. Hervy *et al.* (1998) offer a CD-ROM giving a comprehensive taxonomic key of *Anopheles* mosquitoes in the Afrotropical Region.

Defining sub-genera is merely of interest to taxonomists. Six sub-genera are recognised (Harbach, 1994): *Anopheles s.s.* (189 species), *Cellia* (239 species), *Nyssorhynchus* (33 species), *Kerteszia* (12 species), *Stethomyia* (5 species) and *Lophopodomyia* (6 species). The last four are all neotropical. The sub-genus *Kerteszia* is highly specialised in ecological terms since its larvae can only develop in the water which accumulates at the base of the foliar axils of epithytic Bromeliaceae; moreover, the females are mainly active during the daytime. No species belonging to either of the sub-genera *Lophopodomyia* or *Stethomyia* are vectors.

Complexes of species

The term species complex or group covers morphologically similar sibling species which can only be differentiated using infertility, cytogenetic, biochemical or molecular criteria. Each sibling species within a given complex will have its own ecology and behaviour patterns, and therefore a distinct degree of efficiency as a vector.

The first such complex defined was that of *An. maculipennis* which comprises eleven palaearctic species (Harbach, 1994). All European experts had observed that the vectorial efficiency of *An. maculipennis s.l.* varied between different European countries and regions. Roubaud (1918) drew attention to the phenomenon of "anophelism without malaria" in certain parts of Europe. Initially, Missiroli *et al.* (1933) distinguished *An. messae* from *An. atroparvus* and *An. maculipennis* on the basis of egg vesiture. This distinction explained why *P. vivax* malaria was more common in coastal regions infested with *An. atroparvus* (which thrives around brackish water deposits) than in inland regions which were colonised by the more zoophilic freshwater species *An. messae* and *An. maculipennis* which rarely transmit the parasite to humans. On the basis of morphological criteria, distinction was made between *An. labranchiae* in North Africa, Italy and Corsica, and *An. sacharovi* in southern Italy, the Balkans and the Middle East; these two species can carry *P. falciparum* as well as *P. vivax*, and are responsible for the historical foci of infection around the Mediterranean Sea. On the basis of morphological or cytogenetic criteria, distinctions were made between: *An. sicaulti* (in Morocco) and *An. labranchiae*; *An. beklemishevi* and *An. messae* in Russia and Siberia; and *An. martinius* and *An. sacharovi* in Central Asia. White's very clear update (1978) is the current reference work but application of the techniques of molecular biology may lead to expansion of the number of taxons.

In 1902, Doenitz had found *An. merus* in Africa and, in 1903, Theobald had classified *An. melas* as a sub-species of *An. gambiae*: these two (which may be one and the same) live around brackish water on, respectively, the east and west coasts of Africa. In 1962, Davidson, who was studying genetics and insecticide resistance, observed that certain populations of *An. gambiae* did not interbreed since hybrid males were sterile. These forms were referred to as "A" and "B" before being classified as distinct species, namely *An. gambiae s.s.* and *An. arabiensis*. A little later in 1964, Paterson reported a zoophilic form of *An. gambiae* in South Africa—this was named *An. quadriannulatus*.

Another closely related species, also zoophilic, was described in Ethiopia (Hunt *et al.*, 1998) and these two became respectively *An. quadriannulatus* A and B. Finally, an anthropophilic form with a restricted role in transmission, occupying the very confined habitat of hot springs in the Semliki forest in Uganda, *An. gambiae* D was described by White (1985) who called it *An. bwambae*. On the basis of cytogenetic and ecological criteria, *An. gambiae s.s.* was sub-divided into five forms: "Forest", "Bissau", "Savanna", "Bamako" and "Mopti", although several experts believe that the last should be classified as a separate species. A new classification was recently proposed, based on DNA sequences encoding ribosomal RNA molecules. This recognises only two different forms, "M" and "S" which do not coincide with the cytogenetic ones. All this illustrates the complexity of modern anopheline taxonomy.

The *An. gambiae* Complex (*Figure 2*) provides a perfect example of the profound differences that can exist between members of a single complex at the epidemiological level: one species, *An. gambiae s.s.* is probably one of the most efficient vectors in the world whereas another, *An. arabiensis*, is only half as efficient in Senegal (Lemasson *et al.*, 1997). However, in Kenya (Joshi *et al.*, 1975), both species which are equally anthropophilic have the same sporozoite rate (s) (7.5-8%) although vector efficiency could be an intraspecific variable. Although they are good vectors too, *An. melas* and *An. merus* are only locally important in coastal regions. *An. bwambae* and *An. quadriannulatus* A and B are not vectors. Many experts continue to talk about *An. gambiae s.l.*; however, this is almost meaningless in both taxonomic and epidemiological terms. The species *An. funestus* and *An. nili* in Africa could also represent complexes. Despite the difficulty involved, it is becoming increasingly important to specify systematically which species of the complex is concerned in any given study with a view to more effective targeting of control operations.

Most vector species are now considered as complexes. In Southeast Asia, *An. balabacensis* was first distinguished from *An. leucosphyrus*, and then divided into three different species, namely *An. balabacensis*, *An. dirus* and *An. takasagoensis*; *An. dirus* was subsequently further divided into seven different species (*see the Chapter on the "Oriental Region"*). The following are also considered as complexes of species: *An. minimus*, *An. fluviatilis*, *An. culicifacies*, *An. philippinensis* and *An. sundaicus* in the Oriental Region, *An. farauti* in the Australasian Region, and *An. pseudopunctipennis* in the Americas.

However, *An. darlingi* in Latin America and *An. stephensi* in Asia seem to be single species even though the former shows significant biological polymorphism.

Each of the various complexes of species will be discussed in detail in the Chapters on the various biogeographical regions.

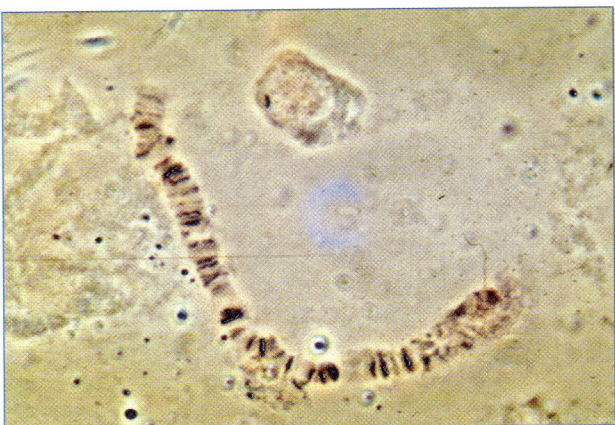

Figure 2. Polytene X chromosome of An. gambiae: microscopic examination of this chromosome allows cytogenomic identification (photograph by Coosemans).

Plasmodium *"capture" by anophelines*

The transmission of malaria depends on a dual biological adaptation of the parasite—to its vertebrate host (Man) and to its vector (*Anopheles*)—as well as ecological adaptation of the vector to the environment in which the host lives.

Why should a given *Plasmodium* species that is specific to one mammalian host (e.g. humans) evolve in a given species of *Anopheles*? No satisfactory answer has been found to this question. However, in the laboratory (but not in nature), sub-populations of vector species (i.e. species that usually transmit malaria) have been isolated which are refractory to *Plasmodium*. This is a focus of active research with the ultimate aim of finding ways to replace local vectors with competing strains of the same species which do not support infection.

Ecological adaptation is closely related to the feeding habits of each species, the availability of suitable larval habitats and its behaviour patterns. Human and ape parasites probably diverged in Africa because of differences in vector ecology, the former thriving in a savannah habitat and the latter in the forest. In practice, *An. gambiae*, the principal vector of human malaria and, to a lesser extent *An. funestus*, are not found in the dense forest interior which apes hardly ever leave.

When malaria spread out from Africa over the whole planet, its expansion is assumed to have involved the "capture" of parasites by *Anopheles* mosquitoes which were already present. In the 17th century, American *Anopheles* which had never previously been exposed to *P. falciparum* very rapidly captured this agent of malaria which had been introduced in the first slaves from Africa. Adaptation was quasi-immediate with intermittent fever representing a serious public health problem on the American continent within one-hundred years of the

Spanish conquest. It was as if there were anopheline species ready to "receive" the new parasites.

The receptivity of various *Anopheles* species to different forms of parasite is a subject in which there is currently great research interest, mainly because of the possibility of being able to select sub-populations which are refractory to *Plasmodium* (possibly as a consequence of genetic modification) and then using them to compete out efficient vectors (*see the Part on* "Malaria Control"). For the time being, such research is far from being applicable on the ground but transgenic mosquitoes are nevertheless all the rage.

In contrast, the results of experiments to investigate whether or not African strains of *P. falciparum* can be transmitted by Euro-Mediterranean *Anopheles* species belonging to the Maculipennis Complex (*An. atroparvus*, *An. labranchiae* and *An. sacharovi*) (*see the Chapter on* the "Palaearctic Region") are unequivocal: they cannot (Zulueta *et al.*, 1975). Nevertheless, these species (especially the last two) were efficient vectors for *P. falciparum* around the Mediterranean in Europe (with this parasite historically causing more than 30% of all cases of malaria in Corsica). No hypothesis has been advanced to account for these results other than there must be some key difference between *P. falciparum* from Africa today and the species that was eradicated in Europe (Bruce-Chwatt & Zulueta, 1980).

Vector species

More than 480 species of *Anopheles* have been found on the planet (*see below*) but only 70-80 appear to be able to transmit malaria. *Table II* shows these according to biogeographical region. The terms "major vector" (or "main vector") and "secondary vector" are often used without any definition of what they mean, e.g. many experts treat *An. moucheti* as a secondary vector in the forests of central Africa although its sporozoite rate is as high as that of *An. gambiae* and it is far denser than that species along waterways. Conversely, many species have been suspected of being vectors without much evidence. A mistake may be perpetuated from expert to expert and finish up in the literature, e.g. Barber & Olinger reported finding infected *An. obscurus* in Nigeria in 1931 whereas in fact, this species does not feed on humans.

Although there is usually consensus about the place of the main vectors (which are, in some cases, confined to limited areas), the importance of secondary vectors has to be made clear. Hamon & Mouchet (1961) proposed making distinctions between broadly distributed "main vectors", "locally important vectors" and "secondary vectors". This terminology is used in *Table II* although no classification system covers all possibilities perfectly.

As a rule, main vectors have a sporozoite rate of over 1% in Africa. Locally important vectors have a sporozoite rate of the same order but on a more geographically confined basis, e.g. *An. paludis* has a sporozoite rate of over 2% in the upper basin of the Congo and the Ubangi rivers whereas elsewhere in Africa, it is rarely found carrying *Plasmodium* (and it may be that the central African population represents a different species). Most secondary vectors have an average sporozoite rate of under 0.1%. In the rest of the world, sporozoite rates are far lower, e.g. in South America, they tend to be below 0.1% (often just 0.01%). Depending on the source and the classification system used, 30-36 species are defined as main vectors, 28 as locally important vectors, and 17-25 as secondary vectors.

The taxonomy, ecology, behaviour and vector efficiency of all the key species will be discussed in detail in the Sections on the various biogeographical regions.

Anopheline biology

In this introductory section, we will review those features of the biology, ecology and behaviour of *Anopheles* which are essential to understanding the parasites' life cycles and the epidemiology of malaria, to be discussed in subsequent Chapters.

Anopheline mosquitoes are dipterous insects (i.e. with two wings). They are holometabolous meaning they undergo complete metamorphosis with four different stages in their life cycle. The first three stages—eggs, larvae and pupae—are referred to as pre-adult, and are exclusively aquatic. The last stage, the adult or imago stage, can fly.

The female lays 40-100 individual eggs on the surface of water. Each egg is 0.5 mm in length and is equipped with floats (*Figure 3*). It hatches 24-48 hours after laying (depending on the temperature) to give rise to a single larva which assumes a position parallel to the surface of the water. Unlike *Aedes* and *Culex* larvae, those of *Anopheles* do not have a siphon for breathing. The larva feeds on detritus at the surface and grows in a discontinuous fashion, moulting four times. During moulting, it sheds its old cuticle and secretes a new, bigger one which allows it to increase in size and volume: the biggest species can grow by 1 mm to 2 cm in length. The fourth moult gives rise to the pupal stage which in most cases lasts less than 48 hours during which the pupa does not feed but undergoes massive morphological remodelling leading to metamorphosis and the emergence of the adult which subsequently flies off.

Adult males live for seven to ten days and females for two to four weeks in the tropics; in temperate zones, the females may live longer as a result of the phenomenon of winter diapause.

As soon as it emerges, the adult rests outside the water for 10-24 hours while its cuticle hardens and its wings are deployed. During this time, the reproductive parts of the male rotate through an angle of 180° to become functional. Depending on the species, mating occurs either in flight in the course of swarming, or on a support. The males have feathery antennae (which are olfactory organs involved in detecting females in the vicinity) whereas the females have

Table II. *Anopheles* which transmit human malaria.

Biogeographical regions*	Main vectors	Locally significant vectors	Secondary or unconfirmed vectors
Afrotropical Region	An. gambiae s.s. An. arabiensis An. funestus An. nili s.l. An. moucheti	An. melas An. merus An. mascarensis An. paludis An. pharoensis	An. brunnipes An. rivulorum An. hargreavesi An. coustani
Australasian Region	An. farauti n°1 An. punctulatus An. koliensis		
Oriental Region	An. minimus A and C An. dirus A and D An. balabacensis An. flavirostris An. maculatus An. sundaicus An. aconitus An. fluviatilis S An. culicifacies A,C,D and E An. stephensi	An. leucosphyrus An. sawadwongporni An. willmori An. pseudowillmori An. dirus B and C An. barbirostris An. letifer An. campestris An. philippinensis An. nivipes An. kumingensis	An. litoralis An. mangyanus An. donaldi An. annularis An. tesselatus An. vagus An. varuna An. subpictus
Palaearctic Region	An. anthropophagus An. sinensis An. labranchiae An. sacharovi An. atroparvus** An. superpictus An. sergentii	An. sicaulti An. messae** An. melanoon** An. maculipennis**	An. claviger** An. plumbeus An. dthali An. hyrcanus An. pulcherrimus
American Region	An. darlingi An. albimanus An. pseudopunctipennis An. aquasalis An. nuneztovari An. quadrimaculatus	An. vestitipennis An. (K.) bellator An. (K.) cruzi An. (K.) homonculus An. (K.) neavei An. freeborni An. hermsi An. deaneorum	An. gabaldoni An. oswaldi An. albitaris An. triannulatus An. braziliensis An. marajoara An. allopha

* Biogeographical region: *see the Chapter on* "Malaria in the Main Biogeographical Regions"
** Species found in places where malaria has been eradicated and which no longer play any role in transmission

---

glabrous antennae so gender can be ascertained with the naked eye. Males mate several times during their lives but females usually mate once (Clements, 1992). The female stores sperm in a special receptacle called the spermatheca from which spermatozoa are released each time she lays eggs. Whereas the male derives all its energy from nectar, the female also seeks a vertebrate from which she takes a blood meal every two or three days. This meal provides her with the protein necessary to produce the vitellin of the oocytes. In the course of the **blood meal**, she will withdraw up to four times her own volume of blood, usually in one meal. But if the female is disturbed, the meal can be interrupted. Such interrupted feeding used to be considered as atypical behaviour until it was observed that fully 15% of *An. gambiae s.s.* individuals could feed on two or more people in succession (Boreham, 1975; Eldin de Pécoulas *et al.*, 1996; Kulkarni & Panda, 1984).

After her blood meal, the female rests, usually close to where she fed. The blood taken in is concentrated and turns black as the aqueous component is exuded over a period of one to two hours. During the digestion process, her oocytes grow to fill most of the abdominal cavity which then appears white.

These abdominal changes in the course of digestion of the blood meal can be followed with the naked eye. Depending on the extent of their repletion, specimens of females are classified as "fasting" or **unfed, engorged** (in which the

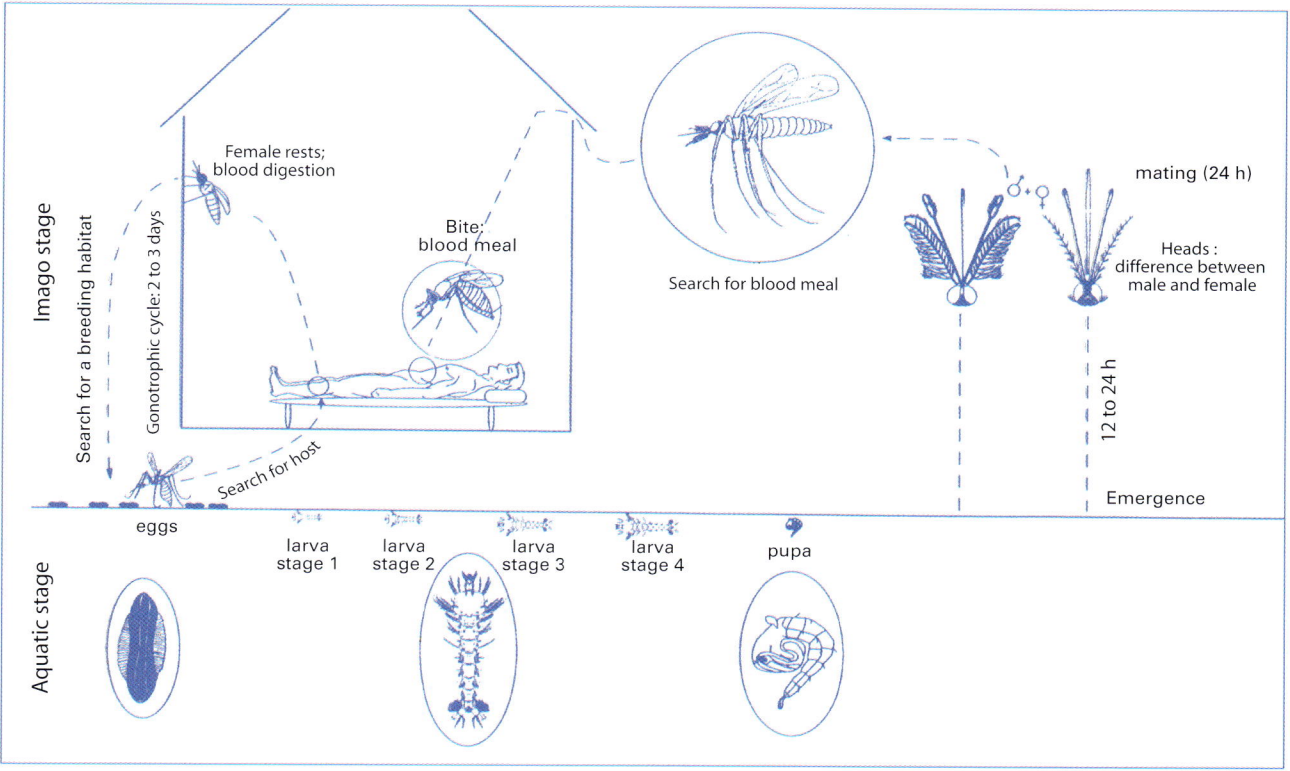

Figure 3. *Anopheline life cycle (drawing J. Finot).*

abdomen is coloured red by the fresh blood it contains), **semi-gravid** (the abdomen black with blood being digested and with a white patch at the top where the ovaries are developing) or **gravid** (in which the abdomen is swollen and white in colour) (*Figure 4*). Once the oocytes are mature, they are laid. During the laying process as the oocyte passes through the oviduct, it is fertilised by spermatozoa stored in the spermatheca to become an egg.

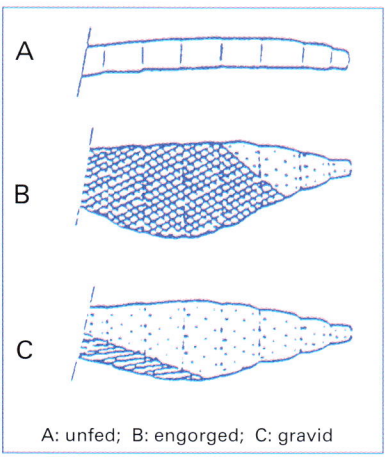

Figure 4. *Abdominal changes in female Anopheles (adapted from WHO, 1961). Reproduced in Danis & Mouchet (1991).*

A: unfed; B: engorged; C: gravid

After laying, the female *Anopheles* looks for a host for another blood meal.

The biological cycle starting with the biting of a vertebrate host, it proceeds through digestion of the blood, oocyte maturation, finding a place to lay the eggs, laying and finally the quest for a new host: this is referred to as the **gonotrophic cycle**.

In tropical and sub-tropical climes, this cycle takes 48-72 hours, depending on species and temperature. In a cold or temperate climate, it may last up to a week and in winter it may be interrupted by a hibernation phase referred to as the **winter diapause**. For example, the Eurasian *An. messae* does not feed at all during diapause but lives on fat bodies built up during the autumn. In other species in Europe and the Middle East, such as *An. atroparvus*, activities are not completely arrested during the winter: the females continue to take occasional blood meals but these do not trigger ovarian development. This phenomenon is called **gonotrophic dissociation** (*see the Chapter on* the "Palaearctic Region").

The gonotrophic cycle is a fundamental physiological process in the life of an *Anopheles* mosquito from which it is possible to estimate a species' life expectancy and the likelihood that it will become infectious (*see below*). Every laying cycle leaves scars in the ovary so, if the duration of the gonotrophic cycle and the number of times the female has laid eggs are both known, the life expectancy of a specimen following its first egg-laying cycle can be calculated which in turn provides an idea of how likely it is that a given *Anopheles* species will become infectious. A simplified method was developed by Detinova (1962) in which the respective proportions of females which have never laid any eggs (nulliparous) and females which have laid at least one batch of eggs (parous) are estimated. These two can be distinguished quickly and simply by microscopic examination because the ends of the tracheoles* of nulliparous females are curled up whereas those of parous females are unwound (*Figure 5*). The percentage of parous females gives the **parous rate** from which it is possible to estimate the daily survival of a population of *Anopheles***.

Because of the central role of *Anopheles* in malaria epidemiology, these insects have been exhaustively studied. An impressive body of research has been dedicated to their physiology (Clements, 1992) as well as their ecology and behaviour.

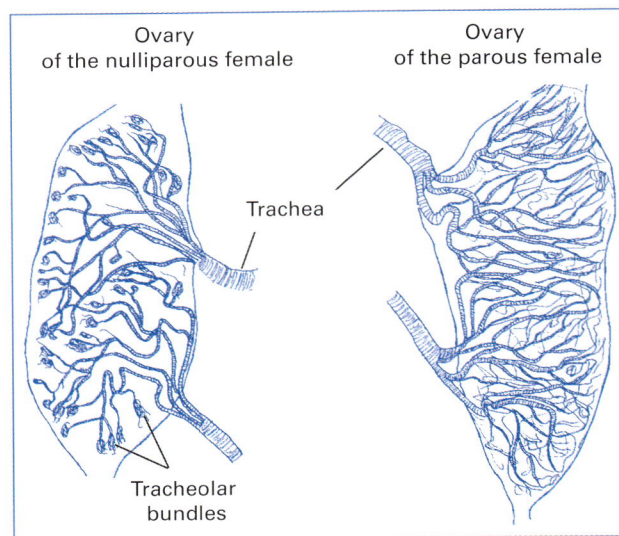

Figure 5. Changes in the terminal ovarian tracheoles of Anopheles *(adapted from Detinova, WHO 1962).*

Anopheline ecology and behaviour

Larval ecology

The various species of *Anopheles* exploit a huge variety of different types of water habitats: flowing torrents or canals (*An. nili* in Africa, *An. minimus* in Southeast Asia), slow-moving river water habitats (*An. moucheti* in Central Africa and *An. darlingi* in Latin America), residual pools (*An. culicifacies* in Asia and *An. pseudopunctipennis* in Latin America), stagnant deposits in sunny spots (members of the *An. gambiae* Complex in Africa), wetlands with emergent plants (*An. funestus* in Africa and *An. albimanus* in Central America), woodland puddles (*An. dirus* and *An. balabacensis* in Southeast Asia), brackish water in coastal zones (*An. sundaicus* in Southeast Asia, *An. melas* and *An. merus* in Africa, and *An. aquasalis* in South America), and axillary accumulations of water on bromeliads (the sub-genus *Kerteszia*). Seasonal changes in flora mean that different species can exploit the same habitat at different times of the year, e.g. in rice paddies, species belonging to the sun-loving *An. gambiae* Complex thrive when the fields are flooded and during planting, whereas once the rice is growing, they give way to species which seek shade from emergent plants such as *An. pharoensis* in West Africa and *An. funestus* in Madagascar.

The choice of oviposition is also a behavioural variable. More than fifty years ago, Muirhead-Thompson (1945) working in Sierra Leone showed that if a sunny area was covered over with vegetation, *An. gambiae* stopped laying its eggs there.

It is important to bear in mind the fact that every species has its own larval sites, be they highly specialised or covering a broad range of different ecological situations, especially when humans have changed environmental conditions. The presence of satisfactory larval habitats determines the spatial distribution of species as well as, to some extent, behaviour patterns. In Southeast Asia, malaria is common in wooded hills and forest areas where shade-loving vectors thrive—*An. minimus* in shady streams and *An. dirus* in woodland water pools; in contrast, there is little malaria on the rice-growing plains where these vectors cannot find places suitable for their larvae. The opposite is seen in Africa with sun-loving *An. gambiae* or *An. arabiensis* found all over the continent apart from in forest areas and at high altitude (above 2,000 metres): because their sunlit larval habitats are relatively unspecialised—being found everywhere in ecological conditions as diverse as footprints and rice paddies—malaria is ubiquitous.

Ecology and behaviour of adults

Apart from the diurnal *Kerteszia* spp. in South America, anophelines are active at night (from sunset to sunrise). Bites during the daytime have often been reported (in houses or in woods) but this is atypical behaviour, sometimes due to the effects of intrusion.

---

* The tracheoles are the terminations of the tracheae at the body surface, whereby air is supplied throughout the insect's body, notably to the ovaries.

** All these methods are described in detail in MacDonald (1957), and developed in Danis & Mouchet (1991).

Some species tend to bite in the early evening but most major vectors are active between 11 p.m. and 3 a.m., after egg-laying. Some individuals, notably nulliparous females who are not delayed by the need to lay eggs, may bite in the early evening. As is true for all aspects of *Anopheles* behaviour, the time of biting varies from population to population (or even from individual to individual), from one site to another, and in different seasons.

Anopheles which feed on humans are said to be **anthropophilic** as opposed to those that are **zoophilic** which prefer biting animals. Some species are known to be strictly anthropophilic, including *An. gambiae s.s.* in the Cameroonian forest* and *An. dirus* A and D in the forests of Southeast Asia. Exclusively zoophilic species—which therefore do not transmit human malaria—are far more common although some of these are commonly found indoors, e.g. *An. rufipes* in West Africa. Many species feed on both humans and livestock, whichever is available, although some have a distinct preference for one or the other. The genetic determinants of feeding behaviour have not yet been clearly defined. How specimens are sampled is extremely important when it comes to elucidating a given species' feeding behaviour: the information obtained may vary enormously according to whether the specimens were gathered in houses, animal sheds or outside. The results of precipitin tests to identify the nature of blood meals should only ever be interpreted in the light of where the specimen was sampled—although many experts restrict their studies to locally dominant tendencies.

If the blood meal is taken inside the house, the mosquito's behaviour is said to be **endophagic** whereas mosquitoes that tend to bite outdoors are described as **exophagic**.

After a blood meal, some *Anopheles* stay inside the house throughout the gonotrophic cycle—these are referred to as **endophilic** (e.g. *An. minimus* A). In contrast, so-called **exophilic** species (e.g. *An. dirus* A in Southeast Asia) leave the house immediately for a safe resting site outside. Between these two extremes, there is a spectrum of behaviour patterns—and behaviour often varies enormously even between individuals of the same species. In hot, dry places where people sleep outside, many vectors actively seek shelter inside houses during the day, e.g. *An. gambiae s.l.* in the Senegalese Sahel (Faye *et al.*, 1997) where resting sites for *Anopheles* outside are relatively rare. The details of houses or dwellings may play an important role, e.g. the wall-less houses of Amazonian Indians favour the exophilic *An. darlingi* and huts in Asia favour *An. dirus*. Exophilic behaviour has often been blamed for the failure of spraying-based vector control programmes although information is often lacking on the degree of exophilic behaviour, be it total or partial. It is vital to make the distinction between the naturally exophilic behaviour of certain anopheline species and the consequences of treatment with DDT or pyrethroid insecticides which tends to drive all types of mosquito out of sprayed houses.

Most other aspects of vector ecology and behaviour are of relatively minor importance compared to feeding and reproduction.

---

* Curiously, *An. gambiae s.s.* do not thrive under the African forest cover. They tend to lay their eggs in water deposits close to villages, on footpaths and along rivers.

Plasmodium Life Cycles in Humans and Anopheline Vectors

Pathogenic malaria complex

Malaria cannot be transmitted directly between humans, apart from in the exceptional cases of medical blood transfusion and mother-to-baby transmission (which are negligible in epidemiological terms). The *Plasmodium* cycle requires development in an invertebrate—an anopheline mosquito—before it is inoculated into a receptive human host.

Human, parasite and *Anopheles* are the three components of an interactive cycle and their mutual functions only proceed if certain climatic and ecological conditions—specific to the different species of parasite and *Anopheles*—pertain. The man/parasite/vector unit which exists only in an environment that promotes transmission of the disease constitutes the **pathogenic malaria complex** (*Figure 1*), to use an already-old term (Sorre, 1943).

Interactions within this complex depend on natural or man-made environmental conditions (deforestation, irrigation, urbanisation, etc.), climate (temperature, rainfall, relative humidity), malaria control measures, migration, and changes in the anopheline fauna as well as other secondary factors. A concatenation of circumstances may result in an increase in transmission and/or in the incidence of malaria in a given place or situation—or a decrease.

Emphasis is readily put on the worsening aspects of the malaria situation across the world resulting from diverse factors such as climatic events (notably floods), the cessation of indoor spraying operations, poorly implemented control programmes, deteriorating health care services, civil war, and resistance—both of *Plasmodium* to drugs and of *Anopheles* to insecticides. Improvements are less often highlighted; nevertheless, between 1950 and 1975, the surface area across which malaria is endemic dropped by 30% and the number of cases outside of tropical Africa fell by over 90% as a direct consequence of eradication operations. At the local level in the Sahel, drought caused a decrease of over 60% in the prevalence of malaria between 1973 and the end of the century (Mouchet *et al.*, 1996). On the other hand, well-organised and implemented malaria control programmes are successful in some countries of Southeast Asia such as Vietnam or China.

Global warming is an obvious concern for all peoples and governments. The media have already talked a great deal about the potential problem of warming-related rises in the prevalence of malaria even though no concrete evidence

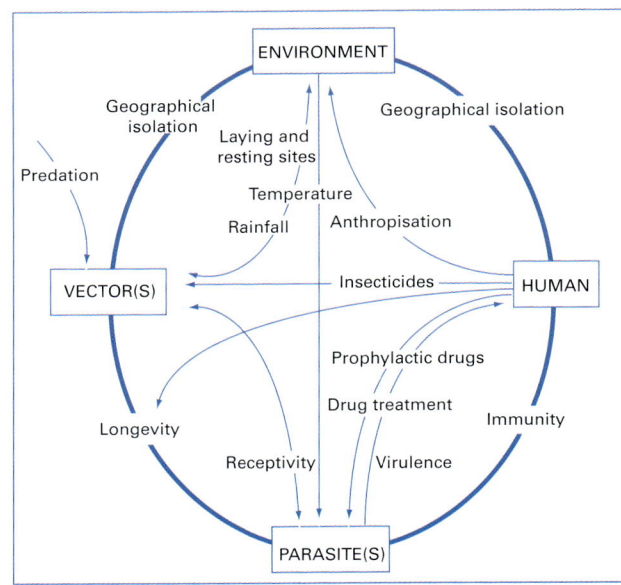

Figure 1. *Key components of the pathogenic malaria complex and interactions (adapted from Julvez, 1993).*

of such rise has yet been observed. Most experts in malaria and meteorology choose not to take up a position before it is clearly understood how the various malaria determinants will be affected. It may indeed be that global warming will be accompanied by an increase in the prevalence of malaria but nobody can be sure that this will definitely occur, nor exactly how or to what extent.

Among the other factors to be taken into account, environmental degradation is a key factor, in both industrialised and developing countries; all epidemiological facies* are concerned and changes could profoundly affect the malaria picture. In Southeast Asia, deforestation is eliminating shade-loving vectors of the *An. dirus* Complex and, to a lesser extent, *An. minimus s.l.*, thereby inducing a drop in transmission and in prevalence of the disease. In Africa in contrast, deforestation is favouring the sun-preferring species of the *An. gambiae* Complex increasing transmission and malaria. Factors related to climate, environment, population movements, the growth of rapid transport and the effects of control programmes are dealt with in the Parts on "Spatiotemporal Dynamics of Malaria" and "Malaria Control". We draw particular attention to the disastrous consequences of the discontinuation of eradication operations or vector control programmes, which take the form of deadly epidemics (e.g. in Madagascar, Swaziland and Sri Lanka) in which the prevalence of malaria can return pre-1950 levels (Mouchet *et al.*, 1998).

Plasmodium cycles

Plasmodium is a sporozoan with a complicated cycle. For transmission from one vertebrate to another, passage through a mosquito is required, during which phase the parasite undergoes sexual reproduction.

Most of the cycles of human plasmodia have been described in specialised treatises (Boyd, 1949; Brumpt, 1949; Bruce-Chwatt, 1980; Russel *et al.*, 1963; Wernsdorfer & McGregor, 1988). All the cycles can be broadly divided into two phases, namely an asexual phase in humans and a sexual phase which begins in the human to be completed in the insect biological vector (*Figure 2*).

Asexual phase in the human host

The cycle of *Plasmodium* in the human begins with an infected mosquito biting and inoculating a plasmodial sporozoite into its host. Sporozoites migrate to the liver within one hour after biting (*Figure 3*). Division of the parasite inside liver cells generates hepatic schizonts, a pre-erythrocytic (i.e. prior to invasion of the red blood cell) or exo-erythrocytic (outside of the red blood cell) stage. After maturation over a period of eight to ten days, the schizont bursts and releases several thousand merozoites into the bloodstream. For *P. falciparum*, every schizont releases about 40,000 merozoites, 15,000 for *P. ovale*, 10,000 for *P. vivax*, and about 2,000 for *P. malariae*.

The merozoite invades a red blood cell inside which it changes into a trophozoite and then an erythrocytic schizont, each of which contains 16-32 nuclei. Every nucleus gives rise to a new merozoite. When the cell ruptures, released merozoites quickly invade a healthy red cell, thereby recommencing the schizogenic cycle. This represents the asexual erythrocytic cycle.

Plasmodium falciparum

Only the beginning of the *P. falciparum* cycle takes place in the peripheral blood; the erythrocytic shizont divides in the internal organs, notably in the placenta in pregnant women.

In the host, all the parasites develop synchronously with an erythrocytic cycle that lasts 48 hours, the rupture of the red blood cells induces the high fever of the paroxysmal attack of the disease, hence the name "malignant tertian fever" by which pernicious or falciparum malaria was known even before the parasite was discovered. After several cycles of asexual reproduction, the patient (if still alive) spontaneously recovers.

After nine to eleven days, male and female **gametocytes** (non-pathogenic, sexual forms) develop. It is believed that gametocytogenesis is triggered by an environmental stimulus linked to the host's immune system (Smalley & Brown, 1981). Gametocytes do not develop further in humans and the cycle thereafter can only continue inside suitable *Anopheles* mosquitoes. Gametocytes can survive in the blood for months, remaining infectious for the vector (Smalley & Sinden, 1977), although the exact duration of infectivity remains controversial.

Plasmodium malariae

The cycle of *P. malariae* is similar to that of *P. falciparum* but it lasts 72 hours and erythrocytic schizogony can occur in the peripheral blood. Asexual forms can persist for a very long time in the host's blood, causing delayed, **clinical relapses**. The parasite density is never nearly as high as that of *P. falciparum*.

---

* An epidemiological facies or stratum corresponds to a group of places in which malaria is transmitted in the same way and that share epidemiological characteristics and similar levels of incidence (Carnevale & Mouchet, 1981).

Biodiversity of Malaria in the World

Plasmodium vivax and *Plasmodium ovale*

The development of *P. vivax* and *P. ovale* differs from that of *P. falciparum*.

Two points merit emphasis:
- the erythrocytic schizont divides in the peripheral blood in which dividing **rosette forms** can be seen (whereas *P. falciparum* schizogony proceeds in internal organs);
- after liver invasion, some of the **sporozoites** transform into hepatic schizonts which continue maturing and launch a cycle that proceeds like that of *P. falciparum*; however, in a variable proportion of the sporozoites, development is arrested resulting in dormant, intracellular forms referred to as **hypnozoites**. After an interval of three to twelve—or perhaps more—months, these hypnozoites start to divide, giving rise to erythrocytic cycles which manifest as **relapsing malaria**. The proportion of sporozoites which develop immediately or become dormant varies between different strains. In cold

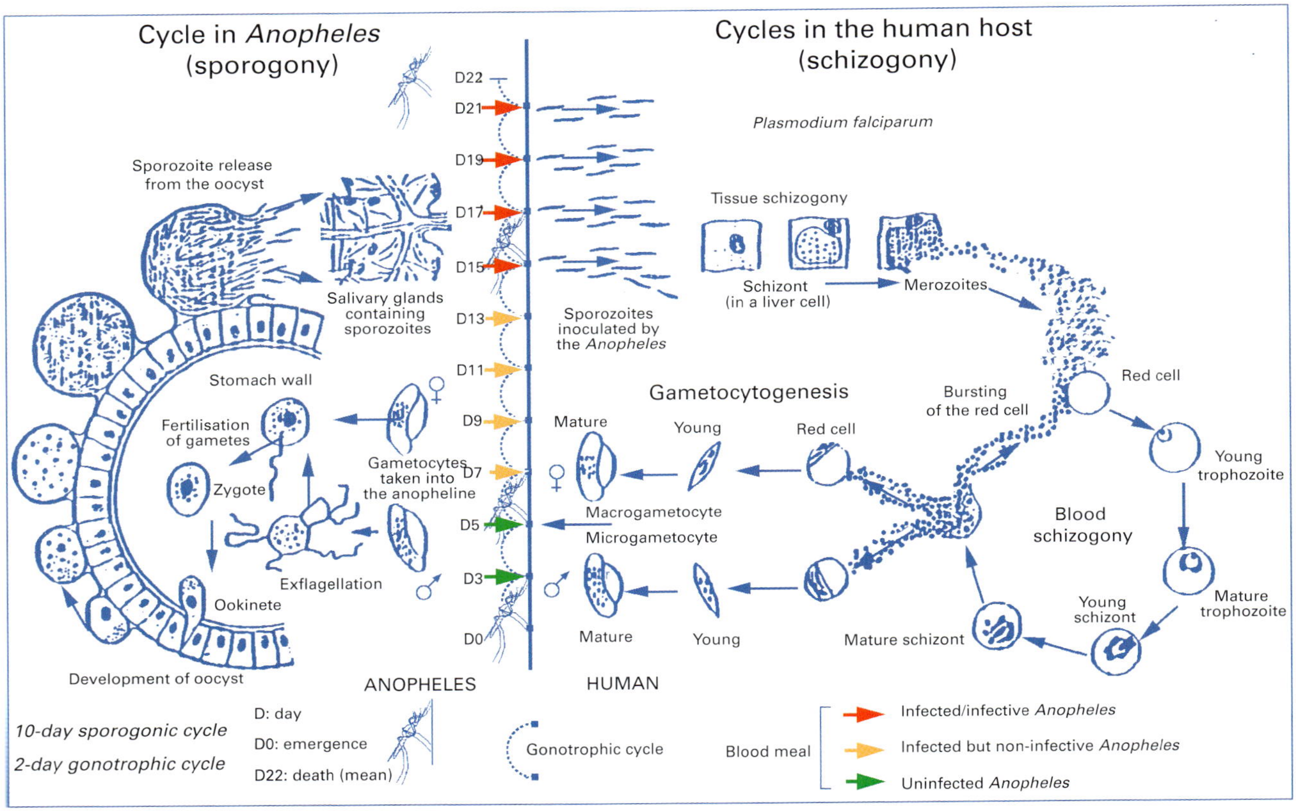

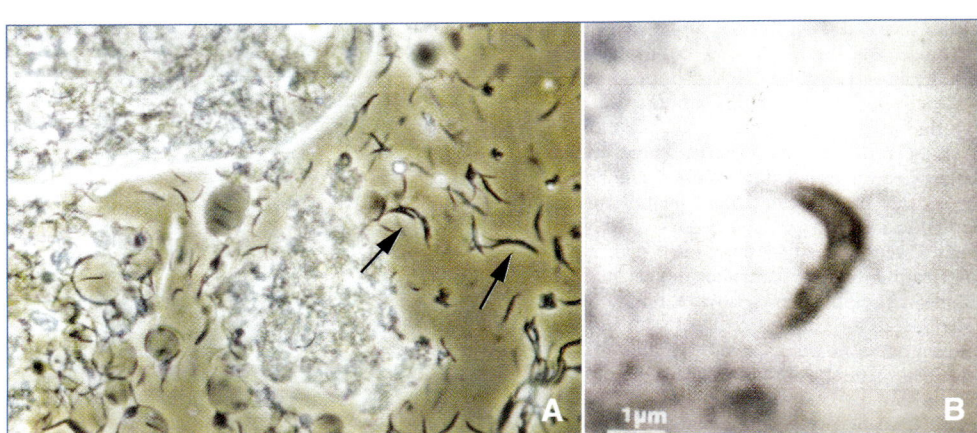

Figure 2. Plasmodial life cycles (reproduced with the permission of P. Carnevale and P. Boussès).

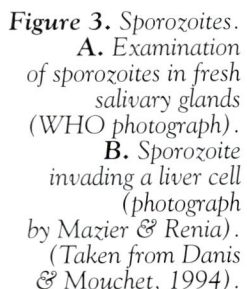

Figure 3. Sporozoites. **A.** Examination of sporozoites in fresh salivary glands (WHO photograph). **B.** Sporozoite invading a liver cell (photograph by Mazier & Renia). (Taken from Danis & Mouchet, 1994).

climates, development can be postponed in up to 100% of *P. vivax* sporozoites and subjects infected in autumn may not experience any attack until the next spring: this has led to the description of *P.vivax* **hibernans** forms (Feighner *et al.*, 1998; Garnham *et al.*, 1975; Lysenko & Kondrashine, 1999; Renkonen, 1944). In contrast, in tropical Southeast Asia, the vast majority of sporozoites go straight into an erythrocytic cycle.

The question can be asked whether the more appropriate term is *P. vivax* or the "*P. vivax* Complex". Studies on the circumsporozoite protein (CSP) have shown the existence of variants of *P. vivax*: VK210 and VK247 (Rosenberg *et al.*, 1989). In 2001, evaluation of the "success" of parasite development in *An. albimanus* led to a distinction between Southeast Asian *P. vivax* strains and a form found in Central America and Colombia which, it was proposed, should be classified as a sub-species, *P. vivax collinsi* (Jun Li *et al.*, 2001). The Asian form cannot be distinguished from the monkey species *P. simium* which was apparently introduced into the Americas on several different occasions: it was probably a strain introduced in about 1500 that gave rise to the modern American form (Mason, 1961).

In addition, in Brazil, Indonesia and Madagascar, a *P. vivax*-like form has been identified which cannot be distinguished from *P. simiovale* found in macaques in Sri Lanka (as mentioned above) (Qari *et al.*, 1993a and b).

Sexual phase in Anopheles

With its blood meal, *Anopheles* takes in male and female **gametocytes**. In its stomach, while asexual forms of the parasite are digested, the gametocytes transform into **gametes**:
- a female macrogametocyte produces a female gamete,
- a male microgametocyte can produce, by exflagellation following nuclear division, eight male gametes.

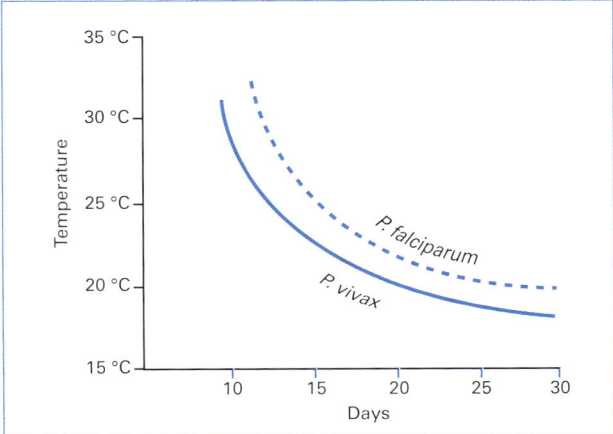

Figure 4. *Duration of the extrinsic cycles of* P. falciparum *and* P. vivax *in Anopheles (in Danis & Mouchet, 1991).*

Males and females conjugate in the insect's stomach (or midgut) to generate a zygote, the **ookinete** which is a motile egg. It crosses the peritrophic membrane (which encloses the blood meal chamber) and the cells of the stomach wall to form an **oocyst** which immediately divides. Meiosis occurs in the course of the first division of the nucleus of the ookinete. Conjugation of a male and a female gamete followed by this meiosis is thus accompanied by genetic recombination. Throughout the rest of its cycle all divisions are mitotic and the *Plasmodium* is **haploid** with a total of thirteen chromosomes. The cells of the oocyst are elongated and transform first into **sporoblasts** and then into **sporozoites**. Once the sporozoites have formed, rupture of the oocyst wall releases them into the insect's principal body cavity where they complete the maturation process, ultimately migrating to the mosquito's salivary glands. Each infected gland can hold hundreds or even thousands of sporozoites which are 2-micron-long, rod-shaped bodies. In a single *An. gambiae* mosquito, up to 250,000 sporozoites per gland have been found in specimens carrying 350 oocysts and in *An. funestus*, 77,000 sporozoites have been reported from 286 oocysts (Pringle, 1966b); however, these are extreme figures—the average for *P. falciparum* is between 2,000 and 4,000 sporozoites per salivary gland but few of them are actually inoculated into the human body.

When the mosquito bites, it "probes" the skin to find the underlying blood vessel and it is at this time that it injects the infectious sporozoites into the dermis (Robert & Brey, 1998).

The cycle in *Anopheles* is referred to as the **sporogonic cycle** and is an essential intermediate in the transmission of the parasite from one human host to the next. It is also essential for the evolution of the parasite since it includes the sexual stage. This cycle is central to the study of malaria if epidemiology is to cover all the phenomena involved in the development and maintenance of a pathogenic complex rather than simply focusing on the features of the disease in human beings.

The duration of the sporogonic cycle of each parasite depends on temperature. At 25 °C, the *P. vivax* cycle takes ten days and that of *P. falciparum* thirteen days. As the temperature drops, the *P. falciparum* sporogonic cycle becomes longer, so at 20 °C it lasts thirty days; at below 18 °C, it is completely stopped. At 20 °C, the *P. vivax* cycle takes twenty-five days, disappearing below 15-16 °C. The calculations of Macdonald (1957) (*Figure 4*) and the formula of Molineaux (*in* Wernsdorfer & McGregor, 1988) make it easy to estimate how long the sporogonic cycles will take at different temperatures. The cycles of *P. malariae* and *P. ovale* are longer—from eighteen to twenty days at 25 °C.

The duration of the sporogonic cycle is a key parameter when it comes to determining the geographical distribution of *Plasmodium* species. Thus, while *P. vivax* can be transmitted in temperate regions (and even in cold regions during the short northern summer), the other species—which require a longer development period at higher temperatures—are confined to tropical and sub-tropical latitudes. Moreover, species with a long cycle (*P. malarie, P. ovale*) can only be transmitted by long-lived vectors, which explains why they are less prevalent even in those places where they are found.

Polymorphism in *Plasmodium falciparum*

Investigation of the plasmodial genome began with the cloning of parasites, notably *P. falciparum* (Walliker, 1981). As of 1994 (Thaithong, 1994), it became apparent that blood samples and even clinical isolates actually contain mixtures of haploid clones (*Table I*).

When *Anopheles* takes in two different clones in a single blood meal, they recombine to generate recombinant clones which are genotypically distinct from either parent with an estimated in-breeding rate of 0.39. In a holo-endemic zone in Tanzania, the *An. gambiae s.s.* vector is highly mobile and in consequence, there is significant gene flow (0.56) between houses in a village in which a great number of distinct clones occur (Babiker *et al.*, 1995, 1997). These clones can be distinguished from one another by analysing the highly polymorphic merozoite surface proteins MSP 1 and MSP 2 (Viriyakosol *et al.*, 1995). For example, in Tanzania, seventeen and twenty three alleles of each of these two proteins respectively have been identified following PCR amplification and the electrophoretic analysis of the corresponding loci. Using these two markers, the number of clones present in any single patient in a given village can be estimated (Hill & Babiker, 1995).

As a general rule, the number of clones and the number of MSP alleles in any subject depends on the incidence of malaria and the rate of inoculation. In Tanzania, people were found to be infected with between one and six clones (mean = 3.5). All the subjects were being regularly inoculated with new clones but many of these were inhibited by specific protection mechanisms directed against genotypes that had been encountered beforehand; this resulted in a constant turnover of clones. Most clones disappear almost as soon as they have appeared. It is the genotypes that persist and are not controlled that provoke paroxysms of malaria. This classic theory comes into the explanation of premunition to malaria (*see the Chapter on "Man Facing Malaria"*) (Babiker *et al.*, 1998, 1999, 2000).

In the dry regions of Sudan where transmission rates are low, the number of clones was far lower (1.3 per subject). Many people were carrying only a single clone although at the end of the rainy season, increased polymorphism was observed (Babiker *et al.*, 1997; Theander, 1998). In these conditions, immunity was low or null and all subjects were susceptible to infection by *P. falciparum.*

Elsewhere in Africa, in Senegal where the Entomological Inoculation Rate (EIR) is 100-200, each infected subject carries 3.9-4.8 clones; in Gambia (EIR = 24), there are 2.9 clones per subject; in Kenya (EIR = 26) the figure is 2, and in Sudan (EIR = 0.6), just 1.3 (Hill & Babiker, 1995).

In a rural region of Thailand where transmission is very low, genomic diversity was nevertheless high (Paul *et al.*, 1998).

In French Guiana where *P. falciparum* was imported four hundred years ago, there was far less polymorphism than in Africa (Ariey, 1996), although the experimental methods used were different from those used in East Africa and Thailand.

Information on this topic is changing rapidly. What it is important to recognise is the extensive recombination between *P. falciparum* clones in holo-endemic regions where malaria is stable, and transmission is continuous and intense. Clone proliferation is modulated by immune defence mechanisms which are overwhelmed by certain genotypes (e.g. due to drug resistance) to give rise to pathological paroxysms. Results from molecular biology are beginning to bring explanations of premunition.

The genomes of other human plasmodia have not been studied in such detail.

Table I. Number of clones of *P. falciparum* per carrier in various parts of Africa.			
Country/region	**Entomological inoculation rate***	**Number of clones**	**Authors**
Senegal	100 à 200 ib/p/yr	3.9-4.8	Trape & Rogier, 1996
Gambia	24 ib/p/yr	2.9	
Kenya	26 ib/p/yr	2.0	
Sudan (arid)	0.6 ib/p/yr	1.3	Hill & Babiker, 1995
* ib/p/yr: infective bite/person/year			

Epidemiological Basis

Requisites for autochthonous malaria

All humans are susceptible to infection with human plasmodia although Melano-Africans are genetically refractory to *P. vivax*. What stops the disease spreading throughout the world is the fact the parasite cannot be transmitted directly from human to human but requires an intermediate, the vector. Introducing an infected man into a place where there is no vector capable of transmitting the parasite amounts to a parasitic cul-de-sac even though he himself will either recover from the disease or die.

The absence of malaria from the islands of Mauritius and Réunion up until the introduction of *Anopheles* between 1860 and 1870 is an illuminating example. Once they were discovered, many carriers of the parasite from Africa and Asia travelled to these islands—Creole people from the region even went there to "regain their health". However, despite what many historians have affirmed, it was not the introduction of such carriers that led to malaria becoming endemic which only occurred following the introduction and acclimatisation of anopheline vectors (Julvez *et al.*, 1990). Humans provide an intermediate vertebrate host and even act as an amplifier but they cannot on their own sustain the disease cycle.

It is therefore the vector—in which the parasite undergoes sexual reproduction—which is the definitive host and the hub of malaria epidemiology. In addition, *Plasmodium* "respects" its vector, only provoking pathology in its vertebrate host, maybe causing death.

If there is to be "autochthonous malaria" in a given region, the presence of the following is necessary:
- anopheline species that are genetically capable of hosting the *Plasmodium* cycle;
- larval habitats for the mosquitoes in sufficient number to sustain a minimum or a "critical" density of *Anopheles* and rate of blood feeding on local people;
- anthropophilic anophelines survive long enough in the local climatic conditions for the *Plasmodium* to complete its sporogonic cycle;
- human subjects carrying infective gametocytes and susceptible to *Plasmodium*.

Whether or not vector insects are present in some natural or man-made environment can currently be determined and the underlying reasons can sometimes be explained; however, their presence cannot be predicted, at least not as yet. The question involves multiple interacting factors—physical, biological and anthropogenic—which determine the distribution of the local fauna. *An. arabiensis* of the *An. gambiae* Complex provides an example: this species which is found in Tropical Africa and south-western Arabia never spread to either Iran or Pakistan to the east, even though climatic conditions there are similar. In contrast, to the west, it crossed the Atlantic Ocean in boats and became established in Brazil in the 1930's (although it has since been eradicated from that country by insecticide treatment); and to the north, it has spread to Egypt but not through the Sahara to other North African countries. Another illuminating example is the absence of *Anopheles* from Oceania east of Vanuatu: this remains an enigma given the fact that it is more than likely that it has been introduced many times into New Caledonia and Fiji.

Malaria indicators

Diagnosing plasmodial infection

Both direct and indirect methods can be used to diagnose malaria. The direct methods are based on detecting the *Plasmodium* itself (e.g. in red blood cells), and the indirect methods may be either immunological (the detection of plasmodial antigens or specific antibodies in the blood) or exploit the techniques of molecular biology (genomic probes).

Biodiversity of Malaria in the World

The microscopic examination of fixed and stained **thin** and **thick blood smears** are the oldest methods still routinely used (*Figures 1, 2* and *3*). A minimum of equipment is required: a staining solution and a microscope with an immersion objective; an electrical light source is not absolutely necessary. However, learning how to perform the examination is difficult and the analysis has to be carried out with rigour. The thin blood smear method is easier and quicker and has a detection limit of 50 *P. falciparum* cells/µl of blood (10^{-5}/l). The various species of parasite can be distinguished without ambiguity. Estimates of the parasite load may not be very exact and a minimum number of fields must be counted. Thick blood smear analysis demands even more rigour (defibrination is obligatory and the diluent must be buffered to preclude artefacts), but it is more sensitive—of the order of 4 *P. falciparum*/µl (10^{-7}-10^{-6}/l). Results are therefore obtained in a shorter time but it is more difficult to distinguish between species mainly at trophozoite stage.

Both methods can be used to estimate parasite load and therefore to distinguish between asymptomatic infection and disease (one of the key criteria in malaria diagnosis).

The two methods are complementary and which is used will depend on the information being sought, e.g. whether the focus is prevalence in human community or diagnosis at individual level.

A test based on **isolating parasitised red blood cells** and staining them with a fluorescent label (acridine) in a capillary tube (the QBC Malaria Test®) is easy to learn and the turn-round time is short. Its sensitivity is comparable to that of thick blood smear analysis. However, the microscope must have a power supply and a UV source, and the disposables are expensive (amounting to $3 per test). The species of *Plasmodium* cannot always be

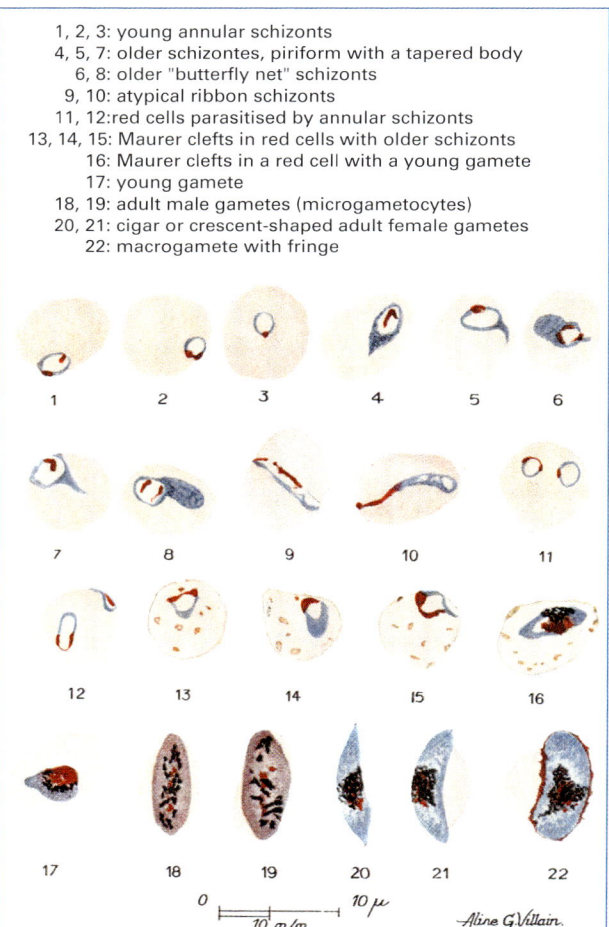

Figure 1. Haematological diagnosis of P. falciparum (*adapted from Villain, 1958*).

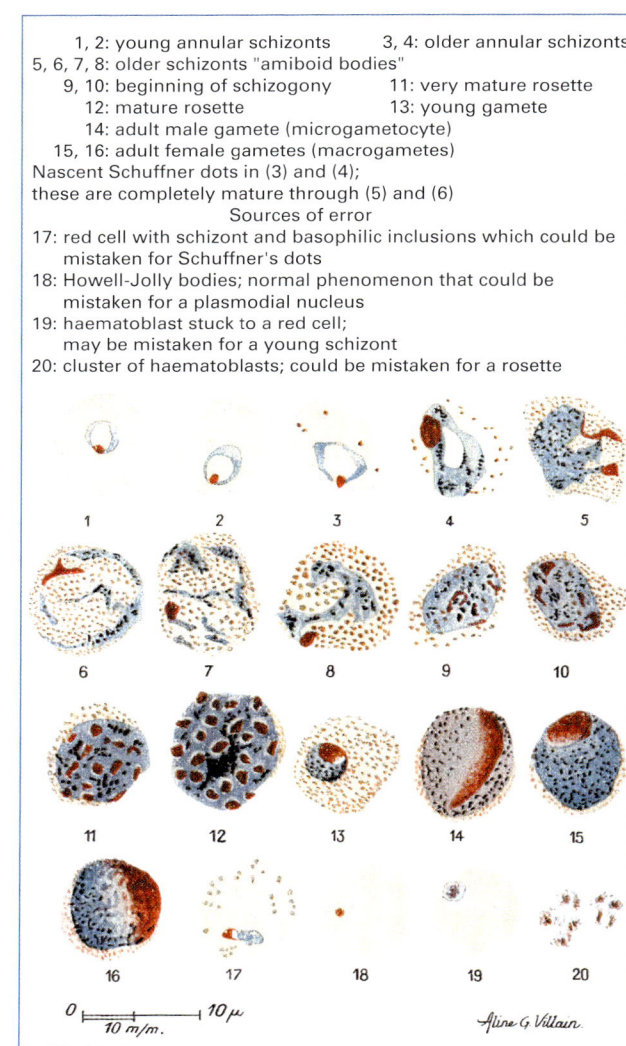

Figure 2. Haematological diagnosis of P. vivax (*adapted from Villain, 1958*).

Epidemiological Basis

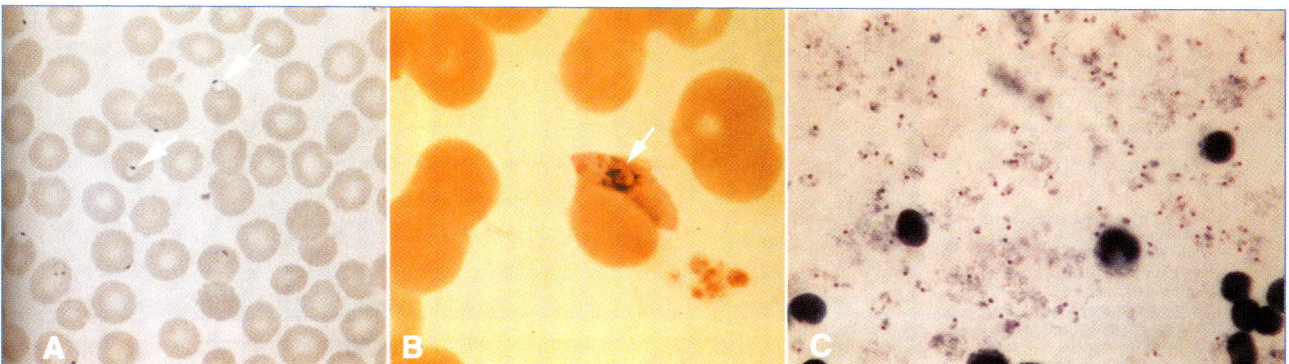

Figure 3. P. falciparum-*parasitised blood.*
A. *Thin smear (trophozoites).* **B.** *Thin smear (gametocyte).* **C.** *Thick smear (taken from Danis & Mouchet, 1991).*

ascertained and infected red blood cells cannot be counted. This technique is no longer in use.

Plasmodial antigens are most commonly assayed using an ELISA (Enzyme Linked ImmunoSorbent Assay) method which has the advantage of being able to detect the parasite in both humans and mosquitoes. Parasite-specific gammaglobulins in the human are assayed using polyclonal or monoclonal antibodies; other antibodies are used for Circumsporozoite Proteins (CSP) in the vector (Rapid Diagnostic Tests – RDT are commercially available such as Parasight F Test®, ICT Malaria Pf Test®, Paracheck Pf®). This method is very sensitive and RDT has been used for malaria diagnoses in places where microscopes are not available. Immuno-chromatographic diagnostic strips have been developed for the detection of a *P. falciparum*-specific antigen found in the blood, the Histidine-Rich Protein (HRP). A "pan-plasmodial antigen" can also be assayed in parallel to HRP in order to distinguish *P. falciparum* infection from other forms of malaria. Most of these tests are relatively specific but their sensitivity (the number of falsely negative results) is highly dependent on parasite density.

Another test is based on the **lactate dehydrogenase** produced by the sexual and asexual forms of *Plasmodium* (Opti Mae Test®).

There are various **serological methods** (immuno-fluorescence, ELISA, etc.) with a wide variety of different antigens (more or less highly purified somatic antigens, secreted or excreted antigens found in culture supernatants, circumsporozoite proteins). These quantitative tests assay antibodies, i.e. whether or not the subject has been exposed to the parasite in the past. They are species-specific but have not been standardised.

Genomic probes have proven highly sensitive in the detection of small parasite loads showing that, in holo-endemic regions, almost all people seem to be infected.

The manifold disadvantages of this type of method preclude its routine use in every laboratory for the time being.

In definitive terms, none of these methods, other than microscopic parasite identification, are routinely applicable in endemic zones, especially in Africa for both epidemiological and logistical reasons. This is largely because they fail to make the crucial distinction between asymptomatic infection and disease. The tests remain difficult to carry out (Ambroise-Thomas *et al.*, 1993) although improvement in the short term can be hoped for, especially in RDT (which will nevertheless remain expensive).

Parasitological indicators

Prevalence

Prevalence corresponds to the proportion of subjects carrying *Plasmodium* at a given location, on a given date, belonging to a given age group—it represents a snap-shot of the situation. However, the prevalence during a particular season can also be important, e.g. during the rainy season (when transmission occurs) or in the dry season, so called "period prevalence"—or in a certain age group. This universal indicator remains the most commonly used parameter to quantify and classify endemic malaria.

For many years, prevalence was determined indirectly on the basis of the number of subjects with **splenomegaly**. Red blood cells that have been killed by the parasite are phagocytosed in the spleen which then becomes enlarged. Splenomegaly used to be considered as pathognomic of plasmodial infection with various systems to assess splenic hypertrophy in use (Boyd, 1949; Schuffner, 1919), notably that of Hackett (1944b) in which the size of the spleen is estimated on a scale of 1-5 with reference to the lower edge of the ribcage (*Figure 4*).

However, such estimates are inaccurate when the spleen is only minimally enlarged (level 1 when the whole of the spleen is confined below the ribs). The measurement is also subjective and can vary significantly from one examiner to another. Spleen Rate (SR) can be measured at

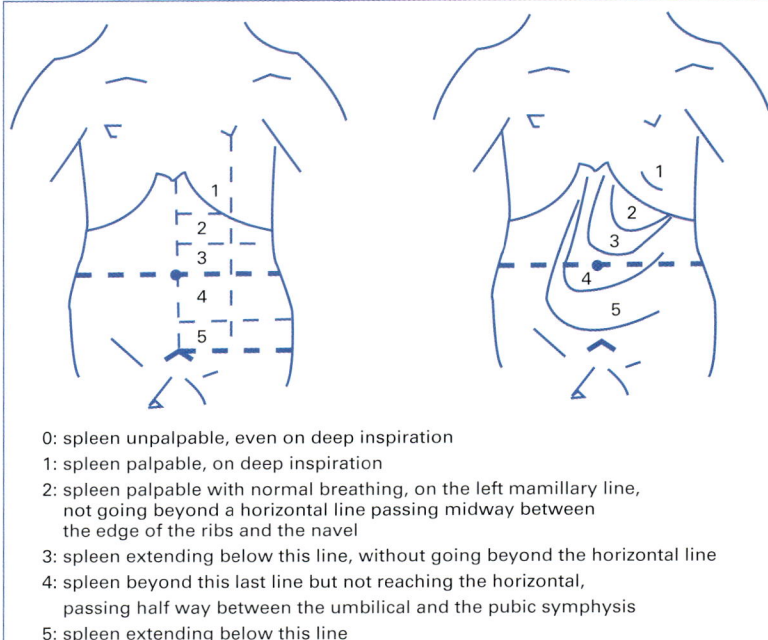

Figure 4.
*Measuring spleen size by palpation:
Hackett's classification system,
WHO, 1963
(adapted from Hackett, 1944b).*

0: spleen unpalpable, even on deep inspiration
1: spleen palpable, on deep inspiration
2: spleen palpable with normal breathing, on the left mamillary line, not going beyond a horizontal line passing midway between the edge of the ribs and the navel
3: spleen extending below this line, without going beyond the horizontal line
4: spleen beyond this last line but not reaching the horizontal, passing half way between the umbilical and the pubic symphysis
5: spleen extending below this line

all ages and analysis of such measurements shows that it tends to change with age: in rural areas in Africa, splenomegaly tends to regress in adults whereas this indicator persists into adulthood in Papua New Guinea. Splenomegaly can also be due to other diseases, such as schistosomiasis and misinterpretation in term of malaria situation may occur

These days, prevalence is more commonly estimated on the basis of the **Parasite Rate** (PR). In a microscopic thick blood smear analysis, any subject with at least one parasite in two-hundred fields is considered as positive, i.e. if the parasitaemia is over 20/µl. Despite standardisation of how the results of the thick blood smear are interpreted, optical detection is relatively insensitive and small parasite loads may be missed. With the methods of molecular biology (notably PCR), very low-level parasitaemia can be detected (Mockenhaupt *et al.*, 2000). When such ultra-sensitive methods are used, prevalence figures rise, reaching close to 100% in holo-endemic zones. This partly erases age-dependent differences since many adults in these areas have very small parasite loads. Similarly, seasonal differences can be masked because these often correspond to a reduction in parasite load rather than sterilisation. Prevalence was the indicator chosen to monitor malaria in eradication programmes of which the target was the complete elimination of all parasites. It loses its relevance in asymptomatic subjects with very low parasite loads.

It has long been recognised that thin and thick blood smear analyses yield different prevalence figures and Schwetz (1942) gives a series of results using both methods: although significant differences were observed, no correlation was established with clinical picture.

Parasite load and pyrogenic threshold

The **parasite load** is the number of parasites per microlitre of blood and it is estimated by counting parasites and calculating the number either: per microscopic field; per a set number of leukocytes (usually 200); or per a set number of red blood cells. It is probably the most important parameter in a community living in a place where malaria is stable because most people would be infected and whether or not they are experiencing symptoms is more dependent on parasite load than on the simple presence of parasites (with over 90% of carriers commonly asymptomatic). An idea that has been used for a long time is that of **pyrogenic threshold*** (Sinton *et al.*, 1931) which differentiates asymptomatic infection from disease, thereby defining the disease state (usually associated with fever) in a parasite carrier. This threshold varies with transmission conditions, age and individual susceptibility. In the Congo, it has been estimated at 19,000 parasitised red cells/µl in children of up to 5; 2,300 in 10-15 year-olds; and 537 in adults (Richard *et al.*, 1988c). Elsewhere, the threshold in adults has been set at 16,000 in Liberia (Miller, 1958), 10,000 in rural Burkina Faso (Baudon *et al.*, 1986b), 5,000 in Tanzania (Smith *et al.*, 1994), and 3,890 in an urban

---

* The pyrogenic threshold, a statistical derivative, is the parasite load above which paroxysmal attacks may occur in a zone of stable malaria and below which most cases are symptomless.

Epidemiological Basis

setting in Nigeria (Bruce-Chwatt, 1952). On Grande Comore, the threshold was 4,000 in babies and 7,000 in children of between 1 and 9 (Blanchy et al., 1990), i.e. the reverse of the pattern seen in the Congo. In Papua New Guinea as in Congo, tolerance to the parasite drops with age, as immunity is acquired (Smith et al., 1994). Results are very scattered and are highly dependent on the method used to calculate the pyrogenic threshold. The parameter is relevant to populations not individuals, and it is out of the question that a patient showing signs of a paroxysm should be denied treatment just because his or her parasitaemia is below the pyrogenic threshold.

Bruce-Chwatt (1980) developed a scale of mean parasite loads to characterise the various communities at risk.

Incidence

Incidence corresponds to the number of new cases (or new infections) in a population or a sub-population or a certain age group over a given time interval. It is usually expressed per 1,000 individuals per annum (longitudinal cumulative data). Unless otherwise stipulated, the figure refers to the **Clinical Incidence**, whether it concerns patients with symptoms that are assumed to be due to malaria or cases that have been parasitologically confirmed. It is important to differentiate this parameter from the **Parasite Incidence** which corresponds to the number of infected subjects regardless of whether or not they are presenting clinical symptoms of the disease. During the eradication period, extensive use was made of the **Annual Parasite Incidence** (API) parameter, i.e. the number of positive slides per 1,000 examinations with, ideally, at least 10% of the population at risk having to be examined.

It is the parasite incidence or **Parasite Inoculation Rate** (PIR) that was used to monitor the progress of eradication campaigns. This criterion is still used, mainly in vector control programmes with Insecticide-Treated Nets (ITN). For example this parameter is measured in a cohort of subjects who were all treated with drugs at a time t_0; subsequently, a record is made of the percentage of the subjects who become infected at t_1, t_2, t_3, comparing those with/without ITN etc. Repeated longitudinal surveys on a representative sample have also been carried out for such evaluation.

It is important to avoid confusion between Parasite Incidence and the **Entomological Inoculation Rate** (EIR) which is an indicator for transmission, not for the presence of the parasite.

Clinical incidence is a direct measure of malaria morbidity. The **number of clinical episodes per person per annum** is another criterion that is in widespread use. In endemic zones where malaria is stable, the figure is usually below 2 in children by virtue of protective immune responses: in Liberia, a rate of 1.6 paroxysms per child per annum has been reported (Miller, 1958); and in a rural zone in Ivory Coast, a rate of 4.5 was measured in children of under 2, while that for children of 2-5 was 2 (Henry et al., 2001). This criterion has also been used to evaluate malaria control programme based upon large scale ITN use.

Gametocyte Rate

The Gametocyte Rate is the proportion of carriers of sexual forms (gametocytes) in a population at a given time. This corresponds to the human population's parasitic potential for infection at that moment. This index has to be formulated for each different plasmodial species. It is one basis for calculation in Macdonald's equations (1957) (*see below*) and can also be calculated on the basis of entomological parameters.

The infectivity of gametocytes (discussed above) has become a topic of interest with active research underway into the possibility of developing a blocking vaccine to inhibit the plasmodial cycle in the vector (*see the Chapter on* "Prevention by Means of Control Vector").

Serological indicators

Theoretical aspects and technical solutions

Serological tests are designed to assay antibodies directed against *Plasmodium*, be they simple markers, circulating or protective antibodies (without it yet being possible to differentiate between these or assign distinct functions to the antibody in question). The sensitivity and specificity of the various methods depend on the quality of the antigenic material used which is a mixture of secreted/excreted molecules derived from *P. falciparum* culture supernatants.

The three methods in most widespread use are **indirect immunofluorescence** (IIF) and, for diagnostic and epidemiological purposes, **passive haemagglutination tests** and **ELISA**.

The acquisition of antimalaria antibodies depends on the frequency of contact between the human host and the parasite. Because responses wane relatively slowly, a cumulative effect is observed as long as exposure to the antigen is fairly regular; thus, the amount of specific antibody in the blood tends to rise with age and will depend on the level of exposure (Ambroise-Thomas, 1974; Lobel et al., 1973). However, the blood antibody concentration does not reflect a subject's resistance to the disease since we cannot distinguish between the various different types of antibody; in fact, **we do not currently have any way of measuring premunition**.

Serology data are the basis for frequency distributions of antibody titres. Subjective, visual readings are based on dilutions which vary from technician to technician (1:16, 1:32, 1:64 or 1:128).

These results can be used to:
- calculate a seropositivity rate in a sample. The theoretical idea of positivity threshold does not pose much of a problem as long as it is established in the light of the purpose of the testing (Ambroise-Thomas, 1974). In effect, diagnosis assumes a reasonable degree of

specificity to minimise the number of falsely positive results (increased threshold), whereas sensitivity (i.e. the exclusion of false negatives) would be more important in the prevention of transfusional malaria. As a general rule, a threshold of 1/80 (or sometimes 1/160) is most commonly used for epidemiological surveys whereas an unambiguously negative result is required for blood transfusion;
- or convert individual into collective data (Mean Geometric Antibody Rate, MGAR)* which can be based on either age group or some geographical unit such as a village, an area or a country). This ratio can be calculated either using only positive data (Bruce-Chwatt et al., 1973), a method which raises the issue of the cut-off point to be applied; or it can be based on all the data—including negative results (Julvez et al., 1986)—to express the overall serological response of the group in question (including any seronegative subjects).

Interpreting results

The statistical treatment of serological results poses a number of problems (Grab & Pull, 1974) of different natures and variable impact. The resultant bias cannot usually be controlled for. It is also important to emphasise that the usefulness of serological data taken in isolation is limited because how they are interpreted—or at least the hypotheses based on such data—depend on other variables, notably entomological and parasitological criteria.

Indirect immunofluorescence has been in use for many years (Ambroise-Thomas, 1974; Voller & Bray, 1962) in the analysis of both individuals and populations, and the resultant data have been useful in three very different fields:
- in diagnosis in non-endemic places, either when parasitaemia is difficult to detect or where there is relapsing malaria or for retrospective confirmation (Ambroise-Thomas et al., 1972) of the blocking of transmission (a kind of "serological aftermath");
- in the prevention of parasite transmission through blood transfusion (Ambroise-Thomas, 1976), cell therapy or organ transplantation as well as in the screening of subjects from areas where *Anopheles* persists without malaria (Ambroise-Thomas, 1981);
- in epidemiology: to estimate transmission rates (Ambroise-Thomas, 1974), to evaluate the efficacy of control measures and monitor a changing situation (Cornille-Brogger et al., 1978), and to confirm the cessation of transmission (Benzerroug & Wery, 1985; Bruce-Chwatt et al., 1973, 1975).

Measuring transmission and estimating infection levels in populations

Sporozoite rate

The **sporozoite rate** (s) is the percentage of anophelines carrying sporozoites in their salivary glands. This can be estimated by direct microscope counts on the freshly dissected salivary glands of mosquitoes captured while biting human subjects or resting inside houses, or by using an ELISA test to detect the circumsporozoite protein (CSP) in the head and thorax of the insect (in which case, the specimen may be dried).

In the latter case, the term **Circumsporozoite rate** (Cs) is used to distinguish it from the s obtained by dissection (which is usually lower, especially in secondary and undefined vectors) (*Figure 5*).

The elements of the sporozoite rate have been modelled by Macdonald (1957) in the equation:

$$s = \frac{ax\, p^n}{(ax - \log_e p)}$$

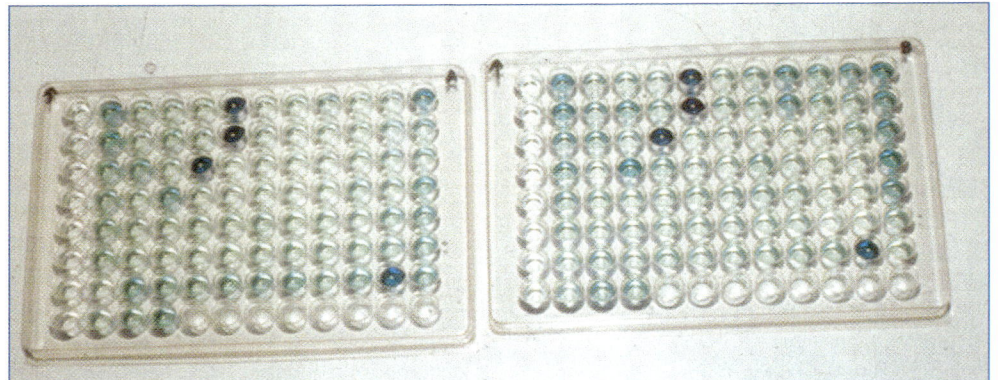

Figure 5. ELISA test for the circumsporozoite protein (photograph by Coosemans).

---

* MGAR = EXP($\sum$ (n_0 log[1] + n_1 log[d_1] + $n_2$log[d_2] + …)/ $\sum$(n_0 + n_1 + n_2 + …) in which n_0 is the number of negative serological results, n_1 the number of serological tests that give a positive result at the first dilution (d_1), n_2 the number of serological tests that give a positive result at the next dilution (d_1/2), etc.

Epidemiological Basis

s: sporozoite rate;

p: the daily probability of an anopheline's survival: this can be calculated in various ways, the simplest being based on the percentage of parous females in the population sampled. After dissection, parous (i.e. those who have laid eggs at least once) and nulliparous females are distinguished on the basis of the morphology of the ovarian tracheoles (which are coiled prior to laying and unravelled afterwards). The parameter p can only be estimated in a stable population, which is rare in nature but it is still largely used;

n: length of the sporogonic cycle which will depend on temperature: this can be worked out from Macdonald's model or calculated using the equation: n = T/(t – tmin). In this equation: n = length of the cycle; T = 105 for *P. vivax*, 161 for *P. falciparum*, and 144 for *P. malariae*; t = temperature in degrees Celsius; tmin = 14.5 for *P. vivax*, and 16 for *P. falciparum* and *P. malariae* (Molineaux, 1998 in Wernsdorfer & McGregor, 1998);

a: average number of people bitten by an anopheline per day, usually between 0.50 and 0.25 (human biting rate/ length of the gonotrophic cycle);

e.g. if the human biting rate is 100% and the gonotrophic cycle takes two days, a = 0.5; if the former is 90% and the latter three days, a = 0.3;

x: percentage of people that are carrying gametocytes;

e: the base of the system of natural logarithms (2.71828).

Two essential conclusions about malaria transmission follow on:
- the shorter the sporogonic cycle, the sooner will a mosquito become infective (i.e. with sporozoites in its salivary glands);
- the longer-lived the anopheline, the more likely that it will inoculate parasite into more victims.

Thus, transmission would be expected to rise with global warming which is supposed to decrease the length of the sporogonic cycle and thus increase the potential of transmission—as long as the other parameters remain constant and do not exert pressure in the opposite direction.

Entomological Inoculation Rate and Parasite Inoculation Rate

Two factors determine transmission dynamics:
- the **number of infective bites** delivered to the subjects (intensity of transmission),
- and the **annual rhythm of these infections**.

These can be used to estimate the risk of infection for subjects introduced into an endemic situation.

Ross, in his *Theory of the Happening* (whence the parameter h), derived the **Entomological Inoculation Rate** (h_e) (EIR) equation to estimate the intensity of transmission (the number of infective bites per individual per time period [usually 24 hours]):

$$h_e = m.a.s$$

m.a.: the number of infective bites delivered to an individual over 24 hours;
s: sporozoite rate.

Macdonald proposed using another parameter, the **Parasite Inoculation Rate** (h_p) (PIR) which takes into account only the number of bites by infected mosquitoes which actually lead to infection of the human host:

$$h_p = b\, h_e = m.a.b.s$$

b: proportion of inocula which lead to parasites in the blood— a parameter which we are still unable to determine.

In practice, the PIR is derived by analysing infection rates in new-born babies or cohorts (*see above*).

These days, it is Ross' equation which is in most widespread use.

The EIR is expressed as the number of infective bites* per subject per unit of time (year, month, day, season, night, etc.), commonly ib/p/yr.

Measuring the number of infected bites at a given spot is the only really valid way of monitoring transmission. This measurement is made less and less often because it is a demanding process and some Ethics Committees disapprove of the use of human-based capture techniques even if the capturers are local people (and are therefore not being bitten more often than they would be anyway) who are given prophylactic drugs. The method is simple compared to trapping, the results of which are skewed and often misleading.

The EIR may exceed one thousand in some holo-endemic regions of the Congo (Carnevale, 1979), while it is below one in hypo-endemic zones in the Sahelo-Saharan Region or in urban settings (Robert *et al.*, 1986).

Moreover, the EIR should be interpreted in the light of the spread of bites over the year, e.g. the consequences of an EIR of 20 ib/p/yr will be quite different according to whether these twenty infective bites per person are spread fairly evenly throughout the year rather than being concentrated over a period of one or two months (and followed by a long transmission-free season). In the first case, regular immunological stimulation is more likely to elicit a protective immune response whereas, in the second pattern which precludes the steady build-up of immunity, bites will not induce protection but will rather result in seasonal flare-ups in the clinical incidence of malaria.

The two factors which determine the inoculation rate are:
- the number of times an individual is bitten by an anopheline mosquito;

---

* The common term "infective bite" is misleading; a better term would be "infected bite" (i.e. containing sporozoites) because the outcome of the sporozoites in the circulation cannot be predicted, i.e. it is not sure that they will give rise to infection.

- the infectivity of these mosquitoes.

The **risk** of receiving at least one infective bite **r** is given by the equation of Krafsur & Armstrong (1978):

$$r = 1 - e^{-h.t}$$

h: entomological inoculation rate;
t: time frame (in days).

For an inoculation rate of 0.01 ib/p/night, i.e. 3.65 ib/p/year, the risk of being infected at least once a year is very close to 100%.

The daily risk has been estimated at 0.94 at Djoumouna in the Congo (Carnevale, 1979) where transmission is constant, whereas it is 0.34 in the Kou rice-growing region of Burkina Faso (Gazin *et al.*, 1985a) where transmission is seasonal, lasting only 4 months; and in the Senegal River Region where all transmission is concentrated into a short season, it is just 0.073 (Vercruysse, 1985).

Birley's equation (1978) has also been used to measure the risk of receiving a number of infected bites although it is in less widespread use:

$$r = 1 (1 - s)^{mat^*}$$

t* is expressed in days.

Stable and unstable malaria

In 1957, Macdonald first evoked the idea of the duality of **stable** and **unstable** malaria, which is based on eight parameters (*Table I*).

Where malaria is stable, transmission (the rate of which is usually high) continues throughout the year or most of it, and is consistent from one year to the next. This elicits resistance in local people and constitutes a kind of symbiosis between parasite and human host.

Protective immunity is acquired during early childhood although at the expense of a heavy tribute in this age group: subsequently, mortality rates in schoolchildren, teenagers and adults are far lower. Epidemics do not occur in those regions of Africa and Papua New Guinea where malaria is stable—only seasonal peaks; malaria indicators (notably prevalence) have not changed over the last forty years (Desowitz & Spark, 1987; Mouchet *et al.*, 1998).

Where malaria is unstable, transmission tends to be low and seasonal, and it varies from year to year. The population acquires little or no immunity. The parasite circulates, causing endemo-epidemic disease, and when conditions favourable to vector growth pertain, an epidemic may break out. Epidemics may be more or less deadly but, due to the absence of acquired protective immunity, all age groups are affected.

In regions of unstable malaria (and sometimes where it is stable), outbreaks of epidemic disease may occur when control measures are interrupted and transmission is no longer being artificially inhibited by a reduction in vector numbers or prophylactic drug treatment.

Stability depends entirely on entomological considerations, namely the preference of local *Anopheles* for human blood, the mosquito's life expectancy, and the length of the gonotrophic cycle. It is represented by Macdonald's **Stability Index (St)** (1957):

$$St = a/- \log_e p$$

- if St > 2.5, malaria is stable;
- if St < 0.5, malaria is unstable and could break out in an epidemic;
- values between 0.5 and 2.5 correspond to borderline stability.

Table I. Classification of malaria according to the stability of its transmission (adapted from Bruce-Chwatt, 1980).

Characteristics	Unstable malaria	Stable malaria
Endemicity	Usually low/moderate. Endemicity may be locally high	Usually very high. Endemicity may be moderate
Reason	Vector not very anthropophilic and short-lived. Short transmission season	Vector highly anthropophilic, longevity moderate or long-lived. Long transmission season
High critical anopheline density	(1-10 or more bites per person per night)	May be very low (less than one bite per person per night)
Seasonal variations	Marked	Not very marked apart from for short dry seasons
Incidence of the parasite	Major fluctuations from year to year. *P. vivax* most common	Not very marked outside of seasonal fluctuations. *P. falciparum* most common
Immunity	Highly variable due to year-to-year fluctuations; very low in certain groups	High, some local variability
Epidemics	Frequent, depending on weather	Very unlikely

With reference to Southeast Asia, Verdrager (1995) introduced the term "permanently epidemic" for situations such as forestry or mining sites in which the constant influx of naive subjects leads to a high incidence of malaria—often severe forms—among a population which is at once highly exposed and immunologically unprotected. In terms of transmission, malaria is stable but the constant turnover of the human reservoir introduces an element of instability.

Vectorial Capacity

Vectorial Capacity (VC) for a population of vectors corresponds to the expected number of new inoculation events **per day, from a single infective human subject** (Garrett-Jones & Shidrawi, 1969) in contact with the anopheline population.

It is estimated using the equation:

$$VC = ma^2 p^n / -\log_e p \quad \text{where}$$

$m.a^2$: human biting rate,
$p^n/-\log_e p$: infective life expectancy,
n: length of the sporogonic cycle of the relevant *Plasmodium*.

VC is therefore highly dependent on both the life expectancy of the *Anopheles* and the length of the parasite's sporogonic cycle. It is an essentially entomological parameter which depends strongly on temperature and therefore season, as well as on local geographical characteristics and on which plasmodial species is under consideration.

It is calculated (for each species separately if more than one is transmitting malaria) at one site or over a given period. VC values are cumulated to generate a Total VC.

Other equations have been developed to estimate the VC for an anopheline population. Commonly in mathematical models, VC is taken as the entomological indicator and compared to parasitological data in order to monitor relative changes between the two in the course of vector-control operations (Dietz & Molineaux *in* Wernsdorfer & McGregor, 1989).

Parasite Propagation Rate

Propagation Rate (= the reproductive rate of the parasite: z).

According to Macdonald's equation (1957), the propagation (or reproductive) rate is given by:

$$z = \frac{ma^2 \, bs \, p^n}{r \, (-\log_e p)}$$

This corresponds to the total number of inoculation events expected from a single infective subject coming from a susceptible anopheline population. This is distinct from the daily inoculation rate indicator discussed in the preceding paragraph because it takes two other parameters into account, namely:
    b: infectivity of the vector,
    r: infectivity of the human subject,
    if **z** > 1, malaria is spreading,
    if **z** < 1, malaria is regressing.

The goal of vector control operations is to reduce z to below 1.

Since it is often very difficult to attribute meaningful values for parameters b and r, one usually stays with the calculation of the **Vectorial Capacity**.

Classifying malaria endemicity

Whatever the vagaries of the indicators used, malaria endemicity was first addressed using the Spleen Rate (SR) estimates for children of 2-9 years in age which was believed to give a fairly good measure of malaria endemicity (Dempster, 1948): Christopher's classification system (*in* Boyd, 1949) was used at the Malaria Conference in Equatorial Africa held in Kampala in 1950 (WHO, 1964). However, the existence of splenomegaly due to reasons other than malaria and the difficulties associated with measuring the parameter led to a switch to the use of Parasite Rate (PR) in the same age group (Metselaar & Van Thiel, 1959) in the classification system selected at the Third African Malaria Conference held in Yaoundé in 1962 (*Table II*).

	Table II. Classification of endemic zones (Metselaar & Van Thiel, 1959).			
	Holo-endemic	Hyperendemic	Meso-endemic	Hypo-endemic & epidemic
Spleen Rate (Kampala, 1950)	Always > 75% reduction of splenomegaly as of the age of 10	Always > 50% in children of 2-9	11-50% in children of 2-9	Under 10% in children of 2-9
Parasite Rate (Yaoundé, 1962)	Always > 75% in children of 6 months to 11 years. Parasite density drops between 2 and 9, more slowly after 10 years of age (Africa, Papua New Guinea)	Always > 50% in children of 2-9	11-50% in children of 2-9	Under 10% in children of 2-9 but may rise in certain seasons as well as during an epidemic

Since then, SR has hardly been used at all, at least in Africa, although it seems to be more popular in Asia and Oceania.

The definition of holo-endemicity, established in Southeast Asia, is based on not only a constant splenomegaly of over 75%, but also on the diminution of this parameter with age. However, in tropical Africa, such an age-related drop is also seen in people living in hyperendemic and even meso-endemic areas; PR also drops with age. Therefore, the definition of holo-endemicity is not very clear in Africa (Miller, 1958) and it is easily confused with hyperendemicity. In Southeast Asia, splenomegaly does not drop with age in certain groups.

These classification systems lose much of their value since they are based on a single parameter and take into account neither the acquisition of immunity with age (which results in a reduced percentage of parasite carriers) nor the vector component. Many authors have pointed out their relative lack of sensitivity (Carnevale, 1979; Carnevale & Mouchet, 1980) and highlighted the need for a review. Nevertheless, such classification systems often constitute the only information available from certain countries.

Other older systems used to take a broader range of parameters into account.

Wilson's system (*in* Boyd, 1949) distinguished between four different malaria "groups" on the basis of the continuity of transmission over the year. Between the extremes of the endemic type with year-round transmission and the epidemic type with sporadic transmission, two other types were characterised by regular transmission lasting either more or less than six months. This system introduced the phenomenon of premunition, thus making it possible to distinguish between endemic and epidemic disease as related to immunity. The approach became dynamic, relating the number of cases to the way in which they appear.

Epidemiological facies and strata

An idea defined in the context of West and Central Africa (Mouchet & Carnevale, 1981) was that of **epidemiological facies** (Carnevale *et al.*, 1984) which attempts to reflect the dynamics of transmission as a function of changes in biotope through a gradient of diversity. A facies is a group of places in which malaria presents the same characteristics of transmission, acquired immunity and pathological manifestations (*see the Chapter on* the "Afrotropical Region"). This combines Wilson's idea of the continuity of transmission affecting host immunity with that of Macdonald pertaining to the various parameters that can be used to characterise vectors and parasites. Different facies can be grouped together into epidemiological strata.

Thus, Africa has been split into different zones according to the endemicity of malaria (Mouchet *et al.*, 1993) (*see the Chapter on* the "Afrotropical Region"), but the method can be applied everywhere, notably to Southeast Asia (*see the chapter on* the "Oriental Region") with data that are already available.

After a few rearguard actions, the idea of malaria diversity—based on local and regional epidemiological features—was accepted at the 1992 Ministerial Conference in Amsterdam: it integrates the dynamic relationships that exist between environment, vector, parasite, and disease.

Stratification—in the WHO sense—depends on not only epidemiological characteristics in different parts of a country, but also the socio-economic, operational and even political criteria that condition control strategies. WHO stratification schemes seek to integrate data from such heterogeneous sources, that the idea of classifying malaria in terms of the dimensions of the disease completely disappears. Nevertheless, the goal of Roll Back Malaria (RBM) programme is to reduce the burden of malaria by 50%.

Epidemics

Macdonald (1957) described an epidemic of malaria as "a flare-up of the disease, with more cases than are usually found in the community". Epidemics only occur where malaria is unstable, when small changes in transmission factors disrupt the normal balance and the local people are not immune.

It is important to make the distinction between epidemics and seasonal outbreaks or seasonal peaks, e.g. those that might occur in the wet season or when ground water subsides, which recur every year at the same time. However, an epidemic may be superimposed on an annual surge, e.g. in a year of especially heavy rainfall as was seen in Uganda in 1995 (Mouchet *et al.*, 1998) (*see the* "Uganda" *section in the Chapter on* the "Afrotropical Region"). In highland areas, abnormally high temperatures —sometimes associated with heavier-than-normal rainfall—can also cause epidemics (Garnham, 1945). To date, global warming has not been implicated (Mouchet & Manguin, 1999).

Changes to the environment and in farming methods (notably rice-growing) have caused epidemics, e.g. in Madagascar at the end of the 19th century (*see the* "Madagascar" *section in the Chapter on* the "Afrotropical Region").

One of the commonest causes of epidemics in the last thirty years has been the discontinuation of indoor spraying programmes (in Sri Lanka, Madagascar, India, Swaziland, etc.) which left a now immunologically naive population completely unprotected.

Epidemics are not completely unpredictable, depending exclusively on meteorological and/or operational factors. In every case that has been studied, notably Uganda, Madagascar and Burundi, the epidemic was preceded by a more or less acute rise in the number of cases, sometimes sustained over a period of several years, during which time the parasite reservoir had the opportunity to build up. Once the reservoir is great enough, the way is paved for the outbreak of an epidemic either spontaneously or consequent on changes in climate or some other key parameters (Coosemans *et al.*, 2003; Mouchet *et al.*, 1998). Preventive measures should probably be implemented at the time of these "harbingers" rather than when the true epidemic breaks out, which may be too late.

Man, carrier of malaria

Although the spread of malaria across the planet is dependent on the presence of vectors (*see the Part on "Spatiotemporal Dynamics of Malaria"*), it has always been and still is contingent on human beings and human activities (Mouchet *et al.*, 1995). We do not know whether the various species of hominids were already spreading parasites through the Old World but it seems likely that as soon as the first men quit their African birthplace, they took their parasites with them. As they moved further and further away, humans encountered *Anopheles* mosquitoes which captured *Plasmodium* and passed it on. It is likely that the Neolithic Revolution—which combined deforestation for the development of arable farming and the raising of livestock with the concentration of populations around significantly-sized dwelling sites (Fenner, 1970)—promoted the emergence of sun-loving vectors and ensured a critical mass for the circulation and long-term installation of the parasite.

The various species of *Anopheles* all had well-defined territories, resulting from their biogeographical evolution; this determined whether or not malaria was present. The ecology of the species and their efficiency as vectors shaped the epidemiology of the disease.

There is no direct proof that malaria originated in Africa and there probably never will be. However, three pieces of circumstantial evidence point in this direction:
- the *Plasmodium* species found in humans are very closely related to those found in African apes, i.e. chimpanzees, bonobos and gorillas;
- there are major differences between malaria in Africa and the disease elsewhere: in the former, it invests more or less the entire continent and local people have developed highly effective defence mechanisms; elsewhere, the disease is found in certain foci and human defence mechanisms are nowhere near as effective;
- the fact that highly efficient vectors are found throughout the Afrotropical Region, in particular *An. gambiae s.s*, *An. arabiensis* and *An. funestus*.

In the Americas, malaria (at least that due to *P. falciparum*) seems to have been introduced with the slave trade in the 17th century. According to Russel *et al.* (1963), the Amerindians who inhabited the continent at that time had arrived *via* the Bering Strait where temperatures were incompatible with the survival of any *P. falciparum* that they might have brought with them from Asia. However, interest in the question was reawakened by the discovery of indigenous foci of *P. malariae* and possibly *P. vivax* in extremely isolated Amerindian groups in Peru (Sulzer *et al.*, 1975) (with *P. brasilianum* and *P. simium* believed to be strains of *P. malariae* and *P. vivax* that have adapted from monkeys).

Anopheles did not used to be found on certain inhabited islands—including Mauritius and La Réunion in the Indian Ocean—where there was obviously no indigenous malaria. The introduction of vectors and parasites by humans in the 19th century resulted in well-documented epidemics (Julvez, 1993; Mouchet *et al.*, 1995).

On the contrary, the evolutionary history of Anophelinae is not compatible with an African origin but rather a New World origin with the basal placement of the Neotropical genus *Chagasia* that belongs to the Anophelinae subfamily, as well as the Neotropical distribution of four out of six subgenera of *Anopheles* (Harbach and Kitching, 1998). The first radiations of *Anopheles* might have taken place approximately 95 million years ago, before the disappearance of the land connection between Africa and South America (Krzywinski & Besansky, 2003).

The distribution and epidemiology of malaria—which largely reflects the biogeography of its vectors—are addressed in the second part of this volume. But first, we will look at how humans react to the parasite.

Man Facing Malaria

Pathogenicity

The four different *Plasmodium* species cause variable symptoms. Most cases involve simple paroxysms but the overall impact of the disease is dominated by severe and complicated forms that is why diagnosing a possible case of malaria always represents an emergency and should never be postponed.

Plasmodium falciparum causes pernicious malaria and is by far the most dangerous species of the four, accounting for the vast majority of deaths and giving rise to a broad range of pathological manifestations. All symptoms must always be viewed with the subsequent development of severe disease in mind and, in immunologically naive subjects, any attack constitutes a potentially **life-threatening situation**. It is *P. falciparum* that causes cerebral malaria and severe anaemia that can lead to death. Spontaneous abortion and low birth weight (especially in first-born babies) are often linked to this parasite. Severe forms are more common in areas where the transmission rate is high but the relationship is not a linear one, e.g. malaria mortality tends to be low in places where transmission is both high-level and year-round, as in the Congo (Richard, 1988c; Trape *et al.*, 1987c). In fact, the proportion of severe cases is often high where transmission is unstable, especially in epidemics. As long as it is adequately treated, *P. falciparum* infection does not present any further danger because this parasite causes neither relapses nor recrudescences. Blackwater fever (malaria haemoglobinuria) may be simply an iatrogenic complication of quinine treatment (Delacollette *et al.*, 1995), although this opinion is not subscribed to by all scientists. Causal links have even been investigated between holo-endemic malaria and Burkitt's lymphoma.

Passage of the parasite across the placenta, as documented in 2-3% of subjects in Nigeria (Bruce-Chwatt, 1952) does not seem to give rise to any pathological consequences in the baby.

Although *P. falciparum* is extremely polymorphic (*see the Chapter on "Plasmodium Life Cycles in Humans and Anopheline Vectors"*), it probably corresponds to a single species everywhere it is found, with minor geographical variations (Beale & Walliker, 1988 *in* Wernsdorfer & McGregor), at least at our present level of understanding.

Although *P. vivax* (Grassi & Feletti, 1890) causes significant symptoms, its short-term pathogenicity is relatively low because parasite loads tend to be small and infections are rarely fatal. The latent hypnozoite phase leads to relapsing malaria (Garnham, 1966). A distinction has been made between, on the one hand, strains with a long incubation time (Garnham *et al.*, 1975)—up to eight months (*P. vivax hibernans*)—which are more common in temperate zones where parasites inoculated in autumn do not cause paroxysms until the following spring; and on the other hand, those with a shorter incubation period—7-23 days—which are found in the Tropics and which cause paroxysms straight away. The latter can also go into a hypnozoite phase and cause relapsing malaria. This chronic, recurrent manifestation of malaria is called malarial cachexia (Garnham, 1966). The consequences of transplacental infection—although less serious than those associated with *P. falciparum*—were recently observed in Thailand (Nosten *et al.*, 1999). Pathogenic differences between the *P. vivax* variants identified since 1989 have not yet been defined.

P. ovale (Stephens 1922) is rare outside Africa (although it has been found in Western New Guinea and Southeast Asia) where its prevalence can exceed 2%. It does not seem to cause severe paroxysms. Infection is transient with the parasite disappearing from the peripheral blood fairly rapidly although it can, like *P. vivax*, cause relapses. After delivery by caesarean section, the mother can experience an attack of malaria after 24 hours, and the baby three weeks later (Jenkins, 1957).

Primary *P. malariae* (Laveran, 1881) infection is often latent but this species can persist in the blood for a very long time—possibly for 40-70 years (Vinetz *et al.*, 1998), although usually with a low parasite density. Reviviscence can occur after a very long interval. *P. malariae* infection is often intercurrent with *P. falciparum* infection which complicates the study of the former species' virulence. Although it is not evenly distributed in geographical terms, it is the third most common species. In Peru, where there is no *P. falciparum*, *P. malariae* used to be responsible for hyperendemic malaria among the Amerindians living in the Andean foothills (Sulzer *et al.*, 1975). In holo-endemic areas, long-term consequences include serious kidney problems which can be fatal: this nephritic syndrome has been studied in detail in Nigeria and seems to be caused by an immune complex (Hendrickse, 1976; Hendrickse & Adeninya, 1979); however, whether or not this condition has a parasitologic etiology is controversial (Pakasa *et al.*, 1993) and some experts have even attributed it to mercury poisoning linked with the use of skin-lightening products.

The human victim

Difficulties in diagnosing and defining malaria disease

A human may be simply **carrying the malaria parasite** or be at the same time a **parasite carrier and sick from malaria**. This will depend on the subject's immune status, the level and seasonal nature of transmission, and the availability of medical treatment. A distinction is therefore made between **malaria-infection** and **malaria-disease**.

In a highly endemic zone, asymptomatic carriage with a low *P. falciparum* load is the rule—sometimes accounting for more than 90% of all carriers. The level of the parasite load is what determines whether or not there is a risk of paroxysm: the clinical (or pyrogenic) threshold will depend on local epidemiological conditions and age. In West and Central Africa where malaria is stable, the pyrogenic threshold has been used to diagnose malaria attacks (Baudon *et al.*, 1986b; Richard *et al.*, 1988c). Knowing the true morbidity of malaria-disease and diagnosing it is therefore a complicated process but a vital one. Defining malaria mortality is all the more difficult due to the multitude of alternative conditions that may be misdiagnosed as malaria, as well as difficulties associated with the gathering of data.

In endemic zones, diagnosis is usually made on the basis of clinical criteria (or sometimes simply on the basis of the family context) in a patient who has a fever and/or who feels sick—laboratory-based parasitologic confirmation being completely out of the question (Ambroise-Thomas *et al.*, 1993). Considering the most remote West African villages, only 12% of people have access to a clinic (the nearest health care centre which will probably not even possess a microscope)—and the mean for the population as a whole is only 30%.

Official statistics often attempt to number the attacks assumed to be "malaria" seen at clinics which are in fact fever or even "hot body". The bald figures are often reported without any further details by various bodies, with major discrepancies between the number of cases reported and the true number.

In reality, when cases diagnosed according to clinical criteria are checked by parasitologic examination, 30-90% are confirmed where malaria is endemic and stable (Baudon *et al.*, 1986b); but where it is unstable, discrepancies can be even higher: Olivar *et al.* (1991) found that 90% of cases of "malaria" during the dry season in northern Niger had in fact a negative thick blood smear.

Simple primary paroxysms, relapses and recrudescence

A **primary paroxysm** (or a **primary attack**) occurs when sporozoites are inoculated into a receptive subject. Such attacks can be caused by any of the *Plasmodium* species which can infect human beings.

A **relapse** is a paroxysm caused by the reawakening of a **hypnozoite** after a quiescent period of variable duration (up to twelve months). Relapsing malaria can be caused by *P. vivax* or *P. ovale*.

A **recrudescence** is an attack due to multiplication of the parasite, the load of which was previously below the clinical threshold. This is seen with *P. malariae* and far less frequently with *P. falciparum*, usually if the parasite is drug-resistant or if a course of treatment has been poorly administered (e.g. artemisinin).

Primary infection is rare in babies of under five months (Bruce-Chwatt, 1952). For a long time, this population was believed to be protected by maternal antibodies or fœtal haemoglobin; however, PCR-based surveys have detected infection in babies of just 1-2 months although admittedly without any symptoms (Kitua *et al.*, 1996).

From the age of six months until the end of his or her life, anybody can get infected although the number of primary infections and their consequences will depend on the species of parasite, the person's immunological status, and the epidemiological context (Danis *in* Danis & Mouchet, 1991).

The symptoms of the attacks caused by all four parasites are similar although the frequency of paroxysm differs: *P. falciparum* and *P. vivax* give rise to febrile paroxysms every three days (hence the Hippocrates' designation **tertian malaria**) and *P. malariae* every four days (**quartan malaria**).

The cycle can be broken down into a series of different stages (Harinasuta & Bunnag *in* Wernsdorfer & McGregor, 1988).

Biodiversity of Malaria in the World

Incubation takes 9-30 days for *P. falciparum* and 18-40 days for *P. malariae*. It can be substantially longer for *P. vivax* in a temperate climate (up to eight months) in which hypnozoites can persist through the winter in a dormant state.

The true **paroxysm** is preceded by a **prodromic phase** lasting one or two days, marked by lethargy and nausea. During this phase, the parasite is multiplying up to reach its "clinical density" or "critical threshold". The true paroxysm onsets suddenly, and this phase can be broken down into three successive stages:
- **chills**: violent shivering and gooseflesh (lasting 15-60 minutes);
- **fever**: the patient's body temperature rises quickly to 40 °C or over; this is the moment of schizogony when asexual forms of the parasite burst open their host erythrocytes. This stage is marked by headache behind the orbital region, intense thirst, vomiting, excitation and sometimes delirium or convulsions (in children). This phase lasts two hours or more;
- **sweating and rest period**: profuse sweating and extreme lethargy are the hallmarks of the end of the paroxysm, with the patient going to sleep. The entire paroxysm lasts 6-10 hours after which the subject recovers until the onset of the next paroxysm (unless treatment is administered).

If a person is infected with more than one plasmodial species, the paroxystic rhythm will not necessarily follow one or other of the classic patterns.

The outcome of a simple primary attack due to *P. vivax*, *P. ovale* or *P. malariae* is usually benign, even if the patient is not treated. However, a paroxysm due to *P. falciparum* can degenerate into a severe attack at any time, especially in children and immunologically naive or depressed subjects.

The diagnosis and treatment of simple attacks are discussed in the Chapters entitled "Patient Care and Malaria Diagnosis" and "Drug and Treatment Policies".

The clinical pictures of relapsing and recrudescent malaria are similar to that of the primary paroxysm but symptoms are usually attenuated.

Severe Plasmodium falciparum *malaria*

In life, threatening malaria in children is defined by 4 key prognostic indicators: impaired consciousness, respiratory distress, hypoglycaemia, and jaundice. Of these, impaired consciousness and respiratory distress identify these children at greatest risk of dying

A list of severe malaria characteristics of *P. falciparum* (WHO 2000b, 2001a) has been addressed by various international initiatives, concretising the idea of pernicious malaria:
- acute febrile encephalopathy with Grade II coma or a Glasgow score of 7 or lower, i.e. **cerebral malaria**;
- generalised, repeated convulsions (also covered by the pernicious paroxysm concept);
- severe anaemia with an haematocrit of below 15% and less than 5.6 g/ml haemoglobin of blood;
- kidney failure with less than 400 ml of urine per day (12 ml/kg/24 hours) and blood creatinine over 265 µmol/l;
- pulmonary œdema or acute respiratory distress syndrome;
- hypoglycaemia < 2.2 mmol/l or 0.4 g/l;
- circulatory collapse;
- diffuse bleeding with disseminated intravascular coagulation;
- massive haemoglobinuria;
- acidosis with the pH of the blood below 7.25 or a HCO_3 concentration of under 15 mmol/l.

Impaired consciousness or prostration, a parasitaemia of over 5% in an immunologically naive subject, clinical jaundice or impaired liver function (blood bilirubin over 50 µmol/l or 30 mg/l) and a fever of over 41 °C or hypothermia of below 36 °C are not enough to confirm a diagnosis of a severe paroxysm.

Severe forms onset either suddenly or gradually succeeding the symptoms of a simple attack. They mainly arise in immunologically naive subjects, with very young African children accounting for 90% of cases (WHO, 2000a). Where transmission is short-lived and irregular so that immunity is not constantly being elicited, those of all ages may experience severe paroxysms.

Onset is usually sudden in a child, almost always taking the form of cerebral malaria or generalised, repeated convulsions. In adults, the symptoms of primary malaria are succeeded by a severe form in which case, any delay or mistake in diagnosis can be fatal.

Without treatment, the paroxysm can lead to death in less than 72 hours.

Impaired immune responsiveness exposes pregnant women to the risk of pernicious paroxysms which are common in the second trimester, especially in primigravide mothers. The most serious consequences are seen in women in labour or immediately following delivery (Danis, *in* Danis & Mouchet, 1991).

Very low parasitaemia

The development of the PCR assay has made it possible to detect very low parasite loads (less than 10 parasites per mm^3). These do not apparently have any direct pathological repercussions although they may sometimes be implicated in gestational anaemia (Mockenhaupt *et al.*, 2000).

Human resistance to malaria parasites

Resistance of Melano-Africans to Plasmodium vivax

Melano-Africans are naturally resistant to *P. vivax* because they do not carry the Duffy blood-group antigen (Miller *et al.*, 1975, 1976) which is the erythrocytic receptor for the *P. vivax* merozoite. Many African-Americans are similarly resistant (Young *et al.*, 1955). It is important to note that the Bushmen of the south of the continent carry this antigen and are therefore susceptible to infection with *P. vivax*, as are Madagascans of Indonesian origin, mountain-living Abyssinians originally from the Yemen area, the Berber peoples (the Touareg and Moors) in the Sahara, and Caucasians living in Africa.

All humans are susceptible to the other three *Plasmodium* species and, in experimental conditions, also to simian *Plasmodium*.

Development of immunity

In 1911, Ross wrote that "the blood of survivors gradually produces something that has the power to inhibit and possibly block parasite invasion". All people living in endemic areas acquire immunity; this immunity develops more or less rapidly, is progressively acquired, is short-lived and is only partial: it is referred to as "premunition" (Sergent, 1950).

Immunological investigations and elucidation of the *P. falciparum* genome have not yet revealed all the mechanisms involved in premunition, a phenomenon which cannot always be measured. As a result, the many and various speculations about the effects of control measures (especially vector control) on 'immunity" remain largely hypothetical; they are often counter-productively polemical and should not be allowed to delay the implementation of control strategies (Lengeler, 1998).

Bruce-Chwatt (1980) considered this "immunity" as the result of a whole set of interactions underlying individual protection. This idea goes well beyond a simple interaction between antibodies and antigens. He observed that infection was rare in babies of under six months of age whereas after this age and up to five, the rate of infection rises. Malaria mortality peaks at between one and two years of age. Defence mechanisms underlie "antitoxic immunity" which protects the subject from death despite a very high parasite load; as of ten years of age, "antiparasite immunity" develops which restricts parasite numbers, ultimately eliminating them from the body or maintaining them at a very low density.

More recent studies—notably investigations in Tanzania where malaria is stable and holo-endemic (Smith *et al.*, 1999; Tanner *et al.*, 1999)—have confirmed this duality of defence mechanisms (although they have significantly modified the details):
- from 0 to 5/6 months, infection is rare, the baby being protected by maternal antibodies and foetal haemoglobin, although infections have been PCR-detected without any symptoms (as far as we know in this controversial field);
- from 6 to 24 months, there is an immunological hiatus and the only effective defence mechanisms against the parasite's blood stages are believed to be high body temperature and cytokines. Experts tend to remain relatively quiet about this period during which immunity is being acquired; nevertheless, this immunity usually prevents the child dying, despite on extremely high parasite load;
- from 2 years on, repeated infection leads to the development of ongoing, low-level protection, which affords cross-protection against new clones. Protection is genotype-specific and does not persist long after the disappearance of the clone. As premunition develops, an infected state is maintained which precludes superinfection. Once the subject is carrying antibodies against all the local genotypes, a state of premunition is established.

If a clone persists without being eliminated, it will induce a malaria attack. As has long been recognised, susceptibility to malaria diminishes with age. In a place where malaria is endemic and stable, severe paroxysms are rare after the age of five, and as of ten (and to an even greater extent fifteen), simple attacks become steadily more benign. In contrast, where very few clones are in circulation (e.g. in the dry parts of Sudan), premunition does not develop (Babiker *et al.*, 2000; Theander, 1998), although adults are nevertheless less susceptible to malaria attacks than children.

Premunition is maintained by repeated antigenic stimulation as a result of infective bites. If the subject leaves the endemic zone, his premunition disappears or at least wanes after a certain time, e.g. African workers or students living in Europe often suffer malaria attacks when they return home. **Premunition does not preclude the carrying of parasites**. It rather represents a truce between the parasite and host defences. The fact that parasites persist in this way means that a partially immune subject provides an excellent reservoir for the parasite.

The residents of regions of low endemicity or where malaria is epidemic acquire little or no immunity and malaria attacks—be they simple or severe—affect all age groups. This is why epidemics are so feared, whether they result from climatic changes, environmental modifications or follow the cessation of control operations (Mouchet *et al.*, 1998).

Genetics and the host-parasite relationship

Melano-Africans are less touched by malaria than other ethnic groups, whatever their pattern or history of exposure to the parasite (Hirsch, 1883); this raises the question of whether all humans are equally susceptible to malaria. In 1870 in the Comoros, Gevrey observed that Europeans and the Grand Comorians (who were of Arab origin) developed severe malaria (with many dying within six months of arrival), whereas those from Mozambique and Madagascar did not. This observation—made by an administrator rather than a physician—was quite clear-cut. In 1931, during an epidemic in the Zulu lands of South Africa, Swellengrebel *et al.* observed that the incidence of malaria was ten-fold lower among Bantus than in Indians, a difference which could not be explained by differences in living conditions (with the former actually being more exposed to infective mosquitoes).

The differences between Africans and others could be explained by selection: in Africans, effective defence mechanisms against malaria have evolved over a long period of cohabitation with the parasite. African emigrants who have spent a long time in France and who get re-infected when they briefly return home tend not to develop a severe form of the disease (Dupasquier, 1980). Similarly, Bamilékés from the malaria-free Cameroon mountains can relocate without any problem to the holo-endemic western plains. However, the exact mechanisms are undefined: their defence mechanisms seem to be more effective and more rapidly developed although what drives this remains unknown.

In Burkina Faso, differences have been documented in the prevalence of malaria and the incidence of cases between the Peul and the Mossi people who occupy the same territory and are exposed to the same holo-endemic malaria (with parasite prevalence lower in the former) (Modiano et al., 1996). In Papua New Guinea, significantly different degrees of splenomegaly were observed in two groups of women from different ethnic groups living in the same place (Brabin et al., 1988b), although it may be that behavioural differences were involved in this otherwise unexplained discrepancy.

In Gambia (Greenwood et al., 1987b), splenomegaly is far more marked among the Peul than in other indigenous groups.

In the Congo, more than 70% of cases in a community were concentrated in just 15% of the children (Richard et al., 1988c), i.e. certain children never got malaria whereas others had repeated attacks. A similar situation has been observed in Cameroon by Abel et al. (1992) who showed that the children of certain families experienced parasitaemia than the children of other families living in the same habitat. Segregation analysis showed that this trait of susceptibility to malaria—which pertained in 21% of all the inhabitants—depended on a major effect, not compatible with a simple Mendelian model, suggesting a more complex mode of inheritance. A strong interaction between major effect and age was noticed, suggesting that the influence of the putative major gene may be more prominent in children than in adults (Rihet et al., 1998).

Segregation analyses performed at Bobo-Dioulasso in Burkina Faso on four hundred individuals belonging to 41 families failed to identify a single major gene (Traoré et al., 1999): control of parasite density seemed to be under the influence of many genes although one gene on chromosome 5—the *Pfil* (*Plasmodium falciparum* infection levels) gene—accounted for 50% of the variance in parasite load. The relevant region of chromosome 5 is known to contain genes for cytokines involved in the regulation of T lymphocyte functions. In this case, no differences were observed between ethnic groups.

Cox (1984) pointed out the difference between Sudanese people who carried an antibody-independent factor inhibiting the invasion of red blood cells by *P. falciparum* (whatever the individual's personal history) and Indonesian people in whom this factor was absent; this points to important genetic differences which might account for differences in the epidemiology of malaria on these two continents.

Two leukocyte antigens shared by West African peoples are associated with substantial protection against severe pernicious malaria (Hill et al., 1991), although it is not known whether this is due to enhanced immunity to the parasite or attenuation of plasmodial pathogenicity (Carter et al., 1992).

Only a small corner of the veil that masks the genetics governing the relationships between humans and malaria has been lifted and many questions remain to be answered if we are ever to understand how we, the host, have evolved together with the parasite (Gilbert et al., 1998). Nevertheless, such knowledge is essential if an effective vaccine is ever to be developed (Williams, 1998).

Haemoglobinopathies

Sickle cell anaemia is a heritable condition in which the normal haemoglobin A is substituted by an altered form, haemoglobin S, the β-chain of which is mutated (with a valine replacing the glutamic acid at position 6). SS homozygotes suffer from a severe haematological disease characterised by sickle-shaped erythrocytes; this used to be fatal before adulthood. Prior to recent medical advances, homozygotes rarely reached the age of reproduction.

However, AS heterozygotes suffer only from sickle cell trait and rarely experience haematological problems—and they are believed to have some protection against malaria. This hypothesis derives from an observation made in Zimbabwe by Allison (1954) who noticed that malaria was less common in children with sickle cell trait than in children in general. Subsequently, it was shown (and confirmed in other studies conducted in Africa) that the difference is not significant but many experts showed that heterozygous carriers rarely experienced severe paroxysms and survived with parasite loads exceeding 100,000 parasites per mm^3. In brief, heterozygotes rarely die from malaria and therefore should have some advantage over other people. This theory explained why a gene that is lethal in the homozygous state nevertheless persists in the human gene pool and geneticists seized on this phenomenon that they interpreted as a concrete example of balanced polymorphism.

Going further, many ethnologists and biologists concluded that the presence of this haemoglobinopathy helped Africans survive in a malaria-ridden environment. This view has to be corrected. In fact, the percentage of AS heterozygotes never exceeds 25% (and is often lower than 10%). Therefore, at least 75% of all Africans carry only normal haemoglobin and they have nevertheless survived in such an environment. Moreover, haemoglobin S is completely absent in certain groups of people, notably the Mandingos of Guinea and Mali; these people carry haemoglobin C which does not appear to afford them any protection against malaria (Storey *et al.*, 1979), although it does seem to protect the Dogon of Mali against severe disease (Argawal *et al.*, 2000).

To date, five haemoglobin S haplotypes have been isolated: the "Senegal" haplotype in West Africa; "Benin" further to the east including Central Africa; "Bantu" in East and South Africa; "Eton" in the middle of Cameroon; and "Arabo-Indian" in Saudi Arabia as well as among the indigenous peoples of the Indochinese and Indian peninsulars (Capellan & Delpech, 1993; Labie, 1992; Nagel & Fleming, 1992). The last haplotype is associated with few pathological complications.

Sickle cell trait therefore seems to protect its carriers against severe malaria but it cannot be considered as the only factor which has allowed Africans to live and thrive in heavily malaria-infested surroundings.

It was also hypothesised that the various forms of α-thalassaemia (in which the α-chain of haemoglobin is mutated) found in the Mediterranean Basin and Southeast Asia might give their carriers some malaria-related advantage over their peers, but no convincing evidence in support of this hypothesis has ever been produced (Mockenhaupt *et al.*, 1999).

Glucose-6-phosphate dehydrogenase (G6PD) deficiency engenders problems when using amino-8-quinolines (Primaquine®) to treat malaria, but whether or not it has any protective effect against the disease remains hypothetical.

In Vietnam, the high frequency of such deficiencies (9-34%) in ethnic minorities in the foothills (who are highly exposed to malaria) supports the idea that they may confer some advantage *vis-à-vis P. falciparum* malaria (Verlé *et al.*, 2000).

In practice, it has to be admitted that human defence mechanisms are still poorly understood despite extensive research.

Recent sequencing of the human genome may open new research avenues in this field.

Malaria mortality

A hangover from an era in which "fever" was a hallmark of poor hygiene and health in many parts of the world, malaria mortality has become one of the most widely used health indicators, e.g. the WHO Roll Back Malaria Programme has set as its primary objective "the reduction of malaria mortality by at least 50%". But measuring this parameter is not so simple and has proven controversial in various aspects.

Measuring mortality

Direct methods

Official State figures

Notifications of deaths due to malaria in hospitals and health centres are often the only data used for the compilation of national and international statistics, although these figures are notoriously under-estimated in the southern hemisphere.

Autopsies

Figures based on autopsy data are closer to the reality. In Nigeria, Whitbourne (1930) estimated that malaria was responsible for 8-10% of all child mortality; studying four hundred autopsies in 1943, Smith attributed 10.8% of babies' deaths and 14.3% of those of young children to malaria; in Lagos in 1952, Bruce-Chwatt analysed 3,088 autopsies and blamed malaria for 8% of deaths in babies, 13% in children of 2-4 years of age, 7.9% in children of 5-7, and 2.3% in children of 8-10. In the Congo, Duren (1951) and later Janssens *et al.* (1966) reported similar figures.

These autopsies were all performed in a hospital setting and cannot therefore be considered as a representative sample of the population as a whole.

Verbal Autopsies

Verbal Autopsies (VA) are based on questionnaires addressed to all the members of a community, usually *via* community health care activists or community leaders (Anker *et al.*, 1999). This type of instrument has been used to estimate mortality at Demographic Surveillance Sites (DSS) established in the framework of the Demographic and Health Surveys (DHS) Project which is currently active in twenty-nine African countries. At each site, parasite prevalence is measured and the results are subsequently compiled by country, by region or on the basis of some other criterion. These sites have been studied since 1980 or 1990.

The verbal autopsy method has been validated in various hospitals in the Afrotropical Region although it is not very sensitive (56%) and its specificity is only 88% due to inadequately precise classification of both diseases (Todd *et al.*, 1994) and causes of death (Chandramohan, 2001). In highly endemic regions, more deaths are caused by malaria anaemia than cerebral malaria, and the former is less well characterised than the latter in the VA system.

Although malaria mortality was higher in West Africa than it was in East Africa from 1980 to 1998, it has since remained stable in the former, whereas in the latter, it has almost doubled in the last ten years, partly due to the spread of resistance, first to chloroquine then later to sulfadoxine-pyrimethamine. In addition, malaria epidemics occur in East Africa, not in West Africa. HIV has not affected infant mortality.

Information from the Demographic Surveillance Sites system is far more reliable than official statistics when it comes to quantifying the various causes of death, including malaria. However, at a site with 65,000 inhabitants—including 10,200 children of under 5—where there are 309 deaths per annum, the reduction in mortality will only become apparent after 7.2 years; if the sample is smaller, it will take even longer for any reduction in mortality to become substantial.

Indirect methods

Since 1955 and the instigation of malaria eradication programmes, it has been possible to compare mortality before and after eradication operations in Sri Lanka and the Americas. It has also become possible to compare differential mortality in treated and untreated zones, e.g. the pilot zones of Pare Taveta in Tanzania, Kisumu in Kenya and Garki in Nigeria. All these observations have been compiled and summarised by Molineaux (1985).

These methods measure both the direct reduction in mortality (due to the elimination of malaria) and the indirect reduction (due to improvements in health care provision, living standards and even action against intercurrent illness). One reason for this being relevant is the fact that the beginning of the eradication policy coincided with the development of sulphamide drugs, antibiotics, rehydration solutions, etc.

Newman (1969 *in* Molineaux, 1985) studied mortality in Sri Lanka from 1930 to 1945 and again from 1946 to 1960 in two districts, one where malaria was highly prevalent (SR > 70%) and another where it was rare (SR < 20%). For a drop in the Overall Mortality Rate (OMR) of 10 points (from 21.8 down to 11.7), the eradication of malaria only accounted for 43%, i.e. 4.3 points. However, a different system developed by Gray (*in* Molineaux, 1985) quantified the reduction due to the eradication of malaria at only 2.7 points: this illustrates how complicated it is to evaluate reductions in mortality between two successive periods during which malaria control initiatives were not the only factor that changed.

In the Americas, the OMR dropped sharply between 1955 and 1967 (Gramiccia & Hempel, 1972) after the launch of eradication programmes:
- Honduras: 11.9 to 8.4 OMR prior to 1955, 1.59 after 1955;
- Nicaragua: 9.2 to 8 OMR prior to 1955, 1.39 after 1955;
- Mexico: 13.6 to 9.2 OMR prior to 1955, 0.64 after 1955;
- Ecuador: 15.5 to 10.6 OMR prior to 1955, 0.38 after 1955.

In the Pare Taveta Scheme in Tanzania, overall mortality and infant mortality were monitored in a sample of 2,500 people for four years after indoor spraying operations. The OMR was 24 in the first year, 23 in the second, 12 in the third, and 16 in the fourth (from 1954 to 1958). The corresponding Infant Mortality Rate (IMR) figures were 165, 260, 78 and 138. Over the six years following the cessation of spraying, the OMR rose back up but only very slowly, and the IMR remained fairly low (Molineaux, 1985). The persistence of low-level transmission was due to the temporary disappearance of one major vector, *An. funestus*.

In the Kisumu Project in Kenya, operations led to a sharp drop in the incidence of the disease—of the order of 96% among babies. After one year, mortality had decreased by 33% more in the treated zone than in an untreated zone, a differential which had risen to 44% after two years. The OMR dropped from 23.9‰ down to 12.3‰, i.e. by almost one-half. In cohorts of babies, the IMR dropped from 157‰, down to 93‰ within one year.

At Garki in Nigeria (Molineaux & Gramiccia, 1980), after 18 months of house spraying with propoxur, the OMR dropped from 23.4‰ to 17.6‰.

Variable mortality rates

Data from Kisumu and Garki—in tropical strata where malaria transmission is seasonal—show malaria to be a leading cause of death, in particular among babies and young children (over 30%). Even if indirect mortality is considered, the weight of malaria mortality remains very high.

However, it is important to avoid trying to generalise these conclusions. In holo-endemic regions where transmission is perennial such as the Congo, malaria mortality seems far lower. In a cohort of 500 children in Linzolo who were followed for five years, Guillo de Bodan (1982) observed only two cases of severe malaria. In the town of Brazzaville, the annual incidence of severe paroxysms was 1.15‰ between 0 and 4 years of age, and malaria mortality in this age group was 0.43‰. These figures were thirty times lower than those reported for Africa as a whole (Trape *et al.*, 1987d). The author attributed this low malaria mortality to the ready availability of chloroquine but this is not totally convincing since chloroquine availability was not a problem in many African towns or villages. In the Paediatric Department of Brazzaville General Hospital which caters for more than 400,000 people, only 30 cases of severe malaria were observed over a two-year period (Vaisse *et al.*, 1981). During sixteen months of monitoring of a group of 500 children in three villages in the Mayombe forest of the Congo, not one single case of severe malaria was seen (Richard *et al.*, 1988c).

The examples of the Congo on one hand, and those of Kisumu and Garki on the other, point up variations in mortality rates within stable, holo-endemic or hyperendemic units. The interruption of transmission during the dry season could inhibit the acquisition of immunity and lead to pathological problems as soon as transmission resumes; this is no more than a hypothesis that is subscribed to by different experts to a greater or lesser extent, and it constitutes a question that warrants further investigation. This is also a crucial question for the timing of house spraying operation and their evaluation.

In all countries of Europe, Asia and the Americas in which vector control has been effectively implemented, malaria mortality has substantially dropped. Deaths are counted in ones or tens, hardly ever hundreds (apart from a few epidemic re-emergence events). Inequalities between endemic zones have largely been erased.

Epidemics and mortality

Epidemics arise in places where malaria transmission is unstable and where local people's immunity is low or absent. They cause serious symptoms and clinical manifestations, resulting in heavy mortality in all age groups. Considered as a natural scourge, epidemics have featured in stories and histories ever since earliest Antiquity.

The root causes of epidemics were reviewed above.

The fatality of certain epidemics can be estimated with a reasonable degree of accuracy. When anophelines were imported into Mauritius in around 1865, a massive epidemic ravaged throughout all the land below 500 m in altitude (Julvez *et al.*, 1990). In 1866 and 1867, the death rate rose by 327% (Meldrum, 1881); ten years later, the epidemics amounted to no more than seasonal outbreaks which caused little mortality (Antelme, 1888).

In Madagascar, 18th and 19th century historians compared the unhealthy coastal regions with the healthy Plateaux until the bloody 1878 epidemic which was probably associated with the introduction of irrigation and rice-growing (Laventure *et al.*, 1996). *An. funestus* found a perfect biotope in the rice paddies. Malaria persisted on the plateaux until it was eliminated in 1962 by eradication operations. After the discontinuation of control measures in 1975, malaria returned to the Hautes Terres in 1986 and the epidemic was exacerbated by the dysfunctionality of the health care services, poor access to medication and general economic hardship (Mouchet *et al.*, 1997). The WHO reported 100,000 deaths per annum and some experts estimated the number at 300,000. Estimates made by the Madagascan Public Health Ministry and French experts put the number between 20,000 and 35,000 deaths per annum, a heavy enough toll in a population of just two million.

It is believed that the establishment of *An. gambiae s.s.* on Grande Comore following water tank construction in the 1920's led to the death of more than 20% of the population (Raynal, 1928).

In Swaziland in 1986, a very severe epidemic broke out following the cessation of indoor spraying operations; almost 10% of the cases were of severe malaria (Fontaine *et al.*, 1987, Rep. WHO; Mouchet, 1987, Rep. WHO).

The 1958 epidemic in Ethiopia following particularly heavy rainfall is believed to have led to over 150,000 deaths (Fontaine *et al.*, 1961). Recent outbreaks, although less deadly, occurred following changes in control modalities at Zwai (1993) in the Rift Valley, at Tigré, and on the plateaux of Bah-Dar and Gondar (Teklehaimanot, 1991, Rep. WHO).

Following heavy rainfall in south-western Uganda in 1995, a very serious epidemic broke out as reflected by a dramatic increase in the number of cases seen at the Kisizi hospital (Mouchet *et al.*, 1998).

Rain associated with the 1998 El Niño southern oscillation caused, at the beginning of the following year, an epidemic that spread through north-eastern Kenya and southern Somalia (WHO, 1999a).

In 1999, there was major flooding in southern Mozambique but we could find no written evidence that this had any health-related repercussions.

In 2000, no climatic, environmental or demographic trigger can be identified for an epidemic that struck a million people in Burundi. Coosemans *et al.* (unpublished data) proposed the hypothesis of saturation of the reservoir (drastic increases of the number of cases) followed by its overflowing in a genuine spiral.

In West Africa around the edges of the Sahara, epidemics are less common and smaller-scale. At the Bilma oasis in Niger where vectors are not usually found, epidemics broke out in 1958 (Bilma Health Centre archives) and in 1991 (Develoux *et al.*, 1994). In Mali, in the circles of Kidal and Tessalit, at Adrar des Iforas, and in the Sahara desert, nearly 3,000 cases were reported in 1999 (Doumbo *et al.*, 1999) although mortality was not evaluated in these outbreaks.

On the Indian Sub-Continent, notably in the Punjab, medical accounts recount irregular epidemics of malaria. In the 1930's, millions of deaths were attributed to each epidemic wave (Bouma, 1995). Most of the epidemics were associated with heavy rainfall following extended dry periods. An end was put to this serial catastrophe by the instigation of indoor spraying with long-acting insecticides (DDT). In Sri Lanka (described above), epidemics tended to break out in dry years when water courses ceased flowing.

The epidemics which followed the introduction of *An. gambiae s.l.* (probably *An. arabiensis*) into Brazil (Soper & Wilson, 1943) and Egypt (Shousha, 1948) were documented in detail. By the time of the eradication of this mosquito, it was estimated to have caused 150,000 deaths in ten years in Brazil, and 40,000 in Egypt over three years.

From the accounts of various epidemics, it is important to note that mortality largely depends on the accessibility and quality of health care (notably malaria drugs). The deadly 1986-1988 epidemic in Madagascar spread against a background of poverty and degraded health care infrastructure, so patients neither had any health care facilities to support them nor the resources to buy drugs. Making chloroquine available to all, even the poorest—through grocers' shops, public institutions, travelling salesmen, etc.—will help counter the immediate pathological consequences of an epidemic even if it does not actually interrupt transmission (Mouchet *et al.*, 1998). In the 1999 Kidal epidemic in Mali, immediate care provision significantly mitigated the consequences (*see the Part on* "Malaria Control").

Medium-term consequences of vector control on malaria mortality: a controversial subject

In places where transmission has been curtailed and the number of malaria attacks has been reduced by vector control measures (notably treated mosquito nets and curtains), certain experts have claimed that the resultant damping of immunity leads to increased infection rates in older children (over 2-3 years of age) that have not developed immunity (Snow *et al.*, 1997; Trape & Rogier, 1996). No such **rebound effect** (Coleman *et al.*, 1999) has ever been clearly demonstrated; rather to the contrary, it has been observed that the simple reporting of the first episodes of an epidemic reduces overall mortality (Molineaux, 1997a, 1997b). It has also been observed that the chances of survival of a young child suffering six attacks over a short period (one year) are lower than those of one who experiences two episodes a year for three years in a village where the rate of malaria transmission is moderate (D'Alessandro & Coosemans, 1997). After an in-depth analysis of all infant mortality data since 1980, Smith *et al.* (2001) arrived at the conclusion that reduced transmission—either through the use of treated curtains (Habluezel *et al.*, 1997) or treated mosquito nets (Armstrong-Schellenberg *et al.*, 2001)—did not lead to any subsequent increase in mortality. These authors concluded that protecting children in these ways is still an excellent way of preventing malaria attacks in hyper- and holo-endemic regions (Lengeler, 1998).

Several other studies on the use of ITNs also showed the absence of this rebound effect on mortality. There was no increase in the proportion of older children (12-59 months old) dying in villages in which ITNs had been in use for 5-6 years (48.1%) compared historically with villages without ITNs (47.9%), after controlling for seasonality (AHR = 1.03, P = 0.834). No evidence was found that sustained ITN use increased the risk of mortality in older children in this area of intense perennial malaria transmission (Eisele *et al.*, 2005). In another study, ITN-decreased exposure reduced IgG responses to pre-erythrocytic antigens, but there was no evidence that two years of ITN use compromised IgG responses to blood stage antigens in these young children (Kariuki *et al.*, 2003). A seven year follow-up (until the end of 2000) found also no indication in any age group of increased mortality in the ITN group after the end of the randomised intervention (Binka *et al.*, 2002).

Malaria morbidity

Measuring morbidity

The malaria attack is defined as an otherwise unexplained fever of over 38 °C in a subject with a parasite load over a certain fixed pyrogenic threshold. Being sure of these criteria means having access to both a thermometer and laboratory services, which is rarely the case in practice—and this does not seem to be improving very quickly outside of urban areas in which the cost efficiency of accurate diagnosis (e.g. investing in a microscope) has been demonstrated (Jonkman *et al.*, 1995).

There is no single method. It depends on the circumstances, epidemiological context, available facilities, and goals. Diagnosis for treatment is one thing and diagnosis for evaluation is another. Rogier *et al.* (2001) provide recent literature and up-to-date information needed to deal with the problem of diagnosing malaria attacks in endemic areas.

Currently, 90% of cases in endemic zones are diagnosed on purely clinical criteria (Najera, 2000, personal communication), usually a temperature of over 38 °C without any specific evidence pointing towards another disease. Whatever skills of the practitioner, this diagnostic method is susceptible to an error rate of at least 50% in those parts of Africa where malaria transmission is stable (Baudon *et al.*, 1986b).

The search for a diagnostic algorithm based on clinical signs (Genton *et al.*, 1994; Redd *et al.*, 1996; Rougemont *et al.*, 1991; Trape *et al.*, 1985) has not yielded results other than the indispensable development of certain alternative treatment or standard protocols for severe forms.

Incidence estimates for a given population are usually based on cohort analysis (Carnevale *et al.*, 1988; Henry *et al.*, 2005).

Malaria morbidity on the different continents

In field conditions of endemic zones, evaluating the morbidity of simple malaria is a difficult enterprise (Baudon *et al.*, 1984; Greenwood, 1987), especially in Tropical Africa. This is why official figures are so imprecise (to say the least).

Entomological data (e.g. the number of infective bites per person per annum) gives no information about morbidity because there is no way of gauging the likelihood of productive infection or its clinical consequences. However, this indicator which represents the maximum theoretical transmission rate (apart from iatrogenic pathways) is a useful parameter when it comes to planning vector control for malaria control programmes.

The data available depend on the accuracy of the notifications of supposed malaria cases by the health authorities. Given the failings of diagnosis at remote health care centres, these figures tend, on the one hand to be overestimated as a result of mistaken diagnoses of non-malaria fever and, on the other underestimated due to the inaccessibility of health care structures and under-reporting. Moreover, many patients rely on self-treatment and traditional medicine—or they just wait to get better... or die.

Estimating the mean number of malaria attacks per child per annum in a stable zone is complicated by the damping effect of immunity. In a holo-endemic zone of Liberia, a figure of 1.6 attacks per child has been recorded (Miller, 1958), but in equally holo-endemic Senegal, the incidence of symptomatic cases was six per subject in the second year of life whereas in a meso-endemic zone, it ended at three per annum (Trape & Rogier, 1996). In a holo-endemic zone in the Gambia, the mean number of attacks per child per annum varied from one to five (Greenwood et al., 1987a). In the forest of western Ivory Coast, the number of attacks was five per annum up to 2 years of age, and two per annum between the ages of 2 and 5 (Henry et al., 2005). In under-5 year-olds, Brenan & Campbell (1988) estimated the rate of febrile episodes in Africa at one to nine per annum, only some of which would have been due to malaria because of inaccurate diagnosis. In Tanzania, Rooth & Bjorkman (1992) estimated the rate at 1.5-3 per annum between 18 months and 2 years of age, with a mean of barely over 1.5 in rural settings. In West Africa, the annual number of attacks is between one and five in under-5 year-olds—a very broad range (Greenwood et al., 1987; Trape et al., 1987d). However how this parameter is calculated is not standardised and it is not inconceivable that the various experts might have used different methods.

In sub-Saharan Africa, information from the *Weekly Epidemiological Record* obtained on country-based malaria reports is unusable because confirmed and tentative diagnoses are mixed up; in addition, over 90% of the data are either incomplete or uninterpretable.

In order to be able to evaluate malaria morbidity in Africa, the number of attacks per person in the various epidemiological conditions has been estimated starting from the hypothesis that 90% of the population is exposed to the risk. Then, the mean number of attacks per person per annum was calculated for different age groups.

For children of over 5 and adults, the only information available (Bruce-Chwatt, 1963) concerns the Lagos suburbs, i.e. an urban setting, where the mean rate was 0.4-0.52 attacks per person per annum.

Year 2000: Time to Take Stock

Malaria and malaria control over the last two centuries

The Primary Health Care System, as defined at the 1978 Alma-Ata Conference, predicted access for all to health care by the year 2000. This slogan—in which few professional health care providers had much confidence at the time—may now raise a few smiles.

In the special case of malaria, it is important to make a distinction between the period up to 1975 during which the impact of disease was on the wane, and the period of subsequent stagnation between 1975 and 2000 following termination of the Global Eradication Programme.

Hackett (in Boyd, 1949) estimated that in 1850 malaria ravaged all lands where climate and ecological conditions were conducive to the transmission and maintenance of the disease. From the end of the 18th century through the following two hundred years, the tendency towards expansion reversed. In Europe and North America, the disease began to regress spontaneously as a result of increased standards of living and habitat improvement. After isolation of the causative parasites in 1880 and discovery that the disease is transmitted by anopheline mosquitoes in 1892, efforts began to be made to target *Plasmodium* and its vectors. Curative and prophylactic "quininisation" was the basis of an effective battle against malaria in Mediterranean Europe, The Netherlands, North Africa, South Africa, the United States of America, the Caribbean, and a few Latin American countries. This was complemented by measures to control anopheline larvae using insecticides (mineral oil and Paris Green) or, more importantly, by draining swamplands (largely undertaken in order to recover arable land). By 1945, the prevalence of malaria had fallen by 90% in Italy (*see the Part on* "Malaria Control"). But these efforts benefited hardly any of the poor tropical countries in which trial projects met with nothing but failure.

The development of DDT and the formulation of an eradication policy designed to protect all social strata was going to change the face of malaria across the globe. Outside of Africa—which was excluded from the Programme—all malaria indicators dropped dramatically. The disease disappeared from 30-50% of the surface area that it had formerly ravaged, and the number of cases dropped by 70-90% in most countries where indoor spraying was implemented.

In consequence, as of that time 85% or more of cases were found in Tropical Africa which became very much the disease's focus.

Since 1975, changes in strategy—notably the curtailment or discontinuation of indoor spraying operations—have been followed by the resumption of local transmission and the outbreak of epidemics. In 1989, Najera concluded that the situation vis-à-vis malaria was deteriorating.

Much was expected from the **Global Malaria Control Strategy** as formulated at the 1992 Amsterdam Conference and now from the Roll Back Malaria Programme (RBM).

An overview of malaria 2000

Malaria is the most common parasitic disease in the world. Over two million human beings are exposed to it, and those at highest risk are young children living in the tropics and sub-tropical regions. Here, we attempt to:
- review **malaria impact on health**, in terms of both morbidity and mortality;
- **map the disease**, towards a new geography of malaria;
- provide a **cost analysis**, including both care costs and an estimate of economic losses.

Health figures

Malaria is generally considered as a disease without sequelae although severe pernicious paroxysms in young children caused by *P. falciparum* can give rise to irreversible neurological and motor deficienciencies. Relapses due to *P. vivax* and recurrent *P. malariae* malaria used to cause progressive visceral malaria, although this has practically disappeared since modern drugs became available, even though similar problems are still sometimes seen with drug-resistant parasites. However, as a general rule, malaria either resolves spontaneously or, in the most extreme cases, kills its victim.

Assessing the impact of the disease must take into account the associated mortality and morbidity, parameters which both vary enormously in different parts of the world.

The WHO regularly compiles and publishes malaria statistics for its member states on the basis of figures supplied by the national authorities derived from data collected at local health centres. Given that fully 90% of the notifications concern unconfirmed diagnoses, these figures are far from reliable. Moreover, fewer than 50% of malaria patients ever attend a health care centre, and many dispensaries fail to submit figures.

In Tropical Africa for example, 10% of cases at the most appear in these statistics although in Asia and the Americas where laboratories are better equipped, figures are more reliable.

Rather than relying on defective official statistics, most experts choose to make estimates and extrapolations on the basis of figures gathered in rigorously studied areas.

How many people die of malaria every year?

The Afrotropical Region is by far the most profoundly affected part of the world, being home to 85-90% of all cases. In places where malaria is stable—either holo- or hyperendemic (in which 60% of African population lives)—the disease is thought to be responsible for 4% of deaths among babies and 25% of those in young children; in meso- and hypo-endemic zones, malaria is believed to account for 10% of mortality in 0-4 year-olds and 6% in over-6 year-olds. Extrapolating from these figures and given a total population of 600 million people, the number of deaths every year due to malaria has been estimated at one million. However, caution is warranted given that the source data were collected in Gambia, Kenya (Kisumu) and Nigeria (Garki) in tropical savannah lands where mortality has always been considered to be particularly high.

As of 1980 and especially since 1990, the Demographic and Health Survey programme which operates in twenty-nine African countries and collects its data at defined Demographic Surveillance Sites by means of the Verbal Autopsy system, has made it possible to refine malaria mortality estimates: according to these, mortality is 7.3 per thousand child years, corresponding to 21% of the 15,665 deaths of under-5 year-olds recorded at these sites. If this is extrapolated to the continent as a whole, the number of deaths in children of this age group would be about 800,000 per annum (Snow *et al.*, 1999).

This figure is substantially lower than the estimates of Najera and Hempel (1996) of 1-2.8 million deaths per annum worldwide, with 95% in Africa.

In the Australasian Region, no overall evaluation has been carried out. In Papua New Guinea, malaria mortality in 1998 was reported at 1.8%, which seems extremely high given that in the Solomon Islands, only 30-40 deaths per annum were reported in 1991 (WHO, personal communication) and mortality was considered low in Vanuatu (Ratard, 1975); in the hyperendemic part of the island of Espiritu Santo, there was apparently no specific mortality (Maitland *et al.*, 1997). In immigration zones on Western New Guinea (Indonesia), an "epidemic" among Javanese immigrants made malaria the second cause of death in the province.

In other parts of the world, malaria mortality is more or less negligible compared with Africa, although forest malaria kills more than five hundred people a year in Vietnam (*see the Chapter on* the "Oriental Region").

In South America, apart from in Amazonia and Guyana, most malaria is due to *P. vivax* and only a few hundred people a year die from the disease.

Malaria morbidity on the different continents

In **Tropical Africa**, application of the criteria described in the preceding chapter leads to the following conclusions:
- in regions where malaria is stable and holo- or hyperendemic (which account for 60% of the population), the number of annual attacks ranges from 0.45-0.65 per person (all ages included);
- in meso- and hypo-endemic regions at risk of epidemics, the number of attacks is 0.25 per person per annum.

Analysis of these figures gives a range of 200-280 million cases annually in a population of 450 million people (WHO, 2000). If population growth is taken into account, this estimate is comparable to that of Baudon & Mouchet (OCCGE Technical Conference, 1972 Bobo-Dioulasso) who estimated a range of 100-200 million cases.

The number of people carrying the parasite is estimated at 300-350 million (WHO, 2000a).

In **Australasia**, the situation is unclear because the figures for the Moluccas and Western New Guinea—where most cases of malaria occur—are included with those from Indonesia (i.e. Asia). In Papua New Guinea, the number ranges from 66,000 to 629,000, depending on whether cases were diagnosed by microscopic examination or on purely clinical criteria. Under 100,000 cases were declared on the Solomon Islands (84,800 in 1996) and only 6,099 in Vanuatu in 1997—although notifications from the latter should be treated with caution.

In **Asia**, 5,288,000 cases were reported in 1997, mostly in India and the Indochinese peninsular. No reliable submissions come from Afghanistan because of the political situation there, although the WHO (Beljaev, personal communication) estimates the number of cases at about 2 million. A similar figure has been reported for Yemen which constitutes an enclave of Africa in the Asian Region. Attention should be drawn to the considerable drop in the incidence of malaria in China, as well as to the re-emergence of the disease in Korea, Tajikistan, Azerbaijan and Armenia, all countries from which malaria was considered to have been eradicated.

Throughout the **Mediterranean Basin** and the **Middle East**, malaria is in regression, apart from Turkey where *P. vivax* causes 50,000-100,000 cases. In North Africa, a few cases of *P. vivax* malaria (under 50) were reported in Algeria (Benzerroug & Wery, 1985) and Egypt (Bassiouny, 2001).

In **Europe**, there has not been any local transmission since 1976, the last case having been reported in Macedonia in 1975. But imported malaria, especially *P. falciparum*, affects about 10,000 people a year, mostly in Western Europe (*see the Part on* "Spatiotemporal Dynamics of Malaria").

In the **Americas**, twenty-one out of thirty-nine countries have reported indigenous malaria: a total of 1,054,000 cases (mostly due to *P. vivax*) were notified in 1997 (WHO, 1999). These are essentially all concentrated in Central America, the Amazonian Basin and the foothills of the Andes.

Towards a new geography of malaria

The disappearance of malaria from temperate zones around the beginning of the 20th century reduced its range to the tropical and sub-tropical belts. From 1950 to 1970, eradication operations further reduced the territory ravaged by the disease and, notably, highlighted the regional variability of endemicity. Africa—home to 90% of all cases worldwide—has thus emerged as the "malaria continent".

As discussed above, geographical disparities must always be taken into account when assessing the impact of malaria.

Maps

Distinction has to be made between maps drawn up at the national or regional scale and less detailed global maps derived from official figures and statistics.

National and regional maps

For many years, such maps were intended to locate disease foci and delineate different zones according to transmission characteristics: holo-, hyper-, meso-, hypo-endemic areas, and epidemic zones. In Africa where the disease extends over almost the entire continent, a distinction is often made between those places where malaria is stable and those where it is unstable (Mouchet *et al.*, 1991).

In Southeast Asia, the Mekong Malaria Project has produced a series of physical maps showing altitude, river network and landcover (forest) onto which are superimposed epidemiological data. In addition, district maps have been drawn up to show the local incidence of the disease and even the relative distribution of *P. falciparum* and *P. vivax*.

In Kenya, remote sensing data combined in a Geographical Information System have been used to draw up quantitative maps (*Figure 1*) with the density of dots reflecting the number of inhabitants superimposed on a background representing transmission modes (Snow *et al.*, 1998b).

To date, these maps have not been useful in predicting epidemics but they give an excellent overview of malaria in south-western Kenya.

Global maps

The WHO has been regularly producing global malaria maps since 1955, simplified representations which were for a long time designed to track the success of eradication operations. Most of these maps separated countries in which malaria was still present from those in which it had either been eradicated or had never existed. The purpose of these maps was principally political and they do not show different levels of endemicity and therefore give no idea of the local impact of the disease.

The MARA programmes developed useful maps with a lot of information on malaria transmission and morbidity throughout Sub-Saharan Africa.

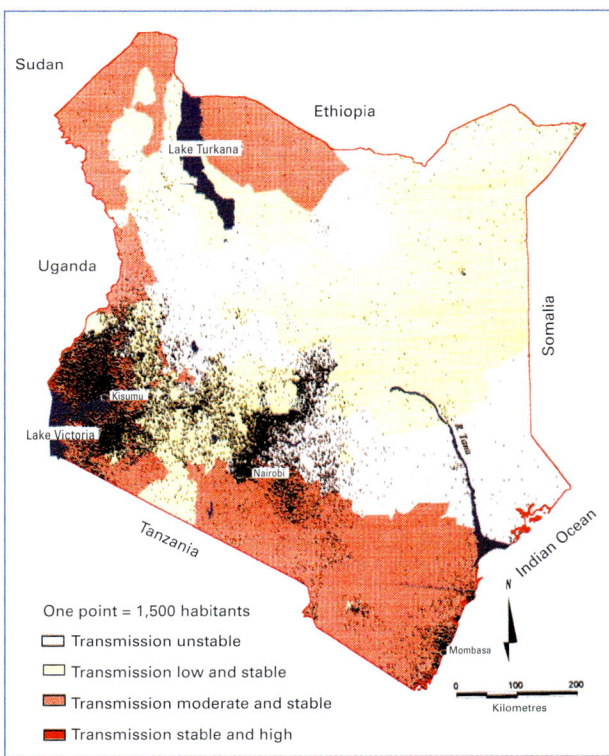

Figure 1. *Population density and endemicity (figure MARA, Mapping Malaria Risk in Africa).*

We have tried to produce a simplified map which clearly delineates the broad endemic zones of Africa and Australasia, the localised foci of Southeast Asia, Latin America and the Middle East, and places where malaria is relatively rare (*Figure 2*).

Epidemiological classification of malaria regions

At this stage, this attempt at classification only aims to give an overview of how the disease is distributed across the planet. In the second part of this book, the epidemiology of malaria is addressed region by region, and country by country. Three different types of situation emerge from this analysis:
- **contiguous areas of high endemicity** where malaria affects all villages;
- **disease foci** fostered by specific ecological or anthropogenic conditions, interspersed with zones in which there is no malaria;
- **zones of low endemicity** around microfoci or sporadic outbreaks.

Areas of high endemicity

They are found in two regions, namely the Afrotropical Region and the Australasian Region.

• *Afrotropical area*

This area corresponds to the biogeographical region of the same name which includes Madagascar, the Comoros and the south-western part of the Arabian Peninsular. Malaria is present in all villages (with the exception of those above 2,200 m in altitude and deserts), i.e. a contiguous area. This is the heartland of pernicious malaria due to *P. falciparum*, the most virulent of the malaria parasites and the one which accounts for the vast majority of mortality from this disease. At least 60% of the population of West, Central and Eastern Africa are exposed to stable, holo- or hyperendemic malaria. People develop strong premunition and most clinical events are seen in children, with the majority of deaths occurring in children of between six months and four years of age.

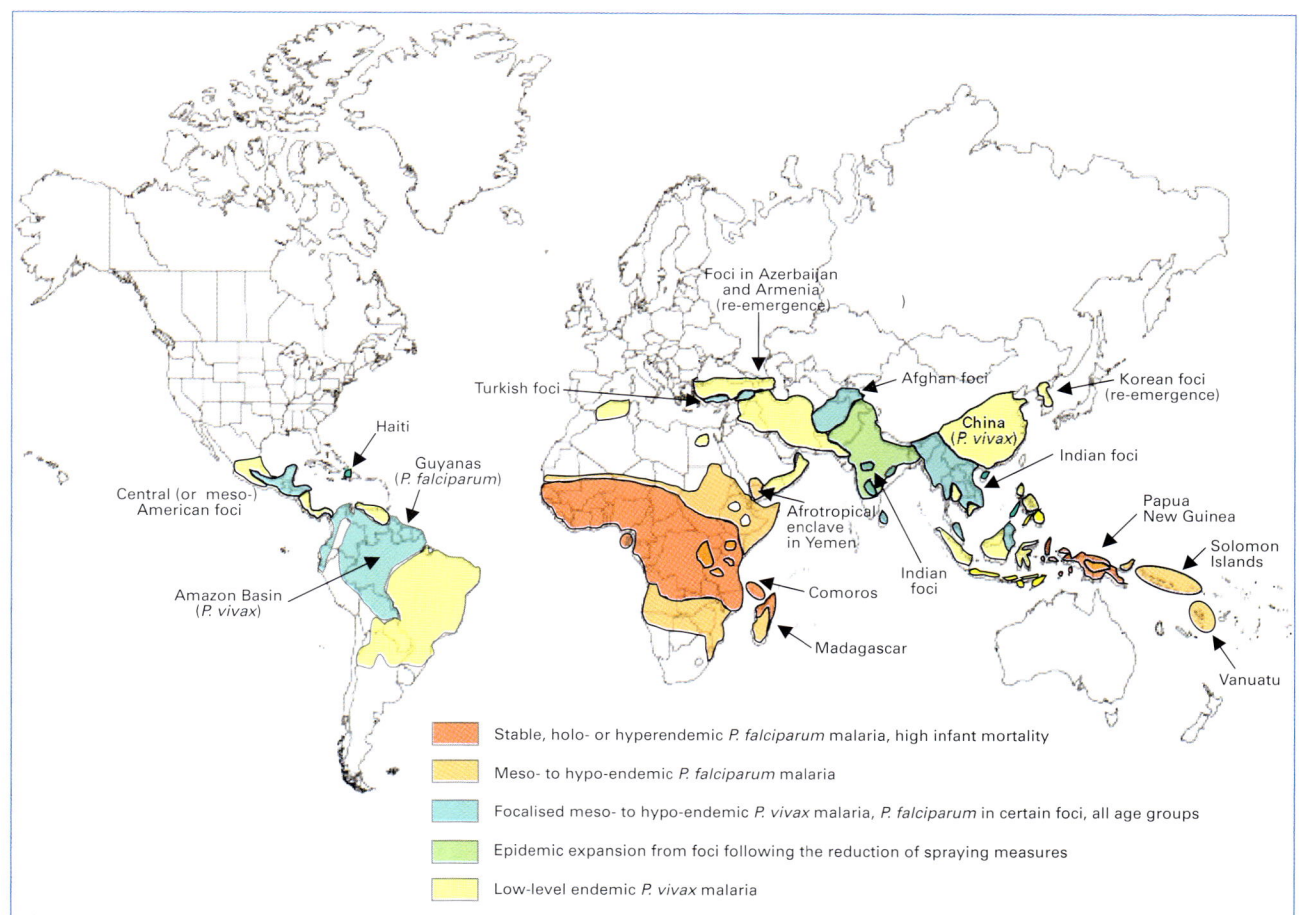

Figure 2. World-wide epidemiological distribution of malaria.

Biodiversity of Malaria in the World

As altitude or aridity increase, malaria indicators steadily drop and the disease becomes meso- or hypo-endemic. Here epidemics may break out, affecting people of all ages, and malaria mortality does not vary much from one place to another.

• *Australasian expanse*

In this region of islands and archipelagos, the only places affected are the Moluccas and Western New Guinea in Indonesia, Papua New Guinea, the Solomon Islands, and Vanuatu. Although this region is classified together with the Afrotropical Region, the number of cases is far lower and severe forms of the disease much rarer. In New Guinea, the stable malaria is holo- or hyperendemic, and even meso-endemic above 600 m. Local people acquire strong premunition. The parasites are *P. falciparum* and/or *P. vivax*. From 600 to 1,200 m in altitude, the incidence of malaria drops and outbreaks become seasonal or are even limited to epidemics.

In the Solomon Islands, malaria control measures have reduced the disease's range and endemicity. In Vanuatu, it is confined to the coastal plains.

Foci

The idea of disease focus is a poorly defined one as a result of the diversity of causes. It means a concentration of malaria cases in one place while the disease is not found in the surrounding area.

• *Southeast Asian forest*

These Indochinese and Indian foci are due to the presence of highly efficient vectors, notably *An. minimus s.l.*, *An. dirus s.l.* and *An. fluviatilis s.l.*, together with *P. vivax* and *P. falciparum*. Most of the people living in these jungle areas belong to ethnic minorities and "forest malaria" is the cause of more than half of all cases of malaria in Indochina (Vietnam, Laos, Cambodia, Thailand, Myanmar, Bangladesh), India (the north-eastern States, Madhya Pradesh, Orissa, Karnakata, Tamil Nadu) and, to a lesser extent, Malaysia (Sabah, Peninsular Malaysia), Indonesia (Kalimantan, Sumatra), and the Philippines (Palawan). Indigenous people are usually fairly resistant to this type of malaria but the immunologically naive—coming from malaria-free areas—fall victim to severe pernicious *P. falciparum* malaria.

• *Historical epidemic foci*

Before the partitioning of India and Pakistan, malaria foci along the Indus Valley in the Punjab gave rise to epidemics involving millions of people and leading to high mortality. These were due to climatic factors, often a period of heavy rainfall following a succession of dry years. They were largely eliminated by means of widespread indoor spraying operations, since which time lesser epidemics have broken out at Karachi in Pakistan, in Rajasthan and north-western India. These regions need to be monitored closely. Malaria is most common along rivers, streams and around irrigated land.

• *Afghanistan and Tajikistan*

This focus developed with the breakdown in health care services in Afghanistan and subsequently spilled over into Tajikistan following post-independence unrest. The proportion of *P. falciparum* has risen sharply in Afghanistan and this species of parasite has now appeared in Tajikistan, a country from which it had been eradicated over thirty years beforehand.

• *Turkey*

This focus—or more exactly the dual foci of Adana and the Upper Euphrates—arose as a result of the vector developing resistance to insecticides used indiscriminately for agricultural purposes. This factor was compounded by operational problems and seasonal migration in search of work. Only *P. vivax* is present, hence the impact of the disease is moderate.

• *Meso-American foci*

Foci of *P. vivax* transmission are found in Mexico, Belize, Guatemala, Honduras, Salvador, and Nicaragua. In contrast, only *P. falciparum* is found in the single focus found in the Caribbean—Haiti and the Dominican Republic.

• *Guyana and its neighbours*

The highest incidences of malaria on the American continent are found in Guyana, Surinam and to a lesser extent French Guiana. *P. falciparum* predominates among those of African descent whereas *P. vivax* is far more common in Amerindians and those of Asiatic origin.

• *The Amazon*

The Amazon is the great reservoir of malaria in the Americas. It encompasses northern and western Brazil, southern Venezuela, southern and eastern Colombia and the east of Ecuador, Peru, and Bolivia. This vast focus is cut up along lines marking incursions into the forest mass. It arises when farmer-settlers enter the forest along the trans-Amazonian roads in Brazil. These very poor people originally settled on cleared forest land in rudimentary settlements where they were directly exposed to vectors and where health care infrastructure was minimal, although they later came together in villages where facilities were improved. During the rush of colonisation which took place between 1980 and 1995, one million people moved into the State of Roraima alone; the States of Acre, Amazonas, Roraima, and Amapa were also concerned, and more or less similar migrations took place into the forest in southern Venezuela, Colombia, Ecuador, Peru, and Bolivia.

Temporary migrations of miners—which were better organised—had less impact on health.

More than one million cases per annum were reported in immigrants between 1985 and 1990, *P. vivax* in most cases, although *P. falciparum* was also present.

Currently, there is a hiatus in immigration into the forest in Brazil but these movements have nevertheless resulted in a return of settlers back to their places of origin, in introducing malaria to a large part of the country where there was none hitherto.

• *North-western Andes*

This focus covers the Pacific side of the Andes from the far north of Peru up through Ecuador, Colombia and western Venezuela. It is due to development of low-altitude forest land. The parasites are *P. vivax* with a greater or lesser fraction of *P. falciparum*.

Regions with very low-level disease

In many places where malaria was present at a low level, eradication operations have eliminated it but there remain regions and countries in which a few hundreds or thousands of cases occur each year, often grouped together in microfoci. The parasite is *P. vivax*.

Such foci are still found in China. At Sarawak in Malaysia, in the Philippines, in Java, Bali, southern Sumatra, Sulawesi, and Flores in Indonesia, the prevalence is very low. In the flood plains and deltas of Indochina (the Red River, the Mekong, the Salouen, the Chao Praya and the Irrawaddi), malaria is not a major problem in foci where it is found. Very little malaria is seen in the valley of the Ganges, the Bengali Delta or the south-eastern Deccan in India.

In the Middle East and Iran, imported malaria is far more common than local transmission. In Syria, and Saudi Arabia, there are a few cases although in Iraq, transmission resumed after the Gulf War. The Caucasus, Armenia and Azerbaijan have been re-infested (*see below*). In North Africa, fewer than one hundred cases per annum are reported (in Algeria and Egypt).

In the Americas, only a small number of cases occur in eastern and southern Brazil (i.e. outside of the Amazon). Similarly, there is very little malaria in Argentina or Paraguay.

"Re-emergent" malaria

The term **emerging** is used to describe diseases that appeared (or were identified) only recently, the prototype being AIDS due to infection with the Human Immunodeficiency Virus (HIV). Other emerging etiologic agents include the Ebola and Marburg filoviruses and the arenavirus of Lassa fever.

The media success of the term has led to its being applied to other diseases that have reappeared after a hiatus of some time. This has been the case with malaria when it has returned in places from which it had been eradicated (or had simply regressed) more than twenty years before

A typical case is that of South Korea to which *P. vivax* has returned more than thirty years after its eradication. Now, the focus extends up into North Korea although whether this is due to re-importation or the reactivation of a latent focus in the country (from which no information has been forthcoming since 1945) is uncertain.

The re-emergence of foci in States of the former Soviet Union (Tajikistan, Azerbaijan and Armenia), from which it was believed to have been eradicated by 1979, resulted from the post-independence degradation of health care infrastructure, although some believe that migrations from neighbouring countries (Tajikistan and Afghanistan) and reactivation of very low-level but still endemic disease (Azerbaijan and Armenia) may have played a role in this recrudescence.

War and social unrest tend to disrupt health care structures and can promote the re-emergence of malaria. However in this context, it is worth noting that not one case has been reported in the former Yugoslavia after years of serious strife.

It has been mistakenly stated that the disease has returned to the Plateaux of Madagascar whereas in fact, the disease never completely disappeared from this region. Similarly, in the mountains of East Africa, the "re-emergence" of malaria was simply an increase in the incidence of cases following environmental changes.

It is tempting to make a link between emergence/re-emergence and global warming but to date, there is no concrete evidence pointing to any such link.

The socio-economic impact of malaria

Ever since the beginning of the 20th century, doctors and economists have been trying to assess the socio-economic impact of malaria, usually to justify investment in patient treatment and disease prevention.

When malaria was rampant in temperate zones, the usefulness of recovered swampland and the recovered productivity were the factors most often taken into account. As of 1955, by which time malaria had been eradicated from the temperate countries and its prevalence had been considerably reduced elsewhere (outside of Africa), interest began to be focused on the tropical belt, especially that in sub-Saharan Africa.

Malaria and poverty

Mean annual per capita income in malaria-infested countries (in Africa and the Indian and Indochinese peninsulas) is less than $2,000 (mean = $1,526) per annum; in countries from which malaria is absent or present only at a low level, it is well over this figure (mean = $8,286) (Gallup & Sachs, 2001). Similarly, whereas economic growth between 1980 and 1995 amounted to only 0.4% in the former countries, it was 2.3% in the others. In thirty-one States in the Afrotropical Region, the cumulative lost growth due to malaria between 1980 and 1995 corresponds to 1.3%, i.e. $73,638 million ($185 per capita), corresponding to 10% of income for 1995 (Sachs & Malaney, 2002). Poverty tends to exacerbate transmission by limiting the control options available, and the disease itself entails adverse economic consequences in turn, constituting a vicious cycle. However, there are numerous exceptions to this rule: in Bangladesh, where malaria is negligible in the delta lands, the per capita Gross

Domestic Product (GDP) is only $1,050 $; in Cuba, from which malaria was eradicated in 1963, it is only $1,500.

In any given village of African holoendemic areas, there is no difference in malaria incidence between richer and poorer families, but the richer populations have a better access to medication and insecticide products.

Although it is true that a map describing poverty corresponds with one depicting the incidence of malaria, underlying cause and effect relationships are difficult to untangle. It would be too hasty to conclude that malaria is responsible for poverty across the world.

Cost of prevention and treatment

Personal medical costs

These costs correspond to all that a family has to spend to prevent and treat malaria, including the purchase price of mosquito nets, doctors' fees, the cost of drugs, travel to the hospital and hospital charges, accommodation costs for family members near the hospital, and loss of the spouse's wages. Although drugs are cheap and hospital stays often free of charge, hospital staff—often low-paid if they are paid at all—sometimes require payment by the family.

Medical costs for health care services

These costs can be broken down into three categories:
- cost of malaria drugs and care provided by the health care centre: the presence of resistance can increase the cost of drugs by over ten-fold if combination therapy including an artemisinin derivative has to be administered. In line with the Bamako initiative, the recovery of the hospital costs should help health care services;
- cost of prophylactic drugs (chloroquine) and the intermittent treatment of pregnant women. In certain circumstances, immunologically naive foreigners and immigrants should be considered;
- vector control operations: indoor spraying remains expensive, whichever insecticide is used. Protecting high-risk subjects using treated mosquito nets has been simplified by the development of ways to produce ready-impregnated fabric which remains active throughout the net's lifetime of about five years (precluding the need for re-treatment).

All the costs involved in treatment and prevention will be detailed in the Part on "Malaria Control".

Infant mortality and birth rates

In most socio-economic surveys, the impact—or rather the cost—of the disease is assessed by estimating the sum that the subject could have earned had he or she lived to a certain age (50-60 in Africa). This calculation makes the cost associated with childhood malaria very high.

Conversely, an indirect compensatory effect of infant mortality results in increased birth rates (Galloway *et al.*, 1998) which entails a reduction in per capita income and compromises the monitoring of births, as well as impairing the condition of women and child care (Sachs & Malaney, loc. cit.).

Productivity

In a highly endemic zone of Kenya, malaria is responsible for 11% of absenteeism in primary school, and 4.3% in secondary school (Brooker *et al.*, 2000).

Between 5% and 20% of children who have survived an episode of cerebral malaria suffer neurological sequelae (Brewster *et al.*, 1990; Murphy & Bremen, 2001) and are subsequently incapable of creative work. Asymptomatic malaria has been found to impair cognitive function in Yemeni schoolchildren (Al Serouri *et al.*, 2000).

Finally children of low birth weight (due to maternal infection) do not seem to perform as well at school (McCormick *et al.*, 1992).

The field of the relationship between malaria and psychological development is a very sensitive one in political terms, and is open to controversy.

Financial needs in the next decade

International funding for malaria-related initiatives has been well below $100 million per annum whereas the WHO estimates the costs of treatment and prevention at $2.5 billion in 2007 ($4 billion by 2015). To mobilise international efforts, the WHO created the Roll Back Malaria programme, the goal of which is to halve the burden of malaria by 2010..

However, the situation should improve with two major current initiatives, the Bill & Melinda Gates Foundation and the President's Malaria Initiative (PMI). The Gates Foundation has announced new grant commitments to combat malaria totalling $83.5 million, including a $7.1 million grant to strengthen the southern Africa subregional network of Roll Back Malaria. The PMI announced by President Bush on June 30, 2005 reaches $1.2 billion for a five-year initiative to control malaria in Africa.

Global review of malaria in the year 2000

- Malaria is confined to the tropical and sub-tropical regions (apart from Korea).

- The Afrotropical Region—which contains only 8% of the world's population—accounts for 85-90% of cases of malaria (200-280 million cases, including 90% due to *P. falciparum*) and 90 % of all carriers of *P. falciparum*. Malaria causes about 800,000 deaths per annum according to the most recent estimates.

- The various foci in Asia, Oceania and the Americas, taken together, account for 10% of cases with less than 100,000 deaths even though they cover a surface area comparable to that of the Afrotropical Region.

- Although low-level transmission occurs in very geographically extended areas, the disease there is relatively benign and the number of direct deaths small.

- Malaria and poverty coexist in many tropical regions, especially in Africa, where they both inhibit growth and development.

- The high infant mortality due to malaria is countered by very high fertility which affects women's social status and complicates education.

- The direct costs in terms of care and medications to prevent and treat malaria are very expensive for both private pockets and public funds. Nevertheless, the funds available for malaria control remain far from sufficient and poor countries have to appeal to other countries or the international community.

- WHO estimates that $2.5 billion will be required in 2007, and 4 billion in 2015 to control malaria.

Epidemiological Biogeography of Malaria

Malaria in the Main Biogeographical Regions

Factors which affect the distribution of malaria

Malaria is a vector-transmitted parasitic disease with a cycle that involves three organisms, humans, the parasite and the anopheline vector.

• The **presence of humans** is not a limiting factor since people are found in all parts of the world.

• **Four species of *Plasmodium*** can infect humans and these can thrive wherever permissive vectors are found and the climate is compatible with their sporogonic cycle. The only exception is that *P. vivax* does not develop in those who do not carry the Duffy antigen (Melano-Africans) and is therefore not found in most of the Afrotropical Region. It does however infect Saharan Berbers, semitic Ethiopians from the high plateau region, Malgasy of Indonesian origin, Caucasian minorities and particularly Bushmen, who are the longest-standing occupants of eastern and southern Africa; all of these peoples carry the Duffy antigen and are thus susceptible to *P. vivax*.

• The genus ***Anopheles*** contains about four-hundred eighty species distributed throughout the world. Of these, fifty or so are able to transmit human plasmodia. As with all life forms, each anopheline species occupies a specific geographical area where it colonises a specific type of larval niche at a specific time of the year. Anopheles existed before human beings and adapted to the new host, capturing parasites from it. It is vector diversity that dictates the malarial potential at a given location but human factors may have played an important role with the expansion of *Homo* species.

All the sites in which parasite-vector exchange conditions (i.e. the conditions which govern malarial transmission) are identical can be grouped together into epidemiological units within a given biogeographical region.

With many and various vectors, malaria is characterised by true biodiversity and this is reflected in its epidemiology (Mouchet & Carnevale, 1998).

Major malaria biogeographical regions

Geographers typically speak of seven different biogeographical regions: the Palaearctic, the Oriental, the Oceanian (or Australasian), the Afrotropical (or Ethiopian), the Neotropical (South and Central American), the Nearctic (North American) and the Antarctic. As the last is uninhabited, it is not affected by malaria.

Originally, Macdonald (1957) distinguished twelve malarial geographical regions on the basis of epidemiological and entomological criteria: we have placed these in the framework of the six regions indicated above.

The Nearctic Region and the Neotropical Region have been grouped together in the American Regions. We have chosen a division based on five regions within which various subregions are distinguished according to epidemiological, ecological and climatic characteristics.

In this book, each country is described in a specific section, the length of which is more or less proportional to the amount of research that has been carried out there. How countries are grouped together into larger geographical units depends on local epidemiological patterns. Thus, the Afrotropical and Oriental Regions are subdivided in different ways, the Australasian Region is treated as a single unit, and the extremely vast Palaearctic Region is fragmented.

Afrotropical (or Ethiopian) Region

This region (*Figure 1*) covers the entire African continent south of a line along the 22nd northern parallel that bisects the Sahara. The Tagant Mountains in Mauritania, the Adrar des Iforas Mountains in Mali, the Aïr Mountains in Nigeria and the Tibesti Mountains in Chad are included in the Afrotropical Region but the northern Saharan mountain ranges, Hoggar and Tassili N'adjers in Algeria, and Fezzan in Libya are excluded. This division is not arbitrary but corresponds to the presence of Afrotropical species in the southern mountain ranges of the Sahara, while those of the north harbour a fauna with Mediterranean affinities.

The south-western portion of the Arabian Peninsula (Yemen and the south-eastern portion of Saudi Arabia) is generally included in the Afrotropical Region which is characterised by the presence of *An. arabiensis*. However, for convenience, the Arabian Peninsula as a whole has been included in the Palaearctic Region.

In Africa, the concentric distribution of plants and animals on either side of the equator makes it difficult to identify sub-regional units since the same species (belonging to the *An. gambiae* Complex and the *An. funestus* Group) are found from the Tropic of Cancer to the Tropic of Capricorn, and from the Atlantic Ocean to the Indian Ocean. The unique nature of the flora and fauna of Madagascar and the islands of the Indian Ocean is not reflected in anopheline vectors which—on the basis of genetic analysis—probably arrived there relatively recently. There is thus no need to create a specific subregion, even if the endemic form *An. mascarensis* is a recognised malarial vector. Anopheles arrived in the Madagascan islands quite recently whereas the older population found in the Comoros Islands is of African origin. No *Anopheles* are found in the Seychelles and imported *An. gambiae* failed to become established there.

Australasian (or Oceanian) Region

The flora and fauna of the Pacific islands east of the Wallace line are very different from those of Indonesia and Southeast Asia. Different boundaries have been proposed

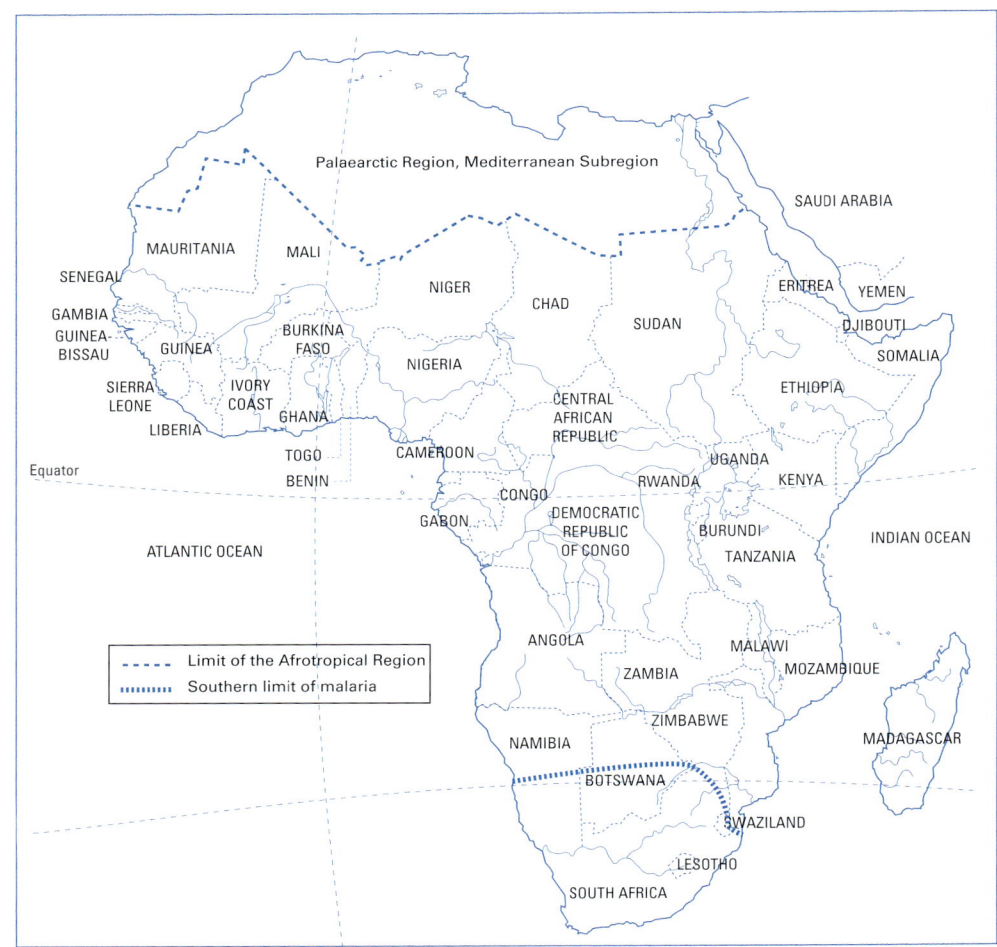

Figure 1.
The Afrotropical Region.

depending on the groups of species under consideration (*see the Chapter on the* "*Australasian Region*"). The boundary is very clear when it comes to anopheles and malaria. The *Anopheles* that characterise the region, namely the *An. punctulatus* Group, extend from the Molucas to Vanuatu, including New Guinea, the Solomon Islands and the north of Australia (*Figure 2*). In this part of the Pacific, only vectors belonging to this group are found. To the east and south of Vanuatu, it is worth pointing to the surprising absence of anopheles in New Caledonia, Fiji, Micronesia, Polynesia and New Zealand. Other anopheline species are present throughout Australia, although they cannot transmit malaria. This "gap" in the distribution of this zoological group is characteristic of the central and eastern Pacific.

Oriental Region

This region can be divided into three highly distinct subregions (*Figure 3*):
- the **Indo-Chinese Subregion** consisting of Vietnam, Laos, Cambodia, Thailand and Myammar as well as the southern Chinese provinces of Yunan, Guangxi and

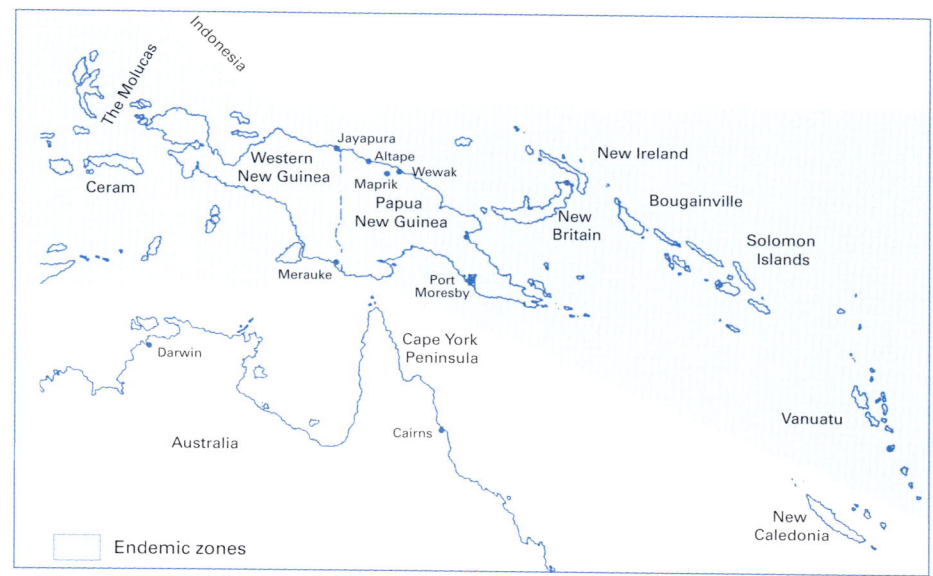

Figure 2.
The Australasian Region.

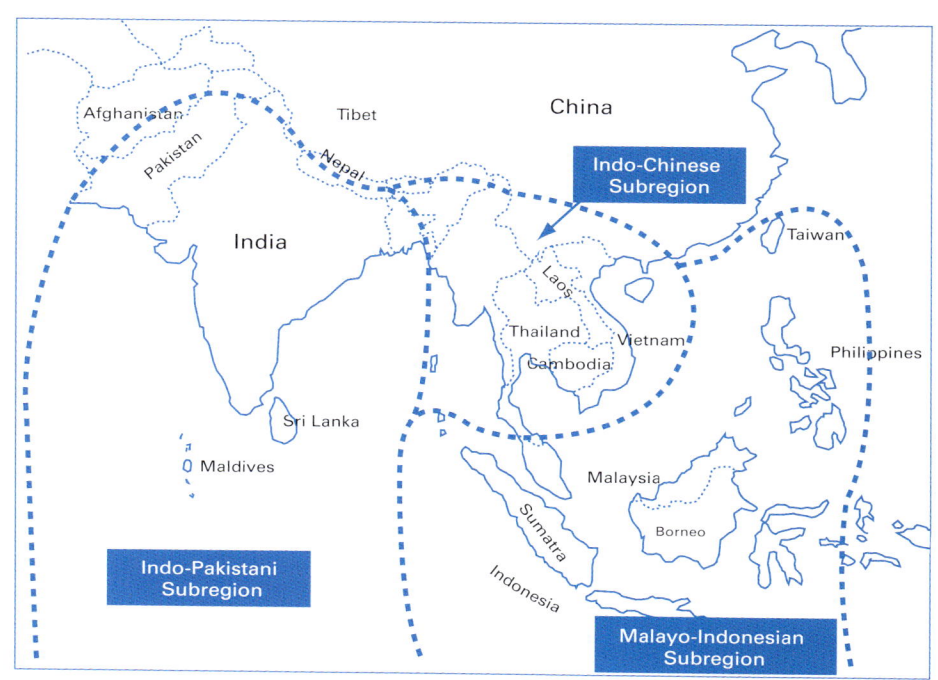

Figure 3.
The Oriental Region.

Hainan, the Ryu-Kyu archipelago in Japan, the States of India to the east of the Brahmaputra, eastern Bangladesh, Nepal and southern Bhutan. The common denominator among these countries is the presence of efficient vector species belonging to the *An. minimus* and *An. dirus* Complexes (which were originally confined to jungle habitats);

- the **Malayo-Indonesian Subregion** includes peninsular Malaysia, the Philippine Islands and the islands of Malaysia and Indonesia (to the west of the Molucas). Several anopheline species with highly variable vectorial capacities have been reported on the various islands and only *An. sundaicus* is consistently found in coastal regions outside the Philippines;
- the **Indo-Pakistani Subregion** extends into the Indian peninsula to the west of the Brahmaputra up to the Hindu Kush mountain range in Afghanistan. The western part of Bangladesh, the island of Sri Lanka and the Maldives archipelago are also included in this subregion. The vectors are *An. stephensi* and species belonging to the *An. culicifacies* and *An. fluviatilis* Complexes. These three species extend beyond the Oriental Region and into the subtropical regions of the Palaearctic Region in Afghanistan, Iran, Iraq and the countries of the southern Arabian Peninsula.

Palaearctic Region

This is the largest of the biogeographical regions. From north to south, it extends from the Arctic Ocean to the deserts of the Sahara and the Himalayan mountain chain. From west to east, it covers most of the land in the northern hemisphere from the Atlantic to the Pacific (*Figure 4*). We have divided this region into four subregions:

- the **Euro-Siberian Subregion** including the **Atlantic-influenced zones of western Europe, the Mediterranean peninsulas** (Iberia, Italy and its islands, and the Balkans), the **continental zones of eastern Europe and Siberia**, and the **countries of the Caucasus**. The vectors are or used to be species of the *An. maculipennis* Complex, namely *An. labranchiae*, *An. sacharovi*, *An. atroparvus*, *An. messae* and *An. superpictus*;
- the **Mediterranean Subregion** with the Maghreb and northern Sahara in Africa, and the regions of the Near East and Turkey in the eastern Mediterranean Region. The vectors are *An. labranchiae* in the west, *An. sacharovi* in the east and *An. sergentii* in the deserts;
- the **Arabo-Iranian** (Arabo-Persian) **Subregion**, with the Arabic Peninsula (except for the Afrotropical part in the south-west), Mesopotamia and the plateaux of western and Central Asia (Iraq, Iran, Afghanistan and the former Soviet republics of Central Asia) as well as western China (Xinjiang Province). This is a transitional subregion which includes Indo-Pakistani vectors in the south (*An. culicifacies*, *An. stephensi*, *An. fluviatilis*) and Palaearctic vectors in the north (*An. sacharovi*, *An. superpictus*). This is why Macdonald (1957) included it in an Indo-Iranian Region;
- the **Chinese Subregion**, including all of China (except for the southern provinces already mentioned and Xinjiang Province), Korea, Japan, Taiwan and the extreme eastern part of Siberia (the coastal province); the vectors are *An. sinensis* throughout the entire subregion and *An. anthropophagus* south of the 35th parallel.

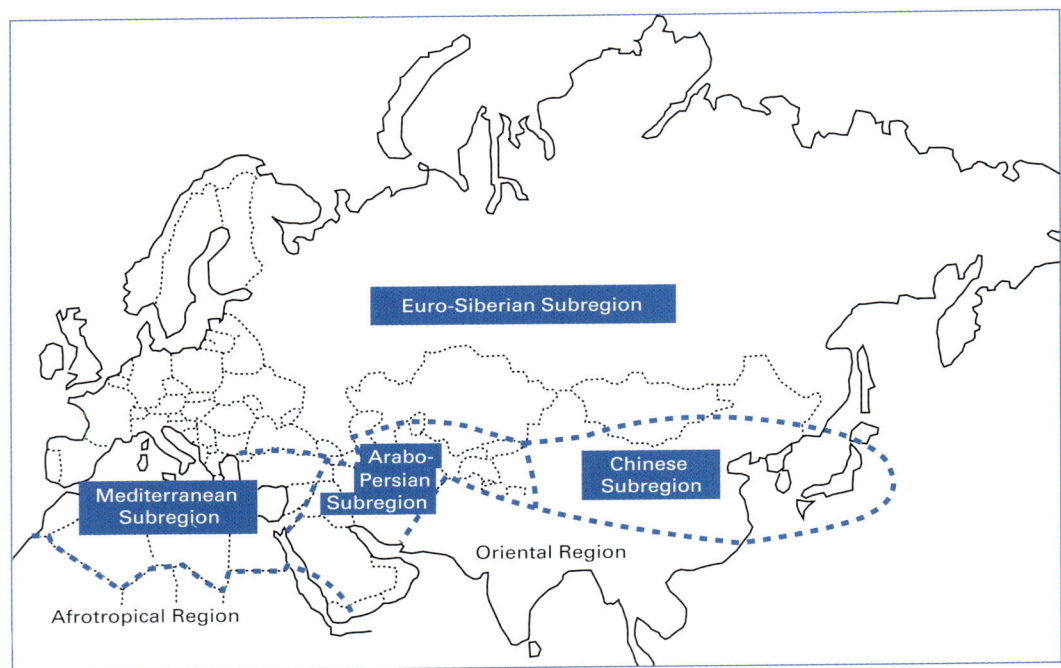

Figure 4. The Palaearctic Region.

Malaria in the Main Biogeographical Regions

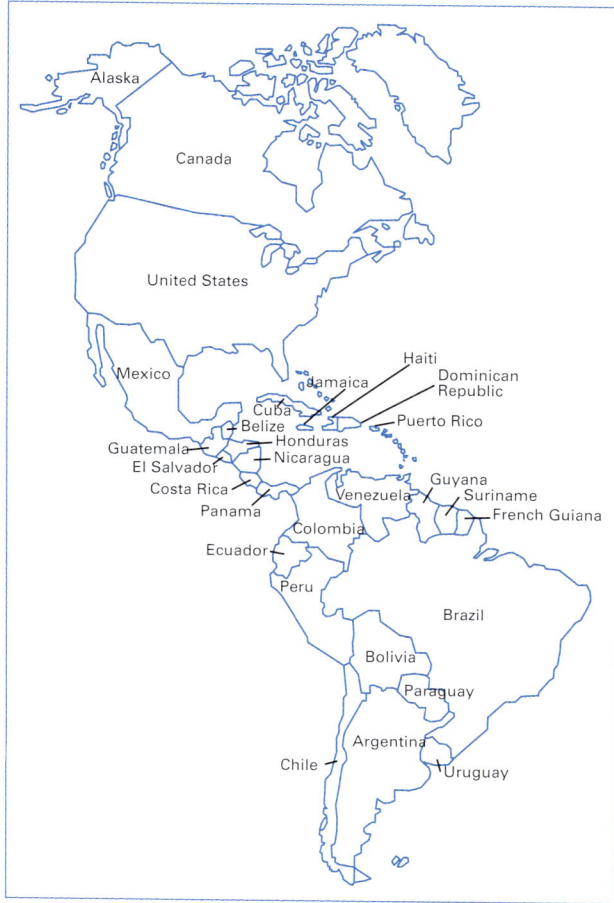

Figure 5. *The American Regions.*

American Regions

In terms of the vectors, the division between the Nearctic and Neotropical Regions is not a very clear one. We propose that the entire American Region be broken down into three subregions (*Figure 5*):
- the **North American Region**: including Canada, the United States and Mexico north of the Tehuantepec Isthmus. As in Europe, the vectors belong to the *An. maculipennis* Complex;
- **Central America and the Caribbean**: including Southern Mexico, all countries of Central America, the Caribbean Islands and the northern parts of Venezuela, Colombia, and Ecuador (the Pacific side of South America to the north and west of the Andes Mountains). *An. albimanus* is characteristic of this subregion, this being one of the two important vectors found on the American continent;
- **South America**: this subregion includes the Andes Regions (where malaria can be transmitted at altitudes of above 2,700 m by *An. pseudopunctipennis*) and the Amazon Region which stretches all the way down to Argentina where *An. darlingi* is the main vector.

Classification of regions

The **Afrotropical Region**, the "cradle of humanity", occupies a special place in the story of malaria. On this continent, malaria is more of an environmental constant than a sickness (Mouchet and Carnevale, 1988). In areas where malaria is endemic, human beings survive only by virtue of their remarkable ability to develop defence mechanisms—which are usually grouped together under the highly imprecise terms of immunity or resistance (Sergent, 1950).

While geographically distant, the epidemiology of the **Australasian Region** is very close to that of the Afrotropical Region with malaria endemic and highly developed resistance seen amongst the indigenous peoples.

The **Oriental Region** stands out due to the contrast between hyper-endemic malarial foci in jungle regions and among minority populations and the low prevalence (or even absence) in the densely populated plains.

The **Palaearctic Region**—the Mediterranean basin in particular—has been ravaged by malaria throughout history. Since the early 19th century however, especially since the arrival of DDT in 1940, malaria has become a historical phenomenon rather than a public health problem in those countries with sufficient resources to protect their populations. Close attention is being paid now to the re-emergence of the disease in Korea, the Caucasus, Turkey and Tajikistan.

In the **Americas**, malaria—at least the form that is caused by *P. falciparum*—is a relatively recent problem, having been imported by slaves brought over from Africa. Just how long *P. vivax* and *P. malariae* have been present is open to debate. A remarkable aspect is the speed with which human plasmodia were "captured" by native anopheles which had never previously encountered the parasite.

In this book, the distribution and impact of malaria is described on the basis of these various regions of the world.

Afrotropical Region

Main characteristics of malaria in the Afrotropical Region

Peoples and countries

The total population of the various countries amounts to almost 600 million people (*Table I*) with more than 500 million living in areas in which malaria is endemic. The majority of Africa is populated by Melano-Africans belonging to a great number of different ethnic groups who have the common trait of not carrying the Duffy antigen and therefore of being resistant to *P. vivax* (*see the Part on* "Malaria, a Vector-Borne Parasitic Disease").

The Pygmies are Melano-African people of small stature who live in and around the great forests.

The Sen who were the first occupants of East and South Africa are now represented by a few relic groups in Tanzania (Hamza), Namibia, Botswana and South Africa (grouped under the name of Bushmen).

Berbers—the Tuareg and the Moors—have been living around the edges of the Sahara desert for as long as Melano-Africans; Yemenites (Semitic people) established themselves on the Abyssinian plateaux around 600 BC; Indonesians began populating Madagascar at the beginning of the Christian era; and the Boers first invaded South Africa in the 17th century: all of these invaders avoided regions where malaria was highly endemic.

Up until the 19th century, Africa developed in isolation, protected from foreign invasion by the omnipresence of stable malaria that deterred the non-immune.

Africans can survive in a highly malarious environment due to their remarkable ability to develop premunition and they also have one of the highest rates of population growth in the world, despite the high infant mortality rate.

Today, the majority of African countries are amongst the poorest in the world and only a few of them are able to afford the costs of a comprehensive and well organised malaria control programme; most need outside assistance on a long term basis.

Geography, elevation, climate, flora and fauna

The African continent arose as a result of the splitting of the continent of Gondwana which, until the Primary Era, included South America, Africa, Madagascar, India, Australia and Antarctica combined. Africa probably continued to drift away from Madagascar throughout the entire Secondary Era, which explains the presence on the island of dinosaur fossils (*Bothriospondylus madagascariensis*) dating from the mid-Jurassic Period to the upper Cretaceous Period. It is estimated that Madagascar definitively separated from Africa 65 to 100 million years ago.

The Rift Valley and the Red Sea originate from the last great tectonic displacements of the Tertiary Era, which shifted a part of Africa towards Arabia at the same time as the Great Lakes were being formed. The large plate (ancient birimian), rich in minerals, rose up along the coast of West Africa, demarcating inland basins such as the Niger-Chad basin in the north (Prehistoric Chad), the Congolese basin in the centre, and the Botswana basin in the south through which flow, respectively, the Shari, the Congo and the Okavango Rivers. The rivers carved out a difficult passage towards the Atlantic (the Niger, the Congo and the Sanaga), and easier ones towards the Indian Ocean (the Zambezi) or the Mediterranean to the north (the Nile). Volcanic changes in East Africa created Mounts Kenya, Kilimanjaro, Elgon, Rwenzori and, more recently in West Africa, Mount Cameroon.

On both sides of the equator, Africa has a symmetrical succession of climatic zones that range from equatorial climates (four seasons) to tropical climates (two seasons, dry and wet) up to the Saharan deserts in the north and down to the Kalahari in the south. This succession of climatic

Table I. Population and surface area of the countries of the Afrotropical Region (according to Wikipedia, 2006).

Country	Size (km²)	Population	Country	Size (km²)	Population
West Africa			**East Africa**		
Benin	112,600	7.6 M	Djibouti	23,200	0.8 M
Burkina Faso	274,200	13.5 M	Eritrea	121,144	4.7 M
Cape Verde	4,000	0.4 M	Ethiopia	1,097,900	73.0 M
Chad	1,284,200	9.2 M	Kenya	582,640	33.8 M
Gambia	11,300	1.5 M	Somalia	637,660	8.2 M
Ghana	238,500	22.0 M	Sudan	2,505,810	40.2 M
Guinea (Rep.)	245,860	9.4 M	Tanzania	945,090	36.8 M
Guinea-Bissau	36,120	1.6 M	Uganda	236,040	27.3 M
Ivory Coast	322,462	17.3 M	**Southern Africa**		
Liberia	111,370	2.9 M			
Mali	1,240,000	11.4 M	Angola	1,246,700	11.8 M
Mauritania	1,030,700	3.0 M	Botswana	600,372	1.8 M
Niger	1,267,000	12.2 M	Lesotho	30,350	2.0 M
Nigeria	923,768	131.5 M	Malawi	118,480	12.7 M
Senegal	196,200	11.7 M	Mozambique	783,080	19.4 M
Sierra Leone	71,746	5.0 M	Namibia	824,790	2.0 M
Togo	56,800	5.4 M	South Africa	1,221,037	46.9 M
			Swaziland	17,360	1.0 M
Central Africa			Zambia	752,610	11.3 M
			Zimbabwe	390,580	12.2 M
Burundi	27,830	7.8 M	**Islands of the Indian Ocean**		
Central African Rep.	622,980	4.0 M			
DR Congo	2 345,409	57.5 M	Comoros	2,170	0.65 M
Equatorial Guinea	28,050	0.5 M	Madagascar	587,040	18.6 M
Gabon	267,670	1.4 M	Mauritius	2,045	1.2 M
Republic of Cameroon	475,440	17.0 M	Mayotte	1,000	0.16 M
Republic of Congo	342,000	3.6 M	Reunion	2,200	0.8 M
Rwanda	26,340	8.6 M	Seychelles	208	0.083 M
São Tomé and Principe	1,000	0.17 M			

zones is very clear in the northern hemisphere while, in East and South Africa, defining latitudes are more dependent on altitude, e.g. the plateaux of Zimbabwe and Zambia are not comparable to those of the Sahel since in the former sub-zero winter temperatures are common above 1,500 m.

The same climatic zones are found in Madagascar with an eastern equatorial coast, a western tropical coast, a Sahel-like dryness in the south, and a plateau with a climate very similar to that of southern Africa.

The flora shows the same north-south stratification as the climate (*Figure 1*):
- equatorial forest (or what is still remaining of it) all along the Gulf of Guinea and in the Central African Massif, i.e. southern Cameroon, Gabon, Congo (Brazzaville), Central African Republic, and central and northern Democratic Republic of Congo all the way to western Uganda (Semliki forest);
- wet savannah in Guinea and then the Sudan, with more than 800–1,000 mm of rainfall during a wet season of six months and more. These are the most populated parts of Africa and millet is the most widespread crop;
- dry savannah (< 500 mm) and the steppes of the Sahel and the Sahara (< 200 mm) used for animal rearing, and finally, the desert (< 100 mm);
- the plateaux of the Southern Cone (Democratic Republic of Congo, Zimbabwe, Zambia, Botswana, Malawi, South Africa) are covered with dry savannah and/or steppe. Large annual variations in rainfall mean massive changes in aspect from one year to the next;
- the plateaux of Madagascar are made up of sparsely covered grassy steppes with rice paddies in any depressions or basins in the landscape;
- the mountainous regions of East Africa—originally covered with high altitude forest—have been for the most part cleared for grazing, banana farming and tea plantations. In the valleys, the papyrus swamps have been replaced with crops.

Biodiversity of Malaria in the World

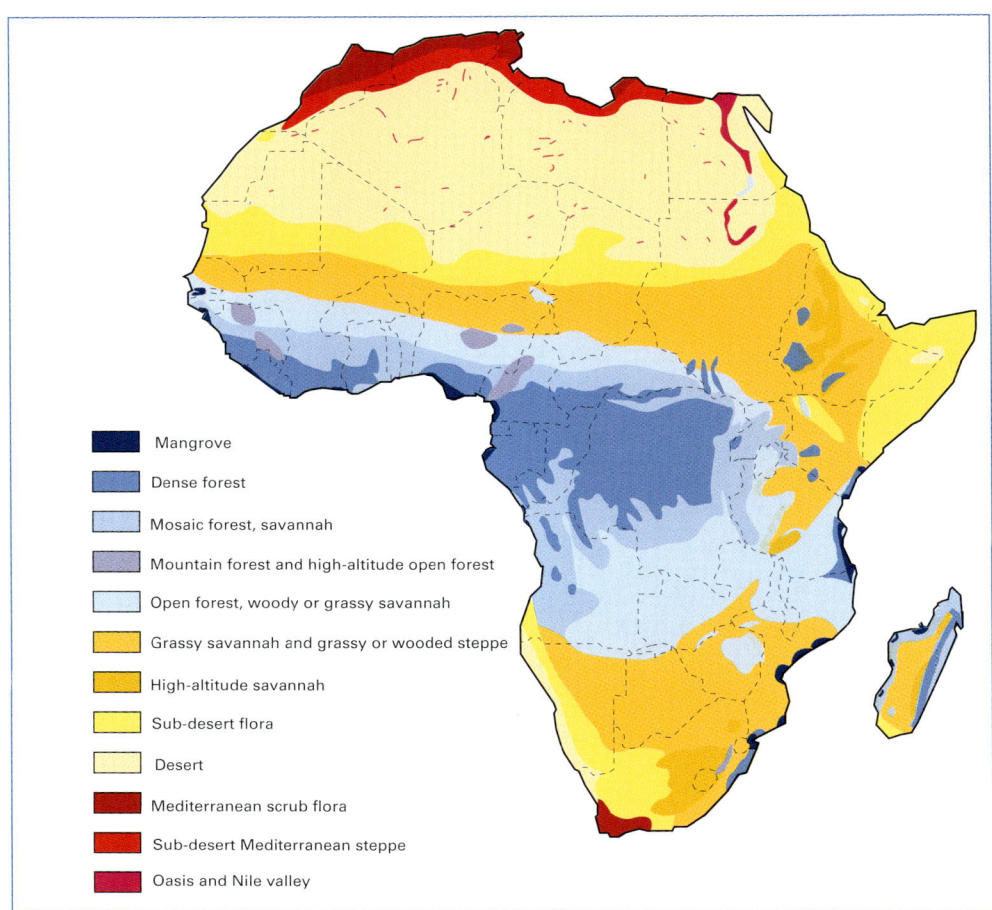

Figure 1.
African vegetation
(adapted from
Mouchet et al., 1993b).

The fauna is quite distinct from those of the other biogeographical regions. The ungulates (elephants, giraffes, rhinoceri, antelopes), formerly found in great numbers, have been massacred by over-hunting and several species survive only in nature reserves. Man has not spared his close relatives either, namely the apes (chimpanzees bonobos, and gorillas) which share a common ancestor with hominids.

The entomological fauna is exceptionally rich, in particular when it comes to the vectors of diseases: tsetse flies which transmit sleeping sickness; *Chrysops* which transmits the filarial worm *Loa loa*; *Simulium* of the *Damnosum* Complex which transmit onchocerciasis; various mosquito species belonging to the genus *Aedes* (*Stegomyia* and *Diceromya*), including the vectors of yellow fever and dengue; *Culex* and *Anopheles* transmit filariasis; the latter one is vector of malaria. Nowhere else in the world is there such a panoply of vectors and nowhere else in the world have parasitic and viral diseases affected the evolution of a continent to such an extent.

On the island of Madagascar, most of the animal and plant species are endemic and were present well before the arrival of man. There are thirteen endemic anopheline species but the majority of vectors, members of the *An. gambiae* Complex and the *An. funestus* Group, reached the island more recently as shown by the close match between the shape of the island and that of the continent (*discussed later*).

Malaria vectors

Only a dozen *Anopheles* species are actual vectors of malaria in the Afrotropical Region (*Table II*), but their efficacy is formidable. They constitute a dense network that covers the entire region with the exception of a few peaks of over 2,000 m in altitude and the extreme southern part of the continent. All inhabitants of the region are exposed to malaria at least during one period of the year and this throughout their entire lives (Mouchet & Carnevale, 1988).

Anopheles gambiae Complex

In current taxonomy, the *An. gambiae* Complex is divided into seven species of which two have larval stages in brackish water and five in freshwater (*Figure 2*).

- Freshwater species:
- *An. gambiae sensu stricto* Giles, 1902,
- *An. arabiensis* Patton, 1905,

Afrotropical Region

Species	Vector efficiency	Distribution
An. gambiae s.s.	+++	Whole region apart from the Horn of Africa
An. arabiensis	++ or +	Whole region - Rare or absent in forest land
An. melas	++	Western coast
An. merus	+	Eastern coast
An. funestus	+++	Whole region
An. nili	+++	South of the 12th parallel
An. moucheti	+++	Central African forest band
An. mascarensis	++	Localised in Madagascar (endemic)
An. paludis	++	Only a vector in Central Africa
An. pharoensis	+	West and East Africa
An. culicifacies	+	Eritrean coast
An. brunnipes	±	Kinshasa
An. hargreavesi	±	Ghana
An. dthali	±	Sudanese coast

Table II. Malaria vectors in the Afrotropical Region.

+++ : highly efficient vectors; ++: efficient vectors, possibly localised; +: secondary vectors; ±: uncertain vectors
Species of the *An. gambiae* Complex which do not transmit malaria are not included on this list

- *An. quadriannulatus* A Theobald, 1911,
- *An. quadriannulatus* B Hunt *et al.*, 1998,
- *An. bwambae* White, 1985;
• Brackish water species:
- *An. melas* Theobald, 1903,
- *An. merus* Donitz, 1902.

Larval habitats for the freshwater species include rainwater pools in sunny spots without vegetation, potholes or footprints, and residual ponds left where streams have dried up. Anthropogenic larval habitats include irrigation ditches, dams and excavated trenches.

Larval habitats for the brackish water species are in full sunshine, including pools left over after spring tides and after the inundation of salt pans during the rainy season (such as the "tales" in Senegal). In South Africa, Mozambique and Madagascar, *An. merus* colonises larval habitats on salt-laden land fairly far from the coastline.

These two brackish water species, which resemble one another, are distinguished from the freshwater species by morphological features: the female palps and the larval pecten.

Only recently has it become possible to differentiate *An. arabiensis* from *An. gambiae s.s.* on the basis of statistical morphometric profiles of adults, the former being slightly larger (Petrarca *et al.*, 1998). In Madagascar, Chauvet (1969) was able to separate these two species on the basis of larval chaetotaxy.

The most reliable methods for identifying the different taxa are cytogenetic analysis of the polytene chromosomes in the salivary glands of the larval stage IV and the nurse cells of the ovarian follicles (stage IIIf) or DNA analysis after amplification by Polymerase Chain Reaction (PCR); the high degree of polymorphism in the Intergenic Spacer (IGS), region between ribosomal DNA (rDNA) genes, makes it possible to differentiate all five of the most widespread species belonging to the *An. gambiae* Complex using multiplex PCR (Scott *et al.*, 1993), a relatively simple method which allows each specimen to be identified individually from a very small sample (e.g. just the legs), frozen, dried, even after years of conservation; one advantage is that specific DNA sequences can be amplified directly from the sample without any preliminary DNA extraction.

Freshwater species breed in sunny rainwater deposits where there is no vegetation, e.g. ruts or footprints and pools left after the draining-off of surface water. Man-made larval habitats include irrigated land, dams, drainage ditches, etc. Brackish water species also prefer sunny larval habitats—pools left by the retraction of marshes or rain-submerged salt fields such as the "tales" in Senegal. In South Africa, Mozambique and Madagascar, *An. merus* breeds in brackish sites far from the coast.

A map detailing the distribution of the different species of the *An. gambiae* Complex has been published recently by Coetzee *et al.* (2000).

Biodiversity of Malaria in the World

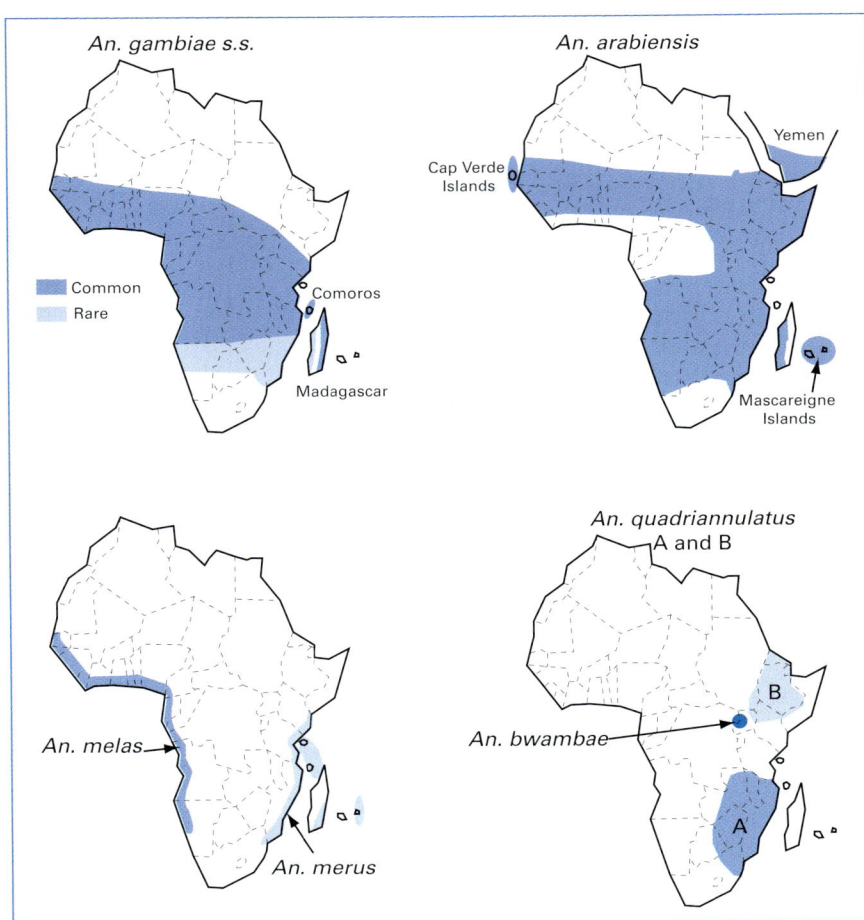

Figure 2. Distribution of species of the An. gambiae Complex.

Anopheles gambiae s.s. *Giles 1902*

In accordance with the polymorphism of chromosomal inversions *An. gambiae* s.s. (= *An. gambiae* A) was divided into five chromosomal forms: "Forest", "Bamako", "Savanna", "Mopti", and "Bissau" (Coluzzi *et al.*, 1985). These chromosomal variants correspond to real ecological markers with the "Mopti" form, adapted to permanent water, the flood zones and rice paddies of West Africa, being associated with low-endemicity malaria on the loop of the Niger; classifying it as a distinct species has even been considered. The "Savanna" form mainly breeds in temporary puddles of water.

Molecular techniques have been developed to identify "Mopti", "Savanna" and "Bamako" forms by Restriction Fragment Length Polymorphism-PCR (RFLP-PCR) of the IGS (Favia *et al.*, 1997) or by PCR of the Internal Transcribed Spacer (ITS) (Favia *et al.*, 2001).

As of 2001, the taxonomy of *An. gambiae* s.s became more complicated with the division of the species into two different molecular forms, namely M and S (Della Torre *et al.*, 2001; Gentile *et al.*, 2001), a classification which is quite independent of that based on the chromosome analysis. In Mali, the "Mopti" forms have an M profile and the "Savanna" and "Bamako" forms have an S profile. In South Cameroon, the "Forest" form was divided into both S and M while only the S form was found in East Africa and Madagascar (Fontenille *et al.*, 2003).

An. gambiae s.s. (*Figures 2 and 3*) is found throughout most of the Afrotropical Region with the exception of the Horn of Africa and the Arabian peninsula (Gillies & Coetzee, 1987). In the Sahel, it is rare above the 500 mm isohyet (Faye *et al.*, 1995b; Julvez *et al.*, 1998) except for the "Mopti" form which penetrates into the Sahara in Mali (Doumbo *et al.*, 1999). To the south of the 15th parallel, it is rare in South Africa, Swaziland, Botswana and Namibia (Coetzee *et al.*, 1993). In Mozambique, it is unusual in the south but dominates in the north (Crook *et al.*, 1994), as well as on the coasts of Tanzania and Kenya.

In all the forest regions of Central and East Africa, the species is almost exclusively represented by the "Forest" form which is also predominant in the wet savannah of West Africa.

On the plateaux of East Africa, southern Congo, Angola and Zambia, both *An. gambiae* s.s. and *An. arabiensis* are found, depending on local ecological characteristics.

On the highlands (up to 1,800-2,000 m) of Kenya (Nandi), Uganda (Kigezi), Rwanda, Burundi, Congo and Tanzania, *An. gambiae s.s* occupies the valleys, particularly where papyrus has been cleared (Mouchet *et al.*, 1998; White, 1972) whereas rice paddies at lower altitudes (900 m) in Burundi (Coosemans, 1985) and Kenya (White, 1972) are occupied by *An. arabiensis*.

An. gambiae s.s. is the dominant species on the eastern and northern coasts of Madagascar; it is less common on the west coast and practically absent from the south and the plateaux (Mouchet *et al.*, 1993a).

In the Comoros as well as in the Atlantic islands of Sao Tomé and Malabo, *An. gambiae s.s.* is the only freshwater species of the complex found.

Trophic preferences vary according to the environment and the hosts available.

In the forest region of Cameroon, the "Forest" form—which is the only one present—feeds on man more than 90% of the time (*Figure 4*). This trophic selection is probably due to an absence of cattle and a scarcity of antelopes in the forest (Livadas *et al.*, 1958). Even though *An. gambiae s.s* is highly attracted to primates, it does not transmit *Plasmodium* between apes as it does not penetrate into the dense forest areas where these animals reside. In big, dense forests, the only natural larval habitats are drying-up river beds (Mouchet, 1962).

In the savannah zones where the "Forest" and "Savanna" forms succeed one another and mix, *An. gambiae s.s.* appears to be increasingly attracted to animals as the density of livestock increases. Some specimens bite both man and livestock indifferently (*Figure 5*), e.g. in Burkina Faso, specimens found feeding on livestock were carrying human sporozoites, direct evidence of their promiscuous feeding habits (Choumara *et al.*, 1959).

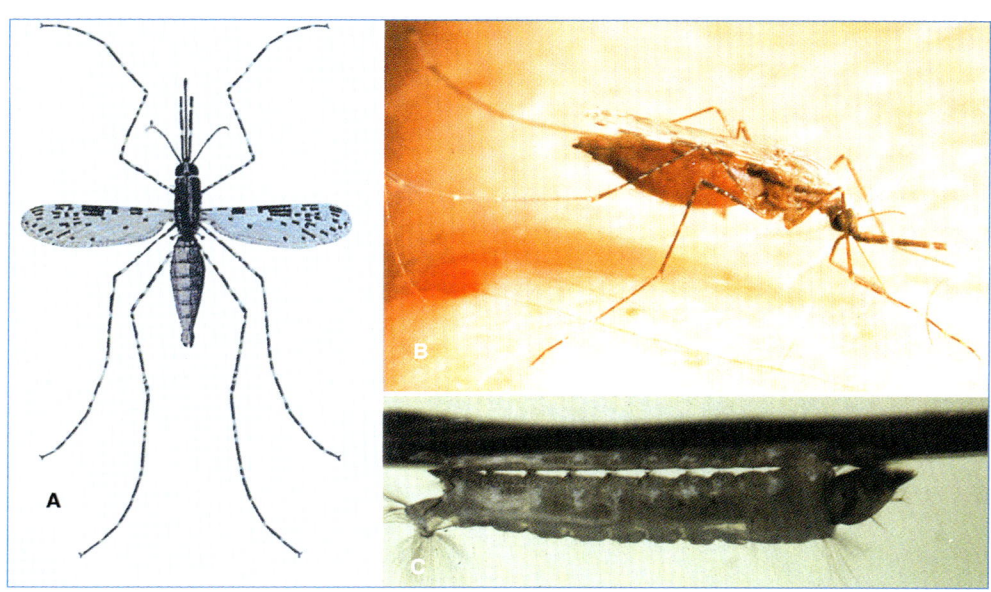

Figure 3.
A. *Female* An. gambiae *s.s. "Forest" form (in Mouchet et al., 1998).*
B. *Female mosquito biting (photograph by Hervy in Danis & Mouchet, 1991).*
C. An. gambiae *larva breathing at the air-water interface (photograph by Hervy in Danis & Mouchet, 1991).*

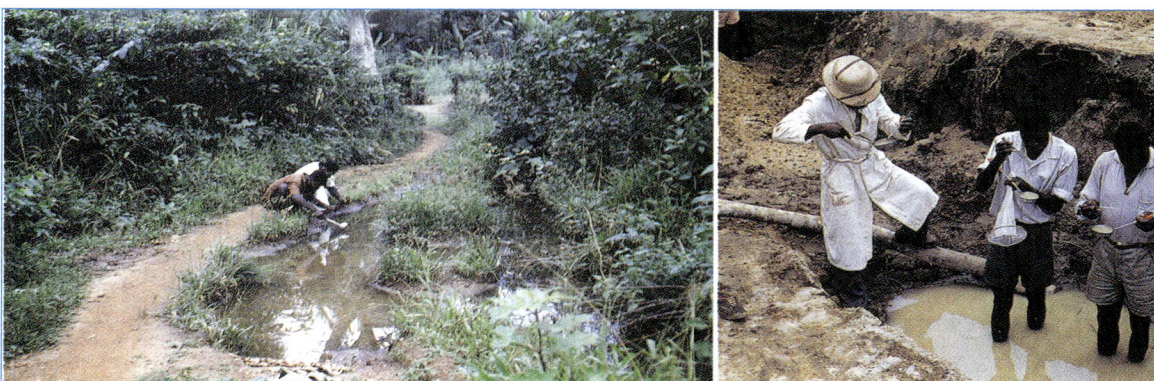

Figure 4. An. gambiae *forest larval habitats (photographs by Mouchet).*

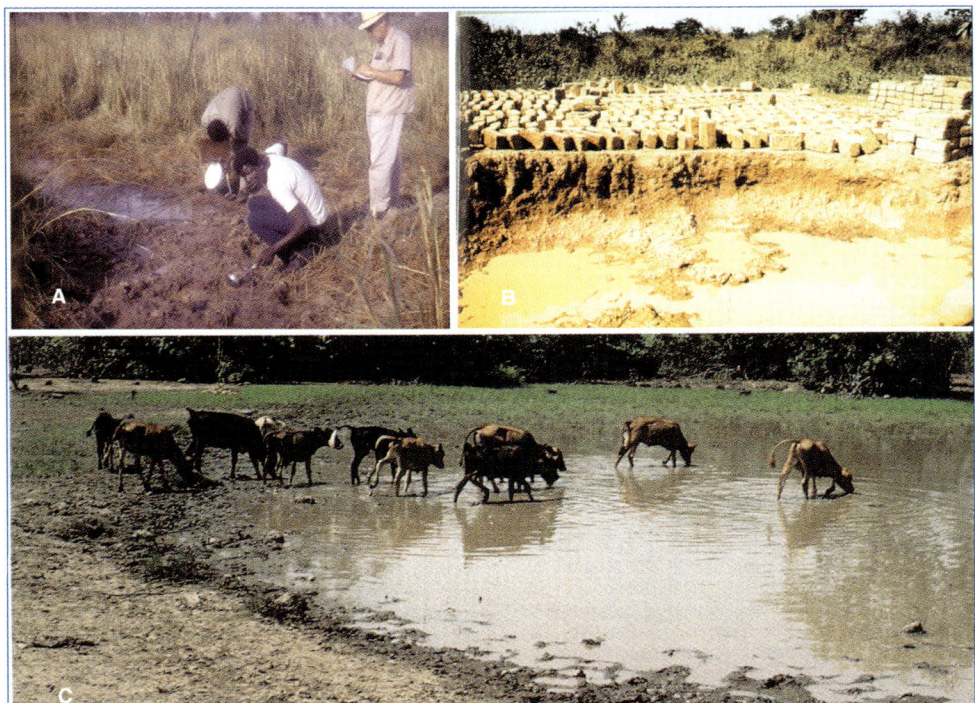

Figure 5.
An. gambiae *savannah larval habitats.*
A. *Footprints in Nigeria*
B. *Brick-making site in Burkina Faso (photograph by Hervy in Danis & Mouchet, 1991).*
C. *Hoof prints close to Bamako (in Touré et al., 1998).*

The endophilic behaviour of *An. gambiae s.s.* is a controversial subject, a controversy which is associated with the existence of different cytotypes. In the forest regions of the eastern coast of Madagascar (Chauvet, 1969) and of southern Cameroon (Mouchet & Gariou, 1957), most of the females left the houses in which they had bitten during the night or the next morning. In the Maroua Region in Cameroon and in Burkina Faso, most stayed at least 24 hours inside the house in which they had fed (Cavalié & Mouchet, 1961; Choumara *et al.*, 1959).

An. gambiae s.s. is considered to be one of the most efficient, if not the most efficient vector in the world with sporozoite rates generally greater than 3%, reaching 10% in Uganda at an altitude of 1,700 m (Mouchet *et al.*, 1998). It should be noted that the "Mopti" form has a sporozoite rate of less than 1% (Robert *et al.*, 1988b) in the rice paddies of Kou Valley in Burkina Faso.

Anopheles arabiensis *Patton 1905*

An. arabiensis (formerly *An. gambiae* B) is found throughout all the savannahs and steppes of the Afrotropical Region (*Figure 2*). In general, it is not found in forests despite its penetration of certain large Nigerian cities such as Benin City (Coluzzi *et al.*, 1979); outside the city (in the forests or bushlands), it is surrounded by *An. gambiae s.s.* It is the only freshwater species of the complex with anthropophilic behaviour in the Horn of Africa and in the south-western part of the Arabic peninsula. In contrast to *An. gambiae s.s.*, *An. arabiensis* has not been divided into genetically distinct forms, e.g. the specimens of Madagascar are not separated from those of East Africa. However, the methods of molecular biology revealed significant polymorphism both within and between the various populations. On a cross-section spanning 4,500 km between Mozambique and Sudan, significant differences were observed in the frequency of genotypes in populations separated by more than 200 km (Donnelly & Townson, 2000). Major genetic disparity was observed between populations of *An. arabiensis* in Senegal and those found in Madagascar, Reunion and Mauritius: in the latter populations, genetic pooling may have resulted from man-mediated migration events (Simard *et al.*, 1999).

The zone covered by *An. arabiensis* and *An. gambiae s.s.* (especially the "Savanna" form) extends over almost all the savannahs of West and East Africa and the Southern Cone. The ratio of *An. arabiensis* to *An. gambiae s.s.* increases with distance from the equator and dense forest. In addition, seasonal variations in the relative frequency of these two species have been observed: in Burkina Faso (Coz, 1973b), the relative proportion of *An. gambiae s.s.* increased during the rainy season and decreased during the dry season.

An. arabiensis is well adapted to the dry climate of the northern Sahel and can be found all the way to the oases of Aïr (Niger). How it manages to survive during dry regions remains an unanswered question although in the northern parts of Nigeria, Cameroon, Niger, and Senegal, small populations were found to be able to survive in favourable sites (springs, permanent ponds, etc.) (Cavalié

& Mouchet, 1961; Hamon *et al.*, 1965). In these regions, genetic studies revealed that anopheline populations continued to survive in the same locations from one year to the next (Taylor *et al.*, 1993; Simard *et al.*, 2000).

Only Omer & Cloudsley-Thompson (1968, 1970) observed females hibernating (or "summering") in inhabited or abandoned houses, burrows, and crevices in Sudan, 20 km to the west of the Nile. Despite numerous investigations, no one else has observed this phenomenon since. However, just 20 km away on the banks of the Nile, *An. arabiensis* was found to be present and active all year round; its larval habitats were residual rainwater pools (Dunkeen & Omer, 1986).

On the other hand, on the edge of the Sahara—where several years can pass without any rainfall at all—we were able to observe *An. arabiensis* in the Tagant in Mauritania, following an absence of two years with the last known permanent larval habitats located 300 km to the south. In Niger in 1990, an outbreak of several hundred cases of malaria occurred at the oasis of Bilma (Develoux *et al.*, 1994) more than 500 km from the closest larval habitat. This epidemic ended spontaneously. Similarly, *An. gambiae s.l.* (*An. arabiensis*) was collected in the oasis of Faya-Largeau in Chad (Rioux *et al.*, 1961) but it seemed to have disappeared from this location by the next year (Saugrain & Taufflieb, 1960). One plausible hypothesis is that *Anopheles* migrates along a south-west/north-west axis with the converging intertropical front. In some years (e.g. 1990), this front actually rises beyond Bilma. It could be that the migrations are caused by monsoon winds at the beginning of the rainy season such as those observed with *Simulium damnosum s.l.* The Tuareg have observed a strong increase in the number of mosquitoes when the front rises and the winds are inverted (Robert, personal communication). It seems unlikely that residual populations can persevere during two or three consecutive years without rain.

An. arabiensis is considered to be much less anthropophilic than *An. gambiae s.s.* In the Sahelo-Sudanese zone, more than 50% of their blood meals were taken from cattle. In Madagascar, its affinity for animals exceeded 90% on the plateaux where it rested in cowsheds (Laventure *et al.*, 1996). In Senegal, however, under identical conditions regarding access to hosts, it attacked man as often as it did livestock (Diatta *et al.*, 1998). There are therefore significant behavioural differences depending on region and environment.

The endophilic behaviour of this species also varies tremendously from one region to the next. On the plateaux of Madagascar (Laventure *et al.*, 1996), it was mostly found in animal shelters. In the Sahel, its behaviour was clearly endophilic. In regions where people sleep outside, such as the north of Senegal (and throughout the Sahel at the end of the dry season), it would take refuge in houses, even in the daytime (Faye *et al.*, 1997). In Burundi in the Imbo, Smits *et al.* (1996) associated endophilic and endophagic behaviour with isozyme frequency of the locus Mdh-2 although the populations of this region were found to be panmictic.

An. arabiensis is generally considered to be a good vector even though its efficiency is intrinsically half that of *An. gambiae s.s.* (Lemasson *et al.*, 1992). Its sporozoite rate, often greater than 1% (Senegalese Sahel), can be much lower: on the plateaux of Madagascar, its behaviour was exophilic and zoophilic, and its sporozoite rate was below 0.5% (Ralisoa Randrianasolo & Coluzzi, 1987); on the eastern coast of the same country, its sporozoite rate was only 0.1% (Coz, personal communication). On the plateau of south-west Kenya around Kisumu, the sporozoite rates of *An. gambiae s.s.* and *An. arabiensis* were almost identical in a place where both species were highly anthropophilic (Joshi *et al.*, 1975). But in the environments where *An. arabiensis* is less anthropophilic in its behaviour (with an average of only 39% of meals taken from humans), and *An gambiae s.s.* is highly anthropophilic (98% of meals taken on humans) the respective sporozoite rates were 0.3% and 5.3% (Highton *et al.*, 1979).

Vector efficiency can be considered to be an intraspecific variable (Coosemans *et al.*, 1992).

Apparently, in natural populations of *An. gambiae s.l.*, no specimens are naturally resistant to *Plasmodium*, at least according to the results of a study conducted in Burkina Faso (Coosemans *et al.*, 1998).

An. arabiensis, when it is the dominant species, is most often associated with unstable malaria in the Southern Cone, the Horn of Africa and the plateaux of Madagascar as well as on the edges of the Sahara; it is in these regions where the most severe epidemics on the continent occur.

Anopheles merus *Dönitz 1902* and Anopheles melas *Theobald 1903*

These two brackish water species have such similar morphological and cytogenetic characteristics that whether or not they represent distinct species remains unresolved.

An. merus occupies the coasts of East Africa from Somalia to South Africa as well as the coastlines of the Comoros, Mauritius, and Madagascar (*Figure 2*). It has been found fairly far inland in South Africa, Swaziland, Zimbabwe and Tanzania as well as in the salt water lakes of the Rift Valley (Coetzee *et al.*, 2000). In southern Madagascar, it was found at high density as far as 50 km inland (Marrama, 1999), but the most important larval sites were located in *Avicennia* mangroves as well as in crab holes in both Mohéli in the Comoros (Blanchy *et al.*, 1987) and Zanzibar. The larvae tolerate freshwater as well and can develop in this environment. It is a proven vector of malaria and of Bancroftian filariasis on the coast of Kenya (Mosha & Petrarca, 1983). Although Pringle (1962) showed that it was receptive to malarial infection on the Tanzanian coast, its sporozoite rate was vanishingly small (compared with the *An. gambiae s.s.* sporozoite rate of 9%) (Muirhead-Thompson, 1951); in Madagascar, of over two hundred samples taken, none collected contained any circumsporozoite protein (Marrama, 1999).

An. melas is found on the west coast and extends all along the Atlantic coastline from the mouth of the Senegal River to Benguela in Angola (*Figure 2*). However, in contrast to its East African "twin", it does not penetrate far inland. The degree of salinity tolerated by the larvae ranges from 5 to 37 g of ClNa/l. It grows in mangrove of *Avicennia* not *Rhizophora*; its development is synchronised with the monthly high tides of great amplitude which leave residual pools of water. Waves of *An. melas* invade local villages every two weeks following the high tides in Gambia (Bryan, 1983; Giglioli, 1964). Along with these almost ideal conditions, rainfall also plays an important role in this mosquito's development. In Senegal, the "tales", or stripped salt plates which fill with water during the rains, also provide excellent larval habitats for *An. melas* (Faye *et al.*, 1994). On the coastline of the Gulf of Guinea where there is heavy rainfall, the rain tends to reduce the salinity of water pools and the relationship between *An. melas* and *An. gambiae s.s.* is greatly disturbed, especially in Cameroon (Mouchet, personal observation) and Benin (Akogbeto, 2000).

The zoophilic behaviour of *An. melas* has often been put forward to explain its low sporozoite rate of 0.3% compared with those of 3% or 4% recorded with freshwater *An. gambiae* in Gambia. In Senegal, in a fishing village with no livestock, the sporozoite rate of *An. melas*, the only species present, was nonetheless 3% whereas in neighbouring villages with livestock where *An. melas* and *An. arabiensis* were breeding side by side, the sporozoite rate of the former was above 1% (Diop *et al.*, 2002). The environment, therefore, greatly affects *An. melas* vector efficiency.

Zoophilic species of the Anopheles gambiae Complex

An. quadriannulatus (Theobald, 1911) was discovered in South Africa when non-anthropophilic *An. gambiae* were persisting in the absence of transmission following DDT indoor spraying. It was believed that a behavioural change had occurred in *An. gambiae* but what had actually taken place was that a different, zoophilic, species of the *An. gambiae* Complex was present. This example shows just how risky it is to talk of behavioural changes in a species, a phenomenon that has never really been proven to occur (*Figure 2*).

An. quadriannulatus B (Hunt *et al.*, 1998) had already been collected in Ethiopia (White, 1980) where it had been mistaken for *An. quadriannulatus A* which has similar behaviour patterns (*Figure 2*).

An. bwambae White 1985 has only been collected in the Semliki forest of Uganda where its larvae develop in thermal springs in the undergrowth; an exception in the Gambiae Complex which is generally attracted to sunlight. This, therefore, explains the presence of *An. gambiae* in buffalo footprints found in forests as reported by Haddow *et al.* (1951) (*Figure 2*).

Anopheles funestus Group

An. funestus has a wide spatial distribution throughout the Afrotropical Region (*Figure 6*) and it is one of the major vectors of human *Plasmodium* on the continent. It belongs to the Funestus Group with species difficult to differentiate on the basis of larval or adult morphological criteria alone (Gillies & Coetzee, 1987; Gillies & de Meillon, 1968) Recent studies showed that the Funestus Group includes five subgroups, two with species from Africa and three from Asia, except *An. leesoni*, an Afrotropical species closely related to *An. minimus* C from Asia that both belong to the Minimus Subgroup (Garros *et al*, 2005; Harbach, 2004). The subgroups with species from Africa are the Funestus Subgroup with *An. aruni, An. confusus, An. funestus, An. parensis* and *An. vaneedeni*; and the Rivulorum Subgroup with *An. brucei, An. fuscivenosus, An. rivulorum* and *An. rivulorum-like* sp. (Garros *et al.*, 2005).

Given the important biological differences between the various species belonging to the Funestus Group, especially their vectorial capacities, accurate identification of its various members is necessary if effective and selective vector control measures are to be implemented. The broad spatial distribution of *An. funestus*—a highly efficient vector—means that it is often found in the same place as other members of the group which are all zoophilic. On the other hand, *An. rivulorum* was found to act as a secondary vector in Tanzania (Wilkes *et al.*, 1996) and *An. vaneedeni* has been successfully infected in the laboratory but does not seem to transmit malaria in natural conditions.

An. funestus itself has never been split even though ecological and behavioural disparities lead us to suspect it

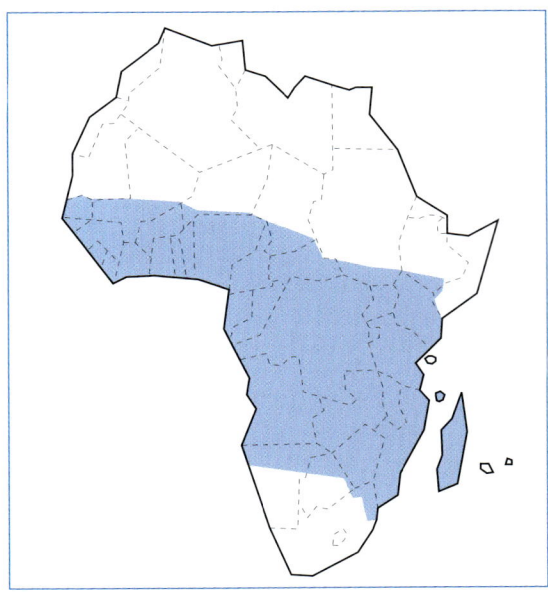

Figure 6. Distribution of An. funestus.

of constituting a species complex. In Senegal along a west-east cline, its anthropophilic and endophilic behaviour perceptibly diminishes (Diatta *et al.*, 1998; Lochouarn *et al.*, 1998) and the degree of polymorphism of inversions is following the same trend (Dia *et al.*, 2000). However, the results of analyses of the cytochrome b gene of the mitochondrial DNA and ribosomal DNA markers are not consistent with the idea that the chromosomal taxa in Senegal are reproductively isolated (Mukabayire *et al.*, 1999).

The ecological differences are no less troubling. In South Africa on the Drakensberg slopes, *An. funestus* used to develop in streams of running water (de Meillon, 1933, 1934) but in 1951, it disappeared from this type of larval habitat when indoor insecticide spraying became common. Its ecology appeared to be different on the plains or plateaux with larval habitats in ponds or swamps left over after rainfall in areas where the vegetation is high and dense.

It should be noted that *An. funestus* has tenaciously persisted in the rice paddies on the plateaux of Madagascar (*Figure 7*) (Laventure *et al.*, 1996), whereas this species scarcely ever breeds in the rice fields of the West African savannah (Robert *et al.*, 1988b). In Ivory Coast, *An. funestus* meets with *An. gambiae* in the villages in the rice producing region of Danané but its presence in the paddies need to be checked as it could also be breeding in the surrounding swamps (Dossou Yovo, personal communication).

In savannah areas *An. funestus* is found in great numbers at the end of the rainy season and the beginning of the dry season where it may be said to prolong the action of *An. gambiae* even though this scenario is not always exact.

An. funestus is found throughout practically all of tropical Africa except for the very dry areas in the northern, southern, and eastern parts of the continent. However, in the great forests, it is highly localised.

In the Sahel, its coverage has shrunk by more than 100 km southwards in Senegal and in Niger (Faye *et al.*, 1995a; Julvez *et al.*, 1997b; Mouchet *et al.*, 1996). In the Niayes of Senegal, where it used to be dominant, the drop occurred in two phases: poor rainfall in 1973 led to the absence of larval habitats and, in addition, the low humidity resulted in the sites being degraded. During the following years, even when the level of rainfall had risen, larval habitats were not recreated because there was no longer any vegetation. This situation lasted until 2000 when the Senegal River valley was developed, leading to the restoration of *An. funestus* larval habitats in newly irrigated farms (Konaté *et al.*, 2001). The regression of *An. funestus* is a phenomenon that has occurred throughout West Africa during dry periods.

An. funestus was previously common in South Africa, Zimbabwe and Swaziland but it was eliminated by indoor spraying. Under pressure from environmentalists, DDT was replaced with pyrethroid-based insecticides (Hargreaves *et al.*, 2000) and resistance to this group of compounds became established. *An. funestus* then re-invaded its territories in the Southern Cone, radiating out from Mozambique where it had never been eliminated. Resistance caused epidemic conditions in these parts of the Southern Cone and DDT was used again to stop it, together with Artemisinin Combination Therapy (ACT).

In mountainous regions of Uganda (Lake Bunyani), Ethiopia, Kenya, Rwanda, and Burundi, *An. funestus* colonises the valleys up to an altitude of 2,000 m (Mouchet *et al.*, 1998).

In the western mountains of Cameroon, it occupied the bottom of the valleys from where it spread to the houses on the surrounding hills (Mouchet & Gariou, 1960); SRs in children were found to be inversely proportional to the distance from the larval habitat, up to 300 m (in elevated areas).

An. funestus is considered to be as efficient a malaria vector as *An. gambiae s.s.* sporozoite rates of over 1% have been observed throughout its area of distribution. *An. funestus* can be associated with either stable or unstable malaria, depending on the local epidemiological context. On the plateaux of Madagascar, it is the main vector in the unstable zones. In West Africa, it is associated (together with *An. gambiae s.s.*) with stable malaria.

Being highly endophilic, *An. funestus* was particularly susceptible to indoor spraying programmes. In Madagascar, it was practically eliminated from villages on the plateaux; treatment stopped in 1960 but the vector's reappearance in 1985-1988 was followed by a highly lethal epidemic. It was also eradicated from South Cameroon, Pare-Taveta in Tanzania, Mauritius (Dowling, 1953) and Mayotte (Julvez & Mouchet, 1998). But in the wet savannah of West Africa—in Cameroon (Cavalié & Mouchet, 1961), Burkina Faso (Choumara *et al.*, 1959) and Nigeria (Bruce-Chwatt

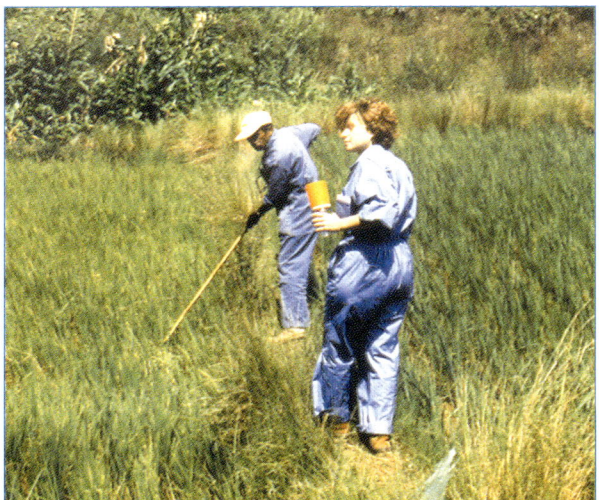

Figure 7. An. funestus *larval habitat (Ankazobe, Madagascar) (photograph by Mouchet).*

& Archibald, 1958)—it was never eliminated, perhaps due to its ability to feed on animals as well as humans. In every country in Africa, it is important to be aware of the status of *An. funestus*.

Anopheles nili Theobald 1904 Group

An. nili (Theobald 1904) (*Figure 8*) belongs to a group of species that includes *An. carnevalei* (Brunhes *et al.*, 1999) and *An. ovengensis* (Kengne *et al.*, 2003).

An. somalicus has been reported in Somalia and Cameroon, the larvae are easily distinguished by their very short clypeal setae (Mouchet & Gariou, 1961); its biology and its epidemiological role are unknown.

An. nili s.l. is distributed throughout all of tropical Africa from the Sudanese savannah as far as Natal in South Africa. It has not been reported in dry regions where streams only flow for short periods (Gillies & de Meillon, 1968); in Burundi, it is found at altitudes of up to 1,000 m (Vermylen, 1967).

Up until recently, no distinction was made between the various different members of the Nili Complex; most of the observations made in the Congo (Brazzaville) (Carnevale, 1974) and in Cameroon (Carnevale *et al.*, 1992a) referred to *An. nili s.s.* The larvae live in small, calm eddies at the edge of the current of fast-flowing streams (*Figure 9*). These larval habitats are very similar to those of *An. minimus* in the Indochinese peninsula. The adults, which are highly anthropophilic in the forest of Cameroon, have a more eclectic diet in the Sudanese savannah. Although endophagous, *An. nili* tends to be exophilic and, after feeding, most females leave the house the same evening (Carnevale *et al.*, 1992a).

In villages in the southern parts of Cameroon and Congo, the species persists year-round whereas on the savannah, it is seasonal (depending as it does on the presence of flowing water) (Choumara *et al.*, 1959).

An. nili is a highly efficient vector of malaria with sporozoite rates greater than 1% in Cameroon (Carnevale *et al.*, 1992; Livadas *et al.*, 1958), Congo (Carnevale *et al.*, 1974), Burkina Faso (Choumara *et al.*, 1959), and the lower parts of Ethiopia (Krafsur, 1970). Gillies & de Meillon (1968) compiled a list of s values.

Anopheles moucheti Evans 1925 Complex

An. moucheti is the natural vector of malaria in the great forest of Central Africa, from Nigeria to Uganda and from the Central African Republic to the Democratic Republic of Congo. The surface area of this habitat is being encroached upon by human activities—farming, timbering (for exotic woods)—but *An. moucheti* continues to survive in gallery forest salients which can be at some distance from the forest itself (*Figure 10*).

The larval habitats are in slow-moving rivers of all sizes, in riverbeds which are often full of floating vegetation (*Pistia*, water hyacinth). In the large rivers, eddies downstream from islands are particularly productive sites.

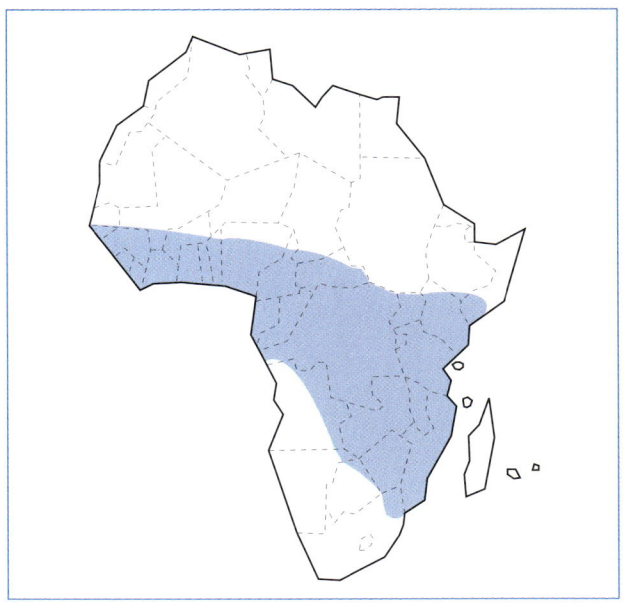

Figure 8. Distribution of An. nili.

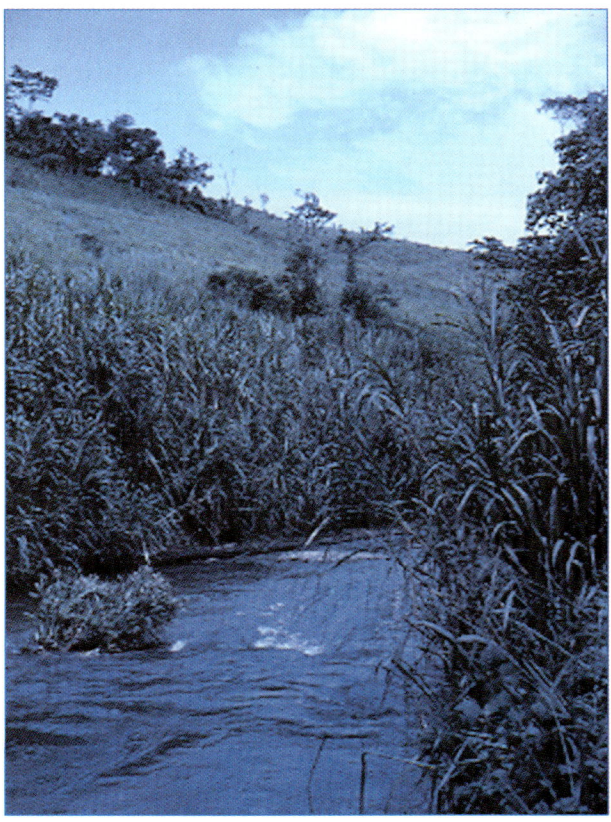

Figure 9. An. nili *larval habitat in the Congo (photograph by Carnevale).*

Afrotropical Region

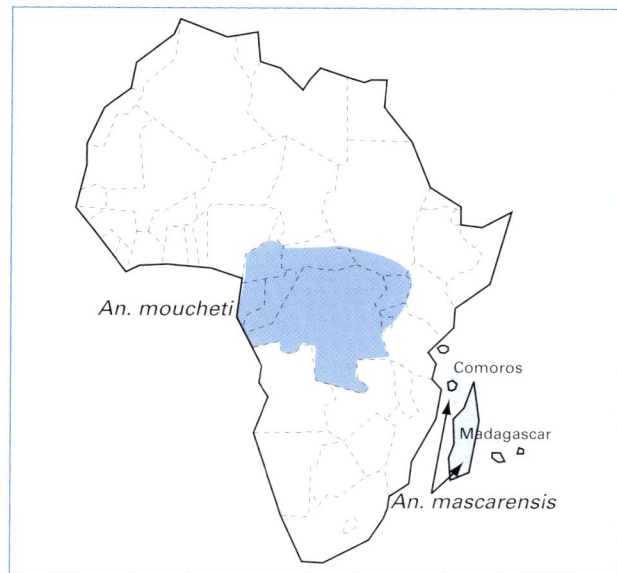

Figure 10. Distribution of An. moucheti and An. mascarensis.

It would seem that a certain amount of incident sunlight is needed on the larval habitats.

The adults are very anthropophilic in their behaviour, a trend reinforced by the absence of livestock in the forest. They are also highly endophilic (Mouchet & Gariou, 1966), staying inside the houses in riverside villages. They can travel up to 3 km between the village and the place where they lay their eggs, which extends their gonotrophic cycle to four days (Njan Nloga et al., 1993a and b). Daily life expectancy is generally greater than 0.9 and peak numbers are reached about two weeks after the river level stabilises or just begins to drop. The density of anophelines in the riverside villages is generally high—at least one hundred per home.

An. moucheti plays as important a role in the transmission of malaria in the forest as *An. gambiae s.s.* and in many riverside villages it is the dominant species. Its sporozoite rate generally varies from 1% to 3% (higher indices have been recorded). It is definitely not a secondary vector: it is a main vector albeit a localised one. Due to its anthropophilic and endophilic behaviour it can easily be controlled by Insecticide Treated Nets or Indoor Residual Spraying.

The *An. moucheti bervoesti* form found in the Democratic Republic of Congo is an independent taxon with a poorly defined role.

Localised species and secondary vectors

An. paludis Theobald 1900 is a forest species that occupies the entire wet equatorial and tropical region of Africa. It is generally exophilic and bites humans in the undergrowth of the great forest, even in the middle of the day (Mouchet & Gariou, 1961). In the northern part of the Congo basin, *An. paludis* behaves differently: it is both endophilic and anthropophilic, and has sporozoite rates of above 1% (Karch & Mouchet, 1992). This was first observed in the early 1960's by Jacob (personal communication) and it suggests that this represents a different form or even another species, quite distinct from the *An. paludis* described in the literature.

An. mascarensis de Meillon 1947 is the only endemic species of Madagascar involved in the transmission of malaria (*Figure 10*) today. Its vector role, discovered on Ile de Sainte-Marie off the east coast of the main island (Fontenille & Campbell, 1992), was confirmed by Marrama (1999) in the surrounding areas of Tolanaro (Fort-Dauphin), in the extreme south-eastern part of the country. *An. mascarensis* was the most abundant species and presented a sporozoite rate of about 1%. The behavioural differences observed in this species in the different regions of Madagascar strongly suggest the existence of a *An. mascarensis* Complex on the island.

An. pharoensis Theobald 1901 has been divided into at least two species (Miles et al., 1983). The form (or species) found in East and South Africa is zoophilic and does not act as a vector. The Sahelo-Sudanese form that covers an area extending from the Atlantic Coast to the Valley of the Nile and to the Middle East displays mixed, opportunistic behaviour. It is found in high numbers in developed rice paddies in Burkina Faso (Kou Valley) and in the Senegal River Delta, it can tolerate a chloride concentration of 0.5-5 g/l. It can fly great distances, e.g. the 70 km between the Nile Delta and the Israeli coast (Saliternik, 1960). Several infected specimens of this anopheline have been found in the halophylic rice-producing borders of the Senegal River Delta (Carrara et al., 1990), in Sudan and in Tanzania.

An. culicifacies, species A, is found in the Horn of Africa in Eritrea, all along the shores of the Red Sea, where it was described under the name of *An. adenensis* by de Meillon (1947). It is a well characterised vector in Asia and the Arabic peninsula but nothing is known about its role in Africa.

Other species have been observed in the Arabian part of the Afrotropical Region such as *An. fluviatilis, An. stephensi,* and *An. sergentii* (Glick, 1992). They will be addressed later on in the Chapter on the "Palaearctic Region".

Infection has also been described in various other species, notably *An. coustani, An. chrystii,* and *An. flavicosta.* These seem to have been isolated events and whether the parasite came from a human being and the quality of the dissections are debatable. In any case, they are of no epidemiological significance.

An. brunnipes Theobald 1910 was confirmed as a vector for the first time in Kinshasa (Coene, 1993) with a sporozoite rate of 0.53%, even though it rarely bites man. It had been reported infected by Lips (personal communication, 1955). Very old reports from Douala based on pre-1955 Cameroon Health Department records have never been confirmed.

An. dthali was commonly found in Djibouti and infected specimens were found in Sudan on the coastline of the Red Sea but its role has not been confirmed (Gillies & de Meillon, 1968).

An. hargreavesi Evans 1927 has been found in Nigeria (Bruce-Chwatt, 1951) and Cameroon. In Ghana, it has been proposed as a possible vector (Vincke, personal communication).

Parasites

All four human *Plasmodium* species are found in the Afrotropical Region, with prevalences which vary enormously from country to country.

Plasmodium falciparum

The most widespread species by far is *P. falciparum* which accounts for 80%-95% of infections and is the main cause of the high level of malarial infant mortality in the Afrotropical Region. Local people show immunological reactions that translate into protective immunity or premunition—and the earlier and more regularly children are bitten, the stronger the immunity. This immunity is acquired at the price of high rates of infant mortality, primarily affecting children between the ages of 6 months and 5 years or between 6 months and 2 years in some areas, seldom older. Because of this protection, most carriers of parasites remain asymptomatic (*see the Chapter on* "Man Facing Malaria").

According to WHO, of the 600 million inhabitants of tropical Africa, 350 to 400 million are carriers of parasites, symptomatic or asymptomatic. Man acts as an enormous reservoir for *P. falciparum* and in stable malaria zones, everyone is infected throughout the year.

P. falciparum is genetically highly heterogeneous. Even in dry regions where transmission only occurs for two or three months of the year, several clones can co-exist in the same subject (*see the Chapter on* "*Plasmodium* Life Cycles in Humans and Anopheline Vectors").

Plasmodium vivax

Melano-Africans who do not carry the Duffy antigen are naturally resistant to *P. vivax* (*see the Chapter on* "Man Facing Malaria"). Hence, this parasite is found in only a few ethnic groups.

The Bushmen or Sen are the oldest inhabitants of East Africa. They only amount to 50,000 in number and are confined to the Kalahari Desert apart from a few tiny groups in Tanzania (Hamza). They possess the Duffy antigen and can become infected with *P. vivax*.

On the plateaux in Ethiopia, a population survey revealed a ratio of 60% *P. falciparum* to 40% *P. vivax*. The latter species was particularly highly represented in populations of Semitic origin. But in Melano-African populations originating in the Nile Region, *P. vivax* was not present (Mathews & Armstrong, 1981). In Somalia (Border Meeting, WHO, 1990), the level of *P. vivax* was established as being at between 1 and 2%.

In Madagascar before eradication, on the plateaux where populations of both African and Indonesian origins live together, Joncour (1956) observed equal prevalences of *P. vivax* and *P. falciparum*, especially among people of Indonesian origin (Merina, Betsileo). Following eradication, the percentage of *P. falciparum* was greater than 90%. In the coastal regions and the south, the percentage of *P. vivax* was lower. In the Androy (the southern part of the island), seven out of twelve infected *An. funestus* salivary glands contained *P. falciparum* while the other five contained *P. vivax*; however, the number of *P. vivax* carriers amounted to just a few per cent (Marrama, 1999). These apparently contradictory observations have not yet been explained to this day.

The Berber populations of the Sahara, the Moors and the Tuareg, are normally susceptible to *P. vivax* but the number of cases remains small. At Niamey University Hospital in Niger, not a single case of *P. vivax* was detected in ten years (Develoux, personal communication).

In Gabon, atypical forms of *P. vivax* have been observed, e.g. with several trophozoites infecting a single red cell (Poiriez *et al.*, 1991). In Central Africa where many different races live side by side, not all the members of the community are non-Duffy antigen carriers and these people are therefore susceptible to *P. vivax* infection. These observations require confirmation but in any case, the number of *P. vivax* cases reported does not exceed 1%.

Plasmodium malariae

This parasite is found throughout the entire Afrotropical Region but its prevalence varies enormously—from 2-45%. In general, it is at its highest prevalence in forest regions. *P. malariae* is almost always associated with *P. falciparum* and infections with only the former are rare.

In mixed infections with *P. malariae* and *P. falciparum*, the former parasite is generally found at much lower density than the latter one, and can even go unnoticed knowing that it is not always easy to identify it in thick smear analysis. Its transmission is weakened by the long time needed for its sporogonic cycle.

Plasmodium ovale

For a long time, this parasite was considered to be rare. In the forest region of Cameroon, its prevalence reached 2% in 1955 (Languillon *et al.*, 1955). Since then, *P. ovale* has been reported at frequencies of between 1 and 5% throughout Africa, with the highest densities in wetter areas.

The presence of this parasite is often transient from one blood sample to the next, and in semi-immune Africans, it often goes unnoticed as it induces hardly any symptoms.

Haemoglobinopathies

This subject is addressed in the "Man Facing Malaria" Chapter.

The S allele of the sickle cell disease is carried by a high percentage of Melano-Africans in West and Central Africa with the exception of the Mandingues of Guinea and Mali and their "relatives", the Samo of Burkina Faso and the Kru of Ivory Coast. In these groups, S haemoglobin is replaced by C haemoglobin which is neither pathogenic, nor protective.

Various different haemoglobinopathies are due to changes in the α chain of haemoglobin. In Congo, almost 50% of the inhabitants are carriers of such mutations (Lallemant *et al.*, 1986) but we understand little about them, neither their roles in pathogenesis nor their relationships with malaria which is still discussed.

Epidemiological strata

Epidemiological facies and strata

Malaria classification systems based on spleen rate or parasite prevalence (*see the Chapter on* "Epidemiological Basis") do not give an accurate picture of the disease in regions where more than 90% of subjects are asymptomatic. Moreover in Africa, the idea of reduction of the spleen rate or the parasitaemia—a criterion reserved for holoendemicity—is valid for hyperendemic and even mesoendemic areas.

Several authors (Carnevale *et al.*, 1984; Mouchet *et al.*, 1993b) have classified Afrotropical malaria according to epidemiological facies by adopting Boyd's classification system (1949) which is based on the dynamics of transmission. An epidemiological facies is a set of places in which the conditions for transmission, the stability of the disease, parasitic prevalence, and the incidence of clinical cases are similar. We have thus been able to group these facies into epidemiological strata that are more or less concentric around the great forest areas of Central and East Africa. These strata correspond to natural boundaries since it is climate, vegetation and the local anopheline fauna that affect transmission and, therefore, determine the parasite prevalence and the incidence of the disease (*Figure 11*).

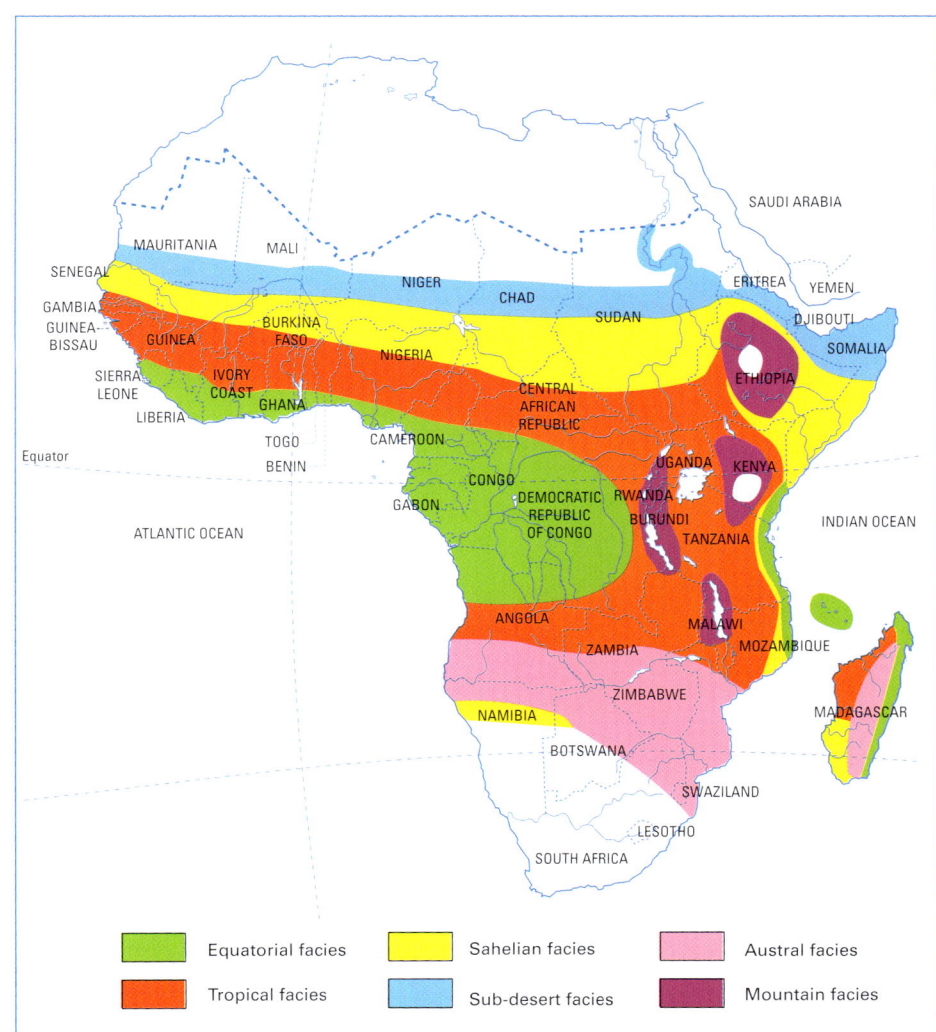

Figure 11.
Epidemiological facies in the Afrotropical Region (adapted from Mouchet et al., 1993).

The Afrotropical Region can be divided into six major strata: Equatorial, Tropical, Sahelian, Sub-desert, Southern, and Mountainous. Onto these primary facies, it is necessary to superimpose local features (relief, rivers, lagoons, soil-type) and anthropogenic factors (irrigation systems, deforestation and urbanisation).

Equatorial stratum

The Equatorial stratum covers the forests and adjacent savannahs of Central and East Africa, from Uganda all the way to Sierra Leone. There are two rainy seasons and two dry seasons each year although no month is really dry (except in Congo where there is a southern winter microclimate of foggy, cool weather) (*Figure 12*).

The main vector is *An. gambiae s.s.* ("Forest" form) which develops in natural or man-made clearings, and in deforested regions with a forest climate. *An. moucheti* inhabits the banks of slow-flowing rivers in the Central African Massif, and *An. nili* is found around fast-flowing rivers. *An. funestus* is limited to parts that have been deforested.

Transmission takes place on a permanent basis with as many as 1,000 infective bites per person per year (ib/p/yr) around Brazzaville in the Congo (Carnevale, 1979). In the Mayombe Region of the same country, the number of bites varied between 80 and 397 ib/p/yr (Richard *et al.*, 1988a), and on the Tanzanian coast, the figure is 35 (Davidson & Draper, 1953; Davidson, 1955). The population is thus being re-infected all year round. The average number of disease episodes per child per year is over 1.5 (Miller, 1958).

The annual incidence of malaria cases in Mayombe was identical between villages where people had close to 400 ib/p/yr and those where people had only 80 ib/p/yr. However, the incidence recorded by clinics was greater during the rainy season (9.6%) when transmission was more efficient than during the dry season (3.6%) (Richard *et al.*, 1988c). Malaria was responsible for 30% of episodes of fever in children.

In a population where more than 80% of the children are carrying the parasite, the detection of *P. falciparum* does not necessarily mean that a feverish attack is due to malaria. It is assumed that the parasite load has to reach a pyrogenic threshold before a fever can be attributed to malaria; in the Congo, this threshold has been estimated at 20,000 parasites per microlitre in babies, although in adults, it is only 5,000 (Richard *et al.*, 1988b).

Most serious malaria attacks take place before 5 years of age and particularly between the ages of 6 months and 2 years. A protective response develops progressively until the age of 10 years by which time the number of attacks decreases although parasite loads do not really begin to drop before the age of 15.

In rural areas of the Congo, serious attacks (cerebral malaria) were observed to be relatively rare. Richard *et al.* (1988c) did not observe one single case in Mayombe in a population of 5,000 people and Guillo du Bodan (1982) observed only two serious cases in a population of 500 children that had been followed for five years. In the Paediatric Department of Brazzaville University Hospital, only twenty cases of pernicious malaria were seen in two years. In Brazzaville, the urban malarial mortality rate for children was thirty times lower than the average for Africa (Trape *et al.*, 1987a). It is difficult to believe that this low mortality rate is due simply to the availability of chloroquine (self-treatment) and it would seem that malarial mortality is lower in places where transmission is ever-

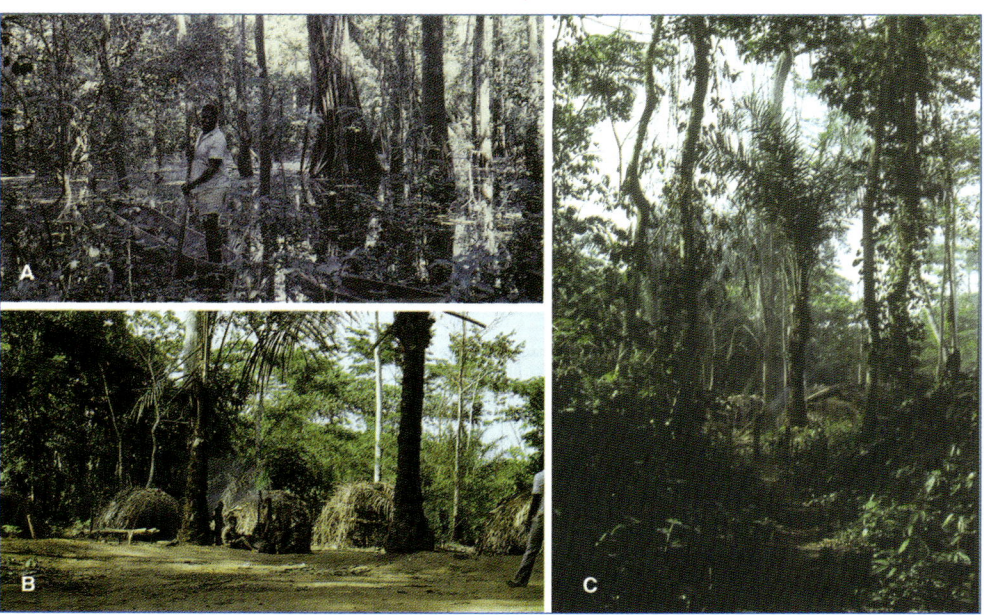

Figure 12.
A. *Flooded forest in Cameroon, vector-free (photograph by Mouchet).*
B. *Pygmies' dwellings at the edge of the great forest, few vectors in the interior (photograph by Mouchet).*
C. *Forest being cleared: An. gambiae larval habitats (photograph by Mouchet).*

present than in the tropical stratum. This is a subject itself that warrants detailed investigation (*see the Chapter on* "Man Facing Malaria").

Equatorial conditions are also prevalent on the coasts of Kenya, Tanzania and Mozambique (north of the Beira). Also included in this stratum is the eastern and northern coast of Madagascar, as well as the Comoros and, in the Atlantic Ocean, Sao Tomé-et-Principé and Malabo.

Tropical stratum

The Tropical stratum extends out to the north, east and south of the Equatorial stratum. In West Africa and to the south of the Democratic Republic of Congo, the two rainy seasons merge into one which alternates with a true dry season lasting at least six months. To the east of the Democratic Republic of Congo, in Kenya, Tanzania and to the north of Mozambique, the four-season climate extends as far as the Indian Ocean but the contrast between the dry and rainy seasons is greater in highlands.

The main vectors are *An. gambiae s.s.*, *An. arabiensis* and *An. funestus*; *An. nili* has a very limited presence. Within the large area of sympatry, the proportion of *An. arabiensis* decreases from north to south towards the equator and *vice versa* in the southern hemisphere. Moreover, the proportion of *An. gambiae s.s.* increases during the rainy season. This variation in the balance between the two species has been observed in Senegal (Faye *et al.*, 1995b), Burkina Faso (Coz, 1973b) and Kenya (Joshi *et al.*, 1975; Service *et al.*, 1978). It is of note that *An. gambiae s.s.* is not found in the tropical regions of the Horn of Africa and is relatively rare in southern Sudan. On the western coast of Madagascar, *An. arabiensis* is the most common species of the *An. gambiae* Complex. In Mauritius and Reunion, it is the only species currently found (Julvez & Mouchet, 1998). The sporozoite rates of all three species are generally over 1% except on the west coast of Madagascar where that of *An. arabiensis* is very low. Malaria is stable throughout the entire stratum despite the fact that transmission is seasonal; this is because it continues for a large part of the year (over 6 months) and is regular. The number of ib/p/yr varies between 100 to 400 in Burkina Faso (Robert *et al.*, 1988), as well as in Nigeria (Molineaux & Gramiccia, 1980); the number of ib/p/yr in Senegal is 200 (Konaté, 1991) and in Gambella, western Ethiopia, it is 97 (Krafsur, 1971).

The annual number of infective bites per person is about the same in this stratum as in the equatorial stratum but these bites all take place during one season as opposed to being spread out throughout the year. The prevalence of malaria in children varies from 30% in the dry season to 80% during the rainy season (Cavalie & Mouchet, 1961; Choumara *et al.*, 1959; Gazin *et al.*, 1985a; Wernsdorfer & Wernsdorfer, 1967). As in the preceding stratum, it decreases progressively in children after the age of 15.

The morbidity rate of malaria is comparable to the rate observed in the equatorial zone. In Burkina Faso, 44% of fevers in children between the ages of 2 and 9 were due to malaria as opposed to only 7% in adults. All the serious malaria attacks observed in the rural clinics of this country involved children of under 4 (Gazin *et al.*, 1988c). The seasonal nature of the transmission means that disease episodes are concentrated (88%) around the end of the rainy season and the beginning of the dry season (Baudon *et al.*, 1985). The average annual number of cases was estimated to be between 0.5 and 3 per child under the age of 5, but these figures are considered to be just a rough estimate given the problems associated with diagnosis.

The mortality rate in this stratum seems very high compared to the rate in the equatorial zone (Gramiccia & Hempel, 1972; Molineaux, 1997a; Najera & Hempel, 1996).

The pyrogenic threshold used to define an episode of malaria was 10,000 parasites per µl in Burkina Faso (Baudon *et al.*, 1988). Most deaths occurred in children under 4 with some degree of premunition being established by the age of 10, even though malarial attacks were still common up till the age of 15.

Sahelian and Sub-desert strata

The Sahelian and Sub-desert strata are addressed together. Annual rainfall drops to 500 mm in the southern Sahel and to just 0.1 mm in the Sahara. The wet season lasts for no more than six months, more commonly less than three. These strata are characterised by sparse vegetation that gets poorer moving northwards. The distribution of vectors follows the same trend. Moreover, the droughts that have ravaged the Sahelo-Saharan Regions since 1970 have profoundly modified the anopheline fauna and the epidemiology of malaria (*Figure 13*).

The Sahelo-Saharan and Sub-desert Region extends from 13° to 20° north at the level of Senegal, from 7° to 16° at the level of the Central African Republic and Sudan, and terminates at the Abyssinian plateau. In East Africa and in the Horn of Africa, this region covers Eritrea, Somalia, southern Ethiopia and northern and north-eastern Kenya.

In the southern hemisphere, the counterpart to this region does not exist due to the altitude and resulting climate differences.

Only *An. arabiensis* and, in some areas, *An. gambiae s.s.* (particularly the "Mopti" form) are involved in the transmission of malaria in the Sahelo-Saharan Region. In the Horn of Africa, *An. arabiensis* is the only vector of the Gambiae Complex. *An. funestus* was considered to be an active vector but its density has considerably diminished and recent information is lacking.

In these regions, there is a problem of parasite maintenance without transmission during a dry season of more than eight months. Even at the end of a long dry season, carriers of gametocytes (and even of erythrocytic forms) are common (Gazin *et al.*, 1988a). Several different genotypes of *P. falciparum* can be found successively in the same subject in Sudan (Arnot, 1998; Theander, 1998).

Vector maintenance during the dry season as well as their sporadic appearance in certain oases were addressed above.

Biodiversity of Malaria in the World

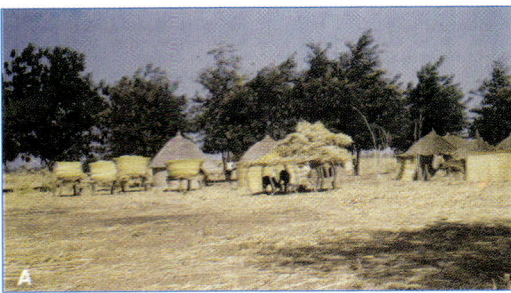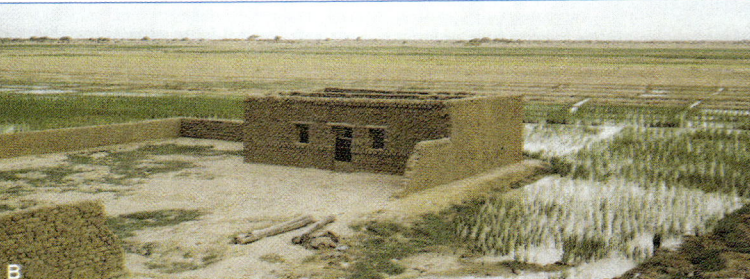

Figure 13. **A**. *Sahelian village in the dry season (photograph by Mouchet).*
B. *Irrigated rice paddies at Diré, Mali (in* Touré *et al., 1998).*

In the Sahel strip, malaria is intermediately stable. Further north on the edge of the Sahara and in the Horn of Africa, it is unstable.

To the north of Burkina Faso in 1965, the anopheline sporozoite rate was low (less than 1%). The number of ib/p/yr was 21 in Dori (Hamon *et al.*, 1965). The parasitic prevalence in children under the age of 5 was 69% during the rainy season and 24% during the dry season; in adults, the corresponding prevalences were 24% and 2%. Despite the small number of infective bites, the decrease of the parasitaemia in adults suggests good immunity. This pattern becomes less marked moving towards the north, ultimately disappearing completely in the semi-desert regions. However, in northern Sudan, adults were observed to be more resistant to epidemic malaria than children (Theander, 1998) as their immune responses were more developed.

The drought that ravaged the region, beginning in 1973 and reaching a second peak in 1983 drastically changed the picture of Sahelian malaria. The scarcity (and often the disappearance) of *An. funestus* coupled with a drop in the numbers of *An. arabiensis* cut transmission down. In the Ferlo in Senegal, only two to four ib/p/yr were recorded (Vercryusse, 1985) and in the Niayes of Senegal, vector density was too low for the number of bites per person per year to be measured. Parasitic prevalence in children dropped from 50% in 1968 to 8% in 1992 (Fayes *et al.*, 1995a) and the number of cases followed a similar pattern. In Niger, Niamey and Zinder, both prevalence and the number of cases likewise dropped (Julvez *et al.*, 1997a and 1997b). The return of *An. funestus* in irrigated fields along the Senegal River is carefully monitored (Konaté *et al.*, 2001).

The climate on the coastline of the Red Sea in Eritrea and the Indian Ocean in Somalia is a sub-desert one. Malaria, which is rare and localised on the coast of the Red Sea, is very unstable in the rest of the lowlands of the Horn of Africa. It is an epidemic zone in which the rivers coming from the Abyssinian plateau (Juba, Uebi Shebelli) are subject to destructive floods which lead to lethal outbreaks of malaria like those of 1998.

The return of *An. arabiensis* and malaria to Djibouti in 1975 (Carteron *et al.*, 1978), after an absence of sixty years, is a remarkable phenomenon that is addressed later on. It warrants investigation on a regional scale, in particular in Berbera (Somalia) where there was not any malaria.

In very dry regions, vectors can survive in bodies of water such as lakes and rivers, especially when the waters recede during the dry season. On the Nile, *An. arabiensis* has been found all the way up to 21° parallel north at the mouth of Lake Nasser (Nasr, 1972). The same is true along the Chari where the zone of transmission during the dry season extended all the way up to Lake Chad (Mouchet, personal observation). The Oursi swamp in Burkina Faso represented a permanent focus of transmission (Gazin *et al.* 1988a), and the same is true of smaller permanent ponds around Zinder (Julvez *et al.*, 1997b). On the other hand, along the Niger River from Tillabery to Niamey in the Niger Republic, the flood waters arising from far upstream in July and precede the rainy season of the following year arising (Baudon *et al.*, 1986a; Julvez *et al.*, 1997a).

In the Sahel, the average temperature rose by 0.5°C between 1982 and 1992 (Fofana & Touré, 1994). Not only did this rise not provoke any increase in the incidence of malaria, it actually caused a decrease as the drought reduced the number and productivity of larval habitats.

Yemen belongs to the same epidemiological stratum and though it is a part of the Afrotropical Region, we will address it in the chapter on the Palaearctic Region, Arabic Peninsula.

Southern stratum

The vegetation zones that cover the Southern Cone of Africa are not homologous to the Sahelo-Saharan strata, despite the fact that the climate gradually changes from the southern Congo and Angolan plateaux up to the Kalahari Desert. This stratum is made up of plateaux that are 1,000 to 2,000 m high, crossed by the valleys of the Zambezi and the Limpopo, and rising from a 100-kilometre wide coastal plain extending along the shores of the Indian Ocean to Mozambique and to Kwazulu-Natal; the plains on the Atlantic side are very narrow. In the middle of these plateaux in Botswana is a huge basin where the Okavango River (which rises in Angola) disappears. Due to the altitude, the climate is cool in winter and in Zambia, Zimbabwe and South Africa, winter frosts are common. It snows in the Drakensberg Mountains in South Africa and in the mountains of Swaziland.

The boundaries of this stratum are ill-defined in the southern parts of Angola and Congo, and Zambia. Apart from the latter, the boundaries include southern Mozambique, Zimbabwe, the northern and eastern parts of South Africa (east of Transvaal and north of Natal) and eastern Swaziland, as well as the northern parts of Namibia and Botswana. To the south of this boundary, there is no malaria in the central and southern parts of Namibia, southern Botswana, most of South Africa or Lesotho. The stratum of the plateaux of Madagascar is very similar to the Southern stratum.

The plateaux are rich in mineral resources, notably gold, diamonds, copper and lead, which has made it possible in several countries—in particular Zimbabwe, South Africa and Swaziland—to carry out highly efficient malarial control campaigns that have changed the profile of malaria in the region. The same was true in Madagascar from 1950 to 1970.

Essentially, there are two vectors, *An. arabiensis* and *An. funestus*. In Mozambique, *An. gambiae s.s.* is the dominant species in the north up until Beira, part of the Tropical stratum, while in the southern part of the country, *An. arabiensis* is dominant or the only vector (Crook *et al.*, 1994). Elsewhere in the Southern Cone, the presence of *An. gambiae s.s.* is unusual at the moment.

An. funestus became very rare after the malaria control campaigns, and almost disappeared from Zimbabwe, South Africa, Swaziland and the plateaux of Madagascar although it is still abundant in Mozambique. After resistance to pyrethroid-based insecticides appeared (Hargreaves *et al.*, 2000), this species came back in abundance to South Africa where the malaria control campaigns restarted using organophosphates and DDT. It seems that the forms currently found in Kwazulu-Natal are different from those observed at the foot of the Drakensberg Mountains by de Meillon (1934) (*see above*). In Madagascar, after eradication operations ceased, *An. funestus* reinvaded the Plateau Region provoking the epidemics of 1985-1988 (Mouchet *et al.*, 1997).

Following Leeson (1931), Zimbabwe was stratified into three altitude zones which shift from one year to the next according to temperature and rainfall, which are key determinants of seasonal outbreaks. Not all experts subscribe to the hypothesis that the intermediate zone is reinvaded on an annual basis (Muirhead-Thomson, 1960). In Madagascar, where conditions are fairly similar to those in Zimbabwe, *An. arabiensis* and *An. funestus* both survive year round (Mouchet *et al.*, 1998).

Malaria in the Southern Cone is unstable, marked by epidemics following periods of drought. A combination of such unpredictable climatic events with the El Niño Southern Oscillation (ENSO) is discussed later on (*see the Part* on "Spatiotemporal Dynamics of Malaria").

Mountainous strata

The Mountainous strata (*Figure 14*) are considered to include regions between 1,400 and 2,200 m in altitude: in these, malaria tends to be concentrated in the valleys.

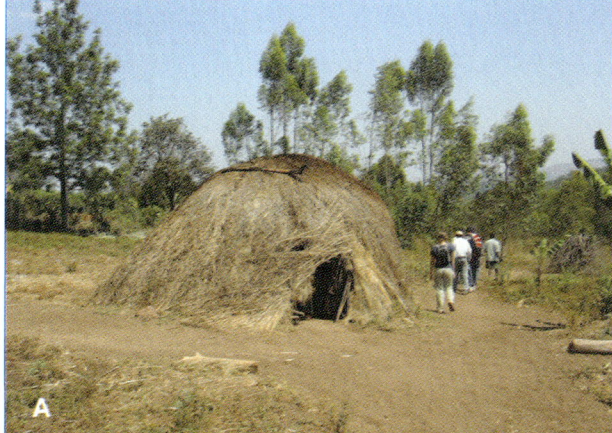
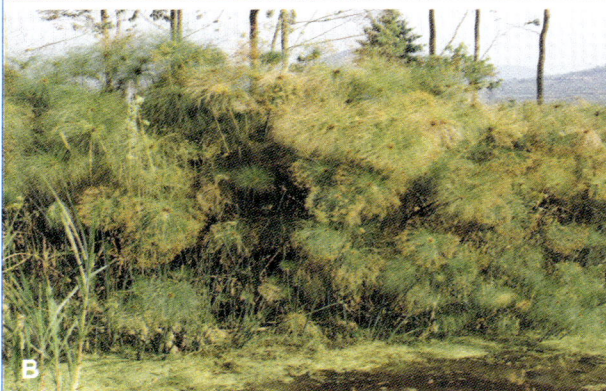
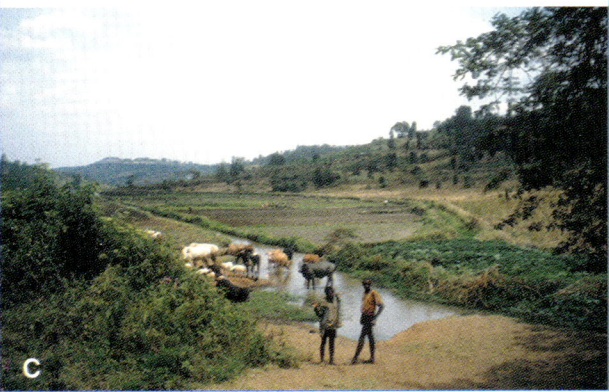

Figure 14. **A.** *Burundi: makeshift dwelling in a zone subject to epidemic malaria (photograph by Coosemans).* **B.** *Papyrus swamp (larva-free) (photograph by Mouchet).* **C.** *Rwanda: excavated water deposit (*An. gambiae s.s. *present) (photograph by Coosemans).*

Distinction is made between the Ethiopian Massif and the massifs of East Africa even though they have many characteristics in common.

In Madagascar, anophelines which are limited to 1,500 m do not really encroach upon the Mountainous stratum. In West Africa, the Nimba Mountains in Guinea and the mountains of West Cameroon (up to 4,000 m) are not affected and belong respectively to the Tropical and Equatorial strata of which they constitute special local facies.

In Kenya and in Uganda, epidemics at altitudes of 2,000 m and higher have been reported since the beginning of the century (Garnham, 1945), e.g. in Nairobi during wet and hot summers.

In Ethiopia, where 17 million people live above the endemic zone, deadly epidemics have been observed, e.g. in 1958 when 3 million cases and 150,000 deaths were recorded (Fontaine *et al.*, 1961). In 1992, an epidemic which lasted until 2000 was declared in Zwai in the Rift Valley at an altitude of 1,800 m. It affected more than 90,000 people and 700 deaths were documented (Desta Alamerew, personal communication). It could have been caused by weak malaria control practices, following political upheavals. A similar event occurred over a large part of Tigray in the northern part of the country.

Stable endemic foci, due to *An. funestus* breeding in reed beds (Zulueta *et al.*, 1964), have been observed at 1,900 m in Uganda around Lake Bunyoni. This environment is very different from the papyrus swamps in the valleys.

In the mountains, the temperature inside houses can be 3 to 5° C higher than that outside which allows the sporogonic cycle to proceed below an ambient temperature of 18° C (Meyus *et al.*, 1963).

In response to the alarmist predictions of Haines *et al.* (1993), Almendares *et al.* (1993) and Dobson & Carter (1993), several experts have attempted to verify whether global warming is causing an increased incidence of malaria. At present, malaria—even epidemics thereof—is not occurring at altitudes higher than those observed at the beginning of the century (Garnham, 1945; Schwetz, 1942). On the other hand, a definite, steady increase in the incidence of the disease has been documented over the last twenty-five years. According to statistics from the Kisizi Hospital in Uganda, the number of cases has increased twenty-fold in 30 years. In Rwanda, the incidence went from 35‰ in 1975 to 180‰ in 1988 (Malaria Control Department of Rwanda); malaria accounted for 42% of infectious disease pathology. Some of this increase may be due to chloroquine resistance but not all of it: in a village near Addis Abeba at an altitude of 1,800 m, Tula (1993) noted a strong increase in the prevalence of malaria over the last decade. It is too soon to conclude that the increase of malaria is a result of global warming. In these mountain regions where the population is exploding (increasing by more than 3% every year), the development of agricultural activity is a key factor. Beginning in 1946, Jadin, first with Herman and later with Fain (1951), observed an increase in malaria incidence in newly exploited valleys; before development, most of the valley bottoms had been covered with papyrus which is an unfavourable habitat for mosquito larvae because the plant secretes an essential oil which forms a film over the water surface and prevents larval development (McCrae, 1975). Once such areas had been cleared, *Anopheles* could survive and develop. In Uganda during the epidemic of 1994, most of the cases originated from newly constructed villages on cleared agricultural land. The vectors were riverbank-dependent *An. gambiae* s.s. and *An. funestus* (with the former having a sporozoite rate of 10%) (Mouchet *et al.*, 1998; White, 1972). But on the plateau of Kisumu in Kenya as in Burundi (Coosemans, 1985), at altitudes of under 1,200 m (i.e. below the Mountainous strata), *An. arabiensis* was the only vector found. Amongst the factors that govern the distribution of the two species of the *An. gambiae* Complex in mountains, rainfall is probably a key factor. Epidemic mechanisms are addressed later on.

In addition, the migration of workers returning from endemic zones may skew the statistics. As the infectious event took place in areas outside the villages where they live, local transmission is not involved (Van der Stuyft *et al.*, 1993).

Epidemics which ravaged populations of gold diggers working at night in Kanugu, Uganda, constitute an example of occupational infection.

In the mountains of south-western Uganda, *Anopheles* numbers peak in June-July (i.e. autumn); this time of year often marks the beginning of malaria outbreaks and epidemics.

Malaria in the mountains varies enormously **from one region to the next** depending on the type of **relief**, **vegetation** and **crops**, and any attempt to generalise should be undertaken with care. But this topic provides an excellent opportunity to study the relationship between climate, local topography and epidemiology.

Local and anthropogenic facies

The term secondary local facies refers to natural or anthropogenic factors that affect malarial epidemiology without modifying the characteristics of the stratum in which they are found.

Relief

Topographical relief modifies epidemiological conditions according to gradient and altitude.

Apart from the Mountainous and the Southern strata where altitude plays a key role (as discussed in the preceding sections), most of elevated regions in West Africa are not high enough to modify vector fauna. It is the gradient of the slopes which mostly affect distribution in a given area. The plateaux of Fouta-Djalon and Mount Nimba in Guinea, of Bamoun in Cameroon, and of Joss in Nigeria are characterised by gentle slopes and have the same fauna, *An. gambiae s.s.* and *An. funestus*, as the strata—equatorial and especially tropical—in which they are located. The malaria is stable, hyper or meso-endemic (Adam & Bailly-Choumara, 1964; Languillon *et al.*, 1956).

In the Mandara Mountains (altitude 1,200 m) in northern Cameroon, a region with steep slopes on the borders of the tropical and Sahelian strata, the vectors—*An. arabiensis* and *An. funestus* primarily—are especially dense during the rainy season in the valleys and plains and fly up to the summits to feed with the help of ascending convection currents. During the dry season, there is practically no transmission. The malaria switches between endemic and epidemic from one year to the next (Cavalié & Mouchet, 1961). The arrival of the rains brings high mortality (according to health centre reports) in a region where very little health care is available.

In the mountains of West Cameroon (the Bamiléké Region) in the equatorial stratum where the relief is marked, *An. funestus* was almost the only species found at the bottom of valleys; the prevalence of malaria drops with distance above larval habitats and there is no malaria towards the peaks, at least in the Bafoussan Region (Mouchet & Gariou, 1960). This situation does not seem to have changed much in the last forty years.

Soil

Depending on its permeability, the land surface can be more or less conducive to the development of *Anopheles* larvae.

In the Congo, sand covers the Batéké Plateaux (to the north of Brazzaville). The region is very sparsely populated precisely because of the lack of water, an atypical situation in the Equatorial region. The only larval habitats found are in valleys whose bottom lies above a crystalline sheet. Malaria is hyperendemic especially in depressions in the relief (Carnevale & Mouchet, 1980).

In the Grande Comore (RFI Comoros), a recent volcanic island, the earth, composed of ash and lava, is very permeable, and does not retain surface water. Malaria did not appear here until 1920 following the construction of water tanks. It is now hyper- or meso-endemic (Blanchy *et al.*, 1987, 1999).

Water systems

Rivers and streams

Rivers and streams provide ways to penetrate into forest regions, just like roads, trails and villages.

Any stream can provide an ideal larval habitat for *An. nili* as long as it is fast-flowing, and for *An. moucheti* if it is slow-moving river. Species of the *An. gambiae* Complex congregate in residual pools after the waters subside (Mouchet, 1962) and a peak in transmission occurs during the dry season, as observed on the Sanaga in Cameroon, on the Logone and Chari in Chad, on the upper Niger in Mali, on the Uebi-Shebeli and Juba in Somalia, and on the upper Zambezi in Zimbabwe, among others.

For certain large rivers, the rainwater does not arrive until the next year and the rising of the water is simultaneous with the rainy season, as occurs on the Niger in Niamey. In northern Sudan and in Egypt, the Nile flows practically through desert but allows *An. arabiensis* to migrate along a corridor all the way to the Egyptian border in the Nubian Desert.

Lakes and lagoons

Despite their size, the great lakes of East Africa in the Rift Valley do not modify the epidemiological strata in which they are situated.

Lake Chad, a remnant of the great Paleo-Chad in West Africa, followed the path of its tributary, the Chari. The drought which has affected the Sahel since 1973 has reduced the surface of the lake by two-thirds. All of the eastern part of Niger has suffered from the drying up of the lake which is now more than 100 km to the south of Nguigmi (previously a harbour). The region's fauna has been greatly affected. Not only has *An. funestus* disappeared, resulting in a massive drop in the incidence of malaria, but the tsetse fly (*Glossina tachinoides*) and sleeping sickness have also disappeared.

A certain number of basins in the interior such as Lake Rukwa in Tanzania or the Okavango Swamps in Botswana are nothing but vast marshlands whose water levels fluctuate with the season and year. In the Okavango Delta, the water arrives in July, a cool season that is unfavourable for the development of anophelines.

The mountain lakes of south-western Uganda, lined with reeds, used to be maintenance sites for endemic *An. funestus* malaria (Zulueta *et al.*, 1964) up to an altitude of 2,000 m.

The brackish lagoons that line the West African coast host more or less large populations of *An. melas* mixed with *An. gambiae s.s.* Until now, it has been impossible to distinguish the exact species responsible for transmitting malaria in southern Benin where the malaria is hyper- or holo-endemic (Akogbeto, 1995 et 2000; Chippaux *et al.*, 1991b).

Anthropogenic modifications of the environment

This topic will be addressed in detail in the Part on the "Spatiotemporal Dynamics of Malaria". In the Afrotropical Region, such changes result from water management projects and irrigation schemes for rice growing. Its impact on malaria varies enormously according to the epidemiological stratum and the stability of the malaria; this type of impact will be discussed country by country.

Deforestation, a true ecological disaster, has done nothing other than help stabilise malaria in the Afrotropical Region.

Urbanisation is becoming ever more anarchic in Africa and the expansion of urban species (belonging to the Gambiae Complex) warrants specific investigation.

Biodiversity of Malaria in the World

The invasion of Brazil by *An. gambiae* (probably *An. arabiensis*) in 1930 (Soper & Wilson, 1943) and of Egypt in 1943 (Shousha, 1948) illustrates risks that we cannot ignore.

The airport malaria that arose from importing *An. gambiae s.s.* to Roissy for example (Karch *et al.*, 2001) was confined to non-receptive regions in Europe but the same thing could occur in Asia or in South America. No country is entirely safe from such importation events, the consequences of which will depend on the local potential for malarial transmission. In the Part "Spatiotemporal Dynamics of Malaria", we address the recent climate changes which are worrying both political and scientific authorities.

Stability of malaria, Sporozoite Rates and Inoculation Rates

To illustrate transmission in the different strata, we have grouped all the reliable data available on malarial stability (*Figure 15*) and present sporozoite rate (s) measurements and Entomological Inoculation Rates (EIR) for some countries (*Table III*).

An attempt to produce s and EIR maps (Hay *et al.* 2000) is very interesting and represents a good source of documents but the authors introduce many variables—such as the type of capture (on man or by the unreliable light trap method) for anthropophilic species, and indoor spraying (in Gambia)—which necessitate a detailed interpretation of each different situation which is not provided in the texts. Currently, these data are not really useful for regional or local descriptions.

Malaria in the different countries of the Afrotropical Region

The conventional practice is to divide Africa into subregions: West Africa, Central Africa, East Africa, Southern Africa and the islands of the Indian Ocean. Each of these subregions is extremely varied, e.g. West Africa extends from the Sahara Desert down to the rain forests of the Gulf of Guinea.

It seems well established that 90% of the world's malaria cases are observed in Africa south of Sahara but this is purely an estimate as the health statistics in this region are not reliable enough to allow for an accurate figure. In regions where malaria is stable, 90% of carriers are asymptomatic and should not be counted other than in the context of an epidemiological study focusing on prevalence. Moreover, the definition of an episode of malaria remains very subjective given a general lack of microscopes. It would seem that in field conditions, 50% of presumed episodes are the result of erroneous diagnosis (Baudon *et al.*, 1986b). A malarial mortality and morbidity report is presented in the Chapter "Year 2000: Time to Take Stock".

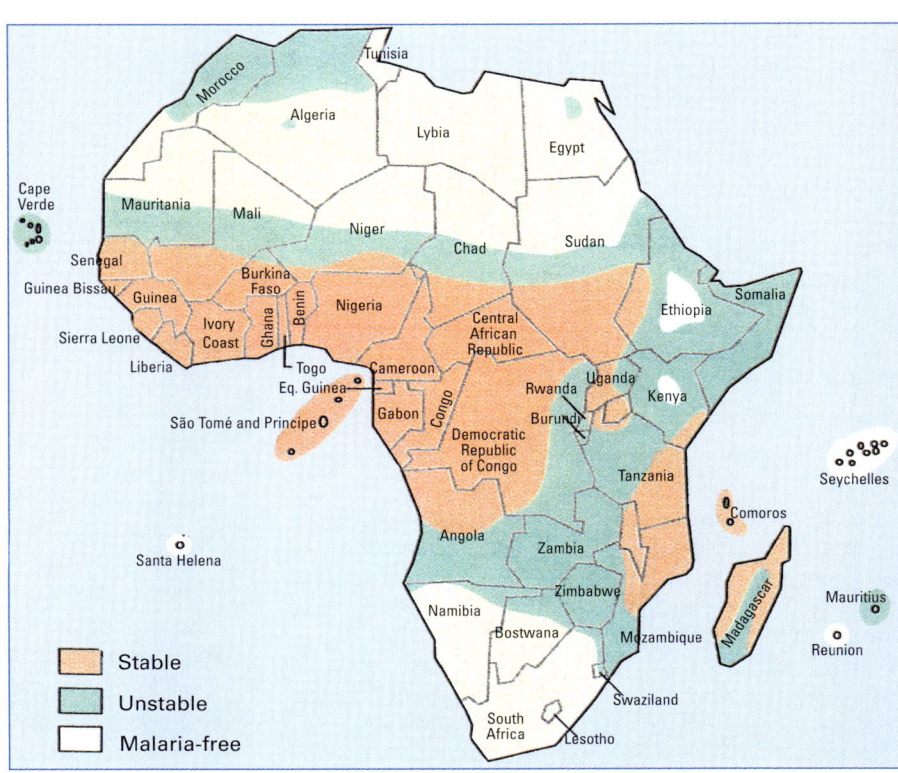

Figure 15. Stable and unstable malaria in Africa (in *Mouchet* et al., 1991).

Table III. Sporozoite rates and entomological inoculation rates reported in Africa.				
Country	Region and environment	Stable versus unstable malaria	s %	EIR
Senegal	Rural, North Sahel Rural, Saloum	Unstable Stable	0.25 1.80-3	9.20 272
Benin	Urban, south Lagoon, south	Stable	1.4-2.8 0.34-0.4	33-58 10-11
Burkina Faso	Bobo-Dioulasso, urban Bobo-Dioulasso, periurban Bobo-Dioulasso, rural Bobo-Dioulasso, rice-growing	Stable	0-0.2 0.4-0.5 1.7-4.5 0.2-0.4	0.1-0.6 4-5 116-440 20-60
	Ouagadougou, urban Ouagadougou, rural	Stable		0-7 113
Burundi	Rural	Intermediate	0.48-3.8	35-600
Cameroun	Urban Rural, forest south	Stable	1.2-8.2 1.2-4	3-30 82-400
Congo RD	Urban Kinshasa Rural	Stable	0.3-1.8 3.1-7.4	3-29 40-612
Congo	Urban Rural	Stable	3.4	22 80-900
Ivory Coast	Rural	Stable	3.2-3.4	200 to > 400
Gambia (all ELISA)	Rural Urban	Stable	0.3-4 0.98	80-70
Sierra Leone	Rural	Stable	3.9-6.8	35-808
Kenya	Rural	Variable Stable to unstable	0.1-10	416-5 (depending on altitude and rainfall)
Tanzania	Rural	Stable	1.3-7.14	122-548
Mozambique	Suburban	Unstable		12
Madagascar	Plateaux East Coast	Unstable Stable	0.14-0.7	0.9 82

s: sporozoite rate; EIR: entomological inoculation rate
For each country mentioned, see the relevant vectors in the section on that country

Malaria is not a static disease and its incidence can rise and fall with variations in climate, environment, and the efficacy of control methods. Its incidence has been rising by 7.3% per annum in Zambia, by 10% in Togo, and by 21% in Rwanda. In contrast, a drop of 14% was observed in Burkina Faso (Sabatinelli et al., 1986a) between 1973 and 1981, although this was followed by a 10% increase over the ten years that followed. A similar decrease was observed in all areas of the Sahel affected by the drought (Mouchet et al., 1996).

West Africa

Natural regions and climatic zones do not necessarily change when crossing the border from one country to the next. Although certain small countries on the coast may belong to one well-demarcated region, most extend over several climatic and phytogeographic zones, from the forest all the way to desert; these zones, parallel to the equator, have already been addressed in the Strata Section which emphasises the concept of epidemiological facies (see above).

We have classified countries according to their geographic proximity and the ecological continua they represent. The following groups were constituted:
- countries on the Atlantic coast: Mauritania, Cape Verde, Senegal, Gambia, Guinea-Bissau, Guinea, Sierra Leone, Liberia: these countries reach the sea by large estuaries;
- enclosed Saharan-Sahelo-Sudanese States: Mali, Burkina Faso, Niger, Chad;
- countries on the northern coast of the Gulf of Guinea: Ivory Coast, Ghana, Togo, Benin, Nigeria.

Countries on the Atlantic Coast

From Liberia to Mauritania over a span of more than 2,000 km, the countries facing the Atlantic extend successively into equatorial forest (Liberia, Sierra Leone), wet savannah (Guinea and southern Senegal), dry savannah (Senegal), scrubby steppe land (northern Senegal and Mauritania), and finally the Mauritanian desert with its oases. Rainfall steadily drops moving from the north to the south with more than 1,500 mm per annum in Guinea, and less than 50 mm in Mauritania.

In Mauritania, the coastline is sandy but in Senegal and beyond, it is pierced by estuaries (Saloun, Gambia, Casamance, Freetown River, etc.) that are lined for dozens of kilometres upriver with lush mangroves. This is the region of southern rivers where European explorers made contact and traded with local people.

The first time Europeans made contact with this tropical world, they described it as an unhealthy land where sickness decimated the seamen. Up until and during the 19th century, Europeans tended not to survive here for very long and most of the governors of Freetown were sent home, if not dead already, before the end of their stay (Carlson, 1984). In memory of this period of time, the government of Sierra Leone created a medal in 1972 in honour of *Anopheles*, their best ally in the fight against imperialists. In reality, the coastline of West Africa was no unhealthier than the hinterland, even if the coastal humidity had contributed to the spreading of the myth of "bad air".

But all of West Africa was home to stable malaria where all non-immune foreigners were, and still are, in mortal danger if they do not take effective prophylactic drugs. In the beginning of the 19th century, only one out of fifty travellers leaving Freetown for Bamako would make it to the destination and even they often arrived in a poor health (Carlson, 1984).

Republic of Cape Verde

The Republic of Cape Verde consists of a chain of about a dozen islands covering a total surface area of 4,000 km², located 500 km off the western coast of Senegal (*Table I*). When they were discovered by the Portuguese in 1460, these islands were uninhabited but they were soon subsequently occupied by West African and European immigrants. Malaria immediately became established and in 1507, the Portuguese authorities discontinued stops in Cape Verde for those heading to India. We do not know if *An. arabiensis*, the only vector found in the archipelago (Cambournac *et al.*, 1982), was already present when the Portuguese arrived but in any case, a chain of transmission was very quickly established. *An. arabiensis* has been found on all the islands except for São Nicolau.

The climate is dry, like that of the Sahel. From 1972 to 1984 during the drought, only 208 mm of rain per annum was recorded. The vegetation in the western islands includes a dry forest very much damaged by farming whereas the ecology of the eastern islands is that of the sub-desert.

The statistics on malaria are already old. In 1930, the disease was hypo- or meso-endemic on the islands of Santiago, Maio, Boa Vista and São Vicente. In 1951, it was meso-endemic in Santiago, the only island surveyed (Cambournac *et al.*, 1984) with epidemic outbreaks occurring in wet years.

From 1937 to 1940 at the hospital of Santiago, malaria was responsible for 36% to 55% of admissions (depending on the year). From 1940 to 1950, the authorities declared an annual death rate of 200 due to malaria.

Beginning in 1952, successful control procedures led to the eradication of *An. arabiensis* from all the islands except Santiago. This mosquito was then reintroduced, probably by plane, from one island to another, and then once again "eradicated". It is thus very difficult to pin down a situation that keeps fluctuating.

Mauritania

This huge country with a surface greater than one million km² has only 3 million inhabitants (*Table I*), of which 80% are concentrated in the southern Sahelian parts and along the Senegal River. This economically productive part of Mauritania contrasts with the vast desert areas which are only interrupted by the Adrar, Tagant and Hogh oases.

Only in the far south does as much as 400 mm of rain fall and the 200 mm isohyet runs close to the 17th parallel. Not only is precipitation low, but it varies considerably from one year to the next. In addition, since 1970 the rainfall has dropped by 30% in the Sahel, causing a long-standing drought.

The information on malaria in Mauritania is not much better than that available on the vectors. In 1935, Farinaud was interested in determining the endemicity of malaria on the riverbanks and in the regularly flooded Gorgol and Brakna plains. Malaria attacks appeared as soon as the wet winter season arrived and every tent had its feverish patients (the population was essentially nomadic). "Black" people appeared less susceptible than were the Moors. Malaria was the second most important cause of morbidity. In the rest of the country, there were only sporadic cases.

In 1948, Sautet *et al.* visited the banks of the river and reported the presence of *An. gambiae* and *An. funestus*. In a very imprecise article, they recorded a prevalence of 17%, based on 307 slides, increasing to 59% in children under the age of 5 in the Gorgol. Needless to say, they observed a predominance of *P. falciparum* (with just 8% *P. vivax*), figures similar to those recorded by Hudleston (1961) at a later date. The prevalence of this plasmodial species is as expected given that about 50% of the population—those of Berber or related origins—carry the Duffy antigen (Lepers *et al.*, 1986).

Hudleston (1961), Maffi, and later Barbié & Timbala (1964) undertook an entire survey of Mauritania. They distinguished three zones:
- **Saharan zone**: in Attar, the PR was 1% or less in the city and zero in rural zones; the possibility that the cases found in the city of Attar had been imported was not ruled out;
- **Sahelian zone** (survey of Tamchakett, Aioun-el-Atrous, Kiffu): hypo-endemic malaria, with PRs of 5.7% in children of 0-2 years, 4.8% in 2-9 year olds, and 2.2% in

teenagers. Since the 1970's, this zone has more or less presented a Sahelo-Saharan facies;
- **River valley**: meso-endemic malaria with a PR of 18.7% in children between 0-2 years, 30.4% in 2-9 year olds, and 9.3% in 10-15 year olds (Kankossa, Kaedi). The Guidi-Makha Region, where Mauritania intersects with Mali and Senegal, was considered to be hyperendemic (bordering meso-endemic) by certain experts (Hudleston, 1961). Differences in prevalence between the rainy season and dry season were great.

This epidemiological "stratification" is still valid but needs updating in the light of the effects of the drought. The survey of Baudon et al. (1986c) on the Gorgol Dam during the dry season revealed very low levels of transmission: only two out of 523 blood samples were found to be infected, specific antibody levels were very low, and no anophelines were caught.

Epidemics were reported in 1989-1990 and in 1994-1995 with a malarial mortality rate of 15% in the hospitals of Boghé, Aleg and Magda-Lahjar.

In 1996 and 1997, Molez & Faye (personal communication) studied a transect from the river (the Boghé) all the way to the stony desert plateau of the Tagant (500 m in altitude). Little rain had fallen in 1996 and it had not rained at all in the centre of the Tagant (Tidjika and Rachid). In 1997, the rain gauge rose to 136 mm in the centre of the Tagant. In 1996, there was no *Anopheles* whatsoever in the oases of the plateau; *An. arabiensis* was only found in a few springs at the base of the plateau. By 1997, the authors observed *An. arabiensis* all the way to Rachid, at the centre of the Tagant; either its site extended gradually, or the mosquito travelled on the wind. We favour the second hypothesis given the distance between the water sources and the shortness of the rainy season. Information on malaria-like fevers is not very reliable (as mentioned by the local health care staff). The presence of malaria in an isolated oasis in the middle of a desert always gives rise to explanations that are speculative rather than based on fact.

In the dry areas, Hudleston (1961) noted a concentration of transmission around the permanent or semi-permanent water sources all the way to the southern boundary of the Tagant. He suggested that *An. gambiae s.l.* and malaria had a northern limit that passed through Boutilimit (PR 2.9%), the north of Aleg, the Tagant (Moudjeria, PR 12%), Aioun el Atrouss, Nema and Tamkachett (PR about 9%).

It has been impossible to obtain reliable figures on malaria in Mauritania since the droughts of the 1970's which persisted until 1995 and perhaps even longer.

For centuries, the rise of the Senegal River—which floods between 100,000 to 500,000 hectares of land (depending on the year)—has determined the agri-pastoral season and conditioned the spread of malaria vectors. Water control projects, notably the Manantali Dam on the Mali border and the Diama Dam near the Senegal Estuary which prevents sea water flowing upstream, have changed the ecology of the valley with, in particular, the development of irrigated farming and rice cultivation. The implications of this development work *vis-à-vis* malaria and its vectors are still not well characterised in Mauritania although this subject has been extensively studied in Senegal.

The anopheline fauna of Mauritania is known from the works of Sautet et al. (1948), Maffi (1964), Hamon et al. (1964), Barbié & Timbala (1964) and, more recently, Faye & Molez (1997, personal communication).

An. funestus, considered as abundant in the Kaolé Region in 1948 (Sautet et al., 1948), was much less abundant by 1964 and was confined to the Assaba (Hamon et al., 1964). Following periods of drought, it had disappeared in 1996 and 1997 (Faye & Molez), as throughout most of the Sahel following the droughts (Mouchet et al., 1996).

An. arabiensis was known to be the main vector in the river region where it was very abundant during the rains and in pools left after the waters had receded. By virtue of expansion of the river's offshoots, this vector spread north of the river into the desert zone. Maffi (1964) observed it all the way to Boutilimit. Faye & Molez (personal communication, 1997) declared that in 1996, a dry year, *An. arabiensis* had not gone beyond Moudjeria at the foot of the Tagant Massif while in 1997, following two bursts of rainfall in August, it could be found in all the valleys up to Tijidja as well as the oasis of Rachid, north of the 19th parallel. This observation confirmed the Vaucel report in 1922 (in Hamon et al., 1964) of malaria outbreaks in Tijidja following the rains.

An. dthali, very abundant in the desert oases (Maffi, 1964), does not seem to transmit malaria in Mauritania even though it is known to act as vector in the Middle East and Arabia.

Senegal and Gambia

Senegal covers an area of 196,200 km² and has a population of 11.7 million people; Gambia covers 11,300 km² and has a population of 1.5 million people (*Table 1*).

The many and various scientific establishments in both Senegal (including the University of Dakar and the Pasteur Institute of Dakar, as well as specialised institutions such as the Institute of Research for Development), and in Gambia (the UK MRC) have contributed to making these flagship countries when it comes to the epidemiology of malaria. This explains the important position that has been given to them.

From the north to the south of Senegal (*Figure 16*) is a succession of ecological strata of a west-east orientation: Sahelian steppes, Sahelo-Sudanese savannah, Sudanese savannah, and Guinean savannah in the far south. These strata are more or less determined by the isohyets, with precipitation ranging from 200 mm in the north to more than 1,000 mm in the south. The coastline is sandy in the north as far as Saloun, after which it is bordered by mangrove to the south. All along the valley of the Senegal River where water flow is controlled, the man-made

Biodiversity of Malaria in the World

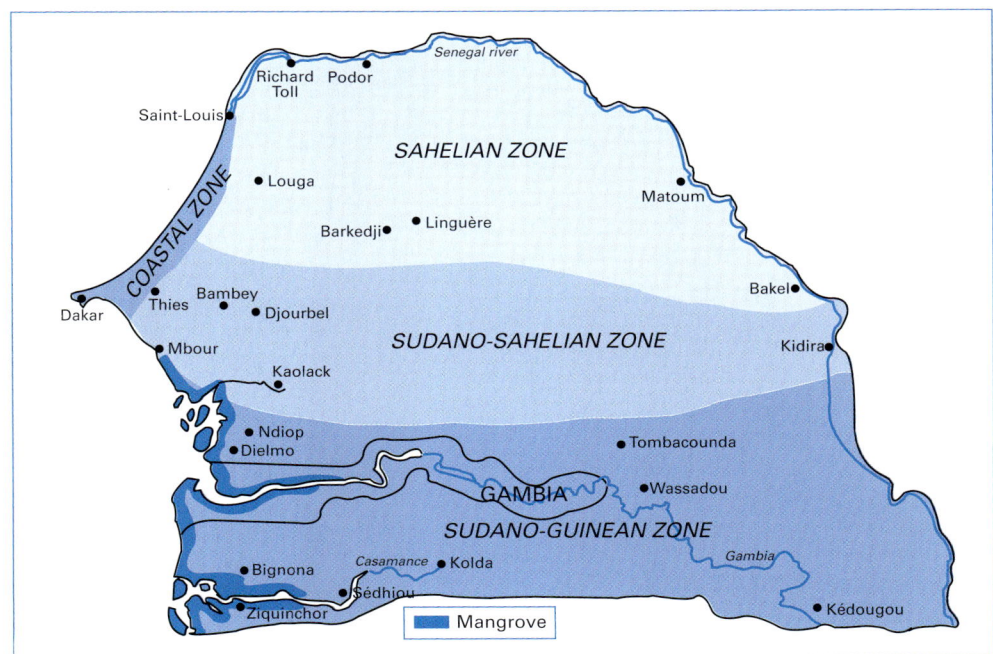

Figure 16.
Senegal and Gambia:
biogeographical zones
(adapted from Faye).

countryside differs enormously from the original countryside.

Since 1970, Senegal has suffered a persistent drought with a 30% deficit in annual rainfall, particularly in the northern regions. In Thiès, at the latitude of Dakar, the average level of precipitation from 1950 to 1959 was 743 mm; this decreased to 594 mm from 1960 to 1969, and to 259 mm in 1992. On the Mauritanian border in Podor, rainfall, already only of 388 mm in 1989, had fallen to 59 mm by 1991.

This drought has drastically changed the ecology and epidemiology of the region. One of the main vectors of malaria, *An. funestus*, disappeared to the north of Dakar. From an epidemiological perspective, the tremendous impact of these changes is considered to be one of the major climatic events of the late 20th century (Mouchet *et al.*, 1996).

It would seem that since 1995 and to an even greater extent since 1998, we are experiencing a return to the situation prior to 1970. Precipitation figures tend to resemble those recorded before 1970. If this trend continues, the output of the Senegal River could markedly increase and water could flow over the Manatali Dam (in Mali) causing the main bed to flood, an event which has not happened for many years.

• *Senegal River Valley*

The Senegal River, 450 km long, acts as the natural border between Senegal and Mauritania and stems from the confluence of two rivers, namely the Bafing and the Bakoy which converge in Bafoulabé in Mali. It enters Senegal upstream from Bakel where the Falémé joins it. It flows through an almost entirely flat valley at an altitude of no more than 20 m, spreading out in a maze of twists and meanders creating many small islands.

Control of its flow has allowed irrigated farming and rice cultivation to develop, with major potential economic benefits.

The river can be divided up into distinct areas: the upper valley upstream from Matoum, the middle valley of Matoum at Richard Toll, and the delta downstream from Richard Toll.

The **delta** is made up of salty land which is partly used for rice paddies and in which *An. pharoensis* (90%) and *An. arabiensis* (10%) breed. Carrara *et al.* (1990) had considered *An. pharoensis* to be the main vector in the delta with a sporozoite rate (CSP) of 0.48%. This was not confirmed by Faye *et al.* (1995c), who did not find a single infected anopheline. In this saline region of the delta, the prevalence of malaria was extremely low, from 0.4% to 0.9% for several hundred subjects investigated. The number of cases was greater than 20% in dispensaries but it cannot be said with any certainty that these subjects had not come from elsewhere; the infected subjects were of all ages.

The **middle valley** is now peppered with irrigated plots. The vectors are *An. gambiae s.s.* (40%) and *An. arabiensis* (60%). In this region where the nights are hot, people sleep outside, often under a mosquito net. But during the day, Gambiae Complex anophelines take refuge inside the houses, a behaviour which is not often mentioned (Faye *et al.*, 1997). In irrigated areas, the density of *An. gambiae s.l.* decreases very rapidly as one gets further away from the cultivated areas (Faye *et al.*, 1998).

An. funestus had completely disappeared from the region but returned in 1999 (Konaté *et al.*, 2001) in the irrigated zones of Keur-Mbaye, even though it remains absent in the Niayes further south.

The EIR was from 0 to 6 ib/p/yr in Diomandé (irrigated zone) (Faye *et al.*, 1998) and from 0.8 to 6.4 in Podor (Vercruysse, 1985) (*Table IV*). PR figures indicate meso-endemicity if not hypo-endemicity: in 1989, they were between 17% and 26% in Podor; in 1990 and 1991, they were between 0% and 16% (Faye *et al.*, 1993b).

• *Sahel*

In the Senegalese Sahel, transmission was low in villages which are not right on the river banks, in the Ferlo especially. Vercruysse (1985) had recorded an EIR of 1 to 7 ib/p/yr, exclusively due to *An. arabiensis* which is only abundant during the wet months. This very low transmission rate was associated with abnormal zootrophic behaviour on the part of the vector as the number of bites on cattle was five times greater than on man.

On the edge of the Sahelo-Sudanese zone in Barkedji, where malaria is almost stable, the EIR was 100 (which is very high for the Sahel). Under identical exposure conditions, the sporozoite rate of *An. gambiae s.s.* was 4.19% whereas for *An. arabiensis* it was 1.8% which suggests that the transmission rate of *An. gambiae* is two times higher than that of *An. arabiensis* (Lemasson *et al.*, 1997). This was the first time that this hypothesis was backed by reliable data.

• *Coastal Sahel: the Niayes*

The Niayes, to the north of Dakar, is a series of dune bars parallel to the coast. Between them are stagnant ponds with standing vegetation whose depths vary depending on the rainfall (Faye *et al.*, 1995b). Before 1960, the annual precipitation amounted to about 600 mm. At that time, the parasite prevalence was between 53% to 59% for children between 2 and 9 years old from a mixture of villages in which malaria was meso- or hyper-endemic. Two-thirds of the transmission was due to *An. funestus*, and one-third due to *An. gambiae s.l.* The sporozoite rates of the former and latter were between 1% and 3.5% respectively, depending on the season.

Beginning in 1970, the situation changed profoundly (Faye *et al.*, 1995a). Rainfall decreased to an average of about 350 mm. Wet depressions dried up and were used to farm vegetables using subterranean moisture. *An. funestus* disappeared and has never reappeared, even when the depressions were submerged again, as occurred in 1995. In fact, cultivation of the lower ground led to the disappearance of the stands of vegetation which are necessary for the development of *An. funestus*. Only *An. gambiae s.l.* (92% *An. arabiensis* and 8% *An. gambiae s.s.*) continued to transmit the disease but at a very low rate and with a very weak sporozoite rate. The EIR was 11 in 1991 and zero or inestimable in 1992 and 1993 in the two study areas of the Niayes. Parasite prevalence was between 3% and 10%. We only recorded four clinical cases from a group of 100 children in the village of Ngadiaga (700 inhabitants) where, in 1967, we had recorded 851 attacks during the rainy season (although this survey might have been overly zealous) (*Table V*).

The Niayes, where malaria suddenly decreased by 80% following a long-standing drought and changes to the

Table IV. Malaria in the Senegal River valley (adapted from Faye *et al.*, 1998; Vercruysse, 1985).

Delta			Middle valley			
PR	Vectors		PR	EIR	Vectors	
0,4-0,9%	*An. arabiensis* 10% *An. pharoensis* 90% s: 0.49%	Podor	17-26%	0.8-6.4	*An. arabiensis* 60% *An. gambiae s.s.* 40%	
		Diomande	0-16%	0.6		

PR: parasite rate; s: sporozoite rate; EIR: entomological inoculation rate

Table V. Drop in malaria in the Niayes of Senegal following drought (adapted from Faye *et al.*, 1995a).

Precipitation		PR		EIR		Vector and s		Incidence	
Before 1970	After 1973	Before 1970	After 1973	Before 1970	After 1973	Before 1970	After 1973	Before 1970	After 1973
600 mm	350 mm	53-59%	3-10%	not calculated at that time	11	*An. funestus* 66% *An. gambiae s.l.* 33% s 1-3%	*An. gambiae s.l.* *An. arabiensis* 92% *An. gambiae s.s.* 8% s cannot be calculated	1,200‰	40‰ (drop of 96%)

environment, represents a unique situation in Africa. Without exaggerating, one could say that similar types of phenomena have occurred all throughout the Sahel and in one part of the Sahelo-Sudanese zone (*see below*).

• *Sudanese zone*

The Sudanese Region, which includes Gambia, occupies a large stratum delineated between the Atlantic and the eastern border of the country from the 12th to the 15th north parallel that is not very well delineated. The expansion of farming land and the effects of drought have largely fashioned the local countryside so that completely different conditions can pertain at sites within a few kilometres of one another, e.g. the situation at Ndiop, a small village cited by Fontenille *et al.* (1997b) located in the Sahelo-Sudanese zone where malaria is meso-endemic and seasonal, is quite different from the very distinctive situation at Dielmo, a village on a permanent flowing river where the disease is holo-endemic and perennial (Trape *et al.*, 1994).

To the east of Dakar, in what was the pilot zone of Thiès, malaria was meso-endemic in most of the villages with PR measurements of between 35% and 38% (*in* Kouznetzov, 1977).

In eastern Senegal (Faye *et al.*, 1995), malaria had all the characteristics of the Sudanese Regions and hardly differed from observations made in Mali, Burkina Faso (Robert, 1988a), Nigeria (Molineaux & Gramiccia, 1980) or Cameroon (Cavalié & Mouchet, 1961).

In **N'diop** (*Table VI*), rainfall varied from 600 mm in 1993 to 860 mm in 1995 and 521 mm in 1996. Most of this fell between July and October. *An. arabiensis* was responsible for 65% of the transmission in 1993, but for only 40% in 1996; *An. gambiae s.s.* accounted for the rest. The two species were 78% anthropophilic in their behaviour. *An. funestus,* probably not originating from the village, was involved 3% of the time and *An. melas* 0.3%. The EIR was 63 in 1993, 17 in 1994, 37 in 1995 (a wet year) and 7 in 1996. Despite the rains being seasonal, anophelines of the Gambiae Complex were present throughout the entire year but in small numbers during the dry season, a constant feature of the Sudanese zone. The amount of rain and of inoculations do not always seem to correlate and rainfall figures are not always a good indicator, as is illustrated in the next example, that of the village of Dielmo.

In N'diop, the incidence of malarial infections was 3 per year per person with a peak incidence in children of between 3 and 6 years of age. It is only with adults that the incidence drops to below 1, which shows how slowly immunity develops (Trape & Rogier, 1996).

In **Dielmo** (*Table VI*), a village that is only 10 km away from N'diop, the rainfall (800 mm per annum) is not significantly different but local ecological conditions are. Malaria was locally holo-endemic and transmission was perennial (Fontenille *et al.*, 1997a; Trape *et al.*, 1994) because of the presence of larval habitats all year round in the river that cuts through the village. Ecologically, Dielmo represents a "local exception" in the Sahelo-Sudanese epidemiological facies. Depending on the year, the most abundant vector was *An. funestus* or *An. arabiensis*; *An. gambiae s.s.* came in third place. The sporozoite rate of *P. falciparum* varied from 0.78% to 2.1% for *An. gambiae s.s.*, 0.75% to 0.54% for *An. arabiensis* and from 3.49% to 1.4% for *An. funestus*. Only *An. gambiae s.s.* was infected with *P. malariae* (from 0.3% to 0.15%). The EIR was 222 in 1992, 78 in 1993 and 139 in 1995, differences of no epidemiological significance. In 1992, *An. funestus* was responsible for 65% of transmission.

In Dielmo, the *P. falciparum* population was genetically highly heterogeneous. Successive clinical episodes experienced by the children were caused by genetically different parasites (*see the Chapter on "Plasmodium* Life Cycles in Humans and Anopheline Vectors").

As in N'diop, the EIR fluctuated over the years despite the high density of the vectors. All the evidence suggested that repeated treatments and over-treatment were causing the

Table VI. Comparison of malaria in a Sahelo-Sudanese village (N'diop) and a holo-endemic village (Dielmo) in Senegal (adapted from Trape *et al.*, 1994; Trape & Rogier, 1996).

	Rainfall and waterways	Ecological localisation	EIR	Vectors	Number of infections per child per year
N'diop	600-850 mm	Sahelo-Sudanese	63 in 1993 7 in 1996	*An. arabiensis* 65% *An. gambiae s.s.* 35% *An. funestus* 3% *An. melas* 0.3%	3 per year per person (peak at 3-6 years of age)
Dielmo	800 m Constantly flowing river	Holo-endemic Exception because of the permanence of the river	222 in 1992 278 in 1993	*An. funestus* s 3.4% *An. gambiae s.s.* s 0.78-2.1% *An. arabiensis* s 0.54-0.75%	6 per person (second year) 0.1-11 years PR: 96% in children

EIR: entomological inoculation rate; PR: parasite rate; s: sporozoite rate parasite reservoir to dwindle. The same phenomenon was reported in Ankazobé (Madagascar) in a study centre of the Pasteur Institute. This aspect has never been considered seriously in epidemiological studies.

In Dielmo, the incidence of cases, symptomatic or not, was 6 per subject during the second year of life, dropping to less than 0.1 from 11 years old (Trape & Rogier, 1996). This profile is very different from the one in N'diop and shows rapid acquisition of immunity, characteristic of perennial transmission zones.

In **Gambia**, outside of the mangrove, *An. gambiae s.s.* was the main vector (90% compared with 8% for *An. arabiensis*, and less than 2% for *An. melas*). There was no report of *An. funestus* (Bryan *et al.*, 1987; Lindsay *et al.*, 1993).

South-eastern Senegal is typically Sudanese. Rainfall was 880 mm in 1992 and 661 mm in 1993. In the village of Wassadou (800 inhabitants) 50 km to the south of Tambacunda, where Faye conducted his studies (1995b), cattle raising is one of the main activities. The dominant vector is *An. gambiae s.s.* (77%), followed by *An. arabiensis* (20%), and *An. funestus* (3%). The EIR was 220, of which 92% occurred during the rainy season. The PR of the children was between 60% and 80%. The region was hyperendemic, or even holo-endemic like the majority of the Sudanese zone. The use of treated mosquito nets (Olyset®) was recently introduced.

• *Casamance*

This is the Senegalese province located between Gambia and Guinea. The lower part is a tangled mass of mangroves while the eastern part has often been associated with the Guinean savannah Region, characterised by only one rainy season that lasts for more than six months. In the saline part of the Casamance (the estuary), *An. gambiae s.s.* and *An. melas* share the role of vector. In the eastern part, *An. funestus* was abundant in 1956 (Hamon *et al.*, 1956a) although now it seems that its numbers have greatly diminished (Faye *et al.*, 1994). Studies done both upriver and downstream from the anti-salt dam of Bignona have shown holo- or hyper-endemic malaria upstream from the dam with a PR of 63% (Gaye *et al.*, 1991). Downstream from the dam in the tidal zone, malaria was meso-endemic with a PR of 33%. EIRs were 20 in the "salty" zone and 39 upstream from the dam.

There is, therefore, a significant difference in terms of both prevalence and transmission between the tidal zone and the area upstream of the dam.

• *Mangrove of the southern rivers*

Mangrove covers the entire coastline of West Africa south of Dakar and penetrates deeply into the estuaries of the Saloum, Gambia, and Casamance in Senegal and Gambia. It is an amphibious environment subject to daily incoming tides. Every month, high tides of great amplitudes leave a collection of residual pools that persist throughout the entire coming month.

The halophytic vegetation, the mangroves (*Rhizophora sp.* and *Avicennia*) and the prairies of *Paspalum* are interspersed with stripped plaques called "tales", the remains of old riverbeds where the salt rises to the surface. These mangrove regions bordering the Atlantic from Senegal to Liberia are referred to by geographers as "the southern rivers" (Cormier-Salem, 1999).

The malaria vectors in this very particular environment are mosquitoes belonging to the Gambiae Complex, namely *An. gambiae s.s.* and *An. arabiensis* in freshwater residual pools, and *An. melas* in brackish water larval habitats (Mouchet *et al.*, 1994). This duality of vectors with intermingling distribution areas often makes it difficult to interpret entomological and epidemiological results in an unambiguous fashion.

Throughout the year in Gambia, *An. melas* swarms for ten to fifteen days in residual pools left by the strong tides; veritable waves of *Anopheles* invade the neighbouring villages (Bryan, 1983; Giglioli, 1964). In contrast, *An. gambiae s.s.* and *An. arabiensis* are dependant on rainfall. *An. melas*, which is mainly zoophilic, has a low life expectancy with a very low sporozoite rate of 0.3%, compared with the indices of 3% recorded with freshwater forms of *An. gambiae*. Meanwhile, we observed that in coastal regions such as those in the rest of Gambia, most episodes of malaria were seen at the end of the rainy season (Greenwood *et al.*, 1987a): in other words, they correlate with the presence of *An. gambiae* from rain-dependent larval habitats.

In the delta of Saloum in Senegal, the scenario is quite different (Diop *et al.*, 2002). The ratio of *An. melas* to *An. arabiensis* (there is little *An. gambiae s.s.*) rose with proximity to the sea. In a fishing village (Differe) without any livestock, *An. melas* (which was almost the only anopheline found) presented a sporozoite rate of 3%, like that in the *An. arabiensis* in neighbouring cattle breeding villages. This obvious contradiction to the observations made in Gambia does not seem to be due to a difference in vector strength but to a difference in the availability of the host, be it human or animal.

We noted above, in the discussion on the Lower Casamance, the differences between the tidal zones and the zones protected from sea water which represent an intermediary situation. The ecological intricacy of mangrove forests makes it difficult to evaluate either malarial prevalence or seasonal anopheline rhythms apart from in certain very specific situations; ill-judged generalisations can lead to major errors of interpretation.

• *Urban malaria*

The new city of Pikine, a satellite of Dakar, has grabbed the attention of experts in the field of hygiene because it represents a highly diverse environment in which plots of cultivated land persist in the middle of the city.

According to studies by Vercryusse & Jancloes (1981) then by Vercryusse *et al.* (1983), the only anopheline present was *An. arabiensis*, a highly seasonal species which is very dependent on rains in August to October (and which persists through December). Given the catch points and their proximity to the watering holes which are the most common larval habitats, the number of bites varied from 70 per person per night in September, to 0.5 in March. Sporozoite rates varied from 0.8% to 1.5% for a 20-day *P. falciparum* sporogonic cycle between January and March, and an 11-day cycle the rest of the year. The stability index was 2.3, i.e. intermediate. The authors spoke of annual epidemics but the term seasonal outbreaks would be more accurate. The PR in children under 10 was 13.5% in January, and 2.2% in August (average 8.9), which suggests hypo-endemicity despite the fact that the EIR had been 13 per person per year. We considered there to be a new infection every 517 days, thus very little antigen stimulation of the immune system—although this remains to be confirmed by comparing children and adults.

Another study in Pikine (Trape *et al.*, 1992) showed that the number of *An. arabiensis* per house decreased with increasing distance to the water source: 80 per house if the distance was 0-160 m, 40 for 160-285 m, 5 for 285-400 m, 2 for 400-600 m, and 0.4 for 600-800 m. The proportion of children between the ages of 8 and 11 that were not carrying antibodies increased from 17% to 75% according to the distance to the larval habitats and the vector density within. The malaria prevalence in the community varied from 1% to 15% (average 6%) and was at its greatest closest to water sources.

A more recent study (Diallo *et al.*, 1998 a and b) in the southern port neighbourhood of Dakar provides a completely different picture of urban malaria in the region. The only vector, *An. arabiensis*, maintained a very low density, i.e. 0.26 bites/person/night and 0.05 females per room. Out of the eighty specimens dissected, not one was infected. Its period of activity had diminished to the three months from September to November. There were few larval habitats as most pools of surface water became polluted soon after the rain. A follow-up of 929 persons, examined and tested every month, confirmed the entomological data. Out of 19,375 blood samples, only 60 were positive for *P. falciparum* for almost the entire period between October and December. The PR varied from 0.1 (for children under 2) to 0.7% (for ages 15-20 years). Parasite incidence was 24 ‰ (22 cases); only one subject in the cohort experienced a simple malaria attack and eight infected subjects remained asymptomatic.

Broadly speaking, therefore, malaria was hypo-endemic and, in many neighbourhoods of the district, not one case had been detected. It was not without a certain amount of astonishment that the authors found that the official statistics indicated that malaria was the leading reason for consultation of a health centre. Once again, we can only doubt the reliability of these figures. In this area of Dakar, the incidence of malaria is therefore eight times less than in the satellite town of Pikine and 17 times less than in another Sudanese city, Bobo-Dioulasso. The results of this study show that, not only is there tremendous climate-dependent variability in urban malaria but also, the **incidence of the disease depends heavily on urban structure** (Dakar and Pikine being in the same climate zone). In this context, the authors pointed to the potential risk of an epidemic following prolonged, heavy rains.

The mortality rate due to malaria has been studied in depth in Gambia with a rate of 4% in children under the age of 7 and 25% in children between 1 and 4 years of age according to autopsy reports based on a post-mortem questionnaire (Greenwood *et al.*, 1987a) (*see the Chapters on* "Man Facing Malaria" *and* "Year 2000: Time to Take Stock"). Most of the deaths caused by malaria and a large proportion of feverish episodes were concentrated at the end of the rainy season: children under the age of 7 presented an average of one clinical attack every year.

These figures were noticeably different from those reported by experts in demographics in Senegal who, without any special clinical investigation, attributed 10% of deaths among children under the age of 5 to malaria (Cantrelle, personal communication).

Guinea-Bissau

To distinguish it from the Republic of Guinea, the former Portuguese Guinea is now called Guinea-Bissau (*Table I*), (after the capital city). This small country of 36,120 km² located between 11° and 12.6° north latitude, stretches along the Atlantic for more than 200 km. Its population increased from 600,000 inhabitants in 1955 to 1.6 million in 1999. The coastline is lined with mangroves while inland is a Guinean savannah, scattered with strips of forest in the south-east. Rainfall ranges from 1,500 to 2,200 mm (depending on distance from the sea) with most falling in a long rainy season which lasts from April to November (with peak rainfall in August) and is followed by a well-defined dry season.

With respect to malaria, the epidemiological facies is of the tropical type, therefore stable, hyper-endemic on the coastal areas and meso-endemic inland. Most of the small amount of epidemiological and entomological information available was compiled in the 1940's. Ferreira *et al.* (1948) measured PR levels greater than 50% in Bissau and its surroundings. Cambournac (1981) recorded a more moderate PR (about 30%) in 3,250 slides prepared from samples taken from children between the ages of 1 and 9 in the course of a survey being carried out throughout the entire country.

The confirmed vectors were *An. melas* on the coast, and *An. gambiae s.s.*, *An. funestus* and *An. nili* inland (Gillies & Coetze, 1987). *An. arabiensis* has never been observed and the role of *An. brunnipes* needs to be investigated. In Bissau (Cruz Ferreira *et al.*, 1948) an *An. gambiae s.s.* sporozoite rate of 1.4% was recorded during the dry season, and one of 2.5% during the rainy season.

Since 1994, several studies have used PCR to identify plasmodial species and measure parasite loads. This method is extremely sensitive but relatively non-specific and therefore of limited relevance (Snounou *et al.*, 1993).

In a study in Prabis, the disease varied between hypo- and holo-endemicity according to the location of villages and farms, and in particular rice paddies (Goncalves *et al.*, 1996). QBC use in urban clinics was well received but this expensive modality was eventually abandoned.

A trial based on treated mosquito nets gave results similar to those observed elsewhere in West Africa (Jaenson *et al.*, 1994).

Guinea

The Republic of Guinea is located between the 8° and 13° parallels north and occupies an area of 245,860 km^2 with 250 km of coastline. It has a population of 9.4 million inhabitants (*Table I*). It is the most mountainous country in West Africa with the massifs of Fouta-Djalon in the north (1,100 to 1,300 m) and Nimba in the south (up to 1,700 m). Rainfall varies between 1,500 to over 2,000 mm, depending on the region, throughout a long rainy season from April to November followed by a well-defined winter dry season. Guinea is the water reservoir of West Africa where rivers such as the Senegal and Niger originate.

The climate is typical of the tropical region. The vegetation is mostly dense wooded savannah that opens up on the plateaux. The forest that used to cover the south has been heavily eroded. The epidemiological facies is that of the tropical stratum with marked seasonal differences. Malaria is stable throughout the whole country.

Few in-depth epidemiological studies have been carried out, and the information available is old, often having been collected in simple surveys. Jonchère & Pfister (1951) thought that Guinea was the most malaria-infested country of the ex-Federation of the AOF, with a PR of 88% in children. The smallness of the number of samples, the absence of information regarding the exact sources, and the dubious sampling methods used all limit the validity of the results. In 1963, Eyraud *et al.* established index levels that were much lower and classified Fouta-Djalon as meso-endemic. *An. gambiae* was twenty times more abundant than *An. funestus*. In October (at the end of the rainy season) at the peak transmission period, the number of infectious bites was 0.3 per person per night for *An. gambiae* compared with 0.1 per person per night for *An. funestus*. The number of anophelines per house was less than 1 and the sporozoite rate was under 1% (1/97 *An. gambiae*).

Bosman *et al.* (1992) revisited the slopes of Fouta-Djalon in 1992: PR measurements indicated holo-endemicity in the villages (78%), a lower prevalence in mid-sized towns (45%), and a far lower prevalence still in the big cities (Labé, 16.7%). The differences in altitude were too small to significantly affect epidemiology. A more recent study (Baldet *et al.*, 2001) confirmed the meso-endemic to hyper-endemic status of the disease in twenty-four villages surveyed for the purpose of building a dam on the slopes of the Fouta-Djalon.

Bespiatov *et al.* (1992) proposed dividing the country into five "malariologic" zones according to landscape, in line with Pavlovsky's theories on the relationships between landscape and epidemiology. They thus distinguished the following:
- river, plain and mountain areas where the PR in children between the ages of 2 and 9 varies from 16% to 45%, reaching 63% in certain sites;
- parts of the wet Sudanese-Guinean savannah where malaria is also considered to be meso- or hyper-endemic;
- more or less heavily wooded mountain areas where malaria is meso-endemic;
- the mixed forest/savannah zones of southern Guinea which carry over into northern Sierra Leone, hyper- or holo-endemic in nature with PR readings in children ranging from 76% to 92%.

The entomological information does not amount to much more than a few lists of species: *An. melas* in Konakry (Toumanoff & Simond, 1956), *An. gambiae s.s.*, *An. funestus* and *An. nili* in the hinterland (Adam & Bailly-Choumara, 1964). There is no proof that *An. arabiensis* is present. Reports of the presence of *An. moucheti*—a species of the Central African forest block—are incorrect. Other anopheline species are of no epidemiological interest.

Sierra Leone

Sierra Leone is a small country with an area of 71,746 km^2 located between 7° and 10° north with about 250 km of coastline. There are 5 million people with a population density of 69.7 inhabitants per km^2 (*Table I*).

It is generally flat with some relief to the east where the altitude reaches 500 m (Kabala Region).

The city of Freetown, initially created to host released slaves, was notorious in the 19th century for fever (Carlson, 1984).

In 1899, Ross made the first on-the-ground observations of *An. gambiae* and *An. funestus* being infected with malarial parasites and it was he who, in Freetown, proposed the earliest vector control measures (Ross *et al.*, 1900).

After this, all the top experts in malaria and in entomology filed into Freetown; Macdonald, Ribbands and Muirhead-Thomson, as of 1945, made this city an extremely active research centre. The School of Tropical Medicine of Liverpool set up its African field research station and it was there that all proposed malaria control measures were tested up until 1945 when the arrival of DDT created a new situation. The history of malariology in Freetown has been documented by Bockarie *et al.* in 1999.

The vegetation includes a much degraded great forest (bush forest) that covers the entire southern part of the country, and wooded savannahs (Guinean) in the north and north-east. The climate is tropical with a long rainy season from March to November. Precipitation levels are among the highest in West Africa with between 2,000 and 3,000 mm of rainfall depending on the region.

• *Malaria in the estuary of Freetown*

It was in Freetown that Theobald, in 1902, described the *An. melas* variety not long after *An. gambiae* had been described. This salt water form was considered to be extremely important in coastal malaria but both the differential identification of the two forms and characterisation of their larval habitats were very vague (Terdre, 1946; Walton, 1947).

Muirhead-Thomson (1945 and 1947) clarified the situation. Once it was recognised that the presence of the four white stripes on the palpi was not a reliable criterion for differentiating *An. melas*, he suggested using larval pecten morphology and especially egg ornamentation to identify this anopheline. This represented a long process since the eggs had to be obtained beforehand but it was the only reliable method up until the development of methods based on cytogenetics and molecular biology.

By studying the eggs, Muirhead-Thomson observed that the F1 male hybrids resulting from the mating of *An. melas* with freshwater *An. gambiae* (probably *An. gambiae s.s.*) were sterile. There was thus genetic isolation which means that the two different forms can each be considered as a separate species.

He located *An. melas* larval habitats in the prairies of *Paspalum* and in stands of *Avicennia sp*. The latter are only covered in water when there is a big spring tide although stagnant pools are left once the waters recede. *An. melas* is never found in *Rhizophora sp*. mangrove. In the villages next to mangrove forests, *An. melas* co-habited with *An. gambiae*. The latter species was especially abundant during the rainy season whereas the rhythm of *An. melas* followed a more or less monthly pattern.

He demonstrated that *An. gambiae*, and to a large extent *An. melas*, laid their eggs in larval habitats exposed to sunlight or moonlight. The presence of vegetation (bushes, grass) at a site discouraged egg-laying, a behaviour pattern that explains why *An. gambiae* does not prosper in the undergrowth of the great forest.

Experimentally, he showed that in identical conditions of host exposure, the sporozoite rate of *An. gambiae* (11%) was far higher than that of *An. melas* (4.5%).

These works were extended by the author in Lagos and in Accra, as well as by other entomologists in many other coastal regions in Africa. In addition, Muirhead-Thomson (1945) demonstrated the important vector role of *An. nili* in the hills surrounding Freetown (s = 3%).

• *Transmission in rural zones*

Studies on malaria in rural zones in the forest region of the south—at least those of which the results have been published—were carried out much later on.

In the great forest of the southern Province near the village of Bayama, the "Forest" form of *An. gambiae s.s.* accounted for more than 99% of the anopheline fauna; its daily life expectancy was rated at 0.85. The EIR in this village was 1,235 ib/p/yr (Bockarie *et al.*, 1995) and the sporozoite rate as evaluated by CSP was 3.9% (Bockarie *et al.*, 1993). *An. gambiae* was almost exclusively anthropophilic and it was partly exophilic, at least in the morning after the blood meal. In addition, it did not breed easily in the rice paddies or marshes, preferring rain water pools (Bockarie *et al.*, 1993).

In a multi-disciplinary study in the region of Bo where the forest is somewhat degraded, the "Forest" form of *An. gambiae s.s.* was 10% associated with *An. funestus*. *An. gambiae* presented a sporozoite rate (CSP) of 7.5% while that of *An. funestus* was 11%. Vector density was low with 9.5 *An. gambiae* and 1 *An. funestus* per person per night. The EIR was 32 ib/p/yr for *An. gambiae* and 2.5 for *An. funestus*, amounting to a global figure of 34.5 (Bockarie *et al.*, 1994). It was pointed out that *An. gambiae* and *An. funestus* tend to bite late at night, after local people had gone to bed, so treated mosquito nets provide good protection (Bockarie *et al.*, 1994).

• *Epidemiology*

From the above-mentioned multi-disciplinary study in the Bo Region where rainfall is very high, the following figures are available:
- the mortality rate of new-borns was 74‰ of live births;
- the infant mortality rate was 25‰;
- the overall mortality rate for children of under 5 years of age was 36‰.

Malaria and malnutrition shared the distinction of being the main causes of the infant mortality rate of 27% (Barnish *et al.*, 1993).

In a population of 900 children under the age of 7, Barnish *et al.* (1993) observed a prevalence of 61% of *P. falciparum*, 12% of *P. malariae* and 1% of *P. ovale*. These figures suggest hyperendemicity. The blood gametocyte load was estimated at 1/5th that of asexual forms. Antibody levels (as measured by ELISA and/or IFAT) were very high in all age groups, suggesting early exposure to malaria.

In the rice paddy regions in the forest, Gbakima (1994) reported a malarial prevalence of 42% and thought that increased rice production had led to a rise in the incidence of malaria, an idea that hardly coincides with observations made on vectors. These conclusions were debatable: a comparison made between the malarial prevalence in rice-growing regions and other rural areas did not show any increase.

In the wet savannah Kabala Region in the north and north-east, malaria is hyper- or holo-endemic depending on the village (Bespiatov *et al.*, 1992).

On an academic level, it should be noted that, in an original study focusing on reptile *Plasmodium* (agama) in West Africa (*P. agamae* and *P. giganteum*), infected specimens were found to be losing their sexual competitiveness, were not obtaining as much to eat, and were dominated in the social hierarchy.

Liberia

Liberia is another small country, covering an area of 111,370 km^2 with a population of 2.9 million people (*Table I*). Its coastline spans about 300 km. The country is made up of a large coastal plain that extends in the north into a series of hills which join up with the mountain systems of South Guinea. At the tip is Mount Nimba (1,750 m) which is located where Liberia, Guinea and Ivory Coast all meet.

The climate falls between equatorial (four seasons) and tropical (a single long wet season). Precipitation levels can exceed 2,000 mm in the mountains. Originally, this area was covered in rain forest although this has since been seriously encroached upon with large plantations (hevea) and uncontrolled farming.

The Republic of Liberia was created in 1847 under the influence of American anti-slavery organisations as a host country for freed slaves. The capital city, Monrovia, is named after President Monroe. The country, therefore, has never been directly under colonial power but the large hevea plantations and the mining companies have a *de facto* control over certain regions.

Two local institutions have been very active in the area of malaria, namely the Liberian Medical Institute in Harbel and the Yepeka Centre in the iron-mining country around Mount Nimba. These two have provided most of the information (since 1950 and 1970 respectively).

In the context of the epidemiology of malaria, Liberia is situated at the boundary of the equatorial stratum (where transmission is perennial) and the tropical stratum (where transmission is seasonal, albeit of extended duration).

In the coastal regions near Monrovia where *An. melas* and *An. gambiae s.s.* coexist, the former is much less efficient than the latter as a vector. Their respective sporozoite rates were 1.4% and 5.7% (Gelfand, 1955). *An. gambiae s.s.*, which is particularly abundant during the rains, was responsible for most transmission events (Burgess, 1960); *An. melas*, which peaks during the dry season, was present year-round, depending on the rhythm of the big tides. These observations confirm the findings of Muirhead-Thomson (1957a) in Sierra Leone.

In Harbel, Muirhead-Thomson (1957b) precisely separated vectors infected with *P. falciparum* from those infected with *P. malariae* on the basis of oocyst size. Thirty years later, we were able to separate the different types of parasite in vectors using the ELISA and later, the techniques of molecular biology.

One of the most interesting research projects in Harbel resulted in an evaluation of the human parasite reservoir in a village in which the infectivity of each age group was taken into account (Miller, 1958; Muirhead-Thomson, 1957b). The study was carried out on 347 individuals and showed that 32 of them (i.e. 9.2%) were infectious for laboratory *An. gambiae s.s.*; 28% of the under-5 year-olds were infected, compared with 12% of 5-15 year-olds, and 3.5% of teenagers and adults. Taking the pyramid of ages into account, under-5 year-olds constituted 4.2% of the parasite reservoir, the group of 5-15 years of age 3%, and adults 3.3%. The percentage of the parasite reservoir constituted by the adults was therefore underestimated.

In 1955, when the eradication program was in its early stages, a pilot project based on indoor DDT spraying was launched in Kpain, 150 km north of Monrovia in a forest region (Guttuso, 1962). Given the strict anthropophilic behaviour of the vectors (*An. gambiae s.s.*) and the absence of livestock as an alternative host, the results were excellent. Not only had the level of holo-endemic malaria dropped to 1% but *An. funestus* and then *An. gambiae* disappeared, just as was seen in the pilot zone of Yaoundé in Cameroon, also a forest region (Livadas *et al.*, 1958).

In the northern part of the country around Mount Nimba, the forest is no longer continuous and the landscape is a mixture of forest and savannah. In a small malaria control campaign around the mining city of Yepeka, *An. gambiae s.s.* was the main vector with a sporozoite rate of 9.3%; the anopheline density per house was 3.8 (Hedman *et al.*, 1979). In a second project in the same region, *An. funestus* was the main species, followed by *An. hanckoki* and *An. gambiae s.s.* (Bjorkman *et al.*, 1985). In the holo-endemic villages that surrounded the city of Yepeka, prevalence was exceptionally high: 82% for *P. falciparum*, 39% for *P. malariae* and 9% for *P. ovale*. Around the city, the EIR varied from less than 3 ib/p/yr to more than 60 ib/p/yr.

Investigations into haemoglobinopathies revealed the presence of HbS, HbC, β-thalassaemia and G6PD deficiency (Willcox & Beckman, 1981). In people of ethnic groups from eastern Liberia, HbS and HbC were rare whereas β-thalassaemia was very common. In the ethnic groups from the western part of the country, the inverse was the case. The prevalence of G6PD deficiency among males was 16%. The rate of malaria infection was somewhat lower in "AS heterozygotes" but the difference was insignificant; carriers of a β-thalassaemic mutation were reported to be relatively resistant to *P. falciparum* (Willcox & Beckman, 1981; Willcox *et al.*, 1983) but this still remains to be confirmed.

Children from holo-endemic villages presented significantly lower hematocrits and HbAe levels than those from hypo-endemic villages. This observation is compatible with the hypothesis that iron deficiency is common in people suffering from chronic malaria (Willcox *et al.*, 1985).

Productivity is always an important issue for mining companies. A comparative study of adult subjects administered prophylactic drugs and untreated subjects showed no difference between the two groups (Pehrson *et al.*, 1984). The question of the economic impact of malaria is an open one: everywhere that malaria is stable, such as Liberia, acquired immunity significantly mitigates the impact of infection in adults.

Nations of the northern coastline of the Gulf of Guinea

Five nations are included in this region: Ivory Coast, Ghana, Togo, Benin, and Nigeria. The latter is the most populous country in Africa with 106 million inhabitants over an area of more than 900,000 km². It is gigantic compared with its immediate neighbours, namely Benin (5.8 million people) and Cameroon (13 million people).

In all of these countries south of the 7th parallel north, the climate is equatorial with four distinct seasons. Moving northwards, the dry season between May and July becomes shorter and shorter and the two rainy seasons begin to merge into one.

The equatorial part in the south is (or was) considered to be an area of dense forest while the tropical north is typically covered with woody savannah. This description is not very accurate considering that areas of savannah covered with Borassus in Ivory Coast descend along the Bandama River almost all the way to the sea: this is known as the "V baoulé", a special phytogeographical enclave. Elsewhere, in Togo and in Benin, the savannah descends all the way to the coast creating "the Dahomey Gap", considered to be a genuine biological and geographical frontier that separates West from Central Africa. With reference to parasitic disease, it has been observed that neither the vectors of loiasis (*Chrysops dimidiata* and *Chrysops silacea*) nor of malaria (*An. moucheti*) cross this "Dahomey barrier", and are therefore confined to Central Africa.

The forest has been seriously damaged by both woodcutters and farmers (especially plantation owners). It is progressively being replaced by a mixture of forest and savannah or by grassland. In locating epidemiological studies, it is important to be aware of the local vegetation because, within a matter of kilometres, one can change from a dense forest environment—where malaria may be meso-endemic—to savannah where the disease will be hyperendemic.

Ivory Coast

• *Description*

The Republic of Ivory Coast is located between 5° and 10° north and covers an area of 322,462 km², including 500 km of coastline on the Gulf of Guinea. The population is 17.3 million (*Table I*). During the last century and in particular over the last fifty years, a large number of workers from Burkina Faso have migrated into Ivory Coast taking permanent or temporary residence. These highly active migrant workers weigh heavily on the country's economy and politics.

Four water systems flowing from north to south sub-divide the country: the Cavally River which borders Liberia; the Sassandra; the Bandama; and the Komoé. All drain into the Gulf of Guinea (*Figure 17*).

As mentioned previously, the southern part of Ivory Coast used to be covered with a magnificent forested massif, the jewel of which was the Taï Forest Reserve in the south-

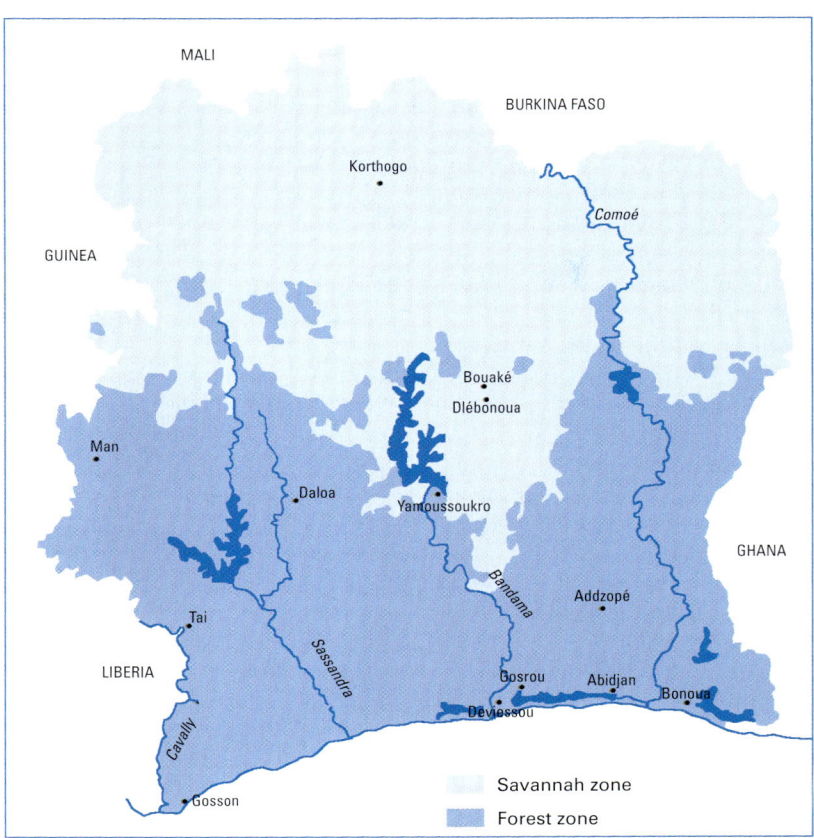

Figure 17. Forest, savannah and waterways in Ivory Coast (adapted from Henry et al., 1998).

west. It is now being transformed into a mosaic of forest and savannah as the forests are being replaced with clearings. All along the Bandama, a Borassus-covered savannah extends all the way to Tiassalé, an area of economic growth. To the north of Bouaké, the Guinean savannah, interspersed with huge stretches of forest, is now a region for cotton growing and food crops.

The difference between the southern forest region and the savannah farms in the north, as in many countries of West Africa, corresponds to more than an ecological divide as people in the south are Christian (with strong animist influences) while most people in the north are Moslem.

• *A long epidemiological history*

Lethal epidemics of yellow fever ravaged the southern part of the Republic of Ivory Coast between 1920 and 1930 until the arrival of a vaccine from the Pasteur Institute of Dakar, which practically wiped out this disease. *Aedes* control measures were so rigorously applied that it was made illegal to grow plants with sheathed leaves such as canas even though these plants are home to only *Aedes simpsoni* larvae, a species which does not bite man in West Africa (as opposed to *A. aegypti*, the public enemy at the time). However, since 1975 small outbreaks have occurred due to lapses in immunisation programmes.

The other scourge which struck African people was sleeping sickness. In order to fight against this terrible endemic disease, mobile teams were created to screen for and treat the disease, and prophylactic drugs were also administered in the so-called "lomidinisation" programme. This treatment was of course very hard but by 1955, most foci had been eliminated. All that remained were a few limited foci, such as in Daloa.

The European fear of "fever", i.e. malaria, was not as frightening as the idea of catching yellow fever. The use of quinine was well accepted and known to be effective and the disease was considered as part of the routine medical landscape—to the extent that it was considered as verging on indecent not to have malaria.

The first general epidemiological study was done by Jonchère & Pfister (1951) who covered six areas. Few blood samples were taken (392 from the whole of Ivory Coast) and the sampling method was not stipulated. Nonetheless, both PRs and SRs were very high, indicating holo-endemic malaria in all the places surveyed, and hyperendemic malaria in the city of Bouaké. Although *P. falciparum* was dominant, the authors recorded a high proportion of *P. malariae*. They reported 1% *P. vivax* (a debatable figure) and *P. ovale* was not mentioned.

The first studies on anopheline vectors were carried out by Holstein (1952), and later studies were conducted by Hamon *et al.* (1956a). They established that *An. gambiae* s.l. and *An. funestus* were present all the time, and in addition that *An. melas* could be found from time to time near the coast. Following sub-classification of the Gambiae Complex, it was *An. gambiae* s.s. that was found throughout most of Ivory Coast. *An. melas* was only found on the coastline. *An. arabiensis* appeared to be absent from the northern part of the country (Dossou-Yovo, personal communication). *An. nili* developed in fast-flowing rivers; *An. carnevalei*, a very similar species that apparently shares habitats with the preceding species, was described in Tiassalé (Brunhes *et al.*, 1999) but we know nothing about the reciprocal roles of these two species.

Beginning in the 1950's, the prospect of being able to control malaria by spraying with long-acting insecticides set off a surge of epidemiological research on malaria. It quickly became evident that the disease was stable in all the sites investigated, whether in the forest or in the wet savannah.

• *Malaria in the southern forest region*

In the **Adzopé Region**, parasitologic surveys revealed PRs of 16% to 52% in subjects under the age of 15, and PRs of 3% to 15% in adults (depending on the season) (Pène & Carrié, 1968).

In the south-western part of the country all along the **lower Sassandra**, the EIR varied from 3.4 ib/p/yr in coastal regions to 1,275 ib/p/yr in relatively degraded forest regions (Coz *et al.*, 1966). According to the authors, the very low EIR in the coastal region was due to the vector being *An. melas*. In contrast, the very high transmission rate in the forest was a result of the combined action of *An. gambiae* s.s. (responsible for two-thirds of transmission events) and *An. funestus* (responsible for one-third) (*Table VII*).

In the **mountainous region of Man**, in the western part of Ivory Coast, more than thirty villages representative of the very diverse ecological features of the region were surveyed twice a year for two years, including evaluations of both entomological and parasitologic parameters (Escudié *et al.*, 1962; Hamon *et al.*, 1962). The vectors were *An. gambiae* and *An. funestus* with *An. nili* found in a few places. The sporozoite rate of both dominant species

Table VII. Parasite rates in Ivory Coast (children of 1-9).					
Southern forest		**Man mountains**		**Wet savannah**	
Adzopé PR: 16-52%	South-western forest PR > 75%	Slopes PR: 43-62%	Mixed land PR: 30-60%	Central savannah PR > 75%	Northern savannah PR: 50-91%
PR: parasite rate in children (0-9)					

was around 1%. The authors categorised the villages into three ecological types (*Table VII*):
- on the mountain slopes, the PR was 43% in January, and 62% in March and September. *An. gambiae* was the only important vector. Malaria was hyper-endemic but in a few very isolated villages, the PR was much lower, suggestive of a hypo-endemic situation;
- in areas where forest and savannah were mixed, *An. gambiae*, backed up by *An. funestus* at the beginning of the dry season, maintained meso- or hyper-endemic disease with PRs of 32% in March and 60% in September;
- in the post-forest savannah lands which are punctuated by projections of forest, both vectors were dense everywhere. The PR, on the order of 75%, indicated holo-endemic disease.

In the **Tomba** Region, to the north of Man and very close to the preceding region, the PR reached 82% and was characteristic of a holo-endemic situation.

As in all the forest areas of Liberia (Guttuso, 1962) and Cameroon (Livadas *et al.*, 1958), it was observed that in Ivory Coast, deforestation created areas with conditions that encouraged the spread of *An. gambiae*, resulting in an increase in the prevalence of malaria. As a result of ongoing deforestation, the level of transmission is continuing to increase as this environmental interference creates heliophilic larval habitats. The EIR, which was measured at 88 in Man (Hamon *et al.*, 1962) and 22 in Sassandra (Coz *et al.*, 1966), had risen to 400 ib/p/yr in the Danané Region (Nzeyimana *et al.*, 2002). "Murder of the forest"—as environmentalists put it—results in an increase in the incidence of malaria.

• *Malaria in the wet savannah*

In the Guinean savannahs of Ivory Coast, malaria is stable as in the preceding facies but transmission is marked by a peak during the rainy season—characteristic of the tropical stratum as defined previously. Transmission occurs year-round but at a lower rate in the dry season.

In the village of Alloukoukro, located in the wet savannah region in the centre of the country, *An. funestus* was responsible for 20% to 30% of malaria transmission with the rest due to *An. gambiae s.s.* (Dossou-Yovo *et al.*, 1995 and 1998c). The biting rate varied from 13 to 20 per day (depending on the season) and *An. funestus* clearly peaked at the end of the rainy season and the beginning of the dry season. In 1991, the EIR was 266 ib/p/yr (204 due to *An. gambiae* and 62 due to *An. funestus*). In 1992, the rate was 196 ib/p/yr (160 *An. gambiae* and 36 *An. funestus*). The PR of pre-school children was over 50% in all places, reaching 91% in certain villages at the end of the rainy season. Indices decreased slightly between the ages of 10 and 14. During the rainy season, peaking in May, the number of episodes of fever (assumed to be malaria) increased sharply (*Table VII*).

• *Bouaké*

Bouaké is a city that has recently expanded. Its administrative and commercial centre dating from 40-50 years ago is surrounded by a series of satellite villages on higher land, often separated by depressions in which rice and other food crops are grown. In this semi-rural environment, the main vector is *An. gambiae s.s.*, the behaviour of which is purely anthropophilic (Dossou-Yovo *et al.*, 1998b). The sporozoite rate of 2% is exceptionally high for an urban area where the EIR varies from 78 to 134 ib/p/yr, depending on the neighbourhood (Dossou-Yovo *et al.*, 1999). For the purposes of comparisons, in Bobo-Dioulasso, a city of the same size in neighbouring Burkina Faso, the EIR ranges from 0.5 to 4.

Therefore, can one really speak of an urban setting in Bouaké? The diversity of these areas within the city centre means that they need to be addressed one by one, taking into account the structure and ecological position of each individually.

In the rice-growing neighbourhoods of the city, the number of bites per person by *An. gambiae* varies according to the phase of rice cultivation. The sporozoite rate ranges from 0.7% to 1% and the EIR ranges from 44 to 50 ib/p/yr. In other words, no different from other neighbourhoods where other food crops are being grown (Dossou-Yovo *et al.*, 1994).

• *Impact of rice farming*

The implantation of farms in the north (the Khorogo Region) greatly increased the density of *An. gambiae s.s.* (x 10) but did not affect either intensity of transmission (150 ib/p/yr) or morbidity (Doannio *et al.*, 2002; Henry *et al.*, 2003).

Rice farming does not, therefore, cause an increase in the incidence of malaria in a stable zone (Carnevale *et al.*, 1999). The molecular form of *An. gambiae* present in the rice paddies area is "S" and not "M" (as it could be expected according to preference in larval ecology), as in neighbouring Burkina Faso. In fact this "S" form possesses the *kdr* gene which confers resistance to DDT and pyrethroids and was selected by large scale use of insecticide for cotton growing.

• *Anopheles gambiae resistance to pyrethroids*

The first time anopheline resistance to pyrethroid-based insecticides was detected was with *An. gambiae s.s.* in Bouaké (Elissa *et al.*, 1993). As mentioned, this resistance (*see the section on* "Malaria Control") is due to the *kdr* (knock-down resistance) gene which affects sodium channels, and was "inherited" from DDT; resistance to this product is determined by the same gene. It has spread throughout a large part of West Africa (Chandre *et al.*, 1999) and the Central African Republic but has not been found, yet, in *An. melas* or *An. arabiensis*, the other species of the complex present in this area. The potential danger of such resistance is mitigated by the fact that pyrethrin owes as much of its efficacy to its repellent activity as to its insecticide activity. In Bouaké, the local *An. gambiae s.s.* have also been shown to be resistant to carbamates, notably propoxur (Chandre *et al.*, 1999; Elissa *et al.*, 1994).

• *Drug resistance*

Initially reported in expatriates by Mahoney (1981) (although at the time he had misgivings), chloroquine resistance is now well established in Ivory Coast (Henry *et al.*, 1996). R3, however, is rare except in the western region occupied by Liberian ex-refugees and in certain plantations where aggressive treatment and prophylaxis measures are implemented (Henry *et al.*, 1998). It seems that only 20-30%, and often less, of patients ever visit health centres. The large majority of people use traditional medicine and self-treatment. The phenomenon of resistance only exacerbates the shunning of formal health centres, and this is associated with a chronic lack of drugs and poor reception of patients by the staff. Rather than mapping new foci of resistance (which is spreading throughout West Africa), the priority today is to find solutions to the problem of community-based treatment.

Several drug trials have been conducted in the university hospitals of Abidjan. There is renewed interest in amodiaquine which, despite resistance in 2% of patients, remains effective against most chloroquine-resistant strains (Adou-Bryn *et al.*, 2000). Sulfadoxine-pyrimethamine was recommended as a second-line drug (Henry *et al.*, 1996) even though cases of resistance to this compound have already been documented.

• *Malaria mortality and morbidity*

One of the only studies undertaken in Ivory Coast was carried out in a district with 240,000 inhabitants in the south-eastern part of the country (Nguessan Diplo *et al.*, 1990). This study focused on the causes of mortality in children of 0-30 months. In one year, a total number of 93 deaths was recorded in this age group, and the causes were as follows: malaria, 21; tetanus, 10; malnutrition, 12; meningitis, 10; diarrhoea, 9; lung disease, 7; obstetric problems and others, 24. This is one of the rare studies in which malaria appears to be the main cause of infant death.

In the region of Danané, four to five attacks per year in children under the age of 2 were observed and between two and three attacks in children between the ages of 2 and 5 (Henry, personal communication).

Ghana

Ghana, formerly known as the Gold Coast, covers an area of 238,500 km^2 with a coastline of about 300 km in length and a population of 22 million (*Table I*). The Akossombo Dam on the Volta led to the creation of a huge artificial lake, Lake Volta which divides the country along a north-south axis that extends over more than 250 km. The slopes are very gentle and none are higher than 500 m. The equatorial, four-season climate of the south gives way to a two-season tropical climate in the north. The great forest that used to cover the south has been cleared for timber and farming and most of the area is now a mixture of forest and savannah, with enclosed savannahs to the west of Lake Volta. To the east of this lake, different types of wooded savannah (bush savannah) and secondary forest extend all the way to the Togo border in the Volta Region. The north is Guinean savannah and in the extreme north, Sudanese savannah. On the southern coast to the east of Takoradi where the cities of Accra and Tena are located is a stretch of coastal savannah with a relatively dry climate (with just 700 mm of rainfall and in the north, about 1,000 mm). Precipitation levels in the north of Ghana have noticeably dropped since 1970 in the context of the Sahelian drought.

• *Malaria in the Accra Region*

The first studies done in Ghana were by Muirhead-Thomson (1954). In a village near Accra, he assessed the size of the parasite reservoir by examining different age groups. Although children between the ages of 5 and 9 constituted the greatest source of infection, adults nevertheless played their part with an infection rate of 7%—which is double that reported later on by the same author in Liberia (Muirhead-Thomson, 1957b).

For almost thirty years, Chinery (1984, 1995) followed urbanisation-dependent changes in the culicine fauna and malaria around Accra. In 1911, 75 culicine species were counted but by 1995, only 28 could be identified. Among those that had "disappeared" was *An. funestus*, which leaves *An. gambiae s.s.* as the only vector apart from *An. arabiensis* and *An. melas* (Appawu *et al.*, 1994).

Even though *An. gambiae s.s.* adapts well to urban settings, especially to polluted surface water, its density was found to decrease as one moved from the city's outskirts towards the city centre, i.e. its distribution was radial. Colbourne & Wright (1955) had noted that the EIR had been 0,1 ib/p/yr in the city centre, 2 or 3 in the intermediate zones and 23 in the suburbs. In the city centre, the PR varied from 32% (1-2 years of age) to 47% (3-7), and in the suburbs, it ranged from 75% (1-2 years) to 89% (3-5). Chinery (1995) observed a very marked decrease in the prevalence of malaria over the last two decades (1980-2000), during which time Bancroftian filariasis had virtually disappeared. He attributed this decrease to the expansion and increasing concentration of people in the city which lowers the life expectancy of exophilic anophelines.

Gardiner *et al.* (1984) compared a group of city residents with country people from outside Accra and observed a PR of 1.7% in the former compared with one of 22% in the latter. Amongst the city people, 40% had no antibodies against *Plasmodium* while fully 97% of the country people did. The "city" effect is thus quite important in Accra.

In a survey of mortality in Accra, Colbourne & Edington (1954) reported an annual death rate due to malaria of 300, most of these being children under the age of 4 (i.e. 9% of infant deaths).

• *Malaria in rural areas*

A series of surveys carried out by Colbourne & Wright (1955) provide a panorama of malaria in the 1950's (*Table VIII*).

Continuing the work done in Accra, Colbourne & Wright (1955) studied two facies typical of the ecology of rural areas (*Table VIII*).

Table VIII. Parasite rates in Ghana between 1950 and 1955 (adapted from Colbourne & Wright, 1955).

	Central Accra					Suburban Accra			
Age	August-September 1952 & 1953		March-April 1954		Age	August-September 1952 & 1953		March-April 1954	
	Examined	PR	Examined	PR		Examined	PR	Examined	PR
0-1	78	11%	40	7%	0-1	149	28%	39	31%
1-2	75	32%	53	8%	1-2	35	89%	49	47%
3-4	77	47%	61	20%	3-4	47	75%	36	61%
5-7	136	43%	39	28%	5-7	211	68%	72	60%
8-10	91	44%	28	29%	8-10	43	67%	13	
11-15	117	44%	30	20%	11-15	41	58%		
Adults	113	26%			Adults	136	24%		

	Bompa - Forest region					Bolgatanga - Northern savannah			
Age	November 1953		February 1954		Age	November 1953		February 1954	
	Examined	PR	Examined	PR		Examined	PR	Examined	PR
0-1	70	67%	53	62%	0-1	46	33%	35	46%
1-2	55	87%	42	83%	1-2	55	69%	35	71%
3-4	41	88%	52	86%	3-4	53	72%	53	87%
5-7	90	86%	52	92%	5-7	102	61%	52	77%
8-10	64	86%	53	70%	8-10	69	42%	50	52%
11-15	76	80%	50	74%	11-15	100	29%	47	28%
Adults M / F	50 / 57	30% / 21%	46	20%	Adults M / F	92 / 147	15% / 20%	36	19%

Examined: number of subjects examined; PR: parasite rate

In the **forest** of the **Ashanti Region**, *An. gambiae s.s.* (notably the "Forest" form) was the main vector (Appawu *et al.*, 1994), accounting for 95% of the samples taken from humans and in homes. All of the other species put together—*An. funestus, An. nili* and *An. hargreavesi*—accounted for only 5% of the samples collected. In *An. gambiae* and *An. funestus*, sporozoite rates were over 15% and 11% respectively. The EIR was 24 ib/p/yr, i.e. quite low for a holo-endemic region where PRs were greater than 80% in children between the ages of 2 and 10. A more recent study conducted by Browne *et al.* (2000) reported identical PIs of 49% and 50% in both degraded forest and savannah.

In the **savannahs of the north** (Navrongo Region) where the climate is tropical, the vectors were *An. gambiae* and *An. funestus*, with sporozoite rates of 25% and 7% respectively—obviously too high for a population in equilibrium. 85% of the *An. gambiae s.l.* were *An. gambiae s.s.*, mainly the "Savanna" form which is also dominant in the coastal savannahs; the other 15% were *An. arabiensis*. The EIR was only 26 ib/p/yr which is very low compared to the corresponding rate in neighbouring Burkina Faso where malaria was holo-endemic with a PR of over 80% in children between the ages of 2 and 10.

Colbourne & Wright (1955) have pointed out inconsistencies in the PR-based classification systems proposed by WHO (*see the Chapter on "Epidemiological Basis"*).

• *Lake Volta and the Volta Region*

Lake Volta is an immense body of water and its epidemiological importance has to be taken into consideration. For example, schistosomiasis has become well established around the lake whereas this disease is rare or non-existent in the forest regions. Very little has been said about the impact of the lake on the incidence of malaria and this for good reason: malaria used to be holo-endemic and stable in all areas around the lake and the situation of the local people has not really changed, as might have been expected. Recommended control measures have always been somewhat vague.

In the **Volta Region**, a **malaria eradication pilot zone** was launched in 1962 (WHO/Mal/Eradic./Pilot/Project/

Ghana I, 1962). This was centred around the city of Ho and targeted an area containing 770,000 inhabitants which stretched all the way to the coast. In 1968 (Rickman, 1968), the work seemed to have hardly gone beyond the preparatory phase. In 1969, WHO changed its policy and the project was closed. The region has coastal savannahs in the south with bush savannah in the north the vectors were *An. gambiae*, *An. funestus*, *An. nili* and *An. hargreavesi*, with respective sporozoite rates of 12%, 10% and 5.5%. Only one *An. hargreavesi* was found to be infected. The PR was between 70% and 89% in children between the ages of 4 and 9, so the region was classified as holo-endemic.

In 1986 and 1987 in the **Central Region**, malaria appeared to be meso-endemic (Afari *et al.*, 1993) with PRs of between 19% and 33% during the dry season, and between 33% and 44% during the rains. Parasite loads of over 3,200 per mm^3 were counted on 30-45% of the positive slides; of the infected children, 7-24% had a parasite load of over 25,600 per mm3.

In retrospect, it appears that counts in the 1950's and 1960's were higher than those recently recorded, possibly because of current self-treatment with chloroquine.

• *Diagnosis and clinical incidence*

New molecular techniques (notably PCR) that can detect very low-level parasitaemia have changed epidemiological pictures in that very low-level infection may not be detected using a microscope-based method, e.g. PR went from 37% to 62% when a PCR-based assay was introduced. The consequences of such low-level infection are poorly understood but it is possible that it could induce some degree of anaemia (Mockenhaupt *et al.*, 2000).

In infants under the age of 6 months, the incidence of malaria is very low, so they must be protected in some way although no specific mechanisms are clearly understood. Nevertheless, episodes of fever with parasite loads of 100 per mm^3 have been observed. The clinical incidence in children under the age of 6 months is thus 0.09 per child/year, increasing to 0.4 between 6 months and 1 year, and to 0.69 between 12 and 23 months; out of sixty-six cases, only three involved babies under the age of 5 months. After the age of 2, the PR reaches 89% (McGuinness *et al.*, 1998)

For a long time it was believed that babies were protected during the first six months of life because of the passive transfer of maternal antibodies, the presence of foetal haemoglobin and, possibly, cytokine production. Studying antibody responses to primary infection, Biggar *et al.* (1980) observed that seroconversion never occurred before the age of five months and was not associated with any symptoms and, more recently, Riley *et al.* (2000) questioned the role of maternal antibodies. So, the mechanisms which protect babies up till the age of six months remain unclear.

• *Control measures*

Here, we do not intend to review all the various control measures implemented apart from mentioning the fact that the large scale use of mosquito nets treated with permethrin between 1993 and 1995 led to a decrease of 17% in the overall mortality in children of between 6 months and 4 years of age (Binka *et al.*, 1996). In addition, the mosquito nets afforded bystander protection to those sleeping close by who did not even have a net (Binka *et al.*, 1998).

Togo

The country of Togo covers an area of 56,800 km^2 with a population of 5.4 million people (*Table I*). Located between the 6th and 11th parallels, it consists of a 100-200 km-wide strip between the eastern border of Ghana and Benin. The

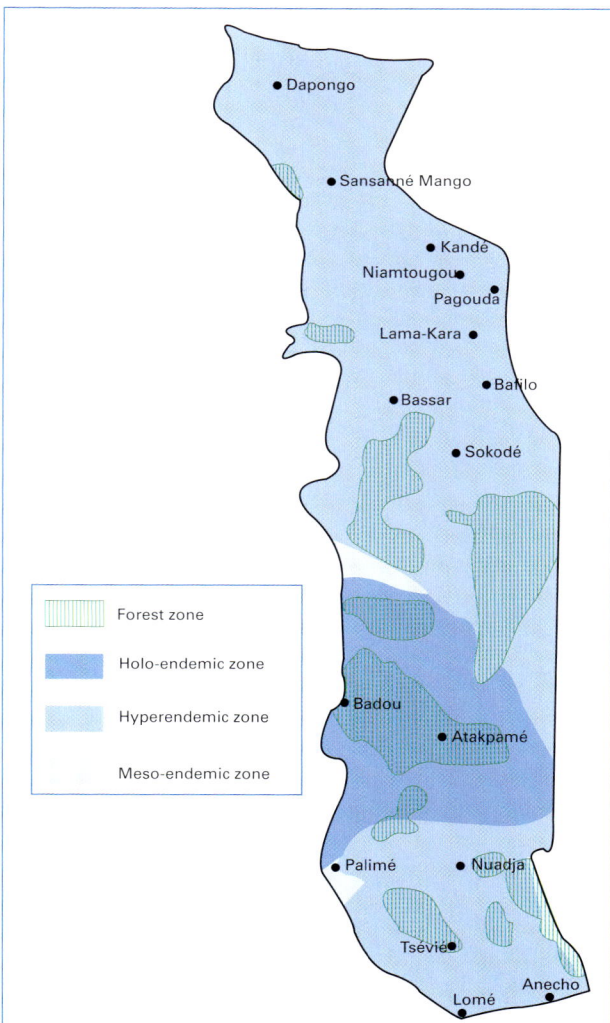

Figure 18. Epidemiological map of Togo (adapted from d'Almeida, 1966).

climate is similar to that of Ghana. Forest (highly degraded) is confined to the western part of the Palimé Region between the 7th and 8th parallels and the rest of the country is covered with different types of savannah that extend all the way to the ocean. Togo and Benin, thus, make up a gap in the forest belt of West Africa which is known as the "Dahomey Gap", as mentioned above.

- *Malaria*

The first global study available was conducted by d'Almeida (1966). He considered that the malaria was stable and hyperendemic throughout the country as a whole with one holo-endemic area between parallels 7.2 and 8 (*Figure 18*). The PRs measured in young children in the northern part of the country varied between 74% and 89%: more than 95% of the parasites were *P. falciparum* with 15% of *P. malariae* (mostly mixed infections). Splenic indices were greater than 80% although they dropped to below 15-20% in adults, indicating holo-endemic disease. The vectors were *An. gambiae s.l.* and *An. funestus* which were infected year-round, thus guaranteeing perennial transmission.

Togo, a former mandatory territory, has benefited from an enormous amount of international expertise and several control projects have been implemented in the country. In the experimental zone of Anecho on the coast, the malaria was hyper- or holo-endemic. In the wooded region of Palimé, the malaria was in between meso- and hyper-endemic with a PR of 50% in pre-school aged children (Bakri & Noguer, 1977). In this last region, a project was undertaken to test the possibility of eliminating *An. funestus* with only one annual treatment of DDT. The goal was achieved but transmission by DDT-resistant *An. gambiae* continued and malarial indicators remained high.

- *Malaria and nutrition*

In a placebo-controlled trial conducted in the southern part of Togo, iron supplements provided to young children did not affect either parasite load or antibody levels (Chippaux *et al.*, 1991c). In addition, Berger *et al.* (2000) concluded that this same type of supplementation had no effect on infection rates, in particular malaria, which confirmed conclusions made by McGregor & Smith (1952) thirty years previously in Gambia.

Benin

Benin (formerly Dahomey) extends 730 km from the Gulf of Guinea in the south to the Niger River in the north between parallels 6.2 and 12.2, spanning 400 km from east to west. The country covers an area of 112,600 km^2 and has a population of 7.6 million with a density of 67.5 per km^2 (*Table I*).

Benin is a flat country that mostly lies below 500 m apart from, in the north-west, the beginning of the Atakora Chain which is no higher than 1,000 m. The climate varies with four seasons in the south, and a more tropical rhythm in the central and northern parts with one dry season and one rainy season. Rainfall varies enormously from year to year but ranges from 1,200 mm in the south to 800 mm in the north.

The coast is lined with a sandbar creating a series of enclosed lagoons with mangroves. Several types of savannah, wooded and then shrubby, succeed one another from south to north and eventually, as in Togo, break into the West African forest strip. Wooded areas are never more than forest galleries or coppices, especially in the Atakora Mountains.

- *Vectors and transmission*

Since the articles of Hamon *et al.* (1956b), no comprehensive surveys of the anophelines of Benin have been published. The authors noted *An. gambiae* (distinguished from *An. melas* before the reclassification of the complex), *An. funestus*, and *An. nili* at high density after the rains. *An. pharoensis* and *An. hargreavesi* remained secondary vectors.

Beginning in 1975, the majority of entomological and epidemiological studies were conducted in the coastal lagoon areas around Cotonou, the economic capital, and Porto-Novo, the administrative capital.

The distributions of *An. gambiae s.s.* and *An. melas*, and their respective roles in malaria transmission, have been studied in various different coastal sites (Akogbeto *et al.*, 1992b; Akogbeto & Romano, 1999). In the northern suburbs of Cotonou along Lake Nokoué, *An. gambiae s.s.* represented 90% of the anophelines collected. Its sporozoite rate varied from 2-3% (3-4% by CSP) (*Table IX*). In the villages to the north and east of Lake Nokoué, *An. melas*

Table IX. Sporozoite rates (s) and CSP rates in seven sites in the lagoon region of Benin.

Zone and region	Site	An. melas		An. gambiae s.s.	
		s	CSP	s	CSP
Cotonou	Ladji	0	0	2	4
	Filadji	0	0	3	3
Lake Nokoué	Ketonou	0.4	0.8	1.6	0
	Ganvie	0.5	1.9	0.5	3.5
	Agbalilame	0.4	0.6	0	4
Grand Popo and Ouidah	Heve	0	0	0.5	5.9
	Djebadji	0	5	1.6	4.1

accounted for 90% of the anophelines but nevertheless, *An. gambiae s.s.* was responsible for most of the transmission. The same was true in the villages near Ouidah and Grand Popo where similar numbers of *An. melas* and *An. gambiae s.s.* were observed.

The lakeside village of Ganvié is of special interest, not so much for its great tourist appeal but by virtue of the complete absence of livestock (Akogbeto, 1995). The sporozoite rate of *An. melas* was 0.5% (1.9% by CSP), of the same order as that of *An. gambiae s.s.* (s = 0.5%, CSP = 3.5%). Transmission was low between March and August on this lake that is subject to flooding, leading to lowered salinity levels and increased percentages of *An. gambiae s.s.* In this village, the EIR was only 33 ib/p/yr, lower than the values recorded in other lagoon sites in Benin and in the city of Cotonou. This could be due to the traditional widespread use of mosquito nets.

In Cotonou, the lagoon was filled in order to allow expansion of the city to the north; this led to *An. melas* being replaced by *An. gambiae*, and increased transmission (Coluzzi, 1993). Therefore, there is more malaria in the city than in the surrounding villages, which is unusual in Africa (Akogbeto, 2000). In the central and northern neighbourhoods, the EIR varied from 29 ib/p/yr to 46 ib/p/yr (depending on the methods used) (Akogbeto *et al.*, 1992a) with transmission highest during the two rainy seasons. In the fishing villages along the beach where the sand is not conducive to the creation of larval habitats, the EIR was only 5 ib/p/yr. The city of Cotonou provides an example of "epidemiological polymorphism" within the same agglomeration.

- *Epidemiology*

In Cotonou, the threshold parasitaemia used to diagnose a malaria attack falls between 3,000 and 6,000 parasites per mm^3 in children and under 1,000 in adults (Chippaux *et al.*, 1991a). In two neighbourhoods that are slightly outside the city centre, PRs ranged from 34-67% where *An. gambiae s.s.* was the only vector, and from 42-70% in a neighbourhood where *An. melas* was dominant. In other words, the parasitologic picture was identical in different places if the indicator used was the PR.

Malaria had been diagnosed in 31.6% of all the patients who visited one of the city clinics: 5% during the dry season and 60% during the rainy season (Chippaux *et al.*, 1991b). A study carried out in the Department of Paediatrics (Boulard *et al.*, 1990) concluded that malaria was responsible for 20% of consultations. The most affected (44%) were infants between the ages of 6 and 23 months. The number of feverish attacks in young children was estimated to be 2.4 per subject per year, of which 33% would be caused by malaria (Velema *et al.*, 1991). The number of attacks peaked in April and in August during the rains. These authors estimated the mortality rate caused by malaria to be 8 ‰ per year. Transplacental transmission of *P. falciparum* was shown in three out of fifty-four children that were being followed in a population of mothers and children and the parasitaemia was under 300 per mm^3. Half of the mothers were infected and parasites were detected in all of the placentas (Chippaux *et al.*, 1991d).

A comparison of subjects with sickle cell trait and those with normal haemoglobin showed a similar parasitic prevalence in both groups but *P. falciparum* densities were significantly lower in HbAS heterozygotes (Chippaux *et al.*, 1992b). Malaria was diagnosed more frequently in those with the HbAA phenotype than in the HbAS population. Finally, malaria mortality associated with severe attacks was 3% in the HbAA population compared with zero in the HbAS population, a pattern which supports the idea that the heterozygous state protects against severe malaria (Chippaux *et al.*, 1992a).

Nigeria

Nigeria is a Federal Republic of 19 States covering an area of 923,768 km^2 (*Figure 19*). It is the most populous country in Africa with 131.5 million people and a population density of 142.4 per km^2 (*Table I*). The country has seen remarkable population growth, from 19 million in 1931 to 24 million in 1948, 57 million in 1975, and 106 million by 1998 (Anonymous *L'État du Monde*, 1999a), i.e. a more than 5.5-fold increase in less than 70 years. Omnipresent hyper- or holo-endemic malaria—only controlled in places and that on an irregular basis—has not slowed down the population boom. Given the way the country has evolved, questions could be asked about the real impact malaria actually has on demographics.

The relief in the southern part of the country never rises above 300 m and the northern part is between 300 and 600 m with two mountain systems, the Bauchi Plateau (maximum altitude 1,800 m) to the north of the Benue River and the eastern mountains (2,300 m) in the south.

Rainfall ranges from 3,500 mm in the south-east to less than 685 in Maiduguri in the north-east. The rains are spread over two wet seasons in the south, and only one in the north. In the south-east, there is no longer any summer dry season between two rainy seasons.

The mangroves along the coastline reach inland a distance of between 2 and 90 km (in the Niger Delta). The mangroves give way to rain forest or degraded forest for a stretch of 80 to 160 km. In the northern part of the country where rainfall is lower, there are various types of savannah—Guinean, Sudanese or Sahelian. The population boom has led to a considerable environmental damage over the last fifty years.

The Niger River is the main waterway and enters the country in the north-west flowing 800 km to finish in an enormous delta at Port Harcourt. Its main tributary is the Benue River that flows in from northern Cameroon. The Cross River is the other large river from the south-west. The tributaries of Lake Chad in the north-east are almost all temporary except for the Komadougou which can flow year-round.

The climatic differences between north and south are reflected at both the ethnic and economic levels. The north is populated by the Haoussas and the Foulani who are Muslim, and the south by the Yoruba, Ibos, and other smaller ethnic groups who are for the most part Christian. The crops in the north are millet, sorghum and peanuts whereas, in the south, the main crops are cocoa beans, bananas, yams, and various other food crops. Since 1960, Nigeria's main source of revenue has been oil which is found in the south and in the sea (offshore). In 1931, 90% of the population were rural while today, 42% live in cities. It is a country that is undergoing massive socio-economic changes.

• *Demographics*

In Lagos, the overall mortality rate dropped from 25 ‰ to 13 ‰ in just one quarter of a century and the birth rate increased from 29 ‰ to 51 ‰ over the same period. Infant mortality (under 5 years) went from 238 ‰ to 105 ‰. In Katsinda, in the far north, the rate of infant mortality dropped from 412 ‰ in 1928 to 173 ‰ in 1946.

In 1998, the rate of infant mortality for the entire country was still 80 ‰ and the average life expectancy was 50 years. There were 0.18 doctors for every thousand people, the highest percentage in all of West Africa (Anonymous *L'État du Monde*, 1999a).

• *Vectors and general characteristics of malaria*

Most of the entomological, parasitological and epidemiological information was collected through numerous malaria control programs.

The first list of anopheline vectors (Barber & Olinger, 1931) created some confusion about the very hypothetical role of several "secondary vectors". For example, *An. obscurus* and *An. rufipes*, which do not bite people, were incorrectly classified as vectors and used without discernment by several experts.

Bruce-Chwatt (1951) had reported that *An. melas* was more or less the only anopheline found in the mangroves, and *An. gambiae* as well as *An. funestus* were said to be present throughout the entire country with sporozoite rates of 5.8% and 4.9% respectively. The presence of *An. nili* was noted in the south and on the Bauchi plateau. *An. flavicosta* was found in some parts of the north, and *An. hargreavesi* in some parts in the south (Gillies & de Meillon, 1968). *An. moucheti nigeriensis* is a form that is taxonomically poorly defined and of no epidemiological interest.

Demonstration of the *An. gambiae* Complex meant that the distribution of these taxa had to be revised. A broad strip that is home to both *An. gambiae s.s.* and *An. arabiensis* was identified in the northern part of Nigeria. The former species was dominant during the rainy season while the latter was dominant during the dry season, as is true throughout all of West Africa (Rishikesh *et al.*, 1985; White & Rosen, 1973). Surprisingly, however, populations of *An. arabiensis* developed in certain urban centres in the

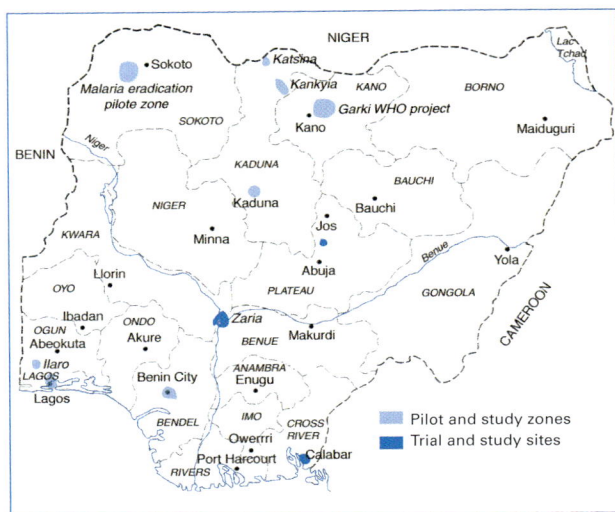

Figure 19.
Malarial research projects in Nigeria.

southern forest region (Benin City) without spreading to the surrounding rural areas (Coluzzi *et al.*, 1979).

Bruce-Chwatt (1951) pointed out the hyperendemic nature of malaria between the coastline and the 245 mm isohyet (during the dry season), but he also noted the presence of hyperendemic foci in Katsina in the far north. There were no malaria epidemics in the Sahelian zone. Splenic indices ranged between 65% and 80% in the south and between 50% and 60% in the north, with peaks of more than 70% at the end of the rainy season. The PR in children was higher in the north than in the south with a range of 15-50% for babies of 6-12 months, 65-90% for 2-10 year-olds, 20-50% for adolescents, and 11-28% for adults.

The proportion of parasites has hardly changed in the last 50 years. In 95% of cases, *P. falciparum* is the dominant species, followed by *P. malariae* (often associated with the former) in 5% to 25% of the cases, and *P. ovale* in less than 1% of the cases. *P. vivax* was considered to be rare (less than 0.5%) even before its actual presence was questioned.

• *Southern Nigeria*

In the Lagos Region, Muirhead-Thomson (1947) focused on the mangrove vectors, continuing the work he had started in Sierra Leone and in Liberia in order to define *An. melas* biotopes in *Paspalum* and *Avicennia* mangroves (excluding stands of *Rhizophora*). He proposed draining the mangroves for malaria control.

The preliminary studies at Ilaro in the south-west indicated that transmission by *An. gambiae* and, in particular, *An. funestus* was perennial. The PR was 33% in babies and 78% in children (Bruce-Chwatt *et al.*, 1955).

In Sapele in the State of Bendel in the Niger Delta, transmission gradually decreased moving from the countryside towards the city centre with the number of infectious bites dropping from 28 ib/p/yr in the forest to 1 ib/p every three years in the city centre (Smith, 1980 *in* Zahar, 1985a). In a forest village in Ologo, the EIR was only 18 ib/p/yr, which is relatively low. Cardenas (1980 *in* Zahar, 1985a) believed malaria to be meso-endemic in urban settings and hyperendemic in rural settings.

In the same State, around Benin City in an area of degraded forest and savannah, the EIR was 63 ib/p/yr for *An. gambiae s.s.* and 31 ib/p/yr for *An. funestus*, i.e. 94 ib/p/yr altogether; transmission was perennial (Payne, 1980 *in* Zahar, 1985a). In the rain forest surrounding Benin City, the PR for children between the ages of 5 and 15 was 64% while it was only 8% in the city (Cardenas, 1980 *in* Zahar, 1985a). In Ibandan in the State of Oyo (*Figure 19*), the PR was 8% in the city as opposed to 23% in the rural suburbs (Ademowo *et al.*, 1995). In the city, only *P. falciparum* was found whereas in the countryside, 20% of the anophelines had *P. malariae*.

Malaria mortality and morbidity have been studied since 1930 in Lagos and the results of these studies are discussed in the Chapter "Man Facing Malaria".

More recently, in the State of Cross River, malaria was considered to be responsible for 29% of infant mortality (children under 5 years), followed by malnutrition, diarrhoea and lung disease (11% each respectively) (Ekanem *et al.*, 1994). This survey, which was based on interviews conducted by community health workers, comes under the oral reports discussed in the Chapter "Man FacingMalaria".

• *Northern savannahs*

The first pilot malaria control project in northern Nigeria was carried out in western Sokoto, from 1954 to 1964 (Bruce-Chwatt & Archibald, 1958; Dodge, 1965), in a region of hyper- or holo-endemic malaria. This project, along with the pilot programmes in Bobo-Dioulasso in Burkina Faso (Choumara *et al.*, 1959) and Maroua in Cameroon (Cavalié & Mouchet, 1961), had a great impact on WHO malaria control policy. This was because they showed how difficult it was to stop malaria transmission in the West African wet savannah by indoor spraying only; in fact, they provided the first indicators of the problems that eventually led to the abandonment of the Global Malaria Eradication Programme. It was in Sokoto in 1955 that the first dieldrin-resistant *An. gambiae* were observed, a resistance which rapidly spread throughout West Africa where this highly effective insecticide is now useless. Also, during the same period in Sokoto, *P. falciparum* resistance to pyrime-thamine was observed.

Several insecticides in combination with various prophylactic regimens were tested in the hope of blocking transmission: dichlorvos in Kankyia (Foll *et al.*, 1965), fenitrothion in Kaduna, and propoxur in Garki (Molineaux & Gramiccia, 1980). Not one provided a solution to the problem. Another project to be added to this list is the study of endemic diseases in Malumfashi (the Plateau State) which was intended to look simultaneously at a range of different health problems (Williamson & Gilles, 1978).

The following entomological points can be concluded from the results of these studies:
- that the Gambiae Complex is omnipresent and a balance exists between *An. gambiae s.s.* and *An. arabiensis*, as pointed out above. In addition, Coluzzi *et al.* (1979) identified the polymorphism of the two species and how the differences correlate with behaviour patterns, particularly endophilic behaviour (in Garki). Furthermore, they demonstrated, on the ground, that the two species are both present throughout the dry season;
- that *An. funestus* is also ubiquitous. Since 1970, with the drought of the Sahel, it has practically disappeared from neighbouring Niger (Julvez *et al.*, 1998). We could not find any information about its current status in Nigeria;
- that *An. nili* is abundant in places in the region of Kaduna;
- the sporozoite rates of *An. gambiae* and *An. funestus* are greater than 5%; 0.8% for *An. nili*, and 2.7% for *An. flavicosta*, which is very much a secondary vector (Service, 1963);
- in Kankyia, Garrett-Jones & Shidrawi (1969) finalised the use of Vectorial Capacity to measure transmission which led Najera (1974) to make very pertinent remarks on the difficulty of using mathematical models in epidemiology; **such models** may be **explanatory** but they are **not predictive**.

In terms of transmission:
- in Garki, the pre-treatment EIR was 145 ib/p/yr, of which 138 were inflicted during the rainy season; 89 (61%) were by *An. gambiae s.l.* and 56 (39%) by *An. funestus* (Molineaux & Gramiccia, 1980). In Kaduna, the EIR was 146 ib/p/yr, of which 101 (69%) were by *An. gambiae* while 45 (31%) were by *An. funestus* (Service, 1965);
- the stability index in Garki amounted to 4.27 for *An. gambiae* and 3.26 for *An. funestus*. Malaria there should therefore be considered highly stable;
- the daily survival rate for the two species ranged from 89% to 90%.

Parasite rates:
- in Garki, the PRs of 79% and 83% in two villages suggested holo-endemic disease, a status which applies to most of villages in northern Nigeria;
- concomitant *P. falciparum* and *P. malariae* infection is more common than infection with *P. malariae* alone. Those with a heavy *P. falciparum* load were more likely to be co-infected with *P. malariae* than those with low-level infection. There were also seasonal fluctuations in the prevalence of the two parasites (Molineaux *et al.*, 1980);
- in all the studies, it should be noted that the results are dependent on the microscopists' skills and the sampling methods, and different teams might obtain highly divergent results in the same village. In addition, should the PR results reported by different authors not be accorded relative reliability weightings? (*see the Chapter on* "Epidemiological Basis").

• *Clinical research*

Various clinical research projects instituted to evaluate malarial morbidity and mortality were discussed above. After 1975, this research constituted an essential part of the activities of several universities and foreign aid organisations. The literature contains more than 200 articles about drug resistance and clinical trials of new drugs: we will restrict this discussion to those works that have a bearing on our concerns.

In Lagos, the trans-placental rate of infection in new-born babies was between 2% and 3%. In babies, the PR reached 20% at the end of the second trimester of their lives, and then rose to 60-70% during the third and fourth trimesters, and up to 80% during the second year (Bruce-Chwatt, 1952). Most primary infections, therefore, occurred after 5 months of age.

In Calabar (State of Cross River), three quarters of the convulsive attacks reported were caused by malaria and 33% were associated with cerebral malaria (Asindi *et al.*, 1993). Anaemia in children in the southern part of Nigeria is more frequently due to malnutrition than to malaria (Azubuike *et al.*, 1977). Although the severity of the anaemia could be linked to the number of plasmodial species carried, the number of *P. falciparum* clones involved (May *et al.*, 1999) and the overall parasite load. In Zaria (State of Benue), the correlation between anaemia and malaria is very weak (Isah *et al.*, 1985).

The nephrotic syndrome which is associated with *P. malariae* infection is caused by an immune complex that once established, is perpetuated (although the mechanisms involved are poorly understood). The prognosis is generally poor (Abdurranan *et al.*, 1981; Hendrickse, 1976; Hendrickse & Adeninyi, 1979). The parasitic pathogenesis of this syndrome as well as the possible causal role played by quinine treatment have been questioned in the Democratic Republic of Congo (Delacollette *et al.*, 1995; Pakasa *et al.*, 1993) and in Malawi, it has been suggested that mercury-based ointments used to lighten the skin are to blame (Brown *et al.*, 1977).

According to Ibadin *et al.* (2000), the correlation between serious diarrhoea and malaria is very high whereas according to Sodeindre *et al.* (1997), there is no relationship at all between the two pathologies.

Research on haemoglobinopathies confirms certain classic concepts. Whereas sickle cell trait is found in 24% of new-born babies, it is found in 28% of 5 year-old children, suggesting that carriers of the trait are more likely to survive this dangerous period (Fleming *et al.*, 1979). In Garki (Molineaux *et al.*, 1979), HbAS heterozygotes seemed to have some degree of protection against the more severe forms of malaria. Haemoglobin C has no protective effect (Storey *et al.*, 1979) and α-thalassaemia (which is very common) causes low-level anaemia without any bearing on malaria (Mockenhaupt *et al.*, 1999). Using PCR, sub-microscopic infections (< 100 parasites per mm^3) can be detected, although these do not appear to have much epidemiological significance (May *et al.*, 1999).

The very high polymorphism in *P. falciparum* was confirmed in Nigeria by analysis of the *msp2* (merozoite surface protein) gene. Each subject tested was carrying an average of four to five different clones (Engelbrecht *et al.*, 2000).

Sahelian States

General characteristics of the Sahelian States

The four countries that constitute the Sahelian States (Mali, Burkina Faso, Niger and Chad) are highly variable from a geographical perspective as they extend from the Sudanese savannahs in the south (8th-9th parallels) all the way to the Sahara Desert (24th parallel). The only country that does not touch the desert is Burkina Faso. In addition, none have any coastline; this puts them at a serious economic disadvantage.

The decrease in rainfall from the south (1,200 mm) to the north (less than 50 mm) is reflected in the stratification of the flora. On the eco-climatic map of Mali (*Figure 20*), six distinct zones of vegetation are defined: Guinean savannah (a mixture of wooded savannahs and sparsely wooded forests) in the extreme south; wooded savannah in the Sudanese area; wooded or shrubby savannah (or steppe according to the botanical definitions) in the Sahelian Region; thorny steppe in the Sahelo-Saharan area; and the desert where vegetation is confined to oases. To this should also be included the distinctive flood zones of the inland Niger Delta in Mali and of the Logone-Chari in Chad.

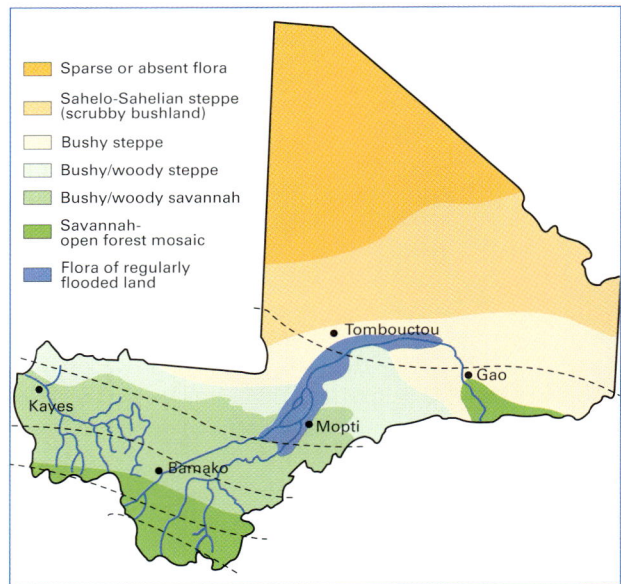

Figure 20. Ecoclimatic map of Mali (adapted from Bissan, 1982).

Since 1970, severe successive droughts have shrunk Lake Chad by two-thirds which has seriously perturbed the balance of both flora and fauna.

On top of this stratification of vegetation, we can superimpose a stratification of endemic malaria that is defined in terms of tropical, Sahelian, Sahelo-Saharan, and desert epidemiological facies (Mouchet et al., 1993) (see above).

Mali

Although the country covers an area of 1,240,000 km^2, Mali only has 11.4 million inhabitants, corresponding to an overall population density of just 9.2 per km^2; more than half of the country is desert (*Table I*). The population is made up of several ethnic groups of Sudanese origin: Bambaras, Dogons, Sonhrais, Peuhls and, more recently, Mossis and Haoussas. The Moors and Tuareg occupy the desert.

Mali is a flat country that lies between 200 and 400 m in altitude. The only hills are the Mandingues Mountains in the west, the foothills of Fouta Djalon, the mountains of Douentza and Hombori in the Niger loop (that rise up to 1,050 m), and the Adrar des Iforas in the Saharan north (which reach about 1,000 m). None of these mountains are high enough to entail any major climatic variation.

The Niger River, which crosses Mali from west to east covering a distance of more than 1,500 km, is the country's lifeline along which long ago the African empires of Mali, Macina and Songhaï were built. The immense inland delta helps mitigate climatic extremes but first and foremost, it provides a fishing resource. From Mopti, dried and smoked fish is exported to all of West Africa. The Office du Niger has developed extensive but underexploited irrigation systems, notably for rice-growing (*Figure 20*).

The drought that has reigned since 1970 has affected Mali to a great extent, reducing fish stocks as well as degrading grazing land in the Sahelo-Saharan and north-Sahelian zones. It has also caused the southward migration of large numbers of people who were previously at little risk of contracting malaria.

• *Epidemiology of malaria*

In Mali, in the Sudanese Zone (between 700 mm and 1,500 mm of rainfall), malaria is hyper- or holo-endemic. Although lower during the dry season, transmission continues year-round (Chabasse et al., 1980). The Sahelian zone is very heterogeneous and is fragmented by the bodies of water of the inland Niger Delta. In the irrigated zones of the southern part of the delta, in the Ségou Region, PRs of 55% during the dry season and 58% during the rainy season were recorded in school children between the ages of 8 and 14 (Maiga et al., 1989a). However, parasite densities were very low with 78% of positive subjects carrying less than 100 parasites per mm^3 of blood. The situation was completely different in the northern part of the delta. In the Diré Circle, south of Timbuktu, Doumbo et al. (1989) measured PRs of 5% on the river banks,

14% around swamps, and 10% far away from bodies of water. This hypo-endemic malaria contrasted greatly with the hyperendemic situation observed in the southern part of the delta, as well as with those meso- or hyperendemic situations observed outside of the flood zones. In the Diré circle, *An. funestus* (< 5%) and *An. arabiensis* (confined to Peuhl encampments) are relatively rare while the "Mopti" form of *An. gambiae s.s.* was found almost everywhere.

At the same latitude, outside of the flood zone, PRs were much higher, indicating hyperendemicity: 66% in Kolokani and 72% in Nara near the border with Mauritania (Doumbo et al., 1989).

In the region of Gourma in the extreme northern part of the Sahelian Zone in the Niger loop, malaria seemed to be meso-endemic with PRs varying from 40% in new-born babies to 20% in adults, whether in the villages or in nomads' camps (Doumbo et al., 1989; Maiga et al., 1989b).

Compared with other desert regions, the Sahara of Mali has been relatively well-studied, notably in the context of a survey carried out prior to the construction of a new Trans-Saharan road in 1988, or during the epidemic that swept through Kidal in 1999. All along the Trans-Saharan transect as far as Tessalit, Doumbo et al. (1991), as well as Koita (1988), recorded a PR of only 1.5% in 2,180 samples (not including Douenza which is not Saharan). The only parasite found was *P. falciparum* and only one case of *P. vivax* was observed and that in a light-skinned little girl. This study was conducted in a particularly "wet" year (with fully 165 mm of precipitation recorded in Tessalit!). It should be noted that there was an almost complete absence of immunity in the population, as would be expected. Entomological investigations revealed low levels of *An. arabiensis* and especially *An. gambiae s.s.*, "Mopti" form, which had never before been found north of the Niger loop.

An epidemic in the Adrar des Iforas, mostly affecting the areas surrounding Kidal and Tessalit, as well as Peulh and Tuareg encampments, raged between July and September 1999 during the rainy season. Records showed 92 cases in July, 112 cases in August, 2,938 cases in September at the peak of the epidemic, and 313 cases from October 1-10. Only 24 deaths were recorded (Doumbo et al., 1999). In the encampments, 265 cases were counted. The population of *Anopheles*, as in 1988, was made up of 15% *An. arabiensis* and 85% *An. gambiae s.s.* among which 28/30 (93%) were of the "Mopti" form and 2/30 (7%) the "Savanna" form. This seems to have been a genuine epidemic like the one in 1988, as opposed to a seasonal outbreak in a region where it may not rain for an entire year.

• *Vectors*

Since 1950, three anophelines have been considered as being responsible for the transmission of malaria in Mali, namely *An. gambiae s.l.*, *An. funestus* and *An. nili* (Hamon *et al.*, 1961; Marneffe & Sautet, 1944; Sautet, 1942). *An. pharaoensis* was cited as a secondary vector.

Following the drought in the Sahel, *An. funestus* numbers plummeted in Senegal, Mauritania and Niger (Mouchet *et al.*, 1996). But very little information on its status in Mali is available apart from that 5% of all the specimens captured in Diré in the northern part of the delta (Doumbo *et al.*, 1989) belonged to this species. Studies on the Gambiae Complex carried out by the Bamako School of Medicine and the Higher Institute of Health of Rome helped clarify the taxonomy of this complex (*Figures 21 and 22*) (*see above*). Two chromosomal forms of *An. gambiae s.s.*, "Mopti" and "Bamako", were thus described in addition to the "Savanna" form (*Figure 22*) already reported in the country (Touré *et al.*, 1998b) and the "Forest" and "Bissau" cytotypes. The "Mopti" form seems to have adapted remarkably well in the irrigated and flooded zones and its peak of reproduction differs from that of the other species of the complex (in which reproduction is more closely synchronised with rainfall). This *Anopheles* travels far north all the way to Tessalit, in the Saharan Region, which today remains unexplained. *An. arabiensis*, which lives in the same place as *An. gambiae s.s.*, is especially abundant in the dry areas outside of the delta flood zones (*Figure 21*).

The following sporozoite rates have been reported (Touré *et al.*, 1986):
- *An. arabiensis* = 4.82%;
- *An. gambiae s.s.*, "Mopti" form = 4.04%;
- *An. gambiae s.s.*, "Savanna" form = 2.68%;
- *An. gambiae s.s.*, "Bamako" form = 0.65%.

Such laboratory results do not always reflect the PR in the population. In Diré, where the **"Mopti" form** is practically

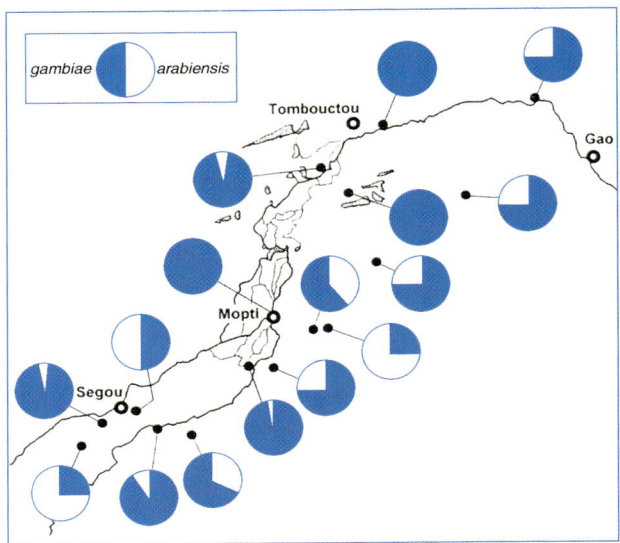

Figure 21. Relative density of An. arabiensis *and* An. gambiae *in the upper Niger Delta (adapted from Touré* et al.*, 1998).*

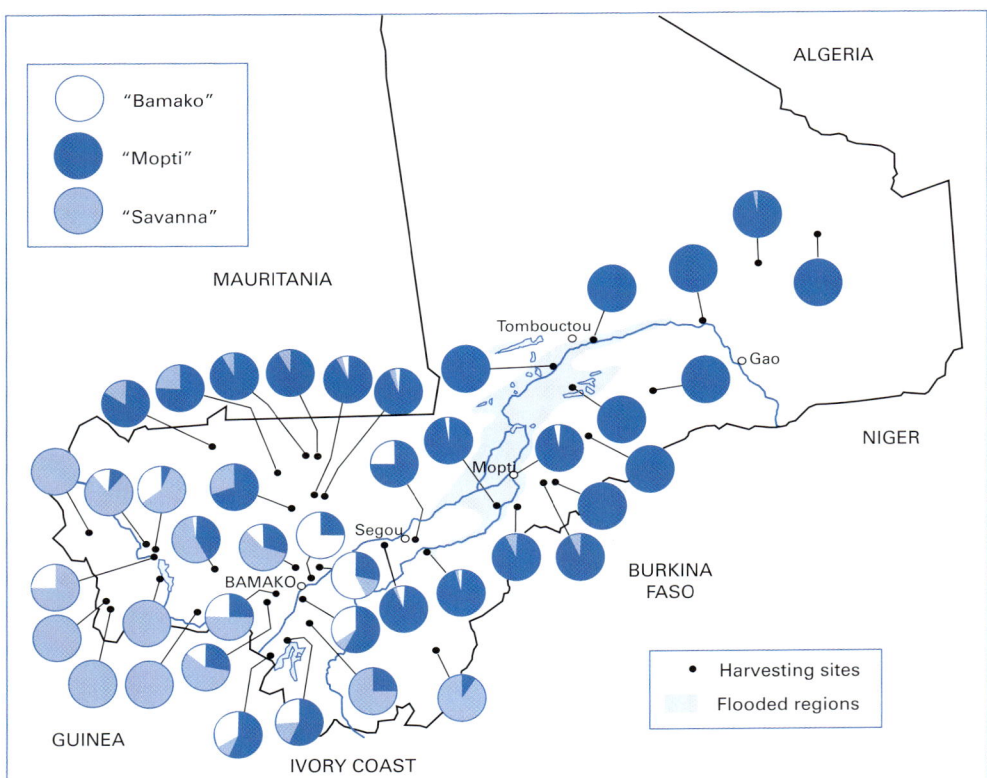

Figure 22. Relative frequencies of the "Bamako", "Savanna" and "Mopti" chromosomal variants of An. gambiae s.s. *(adapted from Touré* et al.*, 1998).*

the only one involved, malaria is hypoendemic while in the region of Koulikoro, far from the river where the **"Savanna" form** is found, malaria is hyperendemic. In Burkina Faso in the rice paddies of the Kou Valley where the "Mopti" form was the only one found, the sporozoite rate was just 0.28% (*see above*). Whether or not this form acts as a vector under natural conditions therefore needs to be reviewed.

Taylor *et al*. (1993) showed that, in the Sahel, *An. gambiae* continued to perpetuate itself during the dry season with very low population densities. The same was observed by Choumara *et al*. (1959) in Burkina Faso and by Cavalié & Mouchet (1962) in northern Cameroon and in the Senegal by Simard *et al*. (2000). Taylor *et al*. (2001) also showed that there is major gene flow within each form. In contrast, in desert regions (where some years it does not rain at all), it is unlikely that *Anopheles* will survive two years without any rainfall, so the possibility of semi-windborne migration on the monsoon front has to be considered.

• *Haemoglobinopathies*

Several populations in Mali, in particular among the Dogon, are heterozygous or homozygous for Haemoglobin C. HbC was identified in 68 out of 391 subjects with uncomplicated malaria, while it was only observed in 3 out of 67 patients with serious malaria: this led Argawal *et al*. (2000) to believe that HbC has a protective effect against severe malaria. This remains to be proven and, in fact, at the hospital in Bamako, Guinet *et al*. (1997) did not find that this allele provided any protection, as has already been observed in Nigeria.

Burkina Faso

This is the only country of the Sahel Region that does not touch the Sahara Desert. It covers an area of 274,200 km^2 with a population of 13.5 million inhabitants (*Table I*). Burkina Faso (formerly Upper Volta) is a flat country made up of two peneplains, the Bobo plateau in the south and the Mossi plateau in the centre, which is separated by the Volta valleys. From south to north, the Sudanese and Sahelian savannahs follow one another. The northern part of the country has been greatly affected by drought. Since 1995, however, the rainfall has been normal.

Thanks to the work carried out by the Centre Muraz of Bobo-Dioulasso, epidemiological problems have been studied thoroughly, particularly from 1957 to 1962, when a pilot eradication zone was established here, and then from 1981 to 1987 in a program supported by the French Ministry of Cooperation, and finally since 1985 with the installation of a study network on the resistance of *P. falciparum*. Since the 1980's, ongoing research on malaria has been conducted in Ouagadougou with the support of the Italian Ministry of Cooperation.

• *Epidemiology of malaria in the Sudanese zone*

The first data available from what used to be the Upper Volta was collected by Jonchères & Pfister (1951) who reported holo-endemic malaria throughout the entire country to the south of Ouagadougou (the only region then investigated). PRs ranged from 75-85% in young children between the ages of 2 and 4 years. During the preliminary studies of the pilot zone of Bobo-Dioulasso, Choumara *et al*. (1959) confirmed this picture. The EIR exceeded 300 ib/p/yr.

All reports attest to a great difference in PR in young children between the dry season (29-40%) and the rainy season (70-85%) (Gazin *et al*., 1985a; Robert *et al*., 1988a). In Karankasso, near Bobo-Dioulasso, SIs of 4.48% and 4.22% were recorded in *An. gambiae s.s.* (30% the "Mopti" form and 70% the "Savanna" form) and in *An. funestus* respectively. Estimates based on the CSP ELISA method put anopheline infection rates 25-50% higher than methods based on salivary gland dissection and microscopic examination. In the village, the EIR was recorded at 263. The prevalence of *P. falciparum* was 35% during the dry season and 82.5% during the rainy season while the corresponding prevalences of *P. malariae* were 3.5% and 25% respectively. It seems that *An. funestus* which is abundant at the beginning of the dry season is a better vector for *P. malariae* than *An. gambiae* (Boudin *et al*., 1991), but this observation cannot be generalised.

A study done in the **rice-producing area** of the Kou Valley near Bobo-Dioulasso brought to light what the authors considered to be a specific epidemiological paradox associated with this form of agriculture (Carnevale *et al*., 1999; Robert *et al*., 1985; Robert *et al*., 1991a): the numbers of the "Mopti" form of *An. gambiae s.s.* (the only vector) were extremely high—six to seven times greater than in the neighbouring savannah villages—but their SI was very low at 0.28% (based on over 7,000 dissections). In villages where farming was confined to the rainy season, only the "Savanna" form of *An. gambiae* was found, growing in rainwater pools. Later in the year, *An. arabiensis* and *An. funestus* arrived. The three species presented sporozoite rates of greater than 3%. The EIR recorded was 55 ib/p/yr in the dry savannah, 133 in the wet savannah, and only 50-60 in the rice-producing region (despite there being 14,000 bites of *An. gambiae* per person per year). In 1991, Robert *et al*. (1991b) observed an EIR of only 29 ib/p/yr in the same rice-producing region. In the rice paddies, the inhabitants were bitten by *Anopheles* much more often than in the wet-season farming villages but these mosquitoes (the "Mopti" form) were hardly infected.

These examples bring to light the epidemiological importance of the various forms of the Gambiae Complex and the danger of extrapolating anopheline density to the intensity of malarial transmission.

Treating local people's mosquito nets with insecticide sharply cut down transmission.

In three villages around Ouagadougou, Sabatinelli *et al*. (1986a) revealed holo-endemic malaria with PRs of 51-88% in young children, like in the southern part of the Sudanese Region.

• *Epidemiology of malaria in the Sahelian zone*

Two series of studies were carried out in the Sahelian zone. One was in the Dori Region in 1961 and 1962 (Hamon *et al.*, 1965) and the other was in the Oursi Pond Region in 1986-1987 (Gazin *et al.*, 1988a). In the second study, *An. funestus* was observed to have disappeared.

A very low sporozoite rate ranging from 0.04-0.15% was recorded in *An. gambiae s.l.* in 1965 and only one specimen out of 157 was found to be infected in 1988. *An. arabiensis* was the dominant member of the Gambiae Complex although this *Anopheles* was hardly present during the dry season, as in the Gourma of Mali (Taylor *et al.*, 1993).

With respect to PR, it should be noted that there are very big differences between the dry and rainy seasons, and also as a function of the distance from a body of water.

In children in the village of Boulay, Gazin *et al.* (1988a and 1988b) recorded PRs of 38% in June (15% *P. malariae* and 3% *P. ovale*), 72% in September (with parasitic densities greater than 10,000 parasites per mm^3), and 60% in March. These figures suggested hyperendemic malaria. In June, a study of school children in Oursi near a permanent pond showed a PR of 41%, while in Deou, far from any ponds, the PR was only 10%. However, by September, the PRs were identical (45%) in both schools.

This region is characteristic of the Sahelian facies where there is a short period of seasonal malaria transmission with the disease borderline stable or, in certain villages, unstable. Malaria was diagnosed in 7% of the patients presenting at the Deou clinic: 75% of these cases were observed between July and November and 90% involved children under the age of 15 years (Gazin *et al.*, 1988b).

• *Urban malaria*

Urban malaria was studied in the country's two major cities: Ouagadougou (700,000-800,000 inhabitants) and Bobo-Dioulasso (500,000).

Bobo-Dioulasso is a city that has grown outwards from its historical centre. *An. gambiae* was the only vector and its density dropped from the suburbs towards the city centre. The EIR was at 0.14 in the city centre (1 infective bite per person every seven years), 4.6 in the suburbs, and at more than 130 in the villages just out of town (Robert *et al.*, 1986). PRs ranged from 9-14% in the city-centre neighbourhoods and from 21-48% in the outskirts (Gazin *et al.*, 1987). The morbidity rate, which was based on a pyrogenic threshold of 15,000 (little difference from 10,000 to 20,000), suggested that malaria was responsible for 50% of fevers during the months of October and November, compared with just 4% from January to May (Baudon *et al.*, 1988; Benasseni *et al.*, 1987).

In Ouagadougou, the prevalence in five city neighbourhoods averaged at 16% as opposed to 51-88% in three villages just outside of town (*Figure 23*). But in the city, some marked foci were identified close to bodies of water, in particular a line of ponds to the west of the city, and some wet ditches. PRs ranged from 3-32% (Sabatinelli *et al.*, 1986a and 1986b). The vectors were *An. gambiae s.s.* ("Mopti" and "Savanna" cytotypes) and *An. funestus* (less than 6%) (Rossi *et al.*, 1986). Malaria was diagnosed in 50% of patients with a fever (Coulibaly *et al.*, 1991). In the city, the average age of patients with severe malaria was 4.8 years, while in the rural areas it was 2.2. Coma occurred in 53% of the cases in the city and in 29% of the

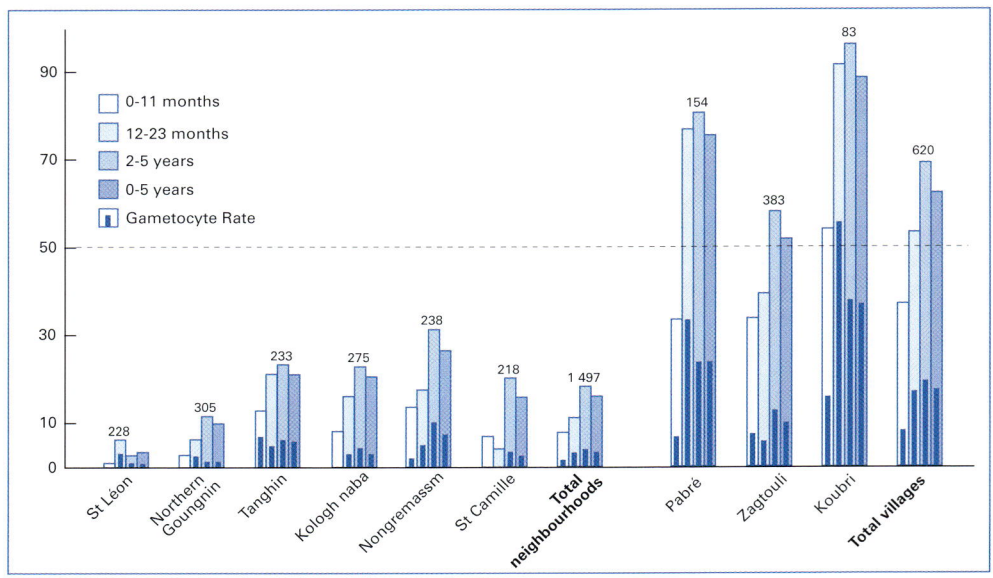

Figure 23. Parasite rates in Ouagadougou and surrounding villages (adapted from Sabatinelli et al., 1986a).

cases in rural areas. The anaemia profile however was the opposite with 15% in town and 47% outside.

• *Entomological research in Burkina Faso*

Studies of *An. funestus* have not yet provided any very clear conclusions. According to Costantini *et al.* (1999), there are two taxonomic entities in Burkina Faso but the work of Mukabayire *et al.* (1999) on ribosomal and mitochondrial DNA showed that there was no reproductively isolated form of *An. funestus*. Hackett *et al.* (2000) concluded that in Burkina Faso, *An. rivulorum* was not the typical form but belonged to a cryptic taxon of the Funestus Group.

Coz & Picq (1972) had shown that *An. gambiae s.s.* (formerly *An. gambiae* A) was a far more efficient vector than *An. arabiensis* (*An. gambiae* B). In Burkina Faso now, the Gambiae Complex includes *An. arabiensis*, a panmictic species, and *An. gambiae s.s.* which is represented by the "Mopti" (in permanent bodies of water) and "Savanna" (in rain water pools) forms (Petrarca *et al.*, 1986; Robert *et al.*, 1989). Coosemans *et al.* (1998) suggested, using a method based on the analysis of two isoenzymes, to differentiate *An. gambiae s.s.* from *An. arabiensis*. A morphometric method can also be used to distinguish the two species as *An. arabiensis* is always larger in size, regardless of its geographic origins (Petrarca *et al.*, 1998).

Coosemans *et al.* (1998) showed that in the natural populations of *An. gambiae s.s.* in the south-western part of Burkina Faso, there was no refractoriness to *P. falciparum* transmission.

• *Human genetics*

In humans, susceptibility to malarial infection does not seem to be determined by a single major gene, as was thought by Abel *et al.* (1992), but is rather multifactorial. The key genes are located in the chromosomes 5/31 – 983 (Abderrazak *et al.*, 1999; Rihet *et al.*, 1998).

Modiano *et al.* (1996, 1998) showed that when exposed to the same level of risk, members of the Peuhl ethnic group were less susceptible to malaria and had fewer attacks than members of the Mossi and Rimaibe ethnic groups. The Peuhl people carry more anti-RESA and anti-Pf332 antibodies. The ethnic origin of the Peuhl people is a controversial subject although they are believed to have some Caucasian ancestry while the Mossis and Rimaibes people come from the Sudanese group.

Niger

Niger covers an area of 1,267,000 km² of which two-thirds is in the desert. The population of 12.2 million people has increased by more than 3% every year for the last thirty years (*Table I*). The country's primary export commodity is uranium, which is mined at Arlit in the far north.

The Niger River flows for 500 km in the southern part of the country, from an altitude of 228 m where it enters the country near Ayourou, down to 161 m where it exits in the central southern part of the country near Gaya. The rest of the country is a peneplain at an altitude of below 400 m. The Aïr is the main mountain range with an average altitude of 600 m but rising up to 2,020 m in the Bagzane Mountains. The Djado Plateau, which extends from the Tassili N'ajer in Algeria, rises to an altitude of 500-600 m.

The vegetation in the south and in the middle valley of the Niger is Sudanese (Say, Maradi) while further north it is Sahelian, and then Sahelo-Saharan before turning into desert in the Ténéré Region (*Figure 24*) (Julvez & Mouchet, 1998b). Several oases marking the former

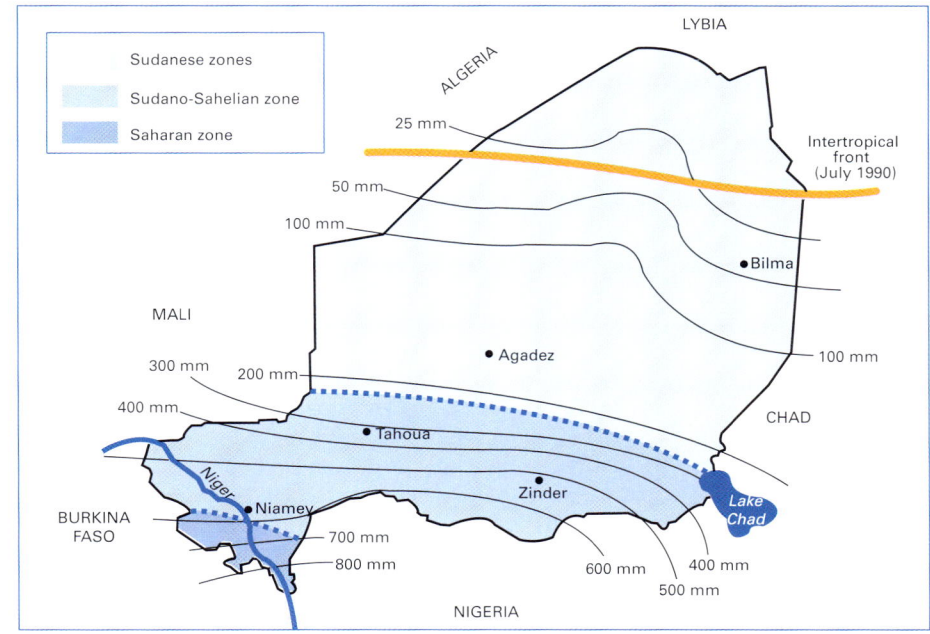

Figure 24.
Isohyets and climatic zones in Niger (adapted from Julvez et al., 1992).

tributaries of Lake Chad are scattered throughout the Aïr Mountains and its surroundings.

The northern part of Niger separates the Mediterranean Palaearctic Region from the Afrotropical Region. In the Aïr Mountains, the fauna in the valleys is Afrotropical while in the mountains it is Mediterranean. The climate is also intermediate, with winter rains. The anopheline vectors are a part of both the African tropical fauna—*An. gambiae s.l.* (*An. arabiensis*) all the way to El Meki and Teguidda Ntekum in the north—and the Mediterranean fauna—*An. hispaniola, An. multicolor, An. dthali* (apparently non-vectors) in the Aïr Mountains and in Djado (Julvez *et al.*, 1998b; Magnaval, 1973; Stafford-Smith, 1981).

The Niger River is also an ethnic crossroads where the Berber Tuareg, Toubus, Haoussa, Kanouri, Djerma (of different Melano-African origins), and Peulh people meet.

• *Epidemiology of malaria*

The stratification of malaria is not different from that of the other Sahelian countries. The Sudanese zone with tropical features is in the extreme southern part of the country and rises to the north more or less along the Niger River. The Sahelian zone, with a dry season lasting less than three months and becoming progressively shorter as one heads north, merges into a Sahelo-Saharan pre-desert zone. These last two strata are characterised by unstable malaria, with seasonal attacks that take on epidemic proportions in some years. In the desert, most of the oases are malaria-free but sporadic episodes may occur (Julvez *et al.*, 1992). It should be noted that *P. vivax* has never been reported in Niger despite the presence of many light-skinned people (the Tuareg).

The epidemiological history of malaria over the last forty years has been dominated by the drought which has reigned over the region since 1973. The anopheline fauna and, therefore, the prevalence of malaria, were affected to such an extent that it is necessary to distinguish pre-1970 PR measurements from those made after 1975. It has to be emphasised that *An. funestus*—once considered as being one of the main vectors (Ochrymowicz *et al.*, 1969)—has disappeared. As in Senegal, this was due to the larval habitats drying up and then being used for farming, thereby depriving the species of its biotopes (Julvez *et al.*, 1998; Mouchet *et al.*, 1996).

In the **Sudanese zone**, PRs were found to be relatively constant near the river at around 50% in Tillabery area (Baudon *et al.*, 1986a), verging on hyper- or meso-endemic disease. The case of the city of Niamey is of particular note; this city grew up as a result of the merging of neighbouring villages and was therefore influenced by the effects of both urbanisation and drought. In 1924 in the village of Goudet, located outside the town at the time, the PR was 66%. In 1994, by which time the village was well within Niamey, the PR was 5% during the dry season, and 30-50% during the rainy season. A serological study showed strong correlation with distance to larval habitats, which happened to be the river (Julvez *et al.*, 1997a). In 1985 in Maradi, on the edge of the Sahelian zone, PRs were between 0.7% and 2.6% in the city and between 22% and 27% in the rural areas (depending on the season). The effects of urbanisation were even more pronounced than in Niamey.

In the **Sahelian zone**, PRs have decreased considerably since 1973. In 1922 in Zinder, PRs of 62-87% were recorded in children. In 1968 surrounding the city, they ranged from 52-73% (Dyemkouma, 1968). In 1994, the PR was 3% during the dry season and 11-30% during the rainy season (Julvez *et al.*, 1997a and 1997b). In October 1994 in Diffa, along the river, the PR was only 7%. The percentage of infected adults was relatively high, which suggests that immunity develops late.

Data from the Sahelo-Saharan zone are rare. All that has been recorded is a PR of 7.6% in N'gourti, just north of Lake Chad, in 1969 (Ochrymowicz, 1969) and one of 4.2% in 1975.

In the **Sahara**, *An. arabiensis* is found just beyond Agadez in latitude, all the way to El Meki in the Aïr Mountains, and Teggida N'tekoum around the mountains (Stafford-Smith, 1981). The presence of other species of the complex requires confirmation. In the oasis of Djado, only Palaearctic species have been recorded: *An. multicolor, An. hispaniola* and *An. dthali*, non-vectors (Magnaval, 1973). *An. sergentii*, the oasis vector, has never been observed in Niger. Information received from health clinics is unreliable due to a lack of microscopes and accessories—and, in the north, even of physicians. In 1958 in Bilma (latitude 18.4° north), a malaria epidemic was declared by a doctor from the Mehari Unit who had laboratory equipment. Until 1991, no doctor had ever been posted to this oasis and upon the arrival of the new physician, 2,310 presumed cases out of a population of 10,500 were reported, i.e. one in five inhabitants. According to serological tests, it would seem that transmission stopped in 1992 (Develoux *et al.*, 1994). In 1995, out of 600 samples, no more positive cases were found but persistent antibodies (at a titre of 1/320) were detected in 24 subjects. Not one vector was found in the homes following indoor spraying with pyrethroid. Only *An. rufipes* was abundant but it is not a vector.

It is difficult to imagine how an epidemic could have occurred in Bilma, which is about 1,000 km away from the closest surface body of water, especially since the cases were confined to the oasis, with the exception of Dirkou, 70 km to the north. One possible hypothesis is that a semi-assisted migration of anophelines from the south took place on an upwelling tropical convergence beyond Bilma in 1990 and 1991 (*Figure 24*), as discussed above. After their arrival, the anophelines can reproduce for a few cycles before disappearing, as permanent bodies of water are not conducive to the species of the Gambiae Complex. This is only a hypothesis but such sporadic outbreaks of malaria can only be explained through the temporary introduction of a vector.

We are still very much in the dark regarding malaria transmission at the northern boundary of the Afrotropical Region. A problem with any study is the unreliable nature of the presumed diagnoses (even microscopic diagnoses) in the absence of equipment and competent personnel. This is said to be true in most African countries but in-depth accounts of these shortcomings have been actually recorded in Niger (Olivar et al., 1991); during the dry season, more than 80% of the diagnoses made were wrong.

A large scale distribution of impregnated mosquito nets is on going with poliomyelitis vaccination (Hoyer, personal communication).

Chad

Chad covers an area of 1,284,000 km^2, and is located between the 8th and 24th parallel north. The population of 9.2 million people is concentrated in the south (*Table I*). Lake Chad's basin—a mere remnant of the Mega Chad from the beginning of Quaternary Era—is at an altitude of under 300 m. The lake is fed by the Chari and the Logone, its tributaries, after it has flowed over the vast flood zones known as the "Yaéré" in Chad and in Cameroon. The low altitude peneplain that makes up the Chad basin is bordered by the Tibesti Mountains (more than 3,000 m) to the north, the Ennedi Mountains (1,450 m) to the east, and the Ouaddai Mountains to the south-east (1,430 m).

As in the other three countries of the Sahel, the southern part as far up as the 11th parallel north is considered to be a part of the Sudanese Region. Rainfall ranges from 1,000-1,500 mm. Further north, the Sahelian zone extends from the 11th to the 14th parallel; then, the Sahelo-Saharan Region which turns into the Sahara, extends all the way to the 24th parallel. Several oases are found in and around the mountain ranges.

• *Epidemiology and entomology*

On the whole, very little is known about the epidemiology of malaria in this huge country. We can, however, construct a map of the epidemiological strata according to vegetation zones whose stratification is fairly constant throughout all of West Africa (Mouchet et al., 1993b). We have also been able to observe a great similarity in prevalence between northern Cameroon and the districts of western Chad, the western Logone, Mayo Kebi, and the Chari Baguirmi (Mouchet, personal observation).

Entomological studies were carried out south of N'Djamena before 1960 (Hamon et al., 1956; Lacan, 1956). The presence of *An. gambiae s.l.* was recorded in all the sites investigated. In the northern part of the country in the Borkou, Rioux et al. (1961) collected *An. gambiae* in Largeau. The authors were retracing the history of malaria in the Sahara of Chad. We still do not know which forms of the Gambiae Complex are present in the country. *An. funestus* was recorded throughout the south and *An. nili* was collected in the Logone and in the Chari.

In 1970, all research came to a halt, with the exception of a few odd surveys in N'Djamena, Mayo-Kébi, and in Moundou.

In N'Djamena in 1960, *An. gambiae s.l.* was very abundant along the Chari River and in residual ponds (Mouchet, personal observation), and the malaria appeared to be severe according to the health authorities at the time. In 1987, however, Merlin et al. recorded a prevalence of only 5% in children, which seems to be an under-estimate.

In the Sudanese zone, where the two vectors were *An. gambiae* and *An. funestus*, Buck et al. (1978) carried out a study on intercurrent parasitic infections (focusing on filariasis) in the Mayo-Kébi. In the same district, Brinkmann & Brinkmann (1991) made projections that had the prevalence of malaria rising in the region although these forecasts are not entirely convincing—no more than their speculations about the economic cost of malaria. In Moundou, in a village outside town, the PR in children was 63% while it was only 15% in a city school (although these latter children might have been given prophylactic drugs) (Traoré et al., 1992). In a hospital in the same city, a nutritional study revealed generalised anaemia in which more than 10% of the cases were considered serious (Renaudin & Lombart, 1994); malaria was considered as a key factor underlying this anaemia.

We have not been able to obtain any recent information on the Sahelian zone.

On the northern border of the Sahelo-Saharan zone, malaria was reported from 1945 to 1956 in Largeau, a garnison city. The possibility of the parasites having been imported from elsewhere was more than likely but in 1955, ninety-five cases were detected in children that had never left the oasis. In 1959, Rioux et al. (1961) discovered *An. gambiae* in larval habitats and in homes during the month of November. However, the local population was not carrying any *Plasmodium*. In 1960, Saugrain & Taufflieb confirmed a lack of both infected subjects and *An. gambiae*. It could have been, as in Bilma (Niger), the malaria had come and gone.

The observed fluctuations in the incidence of malaria and the densities of its vectors on the southern border of the Sahara thus remain largely unexplained and we must be satisfied with hypotheses such as the one suggested for the Bilma oasis in Niger.

Climatic events (in particular, the drought that has reduced the area of Lake Chad by two-thirds) and war have profoundly affected malaria profiles: it is, however, impossible at the moment to understand by just how much, given the absence of reliable information.

Central Africa

Geographical boundaries and general characteristics

The Central African Region includes Cameroon, the Central African Republic, Gabon, Congo, Equatorial Guinea, the Republic of São Tomé and Principe, the Democratic Republic of Congo, Rwanda, and Burundi.

As defined in the French-speaking world, Central Africa covers an area of 4,136,769 km² (of which 2,345,000 km² is within the Democratic Republic of Congo) between the parallels of 13° north and 12° south, from the end of the Gulf of Guinea to the Great Lakes Fault. Central Africa has a total population of 100 million people with 57.5 million in the Democratic Republic of Congo and 17 million in Cameroon. The region corresponds to the geographic centre of Africa.

The four-season equatorial climate in the basin induces a tropical pattern with two contrasting seasons to the north and south of the 5th and 6th parallels. Rain forest still covers most of the Congolese basin and its surroundings up to the 5th northern parallel in Cameroon and the Central African Republic, and down to the 4th southern parallel in Gabon, Congo (Brazzaville) and the Democratic Republic of Congo. To the north and south of the forest block, as one gets further away from the rain forest, the woods thin out to create a mosaic of forest and savannah, sometimes referred to as the "post-forest zone". To the north of the equator in Cameroon and the Central African Republic is a wooded Sudanese savannah; south of the equator, the woodland is gradually replaced by a herbaceous flora in Katanga. In the mountains, forests and prairies are interspersed with papyrus marshes at the bottoms of the valleys.

The forest fauna is highly endemic, including okapi, Giant Forest Hog and Congolese peacock, to name but a few examples. The area represents a final haven for both plain and mountain gorillas, bonobos, and chimpanzees, (although the latter are far more widely distributed). The invertebrate fauna, whose inventory has not yet been completed, is also very rich; all the African malaria vectors are found: *An. gambiae s.s., An. melas, An. arabiensis, An. funestus, An. nili, An. moucheti, An. paludis, An. brunnipes* and *An. pharoensis*. Several other species that do not apparently transmit malaria have been reported.

It was often supposed, without much evidence, that Pygmies were the first occupants of the forest. It should be noted that these peoples come from various origins but none of the groups that have been studied possess the Duffy antigen, which suggests that they are of Melano-African origin. They are tending to mix more and more with the Bantus who occupy the same regions. In the eastern part of the Democratic Republic of Congo, they also mix with the nilotic peoples.

Since 1960, Central Africa's history has been marked by bloody civil wars in the Democratic Republic of Congo, Rwanda, the Central African Republic, Congo (Brazza), and Equatorial Guinea, leading to major destabilisation in these countries. Health care services have suffered greatly as a result, not to mention the complete disappearance of malaria control programmes. Under such circumstances it has been difficult in recent years to obtain reliable malaria data from a number of these countries.

However, the dominant characteristic of the epidemiology of malaria in Central Africa is that the disease is ubiquitous, stable and hyperendemic. The only exceptions to this rule are found in the mountainous regions of West Cameroon, the eastern part of the Democratic Republic of Congo (Kivu), the plateaux of Rwanda and Burundi (above 1,500 m), as well as in a few large cities such as Kinshasa, Brazzaville, Douala, and Yaoundé.

Cameroon

Cameroon (*Table I*) marks the junction between West Africa and Central Africa. Covering a distance of more than 1,500 km from north to south, every type of climate and vegetation zone is represented north of the equator. The fault of the Ngaoundéré escarpment at the 7th parallel north divides the country between the southern part where, beyond the 6th parallel, rain forest gives way to post-forest formations and then into a Guinean savannah in the Adamaoua Mountains, and the northern part with shrubby savannah and thorny steppe. The western mountains have a forest climate in the south, while the northern peaks (Alantikas, Mandara) are savannah-like.

The rainfall decreases from the banks of the Gulf of Guinea (4,000 mm) eastwards (1,400 mm in Yaoundé) and north (500 mm along Lake Chad). Apart from shrinking Lake Chad, the drought that has reigned since 1973 has caused the "yaéré"—submersible prairies in the flood zones of the Chari and Logone Rivers—to temporarily dry up, while the ecologically important forest gallery of the Logone has disappeared entirely. There is little information regarding the impact of these eco-climatic changes on vectors, apart from the disappearance from the far north of *Glossina tachinoides,* vector of sleeping sickness (Cuisance, personal communication).

Cameroon has a very dense network of major rivers such as the Sanaga, the Nyong and the Ntem on the Atlantic side, and the Lom, the Kadei, and the Ngoko which meet up with the Sanga and the Congolese Basin. The north is irrigated by the Benoué, a tributary of the Niger, as well as by the Logone and the Chari Rivers which feed into Lake Chad.

• *Epidemiology*

The first malaria map of Cameroon covered the southern forest (Languillon *et al.*, 1955) and detailed vector distribution; the second (Languillon, 1957) covered the entire country but made no mention of vectors. These were based on surveys and data taken on an *ad hoc* basis. Malaria is hyperendemic throughout most of the country although, in extremely isolated forest villages, the disease tended to be mesoendemic. This was due to the uneven distribution of vectors, mainly *An. gambiae s.s.* In the western mountains, malaria prevalence varied greatly with altitude and, even more importantly, according to the distance of the village from the valley where *Anopheles* was breeding. A great deal of work done since 1955 has only confirmed these general characteristics.

In the **forest region in the central-southern part**, Livadas *et al.* (1958) observed that PR depended on the extent to which the village was contained in the forest. In the very isolated villages of the Mouloundou Region, PRs were lower than 50%; in the Pygmy camps, they were even lower than 30% (in children). In contrast, in bigger villages surrounded by farmland, PRs were hyperendemic (60-70%). Since the main vector *An. gambiae* does not thrive in woodland, most of its larval habitats derive from human activities, especially tracks in which ruts provide a propitious environment for *Anopheles* larvae. *An. moucheti* is the main vector along slow-flowing rivers (Mouchet & Gariou, 1966), and *An. nili* the fast-flowing ones (Carnevale *et al.*, 1992a; Livadas *et al.*, 1958). When water levels are low, *An. gambiae* larvae thrive in residual ponds in exposed sand banks in the middle of the river bed (Mouchet, 1962), entailing transmission in the middle of the dry season all along the Sanaga River.

It should be remembered that, following indoor residual spraying (IRS) with DDT or with dieldrin, anthropophilic vectors such as *An. gambiae s.s.*, *An. nili* and *An. moucheti* disappeared from the pilot zone of Yaoundé where the PR had been less than 2%. Not one *Anopheles* in Yaoundé survived the spraying from 1955-1960 (Livadas *et al.*, 1958). The programme was terminated, *de facto*, in 1962 when resistance to dieldrin appeared. These results allow us to compare the circumstances that prevailed in 1958 to the current situation in Cameroon.

On the basis of work in the central southern part of the country, Ripert *et al.*, (1982-1990) reported meso-endemic PRs well below those reported by Languillon (1957) and Livadas *et al.* (1958), even though de-forestation was supposed to have increased transmission. Widespread self-medication with chloroquine, in addition to the semi-urbanisation of several areas, could explain why the PR dropped. However, in the heart of the forest region near Djoum, malaria remained hyperendemic with PRs over 60% (Josse *et al.*, 1990).

The population of Yaoundé—a city of 60,000 inhabitants in 1958, at which time there were no anophelines—had grown twenty-fold by the year 2000: in 1992, urban malaria represented a major risk with EIRs of 14-30 ib/p/yr (depending on the neighbourhood) (Fondjo *et al.*, 1992; Manga *et al.*, 1993).

In **East Cameroon**, Ripert *et al.* (1991) confirmed the hyperendemicity of malaria at the site of the future Bini Dam on the slopes of the Adamaoua Mountains at an altitude of 1,000 m (PR: 60%). At higher altitudes (1,300 m), Raccurt *et al.* (1993) found meso-endemic disease with a PR of 39%.

In urban or semi-urban sites around the perimeter of the **Bonny's Bay**, at the far end of the Gulf of Guinea, malaria was meso- or hypo-endemic, said to be due to both urbanisation and the almost universal practise of self-medication. Less than 1% of the population was carrying trophozoite densities of over 10,000 per mm^3 of blood (Merlin *et al.*, 1986). In Douala, PRs were substantially lower than those reported thirty years before (Voelckel & Mouchet, 1959). However, in the city of Edea 50 km from the coast, indicators suggestive of holo-endemic situation were documented in a residential neighbourhood (Gazin *et al.*, 1989).

In the **Bamiléké Mountains** in western Cameroon, prevalence rapidly decreased with altitude and distance from *An. funestus* larval habitats at the bottoms of valleys. Certain towns on the ridges, such as Bafoussam, recorded no transmission whatsoever. Traditionally, it was taboo for the residents of this community to spend the night in the valley; it might be supposed that such a restriction arose because there was a risk of catching malaria in the valleys (Mouchet & Gariou, 1960). In the city of Dschang, the presence of the dammed lake explains why transmission occurs in certain, specific neighbourhoods (Cot *et al.*, 1992a). In the mountain regions, environmental conditions and the steepness of the slope seemed to be of greater importance than altitude *per se*. In Nkongsamba, at 1,000 m in altitude halfway up the Manengouba Mountain, the PR was only 12% (Josse *et al.*, 1988b).

In 1961 in **North Cameroon**, malaria was hyper- or holo-endemic (Cavalié & Mouchet, 1961). In 1982 in the city of Maroua, whose population had increased fivefold in the recent past, the disease was found to be hypo-endemic following a survey during the dry season (and therefore not comparable). The pollution of surface waters, due to urbanisation, seriously inhibited anopheline reproduction (Josse *et al.*, 1987b). In the Koza Region, in a hollow of the Mandara Mountains, a survey during the dry season suggested a meso-endemic situation (Ripert *et al.*, 1982).

In North Cameroon, the **lands around rice paddies** on the shores of the Logone (Audibert *et al.*, 1990; Josse *et al.*, 1987a) and the Benoué (Robert *et al.*, 1992) were home mainly to *An. arabiensis* (and not the "Mopti" form of *An. gambiae s.s.* as in Burkina Faso). It does not seem that irrigation greatly modified the local malaria that was already hyperendemic.

Several studies were carried out at future large or small dam sites. However, it is too early to estimate their impact on public health as these structures are still not built, and any forecast seems premature.

• *Entomology*

The duality between the northern and southern parts of Cameroon is characterized by a forest fauna in the south, and a widely dispersed savannah fauna in the north (Mouchet & Gariou, 1961).

The Gambiae Complex is represented by three species: *An. melas* in the coastal mangroves, *An. gambiae s.s.* "Forest" form throughout the entire forest region, and *An. arabiensis*, which is almost the only species found in the rice paddies of the north (Robert *et al.*, 1992). The exact distribution of the two latter species in the northern regions where they live together is unknown: the sporozoite rate of 1-3% coupled with the promiscuous feeding habits of *An. gambiae s.l.* would be conducive to the mixing of these two species (*Table X*).

In areas of interspersed forest and savannah, *An. gambiae s.s.* was scarce in the forest villages whereas it was dense inside homes in villages in deforested areas; the respective EIR measurements were 17 ib/p/yr and 176 ib/p/yr, i.e. a ten-fold difference (Manga *et al.*, 1995 and 1997a; Meunier *et al.*, 1999).

An. funestus was rare in the forest zone, only being found in two out of more than sixty locations surveyed in 1955-1956 (Mouchet & Gariou, 1961). In 1997, following deforestation around Yaoundé, it became very abundant in the deforested shallow marches. It maintained a transmission rate of about 50 ib/p/yr (Manga *et al.*, 1997b). This species acts as an informative marker *vis-à-vis* the region's ecological changes.

In the Sahelo-Sudanese and Sudanese savannahs of North Cameroon, *An. funestus* and *An. gambiae* were responsible for transmission in holo- or hyperendemic regions. Both apparently fed without discrimination on humans and livestock alike; specimens taken off cows sometimes even contained sporozoites. The sporozoite rate was 3% or more. At the end of the rainy season, they were biting even in the middle of the day in the shade (Cavalié & Mouchet, 1961). It should be noted that, in 1960, *An. funestus* was twice as resistant as *An. gambiae* to DDT (Mouchet *et al.*, 1961).

An. moucheti is the "perfect" forest vector. Its pre-imaginal forms develop in slow-flowing rivers once the water level has stabilised. The adults disperse along the rivers, flying up to 3 km, which prolongs their gonotrophic cycle beyond three days. Its sporozoite rate is generally around 1% but can exceed 3%. In a station in Ebogo on the banks of the Nyong, the EIR was 302 ib/p/yr (Le Goff *et al.*, 1993; Mouchet & Gariou, 1966; Njan Nloga *et al.*, 1993a) (*Table X*).

An. nili grows in the backwaters of fast-flowing rivers throughout Cameroon, all the way to the Bénoué and Logone Rivers in the north. With a sporozoite rate greater than 1%, it was the main vector on the shores of the Sanaga where the EIR was 104 ib/p/yr (Carnevale *et al.*, 1992a).

An. nili has already been differentiated from the species *An. somalicus* whose larvae have a distinct type of chetotaxy. Its numbers were high along the Sanaga River but its vector role has never been clearly defined (Mouchet & Gariou, 1961). It appears that *An. nili* is a complex of species, at least four of which have been identified in Cameroon, including *An. carnevalei* (Brunhes *et al.*, 1999) and *An. ovengensis* (Kengne *et al.*, 2003).

An. pharoensis, which bites in early evening, had a sporozoite rate of 2.1% in the Benoué River Region (Robert *et al.*, 1992).

An. paludis, an exophilic species that bites during the day in forest undergrowth (Mouchet, personal observation) is also present in the Democratic Republic of Congo (Karch & Mouchet, 1992) where it is apparently endophilic.

• *Morbidity*

As in most African countries, diagnosing malaria is a matter of concern. In southern Cameroon, out of the twenty-eight centres visited, not one of the seventeen government groups had the equipment to take, perfom and/or read thin or thick blood smear, although ten out of eleven mission groups had adequate equipment. In addition, six out of the twenty-four microscopists did not correctly read the slides (Manga, 1994). Under such conditions, presumptive diagnosis is the only current option.

Much light was shed by a comprehensive study of 903 children examined in clinics around Yaoundé where the parasite prevalence was 33%. Of 903 children, 556 had fevers but only 16% of these tested were positive for *P. falciparum*; 10% of the 903 were found with the parasite and, of these, 12% had a parasitaemia of over 10,000 parasites per mm^3 of blood. In conclusion, high temperature is not synonymous with malaria disease, and the presence of parasites is insufficient to confirm a diagnosis of clinical malaria (Loué *et al.*, 1989) in such endemic situation.

In South Cameroon, more than 50% of cases were self-treated with chloroquine but the dosages administered were often below the recommended levels (Picot *et al.*, 1997), although this did not necessarily preclude cure.

Although there was resistance to chloroquine, amodiaquine continued to work well (Brasseur *et al.*, 1999; Louis *et al.*, 1994; Ringwald *et al.*, 1998a). Various qinghaosu derivatives (Artesunate® and Artéflene®) were tested on *P. ovale* with success (Same-Eboko *et al.*, 1999; Somo-Moyou *et al.*, 1994). Pyronaridine proved to be effective against simple attacks (Ringwald *et al.*, 1998b).

Table X. Sporozoite rates for vectors in Cameroon.						
An. gambiae s.l	An. gambiae s.s.	An. arabiensis	An. funestus	An. nili	An. moucheti	An. pharoensis
1-3%	2-4%	> 1%	3%	1-2%	1-3%	2.1%

KAP (knowledge, attitude & practices) surveys have estimated that 57,000 CFA ($12) is spent per year per household on home insecticides and anti-malarial drugs at Yaoundé and Douala (Desfontaine *et al.*, 1989, 1990; Louis *et al.*, 1992).

• *Mothers and children*

Maternal anaemia and low birth weight were most often linked to infection of the erythrocyte-rich placenta where dividing *P. falciparum* forms are concentrated. In pregnant women, the parasites tended to be more cyto-adherent than in non-pregnant women (Maubert *et al.*, 2000). Children born from mothers with a placental infection had more malaria attacks than those born to uninfected mothers (Cot *et al.*, 1995).

In a semi-rural zone around Ebolowa in South Cameroon, children were infected at a very young age: 7.1% during the first month, 30.9% within the first six months, and 46% within the first year. The first infections were often symptomless (Le Hesran *et al.*, 1995).

• *Genetics*

Abel *et al.* (1992) believed that the level of *P. falciparum* infection was under the control of a single major gene, meaning that the children in certain families would experience more malarial paroxysms than children in other families. Later, these authors revised their opinion and it is now generally accepted that the control of parasitaemia is multifactorial, involving a complex series of diverse mechanisms (Garcia *et al.*, 1998).

In a review of the distribution of HbS haplotypes, Nagel & Fleming (1992) pointed out that so far, the "Eton" haplotype has only ever been found in Central Cameroon to the north of Yaoundé.

• *Gametocytes in the blood*

In the context of a search for a vaccine against the gametocyte stage, laboratory experiments have shown that the percentage of infected mosquitoes is only one-quarter of the number that would be expected on the basis of the parasitaemia in gametocyte carriers (Boudin *et al.*, 1997). Robert *et al.* (1995) emphasised the infectivity of carriers with a very low gametocyte density in the blood.

Central African Republic

The Central African Republic (formerly Oubangui-Chari) is an under-populated country with only 4 million inhabitants covering an area of 600,000 km^2 (*Table I*). The dense forest of the south, located between the 2nd and 4th parallels, extends into a very large strip, a mixture of forest and savannah, and then into a woody Sudanese savannah. The river network includes the Congo Basin in the south (*via* the Oubangi and the Sanga Rivers), the Chad Basin in the north (the Chari River and its tributaries), and the Nile Basin in the far east (Bar el Ghazal). The Central African Republic is a "flat" country where the highest peaks are no higher than 1,300 m—in the Bouar Region in the west.

According to extremely fragmentary local information and assumed parallels with neighbouring countries in the same climatic zones, malaria appears to be stable and hyperendemic throughout most of the territory with the exception of the city of Bangui and the Pygmy camps where the disease is still endemic but lower in prevalence.

• *Epidemiology*

Because of twenty years of political unrest, as well as the fact that most professional health care providers are concentrated in the capital city, the only information available on malaria comes from the city of Bangui, in particular, from the town's University Hospital which focuses on the clinical aspects of the disease. The rest of the country is a *terra incognita* insofar as malaria is concerned.

In the city, the PR remained moderate at 28% in children between the ages of 2 and 4. More than 80% of the population were carrying no parasites, and 9% had between 1,000 and 10,000 parasites per mm^3; only 2.3% had more than 10,000 per mm^3 (Monges *et al.*, 1987). Self-medication with chloroquine was practised by 70% of the population.

In the Pygmy camps of the Lobaye in the southern part of the country, malarial indicators were very low, below 20% (Carnevale, personal observation) as reflected by the scarcity of vectors in huts.

In 1990, in the Paediatrics Department of Bangui University Hospital, the mortality rate was 11.6% out of 8,052 admissions; 60% of the deaths occurred within 24 hours following admission. Malaria and anaemia were considered to be very severe (Lanckriet *et al.*, 1992). In Bangui, out of a population of 500 women, PRs were lower in the 250 who were not pregnant; among pregnant women, higher PRs were seen in primigravidae patients (as is usually the case) (Testa *et al.*, 1987).

• *Entomology*

The *Anopheles* maps of Hamon *et al.* (1956a) and Lacan (1958) are out of date, as the different species of the *An. gambiae* Complex had not been differentiated when they were compiled. *An. gambiae s.s.* is almost certainly present in the southern forest, and *An. arabiensis* in the east and the north.

An. funestus and *An. nili* have been reported throughout the entire country by the preceding authors. *An. moucheti* was collected along all the rivers of the south. *An. paludis* is known to be endophilic in the southern part of the country.

No *Anopheles* have been collected in the Pygmy huts of the Lobaye.

• *Rodent* Plasmodium

Three species of *Plasmodium* have been reported in the rodent *Thamnomys surdaster* in the southern part of the Central African Republic: *P. yoeli*, *P. chabaudi* and *P. vinckei*. The first two ones are closely related to *P. vinckei* and can be used to study the biology of plasmodia and to test anti-malarial drugs. The three species have the same chronosexuality and, in the laboratory, are transmitted by the same *Anopheles* (Gautret *et al.*, 1998).

Equatorial Guinea

Equatorial Guinea consists of the former Spanish colonies of the Gulf of Guinea, i.e. the continental province of Rio Muni between Cameroon and Gabon, and the islands of Bioko (formerly Fernando-Póo) and Annobon (*Table XI*). When the Spanish arrived, the island of Bioko was already inhabited by the Babi and Annobon people from Nigeria. The Rio Muni was inhabited by the Fang people, a Bantu ethnic group that also lives in the northern part of Gabon.

Rio Muni was considered to be a hyperendemic territory. In Nsork, however, the prevalence of 28% in children does not justify this classification (Josseran *et al.*, 1987). A survey carried out in 1956 recorded PRs of between 45-50% in children (Mouchet, personal observation, 1956).

On the island of Bioko, the PR in children used to be above 50% (Merlin *et al.*, 1986) but, by 1991, this had dropped to just 30% (Roche *et al.*, 1991) even though these authors still considered the island to be hyperendemic (*Table XI*).

In the small island of Annobon (1,274 inhabitants), far off the coast of Africa, malaria was holo-endemic with a PR of 80% (Roche *et al.*, 1991 and 1992).

The principal vectors were *An. gambiae s.l., An. melas* and *An. funestus* (Molina *et al.*, 1993) in Bioko. In Rio Muni, the main vector was *An. gambiae s.s.* (Simard, personal observation, 2001) with a sporozoite rate of 12.2% (Toto, personal observation). In Rio Muni, *An. moucheti* was very abundant (Mouchet, personal observation, 1956). In Bioko, the presence of *P. vivax* (detected microscopically) was confirmed by PCR (Rubio *et al.*, 1999). Furthermore, above 10% of the infected subjects were carrying *P. ovale*. Chloroquine-resistant *P. falciparum* were found even though the practice of self-medication was infrequent.

Reports of local centers attributing 30% of deaths to malaria require confirmation.

The environment in the north of the island has been damaged by the petroleum industry whilst deforestation has opened up favourable territories for *An. gambiae*.

The Republic of São Tomé and Principe

The two islands that make up the Republic of São Tomé and Principe are located 250 km off the coast of Gabon. Together they have a population of 170,000 inhabitants (*Table I*). Peaks on the first, which has a volcanic landscape, reach more than 2,000 m. The population is concentrated on the coastline. Principe Island is smaller.

On these islands, which were uninhabited until they were discovered by the Portuguese, malaria became established with the arrival of the first human settlers (Cambournac, personal communication).

Beginning in 1970, a malaria control programme based on indoor DDT spraying was implemented by the Portuguese authorities and malaria was almost eradicated. In 1981, the

Table XI. Parasite rate (children) on the islands of Equatorial Guinea and São Tomé.

Age group	Population surveyed (n)	Parasite rate
Bioko*		
2-4 years	466	26%
5-9 years	664	27%
Annobon*		
2-4 years	102	80%
5-9 years	83	67%
São-Tomé (Guadalupe)**		
2-9 years	190	41%

* adapted from Roche *et al.*, 1991;
** adapted from Ripert *et al.*, 1996

disease reappeared in epidemic form which broke out—it was said at the time—because local people were no longer immune. This "epidemic" was highly publicised by international organisations to discredit eradication policies and promote the development of primary health care systems. However, it is very difficult to obtain objective information about the extent of the epidemic and the associated mortality.

Malaria surveys that were carried out following independence reported PRs of 20% in children in 1978 (Guadalupe Viegas de Ceita, unpublished report), and 40% in 1991 and 1996 (Martet *et al.*, 1991; Ripert *et al.*, 1996). Malaria is therefore meso-endemic on these islands (*Table XI*).

The only vector that has been reported is *An. gambiae s.s.* (Ribeiro *et al.*, 1990) which is particularly abundant in the coastal regions where the population is concentrated. The sporozoite rate was only 0.4% (out of 772 dissections) and the EIR was 1 ib/p/month in São Tomé. No infected anophelines were collected from the island of Principe.

Chloroquine-resistant malaria strains and others with reduced susceptibility to quinine are circulating on these islands (Martet *et al.*, 1991).

Gabon

Gabon is an under-populated country that spans the equator between the 2nd parallel north and the 3rd parallel south. Forest covers 85% of the country and the remaining 15% is made up of post-forest and savannah in the south-west and south-east (*Table I*). Most of the waterways drain into the Oggoué River; the mountains all along the coastline and in the east are below 1,000 m in altitude and hardly affect the equatorial climate which is humid all year round despite a lack of rainfall in August and September. The annual rainfall is more than 2,000 mm of rain per annum fall.

• *Epidemiology*

Richard-Lenoble *et al.* (1987) surveyed malaria throughout the country by analysing blood smears of school children between the ages of 6 and 14. In rural areas, the disease was hyperendemic (PRs of 54-64%) in the estuary, the Woleu Ntem, Doussala; in Mayumbo in the south and Makoukou in the east, malaria was only meso-endemic (*Table XII*).

In the area around the Albert Schweitzer Hospital, near Lambaréné, PRs were very low (8-28%), possibly due to efficient chloroquine distribution. But in the rural areas 50 km from Lambaréné, the prevalence of malaria fluctuated between 68% and 86% (Wildling *et al.*, 1995); *P. falciparum* was found in 96% of infections, a level that was sustained throughout the year.

The studies done by Merlin *et al.* (1990) in the Upper Ogooué near Franceville, in a semi-rural environment in Ngoumé, and in the city of Libreville, only showed meso-endemicity, possibly due to urbanisation and widespread self-medication with chloroquine.

In a group of 158 adults, 19 out of the 20 subjects infected had a parasitaemia below 1,000 trophozoites per mm^3 and without any symptoms (Perret *et al.*, 1991); no conclusions can be drawn as not enough studies have been carried out on adults in hyperendemic areas.

It should also be noted that a sex-ratio imbalance was observed in Lambaréné. In the same place, females were less often infected than males (Widling *et al.*, 1995). No explanation was found for this strange observation apart from the fact that the males would stay up later than the females, but this does not apply to young children.

Walter *et al.* (1981), studying placenta material in Gabon, linked low birth weight with placental damage rather than having a first baby.

Cases of *P. vivax* in Melano-Africans have been regularly reported in Gabon. Irregularities in the development of this parasite were specifically observed in a Gabonese person whose infected red blood cells contained up to six trophozoites each (Poirriez *et al.*, 1991). In this light, the authors emphasised that a few Melano-Africans possess the Duffy antigen, and that the fraction concerned might reach 30% in Rwanda.

In the ape house of the CIRMF in Franceville, *An. gambiae* and *An. funestus* were found to be very aggressive towards chimpanzees and gorillas. As was expected, not one primate was infected even though human parasites had been found in some of the infected *Anopheles*. However, the chimpanzees had significant levels of antibodies directed against sporozoites (Ollomo *et al.*, 1997). It should be remembered that little is known about *An. reichenowi* and *An. schwetzi*, the vectors of African primate malaria.

• *Entomology*

The first lists drawn up by Grjebine (*in* Hamon *et al.*, 1956a) and by Lacan (1958) had already recorded most of the species in Gabon. *An. melas*, *An. gambiae s.l.*, *An. funestus*, *An. nili* and *An. moucheti* were confirmed as vectors. *An. ziemanni*, *An. paludis*, *An. hancocki*, *An. hargreavesi* and *An. wellcomei* were suspected more than they were actually implicated. Of the *An. gambiae* Complex, *An. gambiae s.s.* "Forest" form is the most common vector in the country (Service, 1976; Wildling *et al.*, 1995). These authors also recalled the role of *An. moucheti* already mentioned twenty years before, with a sporozoite rate of 3.7%. *An. nili* was abundant all over the country in numerous foci. *An. funestus* was abundant in deforested zones; Taufflieb (personal communication, 1956) considered it as the main vector for that environment. In the savannah areas of the south-east, it was the dominant species in both the suburban neighbourhoods and the villages (Elissa *et al.*, 1999). In greater Franceville, sporozoite rates were at 3.97%, 2.52% and 3.54% respectively for *An. funestus*, *An. gambiae s.s.* and *An. nili*. In rural environments, the *Anopheles* specimens were more abundant but their sporozoite rates were lower by 1-2% for the three species aforementioned, and by 1% for *An. moucheti*. In the suburban areas of Franceville, every subject received an infective bite once every four days, one bite from *An. funestus* every six days and one bite from *An. gambiae* every seventeen days. In rural environments, on average, every person received one infective bite per night, i.e. one bite from *An. funestus* every two days, one bite from *An. gambiae* every three days, one

Table XII. Distribution of carriers of haematozoa by age and region in Gabon (in Richard-Lenoble *et al.*, 1987).

Region	*Plasmodium* carrier (%) by age (/year)				
	0-1	> 1-4	5-9	10-14	≥ 15
Woleu N'Tem	73%	63.0%	64.0%	65%	–
Ambowe	–	–	25.0%	34%	–
Donguila	–	–	70.2%	46%	25%
Fernan Vaz	–	14.6%	16.7%	–	–
Lebamba Mimongo	–	40.0%	51.0%	37%	–
Doussala	–	–	61.0%	46%	–

(–) = not studied

bite from *An. nili* every six days, and one bite from *An. moucheti* every seventeen days.

The Republic of Congo

The Republic of Congo, which was formerly known as the Middle-Congo of the French Equatorial African Federation, gained independence in 1960, becoming the People's Republic of Congo, before being renamed as the Republic of Congo in 1993. Often it is referred to as Congo-Brazzaville so that it may not be mistaken with the Democratic Republic of Congo, formerly Zaire.

Extending on both sides of the equator, from 3.5° north latitude to 4.2° south latitude, the country has a population of 3.6 million people of which one third live in the capital city Brazzaville, located on the Congo River across from Kinshasa (*Table I*).

The country is made up of a plateau between 500-1,000 m in altitude that culminates in the Mayombe Forest in the west, and which flattens out in the south and to the east to form the northern part of the Congolese Basin. The Congo River stretches out 3 km wide forming the Stanley Pool. Both Brazzaville and Kinshasa are located on its banks. The river then travels over the Crystal Mountains through several spectacular rapids before emerging into the Atlantic Ocean. Upstream from the Pool, the Congo is supplied by tributaries on the right bank, the Sanga and the Oubangi, which are navigable part of the way and which supply not only the Republic of Congo but also the southern parts of both Cameroon and the Central African Republic.

The climate is equatorial with four seasons, with a dry season that is relatively cool and foggy from July to October and which is characteristic of a Brazzavillian middle climate. The great forest that covers the northern part of the country, in addition to the Chaillou and Mayombe Forests, transforms into a mosaic of forest and savannah in the south all the way to the Congo River. North-east of Brazzaville, the arenaceous (sandy) Batéké Plateaux are covered with a steppe-like vegetation that is unusual in equatorial regions, and which is due to the sandy nature of the extremely permeable soil.

• *Epidemiology*

More than 60 years ago, (unpublished) reports from the Pasteur Institute of Brazzaville revealed malaria to be hyperendemic in the Brazzaville Region, with PRs of over 80% in children (*in* Trape, 1987a). The studies carried out by Lacan (1957) had already documented hyperendemic disease in both forest and wooded savannah regions.

On the **Batéké Plateaux** mentioned above, most of the living things and, in particular, mosquito breeding habitats are found in the valley bottoms where the Precambrian platform is visible. Transmission is low-level and seasonal, mostly by *An. gambiae s.s.*, but also by *An. funestus* (just 2%). The EIR was 81 ib/p/yr, concentrated during the wettest three-month period. The PR was of the order of 28% (Carnevale *et al.*, 1985).

In contrast to the preceding situation, a study carried out in Djoumouna, a village in a **mixed area of forest** and savannah surrounded by fish-farming basins, revealed a very high permanent level of transmission with an EIR ranging from 850-1,000 ib/p/yr. The vectors were *An. gambiae s.s.* (90%), *An. moucheti* (7.3%) and *An. funestus* (1.7%). However, the PR of a population of children remained low at 30-45% (Carnevale *et al.*, 1985). These figures were established on the basis of blood smear analyses which tend to ignore low-level parasitaemia and only detect the type of high-level parasitaemia which leads to paroxysms. The objective was to link the dynamics of the transmission to the incidence of high-level parasitaemia and of paroxysms, as recorded at the Djoumouna dispensary. In the same regions, thick blood smear analysis in schoolchildren—with the examination of at least 200 microscopic fields— indicated PRs of 81-94% (*Table XIII*), characteristic of holo-endemicity (Trape, 1987c). In young children, the parasite density was lower than predicted due to widespread self-medication with chloroquine. *An. gambiae s.s.* was the dominant vector with *An. moucheti* and *An. nili* playing very secondary roles. The EIR varied from 200-1,000 ib/p/yr depending on the locality (Trape & Zoulani, 1987a).

In the **Mayombe Forest Region**, studies carried out in four villages outside of Dimonika were described in three articles by Richard *et al.* (1988a, 1988b, 1988c). The principle vector was *An. gambiae s.s.* (96% of specimens). *An. funestus* was significant only during the dry season (3%) and *An. moucheti* never exceeded 1%. The EIR ranged from 80-400 ib/p/yr, depending on the village, with an almost complete absence of transmission during the cool, dry season. The Stability Index (St) was over 2.5 everywhere. Regardless of what the EIR was, malaria was holo-endemic with a PR of 88% in children between the ages of 2-10. The percentages, with a heavy parasite load of over 5,000 trophozoites per mm^3, (the only ones which are significant in clinical terms), dropped from 30% in babies to 17% in 2-5 year-olds, and then down to less than 1% of those over 15, a perfect illustration of premunition.

The PR of *P. malariae* ranged from 13-37% with the highest figures seen in children between the ages of 2 and 5 during the dry season when the reduction in *P. falciparum* density cuts down competition between the two parasites and makes it easier to read the slides!

A number of experts have questioned the usefulness of prevalence as a criterion to evaluate the percentage of infected subjects in holo-endemic areas, since the results are so dependent on the technique used—thick blood smear analysis being far more sensitive than thin blood smears; and the methods of molecular biology (notably PCR) have further enhanced sensitivity. Richard *et al.* (1988c) agree with Bruce-Chwatt (1980) in believing that absolutely all local people are infected, including adults (*Figure 25*). Other factors such as the time taken to examine the slide, the ability of the technician, the quality of the microscope and the other equipment used, as well as the quality of the

Table XIII. Parasite rates by age group in the region of Brazzaville (Linzolo).
Proportion of positive thick film test results in the rainy season (RS) and at the end of the dry season (DS) on the examination of 200 microscopic fields (about 0.5 μl of blood) in inhabitants of the village of Linzolo (adapted from Trape, 1987c).

Age group	P. falciparum (all forms)			P. falciparum (gametocytes)			P. malariae			P. ovale			All species			Number		
	RS	DS	Total (%)	RS	DS	Total (%)	RS	DS	Total (%)	RS	DS	Total (%)	RS	DS	Total (%)	RS	DS	Total (%)
<1	60.7 (34)	–	60.7 (34)	23.2 (13)	–	23.2 (13)	3.6 (2)	–	3.6 (2)	8.9 (5)	–	8.9 (5)	64.3 (36)	–	64.3 (36)	56	–	56
1-4	79.4 (104)	75.0 (66)	77.6 (170)	26.0 (34)	25.0 (22)	25.6 (56)	9.2 (12)	10.2 (9)	9.6 (21)	9.2 (12)	8.0 (7)	8.7 (19)	80.9 (106)	77.3 (68)	79.5 (174)	131	88	219
5-9	76.9 (465)	83.2 (79)	77.7 (544)	23.3 (141)	28.4 (27)	24.0 (168)	16.2 (98)	16.8 (16)	16.3 (114)	5.5 (33)	7.4 (7)	5.7 (40)	78.2 (473)	84.2 (80)	79.0 (533)	605	95	700
10-14	81 (634)	87.5 (42)	81.9 (676)	19.8 (154)	31.3 (15)	20.5 (169)	20.5 (159)	22.9 (11)	20.6 (170)	3.5 (27)	4.2 (2)	3.5 (29)	82.5 (641)	87.5 (42)	82.8 (683)	777	48	825
15-19	68.2 (105)	–	68.2 (105)	19.5 (30)	–	19.5 (30)	16.2 (25)	–	16.2 (25)	0.7 (1)	–	0.7 (1)	70.1 (108)	–	70.1 (108)	154	–	154
20-39	60.9 (42)	–	60.9 (42)	18.8 (13)	–	18.8 (13)	10.1 (7)	–	10.1 (7)	0.0 (0)	–	0.0 (0)	63.8 (44)	–	63.8 (44)	69	–	69
>40	37.0 (57)	–	37.0 (57)	7.8 (12)	–	7.8 (12)	2.6 (4)	–	2.6 (4)	1.3 (2)	–	1.3 (2)	39.0 (60)	–	39.0 (60)	154	–	154

thick smear, will all affect the prevalence figure. The method used to measure prevalence—on which the threshold of positivity will depend—should therefore be chosen according to the objectives of the work.

The pyrogenic threshold was estimated at 20,000 *P. falciparum* parasites/mm^3 in under-5 year-olds, 8,000 in 5-10 year-olds, and 4,500 in adults (Richard *et al.*, 1988b).

The frequency of malaria attacks was 14% per year in babies, 11.7% in children between the ages of 2-5, 9% in children between the ages of 6-10, and 1.2% in adults, and was always greater during the rainy season than during dry periods.

Urban malaria in Brazzaville was addressed in a series of articles in 1987 by Trape, Trape & Zoulani, and Trape *et al.* Since 1960, the city has undergone tremendous growth and is now home to more than one third of the population of Congo, creating a kaleidoscope of situations between well urbanised "old neighbourhoods" and suburban ghettos. Before 1950, according to reports made at the time by the Pasteur Institute of Brazzaville, malaria was holo-endemic in both the city and in the surrounding rural areas (Trape, 1987c). Between 1950-1960, the malaria control programme considerably reduced the incidence of the disease. In 1960, following independence, vector control and chemoprophylactic operations were abandoned and a new type of urban malaria took hold.

The only vector found in the city was *An. gambiae s.s.*, accompanied by *An. moucheti* on rare occasions. The sporozoite rate of *An. gambiae* was at 3.4%. One single infected *An. moucheti* was found. The average EIR in the city was 22 ib/p/yr but the distribution was extremely uneven. Residents of certain surrounding neighbourhoods received more than 100 ib/p/yr while residents in the city centre were infected only once every three years. The construction of a new neighbourhood with its access ditches resulted in *An. gambiae* springing up in abundance. Then, the number of *Anopheles* decreased with land use and with pollution by household waste and drainage. In the end, the vectors gathered around potential larval habitats, which lowered the level of exposure to the rest of the neighbourhood's population. Depending on the level of urbanisation, the PI of school children varied from 0 to 80%. In the neighbourhoods around the city-centre, specific antibodies could not be detected in some children, even by IFI.

• *Morbidity and mortality*

In a holo-endemic **rural environment** in the "Pool" region, the annual incidence of clinical attacks was 3, 2.1, 1.8 and 1.2 for children between the ages of 5-6, 7-8, 9-10, and 11-13 respectively (Trape *et al.*, 1987b). A simplified diagnostic method helped verify if a patient's parasite density was compatible with a malaria attack; in practice, malaria was ruled out if the ratio of the number of parasites to the number of leukocytes was lower than 1.5 (Trape *et al.*, 1985).

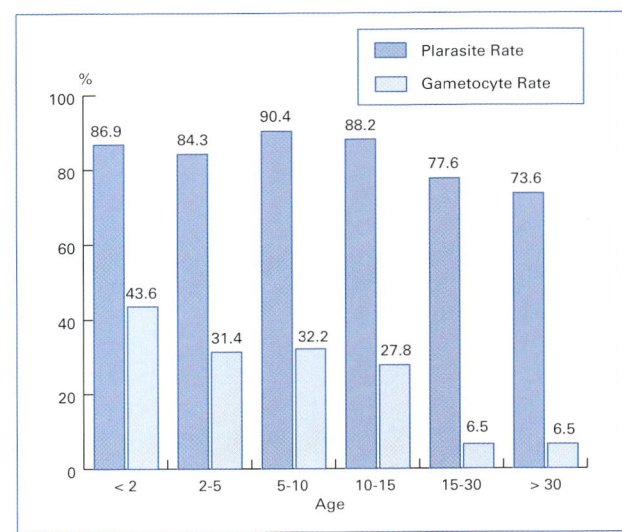

Figure 25. Variation in Plasmodium *rate and* Gametocyte *rate with age in the Mayombe villages of the Congo (Richard et al., 1988).*

In the Mayombe, an isolated fever was the second commonest reason in children under 15 for having a medical consultation but in adults, it was the fifth (*Table XIV*).

In Brazzaville, the **annual incidence of pernicious attacks** was 1.15‰ between the ages of 0-4, 0.25‰ between 5-9, and 0.05‰ between 10-14 years (Trape *et al.*, 1987d). In the Paediatrics Department of the General Hospital, only thirty pernicious cases were recorded in two years; two of these were HbAS heterozygotes (Vaisse *et al.*, 1981).

The malaria mortality rate in the city of Brazzaville was 0.43‰ in children between 0-4 years, and 0.08‰ in children between 5-9 years. These figures are **thirty times less than the malaria mortality rate generally reported in tropical Africa** (Trape, 1987c). In a holo-endemic rural environment, in a **cohort of 500 children** under the age of 5 that were being followed in Linzolo near Brazzaville, **not one death** was directly **attributed to malaria** (Carme *et al.*, 1984; Guillo du Bodan, 1982). Out of 100 successful births, 93 babies had lived through to their first year and 88 had made it to their fifth year; Measles was the main cause of death. Comparable to these observations are those of Richard *et al.* (1988c) who did not diagnose one single case of serious malaria out of a group of 500 children being followed in Mayombe. This **low mortality rate for malaria, in a zone of perennial transmission** in the Congo, is worrisome when we compare it to the figures for West Africa. Widespread self-medication with chloroquine in the Congo cannot account for these differences as it is practised in all of the countries of Central and West Africa, including in the most remote areas. Molineaux (1988) observed this phenomenon but did not give an explanation. In Vanuatu, in a quite different part of the

Afrotropical Region

Table XIV. Reasons for consultation (%) at the Dimonika unit in Mayombe, Congo (adapted from Richard et al., 1988c).

Reasons	< 2 years	2-5 years	6-15 years	Adults
Rhino-pharyngitis, bronchitis, influenza symptoms	16.2	16.1	4.2	2.4
Lung foci	6.3	1.2	0.7	2.1
Isolated cough	16.2	21	16.1	3.5
Diarrhoea, gastroenteritis	25.2	16.1	3.5	1.2
Intestinal parasite infections	4.5	17.9	26.6	7.4
Heart failure	0	0	0	3.2
Hypertension	0	0	0	4.1
Neurological ailments	0	1.2	0	2.4
Rheumatism	0	0	1.4	21.5
Gynaecological ailments	0	0	0.7	8.3
STD	0	0	0	3.2
Burns	0.9	1.2	1.4	1.8
Pyodermitis, fungal skin infections	0	1.2	0.7	1.5
Abscess	3.6	1.2	1.4	0.6
Pruritus	0	0.6	0	14.2
Urogenital disease	0	2.5	0.7	2.4
Serious nutritional disorders	0.9	0	0	0
Ophthalmology	1.8	2.5	2.1	3
Stomatology	0	0.6	1.4	2.4
ENT	2.7	0.9	0	0
Asthenia, diverse subjective problems	0	1.2	2.8	15.9
Isolated fever	18	19.1	24.5	7.4
Headaches	0	0	7.7	13.3
Other	0.9	3.1	4.9	2.1
Total number of consultations	227	326	236	339

world, no malaria deaths occur in a place where malaria is hyperendemic and transmitted year round (Maitland et al., 1997).

• *Entomology*

The five species of vectors in the Congo were already identified in 1956 and are *An. melas*, *An. gambiae s.s.*, *An. funestus*, *An. nili* and *An. moucheti* (Hamon et al., 1956a; Lacan 1958).

An. gambiae s.s. was by far the most important vector in areas of dense forest (Richard et al., 1988a), as well as in areas with mixed forest and savannah (Carnevale et al., 1985), and in Brazzaville (Trape & Zoulani, 1987a). Its sporozoite rate ranged between 1% and 4%. The number of bites received was proportional to the person's skin surface, so young children were bitten half as often as older children who themselves received 2.5 times fewer bites than adults (Carnevale et al., 1978).

An. nili or rather the species of the Nili Complex were very abundant in the hilly regions but their sporozoite rates were very low: one infection out of more than 1,500 dissections (Carnevale, 1974).

An. moucheti develops in most rivers but its density was found to be low in all the sites investigated in the Congo.

An. funestus only assumed a position of importance in deforested areas and during the dry season (Richard et al., 1988a).

In conclusion, the malaria in the Congo is hyper- or holo-endemic, stable with year-round transmission. But its most outstanding characteristic is that the mortality rate for malaria is low, which calls for additional studies.

The Democratic Republic of Congo

The Democratic Republic of Congo (formerly Zaire) has 57.5 million inhabitants, occupying more than half of Central Africa, and is situated between the 5th north and the 13th parallel south, from the Gulf of Guinea to the Great Lakes (*Table I*). The mis-management of the country's politics and economy since its independence has made it one of the poorest countries of Africa with a GNP of 880, despite possessing one of the world's richest mineral deposits.

The country is centred around the central basin (300-500 m in altitude) which is drained by the Congo River and its tributaries. Hills rise up in the west in the Mayombe Region and in the Crystal Mountains (600-900 m in altitude) where the Congo passes through white water rapids before ending up in a deep estuary. In the south, the Katanga Plateaux* at more than 1,500 m in altitude join with the plateaux of southern Africa. But it is mostly in the east that we find peaks resulting from tectonic movements during the Tertiary Period, which border with the "graben", a depression on the western side of the Rift Valley. In Kivu, the Rwenzori are over 5,000 m high and the volcanoes of the Virunga are 3,000 m high. The equatorial climate in the basin becomes tropical to the north and south of the 5th parallel. The altitude and the latitude are both responsible for the introduction of mountain influences in Kivu in the east, and in Katanga in the south. The basin's vegetation is made up of a large tropical forest which transforms in the south into a mosaic of forest and savannah crossed with wide forest galleries. Further south, the herbaceous and shrubby vegetation covers the plateaux. In the north, the vegetation is Sudanese as in the Central African Republic. The fauna is no less varied with several endemic species. The richness of the collection of invertebrate fauna at the Tervueren Museum in Belgium reflects the diversity of the Congolese fauna. The *Anopheles* were amongst the groups that were most studied (Gillies & De Meillon, 1968).

• *History*

The first research on malaria in the Democratic Republic of Congo was carried out at the beginning of the 20th century in Kinshasa (then Leopoldville), when the country was the Independent State of Congo, property of the King of Belgians. Although at first the study was directed towards protecting expatriates, they soon extended to all levels of the native population. From 1920 to 1969, no less than 331 papers dedicated to malaria were published in the *Annales de la Société Belge de Médecine Tropicale*. Several reviews, notably by Duren (1937), Gillet (1953) and Janssens *et al.* (1992) summarise these different studies.

The malaria appeared to be omnipresent except at an altitude above 1,800 m. The following regions were identified:
- regions where transmission was perennial, with the development of a strong immunity by the population, where the serious attacks mainly affected children under the age of 3;
- regions where transmission was seasonal where the increase of clinical cases resulted from seasonal peak of vector bites;
- epidemic regions in the mountains, particularly after the valleys were developed.

From 1930-1960, the major concern of epidemiologists was evaluating the morbidity and mortality rates of malaria.

Before the 1960's, malaria was prevalent throughout the Congo. **Most of the country was hyperendemic** with average PRs of 75% in children under the age of 3, 68% in children between 4-15, and 22% in adults (Duren, 1951). Certain forested areas of the basin were meso-endemic, bordering on hyperendemic. In the Kivu Mountains in the east and in the Katanga Mountains in the south, indices switched from meso- to hypo-endemic with increasing altitude; the disease disappearing entirely at 1,800 m.

Beginning in 1950, the main vectors and their ecology started to be identified. Only after 1962 was the *An. gambiae* Complex delineated.

Even though *P. falciparum* was the most frequent parasite, the role of *P. malariae* was a serious concern. *P. ovale* was a rarity and the polemic surrounding *P. vivax* is never ending.

The discovery of the rodent *Plasmodium*, *P. berghei* and then *P. vinckei* in *Thamnomys surdaster* in Katanga marked an important stage in the study of plasmodial biology (Vincke & Lips, 1948). The availability of a parasite that could infect laboratory mice facilitated research into the factors that govern cycles and provided a valuable *in vivo* model for cheaper testing of candidate antimalaria drugs developed by the pharmaceutical industry.

• *Epidemiology*

In 1942, the **altitudinal malaria limit** in Kivu, in the east of the Congo, was around 1,800 m between Walung (1,750 m) and Kabare (1,850 m). The disease was concentrated in the valleys and disappeared entirely at 2,000 m (Schwetz, 1942). Beyond this limit, *An. christyi*, *An. cinereus* and *An. marshalli* were not vectors. Since then, we have observed malaria transmission at higher altitudes in Ethiopia, Uganda, and in Kenya. The record for Africa seems still to be in Kenya where *An. gambiae* was a vector at 2,600 m (Garnham, 1945).

In **Kivu** (*Table XV*), a longitudinal study of fifteen villages on the shores of Lake Kivu, 1,500 m high, illustrated the unstable nature of meso-endemic malaria (Delacollette *et al.*, 1990a). The average PR varied from 24-44% with season, and from 15-55% from village to village, with a minimum of 7% at 1,750 m in altitude.

The highly particular group of **Pygmies** from the Ituri, in the high forest, presented PIs of 32%, 48%, 22% and 21% respectively in babies, children between the ages of 3-10,

---

* Katanga Province in the south of the Democratic Republic of Congo was called Shaba during the Mobutu régime. It is now called Katanga once more. Lakes Edward and Albert have also been restored to their former names.

Afrotropical Region

Table XV. Parasite rates at Kivu. Numbers examined and malarial indices (%) by age in two regions (Ra & Rb) of the Health Zone. Katana, Democratic Republic of Congo, February 1985 (adapted from Delacollette *et al.*, 1990a)

Age	Number Ra	Number Rb	Parasite rate Ra	Parasite rate Rb
0-11 months	22	18	27.3	27.8
1-4 years	61	60	29.5	38.3
5-9 years	28	32	50.0	25.0
10-19 years	44	43	38.6	41.9
20-29 years	60	45	23.3	44.4
> 29 years	45	58	42.2	41.4

children between the ages of 11-15, and in adults. The Bantus, who lived in the neighbouring villages, presented PRs that were much higher—96%, 50% and 58% for the same age groups (Schwetz *et al.*, 1934). The difference in prevalence reflected the environmental differences between the two communities, just as in Cameroon and the Central African Republic as discussed above (*Table XVI*).

More than 3 million people live in **Greater Kinshasa** (*Figure 26*), which extends along the Congo River for 50 km and 20 km inland at an altitude between 300-500 m high. There are enormous differences in the levels of incidence and prevalence according to the geographical location, the level of urbanisation, and the social standing of the residents of the different neighbourhoods (Wery, 1986). The average level of prevalence was 50% and the incidence of feverish attacks amounted to 500‰ (Mulumba *et al.*, 1990). Babies under one year old were the least infected, relatively speaking. Then, PR increased up to the age of 2, thereafter remaining stable until 10. In the city centre, children received an infective bite once every 128 nights whereas in the surrounding ghettos, they could receive 1.7 infective bites every night during the rainy season (Karch *et al.*, 1992). Similar differences were noted by Coene (1993) who reported EIR of 0.08-1.07 ib/p/night depending on the neighbourhood. The "Forest" form of *An. gambiae s.s.* was responsible for more than 90% of transmission along with the participation of *An. funestus*, *An. nili* and *An. brunnipes*.

• Entomology

The *An. gambiae* Complex is represented by at least three species in this country. The "Forest" form of *An. gambiae s.s.* occupies all of the forest region, the mosaic of forest and savannah, and the forest galleries. In Kinshasa, it is almost the only vector present. Its sporozoite rate was 1.8% in the city centre, and 7.8% in the outskirts (Coene *et al.*, 1993). *An. melas* was reported only at the mouth of the Congo. *An. arabiensis*, the malaria vector in the rice paddies of the Rusizi in Burundi, most certainly crosses the border; it is also probably the vector in Katanga. The presence of *An. quadriannulatus s.l.* in the south and east needs to be verified; in any case, it is not a vector.

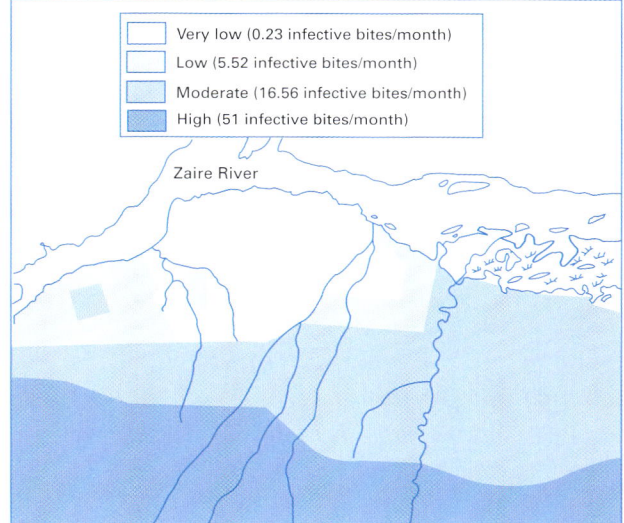

Figure 26. Malaria transmission in Kinshasa (adapted from Karch et al., 1992).

Table XVI. Parasite rates in Pygmies and neighbouring Bantus in the Ituri forest, Democratic Republic of Congo (adapted from Schwetz *et al.*, 1934).

Age group	Pygmies N° of samples	Pygmies Positive results	Pygmies %	Bantus N° of samples	Bantus Positive results	Bantus %
Babies	25	8	32	*		
3-10 years	62	30	48	25	24	96
10-15 years	48	11	22	22	11	50
Adults	165	35	21	39	24	61
Total	300	84	28	86	59	68

* No samples were taken from Bantu babies

An. funestus presented a different ecology in the deforested areas of the west and in the mountain regions of the east; In Kinshasa, although it was uncommon, it had a sporozoite rate of 6.6%.

An. moucheti was described from Congo by Evans in 1926. Its vector role was first demonstrated along the Congo and Kwango Rivers before its presence was discovered all along slow-flowing rivers throughout the entire forest region and in other gallery forest. Parent & Demoulin (1943) correlated the density of the adults in houses with the larval ecology and the level of rivers; this *Anopheles* peaks in conjunction with the stabilisation of river levels.

An. nili is a good vector all along fast-flowing rivers throughout the entire region. Its sporozoite rate was as high as 6.6% in the areas surrounding Kinshasa.

An. paludis is a species of forest regions from the Atlantic to the Indian Ocean. It is generally anthropophilic, as well as exophilic. In northern Congo and in the region of Kinshasa, it is highly endophilic. It is locally a good vector and its sporozoite rate can be as high as 6% (Karch & Mouchet, 1992). Such differences in behaviour could be accompanied by particular taxonomic characteristics.

An. brunnipes was known for a long time to be a vector in Kinshasa where 4% of the specimens were carrying sporozoites (Coene, 1993; Wanson & Berteaux, 1944).

An. marshalli was periodically implicated in transmission in higher altitude regions. In the Kivu Region, sporozoites were observed in 0.24% of the 1,200 specimens dissected (Bafort, 1985). There is still, however, much doubt as to the actual role of this anopheline.

An. dureni has been reported to transmit *P. berghei* to the rodent *Thamnomys surdaster* in the forest galleries of the Katanga Region.

The transmission of primate *Plasmodium* species, *P. reichenowi*, *P. schwetzi* and *P. rodhaini* (= *P. malariae*), still remains unknown despite thorough research carried out by Rodhain (1941).

• *Malaria morbidity and mortality*

Malaria morbidity and **mortality** has varied over time not only according to the modes of transmission but also according to the potential access to health care, the quality of health care, and the development of the malaria control programme. The current political and economic collapse of the country has resulted in the quality of health care declining, so it is difficult today to take stock of the situation.

In the holo-endemic region of the gold mines of Kilo, near Lake Albert, Janssens *et al.* (1966) had carried out 1,800 autopsies on subjects suspected of having malaria. The disease was held responsible for the death of 12.3% of babies, 13% of young children between 1-2 years, 12% of children between 3-5 years, and 11% of children between 6-15 years. The rate of hospitalisation for malaria ranged between 5-15%; malaria morbidity was 100‰; malaria mortality was 40‰ in babies (i.e. 14.7% of the general mortality of this age group). Following the administration of prophylactic drugs, infant mortality decreased from 300‰ to 50‰.

Duren (1951) reported malaria infant mortality to be 7.2% in the Kwango and 28% in the Mayombe, a discrepancy that is most unlikely. In his conclusion, the author stated that out of 11 million inhabitants (the population of Congo at the time), 30,000 died each year of malaria, i.e. 14-17% of deaths of which 47% were in children between the ages of 0-3. The conclusions, however, were not very reliable as the evaluation methods used varied from one observer to the next.

On the shores of Lake Kivu, at 1,500 m in altitude, the mortality specific to malaria was 3‰ of the general population per year, i.e. 18‰ per year in babies and 8‰ in young children between the ages of 1-4 (Delacollette *et al.*, 1989).

In Kinshasa, out of 10,036 child deaths, 13.2% were due to malaria in young children under the age of 3 (Greenberg *et al.*, 1989). In the city, every child under the age of 5 presented an average of 4.6 fever episodes per year; 75% of the feverish patients were carrying trophozoites but only 21% had fever, the others being symptomless (Mulumba *et al.*, 1994).

In the Kivu Region, various etiologies have been ascribed to blackwater fever, including leptospirosis, Haantan virus and G6PD deficiency as well as massive parasitaemia; a role for quinine was excluded, despite the findings of most experts (Delacollette *et al.*, 1995).

In Congo, the causes of nephrotic syndrome have not been completely elucidated but it is not certain that *P. malariae* is responsible for this problem (Pakasa *et al.*, 1993).

Rwanda and Burundi

Rwanda and Burundi, former provinces of German East Africa, became the Rwanda-Urundi Territory after the First World War and placed by the Society of Nations under Belgian mandate. In 1962, following independence, the two countries separated and the Republic of Rwanda in the north, and the Kingdom of Burundi in the south (*Figure 27*) were both founded.

Both countries are situated on a plateau between 1,000-2,200 m of altitude dominated at more than 3,000 m by the Congo-Nile Ridge that runs north-south, and that separates the Congo and Nile basins. The hills gradually slope down to the east and to the north onto the Tanzanian Plateau, and drop abruptly down to the Great Lakes to the west. The Rusizi Valley and Lake Tanganyika form a natural frontier between Burundi and the Democratic Republic of Congo (between 850-1,100 m), while Lake Kivu at 1,500 m separates the Democratic Republic of Congo from Rwanda.

There is an equatorial 4-season climate which is highly affected by the altitude (i.e. it freezes in winter). The rainy season is from March to June and in October-November. The primitive vegetation, high altitude forest, subsists only in a few relict sites, that are more or less protected, in the

Afrotropical Region

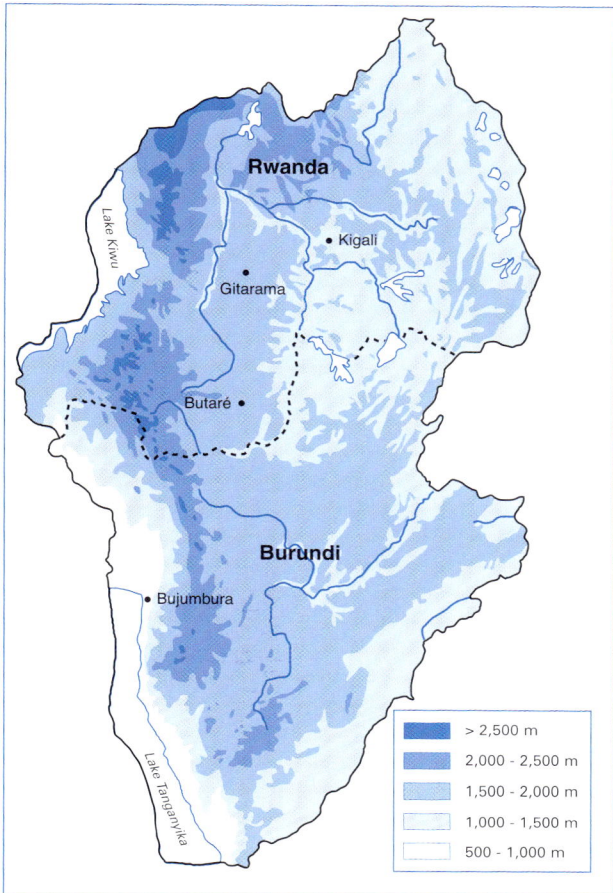

Figure 27. Relief in Rwanda and Burundi.

Virunga Park of Volcanoes where Uganda, Rwanda, and the Democratic Republic of Congo intersect, and where the last surviving mountain gorillas reside. The high altitude prairies, interspersed with papyrus marshland in the valleys, make up the majority of the plant life. The banana plantations take up a large part of the hillsides and provide the population's main staple.

The population is greatly dispersed within these plantations and amounts up to 500 habitants per km^2 (more than 200 people/km^2 on average). The clearing of marshes and their use for farming is a relatively recent phenomenon that dates from the 1940's. The new resources of food crops, fish farming ponds, and now rice paddies have encouraged the population, which was previously scattered in the hills, to settle down near the rivers. These mini-migrations have played a very important role in the development of malaria.

The geographic and administrative unit is the "hill", which is divided into communes. Antagonism between the different ethnic groups, the farming Bantus, the Hutus, and the Nilotic shepherds, the Tutsi, has created an almost permanent state of insecurity since independence, emphasised by massacres and, as in 1994 in Rwanda, genocide that was so sadistic in nature it brings shame to Mankind.

Before 1950, malaria was considered to be meso-endemic below 1,300 m and on the peaks conditions were deemed healthy. The situation greatly changed once the marshland began to be farmed and the valley bottoms populated, along with the strong seasonal migration of farm labourers, bringing their parasites with blood from the two countries.

Against a background of moderately endemic malaria in the valleys and lowlands, Rwanda and Burundi constitute foci of unstable, epidemic disease.

We have first dealt with the information obtained before 1962, when the two countries were under Belgian administration, and then the recent data are concerned individually and by country.

A stratification study came up with the following distinctions:
- in the regions situated below 1,000 m: the valley of the Rusizi and South Imbo along the Tanganyika in Burundi, the shores of Lake Albert in Rwanda, the malaria was meso- to hyperendemic;
- the regions between 1,000-1,500 m high made up a fringe all along the preceding region in Burundi, and on the south-east (Moso) and east (Kagera) rims of the plateau; this zone was generally found to be meso- or hypo-endemic;
- the plateaux between 1,500-2,000 m high were considered to be an epidemic zone;
- the Congo-Nile ridge between 2,000-2,500 m high was entirely free of malaria.

• *Epidemiology*

According to records from religious orders, malaria appeared in Rwanda-Urundi following the passage of troops during the war of 1914-1918. The disease was first recognised in Rwanda in 1929 (Mattlet, 1935).

Schwetz (1942) had admitted that there were no *Anopheles* species capable of transmitting above 1,800 m in altitude. Major cultural changes, however, were to modify the local epidemiology. As Rwanda-Urundi was subject to periodic shortages, the government asked each head of the family to cultivate a parcel of marshland in order to make up for these difficult times. These "bonus" parcels favoured the development of *An. funestus* and *An. gambiae*; in addition, for the purpose of providing more protein to the population, several fish farming basins were created (Jadin & Herman, 1946).

Despite relatively low temperatures, the sporogonic cycles were completed in the endophilic *An. funestus* and *An. gambiae* because the temperature inside houses was 3-5 °C higher than outside (Jadin & Fain, 1951; Meyus *et al.*, 1962). The growth cycle of *P. falciparum* was possible in homes where there were livestock even though outside temperatures barely exceeded 14 °C. In Butaré, 1% of *An. funestus* was infected (at 1,750 m) and the PR was as high

Biodiversity of Malaria in the World

as 65% in children and 41% in adults. Malaria was even found at 1,850 m around Butaré, then known as Astrida (Vincke & Jadin, 1946).

In the area surrounding Butaré (Jadin & Fain, 1951), the global PI varied from 36-65%. The average in babies and children between 5-10 years old was 64% and in adults it was 41% (*Table XVII*). This table reveals both the hyperendemic nature of malaria and the weak premunition in adults.

Epidemics on the plateaux were first reported in 1929 (Mattlet, 1935; Schwetz, 1941); they were considered to be a recurrent phenomenon during which the population acquired hardly any immunity. Rwandan workers expatriated to the neighbour Kivu presented a negligible level of immunity and were extremely vulnerable to fevers (Schwetz & Bauman, 1941).

It should be noted that there was a very high prevalence of *P. malariae* (56%), which was the most common parasite in the Mutara where the global PR was 43%. This is rare in Africa.

In the valley of the Rusizi, malaria brought on through irrigation was meso-endemic; in the savannahs of the east (Moso, Kagera between 1,200-1,500 m high) it was meso- or hyperendemic (Meyus *et al.*, 1962).

In 1952, an indoor insecticide treatment program with DDT was implemented around Butare. The PR, which was at 51% before the spraying, dropped to 7% three years later. On the contrary, in the area which had not been sprayed and which acted as a control, the PR had increased to a holo-endemic level. One remarkable effect of the spraying was the complete disappearance of *An. funestus* (Jadin, 1952).

A map of the vectors reported the presence of *An. gambiae s.l.*, *An. funestus*, *An. moucheti* and *An. nili*; it indicated the catching sites but did not provide any ecological or epidemiological information (Vermylen, 1967).

Rwanda

In 1975, Ivora Cano (1982) collated the information on malaria in Rwanda. He pointed out the very low sporozoite rate of *An. gambiae s.l.* in the Bugarama where this *Anopheles* was nonetheless very anthropophilic.

In 1989, Munyatore observed a level of prevalence from 7-43% in the various regions of the country. He pointed out that several epidemics had been reported by the press and/or the local radio stations but that the nature of these epidemics had never been confirmed.

In 1993, the number of reported cases with fever increased enormously from 24‰ to 183‰. Only 50% were malaria related but as half the cases are not reported in health centres anyway, the figures are considered to represent the true scale of the disease (Schapira & Ravaonjanahary, 1993). The increase of cases reported would be due to an improved coverage of information systems and to the modifications, that are not always explained, of epidemiological determining factors, i.e. changes in the environment and in the location of homes (in the valleys) with respect to farming practises and demographic burdens, an increase in the average temperature over the last ten years, and growth in the number of exchanges and in the circulation of people. Altitude, however, remains the greatest determining factor in the distribution of malaria, with high areas being the least infected (Gisenyi, Kibaye, Rubengi) and the lower areas most affected (Kigali, Butaré, Gitarama). The peak of transmission occurs in June-July,

Table XVII. Parasite rates around Butaré (Jadin & Fain, 1951).

Hills	Number of patients examined	Positive results	%
Nyanza	903	406	43
Mbazi	526	269	51
Kabuga	515	279	54
Save	955	343	35
Kisanze	468	303	64
Musenga	310	119	38
Muyira	500	253	50
Chyarwa	515	295	57
Tumba	504	241	47
Runyniya	500	271	54
Tonga	428	205	47
Chyarwa	492	257	52
Sovu	500	259	51
Rukira	500	298	59
Gatoke	509	230	45
Munazi	521	256	49
Zivu	520	298	57
Shyanda	501	306	61
Musha	516	317	61
Mwulire	536	245	45
Nyakabanda	551	331	60
Rukara	624	301	48
The same rates by age group			
1 year	1,027	666	64
1-5 years	1,352	846	62
5-10 years	1,663	1,085	65
10-15 years	1,408	832	51
Adults	6,444	2,653	41
Total	11,894	6,082	51

at the end of the heavy rains, and in December-January following the little rainy season.

In 1992, there were 1.5 million cases of malaria out of a population of 6.6 million people, including 2,000 related deaths (Schapira & Ravaonjanahary, 1993). The incidence was similar for all age groups, which supports the position of a lack of immunity. In certain neighbourhoods of Kigali, however, 30% of parasite carriers were asymptomatic. Malaria was the main reason for health clinic visits and the main cause of mortality in the country.

Reports from the health services collected by the French Embassy in 1992 showed the average rate of incidence for malaria to be 182‰ (*Figure 28*), and the mortality rate to be 23‰ (*Figure 29*); at high altitudes (Gisenyi) the incidence was 50‰ and at lower altitude, at 1,500 m, it was 280‰ (Kigali).

In Gisenyi, mortality increased from 0.3‰ in 1984 to 1‰ in 1991. Several epidemics had been reported at altitudes above 2,000 m (Pajot, 1991). Malaria had become the most important disease in the country.

Around Kigali at 1,400-1,500 m in altitude, the refugee camps sheltered many people that were originally from high altitude regions greater than 2,000 m. In these camps, there was a high mortality rate due to malaria, amounting to 10‰ per week in children under 5, and transmission was intense with more than two hundred *An. gambiae s.l.* per hut.

The migration of people, which was more and more frequent, even introduced malaria into regions where there was no transmission. In Ngarutara, between 1,800-2,650 m high, 182 cases of malaria were admitted to the hospital in 1982. All but four patients had travelled in the two weeks prior to their hospitalisation. Two thousand children, examined during the same period in the same region, did not have any splenomegaly and, in 686 thick blood smears, none were positive, leading the authors to conclude that these cases had been imported (Gascon *et al.*, 1984).

When global warming became an issue, several scientists attempted to implicate this phenomenon in the increase of disease and, in particular, of malaria. The issue flourished in the media and with futurologists. Often, with one simple correlation, entire scenarios were developed and the more catastrophic they were, the more appreciated they were (*see the Part entitled* "Spatiotemporal Dynamics of Malaria"). In the Health Centre of Meguso (prefecture of Gikongo), Loevinshon (1994) reported that the number of

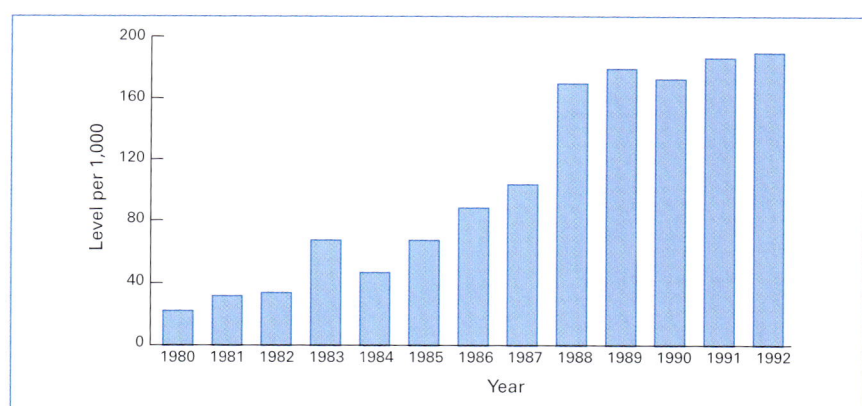

Figure 28.
Changes in the incidence of malaria in Rwanda from 1980 to 1992 (data gathered by the French Embassy) (source SIS).

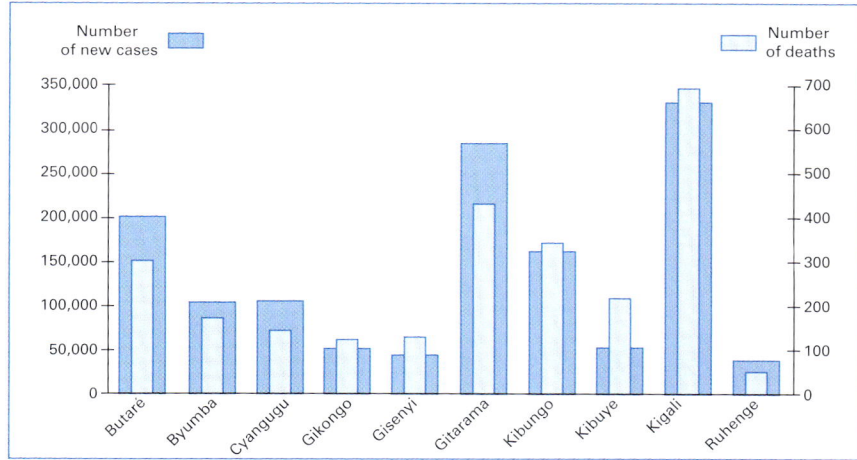

Figure 29.
Crude 1992 morbidity and mortality figures by prefecture in Rwanda (source SIS).

malaria consultations had increased from 100 in 1984, to 200 in 1986, and to 600 in 1987. The temperature (average minimum) had increased by 1.2 °C between 1967 and 1987. This study was used to justify all those who believed that global warming led to a growth of malaria in mountain regions. It should be noted that none of the mathematical models used could in any way justify the correlation between a temperature increase of 1.2 °C with an increase of transmission by 600%. The rainfall deficit in 1984 (-150 mm), and excess in 1987-1988 is enough to explain an increase in transmission. The preceding years (1977-1983) had already been "hotter" than in 1984 and the incidence of malaria remained very low. No reference was made to possible changes in the environment. It is obvious that an epidemiological study that puts into question such an important phenomenon as global warming cannot neglect to take into account all the localised determining factors of the disease.

In conclusion, a study on the cost of malaria that took into account the medication, health fees, and the number of working days missed, concluded that every attack cost 2.88 US$ and that the disease as a whole, with 1,722,271 cases in 1985, amounted to 2.4% of the national budget (Ettling & Shepard, 1991).

Burundi

A study carried out throughout the entire country established the level of endemicity in the various regions of Burundi (*Figure 30*) (Delacollette *et al.*, 1990b). In the Imbo, between 780-1,100 m high, the malaria was generally hyperendemic, with pockets of meso-endemicity in the centre and south. The Moso and the far north were meso-endemic. The disease was hypo-endemic or epidemic on the plateaux. The disease became endemic in several regions where it had previously been epidemic for reasons that are not clear. As in Rwanda, cases of malaria were imported each year by seasonal migrant workers. Their incidence was thus as high as 16‰ in a region above 1,800 m in altitude where there was no indigenous malaria (Van der Stuyft *et al.*, 1993).

• *Endemic disease and epidemics*

The first epidemic reported in the country was disregarded for several months before the departments of the Registry Office took any notice. Since the early 1900's, the valley of the Rusizi was known to be home to meso-endemic malaria in contrast with the healthiness of the neighbouring mountains. Rice-growing, irrigated since the late 1960's, had created an environment that was extremely favourable to the development of *An. arabiensis*; malaria had become hyperendemic (Coosemans *et al.*, 1984; Coosemans, 1985). PRs varied from 69% in June to 25% in January. In the drier cotton plantations, the indices remained between 29% in July and 4.5% in January. In any case, malaria was very unstable, with a Stability Index (St) of 0.7. Clinical incidence was four times higher in the surrounding rice paddies than in the cotton plantations. In the neighbouring city of Bujumbura, the PR amounted to only 5%. The principle vector was *An. arabiensis* (98%) with a scattering of *An. gambiae s.s.* (2%). The role of *An. funestus* was secondary and that of *An. pharoensis* and *An. ziemanni* non-existent. The average sporozoite rate for *An. arabiensis* was 0.45% peaking to 2% at certain times (*Table XVIII*).

Since 1985, malaria epidemics of variable intensity have occurred on the plateaux of Burundi (between 1,400-1,750 m high). The situation was particularly worrisome in November 2000 when 700,000 cases were reported along with several hundred deaths. This latest epidemic cannot easily be explained by climatic events or environmental factors. In the preceding years, a growth of the parasite reservoir had been reported and when it reached a critical point, the epidemic broke out (Coosemans, personal observation). The same seems to be true for many epidemics at high altitude which break out following an increased concentration of the parasite reservoir, regardless of whether or not there are climatic (Uganda) or operational (Madagascar) reasons (Mouchet *et al.*, 1998). The areas located near man-made shallow water (rice paddies, brickworks, etc.) are affected the most. In the past, the papyrus marshlands were especially suitable for the development of *An. christyi*; although certain authors have suspected this *Anopheles* of being able to transmit malaria, there has been no confirmation of this. Intense development

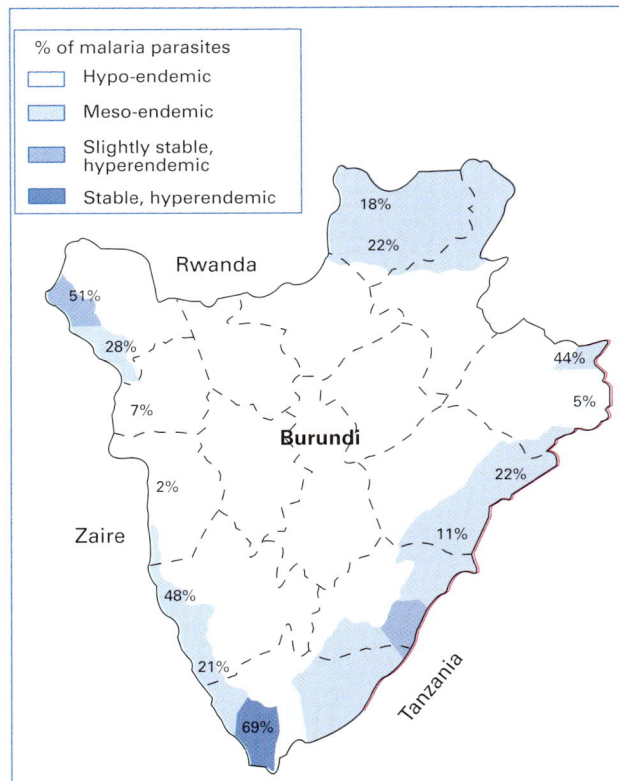

Figure 30. Malaria in Burundi (1989) (*adapted from Delacollette* et al., *1990*).

Table XVIII. Parasite and spleen rates in the villages of Gihanga Mulira and Katumba (adapted from Coosemans, 1985).

Dates	N	PR (%)	GR (%)	Density (%)	Density (n)	SR (%)	SR (n)
Village of Gihanga - Rice-growing							
6 January 1982	136	25.7	6.6	15.2	(33)	–	–
17 February 1982	160	24.4	5.6	10.5	(38)	12.0	(141)
29 March 1982	153	28.7	14.4	25.0	(40)	–	–
11 May 1982	138	38.4	15.2	28.8	(52)	4.6	(86)
22 June 1982	103	60.2	15.5	40.7	(59)	10.5	(95)
3 August 1982	129	64.3	31.8	43.4	(76)	26.4	(121)
21 September 1982	114	60.5	23.7	26.2	(65)	20.7	(106)
2 November 1982	133	48.9	20.3	31.7	(60)	10.0	(130)
21 December 1982	171	36.8	12.9	13.8	(58)	6.4	(156)
3 February 1983	172	46.5	12.8	20.0	(75)	9.6	(156)
15 March 1983	150	53.3	15.3	36.8	(76)	16.1	(149)
10 May 1983	189	60.3	15.9	35.8	(109)	10.2	(187)
21 June 1983	156	69.2	26.9	51.4	(105)	16.4	(165)
14 September 1983	160	66.2	22.5	21.4	(98)	16.7	(150)
3 November 1983	132	62.9	25.0	16.3	(80)	14.5	(131)
21 December 1983	161	59.6	14.9	15.4	(91)	10.2	(157)
Village of Katumba - Cotton-growing							
24 January 1982	265	4.5	1.1	8.3	(12)*	4.1	(169)
9 March 1982	155	4.5	2.6	28.6	(7)*	4.1	(148)
19 April 1982	143	5.6	3.5	37.5	(8)*	4.3	(138)
2 June 1982	100	20.0	4.0	26.3	(19)*	–	–
14 July 1982	54	29.6	14.8	31.2	(16)*	6.8	(44)
30 August 1982	271	23.3	10.7	30.2	(63)	38.5	(13)*
13 October 1982	158	24.7	10.1	30.8	(39)	7.7	(130)
4 December 1982	189	23.8	9.5	38.7	(31)	7.2	(166)

N: number of thick smears examined; PR: parasite rate; GR: gametocyte rate; Density: percentage of samples with 100% of microscopic fields positive for trophozoites, i.e. approximately 400 trophozoites/mm^3 with respect to the number of positive samples (n); SR: spleen rate; (n): number examined
* Note the small number of observations used to establish these percentages

of the marshland for farming purposes (rice) has allowed *An. gambiae s.s.* to settle in progressively on the plateaus of Burundi. This phenomenon is not new and alone cannot be the cause of the epidemics that have occurred in recent years. The epidemic in Kirondo in May 1977 broke out following a period of exceptionally heavy rainfall after a drought (Barutwanayo, personal communication). These exceptional climatological conditions occurring repeatedly over the last decade, along with the transformation of the environment over the last thirty years, large population shifts, and reinforcement of the human gametocyte reservoir, are all factors that favoured a sudden rise in the transmission rate. Although very little has been documented, it is likely that the **transmission was short-lived** each time and that the **vector density was low**. The lack of immunity, increased resistance of *P. falciparum* to chloroquine, poor health coverage, and civil war are also exacerbating the situation. In response, treatment has been improved, indoor spraying is being carried out and, more recently, treated mosquito nets have been distributed. It is difficult to know how effective these measures have been in containing epidemics. It is likely that the vector control measures were applied at the same moment that transmission stopped spontaneously (Coosemans, personal observation).

• *Entomology*

In the southern part of the Imbo, *An. gambiae s.s.* was the only vector, while *An. arabiensis* was observed in rice farm plots in the central part of the Imbo. To distinguish between the two species, an isoenzyme electrophoresis assay was done (Smits *et al.*, 1996). *An. arabiensis* karyotypes were characteristic of wet savannah (Coosemans *et al.*, 1989); this anopheline is capable of gonotrophic dissociation during the dry season.

On plateaux over 1,300 m, *An. gambiae s.s.* appeared to be the main vector, relegating *An. funestus*—long considered to be responsible for transmission in mountains—to the background.

East Africa

Geographical boundaries and general characteristics

East Africa is made up of three distinct geographical entities:
- **Sudan** has the same climatic and phytogeographical zones as West Africa of which it is an eastern extension, from the tropical regions of the south to Sahara Desert;
- the **Horn of Africa (Ethiopia, Eritrea, Djibouti, Somalia)** is a set of plateaux rising up to 3,000 m in altitude; the mountains of the north are separated from those in the south by the Rift Valley which ends in Djibouti. These plateaux drop sharply down to the Red Sea and onto the Sudanese Plain which gradually drops down to the Indian Ocean in the south-east;
- the **plateaux of East Africa (Kenya, Uganda, Tanzania)** include the highest peaks in Africa: Mount Kilimanjaro (5,895 m), Mount Kenya (5,199 m), Mount Elgon (4,321 m), and Mount Ruwenzori (5,119 m). They are cut by fault lines, the two branches of the Rift Valley, with the Nyasa (Malawi), Tanganyika, Kivu and Albert Lakes on the western side, and the Nakuru, Baringo, and Turkana Lakes on the eastern side which leads into Ethiopia. Lake Victoria (= Nyanza) occupies a raised basin located at 1,200 m in altitude between the two branches of the Rift.

The hydrographic system is dominated by the two branches of the Nile, the White Nile which flows out of Lake Victoria, and the Blue Nile which flows out of Lake Tsana in Ethiopia. These create corridors of vegetation across Sudan all the way to the Egyptian border. The Great Lakes are very large bodies of water. Lake Victoria, the biggest in area, intersects Kenya, Uganda and Tanzania. The basin is only 40 m deep whereas the Tanganyika is more than 500 m deep. Each lake has a distinctive icthyological fauna, but the Nile Perch (*Lates niloticus*), which exceeds 100 kg in weight, has taken over Lake Victoria where it is intensely farmed and exported to Europe.

The extent in latitude and altitude provides this subregion of East Africa with a remarkable diversity in climate, flora, and fauna, and contrasts sharply to the ordered and well stratified West Africa. The management of natural reserves has made it possible to preserve several species that would otherwise be on their way to extinction. Tourism in the parks has provided a major source of income to the three countries, and for the maintenance and protection of the reserves.

The hypothesis of the origin of Man in the Rift Valley, two to three million years ago at least, has not yet been refuted. *Australopithecus*, then *Homo habilis*, *Homo ergaster* and *Homo erectus*, followed one another until the emergence of modern Man, *Homo sapiens*. The majority of paleo-anthropologists believe that the latter originated from this part of the world before dispersing across the planet (Coppens & Picq, 2001).

The current population of East Africa is a *melting pot* of Arab, Abyssinian and more recently Indian and Yemenite, and Bantu, Nilotic, Somalian people. A small group of Sen, the Hamza, still found in Tanzania represents a relict of the populations who settled in East Africa before the arrival of the Bantus. The differences, not to mention the rivalry between Muslims, Christians of multiple faiths, and Animists, have fuelled several conflicts that are often of a tribal nature, such as the one in Sudan that has lasted thirty years between Christians and Animists together against the Muslims.

Government policies to open up to the west have led to the development of several research institutes, and in particular, in Nairobi where the headquarters of the UNEP (United Nations Environmental Program) is located.

The epidemiology of malaria is remarkably variable from holo-endemic disease on the coasts of Kenya and Tanzania, passing through an "epidemic" stratum at 1,500-2,000 m in altitude, before reaching a malaria-free area above 2,000 m high. Prevention of these epidemics is a priority of the malaria control programme and is the subject of several research studies that have yet to provide an original solution.

One of the characteristics of East Africa, or of certain countries there, is the presence of *P. vivax*, a consequence of the diversity of populations.

East Africa is a well-studied region since it is one part of the globe susceptible to planetary warming which might manifest itself in a change in the altitudinal limits of malaria.

Sudan

The Republic of Sudan is located between the 4th and 22nd parallels north and is the biggest country in Africa covering an area of 2,500,000 km^2 (*Table I*). Its population of 40.2 million people, with a density of 16 inhabitants per km^2, is unequally distributed between the highly populated valley of the Nile and the deserts, which are almost completely uninhabited, especially in the north.

Since independence, Sudan has been shaken by political troubles between the north and south, which has left millions of victims. The NGOs are practically the only organisation to address public health issues in the south, and to provide a minimum amount of medical coverage particularly in the fight against human trypanosomiasis and visceral leishmaniasis.

The country is divided into 28 provinces of unequal surface area.

The climate is tropical in the south, becoming drier and drier to the north, and in Wadi-Halfa on the Egyptian border, it does not rain (< 5 mm/year). The south is covered with a wooded savannah interspersed with forest galleries and pockets. From south to north, the wooded savannah transforms into a spiny steppe and finally, into the desert. With respect to the climatic and plant strata, Sudan is considered to be the eastern part of West Africa.

The White Nile, which crosses the country from south to north, is both a partly navigable pathway and an ecological corridor. In the marshlands of Jonglei, three fourths of its water is lost. In addition, when the Blue Nile flows into it in Khartoum, the latter has a much greater flow, even after having been used for irrigation in the Project of Gezira. This volume of water results from the Sennar Dam near Ethiopia.

Geographers have identified **five natural regions** (Wernsdorfer & Wernsdorfer, 1967):
- the **clay plain**, which forms a triangle from the southern border to Khartoum. The White Nile drains the "southern" region and crosses large areas of marshland;
- the lateritic **mountains of the south-west**, which are not very high, mark the Continental Divide between the Nile and the Congo Rivers;
- the **Jebel Marra**, in the western-central part on the border with Chad, is the highest point in Sudan with peaks over 3,000 m high;
- the **"Qoz" sandbelt** is between the Jebel Marra and the clay plain (region of El Obeid). The Nuba Mountains which dominate it are not high enough to have an epidemiological incidence;
- the **sands and rocks of the north and east** belong to the Sahara. The altitudes all along the Red Sea do not exceed 1,200 m.

• *Epidemiology*

The only complete epidemiological study carried out was by the Wernsdorfer brothers (1967) between 1961-1965, in the context of an eradication programme that was, in fact, never carried out.

The rainfall, which ranges from 1,300 mm in Juba in the south, to less than 5 mm in Wadi Halfa in the north, is the key to the varying levels of malaria in Sudan, even if the floods of the Nile locally modify the epidemiological landscapes.

The levels of **prevalence** reported by Wernsdorfer (1967) are used as the main indicators to compare the provinces (*Table XIX* and *Figure 31*).

These levels of prevalence are only indicative, given that they result from surveys. But great differences between one site and another were observed within the same province. In the province of Gezira, for example, the prevalence was 5.63%, but in the irrigated surrounding areas PRs of 20% were recorded by Wernsdorfer (1977).

The comparison between one thousand children from ages 2-9 in the northern part of the Khartoum Region, and the same size sample from Juba in the south, showed a difference of prevalence of 1.6% and 62% respectively at the end of the rainy season in 1981 (Taha & Broadhead, 1986). The authors had observed a spleen rate of 36% in the south, whereas this syndrome was non-existent in the north.

In Khartoum, a comparison made between two neighbourhoods, one on the Blue Nile and the other on the White Nile, demonstrated differences in prevalence of 13% and 6%, respectively (El Sayed *et al.*, 2000). According to these authors, the number of declared malaria cases was five times less than the real figure, which was close to 45,000 cases per year; malaria tended towards stability in urban zones.

The parasitic breakdown was similar to that of the Afrotropical Region with 77% of *P. falciparum*, 20% of *P. malariae*, 2.8% of *P. vivax*, 0.3% of *P. ovale*, and several mixed infections of *P. falciparum-P. malariae*. It seems that *P. ovale* was introduced recently to the region of Khartoum. The percentage of *P. vivax* is remarkably low,

Table XIX. Prevalence of malaria (all plasmodial species) in various regions of Sudan (children of 2-9) (adapted from Wernsdorfer, 1967).									
Province	North	Khartoum	Kassala	Blue Nile	Kordofan	Darfur	Upper Nile	Bhar el Ghazal	Equatoria
N° subjects examined	3,786	3,638	5,916	4,115	4,680	2,650	2,750	2,820	3,944
% positive results	0.16	0.03	2.53	5.63	20.6	26.5	47.5	57.41	81
Endemicity	Hypo-endemic			Meso-endemic				Hyperendemic	Holo-endemic

Biodiversity of Malaria in the World

despite the growth potential of this parasite in carriers of the Duffy antigen.

The levels of morbidity and mortality due to malaria were only recorded in a few provinces, based on the clinical diagnoses made in the medical clinics (*Table XX*).

Statistics from the southern provinces, the area most infested, were not available. In Juba, the mortality rate of malaria was reported to be 8% in hospitalised children from 0-7 months, which is hardly representative of the general population (Woodruff *et al.*, 1983).

All the observations made by Wernsdorfer (1967) have been compiled by Zahar (1985c) in *Table XXI*.

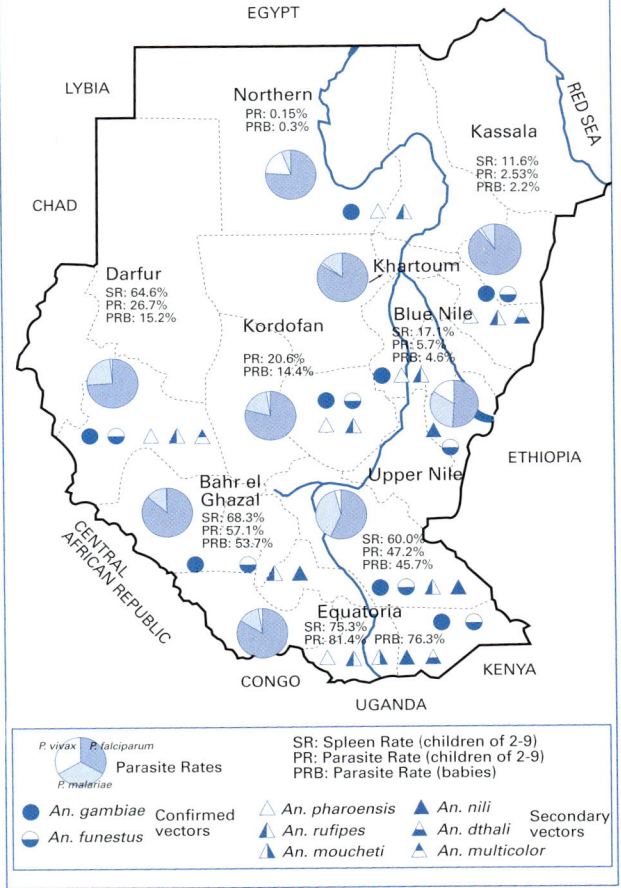

Figure 31. Malaria in Sudan (1961-1963 surveys) (adapted from Wernsdorfer & Wernsdorfer, 1967).

Table XX. Morbidity and mortality (adapted from Wernsdorfer, 1967).			
Region	**Percentage of cases***	**Malaria morbidity p. 100,000**	**Malaria mortality p. 100,000**
North	0.6-4	1,200-2,780	0-1.2
Kordofan	4-12	4,200-9,000	2.6-6.3
Bhar el Ghazal	3-8.5	2,400-4,900	1.2-2.5
* Percentage of malaria cases among dispensary clients			

Table XXI. Epidemiology of malaria in Sudan (adapted from Zahar, 1985).			
Zone	**Endemicity**	**Stability**	**Transmission**
Southern argillaceous plain	Holo- or hyper-endemic	Stable	Perennial
Central argillaceous plain	Meso-endemic	Intermediate	Seasonal
Northern argillaceous plain	Hypo-endemic	Unstable	Seasonal
South-western mountains	Hyperendemic	Stable	Perennial
Jebel Marra	Hyperendemic	Stable	Seasonal
Qoz belt	Meso-endemic	Unstable	Seasonal
Red Sea	Hypo-endemic	Unstable	Seasonal

- *Entomology*

Species distribution

Lewis (1956) published the first monograph of the *Anopheles* of Sudan along with maps listing all of the vectors: *An. gambiae s.l., An. funestus, An. nili* and *An. moucheti*. The role of *An. pharoensis* and *An. dthali* was seriously questioned. *An. moucheti* was localised in the south-west, *An. nili* was in the southern provinces, and *An. funestus* made it all the way up to the Sennar Region in the north; it would seem that it has dropped down towards the south.

Two species of the Gambiae Complex are present in Sudan (Petrarca *et al.*, 2000): *An. gambiae s.s.* is limited to the southern provinces where the rainfall is greater than 1,200 mm; *An. arabiensis* occupies the entire country and, in the south, lives together with *An. gambiae s.s*. The population of *An. arabiensis* in Sudan is polymorphic and panmictic with greater affinity to those in West Africa than East Africa, of which only the Rift Valley separates them (Kamau *et al.*, 1998, 1999; Lehmann *et al.*, 1997).

The ecology of *Anopheles arabiensis* in dry areas

In the northern part of the country where it is desert-like, the conditions on the shores of the Nile favour the perennial development of *An. arabiensis*. The population of this species is at its lowest level from July to October when the river floods, but then it increases from November to mid-June when the water levels drop leaving residual ponds that are highly productive larval habitats. The females are very endophilic, and feed regularly on humans or livestock. Throughout the year, there is gonotrophic concordance, i.e. coordination between blood meals and ovarian development (Dukeen & Omer, 1986).

Twenty kilometres away from the river, surface waters disappear during the dry season but, nonetheless, *An. arabiensis* females could be found throughout the dry season inside houses, abandoned huts, wells, and in ground crevices. These females only took sporadic blood meals and their ovaries grew slowly—over the course of multiple blood meals. Ovarian growth would terminate at the end of the dry season, and the females would subsequently lay their eggs at the beginning of the rainy season. This period of dormancy was based on gonotrophic dissociation, meaning that a blood meal does not lead to full oocyte development, allowing the species to survive through the hostile conditions of the dry season, despite the absence of larval habitats (Omer & Cloudsley-Thompson, 1970). Nobody has yet observed this same phenomenon of semi-diapause in other dry regions in Africa where fewer than 5% of anophelines undergo gonotrophic dissociation (Cavalié & Mouchet, 1961), as occurs elsewhere throughout the year in more humid areas.

In the province of Kassala, *An. arabiensis* had been reported to be highly exophilic following the spraying with DDT (Haridi, 1972). Apparently, this exodus of *Anopheles*, occurring daily, was provoked by the well known irritating effects of DDT.

Northern limit of *Anopheles arabiensis*

The invasion of *An. gambiae s.l.* in Egypt in 1943 caused much trauma to the Public Health officials. Following its eradication, measures were set up to protect the lakes of the Assouan Dam and the new dam of Lake Nasser, which extends for more than 100 km within Sudan, and which has caused the displacement of the city of Wadi-Halfa.

An. gambiae s.l. had already been reported in Wadi-Halfa in the 1930's but in general the northern limit of *An. gambiae s.l.*, which varied from year to year, was said to be between Akasba and Abu Fatma, located respectively between 60-350 km from the Sudanese-Egyptian border (Lewis, 1949). The various programmes conducted to eradicate *An. gambiae*, 100-200 km to the south of Wadi-Halfa, were never fully effective no matter what methods were used.

Shawarbi *et al.* (1967b) fixed the northern limit of *An. gambiae s.l.*, which was in fact *An. arabiensis*, at 192 km to the south of Wadi-Halfa, and Farid (1984) collected this species in Dongola. Gillies (1972) prudently considered that the shores of the Nile, extending for 200 km in Sudan, created favourable conditions for *An. arabiensis*.

Northern Sudan is still a sensitive area that requires surveillance, especially if there are climatic changes or environmental modifications that could provoke new invasions of Afrotropical *Anopheles* into Egypt.

Irrigated zones

The Gezira Project, covering more than one million hectares on the Blue Nile, is the biggest irrigated zone in Sudan and is supplied by the Sennar Dam. It was initially implemented for cotton farming but is currently partly used for rice-growing. These farming developments have encouraged the breeding of both *An. arabiensis* in cleared bodies of water, and *An. pharoensis* in canals with abundant vegetation (El Gaddal *et al.*, 1985). It also encouraged the introduction of meso-endemic malaria. At first it was kept under control through DDT spraying, and then epidemics broke out in 1971, once *An. arabiensis* had developed resistance to this insecticide (Wernsdorfer, 1977). Resistance to organophosphates seems to be an ongoing problem. Novel methods are being tested in this project that serves as a test case.

- *Epidemiology of unstable malaria*

Throughout all of northern Sudan, malaria is unstable. The period of transmission is short, from October to November at the end of the rainy season, during which 90% of the clinical cases occur. In a village of 457 inhabitants near Gedaref, south-east of Khartoum, 430 attacks from *P. falciparum* were recorded over a period of three years (Giha *et al.*, 2000). In the same village, followed over a period of eight years, only one clinical attack was observed per person every two-three years (Arnot, 1998). During particularly dry years, there is practically no transmission or malaria attacks (Theander, 1998).

Biodiversity of Malaria in the World

What happens to parasites during the dry season has been studied using the PCR assay—based on the methods of Bottius et al. (1996) in Senegal—to detect parasites present at levels undetectable by microscopic methods. This showed that parasites were present all year round in the blood of symptomless patients. The prevalence varied from 13-24% (Roper et al., 1996). Many patients who presented clinical attacks remained infected but are symptomless for the rest of the year (Arnot, 1998).

In the north-eastern part of Sudan, the period of exposure to malaria is brief and the number of infective bites is less than one per person per year (Babiker, 1998). Moreover, only half of these inoculations lead to clinical disease because many sporozoites fail to establish infection (Theander, 1998).

In a village near Gedaref (mentioned above), where the prevalence of *P. falciparum* is below 5% in children, 39 isolates were taken from patients. Every isolate was characterised *vis-à-vis* **alleles of the plasmodial surface proteins** *msp1* and *exp1*. In fifteen of twenty-nine patients, the infection was **multiclonal** with **up to three clones per subject**. The means in 1989, 1990 and 1991 were 1.5, 1.4 and 1.1 clone, respectively (Babiker, 1998).

In 1990, no isolate contained exactly the same combination of alleles as any of those of 1989. In 1990, two subjects living in the same house were infected by parasites that were genetically different. *P. falciparum* was therefore highly polymorphic. The coefficient of in-breeding varied from 0.79-0.95, the highest observed so far in any *P. falciparum* population of Africa. Parasites which had caused clinical attacks persisted at a low density through a large part of the dry season. Subjects who experienced new attacks the following year were those who had been infected by new genotypes.

The passage from asymptomatic malaria to a clinical attack could be due to the introduction of a new genotype with which the patient would not have had any previous contact (Arnot, 1998).

In the regions of unstable malaria in Sudan, the subjects did not present any immunity but the adults over 30 years old resisted malaria attacks much better than the younger subjects (Theander, 1998).

With respect to the unstable malaria of *P. falciparum* in Africa, the studies carried out in Sudan are of great value as they have brought a new perspective to malaria in dry regions.

The Horn of Africa

This term refers to a well-defined geographical area in the part of East Africa that is located east of Sudan and north of the equator, and that is lined by the Red Sea, the Gulf of Aden, and the northern coastline of the Indian Ocean. It covers an area of 1,880,000 km^2 and has a population of approximately 86 million people (*Table I*). Ethiopia is the most populated country of this region with 73 million inhabitants living over an area of more than one million km^2. Eritrea gained its independence in 1995 following thirty years of conflict with Ethiopia, and has a population of less than 5 million people spread over an area of 121,000 km^2.

The Republic of Djibouti was the bridgehead of the railroad line to Ethiopia and is now submerged in a flood of refugees fleeing war and famine, with a population of over 790,000 inhabitants.

Somalia is made up of a group of tribes with 8.2 million inhabitants that lack a central government.

The Horn of Africa is dominated by the Abyssinian Plateau that is more than 3,000 m high. The plateau is divided into two blocks, north and south, that are separated by the Rift Valley, a furrow that starts from Lake Turkana in the south-west, and travels all the way to the Gulf of Djibouti. The Valley is at an altitude of 1,500-1,800 m, and is scattered with lakes. In its north-eastern part, its altitude decreases almost to sea level in the Awash Valley and the Afar depression, next to Djibouti.

On the western and northern edges, the Abyssinian (or Ethiopian) Plateau drops down suddenly to the plains of Sudan, and in the north-east to the Red Sea. On the eastern and southern edges, it drops in layers to the Gulf of Aden and to the Indian Ocean. Because of its peaks and its positioning with respect to strong winds from the west, the Horn of Africa has a large variety of climates and vegetation: a tropical and wooded savannah climate in the west on the border with Sudan, a high altitude tropical climate on the plateaux, sub-desert steppes, and a dry climate on the coastal regions which are protected by the mountains from rain.

From 1972 to 1992, temperature has been recorded at three weather stations (information from the Meteorological Department of Ethiopia, 1998), located between 1,900-2,100 m in altitude (Bahir Dar, Gonder and Goro in the southern mountains), to see the effects of **global warming** on malaria. In Bahir Dar, on the banks of Lake Tsana, minimum temperatures had increased from 1.2 °C to 3.4 °C, while the maximum temperatures remained stable. In Gonder and Goro, temperatures remained stable. 1992 was recorded as being the hottest year of the decade. Year-to-year variations between stations were marked.

The Horn of Africa is made up of a mixture of populations: Nilotics and Bantus in southern Ethiopia, Somalians of Hamitic origin (imprecise term), Afars and Danakils in Eritrea, and the Amharas of Yeminite origin (hence Semites) who invaded the plateaux in 1,000 B.C. These ethnic mixtures explain the presence, particularly in the Amharas, of a considerably high proportion of carriers of the Duffy antigen, who are therefore susceptible to *P. vivax*.

The level of malaria, like all the other health parameters, is notably variable according to the altitude and climate. We will examine it country by country despite the fact that there are certain problems in searching documentation. The first studies before 1946 were carried out by the Italians and included Eritrea and Somalia together, whose information needed to be reclassified. In addition, several Italian names of places have now been replaced and no longer appear in current atlases. Finally, it should be observed that the very high percentage (up to 100%) of *P. vivax* reported by Lega *et al.* (1937), is hardly compatible with later studies and, in particular, those of Mara (1950). One should, therefore, regard these old data with great care.

Ethiopia

In Ethiopia, 34-38 million people live in areas that are at risk of malaria (Teklehaimanot, 1991) and 20-25 million people live in high altitude zones above 2,000 m in areas that are considered to be healthy (*Figure 32*).

The most frequently encountered parasite is *P. falciparum* (60-70%), followed by *P. vivax* (30-40%), and *P. malariae* (10%) in the south-west. The presence of *P. ovale* is anecdotal. Among the impressive list of *Anopheles*, *An. arabiensis* is the dominant species, often exclusively. *An. funestus* has a smaller distribution especially in marshy areas. *An. nili* is a species of the plains of the south-west. *An. pharoensis* is one of the most abundant species with a very large distribution (Chand, 1965). It should be remembered that there is no *An. gambiae s.s.* to the east of Sudan.

• *Epidemiology*

The high ground of Ethiopia was and still is considered to be an area of unstable malaria in which epidemics break out during rainy and hot years. The epidemic of 1958 affected 3 million people and caused 150,000 deaths (Fontaine *et al.*, 1961). Indoor DDT spraying eliminated most of the epidemics for a period of about twenty years. However, epidemics seem to be on the rise again due to the problems malaria control programmes encounter today. The 1993 epidemic in Zwai, in the Rift Valley, the Tigray epidemic of 1987 (143,200 cases with 349 deaths), and the epidemics of Bahir Dar and Gonder with 315,000 cases on the plateaux (Teklehaimanot, 1991) seem to be a result, at least in part, of faulty control operations.

Currently, we are witnessing **a strong outbreak of malaria throughout the entire country**. From 1986 to 1991, the incidence of clinical cases was 343‰ per year. In the health centres, 30-40% of fever cases were malaria-related.

In the interior immigration zones of the lowland where malaria was hyper- or holo-endemic (Gambela, Pani, Wellega, Metena, etc.) in 1990-1991, 30% of arrivals had to be treated for malaria in the clinic each month. Out of 564,000 slide samples taken between July 1990 and June 1991, 181,000 were positive. The incidence of 320‰ was of an epidemic scale (Teklehaimanot, 1991). Out of eleven hospitals, 170 deaths due to malaria were recorded out of 2,609 consultations (mortality of 6.5%).

In one area, at 2,000 m in altitude, 50 km east of Addis Abeba, the annual number of cases seen in the clinics had greatly increased between 1980 and 1990. The incidence of *P. falciparum* had increased from 90‰ to 127‰, whereas that of *P. vivax* had decreased from 251‰ to 187‰. This heightened level of malaria was concomitant with an increase of temperature from 1 °C to 3 °C (Tula, 1993). It was not possible to obtain more information on this unclear case, which was considered by its author to be a consequence of global warming. In the Tigray, between 1,800 and 2,250 m high, the proximity of small dams was correlated with the number of cases of malaria in children: 14 episodes out of 1,000 children living within 3 km of a dam as opposed to 1.9 episodes in those living more than 8 km from a dam (Ghebreyesus *et al.*, 1999).

An environmental study done between 1,885 and 2,225 m in altitude covering six risk factors (irrigation, earth roofing, animals in the house, windows, awnings, separate bedrooms) demonstrated through a multivariate analysis that children exposed to zero or one risk factor presented with 2.1% malaria attacks per year, while those exposed to five risk factors presented with 24.9% attacks per year (Ghebreyesus *et al.*, 2000).

In the Rift Valley in the city of Nazareth (1,600 m in altitude, 90 km south of Addis Abeba), the PR was 4% in the outskirts as opposed to 1.1% in the city centre. *P. falciparum* infected 1.6% of the residents and *P. vivax* 1.2%. Prevalence was minimal in older children between the ages of 10 and 14 and maximal in adults between the ages of 31 and 40, which proved both an absence of immunity and the region's susceptibility to epidemics (Mekonnen & Beyene, 1996).

In 1992 in the neighbouring region of Zwai, at 1,800 m in altitude and still in the Rift Valley, which up until then had been well protected with indoor DDT spraying, an epidemic had been observed and persisted. In one village, there were 700 deaths out of 10,000 inhabitants in just a

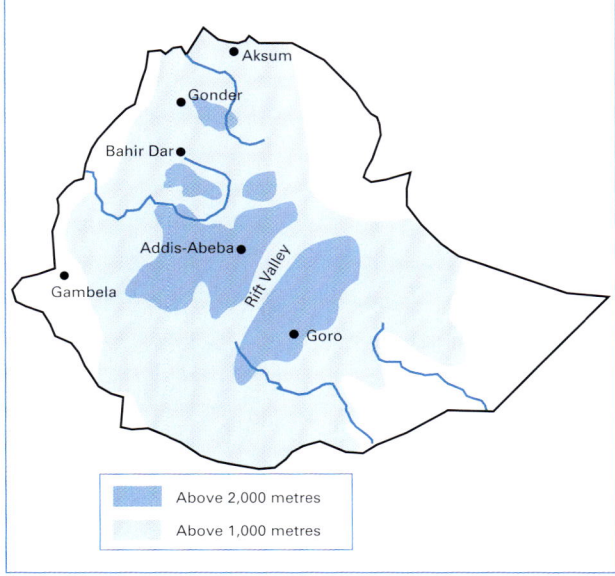

Figure 32. *Relief in Ethiopia.*

few months. The official bodies attributed the epidemic to changes in the water level of two lakes which, having formerly occurred on a seasonal basis, had now become perennial. Operational problems, however, such as the decrease of indoor spraying could not be disregarded. In addition to the presence of *An. arabiensis*, *An. pharoensis*, always the suspect and never again observed, was reported in abundance.

In the southern part of the Rift Valley in Arba Minch (1,600-1,800 m), the PR was 18% (62% *P. falciparum*). The highest prevalences and heaviest parasite loads were seen in babies under 2 years of age. The highest mortality rate for malaria was 56‰ in children under 2 years old, and 28‰ in children under 5. The greatest risk was to children who lived near irrigation canals (Tulu *et al.*, 1993).

In the lowlands of the Gambela Region, the parasite incidence in children was double that in adults (in whom the recovery rate was also three times higher) (Krafsur & Armstrong, 1978). In 1990, the prevalence varied from 3.9% to 39%; the sporozoite rates of *An. gambiae s.l.*, probably *An. arabiensis*, and *An. pharoensis*, were 0.78% and 0.46% respectively, the first time that such a high sporozoite rate was recorded in *An. pharoensis* (Nigatu *et al.*, 1992). Only four ethnic groups were infected by *P. vivax*, including the Amharas and the Anuaks (18% of *P. vivax*). The others were only infected by *P. falciparum* which remained highly dominant in the region (88%). These authors had not observed any *P. malariae* at all, whereas this parasite had appeared in more than 10% of parasitised subjects in 1982; its EIR was 0.4 per human per year, and accounted for 4% of all anopheline salivary gland infections (Krasfur & Armstrong, 1982).

In the semi-dry lowlands of the north in Humera, on the borders of Sudan, Ethiopia and Eritrea, only 12% of children were infected with malaria (5% of *P. vivax* cases). The region was considered to be hypo-endemic. Most of the cases were due to *P. falciparum*, in August-September during the rainy season. *P. vivax* infections were stable throughout the year (Seboxa & Snow, 1997).

• *Entomology*

The entomological fauna of the Horn of Africa has been well studied since the 1940's (Chand, 1965; Giaquinto-Mira, 1950; O'Connor, 1967). All the information was reviewed by Gillies & De Meillon (1968) and completed by Gillies & Coetzee (1987). The principle vectors were *An. gambiae s.l.*, *An. funestus*, *An. nili* and *An. pharoensis*, whose vector role is no longer doubted (Nigatu *et al.*, 1992). The role of *An. dthali* still remains very uncertain.

Following the recognition of the *An. gambiae* Complex, two species from Ethiopia were described: *An. gambiae* B (= *An. arabiensis*) and *An. gambiae* C of Ethiopia, very close to *An. quadriannulatus* of South Africa and now called *An. quadriannulatus* B (Hunt *et al.*, 1998); almost exclusively zoophilic, it does not play any role in transmission (White *et al.*, 1980). *An. arabiensis*, on the other hand, is the main vector in Ethiopia in both high altitude zones, where it is almost the only one present, and lowlands where it plays a role in transmission along with *An. funestus* and *An. nili* (*Figures 33 and 34*).

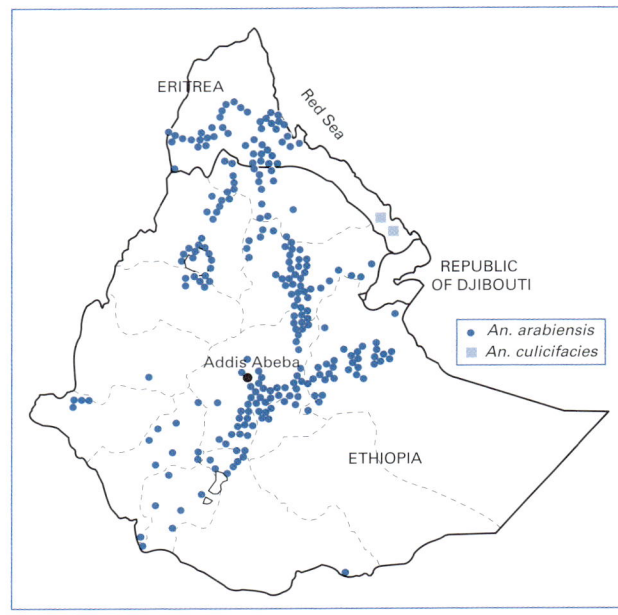

Figure 33. Ethiopia and Eritrea: distribution of An. culicifacies *and* An. arabiensis *(adapted from Cornos, 1967).*

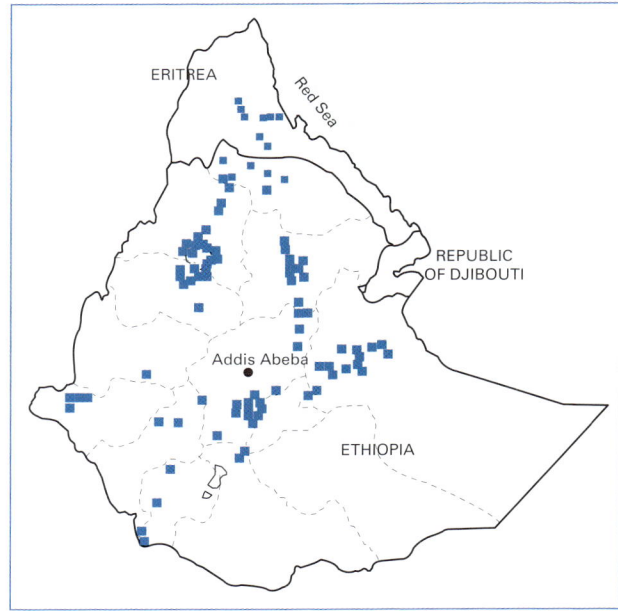

Figure 34. Ethiopia and Eritrea: distribution of An. funestus *(adapted from Cornos, 1967).*

The altitude-based distribution of *An. arabiensis* and malaria is still a big topic of conversation. In Addis Abeba, this *Anopheles* was only found in the low neighbourhoods of the city at about 2,300 m where it had perhaps been imported by train or by truck to the bus station. In Akaki, on the other hand, 25 km from Addis Abeba, it was well established and prospered at altitudes of 2,200-2,300 m (Ovazza & Neri, 1955). The limit of 2,000 m has been exceeded by *An. arabiensis* and a new limit of 2,400 m has been suggested (Tula, 1993). It was *An. arabiensis* that was implicated in the big epidemic of 1958 (Fontaine *et al.*, 1961) and in most of the outbreaks on the plateaux.

The information on *An. funestus* is somewhat limited and imprecise. This *Anopheles* would not go as high in altitude as the preceding species and would have a focal distribution (Chand, 1965). It has only been studied in the plains of Gambella.

An. nili apparently remains to be a species of the lowlands (Krafsur, 1977).

An. pharoensis is very abundant and spreads throughout the entire country; it is cited by all authors for its aggressive behaviour towards humans. It was found to be infected by Ovazza & Neri (1955) and its role was confirmed in Zwai, in the Rift Valley (SNLP of Ethiopia, personal communication), with a sporozoite rate of 0.46%, and in Gambella (Nigatu *et al.*, 1992) with a sporozoite rate of 0.49%. In this part of the world, it is a vector whose abundance compensates for its weak capabilities as a vector.

In Zwai, *An. arabiensis* specimens captured in houses were found to be 88% anthropophilic while those collected in stables were 45%. For *An. pharoensis*, the values were 84% and 9% respectively. *An. funestus*, hardly abundant (Adugna & Petros, 1996), would feed on humans more than 80% of the time.

In Gambela, on the border of Sudan, the fauna hardly differed from that of West Africa: *An. wellcomei*, *An. pharoensis*, *An. nili* and *An. ziemanni* were all exophilic, while *An. arabiensis* and *An. funestus* were endophilic. Sporozoite rates were 1.87%, 1.23% and 1.25% for *An. arabiensis*, *An. funestus* and *An. nili* respectively. The EIR was close to 10 per year in the city of Gambella, and 100 in the villages all along the river (65 ib/p/yr from *An. funestus*, 20.6 from *An. nili* and 10.9 from *An. arabiensis*). In the city, 9.4 ib/p/yr out of 10 samples were from *An. arabiensis*. The highest period of risk was at the end of the rainy season from September to November (Krafsur, 1977).

• *Problems of displaced populations*

In 1984-1985, more than 600,000 people were victims of a famine caused by the drought (*Figure 35*). The government established a resettlement programme in the sparsely populated lowlands which, in some areas, were completely unoccupied. Most of the migrants came from the plateaux and found themselves confronted with pathologies that were new to them: malaria, trypanosomiasis, onchocerciasis, leismaniasis, etc. The introduction of protective measures was laborious and the effectiveness of the programme leaves much to be desired.

The irrigated regions of the Rift Valley and, in particular, of the Awash lowlands suffered greatly from the growth of malaria due to irrigation. The Afar shepherds of the Awash Valley were long used to spending the summer in the mountains to get away from the mosquitoes and malaria (Kloos, 1990). But the new migrants were seriously affected.

Since the country was decentralised in 1995, the WHO has implemented a big mosquito net treatment programme in the Tigray Region, as well as a programme to improve health care coverage of the sick.

Eritrea

Eritrea, an Italian colony at the beginning of the 20th century, was integrated into Italian East Africa from 1936 to 1943 before becoming a province of Ethiopia, and then gained independence definitively in 1995. So, in order to find epidemiological information on this country, we must consult either Italian articles that date before 1945, or works on Ethiopia.

The coastal and low altitude (< 400 m) regions of the north around Massaoua were considered to be meso-endemic with PRs of 30-45%, depending on the locality. From 400-900 m, malaria was hyperendemic (51%) with very high SRs (86%). The mountainous region above 1,900 m and, in particular, the areas surrounding the capital, Asmara (2,370 m), were considered to be free of malaria. The remarks made above concerning the dominant status of *P. vivax* also pertain to Eritrea, even though Mara (1950)

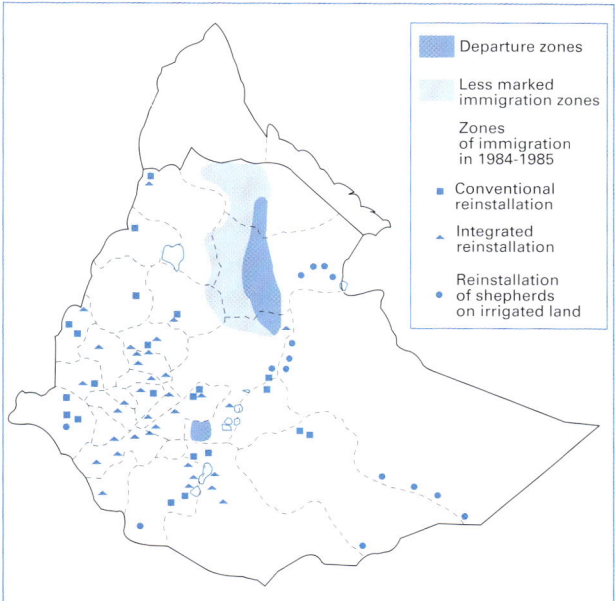

Figure 35. Migrations in Ethiopia during the Reinstallation Programme (1984/1985) (adapted from Kloos, 1990).

had demonstrated that *P. falciparum* was largely dominant (> 70%) in areas of economic development where the PR varied from 3-22%.

The coastline along the Red Sea between Massaoua and the Republic of Djibouti (Danakil Coast) is semi-desert with very little malaria. In the Port of Assab, where the water supply is collected in tanks, malaria seems to be indigenous but very rare (Vyslouzil, 1971).

The maps charting *Anopheles* by Giaquinto-Mira (1950), Chand (1965), O'Connor (1967), as well as Burca & Shah (1943) stipulate the presence of *An. gambiae s.l.* (= *An. arabiensis*), *An. pharoensis*, and *An. dthali*; *An. funestus* was only cited from a dozen larvae captured at 2,500 m but this information remains to be confirmed. One difference in the Eritrean fauna is the presence of *An. culicifacies s.l.* on the coastline of the Red Sea (Mara, 1950); at first, this *Anopheles* was considered to be the sub-species, *An. culicifacies adenensis*, and then a species, before being reinstated as *An. culicifacies sp.* A (Gillies & Coetzee, 1987). This Asian species, which is not found in any other part of the African continent, develops in reservoirs in which control measures based on the larvivorous fish *Aphanius dispar* were strongly promoted by the WHO's Eastern Mediterranean Regional Office.

The principle vector seems to be *An. arabiensis* with a sporozoite rate of 3% (Mara, 1950). Irrigation in the lowlands of the north-east has increased transmission to both the existing population, and to the incoming population of workers.

Republic of Djibouti

The Republic of Djibouti, which was formerly known as the Somalian French Coast at the beginning of the 20th century, and then the French Territory of the Afars and Issas as of 1960, gained its independence in 1975. This small country covering 23,000 km² (*Table I*), located at the outlet of the Rift Valley where the Red Sea and Gulf of Aden intersect, is made up of an alluvial plain with mountain chains rising up in the north (Moussa Ali 2,200 m, Dai 1,400 m). Marshland and salt lakes cover the bottom of the depression (the highly saline Lake Assab). In 1901, the country had a population of 15,000 people, divided half and half between Somalian (Issas) and Afars. Today, there are 793,000 inhabitants, including a large number of Ethiopian and Somalian refugees who have been fleeing armed conflicts and food shortages since 1965.

Malaria fevers were reported in Djibouti in 1901 (*Table XXII*), particularly in the suburbs of Ambouli, on the edge of the "Wadi". In 1905, the entire territory seemed to be infested with malaria (Bouffard, 1905). Around 1910, malaria seemed to have disappeared and up until 1973, it was the only country of intertropical Africa that was considered to be free of the disease. All the cases observed in the health centres were imported, and in particular, from the Djibouti-Dire Dawa rail line. Not one vector was captured in the territory by Courtois & Mouchet (1970) and the only *Anopheles* present were *An. dthali*, highly abundant in lightly mineralised water, and *An. turkudi*.

In 1975, the return of malaria and its vector *An. arabiensis* was confirmed in the suburbs of Djibouti, in Ambouli, where the epidemic of 1901 had taken place (Carteron *et al.*, 1978). From 1973 to 1976, 191 indigenous cases were reported. In 1988-1989, a real epidemic broke out with 3,000 cases out of a national population of 235,000 inhabitants. More than 50% of the cases were in refugees (Louis & Albert, 1988). In 1991, the number of cases increased to 7,500 (Rodier *et al.*, 1995). In 1999, the Republic of Djibouti encountered the biggest malaria epidemic in its history. From the 1st to the 25th of April 1999, 990 cases were confirmed in the city hospital and similar figures were collected for the first trimester (Louis, 1999). These figures, however, were based only on the cases reported in the hospital and do not take into consideration those who practised self-medication without ever setting foot in a medical centre.

Up until now, the only vector identified remains *An. arabiensis* which proliferates wherever water is contained, and notably in watering wells, basins, water tanks, and watering holes in the highly affected Ambouli Region (Carnevale, personal observation 1998).

Malaria vector control is targeted mainly at larvae with Abate® or local fish, *Aphanius dispar*, while spraying was formely done. There have also been trials involving insecticide-impregnation of nets already owned by the population.

Table XXII. *P. falciparum* malaria cases recorded in Djibouti (Army Health Department Report).

Year	Estimated population	Number of cases of malaria recorded	Incidence %
1901	15,000	13	0.086
1963	> 30,000	14	0.046
1964		35	
1965		9	
1973	106,000	16	0.015
1974		28	
1975		96	
1976		51*	
1985	156,000	301	0.192
1986		425	
1988-1989	235,000	3,000	1.276
1991		7,338	
1993	300,000	4,770	1.590
1999	500,000	990 in 1 month (1-25 April 1999)	

* Incomplete data

Malaria is unstable and seems to vary enormously from one year to the next. Rainfall, although abundant for at least a few weeks and leading to floods some years, is more often scarce, if not inexistent, most other years. The question one constantly asks is what led to the establishment of *An. arabiensis* after an absence of more than fifty years. Nobody seems to have truly addressed this question and most experts seem to be satisfied with only reporting the presence of vectors and counting the number of cases. The two following hypotheses should be examined more thoroughly:
- after 1970, a large amount of drilling took place in deep water tables, bringing freshwater to the surface, whereas beforehand, the mineral content of most of the surface water was only compatible with the breeding of *An. dthali*;
- had the water table risen up in a tectonically unstable region, bringing freshwater to the surface?

These are just work suggestions because the question remains currently unanswered, and poses a problem with respect to factors affecting the re-emergence of malaria beyond the Republic of Djibouti.

Somalia

In 1960, the Republic of Somalia was formed through the unification of the formerly British Somaliland, under British protectorate since 1880, and the Italian colony of Somalia (since 1905). It is a country that is culturally homogenous with a generalised use of the Somali language, a strict view of Islam, and a tribal structure. The Somalis, who are also found in Ethiopia, Kenya, and in the Republic of Djibouti, have long been ethnically classified as Hamitic, a rather vague categorisation.

In the north, a low-lying coastline borders the Gulf of Aden and, parallel to the coastline, there are a series of dry cliffs 500-2,000 m high called the "Haud", which make up the country's backbone. They then drop down in the south-west joining into the Ogaden Region of Ethiopia. In the east and south, the Ethiopian Plateau ends in dry steppes below 200 m in altitude that extend all the way to the Indian Ocean. The plain is drained by the Juba in the south, and by the Wabi Scebelli in the centre, which then drains into marshland before reaching the coastline.

The rainfall can vary enormously from year to year and is divided into four seasons with its peak falling between September-November, 50 mm per year on the northern semi-desert coastline, and more than 500 mm in the south in the Juba.

In the northern part (formerly Somaliland), malaria was non-existent or very rare on the coast, localised up to an altitude of 500 m. In the northern foothills, between 500 and 1,000 m high, the disease was endemic with PRs of 18% in children; this is a region covered in temporary rivers which upon drying form residual ponds favouring the development of *An. arabiensis* (Wilson, 1949). The 2,000 m high "Haud" Plateau is dry; since the end of the war, water tanks filled by trucks were spread throughout the "Haud", providing larval habitats for *An. arabiensis*. Pilot biological control projects based on the fish *Oreochromus spilurus* had some degree of success and eliminated malaria in this special setting (Alio *et al.*, 1985). The "Haud" is a hypo-endemic region (PR of 6-10%), and is subject to epidemic outbreaks. In 1951, one outbreak involved 7,500 cases with a death rate of 1-2% (Choumara, 1961) (*Table XXIII*). In the grazing pastures south of the "Haud", between 150-1,000 m high, malaria was rare (Wilson, 1949).

In 1960 in the regions of Mudugh and Migiurtinia in the north-eastern part of Somalia, the "water tank" system had not been set up and the epidemiology among the nomads hardly changed. Malaria was hypo-endemic; seasonal epidemics (Maffi, 1960) broke out in watering holes that had been formed during the rainy season. The *Anopheles* were resting in the tents of the nomads.

There is little recent information on the potential epidemiological impact of the extensive drilling that took place in regions where the rainfall is less than 200 mm (mostly in September-October).

In the southern part of the country, malaria was concentrated in hyperendemic larval habitats all along the Wabi Schebelli and Juba Rivers, and even their tributaries. Away from the rivers in the semi-arid regions, was a rampant seasonal malaria that was unstable hypo or meso-endemic. A weak hypo-endemic malaria reigned over the rest of the country (Anonymous, 1990). Out of 50,000 slides sampled from all of the health centre laboratories, 28-30% were positive.

In 1988-89, epidemics broke out in the refugee camps of the Ogaden Region (Anonymous, 1990). In the Awdal camp near Zeila (far north), the prevalence ranged from 34-74%. In 1986 in Berbera, 600 deaths were reported with no judgement made on the cause of mortality.

An. arabiensis was the principal and often the only vector throughout the entire country. The presence of *An. merus* in Mogadishu has not been confirmed. *An. funestus* and *An. nili* have been reported in the south (Maffi, 1958).

Table XXIII. Malaria in northern Somalia (adapted from Choumara, 1961).		
Age group	Routine tests	
	Spleen rate	Parasite rate
0-11 months	–	10.6 (47)
1-9 years	14.7 (634)	9.3 (605)
Over 10	4.8 (352)	6.1 (684)
Unclassified	–	9.6 (728)
Means + standard deviation	11.3 + 1	8.4 + 0.6

The Plateaux of East Africa

Geographical, climatic and ethnic characteristics

The plateaux of East Africa (Kenya, Uganda, Tanzania) make up a relatively well defined quadrilateral that extends from the Great Lakes in the west to the Indian Ocean in the east, and from Sudan in the north to Mozambique in the south. Rwanda and Burundi could also be considered to be a part of this area but have been included in the region of Central Africa instead.

While West Africa is stratified climatically by west-east longitudinal strips parallel to the equator, in East Africa the strata run from north to south parallel with the Indian Ocean coastline:
- on the east coast, a strip of tropical vegetation extends for less than 100 km inland;
- behind this strip at 50-500 m in altitude, a dry zone of shrubby steppe where the precipitation is irregular extends for 100-300 km. In the 1970's, the devastating droughts in the Tsavo National Park of Kenya resulted in starving elephants massively destroying the vegetation and particularly the baobabs. The same vegetation is found all over the lowlands of Tanzania;
- the plateaux rising up to between 1,000 and 1,400 m high, where the rainfall exceeds 1,000 mm, is the part of the savannah where large animal life used to live in abundance less than a century ago. Now they can only be found in the national parks and reserves. These plateaux meet up with the mountains of Uganda in the south-west (Kigezi Region) and further south with the ridge that borders Lake Tanganyika in Tanzania;
- the highlands, between 1,500 and 2,800 m high, were covered in prairies and regularly swamped forests; a large part of it was cleared for banana, tea, and other food crop and industrial plantations;
- the high mountain slopes above 2,800 m in altitude have a mountain vegetation that is specific to the Afrotropical Region.

This succession of climatic and phytogeographic strips results in there being a variety of epidemiological facies in which the main vectors are essentially *An. gambiae s.s.*, *An. arabiensis* and *An. funestus*. The other species, *An. nili*, *An. moucheti*, and *An. merus* are very localised, and *An. pharoensis* and *An. rivulorum* are of secondary importance.

Kenya

• *Epidemiology*

The main epidemiological features of malaria in Kenya had already been established before the Second World War. The Indian Ocean coastline and the plateaux of the north-west between 1,100 and 1,300 m high were considered to be larval habitats of a strong endemic nature. In the mountains between 1,500 and 2,400 m high, the hot and rainy years were marked with epidemics (Garnham, 1945). In the semi-dry steppes of the north, outbreaks of malaria occurred following periods of excessive rain (Heisch, 1947). These simple models were gradually adjusted according to the geographic characteristics of the various regions of the country.

• *Hyperendemic plateaux*

The plateaux, on which Lake Victoria is situated, reach an altitude of about 1,200 m high and constitute a region of stable hyperendemic malaria in Kenya, as well as in Uganda and Tanzania. From 1976 to 1978, in the area surrounding Kisumu, WHO implemented a malaria control programme based on indoor spraying with an organo-phosphate insecticide called fenitrothion. The results showed that on top of the prohibitive cost of treatment with this insecticide, it was not possible to completely stop transmission even though the population of vectors was drastically reduced (Fontaine *et al.*, 1978). The programme was implemented following an entomological and epidemiological study that revealed the hyperendemic nature of the disease (Rickmann *et al.*, 1972). During the pre-spraying phase, the daily parasite inoculation rate was 0.00958 in young children; after spraying, this parameter had dropped to 0.00037, i.e. by a factor of thirty (Fontaine *et al.*, 1978).

A more recent study confirmed the epidemiological findings from before 1978. The PRs of children varied from 85% in young children between ages 1-4, to 60% in children between ages 10 and 14. The prevalence of heavy parasitaemia decreased from 37% to 1% in the two aforementioned age groups. Clinical manifestations of up to a rate of 20% in babies between 12-23 months fell to 0.3% in children between the ages of 10 and 14. The percentage of anaemia, which was 55% in infants under the age of one, gradually decreased up to the age of 10. Children under 5 years old and particularly under 2 were the main group at-risk (Bloland *et al.*, 1999) (*Figures 36 and 37*).

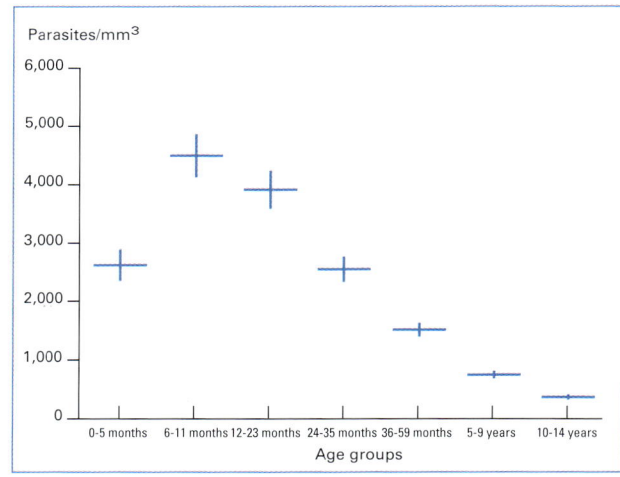

Figure 36. Mean parasite density at different ages on the plateaux of western Kenya (adapted from Bloland et al., 1999).

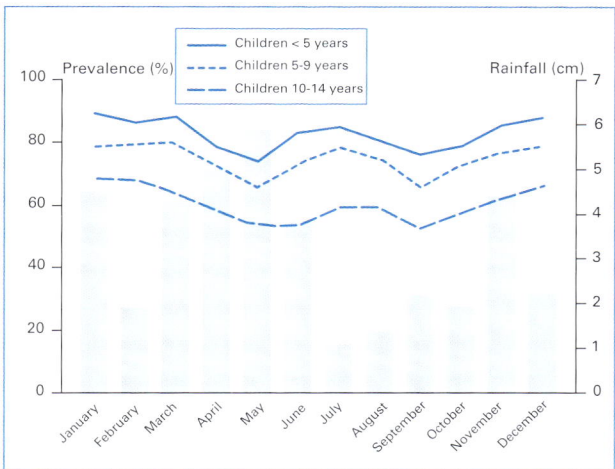

Figure 37. Parasite prevalence on the plateaux of western Kenya (adapted from Bloland et al., 1999).

In the same region, 72% of infections were in children under the age of 10 while 12% were in children from ages 12 to 21, and 16% were in adults. Children between the ages of one and 10 constituted the principal carriers of infection. Not one baby under the age of one was found to be infected (Githeko et al., 1992).

• *Coastal regions*

In the region of Kilifi (60 km to the north of Mombasa), the parasite prevalence in children between 0-9 years old was 34%: transmission was seasonal and the EIR less than 10 ib/p/yr. At their worst, serious cases presented as discreet mini-epidemics concentrated in certain sites, but the prevalence in the community as a whole did not vary (Snow et al., 1993, 1998a). The number of serious cases seemed to correlate with rainfall and, therefore, with the moment of transmission, but there was no statistical difference between the distribution of serious and uncomplicated cases. The presence of a high density of population within 250 m of a house seemed to reduce the risk of serious cases (dilution of bites?). The risk also decreased with the use of fumigants and insecticide aerosols. From an epidemiological point of view, the rationale for separating clinically serious cases from the simple ones is not easily done as transmission remains identical in both cases.

The Kenya coastline south of Malindi was considered to be meso- or hyperendemic (Subra, personal communication, 1975).

• *Mountain epidemics*

In **Nairobi**, malaria first appeared when the city was built in 1907. In 1908, 787 cases and 28 deaths were reported; out of 700 Europeans, 10% were affected. In 1913, a serious epidemic outbreak occurred with 14,000 cases and 60 deaths. During the war of 1914-1918, *P. vivax* was imported by Indian troops but then disappeared spontaneously. In 1938, the prevalence of *P. falciparum* in African children reached 30%. After 1940, following the expansion of the city and urban construction, malaria disappeared from Nairobi (Symes, 1940). The sporozoite rate of the vector, probably *An. arabiensis*, was very low at 0.5%, despite an elevated prevalence of the parasite (Roberts, 1949).

In the **mountains of south-west Kenya**, which were considered to be free of malaria, an epidemic was reported in Londiani near a military camp, located between 2,500 and 2,600 m in altitude, and lasted three years. Most cases appeared from May to July and then disappeared in August, which corresponds with the peak and then the decrease of *An. gambiae s.l.* during the winter in the southern hemisphere. The episodes were localised in space and time due to the vector's distribution and its short period of activity. The temperatures in homes were 3-5 °C higher than outdoors, which made it possible for *An. gambiae* to compete the sporogonic cycle of *P. falciparum* in a region where it would not have been possible outdoors (Garnham, 1945, 1948).

On the **Nandi Plateau** in Kericho, *An. funestus* appeared to be the principal vector (with a sporozoite rate of 1.7%) whereas *An. gambiae* was not infected. The overall malaria prevalence was 7% in May as opposed to 38% in September (Heisch & Harper, 1949).

At the beginning of the 20th century, the Nandi Plateau was considered to be free of malaria. The disease is thought to have been introduced by soldiers returning from the war in 1918-1919. It should be remembered that the vectors had to have been present for part of the year at the very least to support indigenous transmission. Since then, however, the countryside has changed with deforestation. The vectors would then gradually adapt to the environment of the Nandi Plateau (Matson, 1957) (*Table XXIV*).

On the Nandi Plateau in the beginning of the 1960's, in an area around Kericho with a population of 120,000 inhabitants, located between 1,800 and 2,300 m in altitude, the main vector was *An. gambiae s.s.*, whose peak occurred during May-June; *An. funestus* was not very abunddant. According to a pre-spraying investigation, malaria in children between 1-10 years old was meso-, if not, hyperendemic (PI of 78%) in certain exposed sites. There was no decrease in prevalence in adults, which suggested that the population had little immunity. In 1960, the malaria control programme based on indoor DDT spraying was effective as malaria disappeared until 1980 (Malakooti et al., 1998). From 1990 to 1997, 704 deaths (of which 30% were due to malaria) were reported by the hospital of Kericho. During the same period, the rate of tea plantation workers victim to clinical malaria reached 50%.

The re-emergence of malaria would not be due to increased temperatures, but to a change in the environment, particularly deforestation, the decline of health care services, amplified by the resistance of *P. falciparum* to medication, and the abandoned programmes of indoor DDT spraying (Malakooti et al., 1998).

In the district of Uasin Gishu, an outbreak erupted in May-June 1993. at an altitude of 1,500-2,100 m; it more or less extended all the way to the mountainous regions of south-west Kenya. In the hospital of Eldoret during the first nine months of the year, 2,195 patients were admitted for malaria and 146 did not survive (mortality rate of 6.6%). It seems more likely to have been a seasonal outbreak as opposed to an epidemic (Some, 1994) (*Table XXV*).

A more recent publication by Oloo *et al.* (1996) summarises the situation of malaria in south-west Kenya:
- between 1,100-1,300 m, malaria is stable hyper- or holo-endemic;
- between 1,300-1,700 m, malaria is seasonal of medium stability, and meso-endemic with prevalences of 30-50%;
- between 1,700-2,300 m, malaria is unstable and epidemic in nature following heavy rain and during "hot" years.

P. falciparum was responsible for 90% of the infections, *P. malariae* for less than 10%, *P. ovale* was rare, and *P. vivax* was exceptional.

On the plateau, the EIR reached 300 ib/p/yr below 1,300 m. Only 30% of the clinical cases were confirmed microscopically. The rate of resistance to chloroquine (RII and RIII) reached 75%. More than 30% of the deaths occurred in patients treated with chloroquine whereas 10% occurred in patients treated with SP (sulfadoxine-pyrimethamine). Artemisinin, halofantrine and mefloquine

Table XXIV. Prevalence of malaria on the Nandi Plateau in Kenya before the indoor spraying campaign (Roberts, 1964).

Place surveyed	1951 survey				1952 survey			
	Month	Prevalence by age group			Month	Prevalence by age		
		0-10	11-20	> 21		0-10	10-20	> 21
Arwos	February	5	4	6				
	August	58	–	45				
Kapkangani	February	12	8	6				
	September	–	56	45				
Serem	March	41	24	6	November	31	–	–
	June	50	43	54				
Chepterit	October	3	–	6	April	10	–	–
Kibwareng	October	47	36	13	April	77	33	18
Kaptumo	September	33	–	–	May	14	–	–
Kaibo	September	10	14	14				
Chepterwa	September	76		46				
Kesenge					November	34		
Kaptkolei					November	15	10	6

Table XXV. Admissions and deaths, before and after the 1993 malaria epidemic in Eldoret, Kenya (adapted from Some, 1994).

	January	Febr.	March	April	May	June	July	August	Sept.	9 month total
All admissions	1,251	1,888	1,500	1,314	1,585	2,200	1,599	1,606	1,580	14,523
Admissions for malaria	76	119	152	110	153	922	364	184	115	2,195
Total deaths	21	39	33	50	48	85	43	46	38	403
Deaths from malaria	5	6	10	6	10	64	20	16	9	146
Proportion of malarial mortality	23.8	15.4	30.3	12.0	20.8	75.3	46.3	43.8	23.7	36.2
Fatality rate (%)	6.6	5	6.6	5.5	6.5	6.9	5.5	8.7	7.8	6.6

remained effective. **Drug resistance** plays an important role in the **seriousness** of malaria in the **highlands of Kenya** (Shanks *et al.*, 2000).

• *Epidemics of the semi-dry regions and the effects of El Niño*

In the semi-dry regions of north-east Kenya, which are mostly populated by Somali nomads, the scarce and irregular rainfall (306 mm on average), from one year to the next, occurs from March to May, and from October to December. In 1930, after heavy rains, the entire population of the encampments suffered from malaria. In 1947, following a rainy spell, more than 25% of the population of several encampments were infected. In Buna, the global prevalence of 6% was characteristic of hypo-endemic disease (Heisch, 1947). The Somalis did not have any immunity. In 1961-1962, following the flooding of the Tana River, the hospital of Wajir increased their consultations by 70%.

In 1996 and in the beginning of 1997, the drought had destroyed the entire harvest. Beginning in October 1997, the effects of El Niño (*see Part* "Spatiotemporal Dynamics of Malaria") translated into torrential rains from October 1997 to January 1998; the height was in November with 489 mm of rainfall. These rains and flooding destroyed the road network, and drowned 80% of the goats and 50% of the camels. The population migrated towards areas that were not flooded. The epidemic broke out at the end of December during the Christmas holidays when the health services employees were absent. It was only in February 1998 that malaria was identified to be the cause of the epidemic (Brown *et al.*, 1998). The hospital of Wajir treated 20,000 of the 60,000 estimated cases. In three months, the incidence of malaria had risen to 33‰. The total mortality rate was estimated to have been 7.2‰ per day at the peak of the epidemic (Allan *et al.*, 1998). The only vector identified was *An. arabiensis* (*Figure 38*).

The effects of ENSO (El Niño Southern Oscillation) were felt throughout almost all of Kenya, Uganda, southern Somalia, and Ethiopia in 1997-1998.

• *Entomology, taxonomy, and ecology*

In Kenya, almost all the malaria transmission is carried out by *An. funestus* and three species of the *An. gambiae* Complex: *An. gambiae s.s.*, *An. arabiensis* and *An. merus*. *An. pharoensis* only has a localised role.

An. merus, a halophilic species, is localised in a few spots on the Kenyan coast from which it hardly moves (Mosha & Subra, 1982). In Jumbo, it represented 96% of the species of the complex along with *An. arabiensis* (2.5%) and *An. gambiae s.s.* (0.8%). It was a not very effective vector of malaria and Bancroftian filiariasis that apparently was not very effective (Mosha & Petrarca, 1983).

An. gambiae s.s. and *An. arabiensis* are sympatric in extremely variable proportions throughout most of the territory, with the exception of the highlands above 1,600 m where *An. gambiae s.s.* alone is present, and in the semi-dry regions of the north and north-east where *An. arabiensis* alone is present. In south-western Kenya, it has been possible to establish the distribution of each species of the complex and of *An. funestus* according to the altitude and the ecological characteristics of the region (Joshi *et al.*, 1975; White, 1972) (*Table XXVI*).

A study of the larval habitats of *An. arabiensis* has helped establish life tables. The mortality rate, from egg hatching to adulthood was 98%. This mortality rate remained constant in the rice paddies throughout all the stages whereas, in rainwater deposits, it accelerated during the final larval stages as a result of infection with a microsporidium belonging to the genus *Coelomomyces* (Service, 1977).

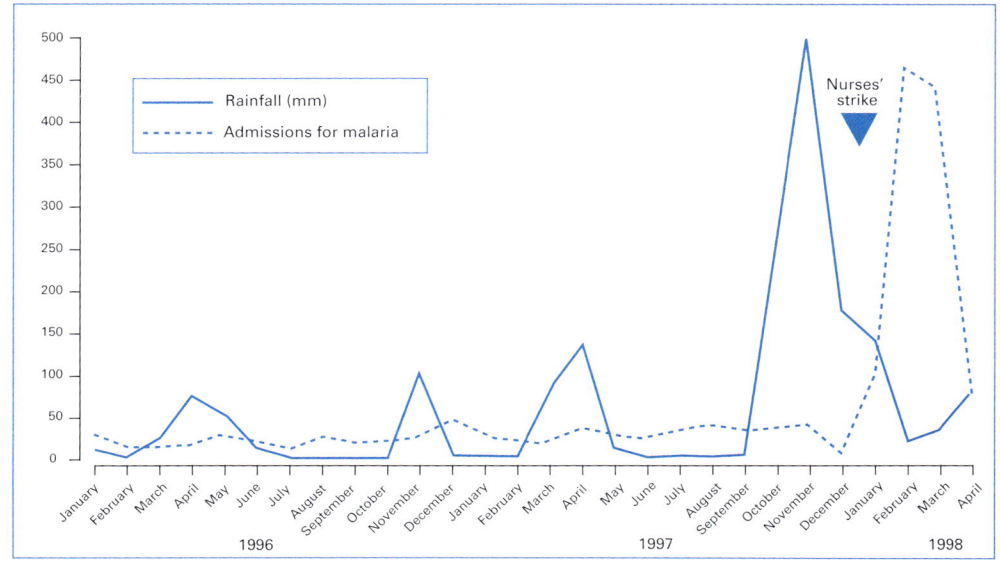

Figure 38. El Niño and the epidemic of January 1998 in north-eastern Kenya (*adapted from* Brown et al., 1998).

Biodiversity of Malaria in the World

Table XXVI. Distribution of the *An. gambiae* Complex and *An. funestus* in south-western Kenya (the Kisumu Region and the Nandi plateau).

Biotopes	*An. gambiae s.s.*	*An. arabiensis*	*An. funestus*
Banks of Lake Victoria, 1,200 m	Very rare	Low density	High density
Unirrigated plateau, 1,200 m	Rare	High density	High density - dominant
Irrigated plateau, 1,200 m	Absent	High density	High density
Foothills, 1,300-1,600 m	Dominant but low density	Minor	Not stipulated
Mountains > 1,600 m	Dense	Absent	Present in places

In south-western Kenya, *An. funestus* is the dominant species in the reeds on the Lake Victoria shores, as well as in the marshy areas on the plateau between 1,200 and 1,300 m high. In mountainous regions, it was considered to be the main vector before *An. gambiae s.s.* took its place. In the dry regions, it is becoming quite rare and is completely absent in north-eastern Kenya.

In 1958, fish farming was introduced into the Nyanga District and, having been poorly managed, resulted in a proliferation of *An. gambiae s.l.*, and then *An. funestus* as vegetation developed in the farm ponds. *An. funestus* represented 83% of the mosquitoes around the fish ponds; contrary to what may have been written, *Tilapia* is not a predator of anopheline larvae (Lockhart *et al.*, 1969).

The role of rice paddies in the development of *An. arabiensis* (45%), *An. funestus* (6%), and *An. pharoensis* has been the object of several studies (Chandler & Highton, 1975; Chandler *et al.*, 1975b, 1976; Mukiama & Mwengi, 1989; Surtees, 1970), which are hardly conclusive from an epidemiological point of view.

In central Kenya, where natural rainfall takes over from irrigation, the role of *An. pharoensis* (which is so often contested) is demonstrated by a sporozoite rate of 1.3% (according to the circumsporozoite antigen assay) and 0.68 (by dissection); the sporozoite rate of *An. funestus* taken from the same biotopes using the same methods is 1.7% and 1.2% respectively (Mukiama & Mwangi, 1989).

The role of houses as safe resting spots was already mentioned above. Also of note is the importance of millet lofts, where *An. arabiensis* is found more frequently than in houses, contrary to *An. gambiae s.s.* (Clarke *et al.*, 1980).

• *Transmission*

In the mountains of south-western Kenya, the EIR was 29 ib/p/yr for *An. gambiae s.s.* and 17 ib/p/yr for *An. funestus*, with respective sporozoite rates of 6.3% and 9.5%. Transmission, however, remained limited to the proximity of larval habitats (valley bottoms). The presence of 55% of symptomless cases amongst parasite carriers demonstrated a tendency towards stability (Shililu *et al.*, 1998).

In the region of Kisumu, once the malaria control programme had ended in 1980, the sporozoite rates were 9.6%, 0.4% and 6.1% for *An. gambiae s.s.*, *An. arabiensis*, and *An. funestus* respectively (Taylor *et al.*, 1990). This very big difference in sporozoite rates between the two species of the *An. gambiae* Complex confirms that *An. arabiensis* is the weaker vector (Lemasson *et al.*, 1997).

In the dry region of Lake Baringo (rainfall between 500-600 mm) in the Rift Valley, the EIR ranged from 14 to 16 ib/p/yr for *An. gambiae s.l.* (probably *An. arabiensis*) and was 3.5 ib/p/yr for *An. funestus*. In a group of children between the ages of 5 and 9, each subject received one infective bite by *An. gambiae* every 5.3 days and one infective bite by *An. funestus* every 47 days in October and November (Aniedu, 1997).

• *Mapping malaria and predicting epidemics*

The number of malaria epidemics (or seasonal outbreaks) has increased considerably in Kenya over the last twelve years during which fifteen epidemics were recorded. The prevalence of malaria has therefore increased from 20% to 60% and the death rate of people with this disease has reached 7.5% in the medical centres. The problem facing the medical services is to know and foresee where and when the epidemics will occur.

In the dry regions of the north-east, malaria outbreaks usually occur in July-August after the rains. But with the effects of El Niño in 1997-1998, heavy rainfall occurred from October to January, setting off an epidemic that lasted from December 1997 to March 1998, i.e. starting one to two months after the peak of rainfall. This phenomenon has therefore increased the epidemic season to six months. It would seem that as of May 1997, one could have predicted six months beforehand the effects of ENSO, but the seriousness of the situation was underestimated considering that the year was predicted to be a good harvest year.

In the mountains of south-west Kenya, one could expect epidemics if the temperature (usually over 18 °C) increased by 3 °C and if the monthly rainfall exceeded 150 mm at 1,500 m in altitude (Githeko & Ndegwa, 2001). These simple signs allow predictions but provide very little forewarning once the elements that set off the rise in transmission are in place. The time left to set up preventive measures is therefore often insufficient. It should be noted that during certain dry years, contrary to epidemic periods, there is a real lack of transmission during which immunity, even limited, tends to diminish, perhaps increasing the risk of future epidemics in such unstable malaria settings.

Measuring soil humidity, as opposed to rainfall, is considered to be a better way of predicting the density of mosquitoes (Patz *et al.*, 1998). Based on the humidity of the soil, it would be possible to predict the theoretical number of bites by *An. gambiae* that an individual in a given place and time might receive. The variability of the density of bites is 45% dependent on humidity and 8% on precipitation. The correlation with temperature is less certain. These models are predictive only on a very short term basis.

In Kenya, because of the variability of temperatures and/or rainfall, it has been possible to stratify the **regions of unstable malaria** which are home to eight million people, and the **regions of stable malaria**. The latter has been classified into three categories according to the malaria prevalence in children under the age of 9: low endemicity with a PR of under 20%, medium with a PR from 20-70% and high with a PR of over 70%. The model was applied to satellite data using a Geographical Information System (GIS). Data on the mortality and morbidity rates were obtained from all available sources (Snow *et al.*, 1998b).

The authors calculated that seventy-two children under the age of 5 die of malaria in Kenya every day and that four hundred develop clinical forms of the disease. The mortality rate of malaria cases, based on health centre statistics, is one of the highest ever reported.

The enormous potential of GIS-coupled satellite data has encouraged several experts to produce **large-scale epidemiological maps**, adjusted according to the season. Determining the areas at-risk according to the season does nothing but reinforce information that has been available for a long time (Hay *et al.*, 1998). One map indicating transmission in Kenya adopts the classification by Snow *et al.* (1998b) of the endemic zones (Omumbo *et al.*, 1998) in the context of the MARA (Mapping Malaria Risk in Africa) project. These maps provide an instant picture but are not tools that can be used for making predictions (*see Figure 1, page 50*).

A large-scale map of the Kisumu Region shows, side by side, the houses and public buildings along with the large *Anopheles* larval habitats, georeferenced by GPS (Global Positioning System) (Hightower *et al.*, 1998). It has become evident that in a small area of a stable zone, the distance from the house to the larval habitat has no effect on the number of *Anopheles* in the homes. But the maps do not point out the rain-fed larval habitats of *An. gambiae*, which are small in size but highly abundant during the rainy season, and which are the best suppliers of *Anopheles*.

Currently, major research on malaria is being conducted in Kenya for the purpose of adapting state-of-the-art techniques to the reality of the field and then integrating them with the more conventional techniques.

Uganda

• *Natural regions and endemicity*

Uganda is an enclosed country with a large variety of landscapes and an epidemiology that reflects this variability (McCrae, 1975). In the wooded savannah and the mosaic of forest and savannah in the north and to the west of Lake Victoria, malaria is hyper- or meso-endemic (1,100-1,300 m in altitude). Malaria is hyperendemic in all the northern savannah lands. In the west, on the shores of the Great Lakes (Lake Edward, Lake George, Lake Albert) on the western branch of the Rift Valley between 900 and 1,300 m in altitude, the malaria is hyperendemic, but rapidly becomes meso-endemic between 1,300-1,500 m. For a long time, it was believed that there was no longer any endemic malaria above 1,500 m in the south-west, with the exception of a few larval habitats on the lakeshores (Lake Bunyoni). This opinion is currently changing as more and more malaria cases are observed in the health centres of the south-west mountains at 1,800 m in altitude, and in particular, on the slopes of the Ruwenzori and Elgon Mountains. This trend corresponds to a strong population increase and the resulting farming development of new areas.

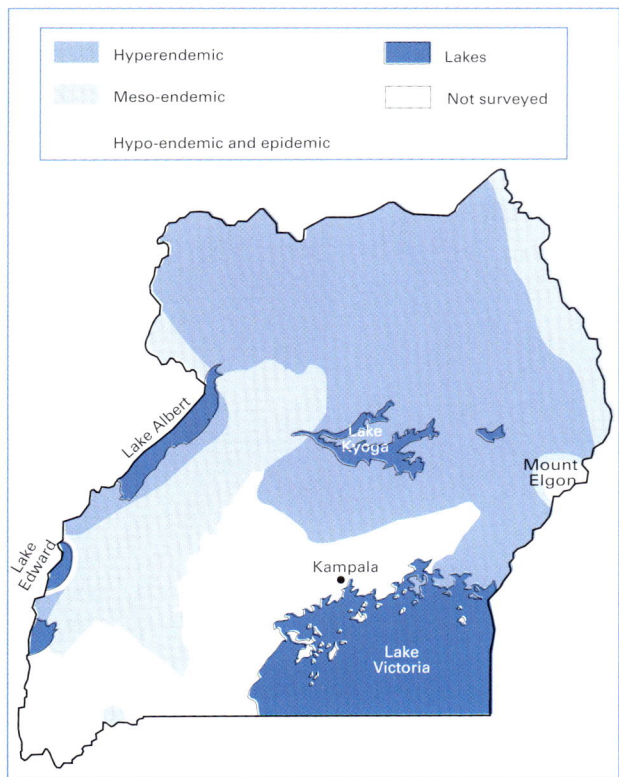

Figure 39. Endemic malaria in Uganda (adapted from McCrae, 1975).

Although it needs an updating, the map by McCrae (1975) provides a fair picture of the endemicity throughout the various regions of the country (*Figure 39*).

• *Vectors*

One of the first studies on vectors in Uganda was carried out by Gibbins (1932). *An. gambiae s.l.*, then *An. costalis*, was the main vector with a very high sporozoite rate from 14-25% in Kampala, whereas in Fort Portal (1,500 m in altitude) this species was not infected. The sporozoite rates of *An. funestus* were 13-17% in Kampala and 1.4% in Fort Portal. The sporozoite rate of *An. moucheti* varied from 1.6-4.3%; that of *An. pharoensis* was 0.7% and that of *An. hancocki* was 0.2% in the central-southern part of the country.

Following the division of the *An. gambiae* Complex, 3 species were identified in Uganda: *An. gambiae s.s.* was in the humid regions on the shores of Lake Victoria (Onori & Benthein, 1969), and was the only species of the complex found in the high altitude regions of the south-west (Mouchet *et al.*, 1998); *An. arabiensis* was in the more or less dry savannah regions of the north (McCrae, 1975; Onori, 1969); *An. bwambae*, an endemic species of Uganda as described by White (1985) whose larvae developed in mineral springs of the Semliki National Park (Harbach *et al.*, 1997), was very abundant in the Bwamba District and was particularly anthropophilic but this species did not appear to play an important role in transmission, only a local role. However, of 278 dissections, sporozoites were found in two specimens.

Goma (1960a and b) demonstrated that *An. gambiae* did not develop in the papyrus marshland that covered the high altitude valley bottoms. It seems that the same was true for *An. funestus*, even though it is highly abundant in the reeds such as found near Lake Bunyoni. McCrae (1975) showed that papyrus secretes an essential oil that forms an iridescent film that covers the marshland surface and prevents mosquito larvae from breathing.

• *Regional epidemiology*

For the purpose of eradicating malaria, regional epidemiological studies were launched by the WHO at the end of the 1960's. Their goal was not achieved but the research carried out until 1967 did provide valuable information on malaria in the different regions of Uganda.

In the Karamoja District, in the north-east on the border of Kenya, a savannah region at 1,000-1,400 m in altitude, malaria was meso-, hyper- or holo-endemic depending on how close the vector sources were (Onori, 1969). In school children between the ages of 5-15, the PR varied from 10-94%. Although transmission was seen throughout the entire year, the seasonal fluctuations were extremely noticeable. The only vector cited was *An. arabiensis* with a sporozoite rate of 3% during the rains, and of 1% during the dry season (*Table XXVII*).

P. malariae had been suspected of causing severe disease by Jeliffe (*in* Onori, 1969) who attributed 75% of malaria cases to this parasite. This estimated figure was substantially cut by Onori (1967a) but *P. malariae* was nevertheless found in 30% of the positive slides. The percentage of *P. ovale* remained stable between 1-2% (Onori, 1967b).

Table XXVII. Results of malaria surveys in schoolchildren (5-15) in Karamoja District, Uganda, May-July 1965 (Onori, 1969).

Place	N° examined	Spleen rate	Parasite rate	Gametocyte rate
Moruita	78	57.7	38.5	9.0
Loro	90	32.2	10.0	1.1
Namalu	102	68.6	71.6	18.6
Lolachat	70	73.0	50.0	1.4
Lorengedwat	78	79.5	53.0	41.1
Moroto	160	45.0	20.6	5.0
Nyakwei	85	85.0	94.1	34.1
Atunga	72	62.5	70.8	27.8
Alerek	52	90.4	94.2	48.1
Panyangara	90	70.0	50.2	21.1
Kapelimoro	66	66.7	72.7	25.8
Kacheri	35	94.3	74.3	28.6
Karenga	200	76.0	60.0	19.5
Nalakas	58	62.1	44.8	12.1
Loyoro	64	21.9	15.6	3.1
Total	1,300	64.0	51.5	16.5

The Busoga District is in the central southern part of the country and is bordered by Lake Victoria, the Nile, and Lake Kyoga, with an average altitude of 1,100-1,200 m. In this area, covered with a mosaic of forest and savannah, wooded savannah, and farmland, malaria was hyper- or holo-endemic all along the lakes, and meso-endemic between the lakes. Neither the climate nor the homogenous vegetation can explain this difference in endemicity. The average PR was 52% in children between the ages of 2-4, 47% in children from 10-14 years, and 17% in adults. The vectors were *An. gambiae s.s.* with a sporozoite rate of 0.15-1.4%, and *An. funestus* with a sporozoite rate of 1% (Onori & Benthein, 1969). Since 1975, the Busoga District has been ravaged by a devastating epidemic of sleeping sickness due to *Trypanosoma rhodesiense*, which was subsequently brought under control by the trapping of tse-tse flies (Lancien, 1991).

In the Masaka District west of Lake Victoria, on the border of Tanzania (1,100-1,450 m in altitude), malaria was tracked in two counties* in 1960 and 1961. In Rakai, a savannah region where homes are widely dispersed, the situation fluctuated between hyper- and meso-endemic. In Buddu, a highly farmed region that is densely populated, the situation was meso-endemic (*Table XXVIII*) (Zulueta *et al*., 1963). Two successive years—1960 and 1961—of extremely low rainfall probably contributed to maintaining the malaria indicators below their normal level. In this district below the equator, the purpose of the study was to show that malaria could vary enormously—between hyper- and meso-endemic—according to human density and crop surfaces. In one part of this district, a study on indoor spraying with an organophosphate insecticide (malathion for 3 cycles/year) was carried out. In the central part of the trial zone, malaria transmission was at least temporarily stopped (Najera *et al*. 1967).

The **Kigezi Region**, often cited in malaria literature, includes all of south-western Uganda from Lake Edward to the Rwandan border. It is divided into four districts: Kabale, Kisoro, Rukungiri and Bushenyi. In the northern part of ex-Kigezi (Rukungiri) on the shores of Lakes Edward, George and Albert, malaria was hyperendemic at 950-1,250 m in altitude with PRs of 40%, 53% and 8% respectively in children between the ages of 1-2, ages 5-9, and adults. At 1,250-1,500 m, the disease was just meso-endemic (Zulueta *et al*., 1961). In Bachiga, a malaria control programme was set up in 1959 to protect the colony of settlers who had come from the over-populated South. *An. gambiae s.l.,* the vector in May-June, was replaced by *An. funestus* from February to July. After only one cycle of indoor DDT spraying, malaria was on its way to disappearing in this very limited area (WHO, 1961).

In the **Kigezi Mountains**, areas above 1,500 m in altitude, were considered to be free of endemic malaria but there seems to have been more exceptions to this rule than confirmations. Around the mountain **lakes** and, in particular, Lake Bunyoni (2,000 m in altitude), highly endemic sites maintained by *An. funestus*, which lived in the lakeshore reeds, were reported by Garnham *et al*. (1948). The SR was 80% and **malaria** was considered to be stable. During a pre-eradication study, the PR was from 30-35% in children between ages 2-9 (Zulueta *et al*., 1964). Other sites were reported around the Mutanda and Kibungo

Table XXVIII. Prevalence of malaria in the Masaka Region in Uganda (adapted from Zulueta *et al.*, 1963).

Age group	Rakai Region (1959)							Kyanamakuka Region (1959)						
	Number	*P. falciparum*	*P. malariae*	Gametocytes	Mixture	Total parasites	PR	Number	*P. falciparum*	*P. malariae*	Gametocytes	Mixture	Total parasites	PR
0-11 months	37	10	2	5	1	11	29.6	42	4	2	2	1	5	11.9
12-23 months	21	9	6	8	2	13	61.9	31	5	5	6	1	9	29.0
2-4 years	9	4	1	1	1	4	44.5	41	12	9	10	4	17	41.0
5-9 years	64	31	5	10	1	35	54.7	143	40	6	13	3	43	30.1
10-14 years	134	49	8	15	1	56	41.8	186	28	4	7	–	32	17.2
15-19 years	31	8	1	5	–	9	29.0	8	1	–	–	–	1	12.7
> 20 years	49	4	–	–	–	4	8.2	1	1					
Total	345	115	23	44	6	132	38.5	452	90	26	38	9	107	23.7

* The county in Uganda is an administrative delineation between parish and district.

Lakes. In the valleys, the papyrus marshland was hardly conducive to vector development. Meanwhile, however, *An. gambiae s.s.* developed in clearings and around fish farm ponds and thus seems to have been responsible for the epidemic in the Kabale Valley (Garnham *et al.*, 1948). In this valley, located at 1,650-1,800 m in altitude, a steady increase in the number of malaria cases was observed in the hospital of Kisizi from 1968 to 1994 (according to the number of consultations). From 1968 to 1975, this figure increased seven-fold and, from 1975 to 1993, increased thirteen-fold (*Figure 40*). This steady rise of case numbers in this valley seems to be related to environmental changes notably land clearing and fish-farming, and population migration to the valley bottoms, where it is easier to farm. In May and June, the principle vector was *An. gambiae s.s.*, with a sporozoite rate of more than 10%. Mosquito captures in November and then in February gave negative result but this does not mean that *An. gambiae* disappeared from the valley at any period of the year (Mouchet *et al.*, 1998). A recent rise in malaria was reported in all the valleys of the Kabale and Rukunguri Districts (reports from the district health centres), and of neighbouring Rwanda.

Local environmental changes, as well as growing population densities are definitely responsible to some degree for these epidemiological changes. Temperature increases can hardly be used to explain these changes given that meteorological readings from the Kabale weather station (1,980 m in altitude) only show a difference of 1.2°C between the "coldest" year (1965 with 16.6°C) and the "hottest" year (1994 with 17.8°C), plus 1.8°C to compensate for the altitude of Kisizi.

On the other hand, the cause of the **epidemics** that broke out in the Kabale and Kisizi Regions in **1994**, from July to October, appears to be very clear (Mouchet *et al.*, 1998).

They were due to **excessive rainfall** (approximately two-fold higher than normal) during the first semester of 1994. In July 1994, 1,684 patients were admitted to the hospital of Kisizi with a diagnosis (microscopically confirmed) of malaria, as opposed to 200 in July 1993, and 225 in 1995. For the entire year, the number of cases reported in this hospital totalled 3,800, as opposed to 2,500 in 1993, and less than 2,000 in 1995. But this epidemic broke out due to the increase, since at least 1982, in the parasite reservoir as can be seen from the Kisizi Hospital statistics. This confirms the hypothesis developed by Coosemans *et al.* (unpublished results) concerning the epidemic of Burundi, that outbreaks follow growths in parasite reservoirs.

Around Kabale, the ENSO episode of 1997-1998 resulted in a malaria epidemic that lasted from February to April 1998. It broke out following heavy rains during the fourth trimester of 1997 that caused *An. gambiae s.s.* to proliferate in January and February 1998 (Lindblade *et al.*, 1999). During El Niño, the "humid phase" of the ENSO episode, the temperature was 1-2.5°C greater than the average for East Africa (Ropelewski & Halpert, 1987). Given the very limited number of vectors, the EIR could not be calculated until January and February 1998. It was at a rate of 0.48 ib/p/month in January and 2.4 ib/p during the first two weeks of February, which remains very low. In February, 41% of the infections were transmitted, and in April-May, the number of clinical cases was at its peak.

At the hospital of Kabarole, also in the south-western part of Uganda, the ENSO resulted, in February 1998, in the number of clinical cases doubling compared to 1997 (Kilian *et al.*, 1999). The authors considered the rains that marked the humid phase of El Niño to be a late indicator of malaria epidemics related to this phenomenon.

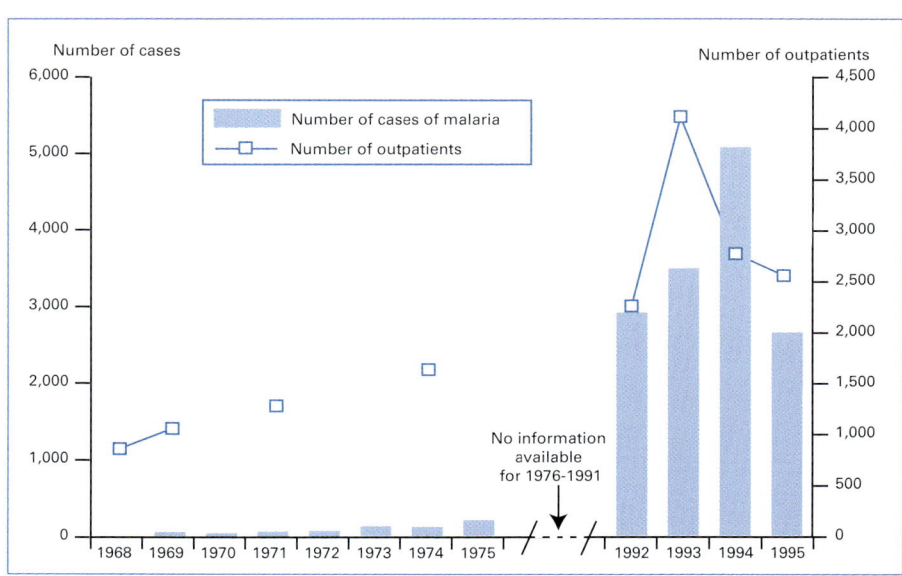

Figure 40.
Rise in the number of cases of malaria at the Kisizi Hospital between 1968 and 1995. Due to changes in the reporting system, the figures for 1976-1991 are missing (adapted from Mouchet et al., 1998).

In south-western Uganda, *An. gambiae s.s.* is very localised in the valley bottoms from where the adults hardly ever seem to stray. The perennial nature of this *Anopheles* during cold periods is a question that still remains unanswered.

• *Occupational malaria*

In the Rukungiri District, in Kanungu and in Kiziba especially, epidemics have broken out above 2,000 m amongst the gold diggers that work illegally at night, while the rest of the village population was not affected. The mining excavation works caused *An. gambiae* larval habitats to multiply and the workers were directly contaminated in their place of work. But given the night-time temperatures in these high altitude regions, transmission still remains a mystery.

• *Refugee camps*

In the Sudanese refugee camps in Uganda, the principle causes of death are diarrhoea (21%), respiratory illnesses (11%), and malaria (10%) although the latter does not appear among the causes of mortality in the camps because of effective treatment (Orach, 1999).

Tanzania

The United Republic of Tanzania (*Table I*) was formed in 1964 by the unification of the Republic of Tanganyika and the Republic of Zanzibar, both independent since 1961. Prior to this date, malaria research and control programmes in both countries were carried out independently.

• *Epidemiology*

The first information on malaria in Tanganyika was collected by German physicians from 1894-1919. The studies of Koch (1898), Wiedemann (1894), Panse (1902), and Taute (1919) in particular were used by Clyde (1965, 1967) to build an epidemiological inventory of the country.

In 1934, following the creation of the Malaria Institute in Amani, in the Usambara Mountains, Wilson & Wilson began an epidemiological survey in the north-eastern part of the country. After the end of the Second World War, they reported a general decrease in the parasite prevalence due to improved living conditions, which allowed the population to buy medication and, in particular, chloroquine (Wilson & Wilson, 1962).

Beginning in 1962, Clyde, along with various collaborators, began to review the malaria situation for the various regions of the Tanganyika territory (Clyde, 1962; Clyde & Msangi, 1963; Clyde & Mzoo, 1964; Clyde & Mluba, 1964; Clyde & Elibariki, 1965; Clyde, 1965). This work is one of the most complete descriptions ever made of an entire country. A large part of the data was also included in Clyde's comprehensive work, *Malaria in Tanzania* (1967). The identification of endemic zones was based on PRs in children under the age of 10, in particular, those of between 1 and 2. The distinction made between holo- and hyperendemic disease was often played down, and rightly so.

These authors identified:
- the **highly endemic zones** (PR of children > 50%) which included the coastal and sub-coastal plains, all the way to the foot of the Usamba Mountains in the north, the mountains of central and southern Tanzania, the shores of Lakes Nyasa, Tanganyika and Victoria, the plateaux of Tabora, Npala, Siginda, and the Serengeti Plain, i.e. an area covering more than 50% of the country;
- the **meso-endemic zones** which included the Masai Steppe in the Rift Valley, the dry region which borders the Tanzanian Plateau in the west (Dodoma), the foothills of the main mountain vary between 850 and 1,250 m (Kilimanjaro);
- the **hypo-endemic areas** which included the mountainous regions of Usambara, Arusha, and Kilimanjaro (between 1,250-1,500 m) in the north, the Subawamga Mountains in the north-west, and Njombe in the south-west.

The areas considered to be **malaria-free** included the high ground of Kilimanjaro (above 1,500 m), the Gera Highlands to the west of Lake Victoria, the Njombe Highlands parallel to Lake Tanganyika, the Meia Region in the south, and the Iringa Region in the centre. Epidemics were observed in the latter two regions as well as in Derema, near Amani in the Usambara Mountains.

This list is far from being complete and determining the exact boundaries of the endemic zones requires consulting the original works cited above, along with the extremely precise maps of the areas sampled. But almost forty years after having been established, this situation analysis is still representative of the basic distribution of malaria in continental Tanzania.

Massive changes have recently occurred in both rural and urban environments, and resistance of plasmodia to drugs and *Anopheles* to insecticides has developed throughout the country. In Dar Es Salaam, urbanisation has transformed stable holo-endemic disease into weak meso-endemic, if not hypo-endemic disease (Clyde, 1967). In addition, the coastal brackish water larval habitats in which *An. merus* lived were absorbed by the city. On the contrary, the deforestation of the Usambara Mountains created a meso-endemic situation in Amani, an area formerly malaria-free (Matola *et al*., 1987). The authors did not invoke global warming but believed that the development of malaria was a result of environmental changes. The tendency towards a lowered prevalence, reported by Wilson & Wilson (1962) and Pringle (1969), may very well reverse with the development of resistance to anti-malarial drugs and, particularly, to chloroquine and proguanil.

In 1958, malaria fluctuated between meso- and hyperendemicity on the two islands of Zanzibar (now Unguya) and Pemba. The PRs were 47% and 52% on Zanzibar and Pemba respectively (in Zahar, 1985b). In 1961, a classic eradication programme was implemented on the two islands which apparently brought the malaria to a very low level. In 1970 it was suspended. Then, in

1973, spraying was resumed when a high mortality rate due to malaria was observed in the medical centres. Up until 1982, numerous experts from the regional office of the WHO/AFRO acted as consultants to the programme, but we have not been able to find out what conclusions were made. In 1984, a thorough report made by Giri *et al.* (1984) stated that the PRs had almost returned to their initial levels, i.e. 42% and 57% for Unguya and Pemba respectively. The authors suggested that the immunity of the population must have lowered as the number of serious, if not fatal, cases was high, with more than 300 recorded in one year in the hospitals of both islands.

• *Research on transmission*

In Amani, the length of the sporogonic cycle of *An. gambiae* was estimated to be 13 days at 25.8 °C with sporozoite numbers peaking between 11 and 13 days (Davidson & Draper, 1953). In the Usambara Valleys, the same experts also compared the incidence of parasitologically detectable infection (a new infection every one-hundred days) and the entomological infection rate (an infected bite every ten days): they concluded that most sporozoites were killed before they could establish a parasitaemia in babies. The same type of study was carried out by Pringle & Avery-Jones (1966) in very young children but these experts found that the parasitological and entomological infection rates were very close and followed the same pattern. With age and the acquisition of immunity, the two patterns diverged, with the parasitological rate remaining stable while the EIR rose.

In the hyperendemic region of Tanga, Pringle (1966a) had estimated the number of sporozoites in the salivary glands in *An. gambiae* (probably *An. gambiae s.s.*) and *An. funestus*. The mean numbers per gland were between 2,000 and 4,000 with a maximum of 250,000 (with 350 oocyts) in *An. gambiae*, and 77,000 with 280 oocysts in *An. funestus*. The same author reported that, from 1934-1965, the sporozoite rates dropped following widespread chloroquine treatment (Pringle, 1966b). This observation is difficult to interpret knowing that chloroquine has no action on gametocytes.

• *Entomology*

Four species of the *An. gambiae* Complex were reported in Tanzania: *An. gambiae s.s.*, *An. arabiensis*, *An. merus*, and *An. quadriannulatus*. This last species (or a similar one), found in Zanzibar, Pemba (Odotoyimbo & Davidson, 1968), and other places in Tanzania, plays no role whatsoever in transmission. *An. merus*, highly confined to the coastline, had a sporozoite rate of 0.8% (Muirhead-Thompson, 1951). It would grow in the outer limits of the marshland in the flooded prairies of *Paspalum* where the salinity did not exceed 15 g/litre. In Pemba, *An. merus*, highly zoophilic, was the dominant species and the larvae were collected in crab holes (Odotoyimbo & Davidson, 1968). *An. gambiae s.s.* and *An. arabiensis* lived together in most of the Tanzanian territory but the proportion of both species varied enormously according to the topography, the climate, the season, the vegetation, and the anthropogeny of the environment.

In the coastal region, *An. gambiae s.s.* was the dominant species followed by *An. funestus*, *An. arabiensis* and *An. merus* (*Table XXIX*). The levels of infection of *An. gambiae s.s.* and *An. merus* were identical (according to the CSP) and the number of sporozoites per infected specimen amounted to less than 2,000 (Temu *et al.*, 1998). In 1970, in the region of Tanga, 60 km from the coast, there was a greater density of *An. arabiensis* than of *An. gambiae s.s.* during the dry season, but this latter species was largely predominant during the rains. This alternation occurs in most of continental Africa. The sporozoite rate of *An. gambiae s.s.* (4.23%) was more than ten times greater than that of *An. arabiensis* (0.32%) (White *et al.*, 1972).

Investigation of the genetics of *An. arabiensis* revealed a greater degree of heterozygosity in Tanzania than in Mozambique, suggesting distinct populations rather than ongoing, mass migration (Donnelly *et al.*, 1999).

Following indoor spraying with dieldrin, *An. funestus* disappeared in Zanzibar and Pemba (Odetoyimbo & Davidson, 1968) just as in the Pare Taveta Scheme (Smith & Draper, 1959b). It was then that various species of the *An. funestus* Group were observed, more or less anthropophilic: *An. parensis n.sp.*, *An. confusus*, and *An. rivulorum* in Pare (Gillies & Smith A, 1960), and *An. aruni*, *An. rivulorum*, and *An. leesoni* in Zanzibar (Odotoyimbo & Davidson, 1968). *An. rivulorum* is the only species of the *An. funestus* Complex, apart from *An. funestus* itself, that was found to be infected in the central eastern part of Tanzania (Wilkes *et al.*, 1996).

When spraying ceased in 1959, the anopheline re-colonisation of the Pare Taveta Scheme (which had been sprayed with dieldrin for almost two years) was monitored until 1967. Before spraying in the Pare Plain, *An. funestus* was the main vector, both in its numbers and in its level of anthropophilic behaviour, whereas *An. gambiae s.l.* was largely zoophilic. The sporozoite rate of the two species,

Table XXIX. Anthropophilicity and sporozoite rates for *An. funestus*, *An. gambiae* & *An. arabiensis* in the Tanga Region in Tanzania (adapted from White *et al.*, 1972).

	An. funestus	*An. gambiae s.s.*	*An. arabiensis*
Percentage of specimens engorged with human blood	97% (n = 508)	91% (n = 1,121)	60% (n = 1,277)
Sporozoite rates	1.6% (n = 2,094)	4.2% (n = 3,169)	0.32% (n = 1,578)

however, was very low at 0.7% and 0.6% respectively (Smith & Draper, 1959a). In 1959, after seven months of spraying, *An. funestus* disappeared and the density of *An. gambiae* decreased by 80% (Smith & Draper, 1959b). In 1962, three years after spraying had ceased, *An. gambiae* regained its initial density but *An. funestus* was still not present. On the other hand, *An. confusus,* of the same group, was abundant (Smith, 1962). In 1966, *An. funestus* resurfaced at the same density and with the same behaviour as before the spraying (Smith, 1966). The Pare Taveta Project was one of the only programmes where we were able to observe the reconstruction of the fauna following its elimination by insecticides The project also provided several observations on the ecology and the behaviour of the vectors. The presence of *An. gambiae* resting in ground crevasses, reported only in Sudan, is one of the rare observations that confirm this type of behaviour. In the same region, *An. pharoensis* was observed resting on the grass in the savannah (Smith, 1961). In the Rift Valley, south of Lake Manyara in the Masai Steppe, *An. gambiae s.l.*, whose presence was very seasonal depending on the rains, was hardly anthropophilic for a region of abundant animal breeding. It was noticeably exophilic with more than 50% of the specimens leaving houses while they were still full of fresh blood. Its sporozoite rate was nevertheless very high. *An. funestus* was rare.

Malaria represented 58% of admissions in health centres during the dry season, and 78% during the rainy season (Smith, 1964). In a holo-endemic region in Tanga (Gillies, 1955 & 1961), the density per acre (= 0.4 hectares) of *An. gambiae* and *An. funestus* was measured by the mark-release-recapture method and amounted respectively to 5-48 and 0.5-78 females per acre. These observations suggested that a very high level of transmission could be achieved with a relatively low number of vectors in a region where there was no livestock.

A study on the different aspects of exophilic behaviour in *An. gambiae* already put genetic factors into question (Gillies, 1956). This hypothesis was largely proven following the division of the *An. gambiae* Complex.

• *Malaria control programmes*

Malaria control programmes are addressed in the Part "Malaria Control". It should be noted, however, that the control programmes in Zanzibar, as in the Pare Taveta Scheme, were carried out with dieldrin (an organochlorine insecticide). The effectiveness of this insecticide caused *An. funestus* to disappear in both programmes, as well as to drastically lower the density of *An. gambiae*.

Despite encouraging results from an entomological point of view, transmission nevertheless quietly persisted (Draper & Smith, 1960), as shown by the presence of infection in infants. This transmission was due to the presence of new unsprayed homes, to the behaviour of the population who slept outside, and to the persistent nature for more than two years of *P. falciparum* in infected subjects. Eleven years after spraying had ceased in 1970, the EIR had returned to the same level as prior to the programme (Draper *et al.*, 1972) but without any epidemic episodes as feared by someone opposed to vector control operations. The programme was beneficial to the population, with a noticeable improvement in the fundamental rates of morbidity, mortality, and fertility (Pringle, 1969).

In Zanzibar, transmission never entirely stopped in the rice paddies. In Pemba, the PR dropped to 1.7% and it is not certain whether the cases reported were of an indigenous nature.

• *Plasmodial biology*

A comparison made between the region of Kilifi on the Kenyan coast, where transmission was low and seasonal, and the region of Ifakara in Tanzania, where transmission was very high and perennial, showed that there was very little difference in the number of serious malaria attacks with 46‰ and 51‰ respectively. The percentage of cerebral malaria cases was four times greater in the first case than in the second. If transmission was reduced by 95% in Ifakara (e.g. using insecticide treated mosquito nets), the level would be comparable in both cases, with a risk of seeing malaria develop later on in the life of children ("rebound mortality"). The mortality rate in both cases would therefore be identical and there would be no gain in survival. This hypothesis, put forward by Snow *et al.* (1994), received some support elsewhere and opened some controversies but has not been confirmed over several years of insecticide-treated net (ITN) use (and of other treated materials) in Ghana, Burkina Faso, etc.

In the region of Ifakara, where the EIR exceeds one ib/p/night, each tenfold increase in EIR corresponds to a 1.6-fold increase in malaria incidence (fever + parasites). Incidence has little relationship with the number of infective bites received since birth, but it drops with the length of time that trophozoites have been present in the blood. This would suggest that protective immunity depends on the degree of exposure to blood stages of the parasite rather than on the cumulative number of parasites inoculated. Therefore, a temporary decrease in human-vector contact would not translate into an increase in morbidity when control ceases. Mosquito nets remain a useful method of malaria prevention (Smith *et al.*, 1998). These conclusions—in contrast to the preceding ones—are subscribed to by a very large number of malaria specialists and are supported by several years use of ITNs in West African countries (Binka *et al.*, 1996, 1998; Habluetzel *et al.*, 1997).

Large scale social marketing of ITNs was recently implemented with some success in Tanzania (Killeen *et al.*, 2006; Tami *et al.*, 2004).

Studies on the biology of *P. falciparum* carried out in Ifakara (Babiker *et al.*, 1997) are addressed in the Chapter "*Plasmodium* Life Cycles in Humans and Anopheline Vectors".

In Ifakara, a longitudinal study on *P. falciparum* in babies during their first year of life (based on 1,356 slides of which

51% were positive for *P. falciparum*) demonstrated an absence of a period of initial protection in new born babies. The daily parasite inoculation rate was 0.029 and the duration of infection was 64 days. Passively transferred maternal immunity was mainly expressed against asexual stages (Kitua *et al.*, 1996). In the first months of life, before the acquisition of their own immune response, young children are somewhat protected by the high temperatures associated with the fever and by cytokines.

Southern Africa

Boundaries and characteristics of Southern Africa

Located south of the equator, between 6° and 35° south, southern Africa is a compact block covering 6 million km² with a population of approximately 121 million people, i.e. a population density of 20.2 inhabitants per km². Ten countries are included in this southern cone of continental Africa and are, in order of decreasing size: Angola, South Africa, Namibia, Mozambique, Zambia, Botswana, Zimbabwe, Malawi, Lesotho, and Swaziland (*Table I*).

Southern Africa is made up of a giant plateau between 800-2,000 m in altitude that culminates 3,000 m high in the Drakensberg Mountains in both Lesotho and South Africa. The central part in Botswana includes a large basin that is fed by the Okavango River which flows from Angola. The plateau is notched with valleys cut out by the Zambeze, Limpopo and Save Rivers which flow towards the Indian Ocean, and by the Orange River which flows towards the Atlantic Ocean. The coastal plains that border the Indian Ocean in Mozambique, Swaziland and South Africa are more than 300 km wide. Those that border the Atlantic in Angola, Namibia, and South Africa are narrower.

The climate, which is equatorial to the north of Angola and Mozambique and tropical in the rest of southern Africa, is highly affected by the altitude. In South Africa and Zimbabwe, it freezes and even snows above 1,300 m in altitude. In southern South Africa, where there is no malaria, the climate is basically "Mediterranean". Levels of precipitation decrease from north to south and from east to west; they are very low all along the Atlantic where the cold Benguella Current prevents oceanic air masses from penetrating. The vegetation is in line with the precipitation. The wooded savannahs of the southern equatorial belt lead into shrubby savannahs, and then into spiny steppes which cover the Kalahari in Botswana. The deserts of Namibia and South Africa are particularly dry.

The southern boundary of malaria was set between the 20th and 21st parallel south in Namibia and Botswana. In South Africa, it shifted towards the south and included the northern part of Mulamanga* and the biggest part of Kwazulu-Natal. Since 1950 in South Africa, indoor spraying treatment programmes with DDT significantly reduced the number of malaria-ridden areas in the Middleveld**. These boundaries, however, cannot be considered to be permanent and may change at any time.

Angola

There is a big gap in information on malaria in Angola due to the long civil war (25 years) which stopped in 2002. There are few recent articles on parasite susceptibility to chloroquine, on *An.gambiae* distribution (Cuamba *et al.*, 2006) and malaria morbidity in the Health Department of the Sonamet Society in Lobito (Besnard *et al.*, 2006).

Epidemiological works covering Angola as a whole were formely done by Mesquita (1942, 1952), who collected results obtained from all over the country. He divided the country into three zones:
- the equatorial one, which included the Cabinda and the Bacongo, and which had a lot of rainfall all year round apart from during the winter season in August and September when precipitation levels would lower;
- the tropical one, from the mouth of the Congo all the way to the southern part of the Benguela District, with two rainy seasons in November-December and April-May. The dry season from May to October is foggy as the sea breeze linked to the Benguela Current lowers the temperatures and the precipitation levels on the coastline;
- the subtropical one, in the southern part of the country, where the climate is sub-arid, similar to that of Namibia and the Kalahari.

Angola is a highly endemic country and malaria is the first cause of death among Angolans. Annually 25,000 deaths are registered. In 2005, 11,648 people died from malaria, out of 2.1 million infected people from January to October with the main victims being children under the age of five and pregnant women (*Angola Press Agency*, Luanda, published on April 24, 2006).

The number of malaria cases established according to the country's official statistics was 60,000 cases with 600 deaths per year. Children under the age of 2 were the most affected. As elsewhere in Africa, it is likely that the official statistics of the number of cases are understated by more than ten times the number (*Figure 41*).

In the Health Department of a private-public company (Sonamet) in Lobito, malaria was diagnosed in 17.5% of overall medical consultations in 2002 and it dropped in 2004 to 4% after implementation of microscopical observations (Besnard *et al.*, 2006) and 3% in 2005 after

---

* New name of the Transvaal.

** Middleveld: in South Africa and neighbouring States, the country is divided into the Lowveld (lowlands below 600 m), the Middleveld (between 600 and 1,100 or 1 200 m) and the Highveld (over 1,000 1,200 m depending on the latitude).

implementation of Long Lasting Nets among workers of the company.

Cambournac et al. (1955), after having consulted the information from the various districts, highlighted the difference in prevalence, from 5% to 80%, between localities within the same province of Bié (*Figure 42*). It was therefore difficult to stratify the endemic areas in Angola. The disease oscillated between meso- and hyperendemicity with a few hypo-endemic spots along the coastline—but the disease was present everywhere. This was the only comprehensive study available (*Figure 41*).

On the coast in Lobito and Luanda, where due to the presence of the cold Benguella Current the rainfall is only 237 and 362 mm in each respective city, studies showed malaria to be sporadic in Lobito with a PR of 0.64% and hypo-endemic in Luanda with PRs of 2.11% and 4.22% (Ribeiro *et al.*, 1964; Ribeiro & Carvalho, 1964). At Labito, the Gambiae Complex species involved was *An. melas*. It would seem that both cities had previously undergone vector control operations.

The dominant parasite found at more than 80% throughout Angola was *P. falciparum*. Cases of *P. vivax* were detected

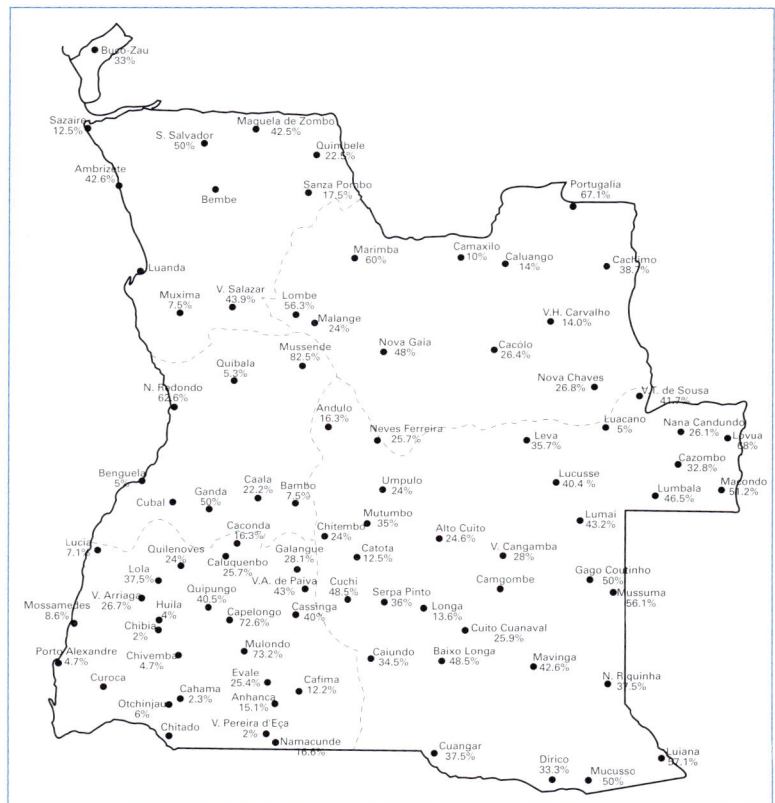

Figure 41. Distribution of malaria in Angola (adapted from Cambournac et al., 1955). Percentage figures refer to parasite rate.

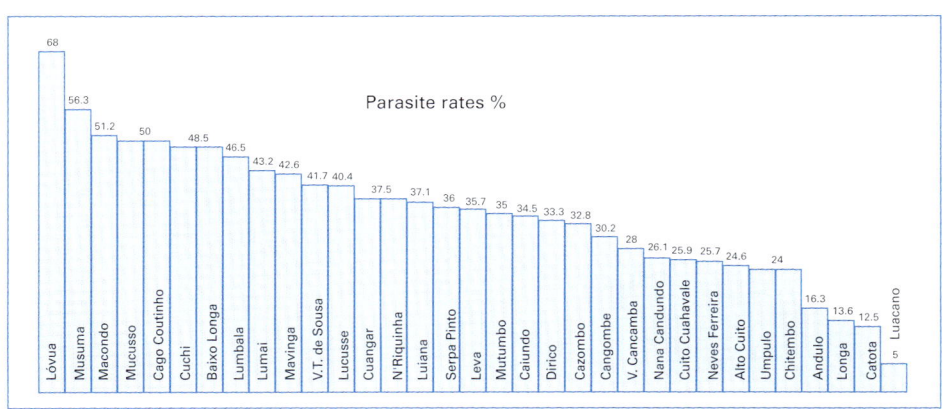

Figure 42. Parasite rate variation in various parts of the Bié province of Angola (adapted from Cambournac et al., 1955).

recently in Russian and Cuban expatriates. Their infection raises some concern as this parasite is absent in Melano-Africans who could therefore not be responsible for these cases.

Several parasitological surveys were recently carried out by Foumane *et al.* (2007) who reported the following observations:
- during the rainy season (November) in Balombo town and surrounding villages the average PR (*P. falciparum*) was about 54.7% but with great variations according to age groups and villages where PRs > 80% were recorded;
- during the rainy season (March) in Lobito-Benguela area PRs in school boys were 26.4% in Asseque, 13.5% in Alto Liro and 3.6% in Fronteira; during the dry season they were respectively 41.3%; 13.4% and 3.6%.

In the Alto Liro urban area, the PR did not change according to the season because, due to the lack of tap water, people stock water in tanks which constitute suitable larval habitats for *An. gambiae* (molecular form "S").

In Asseque rural village, water is needed for agricultural practices and is taken from the river *via* makeshift channels and small pools of stagnant water could constitute suitable larval habitats for *An. gambiae* even during the dry season.

The entomological fauna of Angola has been overseen by Ribeiro & Ramos (1975). *An. gambiae s.s.* was observed throughout the entire northern part; in the south, it lived together with *An. arabiensis*.

The southern boundary of the distribution area of *An. melas* was in Lobito (Ribeiro *et al.*, 1964). This mosquito thrives in the *Paspalum* prairies with salinity from 21-34 g/l. *An. melas* was the dominant species along the coast in the Luanda area but so far it has not been found infected (Ribeiro & Carvalho, 1964). *An. funestus* and *An. nili* were also confirmed vectors in Angola (Gillies & De Meillon, 1968) with sporozoite rates of 2.4% and 3.4% respectively. *An. pharoensis* was considered as a secondary vector.

Recently, Cuamba *et al.* (2006) undertook an indepth study of the Gambiae Complex in Luanda, Benguela and the Province of Huambo which indicated that *An. gambiae s.s.* form "M" was dominant (94%) in permanent larval habitats and form "S" accounted for 6% in small temporary habitats. Forms "M" and "S" were found in sympatry with *An. melas*. In the Liro area, *An. gambiae s.l.* was susceptible to permethrin and deltamethrin (100% mortality with diagnostic dose), but it was resistant to DDT (mortality 73%) and it was suspected to be resistant in Sao Joao (mortality 89%).

Zambia

In the 1970's, there was an extremely active period of malaria control but during the 1980's the programme gradually declined. In 1988, an anonymous report from WHO declared that the incidence of cases had risen from 138‰ in 1978 to 288‰ in 1988. The incidence even reached 584‰ in the Western Province. The specific mortality rate of hospitalised patients had increased from 14‰ to 25‰.

• *Epidemiology*

According to surveys carried out between 1969 and 1972 throughout the entire country (*Table XXX* and *Figure 43*), Wenlock (1978, 1979) had identified the following zones in rural areas:
- **hyperendemic zones**, with a PR of over 50% in children under the age of 10 in the Northern Province (between

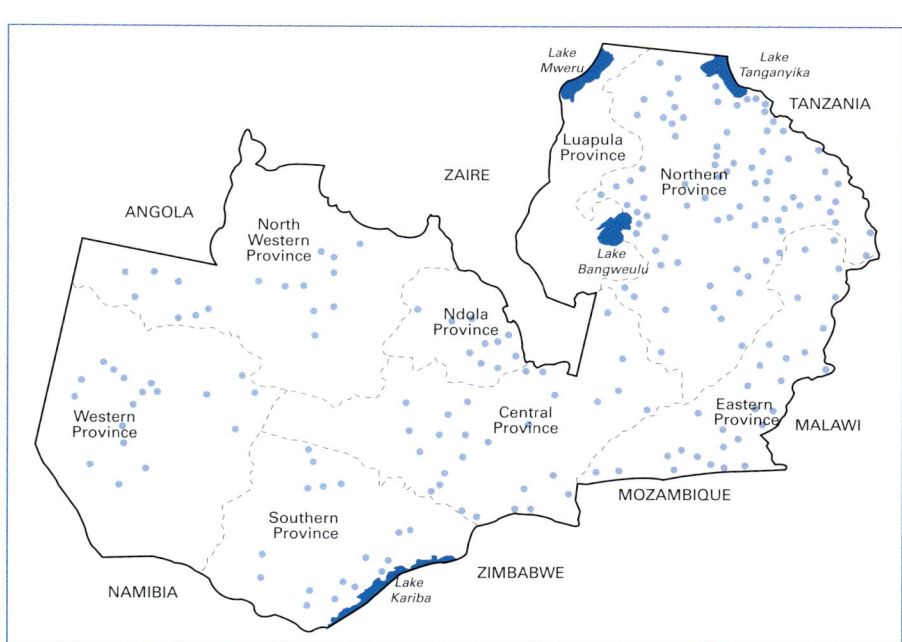

Figure 43.
Malaria estimates in Zambia (adapted from Wenlock, 1979).

Table XXX. Malaria infections by age group in Zambia (adapted from Wenlock, 1979).

Age	Lake Tanganyika Basin n	Lake Tanganyika Basin % pos	Lake Bangweulu Basin n	Lake Bangweulu Basin % pos	Chambeshi River Valley n	Chambeshi River Valley % pos	Highland Plateau Area n	Highland Plateau Area % pos	Eastern Province* n	Eastern Province* % pos	Central Province West n	Central Province West % pos	Central Province East n	Central Province East % pos	Ndola Rural Area n	Ndola Rural Area % pos	North Western Province n	North Western Province % pos	Western Province n	Western Province % pos	Southern Province n	Southern Province % pos
0-5	153	54	182	85	111	64	461	26	175	71	294	13	262	12	305	35	97	25	45	4	125	26
6-10	153	59	79	80	71	48	264	28	37	78	58	19	57	9	209	31	197	19	175	5	85	47
11-15	91	60	70	64	47	38	208	26	21	81	22	5	32	16	177	32	115	17	175	8	33	39
16-20	21	38	33	58	27	30	54	22	14	50	22	5	28	11	40	15	28	11	13	8	25	24
21-25	24	25	39	62	27	11	43	21	12	42	23	4	25	12	33	12	29	7	17	12	26	23
26-30	20	25	22	50	17	18	29	21	6		14	21	26	4	25	12	37	3	11	0	25	8
31-35	24	21	28	43	19	26	50	10	11	18	13	0	20	5	33	6	31	10	13	31	26	19
36-40	18	11	22	41	17	12	55	22	6		23	9	20	5	44	9	37	24	9	0	29	21
41-50	24	25	40	35	27	4	72	14	1		37	8	32	13	52	10	91	3	29	17	39	15
>50	28	4	38	26	25	20	95	14	6		49	12	19	21	44	2	131	5	36	8	53	25
Total	556	47	553	65	388	39	1,331	24	289	66	555	12	521	11	962	27	793	14	524	7	466	28

n = numbers; % pos = percentage positive subjects. *The small numbers for the Eastern Province mean that percentages cannot be established

Lakes Tanganyika and Bangweulu) and in the Eastern Province;
- **meso-endemic zones** in the southern plateaux of the Northern Province, the North Western Province, the Copper Belt and the Southern Province. PRs were comparable in children and adults;
- **hypo-endemic zones** in the high areas of the Central Province and the Western Province; no or very little immunity and all age groups were equally affected by the disease.

A study carried out in 1972 with school children and certain villages had already shown the distribution of malaria to be highly heterogeneous with great disparities between one school and another within the same province. Distinctions between zones did not tally with the altitude, at least under 1,000 m. But all the authors acknowledge that malaria in Zambia was omnipresent (Wolfe, 1968).

This spatial heterogeneity was observed in the Central Province and in the Eastern Province (Bransby-Williams, 1979) where the prevalence varied in each respective province from 23-92% and from 6-66% depending on the geographical location of each place. The prevalence was low on the plateaux, and much higher along waterways. Another variation was the frequency of chloroquine self-medication, which was especially high in and around cities.

In the capital city of Lusaka, the majority of cases were contracted in the neighbouring countryside (Ngandu et al., 1989). In the city centre, children presented with a PR of 2.4%; in areas out-of-town, PRs were between 10% and 27% depending on neighbourhood and season (Watts et al., 1990).

Throughout all of Zambia, *P. falciparum* was responsible for 90% of infections and *P. malariae* for 10%. *P. ovale* accounted for almost 10% of infections in children under the age of 5, becoming less abundant at 2% in older people. *P. vivax* was very rare (Hira & Koularas, 1974; Wolfe, 1968).

In hospitals, malaria was responsible for 9% of admissions and 4% of deaths (Chayabejara et al., 1974a). Morbidity was higher in the Northern and Western Provinces than in the Copperbelt and in the Central Province. At the hospital of Kabwe, the malarial morbidity rate was 9.9% in new born babies (< 1 year), 6.3% in children (1-14 years) and 2.3% in adults. Cases of cerebral malaria were frequent in adults; 90% recovered with chloroquine treatment at that time (Olweny et al., 1986). In children, severe anaemia resulted in as many deaths as with cerebral cases; malnutrition may have contributed to complications developing (Biemba et al., 2000).

• *Entomology*

An. gambiae s.s. seemed to have disappeared or at least became quite rare in the Zambeze Valley following indoor spraying with dieldrin and then DTT (Shelley, 1973) but it was found again in 1993 (Coetzee et al., 1993).

An. arabiensis remains by far the most abundant vector throughout the entire country. The peak of its presence occurs at the beginning of the rainy season and it is maintained at a high level throughout the entire summer season (Shelley, 1973). Its sporozoite rate was found to be very low with zero in Lusaka, and 0.18% throughout the entire Southern Province (Bransby-Williams, 1979). Even in places where it was found to be very anthropophilic (98% of blood meals on humans), similar results were recorded in several regions of Africa without any clear explanation. *An. quadriannulatus* had already been observed by Paterson et al., (1964b); its almost exclusively zoophilic and exophilic behaviour were studied by Shelley (1973) on the shores of the Zambeze. *An. merus* was reported in freshwater habitats in Zambia (in Zahar, 1985b; Kloke, 1997).

Although it is rarely cited, *An. funestus* is indeed a member of the Zambian fauna (Gillies & De Meillon, 1968), but it has been eliminated from several localities, especially in the Zambeze Valley following indoor spraying as usual.

Malawi

Malawi (*Table I*) is a small enclosed country that stretches for almost 1,000 km along the shores of Lake Malawi (= Lake Nyasa) and along the Shire Valley, its spillway, that rejoins the Zambeze. The country's altitude ranges from 1,300 m in the western mountains to 200 m in the south, near Mozambique. The climate is tropical, with the rains occurring from November to April during the summer season.

The malaria studies carried out or collected by Chayabejara et al. (1974b) suggested hyper-, or even holo-endemic disease below 1,000 m in altitude, and a meso-endemic situation above. To our knowledge, however, there is no documentation on high-altitude malaria in Malawi. In fact, most of the studies were carried out around development projects along Lake Malawi or in the Shire Valley. PRs in children between the ages of 2-9 ranged from 65-85%. In 1971 in the city of Lilongwe, it was 18%.

Between 1971-1973, the annual number of malaria cases according to the Health Department, amounted to 151,600 (out of 980,000 consultations) in the Northern Province, 427,000 (out of 2,466,000 consultations) in the centre, and 619,000 (out of 4,280,000 consultations) in the south, i.e. 1,200,000 cases across the country (Chayabejara et al., 1974b). Approximately 50% of the cases were detected in children under 10 years of age. Out of 60,000 slides examined by the monitoring departments in 1971, 28,000 (47%) were positive, as opposed to 20,000 (25%) in 1972 out of 79,000 slides. Out of those hospitalised, the malaria mortality rate was 11.9% in 1971, and 7.6% in 1972. Unless the quality of diagnosing had deteriorated, these figures seem to suggest that between 1971 and 1972, patient care improved.

Various studies dedicated to neonatal and infant mortality were carried out. Out of 3,274 live births, the number of neonatal deaths, post-neonatal deaths, and deaths occurring during the second year of life was 180, 397, and 152 respectively. Malaria was included among those fever cases respectively responsible for 18% and 23% of the deaths (Slutsker *et al.*, 1996b).

At the age of 3 months, 23% of babies were carriers of *P. falciparum*; at 10 months of age, 60-90% were positive. The average parasite density increased every month until 7 months when it reached a plateau. The first infection occurred on average at 199 days (Slutsker *et al.*, 1996a and 1996b). Out of a group of 703 new born babies, 0.7 malaria episodes were seen per child during the first year (Vaathera *et al.*, 2000). A study carried out in two hospitals, one in a zone of perennial transmission, and the other in a region of seasonal transmission, did not reveal a difference in prevalence of cerebral malaria (Nkhoma *et al.*, 1999).

Finally, in Malawi, nephrotic syndrome—which had hitherto been wrongly attributed to *P. malariae*—was linked to mercury poisoning associated with the use of skin-lightening products (Brown *et al.*, 1977).

The entomological information available is very scanty, being limited to references to *An. gambiae s.l.* and *An. funestus* in Malawi (Lehmann *et al.* 2003; Michel *et al.*, 2005).

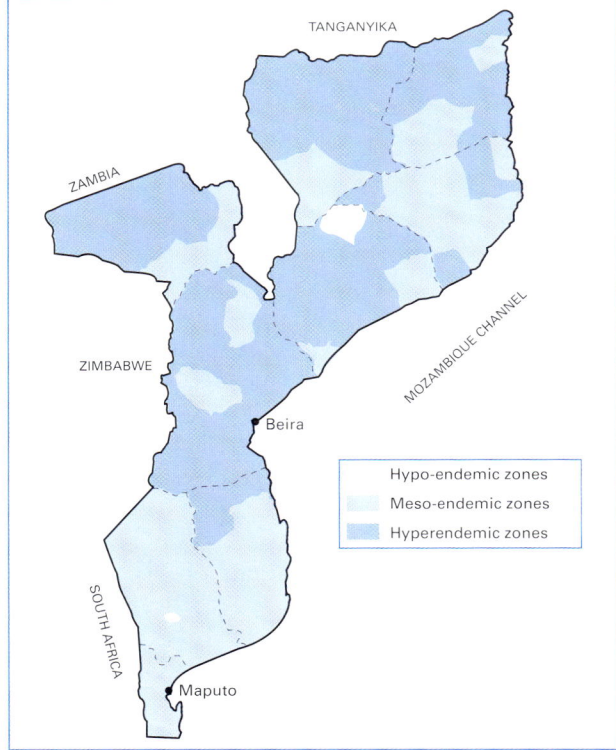

Figure 44. Epidemiological map of malaria in Mozambique (adapted from Soeiro & Morais, 1956).

Mozambique

Mozambique (*Table I*) extends for 1,650 km from north to south along the coast of the Indian Ocean, between the 10th and 26.5th parallel south. Its width ranges from 500 km near Lake Nyasa (= Lake Malawi) to 50 km near the mouth of the Zambeze. The coastal plain has an altitude of under 200 m and occupies 44% of the country; it hills between 200-600 m high occupy 17%. The interior plateau between 600-1,000 m high covers 26%, and the mountains between 1,000-1,500 m high cover 13% (Soeiro, 1956). The country has 2,700 km of shoreline. A network of tributary rivers into the Indian Ocean irrigates the country and includes the Zambeze, Rovuma, Lurio, Save, and Limpopo Rivers. The country's northern region reaches to the eastern shore of Lake Nyasa.

The tropical climate is marked by a reduction in average temperatures from north to south and with altitude. The highest levels of precipitation are recorded in the centre with more than 1,300 mm of rainfall during the southern summer season. July to October is dry, cool, and foggy. The vegetation is mainly wooded savannah, interspersed with forest galleries, that in higher altitudes, becomes steppe-like in appearance.

• *Epidemiology*

A global view of malaria in Mozambique was outlined by Soeiro (1956) as well as by Soeiro & Morais (1959b) (*Figure 44*). This emphasised the regions of Niassa in the north and Maputo in the south. Onori (1982) reviewed all of the available data and drew up a series of maps and a table (*Table XXXI*), district by district. Based on the PR of children between the ages of 2-9, he concluded that **all districts were hyperendemic** with the exception of Manica, which was meso-endemic, and Maputo, which was hypo-endemic. In Maputo, the malaria control programme had considerably reduced the prevalence which was of the order of 6% in 1956. Urbanisation had also contributed to the lowering of malaria indicators (Soeiro, 1956). The mountains, which do not exceed 1,400 m in altitude, did not have a determining influence on the distribution of malaria.

Over the last thirty years, the information on Mozambique has been limited to the regions of Maputo and Limpopo, where development projects were based. Urbanisation made a very strong epidemiological impact in Maputo. The malaria prevalence had nevertheless increased compared with 1956, up to 12%, with a maximum of 42% in the neighbourhoods bordering the larval habitats of *An. arabiensis*, the only vector (Thompson *et al.*, 1997; Thompson & Hogh, 1994). The average incidence was 200‰, with 506‰ in new born babies, 410‰ in children between the ages of 1-5, and 54‰ in adults (Martinenko *et al.*, 1994). Presumptive diagnosis is highly inaccurate in all the countries of Africa; of 432 patients with fever, only 43% were carrying *Plasmodium*, and 38% of clinically negative subjects were infected (Fernandès *et al.*, 1994) (*Table XXXI*).

Table XXXI. Prevalence of malaria in Mozambique by age group (1975-1976 and 1981) (Onori, Rapport WHO, 1982).

Province	0-23 months			2-4 years			5-9 years			10-14 years			> 15 years			Total		
	n	n (+)	% (+)	n	n (+)	% (+)	n	n (+)	% (+)	n	n (+)	% (+)	n	n (+)	% (+)	n	n (+)	% (+)
Maputo (city)	3,926	200	6.1	5,474	284	5.2	5,783	414	7.2	2,938	238	13.5	13,642	933	6.8	31,133	2,238	7
Maputo	5,237	817	15.3	7,228	1,152	15.9	11,993	2,161	18.0	7,924	1,510	19.1	22,109	3,703	16.7	54,581	9,343	17
Gaza	608	248	40.8	659	357	54.2	1,461	697	47.7	1,331	607	45.6	1,580	545	34.5	5,639	2,454	43
Inhambane	576	272	47.2	718	463	64.5	2,723	1,647	60.5	2,690	1,359	50.5	2,960	1,085	36.7	9,667	4,826	49
Sofala	1,507	1,130	75.0	1,195	951	79.6	3,999	3,167	79.2	4,254	3,213	75.5	9,936	5,669	57.1	20,881	14,130	67
Manica	737	312	42.3	1,152	518	45.0	2,616	1,316	50.3	2,552	1,121	43.9	647	287	44.4	7,704	3,554	46
Tete	1,631	1,136	69.7	2,226	1,598	71.8	4,781	3,418	71.5	4,683	3,027	64.6	7,977	4,702	58.9	21,298	13,881	65
Zambezia	2,676	1,828	68.3	1,571	1,167	74.3	5,283	3,560	67.4	8,770	5,431	61.9	13,034	6,828	52.4	31,334	18,814	60
Nampula	3,674	2,330	63.4	2,583	1,631	63.1	8,000	5,019	62.7	8,593	4,854	56.5	31,570	13,456	42.6	54,220	27,290	50
Niassa	2,204	1,519	68.9	2,237	1,616	72.2	5,632	4,032	71.6	3,760	2,444	65.0	9,651	4,614	47.8	23,484	14,225	60
Cabo Delgado	1,699	1,092	64.3	1,118	722	64.6	3,518	2,361	67.1	6,099	3,758	61.6	13,597	6,450	47.4	26,031	14,383	55

n: number of slides examined; n(+): number of positive slides

In the rural areas around Maputo, the prevalence of *P. falciparum* was 15% according to microscopic diagnosis and 36% according to PCR results (Fogg *et al.*, 2000). People with heavy parasite loads were usually carrying more than one clone.

In the city, 20-30‰ of expatriates living among the local population were infected (Martinenko *et al.*, 1994).

Outside of the capital city, information on the malaria situation was rare because of security problems, e.g. we still do not have the results on the impact of the floods of 1999.

In 1997 in Maputo, the mortality rate of mothers reached 3.2‰ and 15% of these deaths would have been caused by malaria. Among the women who died, 19.7% were infected with *P. falciparum*. More than 35% of these deaths—many of which were associated with severe anaemia (Granja *et al.*, 1998)—occurred in teenagers pregnant for the first time.

• *Entomology*

Four members of the Gambiae Complex have been observed in Mozambique: *An. gambiae s.s.*, especially to the north of the Save from the coast to the plateau; *An. arabiensis*, the most abundant vector in the south, present throughout the entire country and often living together with the preceding species; *An. merus*, although halophilic, was not limited to the coastline and was found in several localities inland up to 50 km from the coast; *An. quadriannulatus*, zoophilic and not a vector (Paterson *et al.*, 1964; Petrarca *et al.*, 1984).

An. funestus was present throughout the entire country but its numbers fell after indoor spraying programmes based on DDT and, in a few localities, pyrethroids. Having become resistant to pyrethroids, this species is now a very efficient vector which has also spread to South Africa (Hargreaves *et al.*, 2000) and was involved in the outbreak of malaria following the change from DDT to pyrethroids due to pressure from ecologists.

An. nili has only been reported in the district of Niassa in the north.

An. pharoensis is an inconspicuous vector and since it was divided into two species, we do not know which form is currently present in Mozambique.

Zimbabwe

Zimbabwe, formerly Southern Rhodesia, is made up of a central plateau between 1,200-1,600 m in altitude that gradually drops down, in the north, all the way to the Zambeze Valley (alt. 400-600 m), and in the south, all the way to the Save and Limpopo Valleys, which are tributaries of the Indian Ocean. Geographers have stratified the country into lowlands, or lowveld, at an altitude of 400-600 m with a tropical climate, regions of middle ground, or middleveld, at an altitude of 600-1,200 m, and highlands, or highveld, above 1,200 m in altitude where the winter season is marked by frequent freezing temperatures (Taylor & Mutambu, 1986) and where the altitude affects the temperatures (*Figure 45*).

There are three seasons during the year. The winter season from April to August is dry and cold, August to October is dry and hot, and November to March is hot and humid. Rainfall never exceeds 400 mm in the south-west, near the Kalahari, but reaches 1,200 mm in the north-east on the border with Mozambique.

The gold mines, many of which have closed down, have brought much wealth to the mining companies but today, cattle rearing is the country's principal resource.

• *Epidemiology*

Ever since the first studies carried out by Leeson (1931) and Ross (1932), malaria control has been a priority of the Health Services, at least until recently.

The first research by Ross (1932) demonstrated an absence of malaria in the highlands. Leeson (1931) thought that *An. gambiae s.l.* only reproduced year round at an altitude below 600 m; starting from permanent larval habitats in the lowveld, it would gradually invade the plateaux and make it up to 1,100 m by mid-January. Until 1970, this concept was used as a basis for the malaria control programme and resulted in the development of the "barrier strategy" beginning in 1953-54 (Alves, 1958; Alves & Blair, 1955). De Meillon (1934), however, did not agree with the idea of annual migrations and land reoccupation.

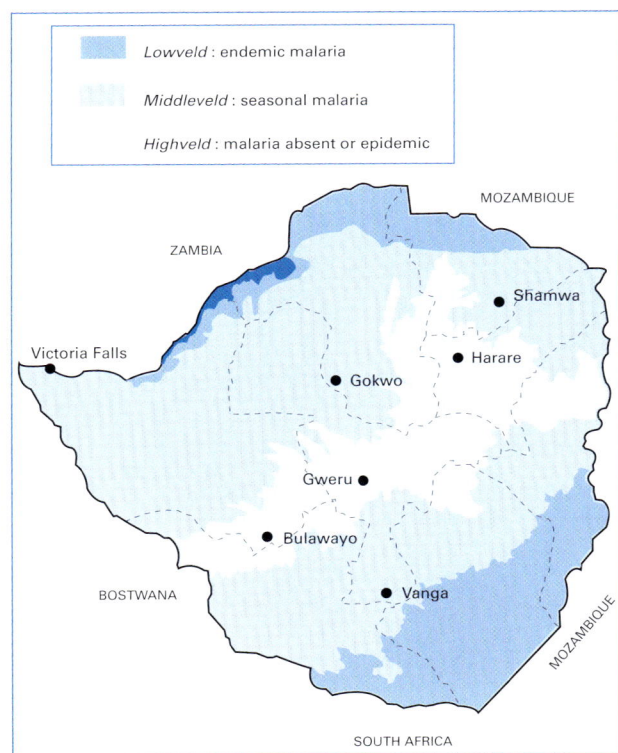

Figure 45. Relief-based stratification of malaria in Zimbabwe (adapted from Taylor & Mutambu, 1986).

Biodiversity of Malaria in the World

This opinion was reinforced by Muirhead-Thomson (1960) who found *An. gambiae* larvae present above 1,000 m in altitude during the winter and on the plateaux.

Malaria control began in 1949 with trial runs of indoor spraying using hexachlorocyclohexane (HCH) in the Mazoe Valley in the north-east. These brought excellent results but the resistance of house flies undermined the population's confidence. In 1953, the barrier strategy was to spray places at around 1,000 m in altitude to prevent invasion of the higher ground. Spraying with HCH took place every three months from October to April. This strategically debatable programme considerably reduced the number of cases and the PR was close to zero in the high altitude areas where the majority of the population resided. *An. funestus* disappeared and *An. gambiae* became exophilic. This phenomenon was later explained by the discovery of *An. quadriannulatus*, which was both exophilic and zoophilic (Paterson et al., 1963), after *An. arabiensis* and *An. gambiae s.s.* had disappeared following house spraying.

Although transmission persisted at a low level, the first malaria control operations were successful (*Table XXXII*). From 1942-1962, the number of patients hospitalised for malaria every year had dropped from 1,250 to 96. The global prevalence of malaria in the native population dropped from 10.6% to 0.3%.

Before the spraying programme, the prevalence was linked to altitude: 30% on the shores of the Zambeze, 1.2% on the plateaux, and 7.2% in the lowlands of the south. In more recent studies (Taylor & Mutambu, 1986), the prevalence below 600 m was found to be only 8.2% in new born babies, and 29% in children between 5-9 years, which then dropped to under 10%. This was far from the 88% recorded in Buba by Alves (1958). Over the last five years, major upheavals have occurred in malaria control centers as they have been integrated into the primary health care services; indoor spraying operations seems to be subject to more and more logistical and budgetary constraints.

Frequencies of the parasites were 97% *P. falciparum*, 2% *P. malariae*, and 0.6% *P. ovale* (Taylor, 1985). Since the disappearance of *An. funestus*, *An. arabiensis* has become the main vector, sympatric with *An. gambiae s.s.*, which is much less common. Malaria is, therefore, linked to fluctuations in rainfall. In the district of Shamva, Mpofu (1985) made a connection between the numbers of anopheline bites and the incidence of cases throughout the year (*Figure 46*).

Along the Zambeze, transmission is perennial between 400-600 m in altitude and seasonal higher up. In the south, given the latitude, the zone between 600-900 m is homologous with the zone between 900-1,200 m in the north. At the same altitudes, the prevalence is lower in the south than in the north.

In the highveld, in Gowké and Umtali, a high level of transmission was reported in April 1972 during the cotton harvest. This was probably due to the importation of gametocytes by seasonal labourers although transmission was subsequently local (Harwin & Goldsmith, 1972).

In the south, near Bulawayo, Wolfe (1964) had observed small family epidemics during which several persons were infected under the same roof, which suggested transmission as a result of interrupted blood meals.

From 1969-1981, the prevalence was under 2% on the highveld, up to 10% in the lowlands of the south, and 30%

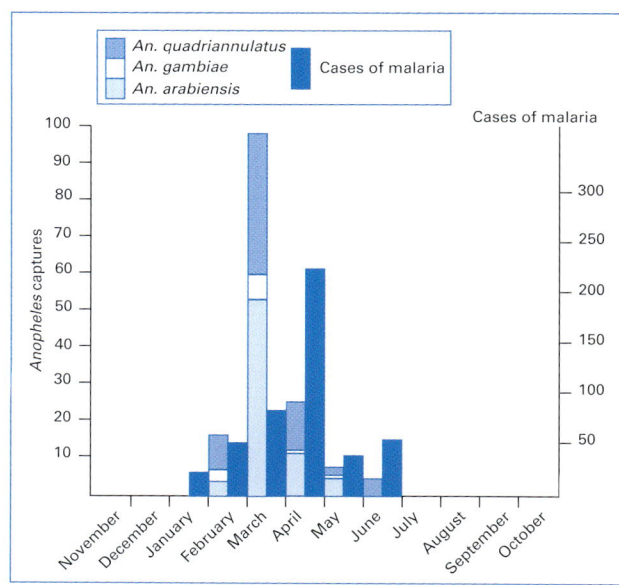

Figure 46. Malaria reports in rural centres around Shamva with human-baited trapping of *An. gambiae s.l.* at Chitengu (adapted from Mpofu, 1985).

Table XXXII. Decline in the number of cases of malaria in Zimbabwe between 1942 and 1962 following control operations (Health Centre statistics) (adapted from Taylor & Mutambu, 1986).

Year	N° of admissions for malaria	Total admissions	Percentage of admissions for malaria
1942	1,256	11,771	10.6%
1952	916	18,321	5.0%
1962	96	29,099	0.3%

in the Zambeze Valley; the incidence was 1-2‰ in the highlands, above 500‰ in the lowlands of the south, and 300‰ in the lowlands of the north (Taylor, 1985) (*Figure 47*).

In 1995 in the south (Vanga, in the Mberengua Region), an epidemic broke out in a community of 30,000 inhabitants who had not witnessed any cases in thirty years. Apart from children and the elderly, the victims were of both sexes between the ages of 15 and 30. It is likely that infection occurred outside of the homes in poachers fishing illegally in a dam reservoir. The parasites could have been introduced by poachers in Gowke, the only place where the parasite was resistant to chloroquine (Mouchet, personal observation), as in Vanga. Even in regions where transmission was relatively high, as in the Zambeze Valley, malaria was, and still is, very unstable, and local people have little, if any, immunity. This unstable nature was masked by the malaria control programme but the lack of protection was evident with local epidemics occurred practically every year (Mouchet *et al.*, 1998).

As shown by serological studies, malaria infection was infrequent above 900 m in altitude, but the inhabitants of the plateaux were not completely protected from epidemic outbreaks (Siziya *et al.*, 1997).

An attempt to predict epidemic outbreaks, or at least periods of increased risk, was made by Freeman & Bradley (1996). Above average temperatures in September, i.e. spring, were predictive of a heightened incidence. The rainy season had no effect except when it occurred following a drought. But in September, it seemed already too late to take appropriate measures against epidemics arising between January and March.

The resources to improve diagnosis on the ground are simply not available. Only 28% of slides prepared from the blood of patients believed to have malaria, according to clinical criteria, give positive results. Taking "disease history" into account has been proposed to improve diagnosis (Bassett *et al.*, 1991).

• *Entomology*

The discovery of the *An. gambiae* Complex was of major importance in explaining transmission in Zimbabwe. A change in behaviour was put forward to explain the exophilic nature of *An. gambiae*, but in fact *An. gambiae*, which had been eliminated by insecticides, had been replaced by *An. quadriannulatus*, which was both zoophilic and exophilic (Paterson, 1964b). In 1985, the proportion of the different species of the complex was established as follows: *An. gambiae s.s.*: 2.5%, *An. arabiensis*: 14.8%, and *An. quadriannulatus*: 83% (Mpofu, 1985); foci of *An. merus* should also be added. All the species of the *An. gambiae* Complex were shown to be at their peak at the beginning of the rainy season which, two months later, led to outbreaks of disease. Human landing collections showed 99.4% *An. arabiensis* and 0.6% *An. quadriannulatus*, whereas larval captures indicated just 5% of the former species as compared with 95% of the latter. Transmission occurred all year round along waterways, but decreased with distance therefrom (Crees, 1996).

Swaziland

The tiny kingdom of Swaziland is the smallest of the three countries enclosed within South Africa. Its phytogeography is divided into three levels (*Table I*):
- the bushveld or lowveld, between 150-500 m high, a thorny savannah zone which used to be highly unproductive, and which is now a rich region due to sugar cane cultivation (in the east);
- the middleveld between 600-1,000 m high;
- the highveld, the eastern ledge of the Drakensberg Mountains between 1,000-1,600 m high (to the west).

In the lowveld, 500-700 mm of rain falls between December-March. The highveld is wetter and gives rise to several rivers that are tributaries of the Indian Ocean, and used for irrigating sugar cane. The rivers' highly irregular rate of flow alternately provokes floods or the drying up of river beds which are both factors in the proliferation of the *An. gambiae* Complex. The subtropical climate is characterised by large variations in temperature and rainfall from one year to the next.

• *Epidemiology*

In 1949, the bushveld was considered to be a hyperendemic region (*see further on*, *Figure 49*) in which the PR of children between 1-10 years reached 78% during the period of transmission from November-March, and 55% during the dry season. In the middleveld, PRs were only 40% and 20% respectively. Malaria was considered to be unstable with frequent epidemics occurring in both the middleveld and the highveld. These epidemics would break out following periods of excessive rain or drought, during which large populations of *An. gambiae* would develop in the residual ponds, once the rivers stopped flowing. *An.*

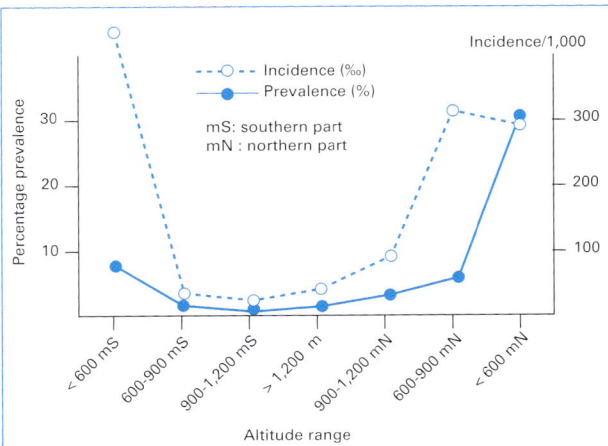

Figure 47. Incidence (per 1,000) and prevalence (per 100) according to altitude from 1969 to 1981 (adapted from Taylor, 1985).

funestus, the other vector, was abundant in the marshy regions at the end of the rains and at the beginning of the dry season (Mastbaum, 1954 and 1957).

In 1949, indoor spraying programmes were implemented using HCH at first, and then DDT. Immediately, malaria indicators began to drop. In 1969 and 1970, the number of cases of malaria dropped to 26 and 10 respectively, out of a protected population of 302,000 (Delfini, 1972).

In 1986 and 1987, due to negligence and a suspension of the programme, malaria made a spectacular comeback on an epidemic scale (Fontaine *et al*., 1987). Official statistics reported 3,000 cases but after consulting clinic records, multiplying these figures by ten was more realistic (Mouchet, 1987a). The situation went back to normal when spraying, financed by South Africa, was resumed (Hansford, personal communication, 1991).

In 1993, on the border with Mozambique, an epidemic was reported when a period of normal rainfall occurred after three years of drought (Coutinho, 1994). Migrant workers from Mozambique or South Africa in Swaziland's sugar cane plantations were considered to be responsible for the return of malaria in the country (Packard, 1986).

- *Entomology*

An. funestus disappeared from the country in 1950 and seemed to have reappeared in small numbers in 1991. It is currently resistant to pyrethroids but not to DDT, the product still being used in Swaziland.

An. gambiae s.s., as well as *An. arabiensis*, *An. merus,* and *An. quadriannulatus* have been reported throughout the entire country (Coetzee *et al*., 1993), the latter three species sharing the same larval habitats.

Botswana

Botswana, formerly Bechuanaland (*Table I*), is an enclosed plateau covering an area of 500,000 km² at an altitude of 1,000 m, which is traversed in the middle by the Ngamiland depression, where the Okavango River from Angola drains. The climate is sub-arid with a thorny steppe vegetation that makes up the Kalahari Desert. The level of rainfall decreases from north to south and from east to west and is extremely irregular from one year to the next.

The southern malaria boundary of Africa, around the 21st southern parallel, goes through Botswana around the level of Francistown. Although malaria is considered to be endemic, it is **very unstable** and takes on **epidemic** proportions when excess rainfall occurs following periods of drought (Chayabejara *et al*., 1975). At the hospital of Kasane in the north, there were 150 cases in February 1986, as opposed to 15 during the same period in 1987, and more than 500 in February 1988 with 70 deaths (Mouchet, personal observation, 1988).

Malaria was meso- or hypo-endemic but reached hyperendemic levels in certain villages of the Chobe (far north). In 1986, the annual number of declared cases was between 1,000-1,500, which was an obvious underestimation. The PR ranged from 33% in Francistown to 7.2% in Maun in the Ngamiland. More than 50% of the cases observed were in adults. Immune status presents a problem with 85% of parasite carriers being symptomless even though the prevalence remained low. These local observations seem to be contradictory.

During the winter, which is dry and cold, there is hardly, if any, transmission.

The vector is mainly *An. arabiensis*; *An. gambiae s.s.* (Ali, personal communication) has been rarely collected. *An. funestus* was considered to be frequent in the Ngamiland but absent in Francistown. The sporozoite rate was 0.5% in *An. gambiae s.l.* (out of 800 dissections), and zero in both *An. funestus* (80 dissections) and *An. pharoensis* (30 dissections) (Chayabejara *et al*., 1975) (the number of dissections is not sufficient to give a significant result).

On an anecdotal basis, it should be noted that in the villages of the Chobe in the far north, which are built on sand, *Ornithodoros moubata* ticks were present in all the huts and the number of cases of recurrent fever was very high (Mouchet, 1987b). The clinic personnel, who lacked proper diagnostic measures and were barely familiar with this rare pathology, classified these cases as being "resistant malaria" and treated them with the medication at hand, i.e. penicillin, which resulted in rapid healing.

Namibia

Namibia (*Figure 48*), a vast desert- or sub-desert-like plateau at an average altitude of 1,000-1,300 m high, has a population of under 2 million people. The majority of the population is Bantu, while the native population of Bushmen in the north-east (Bushmanland) amounts to less than 50,000. The cold Benguela Current, which hugs the coast, cuts off precipitation from the coastal zones. Inland, the amount of rainfall ranges from 600 mm in the north on the Angolan border and in the Caprivi Strip, to 400 mm at the 20th parallel south, to 200 mm at the 24th parallel. The only river is the Okavango, which starts in Angola, and crosses north-eastern Namibia before draining itself into the sands of Botswana. The Oranje River, a tributary of the Atlantic, marks the southern border with South Africa.

Malaria is only endemic north of the 20th parallel south in the provinces of Ovamboland, Okavango, Caprivi, and Bushmanland. Between the 20th and 23rd parallels, epidemics can break out when there is excessive rainfall (De Meillon, 1951; Kassatsky, 1994). Further south, the arid climate prevents any risk of malaria (*Figure 48*).

In Namibia, malaria is very unstable and irregularly distributed according to distances to bodies of water, rivers and lakes, and to how long they are filled. The PRs reported by De Meillon (1951) and Kuschke (1968) suggest meso- or hypo-endemic disease. Out of 14,000 slides examined by Kuschke, i.e. one third of the total population PRs were 27% in the Okavango, 32% in the western Caprivi, and 13% in the Bushmanland (where there were two cases of *P. vivax*). The age group most affected was children between the ages of 4-9. In the Ovamboland in the north-

Afrotropical Region

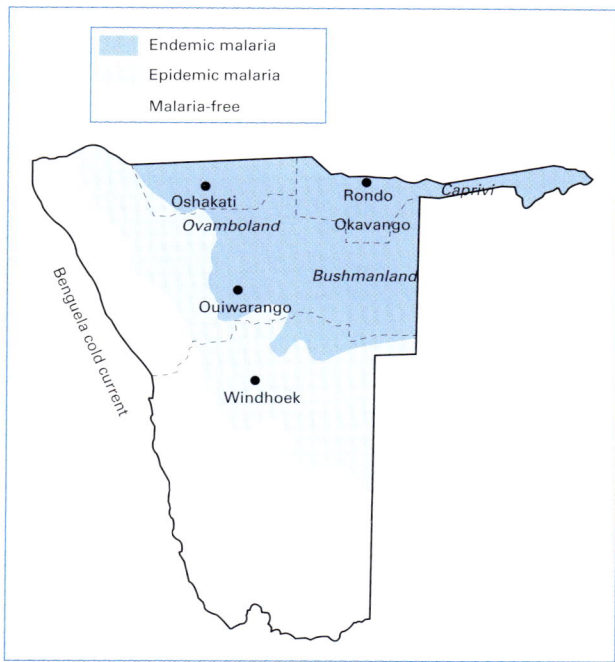

Figure 48. Malaria in Namibia (adapted from Kassatsky, 1994).

west, the PR was only 12%. All age groups were at risk due to the population's weak immunity (Kassatsky, Report OMS/AFRO, 1994). Sixty percent of Namibia's population resides in the northern provinces and are thus at-risk of contracting malaria.

The two vectors were *An. gambiae s.l.*, dependent on the rain, and *An. funestus* in the marshy regions at the end of the rainy season (Kushke, 1968). It seems that this latter species practically disappeared following indoor spraying with dieldrin. On the border with Angola, the species of the *An. gambiae* Complex identified were 4.7% *An. gambiae s.s.*, and 95% *An. arabiensis* while on the Angolan part, it was 36% *An. gambiae s.s.* and 64% *An. arabiensis* (Kassatsky, 1994), figures that are questionable.

South Africa

Out of the 1.2 million km² that cover South Africa (*Table I*), only the two provinces of Kwazulu Natal and Mpulamanga (former Transvaal) in the north and northeastern parts of the country are exposed to a malaria risk.

• *History of malaria and the malaria control programme*

The Boers, who avoided the areas at-risk, first mentioned the "fevers" at the end of the 18th century in Transvaal and in Natal. They even identified a marker for these zones, the fever tree (*Acacia xantolacca*), which indeed grows in the humid areas of the lowveld.

In 1905, malaria was reported in Natal (Hill & Haydon, 1905). From 1927-1947, annual reports on malaria in the different parts of the Union were compiled by the Health Department of the Union of South Africa (which later became the Republic of South Africa). In 1928, the Transvaal suffered the worst epidemic since the turn of the century. The middleveld was affected, as was the lowveld; several cases were reported in Pretoria, but Johannesburg did not appear to be affected. In 1929, the epidemic resumed and ended in May after having caused 2,000 deaths. From 1932-1934, epidemics paralysed the economy, especially in the sugar cane plantations of Kwazulu-Natal where absenteeism was at 85%. An investigation carried out by Swellengrebel *et al.* (1931) reported that infection took place at home. In order to interrupt contact between man and vector, these authors suggested carrying out weekly indoor spraying operations with pyrethrin. In addition to these measures, a anti-larval programme was implemented using Paris Green or oil waste, and quinine was made available (for both prophylaxis and treatment). These measures proved effective in the plantations but both the cost and complexity of this programme limited their use. In the endemic regions on the slopes of the Drakensberg Mountains, indoor spraying with pyrethrin gave highly significant results in zones where the vector was *An. funestus*. Beyond the two aforementioned provinces, the Health Department of the Republic of South Africa reported other epidemics along the Orange River, on the border of Namibia in the Cape Province, and along the Molopo River on the border with Botswana in the Orange Province. The scale of these epidemics was not specified.

In 1945, the first trials of indoor spraying using DDT proved to be conclusive, as with those using HCH. In a very short time, the level of malaria was reduced to just a few cases.

The reports of the Malaria Control Programme, whose statistics are among the most reliable for Africa, illustrate a rise in malaria during the last thirty years. The minimum number of cases (230) was recorded in 1971 and 1973, while in 1993, the number had risen to 11,600 cases. The number of deaths due to malaria ranged from 40-48 from 1988-1993. Sony & Sharp (1997) estimated the average annual number of cases to be 644 from 1976-1983, 3,846 cases from 1988-1992, and 30,000 cases in 1996. This recent increase in case numbers has been acknowledged by all malaria specialists. In Kwazulu-Natal, after indoor spraying was stopped, small epidemics occurred in certain regions where the disease had been previously wiped out (Nethercott, 1974). Hansford (1974), after having observed a rise of malaria in the Limpopo Valley, requested that indoor spraying be resumed in the region of Venda. Kustner (1979) reported increased exposure in a population of 100,000 with 16 cases in 1970 rising to 746 cases in 1978, but the causes were poorly defined.

In a review of the malaria situation from 1987-1999, Govere *et al.* (2001) insisted on a serious increase in the number of cases since 1993. In these non-immune

Biodiversity of Malaria in the World

populations, the pattern conforms to the age pyramid. Mortality was 0.5% of cases notified per annum.

In Kruger Park, which was used as an observatory, 4.5 attacks out of 10,000 visitors in April were reported (Durrheim *et al.*, 1998).

Changing the treatment strategy and replacing DDT with deltamethrin in response to pressure from environmentalists may partly explain the increase of malaria in the northern part of Kwazulu-Natal, which was re-infested from Mozambique by pyrethroid-resistant *An. funestus* (Hargreaves *et al.*, 2000). DDT was reintroduced and combined with large scale use of ACT drugs the deadly outbreak was controlled

Several epidemiologists are pessimistic about malaria control operations being transferred from a specialised service to the districts.

• *Epidemiology*

Orographic and climatic factors determine the areas of malaria transmission (*Figure 49*). The high altitude and harsh winters of the Transvaal Plateau and the Drakensberg Mountains prevent vector development almost entirely. In the lower areas of Mpulamanga and Kwazulu-Natal, the latitude determines the southern boundary of malaria. Even during the epidemics of 1928 and 1930, the disease never went beyond Durban. Therefore, three zones of transmission were identified:
- the endemic larval habitats of the foothills of the Drakensberg Mountains in the Transvaal where the vector was *An. funestus*, which occurs in streams running off the mountains;
- the plains of the lowveld and of Kwazulu-Natal where the vector was *An. gambiae s.l.*, highly dependent on the rains and, therefore, seasonal, and subject to great variations from year to year depending on the amount of rain;
- the epidemic zones where *An. gambiae s.l.* could infest the middleveld in years of excessive rainfall (De Meillon, 1934; Hooey, 1974; Olivier & Grobler, 1992; Swellengrebel *et al.*, 1931).

This epidemiological landscape profoundly changed following indoor DDT spraying and/or other long-lasting insecticides. Since 1971, when the lowest levels were recorded, the number of cases increased between 1985-1989, and again in 1993 (*Figure 50*).

The epidemic larval habitats of the foothills disappeared when *An. funestus* was wiped out, and epidemics no longer occured, apart from a few cases, even though *An. arabiensis* was still largely present. One should remember that malaria has never been eradicated in South Africa.

In the extreme northern part of the country all along the Limpopo River, a persistent level of transmission required indoor spraying to be resumed (Hansford, 1974). The absence of vectors in homes led Smith *et al.* (1977) to suspect *An. aruni* (of the Funestus Group) and a similar species of *An. flavicosta* to be responsible for outdoor transmission but this has not been proven.

Since 1999 in Kwazulu-Natal, we have witnessed the arrival of a strain of *An. funestus* that is resistant to pyrethroids (Hargreaves *et al.*, 2000).

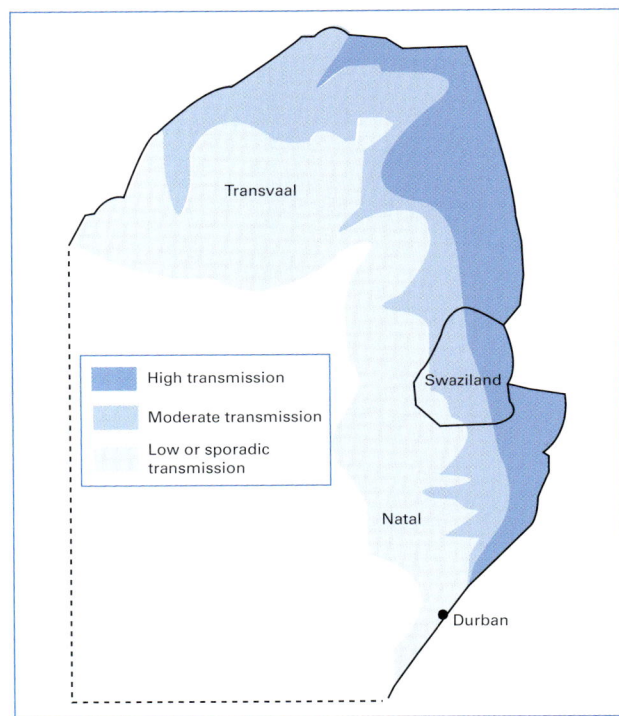

Figure 49. *Malaria in the South African Union and Swaziland in 1928 (adapted from LeSueur et al., 1993).*

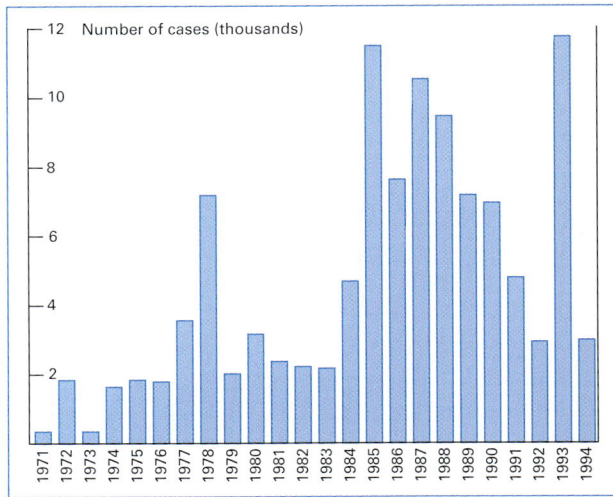

Figure 50. *Incidence of malaria in South Africa (1971-1994) (adapted from LeSueur et al., 1993).*

Despite the pessimism of malaria experts, the malaria death toll remains very low with a mortality rate of 0.5-0.7% in clinically diagnosed subjects (Durrheim *et al.*, 1999).

The publications of Snow *et al.* (1995a) regarding the theory of a potential increase of severe exposure to malaria following a moderate decrease in transmission were contested by South African authors (Moorthy & Wilkinson, 1997; Sony & Sharp, 1997).

In the multi-ethnic country of South Africa, Swellengrebel *et al.* (1931) had drawn attention to the susceptibility of the different ethnic groups to *P. falciparum*. The Indians had three times more malaria attacks than the Bantus, who lived under the same conditions. This lower susceptibility in the Bantus was attributed to their immunity. The same phenomenon was observed in the Comoros (Gevrey, 1870).

- *Entomology*

The principle malaria vectors in South Africa belong to the Gambiae Complex and the Funestus Group. Eight species belong to the Funestus Group and are distributed in three different subgroups. Four species of the Funestus Subgroup are represented by *An. funestus*, *An. confusus*, *An. vaneedeni* and *An. aruni* (Gillies & Coetzee, 1987), three species of the Rivulorum Subgroup include *An. brucei*, *An. fuscivenosus* and *An. rivulorum*; as well as *An. leesoni* which belongs to the Minimus Subgroup (Garros *et al.*, 2005; Harbach, 2004). *An. funestus* is the only species of the group whose vector role in South Africa has been proven, with a sporozoite rate of 4-5% in the Drakensberg Mountains (De Meillon, 1934). It was eliminated from South Africa in 1951 with indoor spraying. In 1999, the populations that reappeared in Kwazulu-Natal (Hargreaves *et al.*, 2000) presented with an ecology that was analogous to that of all the populations of the African savannah, growing in marshland with abundant standing vegetation at the end of the rainy season. Their way of life was, therefore, different from that of the *An. funestus* native to the foothills of the Drakensberg Mountains that had lived in calm streams that were constantly being renewed. The genetic variability of *An. funestus* must be mentioned. *An. aruni*, which can bite humans, was suspected to be involved in exophilic transmission on the Limpopo River. *An. rivulorum* was found infected in Tanzania but not in South Africa (Wilkes *et al.*, 1996).

The *An. gambiae* Complex is represented by four species (Coetzee *et al.*, 1993). *An. gambiae s.s.*, the most efficient vector of the complex, is rare in South Africa. According to Hansford (1974), as it is very endophilic, it may have been victim to the first operations of indoor spraying. This hypothesis has already been put forward in Mauritius. Currently, *An. arabiensis* is the most important vector in the country. *An. merus*, a halophilic species, is not limited to the seaside and is found in numerous places inland (Paterson *et al.*, 1964) and often in great numbers; its role is poorly defined. *An. quadriannulatus* is both zoophilic and exophilic (Paterson, 1964b), and it can be infected in laboratory conditions (Takken *et al.*, 1999) although its role in nature is more than doubtful.

An. marshalli is a complex of three species, of which only the A form bites humans, and has been suspected of being a vector.

South-western islands of the Indian Ocean

Geographical and historical outline

The south-western islands of the Indian Ocean have three origins:
- **continental**: **Madagascar** is a part of the Gondwana Continent that separated from Africa during the Mesozoic Era between 65-100 million years ago. It evolved apart with more than 90% of the species of flora and fauna being endemic;
- **volcanic**: the **Mascarene Islands** and the **Comoros** emerged during the tertiary and quaternary periods. The coral reefs and their lagoons surrounding the oldest islands that have sunk into the sea, trace the ancient perimeters of Mayotte, the Comoros, and Rodriguez in the Mascarene Islands. The youngest islands are the scene of volcanic activity (Khartala in Grande Comore and Fournaise in La Réunion). There have been some important recent introductions into the flora and fauna on these islands, originating from Africa and Madagascar;
- **outcrops of the continental plateau and coral reefs**: the Seychelles are of particular interest as there are no autochthonous vectors.

The human population of these islands is of heterogeneous origin with Africans, Asians, and Europeans origin introduced gradually over the last two thousand years (*Figure 51*). The political status of the islands varies enormously: Madagascar has been an independent republic since 1960, Mauritius and the Seychelles since 1965; the Federal Islamic Republic of the Comoros was established in 1975 and includes three islands: Grande Comore, Moheli, and Anjouan; the latter is more or less in the process of seceding. When independence took place, Mayotte chose to remain as a French Territorial Community, while La Réunion is a French overseas department.

According to local legend, malaria appears to have existed in Madagascar ever since it was first populated. In the Comoros, the unhealthy conditions of Mayotte and Moheli contrasted with the relative healthiness of the northern moorings of Anjouan and the absence of fevers in Grande Comore up until 1920. Mauritius and Réunion were not affected by the fevers until 1865 and 1867 respectively. Rodriguez is still malaria-free, and the Seychelles are outside the malaria zone.

Biodiversity of Malaria in the World

Madagascar

• *Geography*

The island of Madagascar is located between latitudes 12°-27° south and longitudes 43°-50° east, and spans a distance of 1,580 km from north to south and 550 km from east to west. It is positioned on a 587,000 km² pre-Cambrian block covered with 10-80 m of laterite, thus its nickname "the red island". It has an average altitude of 800-2,400 m. On the East Coast, the plateau drops down abruptly to the Indian Ocean while on the West Coast, it falls gradually to the Mozambique Channel through a series of gradations. Volcanic activity during the Tertiary Period resulted in basaltic mountains being created at the same time as collapsed basins (Lake Itasy, Lake Alaotra, Antananarivo Basin, etc.) that are poorly drained and that are rice-growing regions. Permian and Cretaceous sediments cover the southern part of the island (Isalo) (*Figure 52*).

As mentioned above, Madagascar is a part of Africa that separated from the continent at the level of Tanzania, heading east and then south. According to geophysicists, it would seem that initially there was not a complete separation and that the island remained connected with the continent, but these connections would have to have existed a very long time ago, given the level of endemicity.

A number of bio-geographical areas have been identified (Preston-Mafbam, 1982):
- the eastern area, which receives a lot of rainfall all year round (1,500-3,000 mm), and which runs along the entire eastern coastline;
- the western area (north of Morombe), that has a well-marked dry season and where the rainfall decreases from 1,500 to 600 mm from north to south;
- the central Plateaux, sometimes divided into the western and eastern zones, that have a cool winter climate at an altitude of 800-2,600 m;
- the subtropical area of the south where the rainfall ranges between 250-600 mm and with great variations from year to year.

• *History*

That Madagascar was populated by Bushmen from Africa, inspired by various legends of the small Vazimbé people, remains no more than a myth. The first Indonesian migration from the island of Nias near Sumatra dates back to the beginning of the Christian Era and maybe a little before. The Bantus, who had arrived on the African coast around the 2nd or 3rd century, mixed with the Indonesians and up until the 8th century, would have been the only ones to have populated Madagascar. Thereafter, new Indonesian migrations occurred, beginning in the 8th century.

According to certain Malagasy historians (Montagne, 1989), a large part of this latter group, and in particular the Merina, would have migrated onto the Plateaux to get away from malaria. In the absence of written records, the history of this entire period remains unclear. The Arabs from Oman, who invaded the country at the beginning of the 7th century, were barely able to get beyond the coastline.

This historical introduction interests us to the extent that it is linked to the current distribution of the disease. Indeed, the development of rice-growing on the plateaux is itself an example of the spread of disease due to human activity.

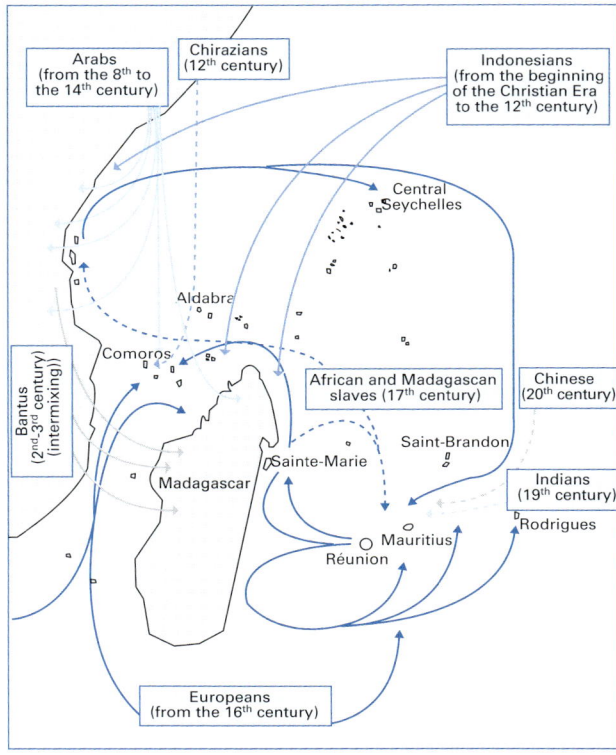

Figure 51. Origins of the populations of the islands of the south-western Indian Ocean (adapted from Julvez et al., 1995).

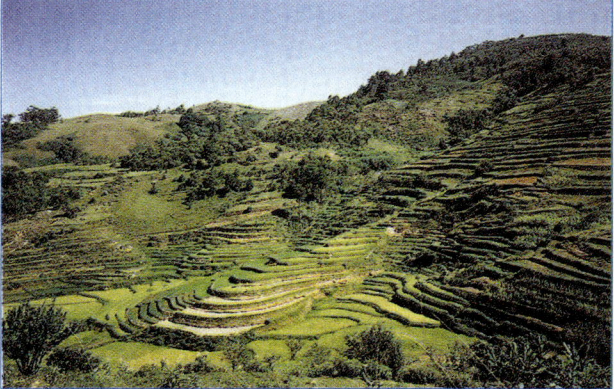

Figure 52. Andina, a district of Ambositra: the lower terraces are used for growing rice and the higher ones for vegetables (photograph by Laventure in Mouchet et al., 1996).

Although the population of Madagascar has diverse origins, they speak the same language with several distinct dialects. Out of a population of 18.6 million people (density of 25 inhabitants per km^2), 80% live in a rural environment. The big cities are Antananarivo (over 1 million people), Mahajanga, Fianarantsoa, and Tamatave.

Less than a century ago, forests covered large parts of the island. They have since seriously diminished in size due to farming and the manufacturing of charcoal, the only available fuel. The highly endemic and exceptional fauna (lemurs, chameleons) is currently endangered due to the destruction of the natural biotopes (Chown, 1990). The arguments of nature conservationists do not weigh heavily on a population that lives below the poverty line.

• *History of epidemics and the malaria control programme*

When Diego Diaz landed in Madagascar in 1500, his crew was decimated by the fevers. All the travellers to the island that followed, up until the middle of the 20th century, have described the unhealthy nature of the Malagasy coastline. In contrast, the same chroniclers boasted of the healthiness of the highlands, and how its inhabitants became rapidly ill if they went down to the coastline (Julvez, 1993).

The first epidemic on the Plateaux broke out in 1878. It coincided with the arrival of labourers from the coast who came to build religious buildings and, in particular, the temple and seminary of the London Mission. The epidemic reached its peak in May, and then came to a stop in winter. The following year, malaria returned again with its peak occurring at the end of the rainy season. The arrival of coastal labourers along with excavation works, allowing *An. gambiae s.l.* larval habitats to multiply, were long considered to be the factors that triggered the epidemic. But closer examination showed that the majority of the cases occurred in May-June following the proliferation of *An. funestus* in the rice paddies six weeks before. During the 19th century, rice-growing had undergone a remarkable growth which, as for any large scale work, required bringing in coastal labourers who were likely to introduce the parasite. In view of how the epidemic progressed, it is obvious that rice-growing was implicated in the epidemic of 1878 (Laventure *et al.*, 1996).

A second epidemic in 1895, which was probably just a continuation or a reactivation of the first one, decimated both the French battle corps and the opposing Hovas troops. The epidemic had the same seasonal characteristics as the first one. In the years that followed, malaria was endemic on a seasonal basis, declining in the winter. All the highlands under 1,500 m in altitude were infected (Blanchy *et al.*, 1993; Laventure *et al.*, 1996). Larval control measures and the seeding of water deposits with *Gambusia* had not even a psychological effect, and most of the quinine distributed went to Europeans and the privileged classes.

In 1949, malaria control operations, which were to develop into a malaria eradication programme, were implemented. The programme involved indoor DDT spraying (or dieldrin) in addition to weekly prophylactic chloroquine treatment for children. In the stable malaria zones of the eastern and western coastlines, the incidence of malaria did indeed decrease but persisted at a significant level. On the Plateaux, one of the principle vectors, *An. funestus*, disappeared and the malaria indicators dropped from 40-50% in 1949 to less than 2% in 1956. In 1961, the rare cases of malaria were confined to just a few sites at-risk in Ankazobé, Lake Itasy, and Anjozolobé (Bernard, 1954; Joncour, 1956; Lumaret, 1962). In 1962, following the disappearance of *An. funestus*, the WHO encouraged local authorities to shift the control programme attack phase to a surveillance phase on the Plateaux (Imerina and Betsileo Provinces). The three sites cited previously to be at-risk were given special attention and continued to benefit from indoor spraying with DDT as indicated by epidemiological surveys.

Progressively, surveillance measures were dropped in the sites at-risk, and the regular distribution of prophylactic treatment no longer took place. At the same time, an unprecedented economic crisis prevented the population from having access to medication. It was in this context that the epidemic of 1985 came to the attention of authorities and the public at-large (Lepers *et al.*, 1990a and 1990b; Lepers *et al.*, 1991; Mouchet & Baudon, 1986). From the outset, mortality was very high due to the population's lack of immunity, difficult access to treatment, and economic poverty. Different ecological phenomena were alluded to such as the repeated cyclones during the two previous years, and even global warming. The most plausible explanation is the gradual increase of incidence since 1980. As the last malaria control measures died down, the disease regained the territory it had lost during the programme since 1950 (Mouchet *et al.*, 1997). This increase of malaria from 1971 to 1995 was recorded by the Analoara Catholic Clinic, one of the only organisations which perform microscopic diagnosis (*Figures 53 and 54*). Their records clearly illustrate the reestablishment of the human parasite reservoir (*Tables XXXIII and XXXIV*) between 1971 and 1981, and then the epidemic explosion of 1985 to 1988. In 1988, chloroquine was taken off the list of prescription drugs and was henceforth available throughout the country at low cost. The epidemic continued but the population was now able to get medication without having to go to the medical clinics that had previously been incapable of providing treatment. In 1993, indoor DDT spraying was resumed on the Plateaux; in one year, the incidence of malaria decreased by 80% and in two years, by 95% (Lantoarilala *et al.*, 1998; Mouchet *et al.*, 1997). Once again at the end of the century, the malaria situation had been brought under control (Jambou *et al.*, 2001), but it could deteriorate again if control is neglected.

In retrospect, global warming cannot have been to blame for the 1985 epidemic because there has not been any significant change in temperature on the Plateaux in thirty years. On the other hand, the impoverishment of the population and failing health care services turned this epidemic into a catastrophe with 30,000-100,000 deaths

Biodiversity of Malaria in the World

per annum for nearly three years (depending on information source and method of calculation) (Mouchet & Baudon, 1986).

• *Epidemiological coverage and stratification*

On the Plateaux before 1950, the proportions of *P. falciparum* and *P. vivax* were identical at around 50% (Joncour, 1956; Lumaret, 1962). In 1993, in these same regions, the proportions of *P. falciparum* and *P. vivax* were 80% and 20% respectively (Blanchy *et al.*, 1993). On the coastlines before 1950, *P. falciparum* was already the dominant species and to this day this proportion has not changed much.

Up until recently, the prevalence and incidence of malaria was recorded only by surveys. Around Antsiranana on the northern coast (Diego Suarez), Wilson (1947) reported a prevalence of 93% in young children, and an incidence of 230‰ among British troops. In 1948, on the Plateaux near Antananarivo, the SR was greater than 50% and the PR close to 50% (Bernard, 1954). By combining the available data, Mouchet *et al.* (1993) have provided an eco-epidemiological stratification of malaria in the "Big Island" that takes into consideration the various "bio-geographical" areas. Most of the epidemiological facies of the African continent are also found on the island (Mouchet *et al.*, 1993a):
- the **Equatorial facies**, on the east coast and far north;
- the **Tropical facies**, on the west coast north of Morondava;
- the **facies of the Plateaux**, similar to the southern African facies
- the **Southern facies**, semi-arid, fairly similar to the Sahelian facies.

It is necessary to review the area and characteristics of the different facies as they define the malaria conditions in the different regions of the island (*Figure 55*).

Equatorial facies

It covers all of the east coast and Sambirano in the north, up to an altitude of approximately 700 m. The rains, of the order of 1,500-3,000 mm, fall over a period of several days, generating a continuity of both vectors and transmission. The vectors are *An. gambiae s.s.*, *An. arabiensis*, *An. funestus*, and *An. mascarensis*. *An. gambiae s.s.* is the dominant species, while the presence of *An. arabiensis* is much less frequent (Chauvet, 1969, subject to the validation of identification methods). In fact, Chauvet had distinguished the A and B species of the *An. gambiae* Complex on the basis of differential larval chetotaxy, a method that is no longer used much. *An. funestus* is much less frequent than *An. gambiae s.s. An. mascarensis*, which is extremely widespread, is a vector only on the island of Sainte-Marie and in the south near Taolanaro (Fort-Dauphin) (Fontenille & Campbell, 1992; Marrama *et al.*, 1999). It seems likely, based on behavioural differences within this supposed species in various regions of the island, that this term actually covers a complex of species.

In Antanakoro (near Tamatave) on the coast, the EIR was 16 ib/p/yr, of which 95% were due to *An. gambiae*; the Stability Index (St) was greater than 2.5. In Vodivohitra, below 100 m in altitude, the EIR was 240 ib/p/yr of which 85% were due to *An. gambiae s.s.* and 15% to *An. funestus*. The St was 3.5.

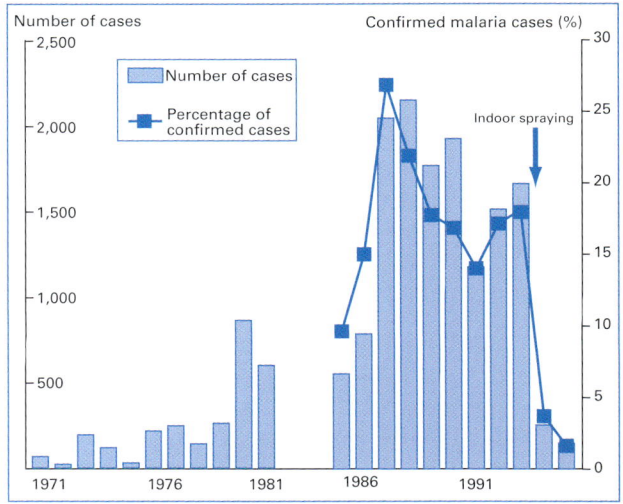

Figure 53. Rising malaria incidence based on the number of cases seen at the dispensary of Analaroa on the Madagascan Plateaux between 1971 and 1995. The number of patients seen between 1971 and 1981 can be estimated at between 5,000 and 10,000 per annum. The figures for 1982-1984 (when the centre was being restructured) were unreliable (adapted from Mouchet, 1998).

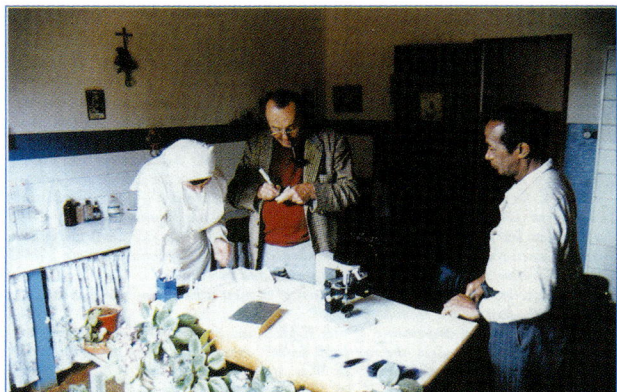

Figure 54. The Analaroa dispensary where the epidemiological data were collected (photograph by Mouchet).

Afrotropical Region

Table XXXIII. Malaria at the Analaroa dispensary from 1971 to 1981: reestablishment of the parasite reservoir (Mouchet et al., 1997).

Month	1971 CS	1971 CC	1972 CS	1972 CC	1973 CS	1973 CC	1974 CS	1974 CC	1975 CS	1975 CC	1976 CS	1976 CC	1977 CS	1977 CC	1978 CS	1978 CC	1979 CS	1979 CC	1980 CS	1980 CC	1981 CS	1981 CC	Total CS	Total CC
January	6	0	18	0	30	14	44	28	33	8	29	6	19	3	16	5	52	17	74	39	117	28	438	148
February	10	1			70	24	35	21	18	6	34	10	21	5	17	5	71	25	121	55	137	85	534	237
March	38	16	30	6	74	43	47	23			28	10	15	3	15	7	72	47	183	111	336	179	838	445
April	42	14	13	13	70	39	56	22	27	7	77	44	81	57	71	21	53	34	299	199	160	89	899	539
May	75	42	5	1	54	39	51	18	11	4	62	84	123	80	130	54	91	57	306	159	176	91	1 084	629
June	29	6	8	2	42	21	42	10	12	8	76	50	97	49	90	36	54	30	284	131	212	106	946	451
July	40	4	9	3	39	14	48	4	7	0	36	14	161	38					249	78	77	18	666	213
August			5	1	11	3	47	0	6	1			66	7	36	8	19	8					176	28
September	18	0	14	1	26	4					18	2	20	0	18	2	71	16	102	32	52	11	339	68
October	13	0	3	0	8	1			8	0	6	0	35	7	18	3	34	7	69	25			194	43
November	10	0	11	0					4	1	28	7	13	5	17	4	28	7	120	30	35	3	266	57
December	8	0	20	6					18	4			32	4	17	5	5	11	87	21			197	51
Total	289	83	136	33	424	202	370	126	144	39	394	227	683	258	445	150	550	259	1 894	880	1 302	610	6 667	2 909
% pos. results	29		19		50		33		25		66		45		43		46		44		55			

CS: clinically suspected malaria cases; CC: parasitologically confirmed cases

(End of nivaquinisation between 1979 and 1980)

In Sainte-Marie, the EIR was 100 ib/p/yr and the St greater than 10; 92% of inocula contained *P. falciparum* and 8% *P. vivax* (Laventure et al., 1995).

In Essana in the far south, *An. mascarensis* was the dominant species (727 captured as opposed to 63 *An. funestus* and 225 *An. gambiae s.s.*). It presented a sporozoite rate of 0.89%. The EIR was 35 ib/p/yr, 23 due to *An. mascarensis*, 3 to *An. funestus*, and 9 to *An. gambiae s.s.* (Marrama et al., 1999). The PR varied from 20-50% in the children of the village (Jambou et al., personal communication).

Tropical facies

It covers the west coast north of Morombe, from the sea up to 900 m. Transmission decreases with altitude and from north to south according to the level of rainfall, from 1,500 to 600 mm. At 600 m in Andriva, the EIR was 6 ib/p/yr with a St of 3. At 200 m in altitude in Andranofositoa, the EIR was 54 ib/p/yr. In Miandrivazo, at 100 m in altitude, the EIR was 32 ib/p/yr with a St greater than 2.5. In all three cases, *An. funestus* was the most efficient vector (Laventure et al., 1995).

In the coastal rice-growing region of Marovoay, the number of infective bites per person per year was 3 inside houses, and 6 outdoors (Rabarison et al., 1999). *An. gambiae s.s.* and *An. arabiensis* shared sites in the northern part of the west coast, whereas in the centre *An. arabiensis* was practically alone (Chauvet, 1969). In Morombe on the edge of the dry zone, *An. arabiensis*, despite being highly anthropophilic, presented a very low sporozoite rate (0.09%) (Coz, 1961).

Facies of the Plateaux (*Figure 56*)

As in the Southern facies, the high altitude tropical climate results in "cool" winters that stop malaria transmission. The *An. arabiensis* and *An. funestus* vectors, however, remain present all year round, such as in Ankazobe (Laventure et al., 1995). An annual re-infestation of the highlands from the lower regions does not seem to be an automatic ecological phenomenon. Transmission stops between 1,500-1,600 m. On the Plateaux, there are great differences in the prevalence and incidence of malaria from one village to the next according to the environment, the altitude, malaria control programme operations, and, to a lesser degree, to the method of stabling livestock, as well as to the economic status of the population which affects the ability to access treatment.

In Manarintsoa, the village near Antananarivo where the epidemic of 1985 was detected, the EIR was very low with 0.9 ib/p/yr due exclusively to *An. arabiensis*, considered to be anthropophilic, perhaps after livestock were stalled in houses to prevent theft. Malaria was very unstable, with a St below 0.25 (Fontenille *et al.*, 1990). The case of this village is unusual because in most sites, the principle vector was *An. funestus*, which develops during the final phases of rice-growing (Marrama *et al.*, 1995), setting off malaria outbreaks from May-June. *An. arabiensis*, which develops during the entire rice cultivation period and during the austral summer season and which is very zoophilic and often exophilic, played a much less important role. In Ankazobe, at 1,200 m in altitude, the EIR was 12 ib/p/yr, due mainly to *An. funestus* from February-June; the St was 2.5 (Fontenille, 1992). In 1996, in the basin of Lake Alaotra at 780-800 m in altitude, the EIR was 0.8 ib/p/yr of which 0.5 was due to *An. arabiensis* and 0.3 to *An. funestus*; in 1997, transmission was almost nil (Rabarison *et al.*, 1999). In Antananarivo, which had not undergone indoor spraying since 1955, the PR remained very low during the epidemic of 1985, so the city was not sprayed. Although there were intramural rice paddies, the PR of 2.5% was due to importation from the countryside (Jambou *et al.*, 1998).

On the Plateaux, the pyrogenic threshold could not be calculated (Boisier & Spiegel, 1999) although it is certain that not every inoculation event gives rise to parasitaemia. At Ankazobé, it would seem that there is one clinical case for every five inoculations (Mouchet, personal observation).

Southern facies

Southern Madagascar west of the Beampingaratra Chain has a subtropical climate that alternates between being dry with 200 mm of rainfall or less, and normal with at least 500 mm of rainfall. The presence of endemic xerophylous plants, such as the Didieriaceae, surrounded by Opuntia and the tiny houses made of Alluaudia wood, give the countryside a particular look.

Permanently flowing rivers are rare. In Beara, a dam supplies the largest irrigated area of the far south. This rice-growing area is exceptional in this region, given the ecological transformation it has undergone, and must be addressed separately from the other dry places in the south. *An. funestus* is the principle vector and is responsible for the EIR of 0.24 ib/p/night in May. Its sporozoite rate was approximately 1% with an equivalent number of infections by *P. vivax* and *P. falciparum*, even though the latter parasite was twenty times more

Table XXXIV. Malaria at the Analaroa dispensary from 1985 to 1996: the epidemic and its management (Mouchet *et al.*, 1997).

Month	1985		1986		1987		1988		1989		1990		1991		1992		1993		1994		1995		1996	
	NP	PCP	NP	PCP	NP	PCP	NP	PCP	NP	PCP	NP	PCP	NP	PCP	NP	PCP	NP	PCP	NP	PCP	NP	PCP	NP	PCP
January	71	15.1	20	6.0	120	26.6	122	20.4	92	12.5	123	15.1	74	9.4	130	27.0	81	11.4	33	6.4	21	2.7	9	1.3
February	62	11.5	47	14.4	227	33.1	274	27.7	173	24.5	174	19.7	100	15.0	185	13.8	131	20.0	25	5.4	19	2.2	12	1.6
March	72	14.2	90	23.0	203	20.0	389	34.4	146	23.2	399	28.2	142	15.6	301	28.0	279	28.6	27	4.7	27	2.6		
April	134	20.0	143	23.2	375	38.5	395	37.0	330	27.1	379	30.0	266	22.9	238	25.5	270	27.5	62	7.2	11	0.9		
May	99	11.9	217	26.9	306	35.2	455	33.0	379	23.8	479	30.3	221	18.4	318	28.8	382	31.4	13	1.3	22	1.7		
June	43	7.7	113	20.6	273	31.3	199	22.4	232	21.7	182	18.3	137	16.7	143	15.9	241	23.0	37	3.6	17	1.5		
July	36	5.2	45	8.9	198	22.6	114	13.5	220	18.4	84	7.5	50	5.6	32	5.2	116	13.7	30	3.1	25	3.1		
August									Dispensary closed												Dispensary closed			
September	25	4.7	26	4.5	101	20.0	70	9.7	40	4.5	16	2.4	33	5.4	26	3.7	22	3.4	8	0.9	8	1.0		
October	24	4.5	40	8.5	88	13.2	48	7.8	69	7.9	23	2.8	66	8.6	43	7.2	19	2.2	17	1.8	2	0.2		
November	5	1.3	23	5.0	84	12.1	60	8.9	54	6.5	44	5.9	65	10.0	42	7.5	69	8.4	10	1.0	0	0		
December	4	1.5	34	12.2	77	14.3	32	7.6	41	7.4	36	10.0	46	12.7	59	11.3	70	9.5	5	0.9	0	0		
Total	575	9.7	798	15	2,052	27	2,158	22	1,776	17.8	1,939	17	1,200	14.0	1,517	17	1,680	18	267	3.6	152	1.6		

NP: number of cases; PCP: percentage of patients with confirmed malaria

(DDT treatment applied through 1994)

Afrotropical Region

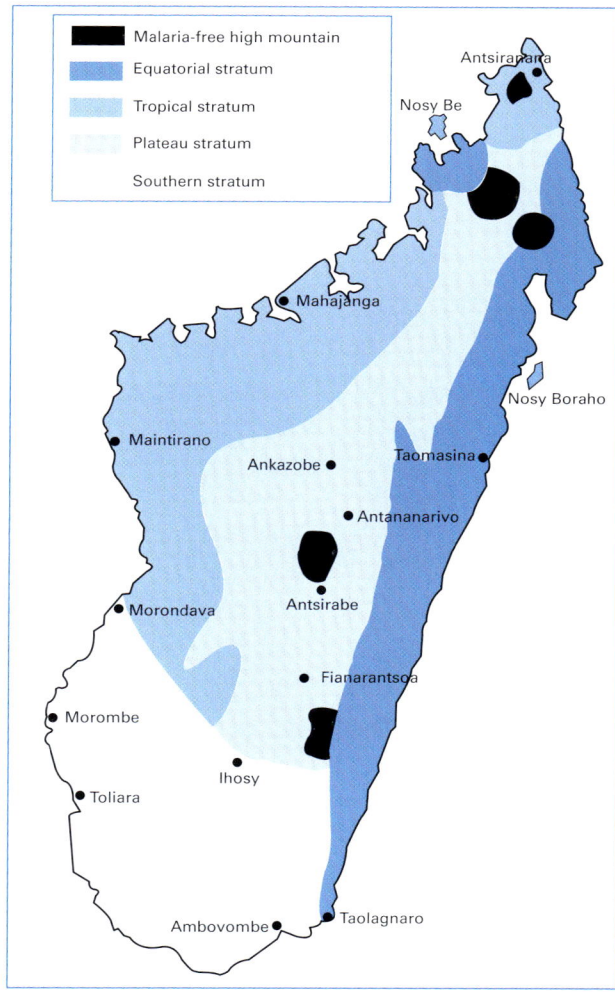

Figure 55. Epidemiological stratification of malaria in Madagascar (adapted from Mouchet et al., 1993a).

This review of malaria in Madagascar illustrates the great diversity of situations and this is reflected in the results of indoor spraying campaigns. Where malaria was stable, tranmission continued, whereas where the disease was unstable, indices dropped sharply and the disease has even been eliminated from the vast expanses of the High Plateaux.

• *Entomology*

Three points dominate the entomology of malaria in Madagascar: *An. funestus* ecology in the rice-growing regions; the distribution and behaviour of members of the *An. gambiae* Complex; and the role and taxonomy of indigenous anophelines.

On the Plateaux, 90% of the larval habitats of *An. funestus* are found in rice paddies towards the end of the growing cycle (maturation and harvest) or on fallow land (Marrama *et al.*, 1995). This anopheline is the main vector, notably having been responsible for reconquest of the highlands where the relationship between rice paddies and malaria is very strong (Laventure *et al.*, 1996). The same relationship exists in the south (Marrama, 1999) but it is not so obvious in the coastal lowlands (Laventure *et al.*, 1995).

For many localities, the study of Chauvet (1969) is the only source of information on the distribution of the two species of the Gambiae Complex. Since 1980, the methods of cytogenetics and molecular biology (notably PCR) have substantially simplifed the identification process. On the plateaux, *An. arabiensis* was the only species of the complex observed by Ralisoa & Coluzzi (1987). Chauvet (1969) put forward the hypotheses that the disappearance of *An. gambiae s.s.* from the highlands was due to indoor DDT spraying. He had even observed a few specimens of *An. gambiae s.s.*—identified on the basis of chetotaxy—in the area around Antananarivo. During the epidemic of 1985, only *An. arabiensis* was found. On the other hand, it seems that the two freshwater species of the *An. gambiae* Complex live together throughout all the coastal regions and in southern Madagascar, but the proportion of each has rarely been determined and all that is known is that *An. gambiae s.s.* is dominant in the north and east, and *An. arabiensis* is most abundant in the west and south. *An. merus* is the most abundant *Anopheles* in the Androy, which is consistent with the level of salt in the soil; no infected specimen, however, has been observed in Madagascar.

Only one endemic species, *An. mascarensis*, has a distribution that goes beyond Madagascar, to the Comoros. Its vector role was observed on the east coast in Sainte-Marie (Fontenille & Campbell, 1992) and near Tolanaro (Fort-Dauphin) (Marrama *et al.*, 1999). In this latter place, the females that bite throughout the night were highly anthropophilic and endophagous but would leave the houses during the night or at dawn. In most places in Madagascar, *An. mascarensis* is highly zoophilic and exophilic.

frequent than the first in villages where the PR of children between the ages of 2-4 exceeded 60%. The *An. gambiae* Complex (96% *An. arabiensis*, 2% *An. gambiae s.s.*, 2% *An. merus*) was equivalent in numbers to *An. funestus* but not a single specimen was found infected (Marrama *et al.*, 1999).

In the Androy, an ancient dried-up sea gulf, the PR varied from 2-20%. The incidence of attacks was 10% in 1996, but less than 5% in 1997 (Jambou, personal communication). In the six villages surveyed, *An. funestus* represented 3% of the samples collected and the Gambiae Complex 97% (70% *An. merus*, 28% *An. arabiensis* and 2% *An. gambiae s.s.*). Considerable differences in rainfall (e.g. between 1995 and 1999) do not seem to have been associated with epidemics (Marrama *et al.*, 1999).

Biodiversity of Malaria in the World

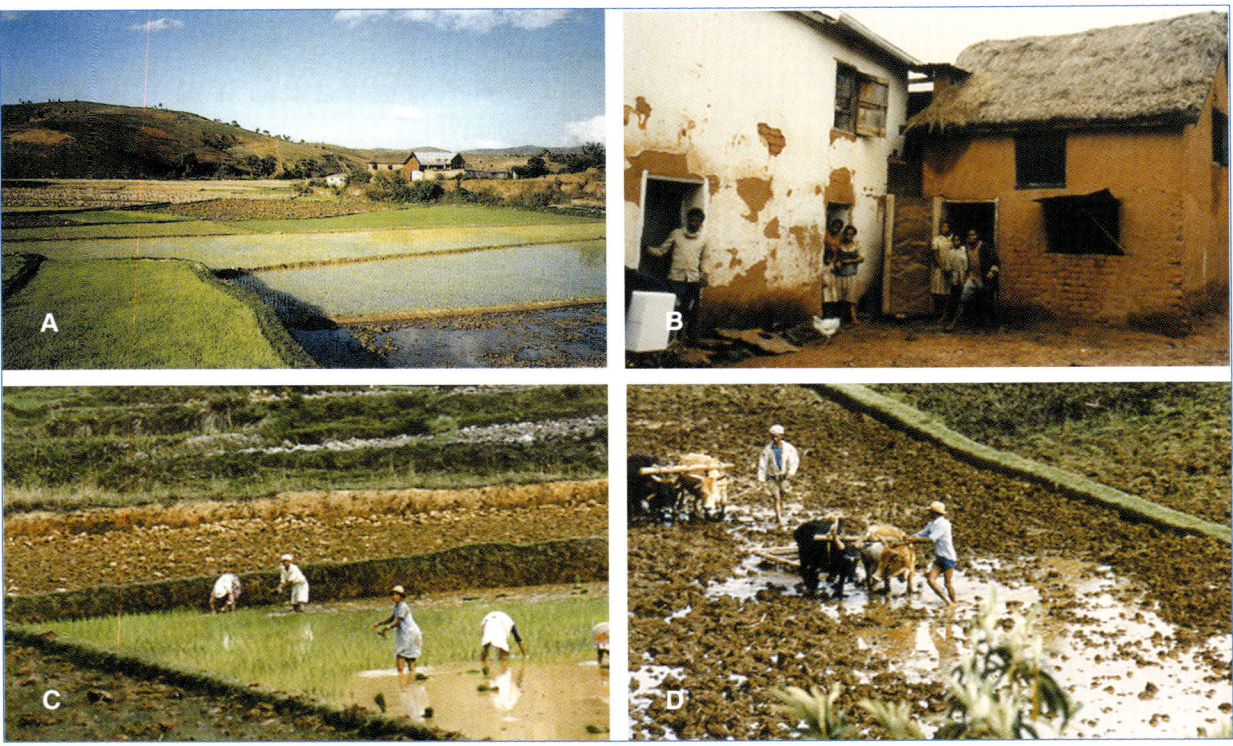

Figure 56. Madagascar Plateaux.
A. Rice paddies at different stages, 60 kilometres south of Antananarivo (photograph by Laventure).
B. Rural house: livestock is kept on the ground floor to discourage thieves (photograph by Mouchet).
C. Replanting of the rice plant (An. arabiensis larval habitats) (photograph by Mouchet).
D. Ploughing (photograph by Mouchet).

While the anthropophilic and endophilic behaviour of *An. funestus* is not disputed, the same cannot be said for the behaviour of the *An. gambiae* Complex, which presents no morphological differences between its species, making it very difficult to interpret the texts of those authors working during the eradication period. On the east coast in the forest regions, *An. gambiae s.s.* was considered to be endophagic and relatively exophilic, with most of the females leaving the houses where they fed before dawn; the fauna remaining in the houses was, therefore, minimal (Chauvet, 1969). On the Plateaux, *An. arabiensis* was zoophilic and exophilic (Fontenille, 1992). On the west coast in Morombe, it was anthropophilic (in the absence of livestock) and exophilic but presented with a very low sporozoite rate under 0.1% (Coz, 1960).

An. arabiensis was considered to be genetically very close to the East African forms. A more in-depth analysis of the polymorphism showed differences between specimens from Senegal, Madagascar, and the Mascarene Islands. This could have been due to a drift during the historical era caused by the geographical separation of populations, and not to mutations. The size of the genetic pool would have drastically decreased when migrations from the continent to the islands occurred, the well-known bottleneck mechanism (Simard *et al.*, 1999).

Comoros Islands

The Comoros Islands, located between 11°-13° south latitude and 42°-45° east longitude, is made up of four islands, Grande Comore, Moheli, Anjouan, and Mayotte, and a series of uninhabited reefs known as the Iles Glorieuses. The total land above sea-level covers an area of 2,170 km^2 with a total population of 646,000.

All these islands are of volcanic origin and have emerged over time as described previously. The Iles Glorieuses are reefs that rise just above the surface of the water. Mayotte (374 km^2), the oldest island, has an eroded relief with a maximum altitude of just over 500 m; it is surrounded by a large lagoon. Moheli (211 km^2) has the same type of relief as Mayotte. Anjouan (424 km^2), a much younger island, rises up to an altitude of 1,600 m on Mount Ntingui; it is shaped like a 3-point star whose ridges circumscribe three basins. The Grande Comore (1,146 km^2), the biggest and the youngest island, emerged during the Quaternary Period and still has an active volcano, Karthala, 2,355 m high. The island is covered with recent, highly permeable lava flows.

The result is that there is no surface water on the island apart from water tanks and basins for washing, even though the rainfall ranges between 1,500-3,000 mm.

• *History of malaria*

The first trace of settlers in the Comoros dates back to the occupation by Arabs from the Persian Gulf that may have come *via* Zanzibar. They brought with them Africans from the continent which are referred to locally as Mozambicans. In the 18th century, "Malagasy pirates" settled in Mayotte and Moheli and continued to speak their language while the rest of the population spoke Swahili. Apart from the Grande Comore, the date that malaria was first introduced into the rest of the Comoros remains hypothetical, if not imaginary. During the 18th century, the moorings of Anjouan were said to be disease-free but at the same time, the Comoros Islands in general were considered to be particularly disease-ridden where half of Europeans and Creoles would die within the first six months of arriving (Gevrey, 1870; Julvez, 1993, 1995). In fact, given the information currently available, it is impossible to know when transmission of malaria first occurred on these islands.

Grande Comore on the other hand was considered to be a hygienic place without *Anopheles* because there was no surface water. The first cases of malaria arose in 1920, before taking on epidemic proportions between 1922-1924 in regions below 500 m in altitude. From an immunological perspective the population was "naïve", and the mortality rate was very high. Up to one quarter of the population may have been victim to this epidemic (Raynal, 1928). The origin of the epidemic was attributed to the construction of freshwater cisterns which provided optimal conditions for the reproduction of *An. gambiae s.s.* This wave of development resulted from the vanilla boom, which had considerably improved the quality of life of a population that, up until then, had relied on brackish well water. Malaria rapidly became hyperendemic on the island.

• *Stratification and diversity of malaria on the four islands*

The Comoros Islands are only a few hundred kilometres apart. They are each, however, very different from a geological, geographical, historical and epidemiological standpoint. Within each island, wind exposure and rainfall have created differences in the flora, fauna, and hydrography. It is, therefore, necessary to address each island individually (Blanchy *et al.*, 1987; Blanchy *et al.*, 1999; Julvez *et al.*, 1986).

Mayotte

Mayotte, the "oldest" of the four islands, has rounded hills under 500 m in altitude. The island is surrounded by a lagoon very rich in fish that is enclosed by coral reefs. The annual rainfall of 1,200-1,800 mm forms various rivers (28 hillside basins) that join the sea through estuaries that block up during the dry season. These estuaries constituted the principle larval habitats for *An. gambiae* (Brunhes, 1977; Subra & Hebrard, 1974) but the development of villages and waste disposal has polluted these sites which have become open-air sewers infested with *Culex quinquefasciatus*. On the other hand, the development of construction and civil engineering works has multiplied the number of man-made *An. gambiae s.s.* larval habitats (ditches, potholes). Before 1976, malaria was considered to be stable and hyperendemic. PRs were greater than 50% in children and only 6% in adults. Perennial transmission occurred through *An. gambiae s.s.* and *An. funestus* (Julvez *et al.*, 1987) (*Figure 57*).

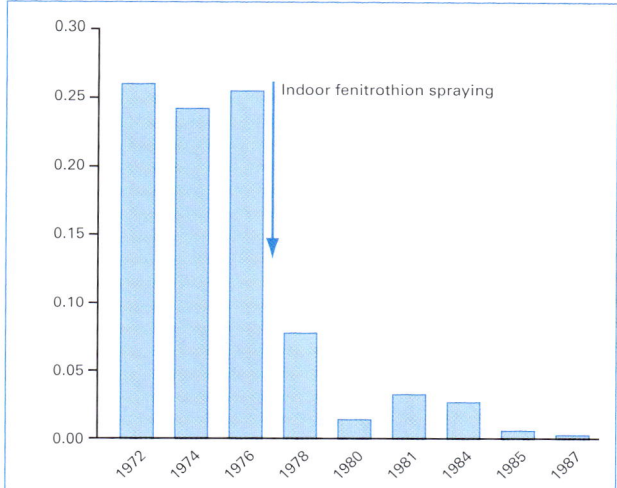

Figure 57. Changes in parasite rate in Mayotte after indoor fenitrothion spraying (adapted from Julvez et al., 1987).

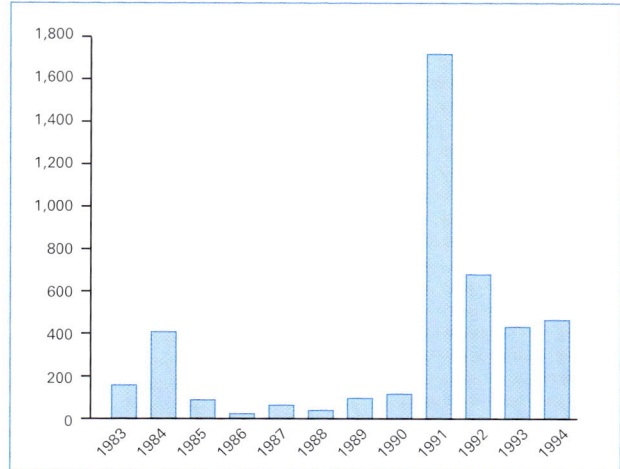

Figure 58. Number of cases of malaria in Mayotte (1983-1994): epidemic resurgence in 1991 (adapted from Ali Halidi, 1995).

In 1976, a malaria control programme based on indoor spraying with fenitrothion (organophosphorus) was implemented and considerably lowered the prevalence of the disease, almost eliminating it entirely. Resurgences in

Biodiversity of Malaria in the World

1984 and 1991 were due to lapses in the indoor spraying programme (*Figure 58*). In 1997, a sero-epidemiological survey demonstrated the drop as well as the disease's recrudescences (Ali Halidi, 1995; Julvez & Mouchet, 1998a). To conclude, *An. funestus* disappeared from the island in 1980 (*Table XXXV*).

Moheli

This island also emerged during the tertiary period, and has an eroded relief no higher than 700 m in altitude. The rainfall of 800-1,200 mm maintains a very dense hydrographic network with most of its rivers ending up in estuaries that block up during the dry season. In contrast to what happens in Mayotte, the estuaries are not polluted and maintain a very high rate of transmission during the dry season by *An. gambiae s.s. An. funestus*, however, is still the most abundant vector on the island. The presence of *An. merus* in crab holes does not seem to have any epidemiological significance. The global PRs were 46% during the dry season and 23% during the rains, but in children under 10 years of age, they were well above 50%, suggestive of hyperendemic or even meso-endemic disease depending on the village (Blanchy *et al.*, 1987; Blanchy *et al.*, 1999) (*Table XXXVI*).

Anjouan

This island is much "younger" with steep mountains that go up to 1,600 m in altitude on Mount Ntingui. The three mountain chains that lead off divide the island into three geographical entities: the northern coast, the south-west coast, and the east coast. The rainfall measures 1,000-2,000 mm on the coast, 2,000-2,500 mm in the hills, and 600 mm on the northern peninsula. Half of the population live on the slopes of which 13% are on the high ground above 600 m in altitude, while 13% live in the plains.

The northern coast has long been considered to be a healthy place with only *An. gambiae s.s.* present and a very low rate of transmission (*Table XXXVI*). In the wet and marshy south-west coast, malaria is hyperendemic, transmitted by *An. gambiae* and *An. funestus*. The situation on the east coast is somewhere between the two (Blanchy *et al.*, 1999).

Grande Comore (*Figure 59*)

This island only emerged during the Quaternary Period and has an active volcano, Karthala (altitude 2,355 m) whose lava has covered all the substrata. This highly permeable covering absorbs all the surface water. As a result, there is a longstanding generalised practise of building rainwater cisterns but their use is decreasing with established water conveyance systems, especially around the capital city of Moroni. The abandoned cisterns make

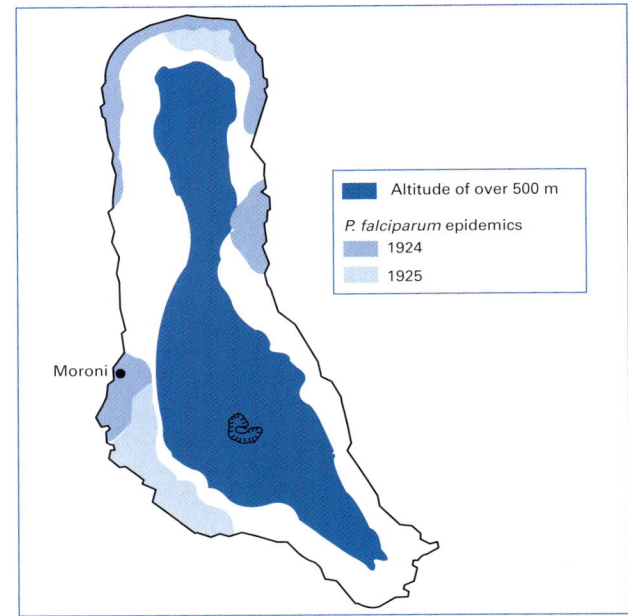

Figure 59. Malaria epidemics on Grande Comore (adapted from Blanchy et al., 1999).

Table XXXV. Parasite rates by species and gametocyte rates in the three islands of the RFI Comoros.								
Island	NE	PRf	PRm	PRv	PRo	Mixed	PR	GR
Grande Comore	3,370	40.9	4.07	1.6	0.03	0.02	46.6	2.14
Anjouan	1,788	20.5	3.58	0.11	0	0	24.2	2.18
Moheli	1,294	43.2	2.09	0.46	0	0.01	45.7	1.62

NE: number of subjects examined; PRf: parasite rate/*Plasmodium falciparum*; PRm: rate/*P. malariae*; PRv: rate/*P. vivax*; PRo: rate/*P. ovale*; PR: parasite rate; GR: gametocyte rate

Table XXXVI. Parasite rates at Anjouan.				
Geographical sector	Northern coast	South-western coast	Eastern coast	Highlands
Parasite rates	9.8%	55%	23%	13%

excellent larval habitats for *An. gambiae s.s.* if the water remains clean but with household pollutants, they have been transformed into breeding factories of *Culex quinquefasciatus*. Wash basins in the mosques, where the water is very clean, constitute the other anopheline larval habitats throughout the entire island (Blanchy *et al.*, 1999). The malaria is stable and hyperendemic with a PR of 55% in children between 1-2 years old (Blanchy *et al.*, 1990). On the west coast, the most humid part of the island where the water conveyance system has largely replaced the use of cisterns, the PR varied from 43-80% depending on the village (Sabatinelli *et al.*, 1988). The pyrogenic threshold was set at 3,200 parasites per mm^3 of blood in babies, and at 6,400 in children (Blanchy *et al.*, 1990). The EIR was 0.055 ib/p/night, i.e. one inoculation every 18 days (Sabatinelli *et al.*, 1991). Malaria was the second highest cause of death and responsible for 18% of consultations; 38% of carriers of parasites were feverish. Ten deaths caused by malaria are declared each year in Grande Comore (Blanchy *et al.*, 1990).

- *Malaria vectors in the Comoros*

Six *Anopheles* species have been identified in the Comoros (Brunhes, 1977; Subra & Hébrard, 1974). One of the species, *An. mascarensis*, originally comes from Madagascar, while the five others are common throughout the entire African continent. The Gambiae Complex is represented by *An. gambiae s.s.*, the "Forest" form, similar to the specimens found in Central Africa (Petrarca *et al.*, 1990; Coetzee *et al.*, 2000), and *An. merus*, found in crab holes in Moheli (Sabatinelli *et al.*, 1988b). *An. gambiae s.s.* and *An. pretoriensis* have been observed on all four islands; the other four species, *An. funestus, An. coustani, An. maculipalpis* and *An. mascarensis* are found on the three other islands. The two sole vectors are *An. gambiae s.s.* and *An. funestus*.

Recent changes include the disappearance of *An. funestus* in Mayotte resulting from indoor spraying with fenitrothion, the development of water convergence systems and the reduced use of cisterns in Grande Comore, the pollution of estuaries, and the development of man-made larval habitats (construction ditches, potholes, changes in farming methods). The impact of these modifications in the near future should be seriously monitored as they could be precious indicators to how malaria will evolve in Africa.

Mascarene Islands

The Mascarene Islands are located between 20°-30° south latitude and 55°-63° east longitude. They include three islands: La Réunion, an overseas French department covering an area of 2,500 km^2 with a population of 780,000 inhabitants, and Mauritius and Rodriguez, which belong to the Mauritian Republic that has sovereignty over the small islands of Saint Brandon and Chagos, covering a total area of 2,045 km^2 with a population of 1,265,000 inhabitants.

These islands are of volcanic origin. La Réunion (2,500 km^2), the most recent one, rises up to more than 3,000 m in altitude and has a highly active volcano called La Fournaise (2,525 m); Mauritius (2,000 km^2) barely exceeds 800 m in altitude and has an eroded relief; Rodriguez (109 km^2) is flat and surrounded by a lagoon.

When the Europeans arrived on these islands, they were uninhabited. The native fauna, such as the endemic "dodo" bird of Mauritius and the turtles of La Réunion, were decimated and several species were imported. The mosquitoes known as "pigailles" did not arrive until the 18th century; the *Anopheles* arrived around 1865. Up until then, the healthiness of these islands was renowned throughout the region and they had become convalescence resorts. Malaria was present but the patients healed spontaneously. Around that time and to the detriment of forests, semi-industrial sugar cane farming was rapidly developing and labourers were imported. It is in this reportedly idyllic context that malaria arrived and established itself in Mauritius in 1865, and in La Réunion two years later. Rodriguez still remains free of *Anopheles* and malaria.

Epidemics and how malaria became endemic in Mauritius

In 1865, the malaria epidemic began in the Albion plantation south of Port-Louis. The disease spread gradually, covering all areas below 300 m in altitude in less than three years (*Figure 60*). Higher regions such as Curepipe, at 550 m, were not affected until 1868 and even then, the disease only affected a small part of the population (Regnaud *et al.*, 1868). The mortality rate reached 18‰ in Port-Louis, 10‰ in Moka and 7.8‰ in Rivière-Rempart. Then, the disease became endemic and the mortality rate

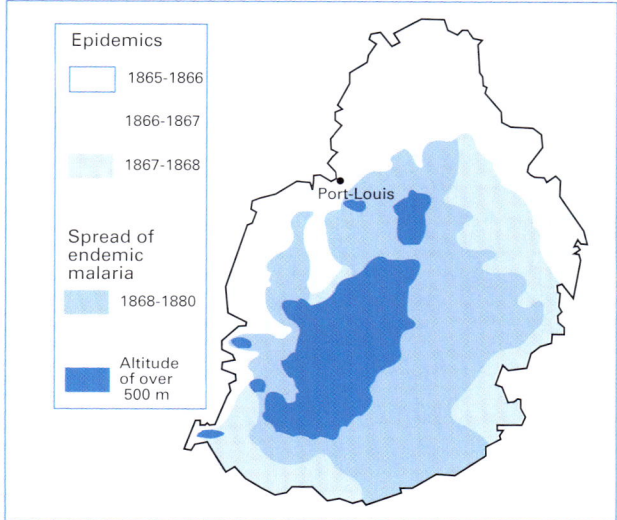

Figure 60. Malaria epidemics on Mauritius (adapted from Blanchy et al., 1999).

of 15.8‰ from 1905-1909 dropped to 5.1‰ from 1925-1929, and to 6.4‰ from 1940-1944 (Lavoipierre & Viader, 1948). This decrease in mortality was due to the massive use of quinine for both prevention and treatment.

In 1947, the malaria was still hyperendemic below 300 m in altitude; PRs varied from 67% in Fernay to 54% in Pamplemousse. But in Curepipe, the disease was hypoendemic with a PR of 6% (Dowling, 1949). Before 1949, the parasitic breakdown varied enormously over time from 68% of *P. falciparum* as opposed to 28% of *P. vivax* in 1906, to 23% and 74% respectively in 1931, and to 38% and 44% in 1948. The frequency of *P. vivax* coincided with the high proportion of Indian and Caucasian populations. It was believed that there was the same percentage of *P. falciparum* transmitted by *An. gambiae* during the summer rainy season as there was *P. vivax* transmitted by *An. funestus* in autumn and winter (Dowling, 1949).

Daruty de Grandpré & d'Emmerey de Charmoy (1900) recorded the presence of *An. gambiae* (then *An. costalis*), *An. coustani* and *An. maculipalpis*. Although it was very abundant, *An. funestus* was not reported until 1932, after having been mistaken for *An. mascarensis* (McGregor *in* Dowling, 1953). *An. funestus* disappeared in 1950 when eradication first began. *An. arabiensis* is currently the only vector (Coetzee *et al.*, 2000; Gopaul & Konfortion, 1988). *An. merus* remains as a potential vector; *An. gambiae s.s.*, suspected of having been at the origin of the 1865 epidemic, has still not been found; this hypothesis, put forward by Paterson (1964a) remains to be confirmed.

• *Eradication and re-introduction*

From 1948-1952, eradication operations based on indoor DDT spraying practically eliminated the parasite. In 1948, PRs were at an average of 9.5%, in 1950 they were 2.4%, in 1951 they were 0.1%, and in 1952 they were 0.05%. In 1973, endemic malaria was officially considered to be eradicated (Bruce-Chwatt *et al.*, 1973) as the only cases detected had been imported. Recent sero-epidemiological surveys have confirmed this (Ambroise-Thomas, 1981). Mauritius is the first country of the Afrotropical Region to have eliminated malaria and has become a model of eradication, obliterating the fact that in its case the malaria was imported into an insular environment, which significantly lowers its standing as a role model for the African continent.

In 1975, transmission resumed resulting in 600 cases in 1982 (Ragawoodoo, 1984), all due to *P. vivax*, which suggests an introduction from the Indian sub-continent. A new eradication programme of indoor spraying along with surveillance measures was implemented in 1990. Once again, malaria has been eradicated in Mauritius (Ragawoodoo, 1995).

• *Why malaria became established in Mauritius*

During the Mauritius epidemic of 1865, neither the etiologic agent nor the role of mosquitoes were known and the disease was referred to as "intermittent or epidemic fever", as described by Regnaud *et al.* in 1868. The etiologic agent, unidentified and sometimes referred to under the vague term of "miasma" could have been introduced from either Africa or India as labourers from both were arriving by the thousand. In any case, it is certain that parasites were imported from both continents well before 1865 without provoking any epidemics. Up until 1864, the voyage from Madagascar to Mauritius meant travelling against the wind and took a long time. At this time, a steamer service from Tamatave to Port-Louis was put in place, reducing the travel time to 4-5 days. This time period became compatible with the survival of *Anopheles*, which did not reproduce on the boats. It was at this moment that local transmission of malaria was observed at the Albion plantation near Port-Louis. It is also this port that seems to have been the epicentre of the epidemic (Julvez *et al.*, 1990). The presence of *Anopheles* was confirmed shortly thereafter. *A posteriori*, the transport of vectors by steamers seemed to be the only probable source of the 1865 epidemic. The installation of vectors, particularly *An. gambiae s.l.*, was probably optimised by the deforestation that occurred for sugar cane plantations.

The second epidemic of 1975 does not have the same origin since *An. arabiensis* was already present. Some of the possible explanations put forward were the cyclones, which provoke the proliferation of larval habitats, as well as changes to the habitat. The construction of flat roofs on which there is poor water drainage, would have allowed *An. arabiensis* larval habitats to multiply (Gopaul & Konfortion, 1988).

Epidemics and how malaria became endemic in La Réunion

In February 1869, the first cases of endemic malaria in La Réunion were observed in Sainte-Suzanne in the northeastern part of the island. The disease was already well-known on the island, so being diagnosed with "intermittent fevers" was accepted with relative ease as opposed to in Mauritius, where the diagnosis traumatised public opinion. Bassignot (1869 *in* Julvez, 1993) came to the conclusion that the disease was endemic in origin but Barat (1869 *in* Julvez, 1993) suspected that the cyclone of March 11-13 in 1868 was responsible for introducing a germ yet unknown at the time. Indeed, the contaminated zone was downwind from Mauritius, from where the cyclone came, and did not reach the usual moorings located on the opposite side of island. This hypothesis of wind-driven infected *Anopheles* is still the most plausible explanation. After every cool season, the disease expanded further, sometimes in a discontinuous fashion. Anopheles swarming from one larval habitat to another *via* lorries was also considered. In 1872, most of the regions below 500 m in altitude were more or less affected (*Figure 61*).

The impact on health was controlled from the outset with the use of quinine. The mortality from malaria seemed to be less than that from the recurrent typhus a few months earlier. However, between 1876-1880 in Saint-Denis, the general mortality rate reached 4.02%, where it had been

Afrotropical Region

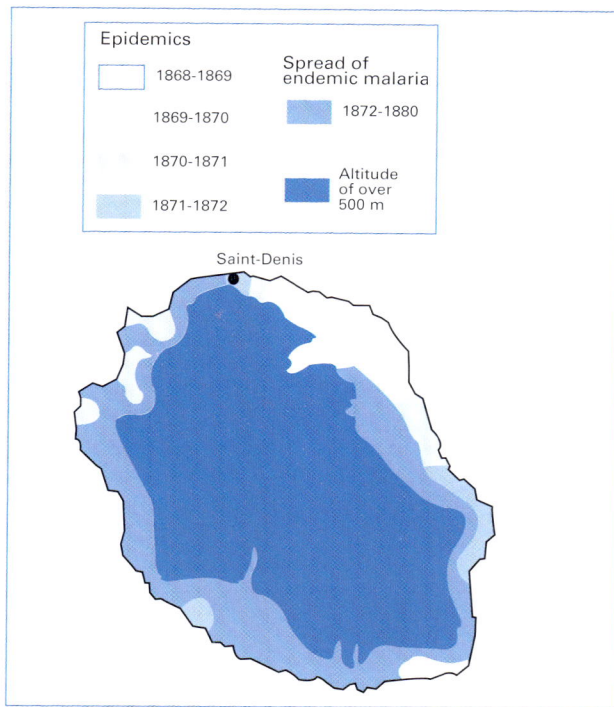

Figure 61. Malaria epidemics on La Réunion (adapted from Blanchy et al., 19999).

only 3.15% before the epidemic, i.e. a very large increase (Delteil, 1881).

Whereas mortality was the same every month of the year before 1868, after 1870 it took on a seasonal rhythm with maximum rates during March-April. This seasonal change in mortality led Merveilleux (*in* Julvez, 1993) to prove, *a posteriori*, the absence of malaria in La Réunion before 1868. Similar conclusions were drawn for Mauritius. In 1926 (Julvez, 1993), according to SRs, the island was divided into five endemic zones: holo-endemic (over 75% with splenomegaly) in Saint-Paul and Saint-Philippe, hyperendemic (SR of 50-79%) in Saint-Denis on the west and south coasts, meso-endemic (SR of 10-50%) on the north and east coasts, and hypo-endemic (SR below 10%) bordering the highlands. Highlands of over 500 m in altitude (and often as of 300 m) were free of malaria. In the same regions, PRs were much lower than the SR and the holo-endemicity gave way to meso-endemicity. In 1952, Hamon (personal communication) thought that the indices, and even more so the malaria mortality rate, had been overestimated.

The eradication of malaria began in 1949 (Hamon & Dufour, 1954) and the last endemic case recorded was in 1966 in a very isolated village in the Mafate Circle. In 1964, the disease was considered to have been eradicated, a situation that has been maintained due to an extremely onerous surveillance system (Girod *et al.*, 1995); the situation is periodically verified through sero-epidemiological surveys of the population (Michault *et al.*, 1985).

An. arabiensis, the only vector on the island (Coetzee *et al.*, 2000; Girod *et al.*, 1995; Julvez *et al.*, 1982), lives throughout the island but the current vector population is highly exophilic and zoophilic in nature. This exophilic behaviour could be a consequence of the improved habitats that followed departmentalisation. These new airy sites are not ideal resting sites for *Anopheles* which prefer dark places. Exophilic behaviour is conducive to lowering the daily rate of survival of *Anopheles* and therefore good for maintaining their eradication (Girod, 2001); it is in any case the most plausible hypothesis. In 1953, Hamon could not confirm the presence of *An. funestus*, of which only one larva had been collected in 1949 by Dowling in the Palmistes Plain. Similarly, the presence of *An. gambiae s.s.* before eradication is speculative. All the specimens collected by Hamon in 1953 were found to be *An. arabiensis* after PCR analysis.

Seychelles

According to WHO, the Seychelles are considered to be malaria-free. They were, and still are, a place where sailors land to recover from illness. In 1932, after a ship had passed through (Mathew & Bradley, 1932), the presence of *An. gambiae* and a few cases of malaria were reported on the islands of Aldabra and Assumption, the closest ones to the Comoros. These were the only islands to have been infested but the vector did not survive. The risk of the Seychelles being infested is very low since the *Anopheles* that had previously been introduced there did not continue to breed (Bruce-Chwatt, 1976).

Australasian Region

Geography and malaria prevalence

From the point of view of fauna and flora, the Australasian Region (or the Australian Region according to some definitions) is a biogeographical entity which is distinct from the Oriental Region to which the islands of Western Indonesia and the Philippines are attributed (*Figure 1*).

From Wallace (1864) to Belyshew (1971), different experts have proposed frontiers which pass either to the east of Sulawesi or to its west, depending on which animal and plant families are used as markers (Nguyen Thi Hong, 1987).

The Australasian Region extends into the Pacific Ocean and has been divided into four or five subregions depending on the experts. Malarial vectors are only found in the western part which includes the eastern provinces of Indonesia (the Molucas and Western New Guinea), Papua New Guinea, Australia (north of the 19th parallel), the Solomon Isles and Vanuatu (*Figure 1*).

Until relatively recently (about 10,000 years ago), the island of New Guinea was contiguous with Australia in the Sahul continent or platform which at certain times also included the Solomon Islands and the Molucas. These links account for the similarity of anopheline profiles across the three island systems, all dominated by the group *Anopheles punctulatus*. On the volcanic Vanuatu Islands (which formed within the last two million years), only one species is found, namely *An. farauti* N° 1. Similarly, only two or three species belonging to this complex have reached northern Australia.

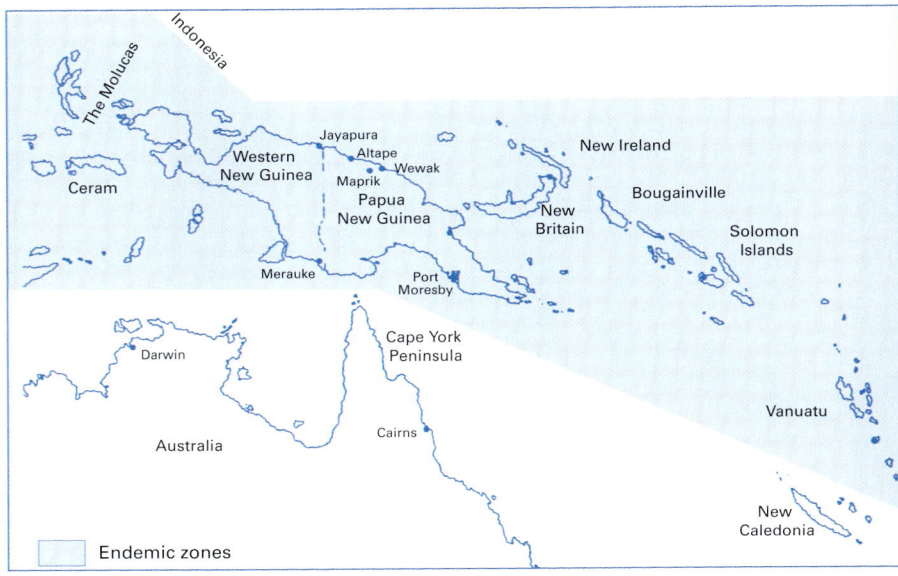

Figure 1. *The Australasian Region.*

Two features characterise malaria in this part of the world:
- the superimposition of malaria with a single group of anopheline vectors, those of the *An. punctulatus* Group, geographically limited;
- the relative isolation of these island systems from Asia, Australia and Micronesia, coupled with the existence of a hyperendemic focus separated by a distance of over 3,000 km from the Afrotropical Region.

In Indonesia, species belonging to the *An. punctulatus* Group have not spread westwards to either Timor (Azevedo, 1958b), Flores or Sulawesi (Kirnowardoyo, 1987). In Australia, they are confined to the north of Cape York Peninsula (and do not transmit malaria). Various anopheline species have been introduced at Guam Airport in the Mariana Islands, but none belonging to the *An. punctulatus* Group (Ward & Jordan, 1979; Ward *et al.*, 1976). There is no evidence that any *Anopheles* has ever been introduced into New Caledonia or Fiji despite regular air and sea traffic.

The endemic zone of Australasia covers just over one million km^2 and is home to seven million inhabitants. The surface area is therefore small but the epidemiological particularities of this zone justify its classification as a distinct malarial region (*Table I*).

Anopheline vectors

Taxonomy and distribution (Table II)

The earliest in-depth work on the region was carried out by Bone-Wepster & Swellengrebel (1953) who also covered all of Indonesia. In 1966, Steffan compiled a list of the *Culicidae* of the Papuan Region. These early surveys already identified members of the *An. punctulatus* Group as the predominant malarial vectors, including *An. punctulatus* itself together with *An. koliensis* and *An. farauti*. On the basis of morphological characters and later isoenzyme analyses, *An. farauti* was further broken down into nine species which were not assigned distinct names but are referred to by number (Bryan, 1973; Foley *et al.*, 1993; Foley *et al.*, 1994; Mahon & Miethke, 1982). Moreover, another "*near-punctulatus*" species has been reported in Papua (Foley *et al.*, 1995). Where these various species or forms are found is shown in *Table II*. Despite the taxonomic complexity revealed by this research, it would seem that the only important malarial vectors are *An. punctulatus s.s.*, *An. koliensis* and *An. farauti* N° 1. Sweeney (1980) suggested that *An. farauti* N° 2 might have transmitted malaria in Australia prior to 1944. *An. farauti* N° 1 is probably the form described as *An. farauti* by Laveran in 1902 because it is the only form found around Port-Vila in the Vanuatan island of Efate where the relevant specimens were collected.

Other species have been suspected to be vectors, especially in Western New Guinea and the Molucas, namely *An. karwari*, *An. subpictus* and *An. barbumbrosus* although the role of these has only ever been secondary and whether or not they are actually present is controversial: at most, their foci are very confined and they have disappeared from many of the places in which they were previously reported.

Larval ecology

An. farauti is remarkably adaptable, growing in fresh as well as in brackish water (up to 80% marine salinity) (Spencer *et al.*, 1975). Only *An. farauti* N° 1 appears to be resistant to salt, which distinguishes it from *An. farauti* N° 2 and N° 3 (Sweeney, 1987). Thus, *An. farauti* N° 1 colonises brackish coastal marshes as well as the low parts of valleys, and man-made biotopes such as ruts in the road, irrigation ditches and taro patches (Rageau & Vervent, 1959).

An. punctulatus s.s. cannot develop in brackish water. It breeds only in fresh water sites which are sun-exposed for at least half the day (which excludes them from woodlands). Such habitats may be natural (e.g. rain pools or residual pools in riverbed) or man-made (e.g. ruts and ditches). This species can become established in cleared woodland as happened following migrations in Western

Table I. Zones of endemic malaria in the Australasian Region (Wikipedia, 2006).		
Country	Size (km^2)	Population
Indonesia		
Molucas (or Maluku)	75,000	2,100,000
Western New Guinea	422,000	2,646,500
Papua New Guinea	462,000	5,887,000
Solomon Islands	28,000	478,000
Vanuatu	14,760/12,336	193,000 (2002)
TOTAL	1,001,760	11,304,500
Australia	Malaria was eradicated from Australia at the end of the Second World War. It only affected the northern part of the country and, particularly, the sparsely populated Cape York Peninsula; above the 19th parallel, the country is receptive	

Species	Indonesia		Papua New Guinea	Solomon Islands	Vanuatu	Australia	Vector	Description and observation
	The Molucas	Western New Guinea						
An. koliensis		+	+	+			+	Owen, 1945
An. punctulatus	+	+	+	+			+	Doenitz, 1901
An. var. punctulatus			+					Foley et al., 1995
An. farauti	+	+	+	+	+	+	+	Laveran, 1902; described from Efate in Vanuatu
An. farauti n°1	+	+	+	+	+	+	+	Bryan, 1973; probably Laveran's type
An. farauti n°2				+		+	−	Bryan, 1973; not anthropophilic, Sweeney, 1977
An. farauti n°3						+	−	Mahon & Miethke, 1982
An. farauti n°4			+				−	Foley et al., 1993
An. farauti n°5			+				−	Foley et al., 1993
An. farauti n°6			+				−	Foley et al., 1993
An. farauti n°7				+			−	Foley, Meck, Bryan, 1994; not anthropophilic
An. clowi		+					−	Rozeboom & Knight, 1946
An. rennelensis				+			−	
An. bancrofti		+	+			+		Giles, 1902; wrongly considered a vector
An. annulipes		+	+			+	−	Walker, 1856; vector of myxomatosis in Australia
An. barbumbrosus	+	+					−	Strickland & Chowdhry; not a vector in Australia
An. subpictus	+	+					?	Grassi, 1899; very localised, possibly a vector of P. vivax
An. karwari		+					−	James, 1902; disappeared and very rare in Western New Guinea

Table II. *Anopheles* of Australasia.

New Guinea (Church *et al.*, 1996), and it often profits when a village is set up or expands.

An. koliensis is mainly found in temporary pools under dense vegetation at the fringe of jungle, but never in woodland (Church *et al.*, 1996). It has a patchy distribution but locally it can be very abundant.

Larval ecology is a key factor governing the distribution of species. Spencer *et al.* (1974) compiled an ecological stratification of vectors in Papua and Western New Guinea.

On coral islands, *An. farauti* N° 1 colonises marshlands which are often brackish. This species is by far the most common, especially in and around villages where it can feed. *An. punctulatus* which accounts for only 1-2% of vector activity is found as small populations although its density can explode at the end of the rainy season or following jungle clearance. In mangroves, it can become established on emerging lands washed away by heavy rains. In lowland valleys *An. farauti* predominates but *An. punctulatus* is common on lower slopes if not too steep for creation of pools. Similarly on higher land, *An. farauti* is found at the bottom of the valleys and *An. punctulatus* in any pools that accumulate on the lower slopes.

In mountainous areas, *An. farauti* is again found at the bottom of valleys and *An. punctulatus* in semi-permanent pools.

An. koliensis is the least common and is only found in limited areas.

The altitude above which vectors are no longer found ranges from 1,300-1,800 m depending on exposure, local relief and human activity.

In the Solomon Islands, it is considered that *An. farauti* is the vector in coastal areas, and *An. punctulatus*—sometimes together with *An. koliensis*—is responsible for transmission inland (Samarawickrema, personal communication, 1995).

In Vanuatu, *An. farauti* N° 1 occupies lower land and is rarely found at altitudes of over 600 metres (Rageau & Vervent, 1959; Ratard, 1975).

Adult ecology and behavioural changes

All three species, *An. farauti*, *An. koliensis* and *An. punctulatus* are ubiquitous feeders and will bite whichever host is available, be it human, porcine or canine—and even bovine inside villages. Moreover, these species are sometimes present in great numbers in uninhabited zones where mammals are rare, suggesting that they can survive on a wide variety of different hosts (Charlwood *et al.*, 1986; Sloof, 1961).

An. farauti tends to feed very close to the ground, leading Charlwood *et al.* (1984) to recommend raising sleeping quarters in order to reduce the incidence of malaria. In fact, in the region, it is common to construct houses on stilts (although we would not go so far as to affirm that this is in order to prevent mosquito bites) and keeping pigs down below may constitute a sort of zooprophylaxis.

Early studies suggested that *An. farauti* activity is characterised by two peaks, one from 8 p.m. to 9 p.m. and another between 11 p.m. and 3 a.m. In Western New Guinea, Sloof (1964) observed that the second peak was eliminated after indoor DDT treatments, so this mosquito was mainly biting early in the evening. The same observations were made in Papua (Charlwood & Graves, 1987) and in the Solomon Islands where a similar pattern was also observed for *An. koliensis* (Taylor, 1975). In the light of the known polymorphism of this species, White (1974) hypothesised that DDT might selectively kill genotypes that tend to bite in the middle of the night.

In contrast, DDT treatment did not seem to induce any behavioural changes in *An. punctulatus* in the Solomon Islands (Samarawickrema *et al.*, 1992) For 76 females of this species infected with *Plasmodium vivax*, Bockarie *et al.* (1996) observed only one bite before 9 p.m.

This point is very relevant when it comes to using pyrethroid-treated mosquito nets for malaria control because in practice, few people go to bed before 9 p.m., so the majority of local inhabitants are unprotected at a time when the risk of infection was hitherto considered as very low. Thus, a behavioural change could compromise the efficacy of one of the few tools in the anti-malarial arsenal. Counter to this pessimistic scenario, it is worth remembering that in Vanuatu—where *An. farauti* is the sole vector—the widespread use of treated nets reduced the incidence of malarial attacks by 80% (Health Ministry, Vanuatu, 1996).

Before DDT treatment, all three species were considered as very endophilic although this was less marked with *An. farauti*. The irritant activity of DDT and/or pyrethroids may alter the resting behaviour of anophelines which currently depends on present or historical insecticide use.

Vectorial capacity and vector longevity

All three of the above-mentioned species are highly efficient vectors with sporozoite rates between 0.3% and 5% depending on location and season (Burkot *et al.*, 1989; Church *et al.*, 1996). In Papua, Bockarie *et al.* (1996) reported a higher rate for *P. falciparum* (1.9%) than for *P. vivax* (1.4%) in *An. punctulatus* although this may simply reflects the proportion of the two parasite species in the carrier population. In the same study, the number of *P. falciparum* sporozoites per mosquito was estimated at 6,300 in all three species whereas the corresponding numbers of *P. vivax* sporozoites were 1,100 in *An. punctulatus*, 330 in *An. farauti* and 250 in *An. koliensis*.

These high sporozoite rate values result from the magnitude of the gametocyte reservoir coupled with vector longevity. In a series of mark-release-recapture experiments in Papua, Charlwood & Bryan (1987) estimated *An. punctulatus* daily life expectancy at 0.75 to 0.77. This would mean that in theory, 2% of females live long enough to transmit *P. falciparum* and 6% long enough to transmit *P. vivax*. However, as pointed out in the article, these are necessarily over-estimates because only a minority of females would take their first blood meal from a gametocyte-carrier. In Vanuatu, *An. farauti*, has a daily survival rate (calculated according to the parous rate) ranging from 0.88 in May during the rainy season to 0.76 in November during the dry season (Ratard, 1975).

It is important to note that some members of the *An. farauti* Complex do not seem to be malaria vectors, in most cases because they do not feed on humans (*Table II*). This must be taken into account when interpreting the results of entomological surveys.

Parasites and immunity

All four human *Plasmodium* species are present in this region. Prior to 1970, *P. vivax* was the most common species but that has changed and now it is *P. falciparum* which predominates. In Papua before 1970, *P. vivax* accounted for 49% of infections, *P. falciparum* 47% and *P. malariae* 2% whereas by 1993, this profile had changed to 22% *P. vivax*, 75% *P. falciparum* with *P. malariae* unchanged at 2% (Palmer, 1993). In the Solomon Islands, Avery (1974) recorded 65% *P. falciparum*. Until 1957, *P. vivax* was by far the most common species in Vanuatu but in the 1960's, the level of *P. falciparum* began to increase (Ratard, 1957) and it is now the most common parasite (Health Ministry, 1997).

A similar shift in the balance of plasmodial species has been observed throughout Southeast Asia. In the opinion of Desowitz & Spark (1987) and many others, this is due to *P. falciparum* resistance to chloroquine although this explanation is not entirely convincing. In Vanuatu, the changes began in 1970 before chloroquine resistance was widespread (Ratard, 1975); at Maprik in Papua, the shift began in 1976 when homes were being treated with DDT but before drug resistance had spread (Palmer, 1993); in Vietnam during the period of eradication, *P. vivax* disappeared before *P. falciparum* (Nguyen Tho Vien, personal communication). *P. ovale* is rare in this region and the level of *P. malariae* remains below 5%.

The geographical isolation of the Solomon Islands does not seem to have affected the genomic diversity of its *P. falciparum* population which is comparable to those observed in Papua and Thailand (Prescott *et al.*, 1994).

Chloroquine-resistance in *P. falciparum* is found throughout the region although its prevalence and level vary enormously from place to place. In the Solomon Islands, Vanuatu and Papua New Guinea, chloroquine remains the first-line drug of choice according to all the relevant authorities. There is some resistance to amodiaquine in Papua but the level remains low (Schuurkamp, 1992).

P. vivax resistance to amino-4-quinoline in the region is now a well-established phenomenon although the public health impact of this resistance has not yet been assessed (Palmer, 1993; Schuurkamp, 1992).

Between 8% and 40% of people in Vanuatu suffer from glucose-6-phosphate dehydrogenase deficiency and this appears to be linked with the prevalence of malaria (Ganczakowski *et al.*, 1995). The consequences of this type of deficiency are poorly understood but it is known that problems arise when it comes to taking amino-8-quinoline (especially for *P. vivax* malaria).

That people in this region develop immunity to both parasites (*P. falciparum* and *P. vivax*) has been known for a long time (Black, 1958; Metselaar, 1961) with age-related attenuation of both the parasite load in the blood and splenomegaly. The latter parameter was taken into account when Metselaar & Van Thiel (1959) developed their classification system for endemic zones in Western New Guinea. Regression of splenomegaly happens long before the drop in parasitaemia and this phenomenon is more marked in Australasia than in Tropical Africa.

The development of immunity in Australasia is similar to that observed in Tropical Africa.

Immigrants from Java are highly susceptible when they arrive in Western New Guinea and Baird *et al.* (1993) showed that, among those who had arrived within the previous year, the prevalence of malaria was not affected by age, suggesting that they had not acquired any immunity. On the other hand, among those who had been living in Western New Guinea for sixteen months or more, the prevalence dropped with age in 6-10 year-olds and 10-14 year-olds. They concluded that, after two years in Western New Guinea, the immigrants' immune responses were as protective as those of the indigenous people.

The malaria situation in the island groups (*Figure 1*)

Taking ecological similarities into account, we have divided the region into four island groups:
- the Molucas,
- Western New Guinea and Papua New Guinea,
- the Solomon Islands,
- Vanuatu.

The Molucas or Maluku

With a surface area of 75,000 km^2, the population of the Molucas raised to 2,6 million inhabitants. Its three main islands are Seram, Ambon and Halmahera (together with numerous smaller islands).

There is a significant lack of recent information about this Indonesian province. *An. punctulatus* and *An. farauti* are present (Knight & Stone, 1977), but *An. koliensis* is not mentioned in the catalogue or its supplements. Kirnowardoyo (1985) made no reference to Molucan species in his review of *Anopheles* in Indonesia.

Western New Guinea and Papua New Guinea

The island of New Guinea is divided into Western New Guinea and the Republic of Papua New Guinea in the east. Papua New Guinea also includes the islands of New Britain, New Ireland, Manus, Bougainville, D'Entrecasteaux, the Milne Bay Islands and a few smaller land masses. The Western New Guinea (former Irian Jaya until 2000) – Papua New Guinea group forms a geographic, ecological and ethnic entity extending over more than 800,000 km^2 that must be considered as a whole.

The northwest monsoon (from October to April) brings the summer rains. Rainfall is more abundant on the northern windward coasts (with more than 2,000 mm per annum) than on the southern leeward coasts (less than 1,500 mm). This phenomenon which applies to all the islands in question affects vector density and therefore, the prevalence of malaria.

An epidemiological stratification system for malaria proposed by Parkinson (1974) for Papua (*Figure 2*) can easily be extrapolated to Western New Guinea (Black, 1958):
- along the northern coasts, malaria is hyperendemic and even holoendemic in certain areas (east of Sepik). People in this region develop immunity as reflected in a lower prevalence of splenomegaly before the age of 6 years, and lower parasite loads in the blood by the age of 10. Malaria is very stable. The prevalence decreases on the inland slopes to become mesoendemic at an altitude of 600 m;
- on the southern, less humid coast, malaria is mesoendemic in the area around the capital, Port-Moresby;
- between 600 and 1,300 m, malaria is hypoendemic or epidemic; certain experts contend that the population density in these areas is as low as it is because of malaria (Parkinson, 1974);
- malaria is no longer endemic above 1,300 m but epidemics may occur up to 1,800 m. Black (1958) set

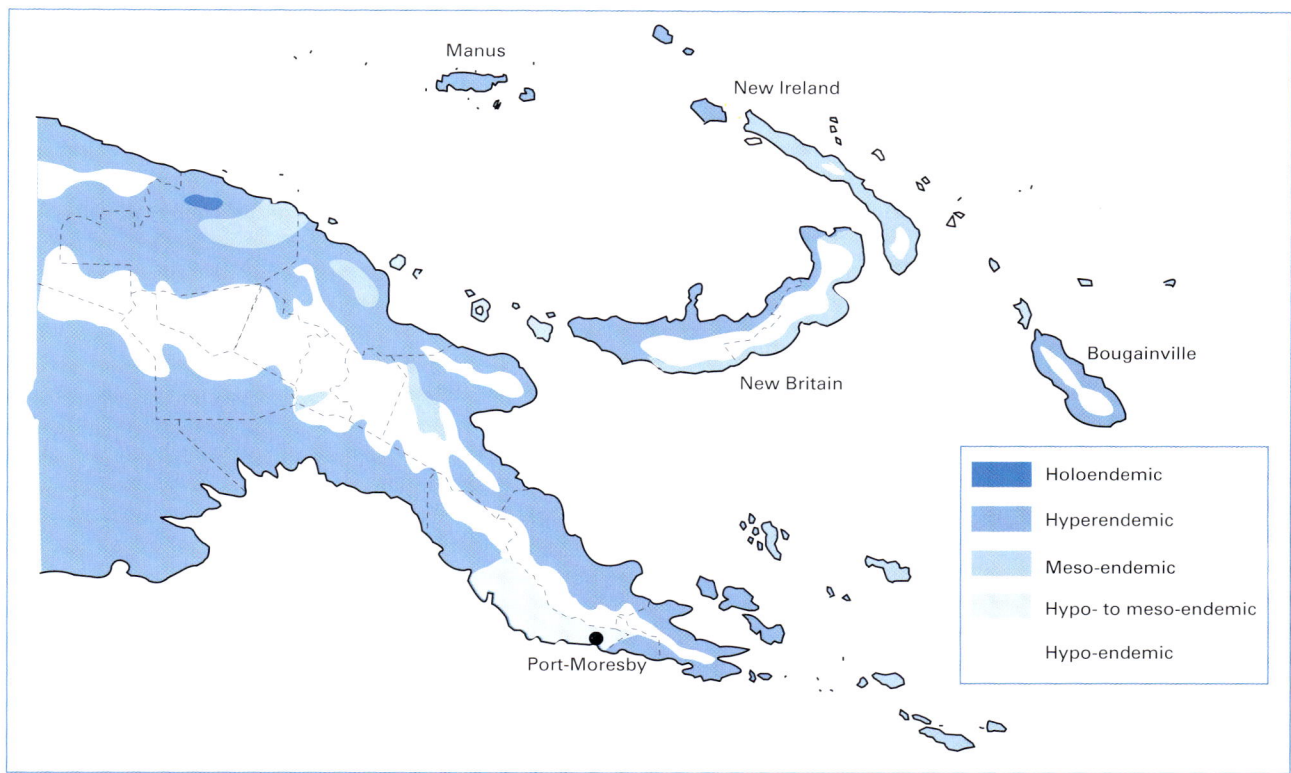

Figure 2. Endemic malaria in Papua New Guinea (estimated) (adapted from Parkinson, 1974).

the upper limit for malaria in Western New Guinea at this altitude. In Goroka at an altitude of over 2,000 m in the Eastern Highlands of Papua New Guinea, most cases are seen in people who have visited the coast (Bashford and Richens, 1992).

In the archipelagos, the situation is hyperendemic at D'Entrecasteaux, Manus, along the northern coast of New Britain and in the coastal areas of Bougainville. It is mesoendemic on the southern coast of New Britain, New Ireland and the islands of Milne Bay. The peaks of some of the large islands, such as New Ireland, New Britain and Bougainville, are malaria-free.

Malaria has changed slightly in the holoendemic zones of East Sepik over the last thirty-five years. Prevalence has dropped from 62% to 50% (from 90% to 78% among children under 6 years old, and from 38% to 30% among adults) (Desowitz & Spark, 1987). This remarkable stability is comparable to that observed in Western and Central Africa (Mouchet *et al.*, 1998).

In 1994, the incidence of cases was 0.53 per person, all age groups included, but it reached 2 per person per year in 2-4 year-olds (Smith *et al.*, 1994).

Environmental changes—particularly deforestation for founding or expanding villages—create larval habitats for *An. punctulatus* and lead to increased transmission by this vector (Church *et al.*, 1996). In the transmigration zones of Western New Guinea where 39,000 non-immune Javanese were installed, full-blown epidemics occurred among newcomers following jungle clearance operations, as the parasites were continually being introduced by the indigenous Papuan population. Malaria has become the leading reason for visiting a health centre and the second cause of mortality in the province (Baird *et al.*, 1993). However, it appears that the migrants had developed good defences after two years in the area (*see above*).

As a result of population growth (3.4% per annum), the search for new arable land could drive people from malaria-free mountain areas down to the more sparsely populated regions at altitudes of between 600 and 1,300 m. The inevitable clearing operations could then lead to increased transmission and trigger epidemics.

Quantitative information about prevalence prior to eradication operations is scarce. Metselaar (1961) reported a prevalence of 46% at Sentani Lake in Western New Guinea.

According to the official figures (not necessarily reliable), the percentage of malaria among individuals examined at health centres in Papua rose from 6% in 1971 to 13.8% in

1991. Malarial deaths rose from 1.1% in 1971 to 1.8% of all deaths in 1998 (Palmer, 1993). This low malaria mortality is attributed to an efficient drug distribution system and the immunity of the inhabitants of highly endemic areas.

Solomon Islands

According to the 1986 census, the Solomon Islands has a population of 478,000 across 28,000 km². The population has been growing steadily (> 3% per year) over the last twenty-five years. Malaria is present on all of the archipelago's inhabited islands, including the easternmost such as Vanikoro which used to be considered the least affected (Maffi & McDonnell, 1971).

Eradication operations based on indoor DDT spraying began in 1970 (Avery, 1974). Since that time, malaria has fluctuated according to the efficacy of control measures.

Prior to 1970, malaria was hyperendemic on the coasts where *An. farauti* transmitted the disease all year-round. Inland, malaria was also transmitted by *An. punctulatus* and, in certain areas, by *An. koliensis*. This transmission tends to be more seasonal as densities of these two species explode with rainfall. This basic scenario still pertains today.

Eradication operations began with success until 1975 in which year only 3,500 cases were reported throughout the islands. However, operations were decentralised in 1976 and in 1981, 60,000 cases were reported. In 1991, the incidence rose to 400‰. As of 1997, the use of impregnated mosquito nets became widespread and in that year, the incidence dropped to 350‰* with 5% of severe cases (Madeley, 1998). *P. falciparum* was responsible for 69% of cases in 1990 and by 1993, with the generalised use of nets, the parasite was responsible for only 49% of all cases (Samarawickrema et al., 1992).

Malaria mortality was very low, with just 30-40 deaths in 1991. According to the WHO Malariologist, this low rate was due to effective immunity, but if this is so, it is difficult to understand why attacks are as common in adults as in children and why there are so few asymptomatic carriers.

Control operations were highly effective up to 1975 and completely changed the epidemiological landscape. It is difficult to interpret the current situation as the country has been used as a test ground for experimental control methods since 1980.

Vanuatu

The island republic of Vanuatu (a former Anglo-French condominium known as the New Hebrides) is made up of 80 very young volcanic islands (less than 2 million years old). They were never joined to the Sahul continent, which might account for the poverty of their fauna. *An. farauti* N° 1 is the only malarial vector. The islands have a surface area of 14,760 km² and a population of 193,000 (2002), i.e. a population density of 13 people per km².

Malaria is indigenous throughout all the islands except Futuna to the south-east of the archipelago where there are no *Anopheles*. Epidemiological analysis reveals four distinct types of situation:
- in villages along the coast and up estuaries, a prevalence of 50% (at the borderline of hyperendemicity) is reached at numerous sites;
- in villages, along temporary streams, malaria is meso-endemic;
- in foothill villages, below an altitude of 600 meters, malaria is hypoendemic. Since the inhabitants of these regions, including women and children, often come down to river banks or the sea to fish, it is hard to say if the cases are indigenous or imported. Vectors are rare although the local entomology has not been extensively studied. Rageau & Vervent (1959) collected *An. farauti* larvae in irrigated taro patches. The two possibilities are not mutually exclusive;
- on inhabited islands, malaria is hypoendemic and of little importance save where *Anopheles* can develop in marshlands near lagoons. It is thus meso-endemic.

The earliest traces of human presence in Vanuatu date back to 4,000 years ago with the Lapita civilisation. When Europeans first came to the islands in 1595, all of the Melanesian inhabitants were cultivating the inland areas rather than living and working on the coast. Subsequently, the highly influential missions which acted as a magnet for local people were set up near the coastal moorings. Ethnologists are interested in the question of whether the Melanesians are descendants of the Lapita civilisation who migrated inland in an attempt to flee malaria, or if they arrived during other migratory movements.

The coastal areas were exploited by the Europeans who established coconut groves and raised cattle in the virgin jungle at Santo, Efate and Malikolo, draining the soil and destroying anopheline larval habitats. The incidence of malaria is currently very low in these areas.

Throughout Vanuatu, a malaria incidence of 196‰ in 1990 has fallen to 33‰ in 1996 with the use of permethrin impregnated mosquito nets (statistics from the Health Ministry, 1997; Ichimori, 1997, personal communication). However, the accuracy of the statistics has not been checked in the field, and the use of mosquito nets is somewhat inconsistent.

---

* The incidence figure needs clarification since 373,000 cases per annum were reported in a population of 300,000, i.e. an incidence of over 1,000‰.

Ratard (1975) reported solid immunity by the age of 6 in areas of high endemicity. As in Papua, SRs dropped faster than parasite prevalence.

Malarial deaths were low and even zero in a hyperendemic area of Santo (Maitland *et al.*, 1997). Nevertheless, at the hospital in Port-Vila, the capital on the island of Efate, malaria was considered to be the primary cause of mortality (Port-Vila Hospital statistics, 1996). The majority of the patients arrived at the hospital in a coma after having been treated for several days by traditional practitioners, who are highly respected by local people.

Until 1975, the majority of cases were due to *P. vivax* (Ratard, 1975) but this balance shifted in favour of *P. falciparum*. The suggested explanation is chloroquine resistance even though it is infrequent and at low level: there is no R3 and chloroquine is still the first-line drug recommended by health officials—and often the only one available.

Australia

In Australia, malaria has never spread down below the 19° parallel. The region concerned the most was the York Peninsula, Queensland. Malaria was eliminated from this region during World War II and the last epidemic was reported in Cairns in 1942 (Macdonald, 1957).

The cases, mostly attributable to *P. vivax*, were located in the coastal area where *An. farauti* N° 1 and *An. farauti* N° 2 (suspected by Sweeney [1980] as being a vector) are found.

Currently, Sweeney (1983) considers the north of Australia to be a malaria-receptive zone owing to the presence of efficient vectors and the importation of parasites by miners from Papua.

Walker (1988) believes that Australia is an ideal region to monitor for the re-emergence of malaria with the expected increase in temperature of 0.4-0.8 °C by 2030. A simulation has indicated that *An. farauti* could spread if the temperature increases by 1.5 °C and rainfall by 10% by 2030; in this case, the risk of malaria would be significantly exacerbated.

Conclusion

Australasia represents the easternmost point of penetration of the South-West Pacific by *Anopheles* and malaria. All malarial vectors in Australasia belong to the *An. punctulatus* Group which remains focused in this part of the world, a remnant of the ancient continent of Sahul.

The most common species, *An. farauti* N° 1, has a remarkable ecological plasticity. Its tolerance to salt (up to 80% sea water) allows it to colonise all coastal areas, low valleys and even inland where its role is complemented or taken over by *An. punctulatus* and *An. koliensis*.

The prevalence of malaria—hyper and holoendemic on the coast—drops at higher altitudes and, above 600 m, the disease tends to be hypoendemic or epidemic. In New Guinea, *Anopheles* does not seem to be found above 1,700-1,800 m, although malaria is epidemic above 1,300 m.

Proximity and modern means of transportation make population exchanges easier between the coast and the interior which was relatively isolated for a long time. The permanent importation of parasites makes it difficult to differentiate transmission zones from import zones.

The inhabitants of hyper and holoendemic zones develop solid immunity which is reflected by a decreased prevalence of splenomegaly by the age of 6 and a reduction in parasite load by the age of 14 (as seen in Tropical Africa).

People living at higher altitudes do not seem to develop defence mechanisms against malaria owing to the low level of transmission. Areas between 600 and 1,300 m are underpopulated.

Jungle clearance operations following migrations or as a consequence of population growth have created larval habitats for *Anopheles* (particularly *An. punctulatus*) thereby worsening the malaria situation. The phenomenon is particularly marked among Javanese immigrants in Western New Guinea.

P. vivax dominated until 1960. Since that time, *P. falciparum* is the species the most frequently reported (accounting for up to 80% of cases). The reason proposed for this shift in the parasite balance is chloroquine resistance although this explanation is not completely satisfactory and DDT indoor spraying may have played a role.

All of the experts report a low malaria mortality rate which they attribute to the availability of drugs and effective immune responses. It is not excluded, however, that the perennial nature of transmission in highly endemic areas promotes the acquisition of immunity, as in Equatorial Africa.

An analysis of malaria in Australasia shows close parallels with the disease in Tropical Africa.

Oriental Region

Limits and subdivisions of the Oriental Region

For the majority of biogeographers, the Oriental Region extends from the Hindu Kush in south-east of Afghanistan to the Moluccas in Indonesia (where it borders the Australasian Region).

The Oriental Region is divided into three subregions:
- the **Indo-Chinese Subregion** which includes the Japanese archipelago of Ryukyu (Tsuda *et al.*, 1999), Taiwan, Vietnam, Laos, Cambodia, Thailand, Myanmar, Bangladesh, China south of the 23rd parallel (including the provinces of Yunnan, Guangxi, Guangdong and Hainan), India (east of the Brahmaputra), Bhutan and Nepal (eastern part). The boundaries between the Indochinese fauna and the palaearctic Chinese fauna between the 20th and the 23rd parallels overlap in four Chinese Provinces (Zhou Zu Jie, 1981);
- the **Malayo-Indonesian Subregion** that includes Indonesia (to the west of the Moluccas), the Philippines, Malaysia (including Peninsular Malaysia), Singapore, Brunei and East Timor. As far as vectors are concerned, this subregion is quite distinct from the Australasian Region;
- the **Indo-Pakistani Subregion** which includes India (to the west of the Brahmaputra), Pakistan, Sri Lanka, the Maldives, Nepal (western part) and Afghanistan (to the east of the Hindu Kush). India is divided on the basis of vector distribution, mainly the presence east of the Brahmaputra of *Anopheles minimus* and *An. dirus*, the most efficient vectors in Asia and part of the Indochinese fauna (*Figure 1*).

The biogeographic status of the part of Asia to the west of the Hindu Kush Mountain range—including Afghanistan, Iran, Iraq and the Arabian Peninsula—is controversial. In the southern parts of these countries, the vectors are Indo-Pakistani, namely *An. culicifacies, An. stephensi* and *An. fluviatilis*; in the north, they are Mediterranean Palaearctic, namely. *An. sacharovi, An. maculipennis, An. hyrcanus, An. superpictus, An. pulcherrimus* and *An. sergentii*; and, in the south-west, they are Afrotropical, notably *An. arabiensis*. Macdonald (1957) joined the Middle East with India proposing an Indo-Iranian Region. In our more biogeographic perspective, we will limit the Oriental Region to the Hindu Kush, as proposed by Rao (1984), and the countries of the Middle East will be considered in the context of the Palaearctic Region.

In the Oriental Region, the variety of climates and weather patterns entails a great diversity of faunal and floral facies from the Indo-Pakistani deserts to the tropical jungles of Borneo, and from the sub-Himalayan steppes to the immense deltas of the Ganges, Indus and Mekong. This region has probably the greatest number of plant and animal species, and more than thirty vector species for malaria parasites (*Table I*) (compared to less than ten in the Afrotropical Region). However, the region has experienced the most devastating ecological damage since the Second World War owing to staggering population growth (India's population now exceeds one billion!) and uncontrolled exploitation of natural resources with modern technologies. This biodiversity is currently threatened with extinction of large animals such as orangutangs, gibbons, rhinoceroses, elephants and tigers—to mention only the most spectacular—already only surviving in reserves or protected areas.

Throughout all of Asia, sparsely inhabited jungles alternate with densely populated plains (extensively occupied by rice paddies). First Chinese and later European colonists accentuated this ecological duality, considering the jungle as "unhealthy" by which they meant malaria-ridden (because of the presence of highly efficient vectors). Two-thousand years ago, among the Han in southern China, it was prohibited to spend the night in the jungle and a link between mosquito and disease was the underpinning of many beliefs.

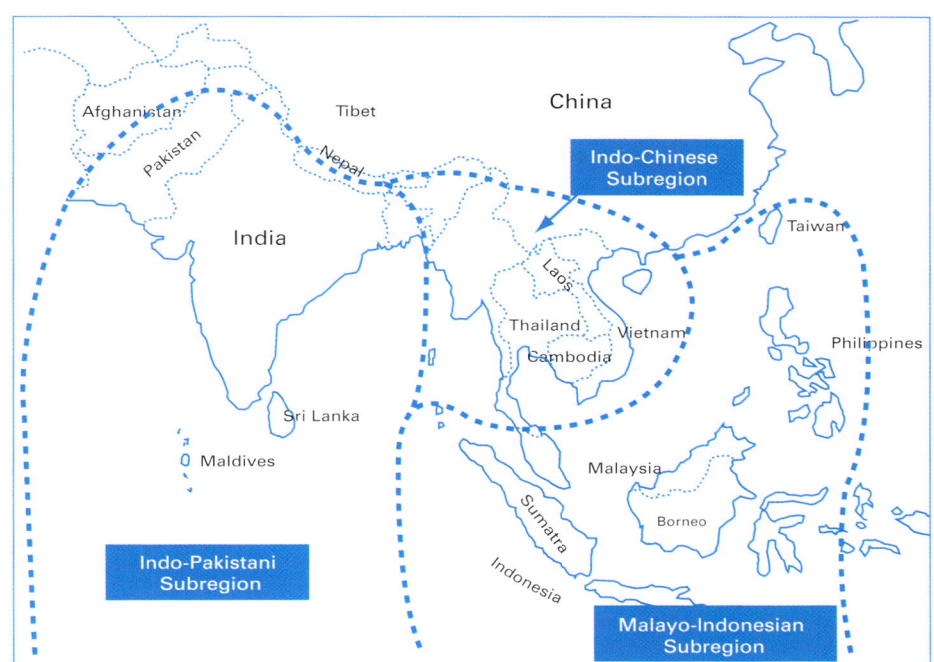

Figure 1.
The Oriental Region.

Table I. *Anopheles* of the Oriental Region (adapted from Harbach, 1994).			
Subgenus *Anopheles*		**Subgenus *Cellia***	
An. lesteri	***	An. aconitus	***
An. barbirostris	*	An. annularis	*
An. campestris	*	An. balabacensis	***
An. donaldi	*	An. culicifacies ABCDE	***
An. kunmigensis	**	An. dirus ABCDE	***
An. letifer	*	An. flavirostris	***
An. nimpe	*	An. fluviatilis STU	***
An. sinensis	***	An. jeyporiensis	**
		An. leucosphyrus A and B	***
		An. litoralis	*
		An. maculatus	***
		An. mangyanus	*
		An. minimus A and C	***
		An. nivipes	**
		An. philippinensis	**
		An. pseudowillmori	**
		An. pulcherrimus	*
		An. sawadwongporni	**
		An. stephensi	***
		An. subpictus	**
		An. sundaicus	***
		An. superpictus	***
		An. tessellatus	*
		An. vagus	*
		An. varuna	*
		An. willmori	**

*** Major vector
** Confirmed vector of local importance
* Secondary or suspected vector

The jungle was originally exploited by hunter-gatherers and nomadic slash-and-burn farmers but our ideas about the prehuman vegetation remain speculative since only a few swaths of primary jungle remain, e.g. in the Mekong Valley in Laos (Vidal, 2000, personal communication) and in Angkor Cambodia.

Over the last thirty years or so, the ecological situation has been changing, and not for the better: slash-and-burn farming intensified with population growth and jungles were felled at the demand of industrialised countries, Japan in particular. The combination of these two practices resulted in the complete devastation of the vegetation. Forest malaria as described by epidemiologists is not a new phenomenon, although one of the results of the anarchic exploitation of jungle resources is exposure of the new forestry workers leading to semi-epidemic disease (Verdrager, 1995).

To the west of the Brahmaputra, the jungle is confined to the highlands where it is steadily being encroached upon for arable land. Rainfall decreases to the west, and both western India and southern Pakistan are characterised by a barren, steppe landscape.

Populations and ethnic minorities

The Oriental Region has a population of nearly two billion people, roughly one third that of the planet. With nearly one billion inhabitants living in its 3,268,000 km^2 of territory, India has a population density of more than 300 inhabitants per square kilometre. There are significant population density differences from one country to another, e.g. in Laos (237,000 km^2), the population density is just 29/km^2 whereas it is nearly ten times that in neighbouring Vietnam (335,000 km^2) with 226/km^2 (*Table II*).

There may also be considerable differences from one part of a country to another, e.g. in Indonesia, the population density is nearly 1,000/km^2 in Java compared with 15/km^2 in Kalimantan and less than 10/km^2 in Western New Guinea. In its efforts to restructure land usage, the Indonesian government has organised apparently voluntary programmed migration between Java, Kalimantan and Western New Guinea. New arrivals have experienced significant problems in malaria-ridden regions, especially people from Western New Guinea (Baird *et al.*, 1993) (*see the Chapter on the* "Australasian Region").

Over the last few decades, Southeast Asia has witnessed remarkable economic growth although the standard of living in a few countries such as Vietnam, Cambodia and Bangladesh is still very low. GNP aside, major differences are seen between certain different social or ethnic groups. "Minorities" in the socialist countries and the tribal peoples of India are greatly disadvantaged in terms of their ability to keep up with technological progress and land rights. The reasons for the isolation of these groups are largely historical; they are descendants of the earliest Southeast Asia humans who are now grouped together as poorly-defined entities such as the Palaeo-Dravidians, the Palaeo-Indo-Chinese and the Malayo-Indonesians.

Starting in the second millennium, Indo-Europeans, arriving from the Iranian plateau, invaded the Indian Peninsula. They introduced Hinduism there and gradually mixed with the Dravidian Peoples of the Deccan Plateau.

During the first millennium AD and up to the 15th century, the Birmans at the outermost bounds of Tibet and the Lao of southern China occupied the plains of Myanmar and Thailand respectively, as well as the Mekong Valley. These peoples introduced Buddhism in these regions. Beginning in the 10th century, the Khins migrated into southern Vietnam, pushing back the Khmers who had settled there previously. People of Malaysian origin occupied the archipelagos of Indonesia, Malaysia and the Philippines.

Indigenous people either intermarried with the invaders or kept their identity and culture (generally animistic), withdrawing into regions of low agronomic value which were difficult to access and/or unhealthy. Among almost **all aboriginal minorities, the incidence of malaria is higher than that in the majority population. Constant immunological stimulation renders those living in areas where malaria is endemic relatively resistant to the disease** because of reduced susceptibility to attacks.

As early as 1914, Perry considered that malaria in the mountains of the State of Orissa had protected the local population against total Hindu domination. Since that time, high prevalences have been documented in Indian minority populations although the data are limited since such questions are considered to be politically sensitive. Broadly speaking, two explanations are possible: either minorities remained confined to territories of little economic interest or difficult to access; or endemic malaria discouraged susceptible invaders. However, other factors may also be important and the debate remains open.

Most of the land occupied by aboriginals is covered in forest which provides both shelter and food. These areas are home to the most dangerous malarial vectors of the Oriental Region (*An. minimus, An. dirus, An. fluviatilis,* and *An. balabacensis*). There is some confusion between "forest malaria" and "tribal" or "minority" malaria.

Minority ethnic groups generally have a very low standard of living (*Figure 2*), much lower than those of the majority ethnic groups living in neighbouring regions or even in the same villages, e.g. in Vietnam (Marchand, *et al.*, 1997), aboriginal Malayo-Indonesians—the Rac Lay of the Danang Region—do not own bicycles, radios,

Table II. Population and size of the countries of the Oriental Region (according to Wikipedia, 2006).					
Country	Size (km^2)	Population (millions)	Country	Size (km^2)	Population (millions)
Bangladesh	143,000	147	Maldives	300	0.3
Bhutan	47,000	2.1	Myanmar	678,000	47.7
Brunei	5,000	0.3	Nepal	140,000	27.7
Cambodia	181,000	13.9	Pakistan	803,000	166
China (Yunnan, Guangxi, Hainan)	552,000	101	Philippines	300,000	89
India	3,268,000	1,120	Singapore	600	4.5
Indonesia (except the Molucas and Western New Guinea)	1,400,000	222	Sri Lanka	66,000	20
Laos	237,000	7	East Timor	15,000	0.9
Malaysia	330,000	27	Vietnam	335,000	85
			TOTAL	8,500,900	2,081.1

Oriental Region

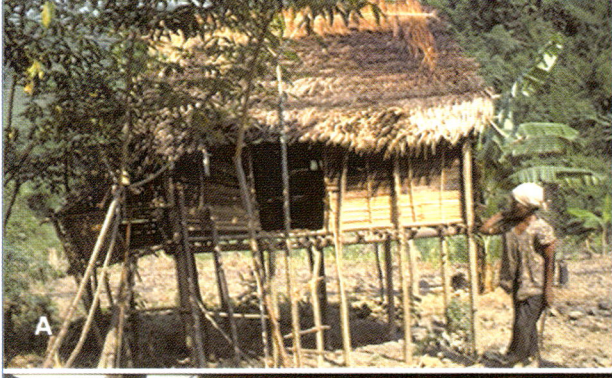
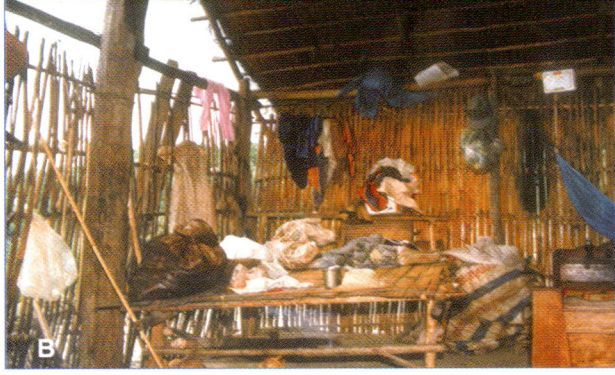

*Figure 2. Vietnam. **A.** An isolated jungle house inhabited by ethnic minorities. **B.** Ethnic minority home (Rac Lay ethnic group), very open to Anopheles. Note the sparse furniture (photograph by Marchand).*

furniture or mosquito nets. They are highly exposed to malaria and do not have the means or money to protect themselves. They suffer five times more malarial paroxysms than Khins (the majority ethnic group) living in the same village.

All the published reports attest to this kind of poverty: in the Koraput District (Orissa, India), the monthly salary of the Boda was 250 rupees in 1988 and their social status was that of agricultural labourers; their literacy rate did not exceed 2-5% (Rajagopalan *et al.*, 1990).

In Malaysia, the semi-nomadic Orang Asli jungle people are more malaria-stricken than the rest of the population (Bolton, 1972). Due to the permanent exposure, the aboriginal people develop immunity or some form of resistance to malaria.

Among the Tharu of the Terai in Nepal, the number of episodes of clinical malaria is seven times lower than in the rest of the population (Terrenato *et al.*, 1988) and malarial morbidity is ten times lower: this is due to the very high frequency of homozygotic α-thalassaemia in this population (Modiano *et al.*, 1991), an allele which may be selected for by the presence of holo-endemic malaria although it has never been conclusively demonstrated that this type of haemoglobinopathy affords any protection.

There are more than fifty minorities in Vietnam along with the Lao Theung of Laos, and they all experience as many malarial attacks as the rest of the population although the paroxysms are generally less severe (Nguyen Tang Am, personal communication).

The frequency of glucose-6-phosphate dehydrogenase deficiency (G-6PD) varies considerably from one ethnic group to another. It is very low among the Khins of Vietnam and the Hmongs of the highlands (< 1%) and reaches 31% among the Muong (Meo) living in the plateau regions. In these latter groups, co-evolution of man with the parasite seems to have resulted in the selection of an advantageous genetic trait (Verlé *et al.*, 2000) although actual evidence about this advantage remains weak.

Governments have pursued different policies *vis-à-vis* their particular minority populations. In China, "minorities" live in the autonomous Yunnan and Guangxi Regions as well as the autonomous counties of Miao and Li in Hainan. In India, the north-eastern States (Nagaland, Aranuchal Pradesh, Mizoram, Tripura and Manipur) are for the most part inhabited by so-called tribal peoples, who are in latent revolt against the central government; the highly represented "minorities" of the Madhya Pradesh, Orissa (Boda-Koraput), Tamil Nadu (Nilgiris) and the Nicobar Islands do not enjoy any particular status. In Myanmar, the Shan and Karen minorities persist in a guerrilla state. In Vietnam, Laos and Cambodia, aboriginal people do not have any special status although they are relatively economically disadvantaged (in a population that is already extremely poor).

There is very little information available about malaria among the Dayaks of Borneo, the aboriginal people of Sumatra and Sulawesi in Indonesia, or those of the Philippines. In Bangladesh and Pakistan, minorities do not seem to pose any ethnic problem or, at least, no mention is made of it; in this context, Islam has a unifying influence.

Many minorities—which have been subordinate to and ignored by the dominant powers for centuries—are reclaiming their political and cultural identities by reviving their traditional religions; others are cohering around the Christian missions founded in the latter part of last century by the colonial powers, or Islam. It is important to remember that malaria is **more prevalent in such peoples than in other ethnic groups** living in the same place, and **their immunity means that they experience fewer clinical paroxysms and fewer episodes**.

Forest malaria and migration

Up to the middle of the 20th century, Southeast Asia, notably the Indo-Chinese and Malayo-Indonesian Subregions, were covered in jungle. The jungle began to thin out to the west in the Indo-Pakistani Subregion.

Biodiversity of Malaria in the World

Nearly one hundred years ago, it was known that there was far more malaria in the jungle than in the arable plains, even before the epidemiology of the disease had been characterised. Following "eradication" campaigns, the jungle remained the only endemic area and malaria experts coined the term "forest malaria". As far as Southeast Asia is concerned, this term is redundant as malaria is concentrated in the jungles as a result of the vectors' ecological niche, as will be discussed extensively further on.

Relationships between malaria and the jungle can be considered under four headings: traditional jungle exploitation; the industrial exploitation of jungle resources; permanent settlements within the jungle; and degradation of the jungle.

Traditional jungle exploitation

Until recently, the jungle was inhabited by minority ethnic groups who engaged in more or less nomadic slash-and-burn agriculture (shifting cultivation). The low population density meant that crops could be rotated every twenty years or so, allowing for progressive regeneration of the natural environment in which aboriginal people lived in harmony. The status of these people with respect to malarial disease was discussed earlier.

The situation has changed since the end of the World War II. The population has grown, so that the natural environment does not necessarily have enough time to regenerate itself after burning. At the same time, as a consequence of the population explosion, "colonists" came searching for available spaces in the jungle where they could settle (*Figure 3*). Sedentary agriculture, rice-growing in particular, replaced shifting cultivation methods and the number of people living in permanent clearings increased.

Rubber plantations have been expanding since 1930 and now provide a secondary jungle habitat where *An. dirus* thrives (*Figure 4*).

Industrial exploitation of jungle resources

Forestry has become a lucrative business in dealing with the demand for structural timber and paper pulp in industrialized countries, particularly Japan and South Korea. The labour employed in these activities often comes from non-endemic regions or cities (*Figure 5*). Without any immunity whatsoever, the labourers are at very high risk and severe malarial attacks are frequent among them although they seemed to be relatively rare among established jungle inhabitants. In Thailand for example, forestry is often a semi-clandestine activity where the workers live in deplorable conditions in makeshift shelters where they are directly exposed to the vectors. In Cambodia, the use of treated mosquito nets has been encouraged to protect these workers. As they are aware of the risk, the workers go to the corner

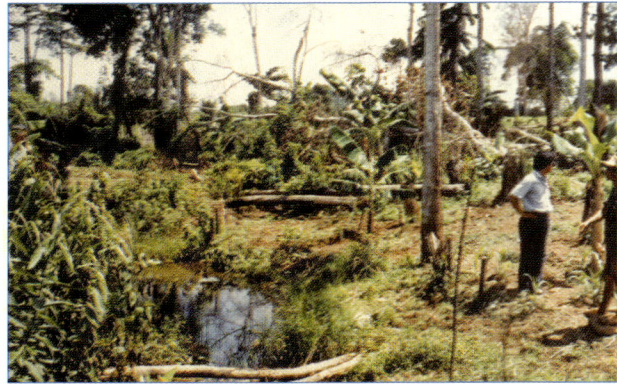

Figure 3. *Vietnam, southern plateaux: clearing of the forest for cultivation (photograph by Mouchet).*

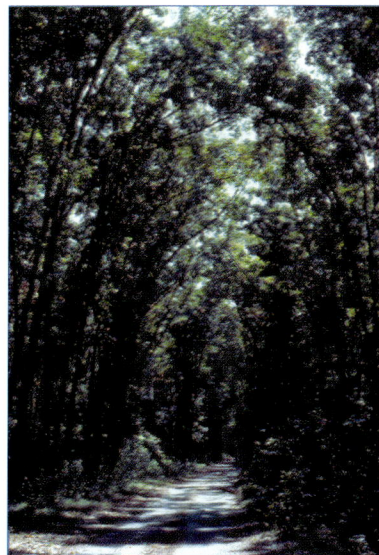

Figure 4. *Cambodia, southern forests: rubber plantation (An. dirus larval habitats) (photograph by Manguin).*

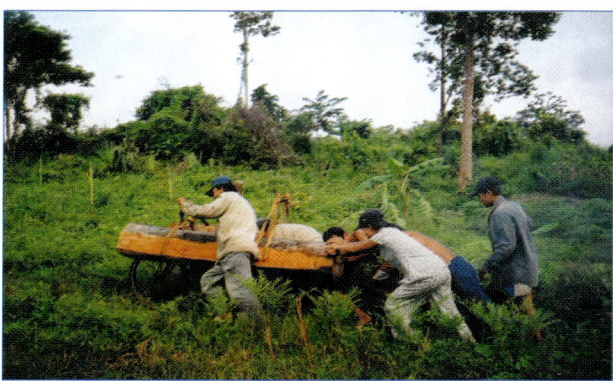

Figure 5. *Vietnam: lumberjacks, a high-risk group (photograph by Coosemans).*

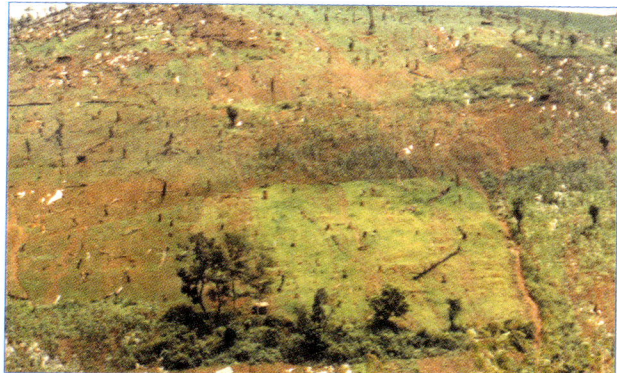

Figure 6. Laos, Plain of Jarres: jungle clearance *(photograph by Mouchet).*

shop to buy remedies, the composition of which is unknown to both user and shopkeeper.

The other jungle activity-related risk throughout the whole of Indochina is the search for precious stones, particularly sapphires and rubies. This activity is often illegal and is practiced in very rudimentary conditions. In southern Vietnam, cases of severe malaria have been recorded in the mangrove jungle among crab and shell gatherers (Nguyen Tang Am, personal communication, 1996).

Permanent settlements within the jungle

The "colonisation" of the jungle by immigrants proceeded either in accordance with planned schemes (e.g. the transmigration program in Indonesia) or, in many instances, through anarchic occupation of the land.

The first step consists in building housing, generally rudimentary, in the centre of the cleared field. Farmers are in more or less direct contact with the vectors from the surrounding jungle, i.e. they are as exposed as the indigenous population (Marchand *et al.,* 1997).

The second step is the construction of villages with huts in the fields where workers can shelter from inclement weather. In Thailand, the prevalence of infection is three times higher in farmers who spend part of the year in such huts than it is in sedentary villagers (Somboon, *et al.,* 1994); similar observations have been reported in Vietnam (Marchand *et al.,* 1997) and Bangladesh (Rosenberg & Maheswary, 1982).

Programmed installations generally include health centres that provide the migrants with medical assistance and sometimes vector control resources. Unfortunately, the "colonists" often depend on a parallel market of peddlers who supply medications, the quality of which is often doubtful and which are not always matched to the problem. More than 30% of the peddlers—who had no formal medical training—prescribed Vitamin C for malaria and only 40-50% proposed antimalarial drugs (MacDonald, personal communication, 1996).

Degradation of the jungle

The new post-jungle landscape of Southeast Asia consists of more or less extensive gaps between stands of jungle marked by plumes of smoke, bearing witness to slash-and-burn operations. The end stage is total disappearance of tree cover as is already the case throughout vast zones of Thailand, Vietnam, Malaysia and Indonesia and, to a lesser extent, Laos and Cambodia (*Figure 6*). Even though the governments concerned recognise deforestation as an ecological catastrophe, the measures implemented to combat it appear rather half-hearted given the magnitude of the problem.

When the two jungle vectors persist, *An. dirus* often dominates *An. minimus* (Meek, 1995). A significant place should be made however for the Maculatus Group—*An. maculatus, An. sawadwongporni* and *An. pseudowillmori*—in recently deforested areas (Harbach *et al.,* 1987b; Rattanarithikul *et al.,* 1996b).

It is difficult to predict the effects of deforestation on the anopheline fauna although, already, the vector role of the Maculatus Group is developing, with sporozoite rates identical to or even higher than those of *An. minimus* and *An. dirus*.

Occupational malaria. Temporary labour

Occupational malaria has been long recognised in India, notably in the tea plantations in Assam, to which people from regions with little or no malaria transmission come as seasonal labourers. As it is often performed by temporary workers from non-endemic cities or zones, forestry is currently one of the main factors in the incidence of severe malaria in Thailand, Cambodia and Vietnam in particular. The sickness affects primarily adults (Harinasuta & Reynolds, 1985; Kondrashin, 1992; Phan, 1998). The same situation is encountered among gemstone hunters (*Figure 7*).

Seasonal labourers are often at very high risk and they rarely have any substantial social support or health insurance.

Population displacements and migration

Kondrashin (1992) proposed a classification of various forms of migration or, more generally, population displacements.

At the district level, migrations are relatively local phenomena, with people moving from the countryside to the city in search of employment; this trend is referred to as the rural exodus. People may also move from the city to the countryside in search of space, or to colonise new land. These migrations can be of relatively short duration, lasting just a few days or weeks; more long term—sometimes definitive—displacements involve a change of residence and result in a sustained change in the environment.

The legal or illegal crossing of borders often involves a stop and sometimes a health inspection. In the Yunnan and Guangxi Provinces of China, a large majority of the malaria cases are detected along the borders with Myanmar, Laos and Vietnam (Hu *et al.*, 1998; Xu & Liu, 1997).

Extensive studies (including drug resistance profiles) have been conducted on refugees coming into Thailand from Myanmar and Cambodia because these migrants are readily accessible (Luxemburger *et al.*, 1996; Meek, 1988). The massive treatment which the refugees had been given was considered a factor in promoting the development of multiresistant strains of *Plasmodium*.

Little has been said in the literature about the malaria epidemic which occurred among Cambodians deported to forced labour camps by the Khmer Rouge. Many of these people were from the non-endemic region of Phnom Penh and mortality was massive although real figures were never accurately gauged. This is not an isolated case and deportees to re-education camps in many countries have sustained devastating losses. Given the renewed interest in pursuing war criminals, light needs to be shed on these dark periods during which various diseases—poorly treated or totally ignored by camp commandants—were a major cause of mortality; in this context, malaria cannot be ignored.

Kondrashin (1992) considers religious pilgrimages and tourist trips as a relevant problem although, on the basis of available medical statistics, these risks can probably be discounted. In the other direction, immigrant labourers, particularly from Pakistan, India and the Philippines, could introduce malaria into the countries of Europe, the United States and the Persian Gulf (where malaria is absent or rare). However, the highly-developed health care structures in these countries ensure that any cases are quickly treated.

Parasites

Plasmodial species

All four species of human *Plasmodium* are found in the Oriental Region although their frequencies vary enormously.

Plasmodium ovale is rare, with single reports from India, Vietnam and Thailand. A variant was observed in a Vietnamese man and in five Japanese subjects who had been infected in Vietnam (Miyake *et al.*, 1997). These morphologically indistinguishable variants can be distinguished on the basis of their ribosomal DNA.

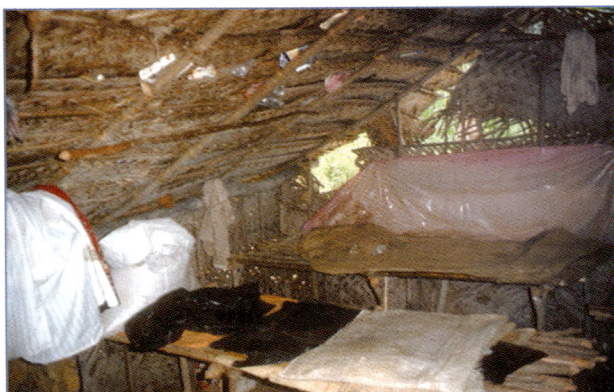

Figure 7. Sri Lanka: temporary shelter for gemstone searchers (photograph by Coosemans).

The frequency of *P. malariae* is generally less than 2%. It was found in 1-2% of cases in Vietnam (Marchand *et al.*, 1997; Phan, 1998), 1.3% of cases in Thailand (Somboon *et al.*, 1998), 1.1% in India (Yadav *et al.*, 1990) and sporadically in China (Zhou Zu-Jie, 1981). Owing to the length of its sporogonic cycle (generally over twenty days), it can only propagate in Oriental Region anophelines with a very high life expectancy, namely *An. minimus, An. dirus, An. sundaicus* or *An. fluviatilis*.

P. vivax and *P. falciparum* are the dominant parasites throughout the entire zone although the relative frequency of the two species varies considerably with environment and vector (Yadava & Sharma, 1995).

P. vivax is the dominant—and sometimes unique—species in the Indo-Pakistani Subregion as well as on the plains of the Indo-Chinese Subregion where it is often responsible for hypo-endemic or epidemic malaria. In contrast, in the Indo-Chinese and Malayo-Indonesian Subregions (where the vectors are *An. minimus, An. dirus, An. balabacensis* and *An. sundaicus*), *P. falciparum* is the dominant parasite and the disease is correspondingly more severe.

In Vietnam, official statistics report 72% *P. falciparum* and 28% *P. vivax* (Morillon *et al.*, 1996). In Luang Prabang, Laos, the proportions were identical (Pholsena, personal communication) but in the Mekong plain, around Vientiane, the proportions were reversed (Southammavong, 1997). In Thailand, the proportion of *P. falciparum* to *P. vivax* was 80% from 1965 to 1973, then 55% to 45% from 1976 to 1992. The relative increase of *P. vivax* occurred despite the development of drug resistance which would supposedly favour *P. falciparum* (Prasittisuk, 1985). In Bhutan, 4,000 *P. falciparum* were recorded for 3,000 *P. vivax* (Rajagopal, 1985). In Assam, India, the proportion of the two parasites was 50/50 bordering the plain but, in the Bangladesh River Delta, *P. vivax* was basically the only species present. In Pakistan (Farid, 1987), 29,000 *P. falciparum* were recorded on 90,000 positive slides. The percentage of each species is greatly influenced by vector control operations which had a greater impact on *P. falciparum* than on *P. vivax* (which can persist in the hypnozoite form).

The average relapse rate of *P. vivax* in India was 40% (Sharma *et al.*, 1990) and 54% in Nepal, with a higher rate in the highlands than in the lowlands (Kondrashin & Sakya, 1981). All reports highlight the difficulties of treating *P. vivax* malaria with primaquine among people with glucose-6-phosphate dehydrogenase deficiency.

Rosenberg *et al.* (1989) showed heterogeneity in *P. vivax* sporozoites. Approximately 14% of infected subjects were producing sporozoites immunologically distinct from those identified during a circumsporozoite protein test. *P. vivax* variants based on CircumSporozoite Protein (CSP) differences have also been studied recently in Brazil (*see the Chapter on the* "American Regions").

In parts of Thailand where transmission is low, *P. falciparum* was genetically diverse with many different genotypes observed (Paul *et al.*, 1998; Thaithong, 1994), heterogeneity being promoted by cross-border exchanges with Myanmar. The same enzyme polymorphism is observed in India (Joshi *et al.*, 1989) and the phenomenon has been extensively probed in numerous studies in Tropical Africa.

Mention should also be made of the fact that *P. cynomolgi bastianelli* has been isolated in humans in the Oriental Region (in Malaysia). This discovery led to a lot of discussions with many authors questioning whether or not this parasite is a zoonosis which could compromise eradication strategies (Coatney *et al.*, 1971). Recently, it was observed that *P. simiovale* in Sri Lankan macaques could not be distinguished from the human *P. vivax*-like parasite in Brazil (*see the Chapter on the* "American Regions").

Asymptomatic malaria

To a certain degree, the presence of asymptomatic, infected carriers is considered as proof of the existence of protective immune responses. In the holo-endemic zones of the Afrotropical Region, the proportion of asymptomatic carriers exceeds 90% suggesting that adults and even teenagers are strongly protected. In the Oriental Region, the number of asymptomatic-carriers varies enormously and it is impossible to gauge the significance of this parameter in terms of protection against the disease. The discussion hereafter is limited to the currently available data.

Among a group of Karen refugees from Myanmar living in Thailand, 68% of 4-14 year-olds were symptomatic with an average of 1.5 attacks per annum. The pyrogenic threshold was 1,460 *P. falciparum* per microlitre of blood and 180 *P. vivax* per microlitre; this is significantly lower than in Africa where it is at least 5,000 and up to 10,000 (Luxemburger *et al.*, 1998).

In Thailand, Prasittisuk *et al.* (1994) recorded 5.1% of asymptomatic carriers as opposed to 3.2% with symptoms.

In Vietnam, among the "minorities" considered to be malaria-tolerant, half of the cases were considered as asymptomatic (Phan, 1998); according to Marchand *et al.* (1997), 90% of individuals in the Rac Lay ethnic group were asymptomatic compared with just 30% among the majority Kinh people.

In Pakistan, attacks are seen in teenagers and adults with parasite loads of below 1,000 per µl (Prybylski *et al.*, 1999).

Vectors

General information about the anopheline fauna of the Oriental Region

The anopheline fauna of the Oriental Region is extremely diverse with about thirty species that have been designated as vectors. In *Table I*, Harbach's classification (1994, 2004) has been adopted in which two subgenera, *Anopheles* and *Cellia*, invest the region. Recent genetic research has led to the splitting of certain taxonomic units into different forms which are morphologically very similar or even identical: these different forms are designated by the letters A, B, C, D, etc., following the former name of the species. This remains a provisional naming system since every species will have to be designated by genus and species names attributed in the adopted international binominal classification.

Priority has thus been given to the most epidemiologically important vectors while brief mention is made of some species of local interest and secondary vectors (the role of some of which remains controversial).

Certain Palaearctic species encroach upon the Oriental Region only at its northern borders, notably *An. superpictus* and *An. pulcherrimus* in Pakistan and India, and *An. sinensis* and *An. anthropophagus* in southern China. To the east, however, the border with the Australasian Region is well defined.

Minimus Complex (Figure 8)

An. minimus Theobald 1901 was described in Hong Kong from where it seems to have disappeared with urbanisation. It is the major vector of the Indo-Chinese Subregion and its range corresponds exactly to this geographic entity. It has been reported to the east of Nepal (Shrestha 1966), in all States of north-eastern India (Rao, 1984), Bhutan (Rajagopal, 1985), Bangladesh (Khan & Talibi, 1972), Myanmar (Khin-Maung-Kyi, 1971), Thailand (Harinasuta *et al.*, 1976), Laos (Pholsena, 1992), Vietnam (Phan, 1998), Cambodia (Chow, 1970), China, south of the 23rd parallel (Chow, 1948; Zhou-Zu-Jie, 1981), Taiwan (Chang *et al.*, 1950) and in the Ryukyu Islands, Japan (Tsuda *et al.*, 1999) (*Figure 9*).

Since malaria eradication indoor DDT spraying campaigns began in 1950, *An. minimus* seems to have disappeared from Nepal (Parajuli *et al.*, 1981), and its numbers have

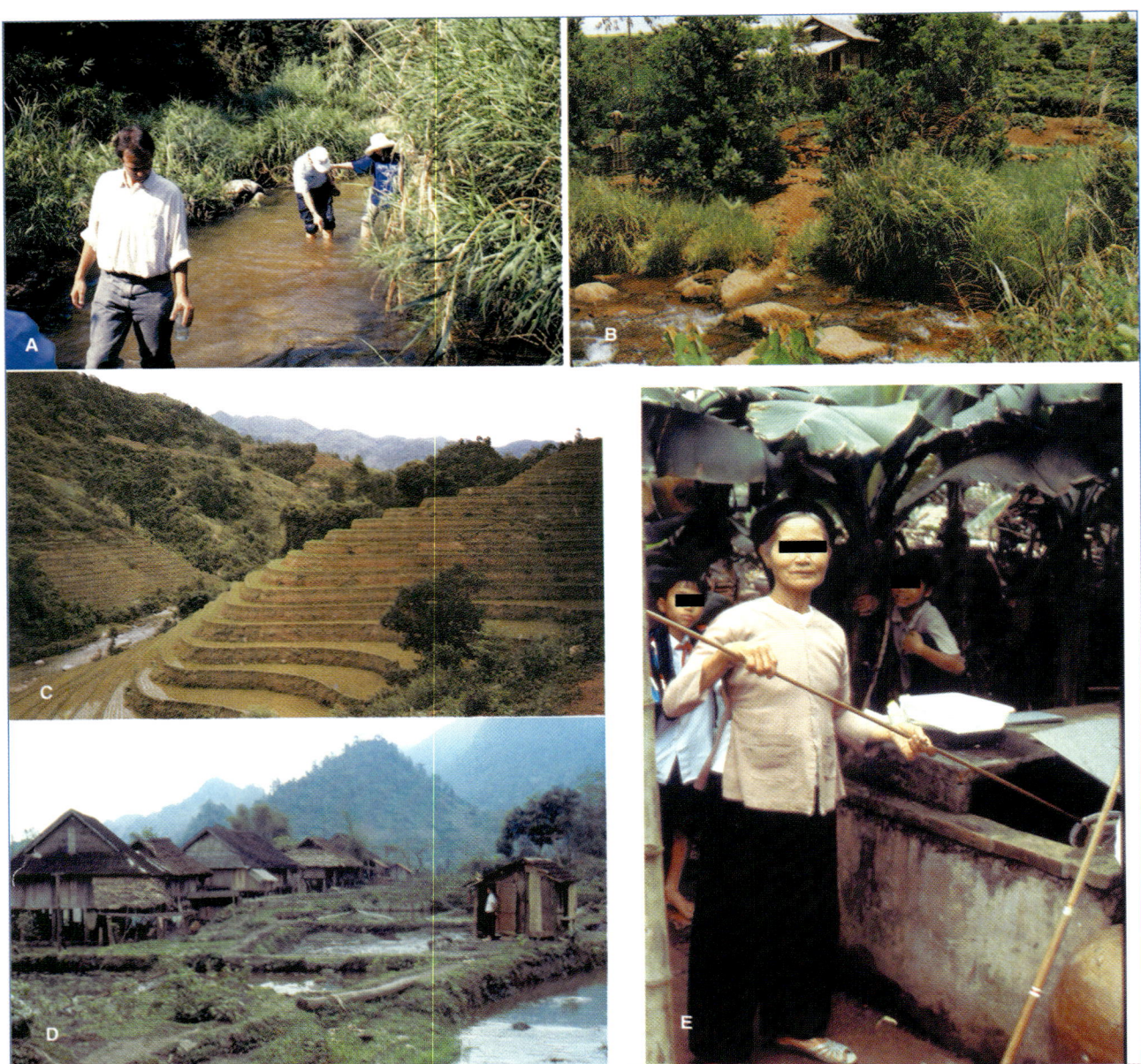

Figure 8. An. minimus *larval habitats.*
A. Stream in northern Vietnam (photograph by Coosemans). B. Stream near a home (photograph by Nguyen Duc Can in Vu Ti Phan, 1998). C. Terraced rice paddies in the mountains (photograph by May Hoanh in Vu Thi Phan, 1998). D. Hillside rice paddy canals, Hoa Binh, Vietnam (photograph by Manguin). E. Water tank, Hanoi (photograph by Manguin).

been considerably reduced in both north-eastern India (Das *et al.*, 1990; Malakar *et al.*, 1995; Rajagopal, 1976) and southern China.

The larvae of this species develop in clearwater streams flowing at speeds of below two m/sec and bordered by aquatic vegetation providing moderate shade. They adapt well to terraced hillside rice paddies in which the water is renewed continually. They occupy hilly regions below 800 m in northern Vietnam, and below 1,500 m in the south (Phan, 1998; Tho Vien *et al.*, 1996). Larval habitats are located in the lowest areas (Hu *et al.*, 1998) of Yunnan Province in China, where the temperature changes by 0.6°C with every 100 m rise in elevation. *An. minimus* has persisted in deforested areas throughout most of its range.

An. minimus larvae have also been collected in stagnant water in the suburbs of Hanoi in northern Vietnam (Phan,

Oriental Region

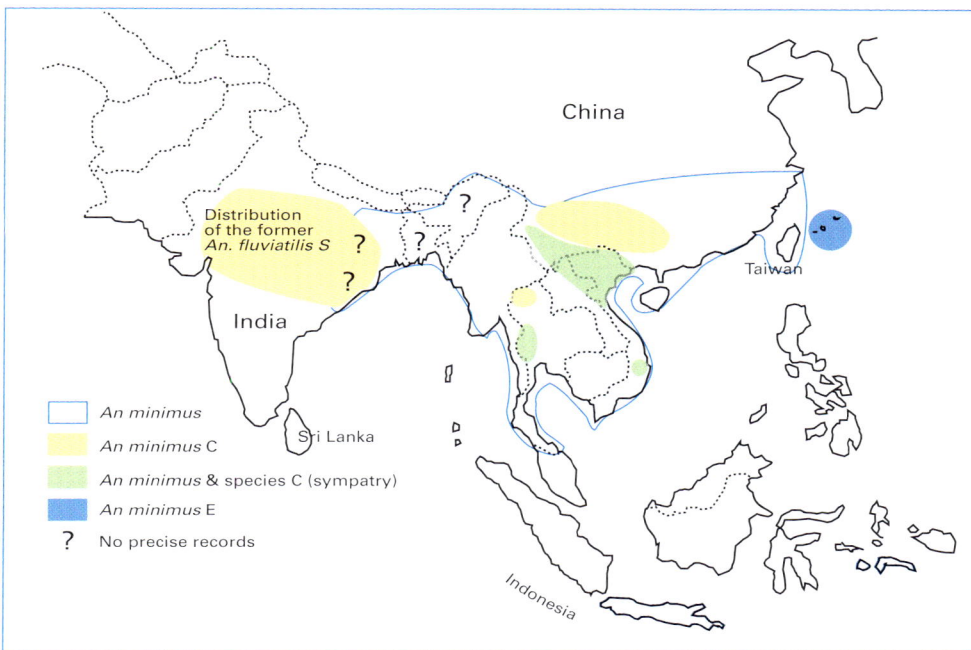

Figure 9.
Distribution of the three species of the An. minimus Complex (adapted from Garros et al., 2006) in Southeast Asia with the Indian extension of the suspected An. minimus C, synonymous with An. fluviatilis S (adapted from Harbach et al., 2004).

1998; Tho Vien, 1992a), although they do not appear to have been transmitting malaria.

An. minimus is known for its endophilic and anthropophilic behaviour and was known to bite throughout the night (Rattanarithikul *et al.*, 1996a), especially the second part (Rao, 1984). This behaviour made it a highly vulnerable target for indoor spraying (and insecticide treated mosquito nets) which explains why it became increasingly scarce, and even disappeared in many places.

An upsurge in the numbers of this species and a change in its behaviour was observed beginning in 1975, in northern Thailand (Ismail *et al.*, 1975, 1978). An increase was noted in the percentage of specimens feeding on animals outside homes (Rattanarithikul *et al.*, 1996a) and it was observed that they soon leave the areas where they have been feeding to search for external shelter (Nutsathapana *et al.*, 1986a); furthermore, they bite earlier at night (Harbach *et al.*, 1987b). Similar observations were made in Vietnam (Phan, 1998; Tho Vien *et al.*, 1996) and Myanmar (Myo Paing *et al.*, 1988).

These behavioural differences suggest the existence of a species complex within *An. minimus* (Nutsathapana *et al.*, 1986b). Proof was provided in Thailand (Sucharit *et al.*, 1988), Vietnam (Van Bortel *et al.*, 1999) and China (Chen *et al.*, 2002) where two distinct species, A and C, were identified. *An. minimus s.s.* (formerly species A)—endophilic and anthropophilic—behaves like the classic *An. minimus* as described prior to vector control campaigns. Species C is three times less frequent in homes and more zoophilic. To date, these two species have been sympatric although studies of their distributions, ecologies and respective vector roles has only just begun. A third species, *An. minimus* E, has also been described on Ishigaki Island in the Ryukyu Archipelago of Japan, a malaria-free region (Somboon *et al.*, 2001, 2005). Experiments have shown that F1 crosses between species A and E, and species C and E are sterile (Somboon *et al.* 2001; 2005). Both studies showed hybrid male sterility, which is generally accepted as very clear evidence of distinct species. Therefore to date, three sibling species, *An. minimus s.s.*, species C and species E, are currently recognised within the Minimus Complex (Garros *et al.* 2006; Harbach 2004) although they cannot be reliably distinguished on the basis of any morphological criteria. This Minimus Complex belongs to the Minimus Subgroup, itself part of the Funestus Group which includes four other subgroups with species distributed in either Asia or tropical Africa (Garros *et al.* 2005; Harbach 2004).

In China, in the Yunnan and Guangxi Provinces (Sawabe *et al.*, 1997) and on the island of Hainan (Yuan Yu, 1987), two forms, A and B, have been described. Recently, Chen *et al.* (2002) showed that these two forms A and B are morphological variants of *An. minimus s.s.* (formerly species A).

The stagnant water forms in northern Vietnam have been identified through genetic and isoenzyme analysis as belonging to *An. minimus s.s.*(species A).

Very high sporozoite rates—of the order of 5%—were recorded in Vietnam in 1936 (Toumanoff, 1936) and in India in the 1950's (Rao, 1984). Recently, lower sporozoite rates (0.3-1%) have been reported in Thailand (Gingrich *et al.*, 1990; Harbach *et al.*, 1987b). No infection was recorded in the refugee camps along the Thai-Khmer border (Meek, 1988).

According to more recent information, it appears that the vector capacity of *An. minimus s.s.* is greater than that of species C in Thailand (Somboon *et al.*, 1998). In central Vietnam, Marchand *et al.* (1997) reported sporozoite rates of 3.6%, very close to those observed prior to eradication operations, these were associated with strongly anthropophilic and endophilic behaviour. In several countries of the subregion, *An. minimus* is coming back, apparently due to relaxation or suppression of vector control measures.

Available information indicates that both *An. minimus* species A and C exhibit considerable behavioural and ecological plasticity; sympatry was underestimated and it seems that species C is more widely distributed on the Asian continent than suspected; and high biological heterogeneity is evident depending on the geographic location, abundance of cattle, and the density of houses (Garros *et al.*, 2006). However, the relative importance of the individual species in malaria transmission, as well as the specific biological variability of their bionomics, should be further analysed using molecular methods over their ranges of distribution.

Leucosphyrus Group

An. leucosphyrus had been reported as early as 1926 in the rubber plantations of southern Vietnam (Borel, 1926a). In 1936, Baisas was identifying *An. balabacensis* that he distinguished from *An. leucosphyrus* whose distribution range was reduced to the Malayo-Indonesian Subregion.

In 1979, Peyton & Harrison divided *An. balabacensis* into three species: *An. balabacensis s.s.* of the Malayo-Indonesian Subregion, *An. dirus* of the Indo-Chinese and Indo-Pakistani Subregions and *An. takasagoensis* in Taiwan.

Beginning in 1988, Baimai (1988), Baimai *et al.* (1988a and b) and Peyton (1990) divided the Leucosphyrus Group into the Leucosphyrus Complex and the Dirus Complex.

The former (Sallum *et al.*, 2005) includes *An. latens* (species A), *An. leucosphyrus* (species B of Baimai *et al.*, 1988), *An. balabacensis* of the Malayo-Indonesian Subregion and *An. introlatus*, a vector of plasmodies simiennes in Malaysia. The latter complex includes seven species, *An. dirus* A, B, C, D, E, *An. nemophilus* (species F, a zoophilic species) and *An. takasagoensis* (Baimai *et al.*, 1988b).

Dirus Complex (*Figure 10*)

The five species of the *An.dirus* Complex designated by letters have recently been named as follows: *An. dirus* (species A), *An. cracens* (species B), *An. scanloni* (species C), *An. baimai* (species D), *An. elegans* (species E) by Sallum *et al.* (2005).

An. dirus and *An. baimai* (species A and D respectively) appear to share Indochina: the first is found to the east of a central line that splits Thailand and includes Laos, Cambodia, Vietnam (south of the Red River), the island of Hainan and probably the Ryukyu Islands; the second predominates to the west of Thailand, including Myanmar, Bhutan, Bangladesh and the States of north-eastern India (*Figure 11*).

An. cracens (species B), previously known as the "Perlis" form (named after the city in Malaysia), invests the Malaysian peninsula, principally on either side of the border with Thailand.

An. scanloni (species C) has been observed on the eastern coast of the Thai peninsula and near the Myanmar border; its behaviour is different from other species in the complex and it bites at nightfall.

An. elegans (species E) has an eccentric distribution, in the regions of Western Ghats in south-western India, in the States of Karnataka and Tamil Nadu (Bhat, 1988; Kalra &

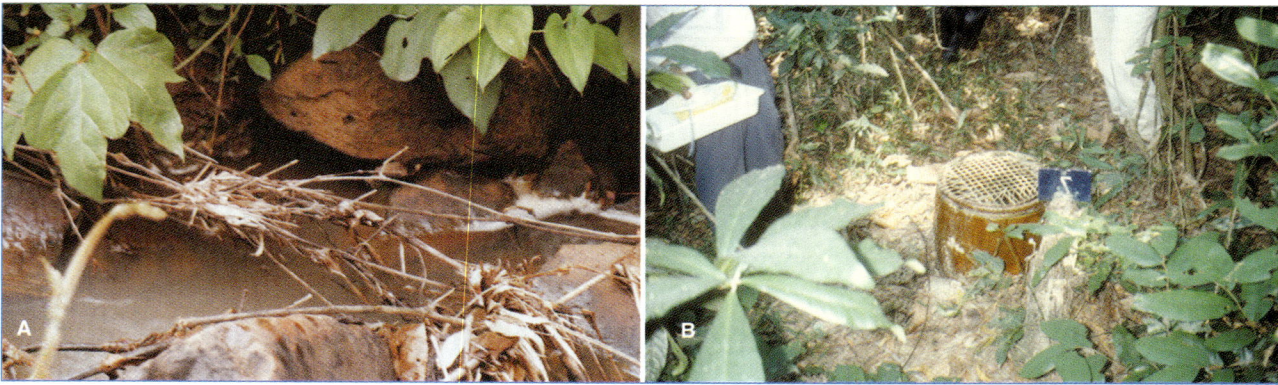

Figure 10. **A.** *Stagnant water near streams in the forest,* An. dirus *larval habitats (photograph by Nguyen Duc Can in Vu Thin Phan, 1998).* **B.** An. dirus *egg traps (photograph by Coosemans).*

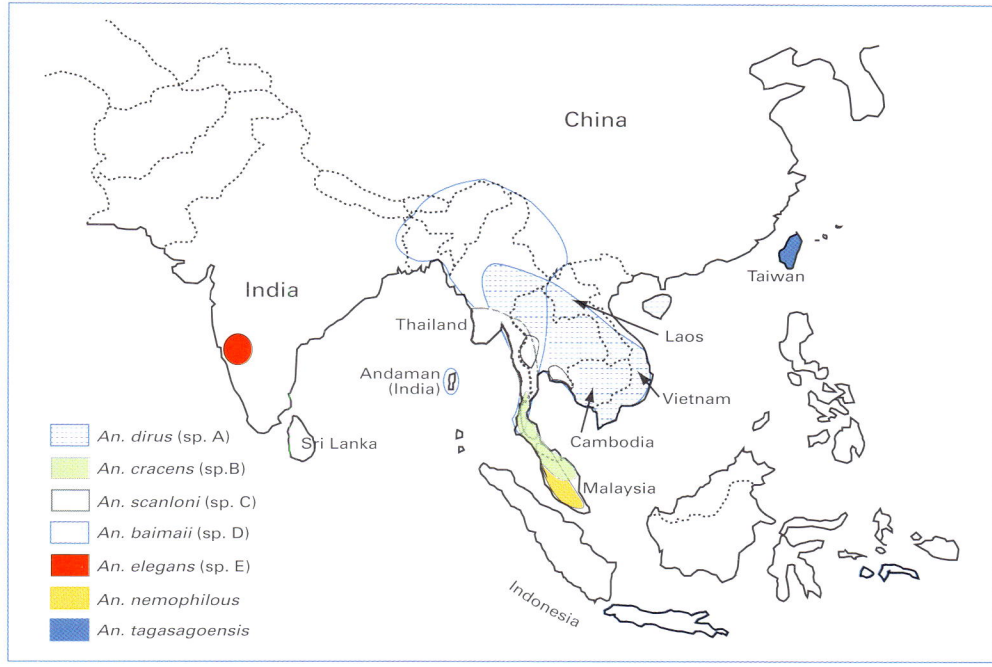

Figure 11.
Distribution of the seven species of the An. dirus *Complex (adapted from Obsomer et al., 2007 and Sallum et al., 2005).*

Watal, 1962; Sawadipanich *et al.*, 1990; Tewari *et al.*, 1987).

In China, outside the island of Hainan, the significance and typology of the small populations above 1,000 m in Yunnan Province warrant special investigation; nor is the taxonomic status of the specimens of the Indian Andaman Islands known (Nagpal & Sharma, 1983). Finally, the unexplained absence of *An. dirus s.l.* north of Danang, Vietnam should also be emphasised (Phan, 1998).

Since the 1960's when it was known as *An. balabacensis*, *An. dirus* was considered as the "*bête noire*" in malaria eradication in Southeast Asia, following the reduction in numbers and even disappearance of *An. minimus*. The work conducted by Rodenfeldt, Kow Phan & Cervone in 1963 (cited by Sloof & Verdrager, 1972), at the Snuol experimental station in Cambodia, showed that *An. dirus* tends to exit the house once it has fed. After nine weeks, the mortality in homes treated with DDT was only 48%, while the daily life expectancy of *An. dirus* was still 0.89 in untreated villages. This thus explains the relative failure of conventional Indoor Residual Spraying (IRS) of human houses with DDT.

Since 1965 (Scanlon & Sandhinand, 1965), many articles have been published on the exophilic behaviour of *An. dirus* and its consequences. Not only does its behaviour complicate insecticide treatment but also its jungle and rural habitat means that it tends to bite outside villages inside temporary, rudimentary dwelling structures. In fact, it is three times more aggressive in these huts than in village homes (Marchand *et al.*, 1997; Somboon *et al.*, 1998). Furthermore, *An. dirus* has adapted very well to rubber plantations (Tang Am, personal communication) in southern Vietnam.

Jungle farmers, often belonging to ethnic minorities, are the most exposed. These people engage in nomadic slash-and-burn farming methods and live in poor conditions (Marchand *et al.*, 1997). To this group should be added the temporary jungle workers, seasonal labourers, rubber workers, and all low wage-earning groups who do not have the means to protect themselves against the vectors or buy drugs.

It is worth noting that the affinity of *An. dirus* for humans is matched by its affinity for monkeys (Eyles *et al.*, 1964), reservoirs for Simian *Plasmodium*.

Assuming that the larval habitats of each species have been correctly identified, the larvae develop in puddles of stagnant water in the undergrowth, and sometimes in tree trunks and hollow stumps. In Myanmar, larvae have been observed in cisterns and wells (Htay-Aung *et al.*, 1999; Tin, 1992; Tun-Lin *et al.*, 1987).

Sporozoite rates of 1-1.6% have been recorded in India (Pradesh *et al.*, 1997; Rajagopal, 1976), 3.8% in Bangladesh (Rosenberg & Maheswary, 1982), 2.9-7% in Cambodia (Sloof & Verdrager, 1972), 3.6% in Myanmar (Khin-Maung-Kyi & Winn, 1976), up to 6% in Thailand (Scanlon & Sandhinand, 1965), and 2-3.9% in Vietnam (Marchand *et al.*, 1997; Phan, 1998).

An. dirus s.l. is now the main vector of malaria in the Indo-Chinese Subregion. Much remains to be done, however, to determine the spatial distribution, ecology and vector efficiency of each species.

Leucosphyrus Complex

Anopheles balabacensis

Currently, its range of distribution includes the jungle regions of Sarawak and Sabah in Malaysia, eastern and central Kalimantan in Indonesia, the island of Palawan and the neighbouring islands (including Balabac from where the species gets its name) in the Philippines. Earlier reports from Java and Sumatra are doubtful and require confirmation. In Borneo, there is a large overlapping area with *An. latens* (species A) (Harbach *et al.*, 1987a) running from the west to the east (*Figure 12*).

There are many analogies with the ecology of *An. dirus*. *An. balabacensis* larvae live in the undergrowth and the adults are strong exophilic, as already reported by McArthur (1947) in Sabah Province. This author reported very high sporozoite rates (between 2% and 20%).

Harbach *et al.* (1987a) reported a more modest level of only 1.3%, which is nevertheless high enough to make it an efficient vector.

Anopheles latens

An. latens (species A) occupies Thailand, Peninsular Malaysia and the western part of the island of Borneo (Baimai *et al.*, 1988b; Sarawak & Kalimantan) where it is sympatric with *An. balabacensis* (Chooi, 1985). It appears to be an effective malaria vector on the island of Borneo, with a sporozoite rate of 1% (Harbach *et al.*, 1987a) (*Figure 12*).

Anopheles leucosphyrus

An. leucosphyrus (species B) (Baimai *et al.*, 1988b) is known only in Sumatra, although there is no information about its role there.

Maculatus Group

An. maculatus was described by Theobald in 1901 in specimens collected in Hong-Kong. It is, or rather was, a species with a wide range of distribution, from Pakistan to Indonesia (Rao, 1984). Prior to 1980, a certain number of subspecies or forms had already been described. Today, the Maculatus Group includes two subgroups for a total of eight species (Harbach 2004), including *An. dispar, An. greeni, An. pseudowillmori* and *An. willmori*; as well as the Maculatus Subgroup which includes *An. dravidicus* and *An. maculatus*; and also the Sawadwongporni Subgroup with *An. notanandai* and *An. sawadwongporni* (*Figure 13*). Chromosomal form K, with its unique ITS2

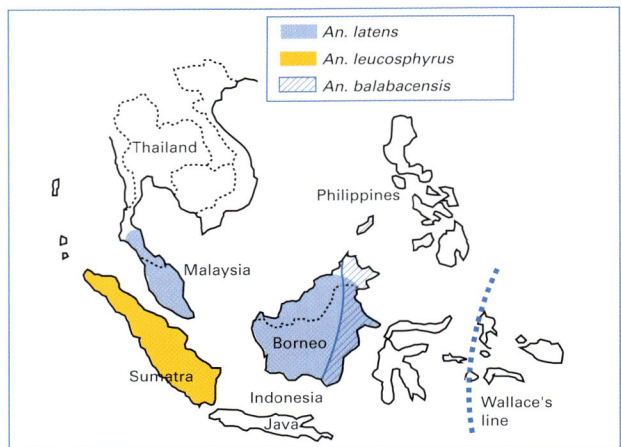

Figure 12. Distribution of An. balabacensis, An. latens and An. leucosphyrus, *three species of the* An. leucosphyrus *Complex.*

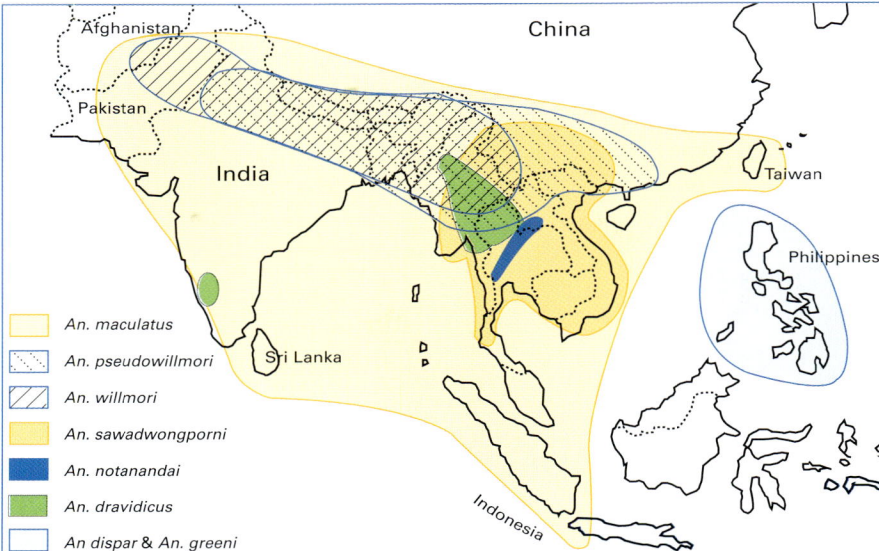

Figure 13. *Distribution of the eight species of the* An. maculatus *Group.*

sequence, is probably another species belonging to the group (Walton *et al.*, 2006).

An. maculatus is a confirmed vector from eastern India to Peninsular Malaysia. In this last region, forms B and E (Loong *et al.*, 1988) are probably not different from *An. maculatus s.s.* in Thailand (Rongnoparut *et al.*, 1999). In Malaysia and Indonesia, it is very abundant in Sabah (McArthur, 1947), Kalimantan, Sumatra and in East Timor (Azevedo *et al.*, 1958b) where it does not appear to be a vector.

Such a fresh water species which prefers a well-exposed, running water habitat, would thrive in deforested areas—which is why it is becoming so important in the context of current ecological changes (Las Llagas, 1985). While relatively zoophilic, *An. maculatus* is considered to be the main vector of malaria in Peninsular Malaysia.

An. sawadwongporni (Rattanarithikul & Green, 1986) is a twin species, very close to *An. maculatus*. It is also a confirmed vector in Thailand where it has comparable sporozoite rates of between 1% and 2% (Rattanarhitikul *et al.*, 1996c; Somboon *et al.*, 1998; Upatham *et al.*, 1988). In Thailand, both species play an important role in the deforested regions (Meek, 1995).

An. willmori (Jaimes in Theobald, 1901) is a high-altitude anopheline in Afghanistan (Glick, 1992), Nepal (Pradhan *et al.*, 1970), Kashmir (Rao, 1984) and the foothills of the Himalayas in Bengal (Bhat, 1975), India and Thailand (Green *et al.*, 1992). The latter authors confirmed its vector role in Thailand (which had already been demonstrated in Nepal) (Pradhan *et al.*, 1970).

An. pseudowillmori Theobald 1910 is known to be a vector in Thailand (Green *et al.*, 1991), and it has also been implicated in malaria transmission in Bengal.

The four other species, *An. dispar, An. dravidicus, An. greeni* and *An. notanandai* have not yet been implicated in malaria transmission.

Taxonomic revision of the Maculatus Complex should be expected as the ecology and vector efficiency of many populations do not seem to be compatible with the characteristics of the species *An. maculatus s.s.*

Sundaicus Complex *(Figure 14)*

An. sundaicus Rodenwalt 1926, a coastal species ranging from the State of Orissa in India to Timor, seems to constitute a complex of species, although this is currently under investigation. *An. sundaicus* from Lundu Province, in Sarawak (Malaysia) has been reported in brackish and freshwater habitats (Linton *et al.*, 2001). *An. epiroticus* (species A) (Linton *et al.*, 2005) seems to occupy niches of brackish water over most of the Continental Asian coast from Orissa in India (from where it has disappeared) to southern Vietnam (below the 11th parallel) down to the Malaysian Peninsula (Dusfour *et al.*, 2004a, 2004b). *An. sundaicus* species D is found in the Andaman and Nicobar Islands, India (Alam *et al.*, 2006; Nanda *et al.*, 2004) and *An. sundaicus* species E is distributed in Sumatra and Java, Indonesia; both species have been found in fresh and brackish water (*Figure 15*). Freshwater habitats have also been reported in Myanmar (Khin-Maung-Kyi, 1971) and continental India (Venkat Rao & Ramakrishna, 1950), although brackish sites are more common. This ecological difference did not point to any distinction between populations, but rather it reflects the range of saline adaptation of *An. sundaicus s.l.* Forms B and C, cytogenetically distinguished in Sumatra and Java, and Sumatra respectively, were found in brackish water, (Sukowati *et al.*, 1999). The taxonomic positions of these two forms are uncertain since they do not correspond to the molecular species cited above.

The majority of *An. sundaicus s.l.* habitats recorded to date are located along the coast in brackish water containing 0.3-25 g NaCl per litre (Nguyen Tang Am *et al.*, 1991, 1993). In Java and Vietnam (Tang Am *et al.*, 1991), the

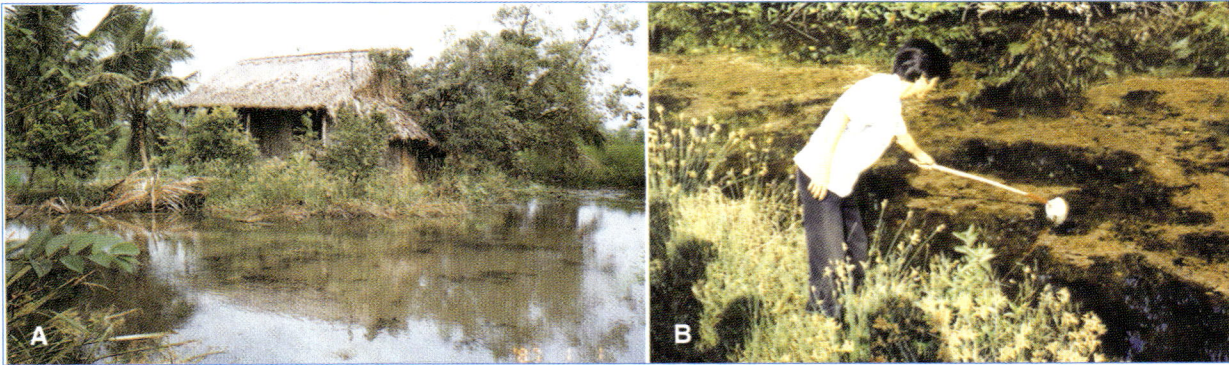

Figure 14. **A.** *Brackish water pond with algae near dwellings,* An. sundaicus *larval habitats (photograph by Sub.IMPE in Ho Chi Minh City).* **B.** An. sundaicus *larval habitats in the suburbs of Saigon (photograph by Mouchet).*

larvae thrive in well-oxygenated water with dense aquatic vegetation, including flowering plants (*Ceratophyllus, Naja*) and green algae. Along the Indochinese coastline, *An. sundaicus s.l.* has adapted to artificial shrimp ponds which are spreading rapidly.

In Bali (Soekirno *et al.*, 1983), a gradient was observed between the coastal area where *An. sundaicus* is the dominant species and the inland area of the island (300 to 1,000 m) where it is rapidly replaced by *An. aconitus*. It should be noted that a sympatric species, *An. subpictus*, extends much further inland.

The behaviour of *An. sundaicus* led to lots of speculation in the 1950's. It is only partly endophilic and after biting, most of the females rested outdoors, or even in caves, resulting in sustained transmission on the southern coast of central Java at Tjiladjap (Sundararaman, 1958).

An. sundaicus s.l. is a highly efficient vector in the Oriental Region with a sporozoite rate of 0.29-4.6%, which explains why *P. falciparum* is endemic in Central Java (Sunderaraman *et al.*, 1957).

In India where the sporozoite rate varies from 0.5-10% according to different experts, Venkat Rao & Ramakrishna (1950) felt that the fresh water populations were better vectors than salt water populations.

In Myanmar, Khin-Maung-Kyi (1971) found no infected specimens.

Information about the vector role of *An. sundaicus s.l.* is patchy and highly variable, and needs to be reviewed in the light of the ecology and taxonomy of the complex.

In southern Vietnam, *An. epiroticus* populations have increased as *An. subpictus* has disappeared, probably due to changes in land usage (Trung *et al.*, 2004). Freshwater rice field cultivation has been progressively replaced by shrimp farming in brackish water which is more propitious for the more saline-tolerant *An. epiroticus* than it is for *An. subpictus*. Studies of *An. epiroticus* in the Mekong Delta showed the absence of circumsporozoites which reflects the weak vector capacity of this species (Trung *et al.*, 2004). However, other species (*An. sundaicus s.l.*) have been suspected of transmitting malaria, including *An. nimpe* and *An. subpictus* (Tang Am *et al.*, 1993).

Vectors of Malaysia, Indonesia and the Philippines

We will not go back over the major vectors which have already been addressed and which are involved in malaria transmission in several subregions, i.e. *An. sundaicus*, and the *An. dirus*, *An. leucosphyrus* and *An. maculatus* Complexes. Rather, in this section, we will focus on a certain number of species endemic to the Malaysian peninsula and archipelagos that play a more or less important role in the local transmission of malaria.

An. flavirostris (Ludlow, 1914) has long been considered a subspecies of *An. minimus*. It now belongs to the Minimus Subgroup along with the *An. minimus* and *An fluviatilis* Complexes and *An. leesoni* from the Afrotropical Region (Garros *et al.*, 2005; Harbach 2004). It is the main vector in the Philippines (Salazar *et al.*, 1988) which overlaps into Malaysia on the islands of Baggi (Hii *et al.*, 1988a) (*Figure 16*). It is shown on the vector map in Sulawesi (Kirnowardoyo, 1985), although the Indonesian locations require confirmation.

The larval habitats are located in the streams in hilly regions, as well as in rice paddy ditches (Salazar *et al.*, 1988).

Peak female activity is between 11 pm and 3 am. The majority of specimens, although endophilic, leave the

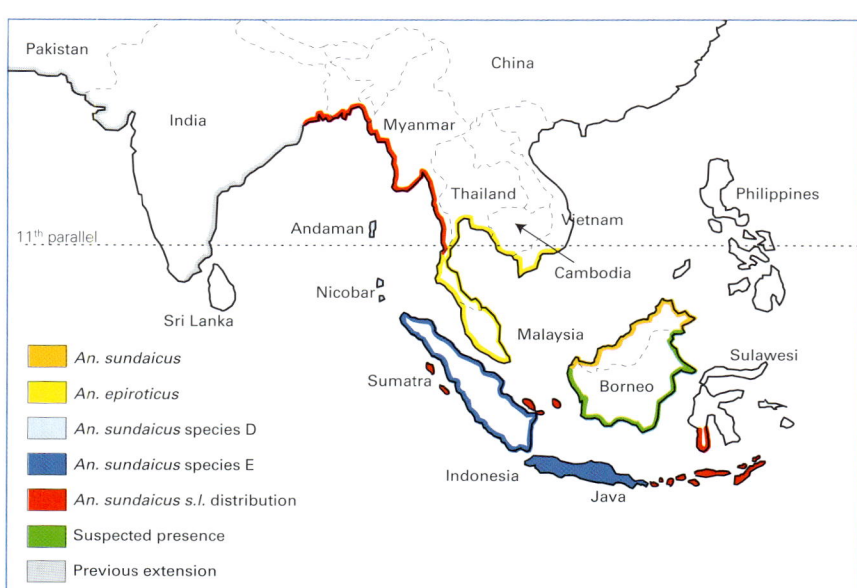

Figure 15. Distribution of the four species of the An. sundaicus Complex (adapted from Dusfour et al., 2007).

homes between 5 am and 6.30 am although indoor spraying in the Philippines killed many *An. flavirostris*. *An. flavirostris* has not reached urban areas due to its ecological particularities. In light of the considerable regression of malaria in the Philippines, little information is available concerning the infection rate in this area. In Malaysia, in Sabah on the island of Baggi, where it is sympatric with *An. balabacensis*, Hii *et al*., (1988a) found two infected specimens in a series of five hundred and thirty-six dissections of *An. flavirostris*, and twelve infections out of three hundred and six dissections of *An. balabacensis* which is apparently a much more important vector.

An. litoralis King 1932 is a coastal halophilic species of the Philippines (Salazar *et al*., 1988) which is also found in Sabah, Malaysia and which was imported to the island of Guam in the Marianne Archipelago (Ward *et al*., 1976). Its role was highlighted only on the island of Sulu, in the southern Philippines, in the absence of any other vector, notably *An. flavirostris*. Its sporozoite rate was 0.11% (Cabrera *et al*., 1970). In eleven specimens, one *P. vivax*-infected gland was detected following a fifteen-day observation period (Darsie *et al*., 1978).

An. mangyanus is a secondary malaria vector in the Philippines (Salazar *et al*., 1988), particularly on the islands of Mindoro and Mindanao. Its importance diminished following deforestation (Las Llagas, 1985). This species along with *An. aconitus*, *An. filipinae*, *An. pampanai* and *An. varuna* belong to the Aconitus Subgroup (Garros *et al*., 2005; Harbach, 2004).

An. aconitus Donitz 1902 is a species with a wide ranging oriental distribution from southern and eastern India to the Wallace line in Indonesia (*Figure 17*). It has not been found in the Philippines or in China. In Kirnowardoyo's very complete map of anopheline vectors in Indonesia (1985), it is not shown outside Java and Bali although it is mentioned in Sumatra, Kalimantan, Sulawesi and Timor (Azevedo *et al*., 1958b; Bonne Wepster & Swellengrebel, 1953). It is a sunny, freshwater species, often confined to rice paddies. The adults bite from 10 pm to 0.30 am (Rahman *et al*., 1993). Although attracted to livestock, their behaviour is mixed and they are fairly anthropophilic.

An. aconitus is the main vector of malaria in Bali, Java and southern Sumatra. In Peninsular Malaysia, it is considered only a secondary vector (Wharton, 1953). In Bangladesh, it has become an important vector following ecological changes associated with massive population growth. When rice paddies replaced the marshlands, *An. aconitus* displaced *An. philippinensis* and/or *An. nivipes* (Maheswary *et al*., 1992).

An. barbirostris Van der Wulp 1884 is a species with a vast range (*Figure 16*) and its behaviour varies considerably from one region to another within this range. In India, it is zoophilic and exophilic whereas it is endophilic and anthropophilic in Sulawesi (Takken *et al*., 1990). The existence of a species complex has been proposed, although the taxonomic situation is not yet clear. Salivary gland infections were reported in Timor (Lien *et al*., 1977) and strongly suspected in Sulawesi (Lien *et al*., 1975).

An. umbrosus (Theobald, 1903) was wrongly considered to be a vector of human malaria. In fact, it transmits only mouse-deer *Plasmodium* in Peninsular Malaysia (Wharton *et al*., 1963).

It is a controversial question as to whether or not *An. donaldi* Reid 1962 is a vector in the coastal plains of Sarawak, Malaysia, where the prevalence of malaria is low. The larvae develop in the rice paddies and open marshes, and the adults are more attracted to livestock than to humans (McArthur, 1947). It was not found to be a sporozoite-carrier in Peninsular Malaysia (Chooi, 1985), although a positive CSP response was obtained (Delorme *et al*., 1989).

An. campestris Reid 1962 is a species of the coastal plain of Malaysia which develops in rice paddies and possibly brackish waters. Owing to its endophilic and anthropophilic

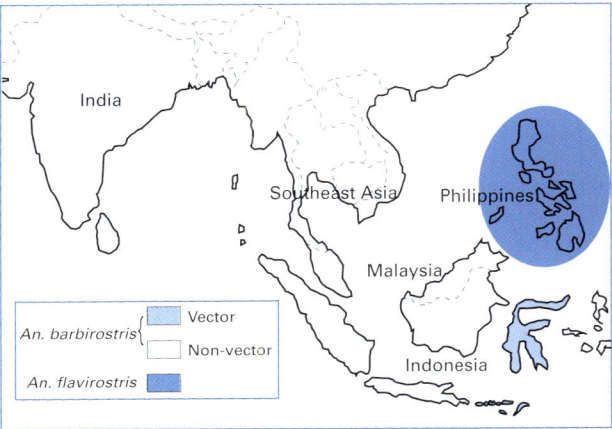

Figure 16. Distribution of An. barbirostris and An. flavirostris.

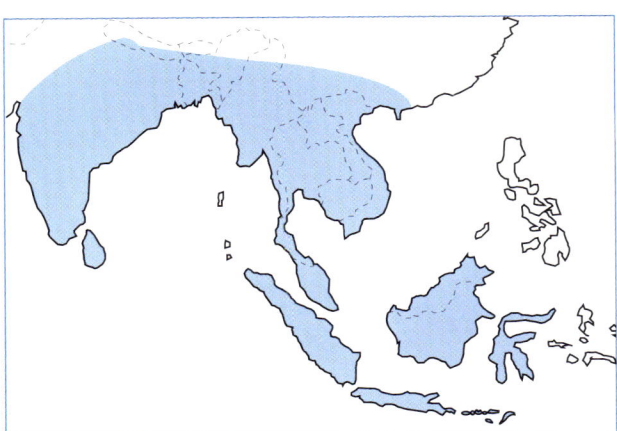

Figure 17. Distribution of An. aconitus.

behaviour, this anopheline disappeared after two indoor spraying campaigns (Chooi, 1985).

An. letifer Sandosham 1944 is known in Thailand, all of Malaysia (Lim, 1992), Sumatra and Sulawesi (Kirnowardoyo, 1985). In Peninsular Malaysia, despite its zoophilic behaviour, it is a vector on the shaded coastal plains (Rahman *et al.*, 1997). It is no longer considered a vector in Sarawak.

Anopheles fluviatilis *James 1902*

The distribution of this species is quite extensive, ranging from Taiwan to Arabia through Bhutan, India, Nepal, Pakistan, Iran and Afghanistan (Glick, 1992; Zahar, 1990) but it does not seem to occur in southern China or east of Myanmar (Chen *et al.*, 2002). *An. fluviatilis* is sympatric with *An. minimus* in Nepal, in north-east India and Myanmar (*Figure 18*).

Originally, *An. fluviatilis* was a complex with three cytogenic species, including species S (Nanda *et al.*, 1996; Sharma *et al.*, 1995; Subbarao *et al.*, 1994), which is anthropophilic and reported as an efficient vector associated with high endemicity. Species T and U, predominantly zoophilic, are respectively little or not at all implicated in malaria transmission (Sharma, 2002; Shukla *et al.*, 1998). Later on, two molecular species were described, X and Y, recognised respectively as cytogenetic species S and T (Manonmani *et al.*, 2001, 2003). Based on morphological data and a recent comparison of the Domain 3 (3D) sequence between *An fluvialitis* S and *An. minimus* C, these two species were thought to be conspecific (Chen *et al.*, 2006; Garros *et al.*, 2005; Harbach, 2004). However, this conclusion was refuted by Singh *et al.* (2006) who found sequence differences when comparing loci ITS2 and 28S-D2/D3 between both species. In conclusion, the current systematic scheme of the Fluviatilis Complex includes three species, *An. fluviatilis* S, T, U, and a form "V" (Singh *et al.*, 2006).

The larvae live in clear, well-oxygenated flowing water (Mulligan & Baily, 1938) and are highly sensitive to pollution (Reisen & Milby, 1986).

As early as 1943, Viswanathan & Rao had made a distinction between anthropophilic, endophilic *An. fluviatilis* populations on the one hand, and zoophilic, exophilic populations on the other; they defined these as distinct "biological races". The first group was found in hilly regions and small mountains while the second group occupied the lower plains. Thus, *An. fluviatilis* was endophilic and anthropophilic in Nepal (Reisen *et al.*, 1993), as well as the State of Orissa (Collins *et al.*, 1990) and Madhya Pradesh in India (Kulkarni, 1987), whereas it was exophilic and zoophilic in Tamil Nadu (Mani *et al.*, 1984; Tewari *et al.*, 1984).

Two types of behaviour were highlighted in the district of Koraput, Orissa, India. In certain villages, *An. fluviatilis* leaves the dwellings within an hour of feeding and has an anthropophilic index of 23% and a daily life expectancy of 0.55. In other villages, this same anopheline spends its entire gonotropic cycle inside the house and has an anthropophilic index of 83% and a daily life expectancy of 0.92 (Gunasekaran, 1994; Gunasekaran *et al.*, 1994).

In India, endophilic forms—probably species S (now *An. minimus* C)—are responsible for the high rate of malaria transmission in the Nilgiris (Russel & Jacob, 1942), in the State of Orissa (Sharma *et al.*, 1995), in Madhya Pradesh (Kulkarni, 1987), in the hills of Darjelling (Malakar *et al.*, 1995) and in Nepal (Reisen *et al.*, 1993). The sporozoite rates reported in these studies were of the order of 2%.

In the plains of southern India, it appears that *An. fluviatilis* is not a vector, species T predominates. In fact, malaria is not encountered in the lower areas of the Tamil Nadu. However, during an epidemic in the plain of the Udaipur District of Rajasthan State, sporozoite rates of 2% were recorded in *An. fluviatilis*, although the index was only 0.39% in *An. culicifacies*.

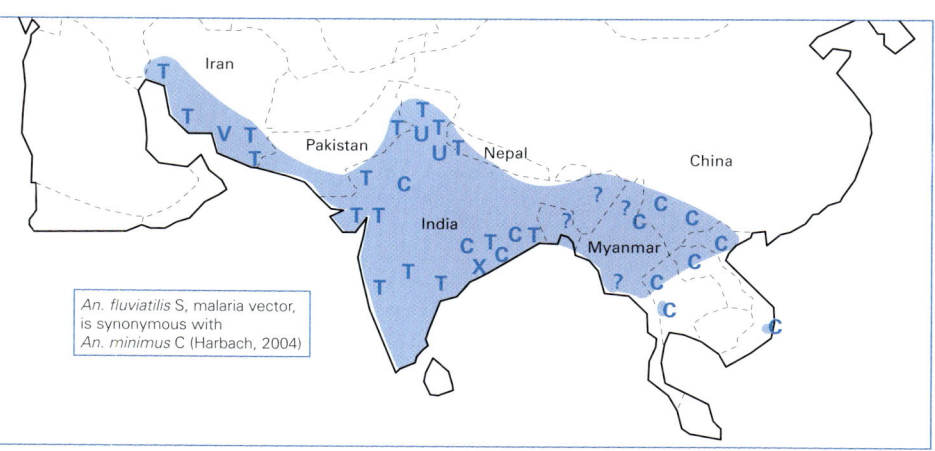

Figure 18. Distribution of the two species (T, U) and two forms (V, X) of the An. fluviatilis *Complex and* An. minimus C (C) *(adapted from Chen et al., 2006).*

In eastern India, *An. fluviatilis*, despite being common, is not believed to be a vector although no species typing has ever been performed.

Anopheles culicifacies *Giles 1901* (Figure 19)

This name covers a more or less sympatric species complex distributed from the Sea of China to Yemen and even as far as Eritrea (*Figure 20*) (Glick, 1992; Rao, 1984; Zahar, 1990).

At least five species are included in this complex: A, B, C, D and E (Green & Miles, 1980; Kar *et al.*, 1999; Subbarao *et al.*, 1988a; Subbarao & Sharma, 1997).

Species A is an efficient vector of malaria in Pakistan, northern India and in the Arabo-Persian Region where the disease is hypo-endemic and epidemics occur from time to time (Subbarao, 1988). The predominantly zoophilic species B has a low vector capacity; there is no malaria in the States of Bihar or Uttar Pradesh, nor in southern India where this form is dominant; it does not seem to transmit malaria in Nepal either (Reisen *et al.*, 1993; Sharma, 2002).

Species C, sympatric with B in Gujerat, may be a vector as well as species D, which is always associated with species A (Subbarao *et al.*,1992).

There is a lack of information about the taxonomic status of the populations in the oriental range of distribution of *An. culicifacies*, particularly in northern Thailand; apparently, it does not seem to be involved in malaria transmission.

In Sri Lanka, *An. culicifacies* B was considered a local vector of malaria; Dewitt *et al.* (1994) had suggested that this Sri Lankan form may be a different species. In fact, there is another species in Sri Lanka, *An. culicifacies* E (Sharma, 2002), recently described on Rameshwaram Island near Sri Lanka (Kar *et al.*, 1999) which is the malaria vector.

Studies prior to 1980 report a mix of species. Also, information about the ecology and the vector role of the *An. culicifacies* Complex may encompass different entities.

In Pakistan, sporozoite rates of 2.3% and 0.84% were reported in Baluchistan and Karachi, respectively. In the Punjab, an initial sporozoite rate of 0.3% rose to 2% if dissection was delayed for 15 days (Mahmood *et al.*, 1984).

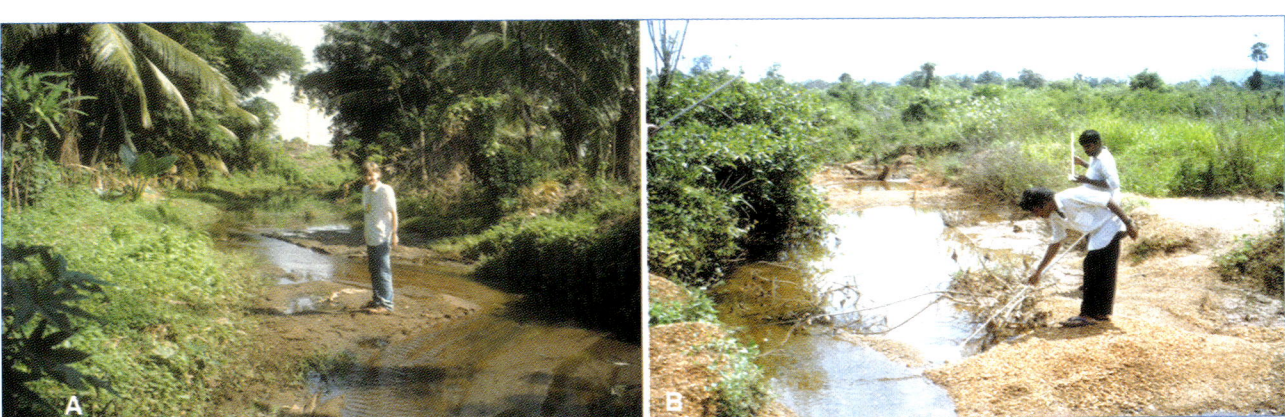

Figure 19. A and B. An. culicifacies *larval habitats in Sri Lanka (photograph by Coosemans).*

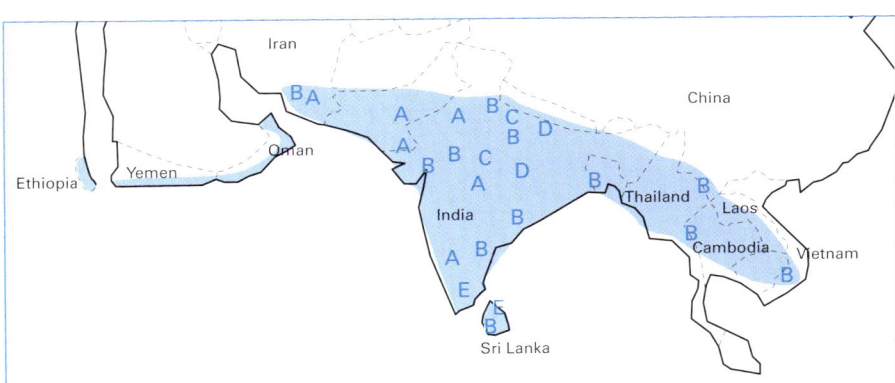

Figure 20. Distribution of the five species of the An. culicifacies Complex.

In India, in the islands of Tamil Nadu, a *P. vivax* s of 0.5% (4,380 dissections) has been reported (Sabesan *et al.*, 1984). The sporozoite rate of 0.59%, particularly concerning *P. vivax* and recorded along the Thenpennai River in the same State, was associated with irrigation (Tewari *et al.*, 1984). In Madhya Pradesh, after the monsoon, *An. culicifacies* was a vector of *P. vivax* (Vaid *et al.*, 1974).

Since 1980, more specific data have been obtained, particularly in India. Around Delhi (Sharma & Uprety, 1982), species A transmits *P. vivax* from May to October and *P. falciparum* from August to December after the monsoon, when the land is covered with residual puddles; species B is not as strong a vector; species C yielded 2 positive CSP1 results (*P. vivax*) out of 148 examinations; species D also gave 2 positive results (*P. vivax* and *P. falciparum*) out of 169 examinations. In northern India, species A gave 44 positive specimens out of 5,386 dissections (0.8%; 28 *P. vivax* and 16 *P. falciparum*) while only one single positive specimen (*P. vivax*) out of 1,208 dissections (0.08%) was observed with species B (Subbarao *et al.*, 1988a). In Nepal, no *An. culicifacies* was infected even though the species was very common (Reisen *et al.*, 1993). Finally, in Sri Lanka, 10 infections (8 *P. falciparum* and 2 *P. vivax*) out of 445 dissections were observed in species E (Dewit *et al.*, 1994); the EIR was 0.95 for *P. falciparum* and 2.55 for *P. vivax*, very low figures compared to those seen in the Afrotropical Region.

An. culicifacies was responsible for past malaria epidemics in the Indian Subcontinent (Shukla *et al.*, 1995). Recent epidemics in Rajasthan, Alwar (1974-1976) (Rahman *et al.*, 1979) and Bikaner (1990) were investigated in depth. After indoor spraying had been discontinued, this anopheline was responsible for post-eradication epidemics, notably in Sri Lanka where several million cases of *P. vivax* malaria were recorded in 1964.

Species B was more resistant to malathion than species A (66% and 2.9% respectively in Delhi) (Raghavendra *et al.*, 1991); species C was even more resistant than B.

The list of the various types of larval habitats (*Figure 19*) given by Rao (1984) is quite impressive. Generally speaking, they are characterised by low organic material content and intense sunshine. Residual pools of rain and run-off water after the monsoon and replanted rice paddies are the most productive larval habitats (Kant *et al.*, 1992; Russel *et al.*, 1963; Sharma & Uprety, 1982). Larvae were even collected in brackish water (Rao, 1984). Each species of the complex has not yet been characterised in terms of their specific habitat, swarming and mating behaviour, or endophily and anthropophily (Reisen, 1978; Reisen & Aslamkhan, 1976; Reisen *et al.*, 1981; Reisen *et al.*, 1982; Reisen & Milby, 1986). The daily life expectancy of *An. culicifacies* is significantly higher than that of *An. stephensi* although any observations about the endophilic or anthropophilic behaviour of this species are complicated by the fact that species are mixed.

In Sri Lanka, *An. culicifacies* E is most active between 8 pm and 11 pm when people are watching television outside; during this time they are not protected by mosquito netting (Dewit *et al.*, 1994).

In Nepal, *An. culicifacies* proliferates in the recently deforested zones of the Terai plain where, as mentioned above, it does not seem to be a malaria vector.

In all the data acquired before 1980 and in many more recent publications, no distinction is made between the various different *An. culicifacies* species, which makes much of the information difficult to interpret. However, a recently developed molecular method able to distinguish each member of the complex will make it possible to study the behaviour of each species, and their respective roles in malaria transmission (Goswami *et al.*, 2006).

Anopheles stephensi *Liston 1901*

Species with a wide oriental distribution from eastern Myanmar to Iraq and the western part of the Arabian Peninsula (*Figure 21*) (Glick, 1992; Rao, 1984; Zahar, 1990); it is not present in Sri Lanka, the State of Kerala in south-western India or the foothills of the Himalayas.

Unlike the majority of vectors in the Oriental Region, *An. stephensi* is a monomorphic species (Reisen & Milby, 1986). According to Knight & Stone (1977), the mysorensis subspecies of India is not considered a valid taxon. The degree of Pgm (phosphoglucomutase) isozyme polymorphism is not sufficient to justify division into distinct species (Bullini *et al.*, 1971), and neither are the observed differences in cuticular carbohydrates (Anyanwu *et al.*, 1993).

It has many rural larval habitats, grassy river banks and residual pools of streams being among the most productive (Rao, 1984). This species' outstanding characteristic, however, is its adaptation to city cisterns and pools that has made it the most important urban vector of malaria in the Indian subcontinent. In Salem, in the southern Indian state of Tamil Nadu, it has been found in wells throughout the year although numbers drop at the end of the dry season

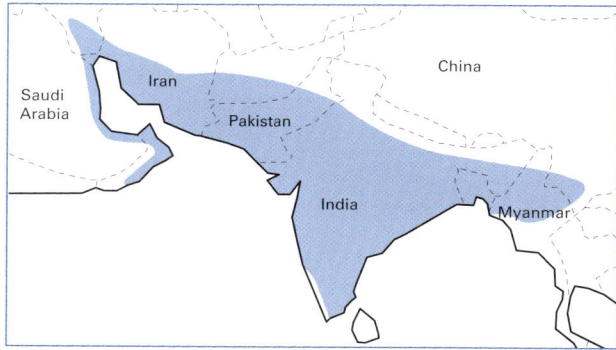

Figure 21. Distribution of An. stephensi.

(Batra & Reuben, 1979). Females captured in homes are endophilic (Batra et al., 1979a). This urban adaptation has been observed in the majority of large Indian cities, including Madras, Bangalore, Calcutta and Delhi (Hati, 1997). In the cities of Tamil Nadu, it lives alongside *An. subpictus*, which is much more abundant although practically never infected (Das et al., 1979). In Salem, one infected *An. stephensi* was found in 145 dissections.

In rural Pakistan, *An. stephensi* and *An. culicifacies* prefer to feed on animals and, although they are endophilic, they are considered to be poor vectors (Bouma, 1995).

An. stephensi numbers peak during and at the end of the monsoon, although they are relatively low during years of especially heavy rainfall associated with El Niño (Bouma, 1995).

A sporozoite rate of 1.19% was found in a rural part of Karachi in Pakistan, although there was no infection in the city in 1956 (Hussain & Talibi, 1956; Rahman & Muttalib, 1967). In Afghanistan, Rao (1951) did not detect any infected specimens of this species even though it was considered to be the main malaria vector.

An. stephensi is an efficient malaria vector throughout most of its range of distribution (Rao, 1984)

Palaearctic species that overflow into the Oriental Region

A certain number of palaearctic species encroach upon the Oriental Region in Afghanistan, Pakistan and India, as well as in southern China.

"Chinese" species

The Hyrcanus Group includes three species in the Chinese Subregion: *An. sinensis* Wiedemann 1928, *An. kunmingensis* Dong & Wang 1985 (synonymous with *An. liangshanensis* Ma et al., 2000) and *An. anthropophagus* Xu & Feng 1981 (synonymous with *An. lesteri* Wilkerson et al., 2003). The range of *An. hyrcanus s.s.* does not appear to extend into the Oriental Region, assuming that the species have been accurately identified.

The distribution of *An. sinensis* is quite vast, ranging from Siberia to Java and from Japan to Afghanistan. It is preferentially zoophilic and bites at nightfall making it a particular menace in rice-growing areas. This vector is recognised in China, Korea and, in the past, Japan. In Taiwan, it was not believed to transmit *P. falciparum* (Lien, 1991). It plays only a highly secondary or random role in the Indo-Chinese Peninsula. In 1984, Beales published a revision of the *An. sinensis* Group.

An. kunmingensis, now *An. liangshanensis*, has proven to be an efficient vector in China, in Yunnan Province, on the Yun River (the upper reach of the Red River) and the border zones of Myanmar, Laos and Vietnam (Dong-Xueshu et al., 1990; Hu et al., 1998; Xu & Liu, 1997).

An. anthropophagus, formerly *An. lesteri,* is an excellent malarial vector in China, south of the Chang Jiang River.

Palaearctic species

The species concerned are essentially *An. pulcherrimus, An. sergentii* and *An. superpictus* which encroach into the Oriental Region in Afghanistan, Pakistan and even India, as mentioned above.

An. superpictus Grassi 1889 invests the whole of Afghanistan and Baluchistan Province in southern Pakistan (Glick, 1992; Zahar, 1990). The species is endophilic and sporozoite rates of 0.4% have been recorded in the district of Laghman (Rao, 1951), 0.3% in Kabul, Afghanistan (Iyengar, 1954) and 1.56% in the north of Baluchistan Province.

An. pulcherrimus Theobald 1902: its range of distribution extends from Turkey and Syria in the west all the way to north-western India. Larval habitats are in the lowlands where there are dense stands of vegetation (reeds), similar to the rice paddy environment. The species becomes quite dense in the irrigated regions of Pakistan. Owing to its relatively short life expectancy, it only really transmits *P. vivax*.

An. sergentii Theobald 1907 is a Saharan species which reaches its eastern limit in southern Pakistan. It is the vector of the Saharo-Arabic deserts.

Vectors of limited significance

This section deals with a number of species that are widely distributed throughout the Oriental Region, which only transmit malaria in very limited parts of their range of distribution, most often *P. vivax*. They are responsible for low-level endemicity or epidemics.

An. nimpe (Nguyen Duc Manh et al., 2000) of the *An. hyrcanus* Group was considered a possible vector in the Mekong Delta (Tang Am et al., 1993).

An. jeyporiensis is widespread in Vietnam (Phan, 1998), Thailand and southern China (Harrison, 1980), with a sporozoite rate of 0.4% in regions close to the jungle. Most reports of this species come from Vietnam and its ecology has not yet been extensively studied.

An. nivipes Theobald 1903 was separated from *An. philippinensis* Ludlow 1903 by Reid (1967). However, they both belong to the Annularis Group along with three other species (including *An. annularis*). The first name applies to the Malaysian form (Knight & Stone, 1977) and the two species appear sympatric from India to Thailand. Broadly speaking, *An. philippinensis* was a well characterised vector in the Brahmaputra River Delta, but it was considered as secondary in Thailand, Cambodia and Vietnam (Rajagopal, 1976). In Bangladesh, it has undergone significant regression after marshlands—where it preferentially breeds—were replaced by rice paddies in response to food shortage. *An. aconitus* subsequently took over in these areas (Elias, 1996; Elias et al., 1983; Maheswary et al., 1992). *An. nivipes* was identified as a vector in Thailand (Harbach et al., 1987b) and suspected in Laos (Kobayashi *et al.*, 2000). Its presence was also reported in north-east India (Nagpal & Sharma, 1987). *An. nivipes* is a complex of two cytogenetic species in Thailand (Harbach, 1994, 2004; Harrison *et al.*, 1990). The distribution and epidemiological role of this complex are to be defined; neither of these two species acts a vector in most of their range of distribution.

An. annularis Van der Wulp 1884 ranges from the Philippines to Afghanistan, and exhibits highly aggressive human host-seeking behaviour. Considered as a secondary vector, with a sporozoite rate of the order of 0.1% (Rao, 1984), it expanded into irrigated areas following deforestation in Nepal (Reisen *et al.*, 1993) and in west Bengal in India (Ghosh *et al.*, 1985).

An. subpictus Grassi 1899, also a widely distributed complex ranging from Iran to New Guinea, is known to be very aggressive at twilight. Suguna *et al.* (1994) highlighted four species: A, B, C and D. In Pondicherry where all four are sympatric, species B, specific to brackish water-seems to be the only malaria vector. The three other species, A, C and D, develop in freshwater habitats and apparently do not participate in transmission. *An. subpictus* was implicated in a malaria epidemic in northern Vietnam (Phan, 1998) and gland infections were recorded positive in Timor (Azevedo *et al.*, 1958), Pondicherry (Panicker *et al.*, 1981) and Madhya Pradesh (Kulkarni, 1983) in India. This anopheline is considered as a menace in the region.

An. tessellatus Theobald 1901, although widespread from the Philippines to Pakistan, was only considered as a vector in the Maldives (Iyengar *et al.*, 1953) after infected salivary glands were observed. It was considered the only vector in the Maldives although in fact, *An. subpictus* was also present. *An. tessellatus* is also the only anopheline of Minicoychas Island in the Laccadives where *P. vivax* infections were discovered in this hitherto "malaria-free" island (Roy *et al.*, 1974).

An. vagus Donitz 1902, present from India to New Guinea, is very aggressive at dusk and has often been reported as being a secondary vector, although on very little evidence.

An. varuna Iyengar 1924 was designated as a vector based on a few dissections carried out in India, and its vector status is still controversial (Rao 1984).

In Japan's Ryukyu Archipelago, *An. saperoi* was believed to have caused an epidemic of *P. vivax* malaria among islanders who took refuge in the jungle to escape the war (Miyagi & Toma, 1990).

The epidemiology of malaria in the Indo-Chinese Subregion

General characteristics and stratification

The landform of the Indo-Chinese Subregion is characterised by a series of folds—oriental extensions of the Himalayas which, after curving southward, define a series of fan-shaped depressions extending in a north-south direction. The peaks, which exceed 4,000 m in China, taper off gradually toward the south into hills and plateaux. The valleys, most of which are less than 300 m above sea level, feature wide rivers terminating in vast deltas, such as the Red River, the Mekong and the Chan Praya which empty into the southern China Sea; and the Salouen, Irraouaddi and Brahmaputra which empty into the Gulf of Bengal.

The entire subregion has a wet, tropical climate, cooler in the north owing to the combined effects of altitude and latitude. In northern Vietnam, the winters are cool and freezing temperatures are common above 1,000 m.

The spatial distribution of the vectors is associated with the vegetation, from highly efficient vectors (*An. minimus* and *An. dirus*) which are the source of highly endemic malaria in the jungles and hills, to less efficient vectors in the hypo-endemic or malaria-free plains.

Two phenomena have modified the epidemiology of malaria over the last thirty years:
- the first is an ecological one, namely deforestation;
- the second is malaria control measures.

The primary vectors still exist in the deforested areas, although the *An. maculatus* Complex is becoming more important. Much of the available information is fragmented and it is not yet possible to assess the geographic distribution and extent of malaria in cleared jungle.

The second factor intervening in the second half of the 20th century was the development of anti-vector measures based on generalisation of indoor spraying. While *An. minimus s.l.* used to be the "marker" species for the Indo-Chinese Subregion (Macdonald, 1957), the numbers of this mosquito have been brought down by indoor spraying and it is currently considered less important than members of the *An. dirus* Complex.

The Indo-Chinese Subregion can be divided into four zones on the basis of the current distribution of malaria and its vectors:
- highland zones: malaria-free above 1,500 m in southern Vietnam and 800 m in the north (Phan, 1998). In central Laos, the limit is roughly 1,200 m; the Hmong minority, highly sensitive to malaria, lives above this limit to avoid sickness (Pholsena, 1992). The altitudinal limit for the transmission of malaria is poorly defined in many countries: in Nepal, *An. minimus* has been reported up to 1,800 m, but *An. willmori* may transmit malaria at altitudes of up to 3,000 m (Pradhan *et al.*, 1970; Shrestha, 1966);
- in jungle belts on hills and plateaux, malaria transmitted by *An. minimus* and *An. dirus* was and still is hyper- or meso-endemic in places. The success of indoor spraying campaigns has made it difficult to gauge accurately the extent of malaria prior to the 1940's. In 1939, on the plateaux of southern Vietnam, a parasite prevalence of 86% (n = 1,835) was reported among the "Mois" (Meo) in children of 6-24 months old; among the Annamites (Khin), Parasite Rate (PR) readings indicated prevalences ranging

from 35-60% among older children (11-15 years old) and Spleen Rates (SR) were also very high. This study, conducted by Farinaud & Prost (1939), now takes on true historical significance. The historical epidemiological patterns can be seen in zones where the programmes were suspended, such as in Vietnam near Nha-Trang (Marchand et al., 1997);
- malaria is absent from the plains or is hypo-endemic with occasional epidemic outbreaks. Although quite dense in rice paddies and marshy areas, the anophelines are poor vectors and most of them only carry *P. vivax*. It has long been recognised that *An. philippinensis* (or *An. nivipes*) is a low-level vector of *P. vivax* in the Ganges Delta (Elias, 1996). In Vientiane, all of the 400 hospitalised cases of malaria came from rural, hillside areas and none from the plains (Southammavong, 1997). Epidemics of *P. vivax*, transmitted by *An. subpictus* in particular, have been reported in the Red River Delta in Vietnam (Phan, 1998);
- in the coastal regions, *An. sundaicus* species A (now named *An. epiroticus*) is encountered from southern Vietnam (below the 11th parallel) to Thailand south to the Malaysian Peninsula. The brackish water larval habitats are continuous with the sea during the high tides and are characterised by the presence of green vegetation, both algae and flowering plants. In southern Vietnam, this species can maintain micro-larval habitats or foci, corresponding to just a few homes, e.g. in suburban Ho Chi Minh city (Nguyen Tang Am et al., 1993). Very active foci are spread along the coasts of Myanmar and Bangladesh, as well as coastal areas of the Andaman and Nicobar Islands; in these islands, *An. sundaicus*, recently named species D, transmits *P. cynomolgi*, among others, which might be passed on to humans (Kalra, 1980). Along the flat and marshy coast of Cambodia, *An. epiroticus* is seldom encountered and endemic malaria is rare; on the other hand, *An. subpictus* is very dense in this region.

Various malaria stratification schemes have been proposed in Vietnam (Phan, 1998), Cambodia (May & Meek, 1992), Myanmar (Postiglione & Venkat Rao, 1956) and Bangladesh (Rosenberg & Maheswary, 1982) but these schemes differ only slightly from the version presented. The review by Kondrashin & Rooney (1992) presented control measures according to drug resistance.

Country by country

Nepal

This country is representative of malaria in the sub-Himalayan zones. The main vectors used to be *An. minimus s.l.* at lower altitudes of below 600 m (from where it has been eliminated by house spraying); *An. fluviatilis s.l.* up to 1,300 m; and *An. willmori* up to 3,000 m (Pradhan et al., 1970; Shrestha, 1966) (*Figure 22*).

The lowland area of the Terai, where malaria was hyper-endemic, was very sparsely populated. The indigenous Tharu population is known for its resistance to the disease (Terrenato et al., 1988); the high frequency of homozygous thalassaemia could be responsible for the observed ten-fold reduction in malarial morbidity (Modiano et al., 1991)*.

Once antimalarial treatment operations had begun, the annual malaria incidence dropped from 2,000,000 in 1965 to 25,000 in 1970 and 14,000 in 1974, after which it stabilised (Sakya, 1981). *An. minimus s.l.* disappeared in the 1960's (Shrestha & Parajuli, 1980) and the density of *An. fluviatilis s.l.* decreased significantly. The explosion of the population in these zones recently "freed" from malaria was accompanied by economic development projects and irrigation schemes which stimulated the spread of a new vector, *An. annularis,* which reinitiated

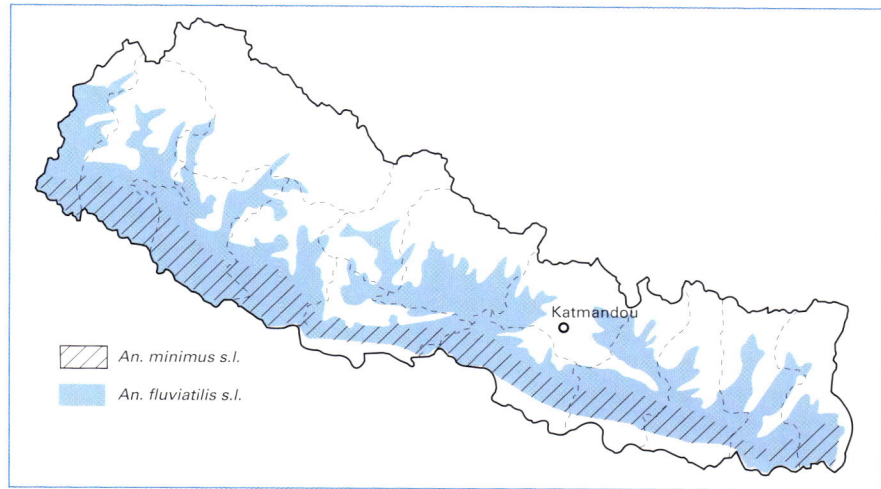

Figure 22.
Vectors of malaria in Nepal (adapted from Shrestha, 1966).

---

* Mention is made of Modiano's speculations about thalassaemia and "resistance" to malaria, although these are far from proven.

transmission, although at a modest level in comparison to the original situation (Shrestha, 1985).

Bhutan

Malaria is present only along its southern border where *An. minimus s.l.* and *An. maculatus s.l.* have been reported (Rajagopal, 1985).

Northeast India

Unstable malaria, often epidemic, used to prevail in the major part of India to the west of the Brahmaputra. Transmission was due to various anophelines, particularly *An. culicifacies s.l.* and *An. stephensi*. On the other hand, malaria in the **north-eastern States** (Tripura, Mizoram, Manipur, Meghalaya, Nagaland, Arunachal Pradesh, Assam, West Bengal and Sikkim) is stable, either hyper- or meso-endemic. Macdonald (1957) intentionally associated these regions with the Indo-Chinese Subregion. The main vector at this time was *An. minimus s.l.* which was, in intervening years, drastically reduced in numbers as a result of indoor spraying programmes, even to the point that it was eradicated from some States. Today, however, it has returned to most of its range (Dev, 1996; Dutta & Baruchi, 1987; Prakash *et al.*, 2000). It was during this intermediate period that the role of *An. dirus s.l.* became evident (Dutta & Bhattacharyya, 1990).

Following eradication, epidemics ensued once indoor spraying programmes had been cut back. In 1992, an epidemic of 1,200 cases was observed in Assam, a region in which malaria had hitherto been thought of as stable (Gogoï *et al.*, 1996). The victims were members of indigenous ethnic groups who were naturally "resistant" to malaria, and the epidemic resulted in only ten deaths.

In the mountains of Sikkim State, where there is no *An. minimus*, malaria is transmitted by *An. fluviatilis s.l.* and, at higher altitudes, by *An. willmori* (Malhotra *et al.*, 1987).

In deforested regions, species belonging to the *An. maculatus* Group have become increasingly important (Dutta & Bhattacharyya, 1990; Misra *et al.*, 1993). In the plains of the Bengali Delta as in neighbouring Bangladesh, *P. vivax* is transmitted by *An. philippinensis* (or *An. nivipes*) and possibly by *An. annularis* as well as by *An. aconitus* in rice-growing areas (Sen *et al.*, 1973).

In the Nicobar and Andaman islands, *An. dirus s.l.* and *An. sundaicus* have both been reported and recent molecular studies identified *An. baimai* (formerly *An. dirus* D) and *An. sundaicus* D (Alam *et al.*, 2006; Sallum *et al.*, 2005).

Bangladesh (*Figure 23*)

Nearly 80% of this State's landmass corresponds to the flood plains of the Ganges and Brahmaputra Rivers, the other 20% being the hills to the east of Chittagong at the India/Myanmar border (which used to be covered in trees). In the plains, the incidence of *P. vivax* malaria was below

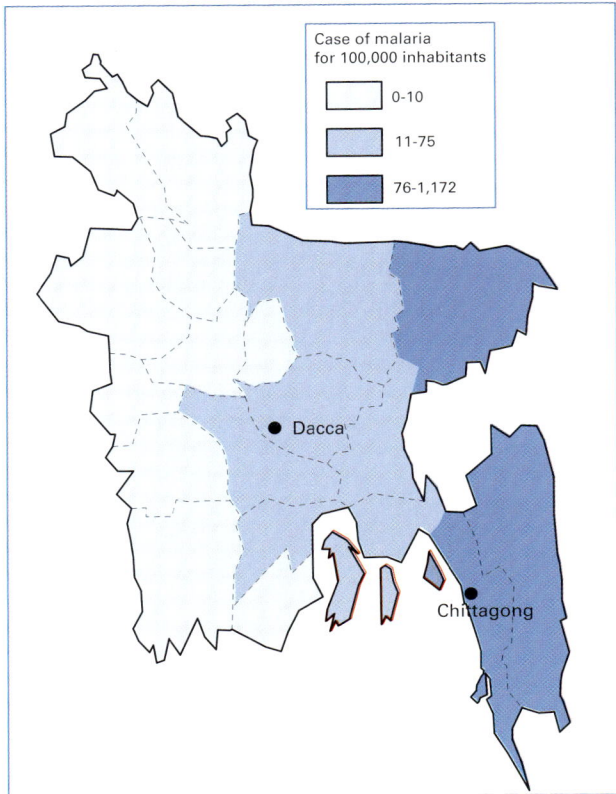

Figure 23. Incidence of malaria in Bangladesh by district and per 100,000 inhabitants: 1969-1971 (adapted from Khan & Talibi, 1972).

5 cases per 100,000 inhabitants and was near eradication in 1968-1970. It was transmitted by *An. philippinensis* (Elias *et al.*, 1983) (or possibly *An. nivipes* following the taxonomic review by Harbach *et al.*, 1994). Overpopulation resulted in agricultural intensification at the expense of marshland, and this triggered the expansion of new vectors, notably *An. aconitus* and *An. annularis*, in the rice-growing areas (Maheswary *et al.*, 1992). In the hilly areas to the east of Chittagong, "jungle" malaria caused by *An. dirus s.l.* most likely species D or *An. baimai*, and especially *An. minimus s.l.*, persists. It was hyper-endemic with 51% prevalence, more than half of which was due to *P. falciparum* (Khan & Talibi, 1972). The incidence was 16‰; the sporozoite rate of *An. minimus s.l.* was 1.3%; the stability index was 4.4; and the yearly Entomological Inoculation Rate (EIR) was 12.8. *An. dirus* appears to be taking over malaria transmission from *An. minimus s.l.*, the density of which was brought down by indoor spraying operations (Rosenberg & Maheswary, 1982).

Myanmar*

Myanmar (formerly Burma) (*Figure 24*) represents a microcosm of Indochinese malaria (as described above). The wooded hilly areas are occupied by minorities (Shan, Karen) while the plains are populated by Burmese people from Tibet. When the eradication program was launched, Postiglione & Venkat Rao (1956) proposed an epidemiological stratification of the country that identified three facies:
- mountains (or rather hills) of below 1,200 m altitude. Malaria was meso- or hyper-endemic, with parasitic prevalences of between 20% and 60%. *An. minimus s.l.* and *An. dirus s.l.*—in all probability sp. D (i.e. *An. baimai*)—had a sporozoite rate of 0.9-1%. The "minority" populations were the most affected (Khin-Maung-Kyi, 1974; Khin-Maung-Kyi & Winn, 1976; Myo Paing *et al.*, 1988; Tin, 1992);
- the extensively agricultural plains which support 41% of the population. These represent the "healthy" part of the country, inhabited by the majority Burmese population; a few epidemic episodes caused by *P. vivax* are transmitted by *An. philippinensis* (or *An. nivipes*), *An. aconitus* and *An. annularis*;
- the coastal regions are divided into the delta, the domain of *An. sundaicus* (most likely *An. epiroticus* but the identification needs to be confirmed), and rocky coasts to the west with features similar to those of the hilly regions mentioned above. The dominant vector, *An. dirus* (or *An. baimai*), had a sporozoite rate of 2.9% and was able to adapt to wells (Tun Lin *et al.*, 1987); malaria was meso- or hyper-endemic (*Figure 24*).

Thailand

As the favourite child of international organisations and the United States in a politically agitated region, Thailand has enjoyed substantial support for its malaria control programme and to develop its research potential.

The global incidence of malaria, which was 300‰ in 1947, dropped to 2.2‰ in 1975, climbed back up to 10‰ in 1981 (Ketrangsee, 1992), then stabilised around 4‰ by 1999. Since 1980, 75% of the cases are found along the borders of Myanmar and Cambodia where the incidence exceeded 500‰ in the first case as opposed to 25‰ in the second. At Mae Sot, in a Karen refugee camp, children 5 to 14 years of age exhibited 1.5 blood parasite peaks per annum, 68% of which were symptomatic: the pyrogenic density was 1,400 parasites/µl for *P. falciparum* and 181 for *P. vivax* (Luxemburger *et al.*, 1996 and 1998). Of 5,776 cases in two years, 303 severe cases led to 11 deaths (0.2%). The other source of infection was isolated jungle villages (Singhanetra-Renard, 1986) where the inhabitants spend part of the year in rudimentary huts in order to work what remains of the jungle (Somboon *et al.*, 1998) (*Figure 24*).

The increased scarcity of *An. minimus* pointed to *An. dirus s.l.* activity (Ismaïl *et al.*, 1975) before an exophilic form of *An. minimus* (sp. C) was discovered. The consequences of intensive deforestation have not yet been fully estimated although certain species, such as members of the Maculatus Group, appear to be taking on an increasingly important role in transmission (Rattanarithikul *et al.*, 1996a; Rosenberg *et al.*, 1990), notably *An. maculatus s.s.*, *An. sawadwongporni* and *An. pseudowillmori*.

Near the borders, rubber plantations and orchards (of lichees, rambutans and mangousteens) are highly conducive to transmission (Singhasivanon *et al.*, 1999).

Cambodia

The malaria control operations that began in 1951 were interrupted in 1971 and were never really resumed.

The epidemiological stratification proposed by Denis & Meek (1992) distinguishes (*Figure 25*):
- a non-endemic zone around Tonle Sap and the lower part of the Mekong;
- a hypo-endemic zone describing a semi-circle around the preceding zone reaching the Gulf of Siam to the south and the Thai border to the north-west;
- a meso-endemic zone covering the majority of the east and north-west of the country;
- highland hyper-endemic zones, in the Cardamone Mountains to the south-west and along the Laotian and Vietnamese borders to the south-east.

Estimates by Denis & Meek (1992), claiming 500,000 cases per annum with 5,000 to 10,000 deaths, are not implausible although they are not based on reliable data, given the decay of the health services and the lack of information on areas under Khmer Rouge control up until recently. In 1998, the incidence exceeded 20‰ in the north-east and the south-west of the country (*Mekong Malaria*, 1999). In 1999, the Phnom Penh branch of WHO estimated that there was no transmission in 979 communities, covering 72.9% of the territory; in 212 communities (10.5%), the risk was low, in 244 (11.9%) it was moderate, and in 126 (4.7%), it was high.

It should be remembered that Rodenfeldt & Cervone (*in* Sloof & Verdrager, 1972) demonstrated the role of *An. dirus* (sp. A) in Cambodia and studied its exophilic behaviour, while *An. minimus* (sp. A) had practically disappeared.

In Cambodia, when Phnom Penh fell to the Khmer Rouge, the population was deported to so-called redevelopment

---

* The countries of the Mekong Region-Myanmar, Thailand, China (to the south), Laos, Vietnam and Cambodia-were dealt with as a single entity in a *Mekong Malaria* monograph in which the main characteristics of the malaria in the various countries of this zone are mapped out (*Figure 24*).

Biodiversity of Malaria in the World

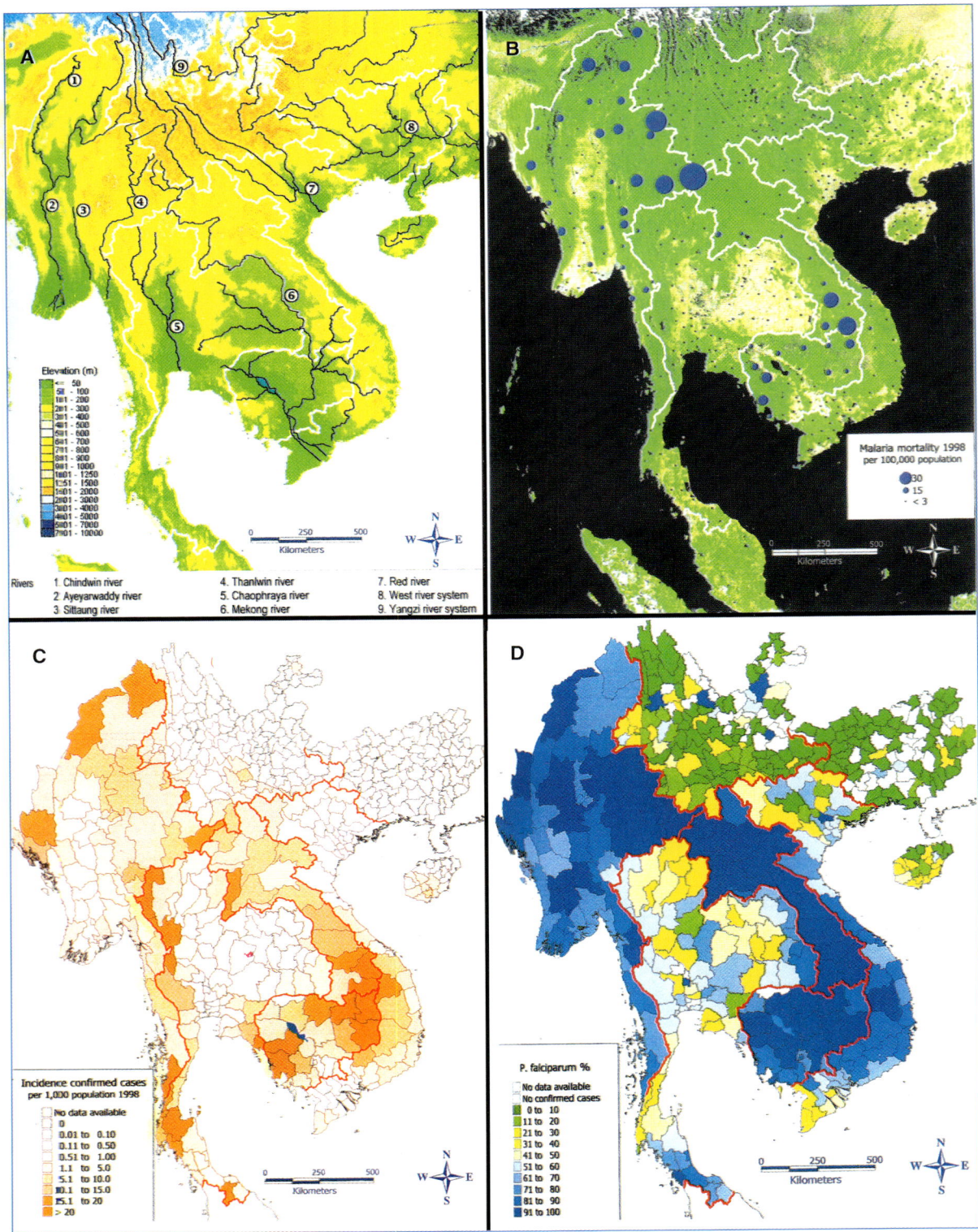

Figure 24. Countries of the Mekong Region (adapted from Mekong Malaria). **A.** Altitudes and rivers. **B.** Malaria mortality according to forest cover. **C.** Incidence of malaria in 1998 by district and per 1,000 inhabitants. **D.** Proportions of P. falciparum versus P. vivax.

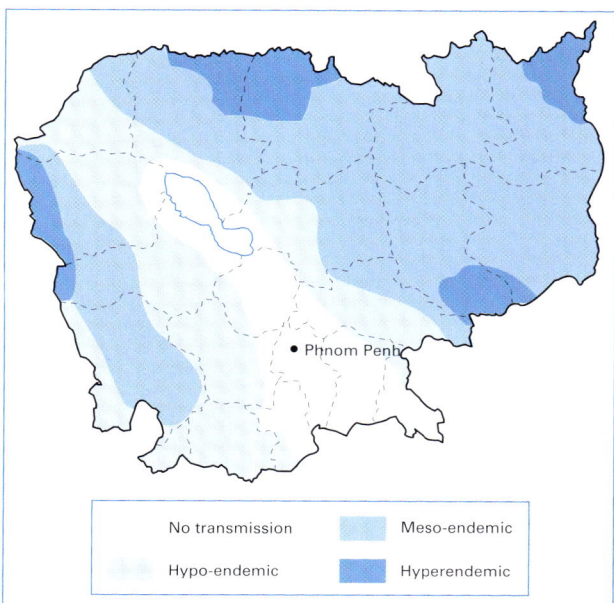

Figure 25. Level of malaria endemicity in Cambodia (from the Antimalarial Department, Ministry of Health, Dr. Lek Sandi).

zones, often located in highly endemic jungle. The deportees were deprived of medication and a large number of them died: malaria became one component in the genocide inflicted by the Khmer Rouge.

Finally, another historical point, the Angkor tragedy; in the 16th century, this capital of the Khmer empire was surrounded by arable land like the entire Tonle Sap plain. It was abandoned a century later leaving behind marvellous monuments. After the site was abandoned following Thai incursions, the ruins were taken over by the jungle, enabling *An. dirus* and malaria to move in, thereby driving out the inhabitants (Verdrager, 1992). At present, there is no transmission of malaria at the Angkor site nor in the neighbouring city of Siam Reap, although the disease is endemic in the hills to the north-east of the city (Lek Sandi, personal communication).

Laos

A small landlocked and peaceful country of 237,000 km², Laos has not been pre-eminent in the history of malaria control which has been limited there to just a few experimental projects. It is currently one of the countries of Asia most affected by malaria which ravages over 70% of the country (*Figure 23*). There are three zones which could be used as the basis for stratification:
- the Mekong plain, 30 to 120 km in width and inhabited by the Lao Loum, a subgroup of the AustroThai people who arrived from China in the 10th century. Malaria here is not endemic. At the Vientiane Hospital, all 400 of the hospitalised patients came from a few wooded regions to the east of the province; none were from the city (Southammavong, 1997). A focus of *P. falciparum* was described in an enclosed area of rice paddies to the east of Savanakhet, inhabited by the Lao Theung (Kobayashi *et al.*, 2000); the suspected vector was *An. nivipes* which is only known to carry *P. vivax*. This atypical epidemiological case requires confirmation;
- jungles at altitudes of between 300 and 1,200 m where malaria is hyper-endemic. The native peoples, particularly the Lao Theung, are relatively "resistant" to the disease. In Luang Prabang Province alone, with 500,000 inhabitants, the number of cases was estimated at more than 100,000 per annum (Sisouphane, personal communication, 1995). The incidence exceeded 10‰ and was as high as 20‰ throughout the mountainous zones;
- at higher altitudes—above 1,200 m—the Hmong, who came from China a century ago, settled on lands above the malaria limit, specifically to avoid the disease (to which they are particularly susceptible).

Their farming methods mean that the Lao Theung and the Hmong move frequently and live a semi-nomadic life; transmission is high at their secondary homes in the jungle.

Recent studies showed that both species of the Minimus Complex, sp. A and C, occur in Laos. They are sympatric in the northern part of the country, whereas only *An. minimus* (sp. A) is found further to the south (Garros *et al.*, 2006). *An dirus* (sp. A) and *An. jeyporiensis* seem to be the most efficient malaria vectors in Laos with sporozoite rates up to 2.5 and 5% respectively (Vythilingam *et al.*, 2003).

Vietnam

Vietnam has a population of more than 85 million over a surface area of 335,000 km². Its population density, greater than 200 per km², is one of the highest in the region.

The Khin ethnic majority, originally from the northern part of the country, gradually took over all of what is now Vietnam, the south of which was for a long time part of the Khmer Empire. The ethnic minorities, driven into the mountainous regions, are the country's "poor" even though they have the same political status; as already noted, they are the main victims of malaria.

The duality—healthy plain and highly endemic wooded hills—was noted by Mathis & Léger (1911), Borel (1926b), Toumanoff (1936) and Farinaud & Prost (1939). Indoor DDT spraying programmes covered 23% of the territory in 1981 but this dropped to just 4% when Soviet aid stopped. The number of cases rose from 135,000 (with 5,120 deaths in 1985) to over one million in 1992 (although the mortality did not rise in proportion). For ten years, the situation seriously deteriorated (*Figure 24c*) but recent data show rapid improvement since 2000 with the use of impregnated mosquito nets and indoor spraying.

The monograph by Phan (1998) emphasises the pre-eminent role of *An. minimus* throughout the entire country; populations of this mosquito, living in stagnant water near Hanoi, belong to species A but do not seem to be involved in the transmission of malaria. The exophilic behaviour of species C was confirmed by Van Bortel *et al.* (1999) and this species occurs in most parts of the country often sympatric with *An. minimus* (sp. A). *An. dirus* (sp. A) appears to be limited to the south of the Red River plain. *An. sundaicus s.l.*, identified as *An. epiroticus*, is found only along the southern coasts (south of Phan Thiet). *An. jeyporiensis* appears to play an important role on the southern plateaux with sporozoite rates of 0.8 -0.4%. *An. subpictus* was implicated in an epidemic of *P. vivax* in the plain of the Red River. The role of numerous other secondary vectors would require confirmation. It should be noted that Phan (1998) included *An. pseudowillmori* of the Maculatus Group in his list of vectors (as in Thailand).

P. falciparum is the dominant parasite throughout the country except in the Red River and Mekong Deltas where *P. vivax* is more common.

A study conducted by Marchand *et al.* (1997) in villages of the Danang Region that had not been treated in the last fifteen years, was used to recreate a table of the effects of malaria prior to eradication efforts. The so-called Khanh Phu study zone included 1,700 inhabitants living in 300 houses. The population consisted of 5% Khins and 95% belonging to the Rac Lay minority (whose economic level is lower even though they live in the same villages). The prevalence varied from 25-45% among the Rac Lay to 6-15% among the Khins. Incidence was 250‰ for *P. falciparum*, 273‰ for *P. vivax* and 31‰ for *P. malariae*, all ethnic groups included. Among the Rac Lay, 90% of infections were asymptomatic as opposed to 30% among the Khins. The prevalence of splenomegaly fell from 70% in 6-15 year-olds down to 20% after 16 years of age. Pyrogenic thresholds were estimated at 200 parasites *P. falciparum* per mm^3 in babies of under one year-old, 800 in 2-4 year-olds, and 12,800 in children over the age of 5; these figures are remarkably low compared to Africa (Richard *et al.*, 1988b) and they tend to rise with age (whereas in the Congo, they drop off). It is quite obvious that pyrogenic thresholds were not calculated in the same way in both cases.

Transmission occurs in the villages although it is higher in temporary dwellings, as in Thailand (Somboon *et al.*, 1998). *An. minimus s.l.* and *An. dirus* (sp. A) are responsible for transmission with sporozoite rates of 3.58% and 3.8% respectively. Other anopheline species were not infected. The EIR was between 50 and 100 infected bites per human per annum, a rate that is now exceptionally high for the Oriental Region. In a given village, the Khins are 75% less exposed to the risk of malaria than are the Rac Lay. The Khanh Phu project, remarkably well-planned and carried out with rigour, gives a good idea of what malaria might have been like in the Indo-Chinese Subregion prior to the "eradication" operations, especially if the results are compared with those collected by Farinaud & Prost prior to 1939 (*as discussed above*).

The persistence of vectors in regions from which malaria disease has disappeared poses a strategic problem in preventing the spread of epidemics (Verlé *et al.*, 1988).

Southern China

In China, the 25th parallel marks the limit between the Palaearctic Region to the north and the Oriental Region to the south, with overlapping zones in Yunnan, Guangxi, Guangdong and Hainan Provinces. The oriental character is affirmed by the presence of *An. minimus* (former species A and C), *An. dirus* (former sp. A on the Hainan Island (*Figure 11*) and D also called *An. baimai*) and *An. jeyporiensis* (Chen *et al.*, 2002; Sallum *et al.*, 2005; Zhou Zu-Jie, 1981) which are responsible for *P. falciparum* malaria.

The palaearctic character is embodied in the presence of *An. sinensis, An. lesteri* (formerly *An. anthropophagus*) and *An. liangshanensis* (formerly *An. kunmingensis*), which usually only carry *P. vivax*. Information on southern China were included in *Mekong Malaria* (*Figure 24*).

The incidence of malaria reaches 500‰ in the Yun River valley and on the southern borders of Yunnan and Hainan. Incidences from 10‰ to 100‰ have been reported at the borders of Guizhou and Guangxi. Elsewhere, the incidence is under 10‰. The use of a Geographic Information System (GIS) reveals the importance of the border problem (Hu *et al.*, 1998) with malaria particularly common on either side. There is extensive traffic across the border between China and Myanmar, a little less across the borders with Laos and Vietnam (Xu & Liu, 1997). On the island of Hainan, where occur *An. minimus* and *An. dirus* (species A for both), malaria is limited to the north of the island which is inhabited by the Li and Miao minorities. The southern part of the island, inhabited by Han people, has little or no malaria.

Taiwan

Malaria was eradicated in Taiwan in the early 1950's. It used to be transmitted by *An. minimus* (Chang *et al.*, 1950) which disappeared from the island in the early 1950's, as it did from Hong-Kong. The results obtained prior to 1950 were collected by Chow *et al.* (1950); they reported sporozoite rates of 0.8%, 1.9% and 2.3% for *An. sinensis, An. tessellatus* and *An. splendidus* respectively, which are not considered as highly efficient vectors. One must be extremely cautious when interpreting these old data. The presence of *An. sundaicus s.l.* is open to debate, as well as the infection rate of 0.45% reported for *An. maculatus*.

Japan

Only a few islands of the Ryukyu Archipelago, south of Japan, harbour *An. minimus* species E (Somboon *et al.*, 2001; Tsuda *et al.*, 1999) and can be considered as being part of the Oriental Region. As malaria had been eradicated from Japan just after the Second World War, these observations are of academic interest only.

It should nevertheless be remembered that, in 1945, there was an epidemic of *P. vivax* caused by *An. saperoi* among people who had sought refuge in the jungles to escape combat areas (Ichiro Miyagi, personal communication).

Epidemics caused by *P. vivax* and *P. falciparum* were also recorded among soldiers who had returned from theatres of operations in 1945 (600,000 cases).

The epidemiology of malaria in the Malayo-Indonesian Subregion

General characteristics

The Malayo-Indonesian Subregion forms the western extremity of the Oriental Region. From the point of view of malarial vectors and epidemiology, it is clearly distinct from the Australasian Region. The subregion is completely insular except for the Malaysian Peninsula. It features more than 10,000 islands, the largest of which are Borneo (750,000 km^2) and Sumatra (430,000 km^2) followed by the Celebes (Indonesian Sulawesi) (189,000 km^2), Java (130,000 km^2), Luzon (108,000 km^2) and Mindanao (99,000 km^2), as well as thousands of smaller islands. Six governments share this subregion: Indonesia, Brunei, East Timor, the Philippines, Malaysia, and Singapore.

The subregion's climate is uniformly tropical. The main factor governing irregular climatic variations is the El Niño Southern Oscillation (ENSO) which either causes drought followed by jungle fires in Indonesia or catastrophic flooding, depending on the year. The primary vegetation used to be tropical jungle, the surface area of which has been inexorably shrinking for many years, a phenomenon common throughout Southeast Asia resulting from forestry operations and agricultural development.

Insular fragmentation is a recent phenomenon with the majority of the islands having been joined in recent geological history. Island formation has led to significant diversification of animal and plant species and each island or group of islands is characterised by the presence of certain well-defined vectors (*Table III*). The only anopheline present through the entire subregion (except for the Philippines) is *An. sundaicus s.l.* or rather the Sundaicus Complex, different members of which are associated with differential degrees of endemicity (from hyper- to hypo-endemic).

Table III. Anopheline vectors (confirmed or secondary) in the island systems of Southeast Asia.									
Anopheline species	Peninsular Malaysia	**Borneo**		Sumatra	Java Bali	**Indonesia**		East Timor	Philippines
		Malaysia Sarawak Sabah	Indonesia Kalimantan			Sulawesi	Eastern islands		
An. aconitus				+	+			+	
An. annularis								+	
An. balabacensis		+	+						+
An. barbirostris D					+	+	+	+	
An. campestris	+								
An. dirus B	+								
An. donaldi		+	+						
An. flavirostris		+							+
An. letifer	+								
An. leucosphyrus		+	+	+					
An. litoralis									+
An. ludlowi						+			
An. maculatus	+			+				+	
An. mangyanus									+
An. sinensis (gr.)						+			
An. subpictus				+	+	+	+	+	
An. sundaicus (Complex)	+		+	+	+	+	+	+	
An. tessellatus								+	
An. vagus								+	

Control insecticide measures implemented during the second half of the 20th century considerably modified the malaria situation in the Philippines, in Malaysia and, to a lesser degree, in Java and Bali. The other islands of Indonesia benefited little or not at all from vector control campaigns.

Country by country

Malaysia

Malaysia consists of a continental part, Peninsular Malaysia, and Sarawak and Sabah Provinces located in the north of the island of Borneo.

Prior to the start of "eradication" operations in 1967, there were an estimated 300,000 cases of malaria in Peninsular Malaysia. The number of cases, which had dropped significantly following indoor spraying operations in the peninsula, as well as Sarawak and Sabah, began to climb back up again in 1979 once treatment operations had stopped, culminating in Sabah Province in 1981. Then the curve began to turn back down again in 1983 (Chooi, 1985) (*Table IV*). In 1990, the average incidence was 2.27‰ (Lim, 1992): 69% of these cases were in Sabah, 27% in the Peninsula and 2.5% in Sarawak. Malaria mortality was only 64 deaths per annum. Two-thirds of infections were attributed to *P. falciparum* and one-third to *P. vivax*. It is worth noting the fact that DDT spraying accelerates the deterioration of roofs made of palm leaves because it kills a wasp which hyperparasitises the caterpillar of the butterfly *Herculia migrivitta*—the caterpillars develop and feed without check since they live in palm stalks in the roof where they are sheltered from the insecticide; in contrast, malathion kills the caterpillar as well as its parasite, so the roof's service life is not compromised (Thevasagayam *et al.*, 1978), thus enhancing confidence in the health crews.

In the Peninsula in 1997 (Rahman *et al.*, 1997), the incidence ranged from 1.5‰ to 4.5‰ depending on the district, with death in 0.9-2.7‰ of confirmed cases (Mak *et al.*, 1992). In the inland jungle regions, prevalence was 25% among the Orang Asli, 25% among wood cutters and only 2% among civil servants, figures that point to the reality of forest malaria (Rahman *et al.*, 1998). As early as 1972 (Bolton, 1972), the prevalence of malaria (confirmed by serological tests) had been shown to be far higher among the Orang Asli, a semi-nomadic ethnic group residing in rudimentary housing than in Malaysian people in neighbouring villages (Mak *et al.*, 1987). Furthermore, indoor spraying was impossible in the wall-less Orang Asli dwellings.

From the coast of Peninsular Malaysia, a series of vectors succeed one another, from *An. epiroticus* (former *An. sundaicus* A) in brackish water, to *An. campestris* and *An. letifer* in the coastal plains, then *An. maculatus* inland with sporozoite rates of 0.4-5% (Loong *et al.*, 1988) and *An. leucosphyrus* A, now designated as *An. latens* (Sallum *et al.*, 2005). *An. dirus* sp. B, now called *An. cracens*, a jungle species, is limited to the Thai border region (Sandosham, 1970) (*Figure 26*).

In Sarawak Province (Rahman, 1982), away from the coastal malaria caused by *An. sundaicus s.s.*, prevalence is very low as the inland vector, *An. donaldi*, is inefficient. The few square kilometres of Brunei are enclosed within the Sarawak and do not have any specific characteristics. On the other hand, malaria is endemic in Sabah Province where *An. balabacensis*, with a sporozoite rate of 2%, maintains stable meso- or hyper-endemic disease. In the east of the province, the vector is *An. flavirostris*, a vector of the Philippines (Hii *et al.*, 1988a); it is sympatric with *An. latens* (= *An. leucosphyrus* A) in the west and the two species overlap along a north-south axis throughout all of Borneo (Harbach *et al.*, 1987a).

Extensive research into monkey malaria has been carried out in the peninsula (Warren *et al.*, 1970).

Malaria has apparently been eradicated from the island of Singapore and from Brunei, so the current situation in these States will not be specifically discussed.

Indonesia

In Indonesia, an estimated 5 million people are at risk. This estimate includes 700,000 in Java and Bali—relatively modest for a population of more than 200 million. The majority of subjects at risk live in the transmigration zones of Kalimantan and Western New Guinea. Currently, 60% of the population of the Outer Islands are medically protected (Arbani, 1992).

Java and Bali

The population of the two islands grew from 59.3 million in 1963 to 105.6 million in 1986. Both islands were included in eradication programs from 1958 to 1975. By 1963, the incidence had dropped to 1.5‰ but after spraying operations were discontinued, it increased back up to 49‰ in 1980 before dropping back down to 2.4‰ in 1986. The number of cases rose from 5,800 in 1963 to 346,000 in 1973, dropping to 20,000 in 1986. Near the sea where malaria was hyper-endemic in the recent past, the coastal vector *An. sundaicus* species E predominated (Dusfour *et al.*, submitted data), while *An. aconitus* was the main vector in inland rice paddies (Atmosoedjono *in* Takken *et al.*,

Table IV. Malaria incidence from 1979 to 1983 in Malaysia (*in* Chooi Chin Khoon, 1985).

Year	Sabah	Sarawak	Peninsula	Total
1979	33,320	1,086	10,540	44,946
1980	34,600	766	9,000	44,366
1981	50,035	745	8,600	59,380
1982	30,650	956	12,400	44,006
1983	11,300	850	10,060	22,210

Oriental Region

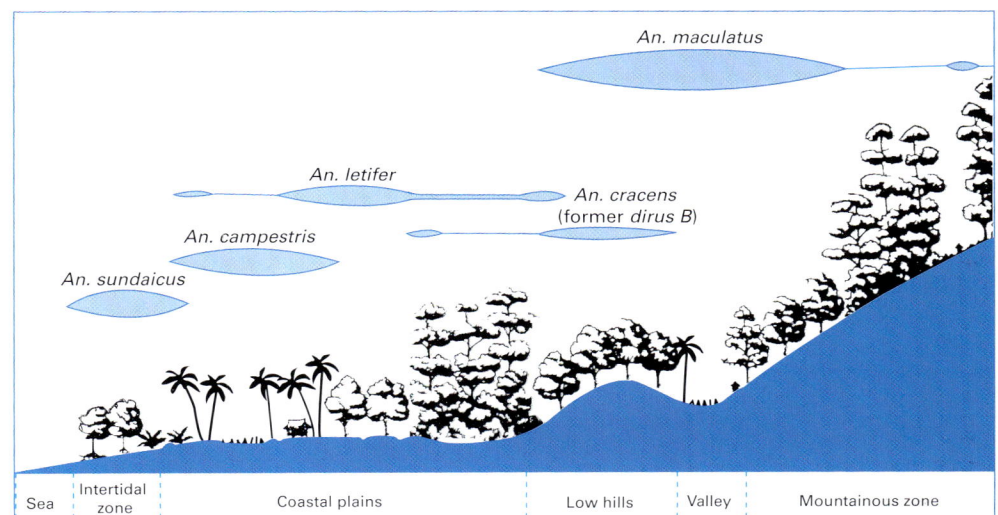

Figure 26. Distribution and density of malaria vectors in the various ecological habitats of Peninsular Malaysia (adapted from Sandersham, 1970).

1990; Soekirno et al., 1983). In 1920, Swellengrebel launched a series of malaria control programmes based on environmental management with some success (in Takken et al., 1990) although pilot zooprophylaxis programmes in Java did not yield conclusive results (Kirnowardoyo & Supalin, 1986).

Sumatra

Little epidemiological information is available about this island in which *An. sundaicus* species E and *An. aconitus* are the two vectors on the coast and inland respectively (Arbani, 1992; Cross et al., 1976; Kambara & Paimjactun, 1983).

Kalimantan

In this southern part of Borneo covered by dense forests, *An. balabacensis* to the east and *An. latens* (= An. *leucosphyrus* A) to the west are the two vectors. They can be found in sympatry, they are predominantly living and biting outside and their respective sporozoite rates are 1.3% and 1.2% (Harbach et al., 1987a). *An. sundaicus s.l.* transmits along the coasts. The presence of such efficient vectors could be expected to be associated with a high level of transmission but in fact, in western Kalimantan, the global prevalence is very low, around 2.8% for each parasite (Cross et al., 1976), although malaria seems to be extremely prevalent in migrant Javanese living in Kalimantan. It is currently difficult to summarise the situation on this large island.

Sulawesi

Located in the south-western part of the island, *An. sundaicus s.l.* transmission has been observed in July-August with a sporozoite rate of 0.09%, although the very abundant *An. subpictus* does not appear to be a vector (Collins et al., 1979). In the south, *Plasmodium* prevalences of 15-32% were reported by Cross et al. (1972) and Partono et al. (1972). *An. barbirostris*, the vector of Bancroftian filariasis (in Lien et al., 1977), was not found to transmit malaria. In general terms, little epidemiological information is available. In the Palu Valley in the centre, prevalence was fairly low, ranging from 3-6% with similar numbers of *P. vivax* and *P. falciparum* infections (Cross et al., 1975).

Lombok, Soembava, Soemba, Flores, West Timor

Not much is known about malaria in the string of small islands (the Outer Islands, of which only the main islands are dealt with here) and the data that have been collected are inconsistent. The annual number of cases varied from 50,000 to 80,000 from 1966 to 1973 (WHO, 1983). In western Timor, *An. subpictus* was infected and no sporozoites have ever been detected in other species (Lien et al., 1975). In the Flores Islands (Lee et al., 1983) where a prevalence of 77% has been recorded in children and one of 20% in adults, the only vectors were *An. subpictus* and *An. barbirostris* with salivary gland infections of 3/275 and 1/126 respectively. Information about the other islands would have to be sought in local reports.

East Timor

East Timor, which gained independence in May 2002, was the most thoroughly investigated island of the region. From 1966 to 1973, the annual number of cases varied from 50,000 to 80,000 (WHO, 1983). According to Azevedo et al. (1958a and 1958b), the parasite prevalence was 46% (among children) below 100 m, 34% between an altitude of 100 and 500 m, and less than 1% above 500 m. The vectors were *An. sundaicus s.l.* and *An. barbirostris*.

Philippines

Malaria is endemic in seventy-two of the country's seventy-five provinces (Asinas, 1992). Malaria morbidity per 100,000 inhabitants had fallen from 1,000 cases in 1946 to 67 by 1971 (Cabrera & Arambulo, 1977) following control measures. It then increased to 202 in 1984. Malaria mortality fell from 91 cases per 100,000 inhabitants in 1946 to 1.6 in 1989. At present, malaria is not listed as one of the ten main causes of mortality (*Figure 27*).

The *P. falciparum/P. vivax* ratio is 65%. At a Manila hospital, 56% of 1,000 positive slides were *P. falciparum*, 38% *P. vivax* and 0.1% *P. malariae* (Salazar, 1989). Out of 562 *P. falciparum* infections, 40 (8%) corresponded to pernicious malaria (Alcantara *et al.*, 1982).

On the island of Palawan, where *An. balabacensis* is the dominant species, 90% of the population had malaria, either as disease or symptomless. On the island of Mindoro, a prevalence of 22% was measured and one of 8% north of Luzon. Malaria was hypo-endemic on the coastal plains and meso-endemic in the hills and foothills where *An. flavirostris*—the country's main vector—thrives. This species also colonised rice paddy irrigation ditches. There was no recorded transmission in population centres which are not conducive to *An. flavirostris* breeding. On the island of Mindoro, the prevalence among children was 7-13% compared with 3-4% among adults: of these, 2.8% were *P. falciparum*, 4.3% *P. vivax* and 0.7% *P. malariae* (Smrkovski *et al.*, 1982).

On Sulu and southern Mindanao, in the absence of the main vectors, a few cases were due to transmission by *An. litoralis* (Cabrera *et al.*, 1970).

On Palawan Island, malaria was meso- or hyper-endemic in certain villages. It is not impossible that *An. balabacensis* is a vector of a primate *Plasmodium* species there (Miyagi, 1973).

The spectacular decline of endemic malaria in the Philippines is a very good example of the success of control operations even if total eradication was not achieved.

The epidemiology of malaria in the Indo-Pakistani Subregion

General characteristics of the subregion

For biogeographers, this subregion extends from the natural barrier of the Hindu Kush in Afghanistan in the west, to the Brahmaputra Delta in India to the east. It encompasses the whole of India apart from the north-eastern part, Nepal (the western part), Sri Lanka (formerly Ceylon), the Maldives, Pakistan, and Afghanistan to the east of the Hindu Kush.

The alluvial basins of the Ganges and the Indus Rivers stretch from the Himalayas down to the Deccan plateau to the south. The latter rises to the west (Western Ghats), to the east (Eastern Ghats), and to the north (Madhya Pradesh). The island of Sri Lanka is fairly hilly with highlands exceeding 2,000 m in the south. The Maldives are flat, sandy islands to the west of Sri Lanka.

Rainfall plays a key role in the incidence of malaria and the outbreak of epidemics.

The entire subregion is directly influenced by the south-western monsoon, which brings summer rains from June to September. The north-eastern monsoon arrives in December on the east coast of the Deccan plateau and

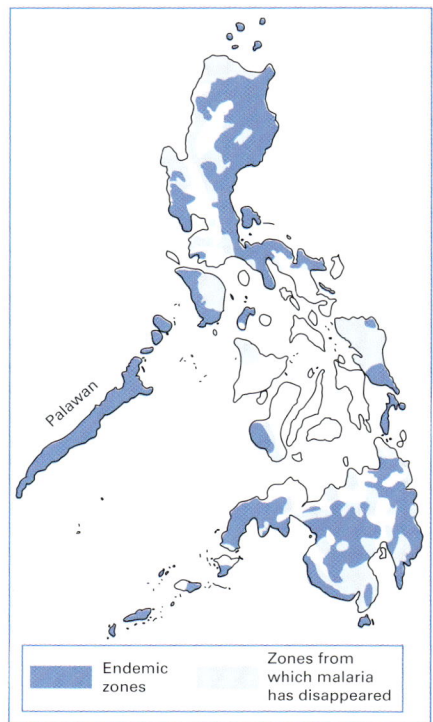

Figure 27. Endemic zones in the Philippines (adapted from Salazar et al., *1988).*

northern Sri Lanka. Rainfall is highly irregular from one year to the next and the ENSO meteorological phenomenon, which affects the temperature of the equatorial ocean masses of the Pacific and Indian Oceans, greatly influences the climate of the whole of Southeast Asia (Bouma, 1995). During El Niño years, precipitation is generally reduced in the Indian subcontinent and in intermediate years—under the influence of La Niña (*see the Part on* "Spatiotemporal Dynamics of Malaria")—it can be excessive.

Aside from these periodic, although irregular, phenomena, a dry zone is observed (less than 250 mm of rainfall per annum) in the south of the Indus Valley, around Baluchistan in Pakistan, and in Rajasthan and Gujarat in India. The foothills of the Himalayas and the Hindu Kush receive considerable rainfall (more than 5,000 mm in Darjeeling) and the Ganges Plain receives more than 1,000 mm. On the Deccan plateaux, far more rain falls on the western slopes than on the eastern ones. In the Nilgiri Hills in the Western Ghats, the western face receives more than 4,000 mm of rain compared to less than 1,000 mm on the eastern face (Russel & Jacob, 1942). In Sri Lanka (Dewit *et al.*, 1994), the humid part in the south-west where annual rainfall exceeds 2,500 mm is somewhat different from the dry northern and eastern parts where precipitation is less than 2,000 mm. This difference in rainfall plays a key role in the incidence of malaria and the outbreak of epidemics.

Considering that the characteristics of malaria changed when it returned following the eradication period,

Pattanayak *et al.* (1994) and Sharma (1996) grouped the various forms into five paradigms: tribal, rural, urban, industrial and border malaria. This classification remains essentially descriptive.

The epidemiology of malaria in this subregion could also be considered in terms of three different facies: **tribal malaria**, **epidemic malaria** and **urban malaria**. Superimposed on this division is the variable balance between *P. vivax* and *P. falciparum* which is often related to climatic variations.

The balance between P. vivax and P. falciparum and haemoglobinopathies

Kondrashin (1992) classified the region into zones where *P. falciparum* dominates, zones where *P. vivax* dominates (with or without G6PD deficiency), and zones in which *P. malariae* is found.

Generally speaking, *P. falciparum* peaks during and at the end of the monsoon (June-November), while *P. vivax* peaks during the same period and also in the spring (February-May) when relapsing malaria occurs. Peak rates can reach 60% (Viswanathan, 1945). Over the last thirty years and particularly after the eradication program was stopped in India, an increase in the *P. falciparum/P. vivax* ratio was observed as well as a decrease in the number of zones considered malaria-free. The percentage of *P. falciparum* reached 70% in the Haryana States (Choudhury & Gosh, 1982; Choudhury *et al.*, 1983), West Bengal (Ghosh *et al.*, 1985) and Uttar Pradesh (Chandrahas & Sharma, 1983). The sporozoite rates of *An. culicifacies* and *An. fluviatilis* rose above 6% in November.

The surface area of malaria-free zones has contracted significantly in northern Pakistan and along the northern border of Afghanistan as shown by a comparison of Christophers' map (1927) (*in* Hehir, 1927) and the Jaffar map (1991 *in* Bouma, 1995). In Punjab, Pakistan, from 1970 to 1975, seventeen *P. vivax* were recorded for every *P. falciparum* but by 1984, this pattern had reversed to just one *P. vivax* for fifty *P. falciparum* (Strickland *et al.*, 1987). In the same country, *P. falciparum* numbers rose from a few hundred in 1983 to 25,000 in 1990 (Bouma *et al.*, 1996a).

According to Bouma *et al.* (1994), this "increase" in *P. falciparum* may have been caused by a lengthened transmission season, following an increase in the temperature in November over seven consecutive years in the North-West Frontier Province of Pakistan. During the period from 1984 to 1990, temperatures in November never fell below 17.5°C; equally high temperatures observed between 1971 and 1974 were accompanied by an increase in the incidence of malaria.

The average November temperature has increased from 16 °C to 18 °C since 1887 (compared with an overall increase of just 0.5 °C in the northern hemisphere). This differential over more than a century, as well as the more recent phenomenon of global warming, requires further investigation.

Various experts have sought immunological explanations for relative variations in *P. falciparum* and *P. vivax*, and others have looked at the influence of various haemoglobinopathies, although their conclusions are not very persuasive.

Strickland *et al.* (1988) compare the strong, long-lasting immunity to *P. vivax* with that against *P. falciparum* which is weak and not sustained from one season to the next (unlike in Africa). These observations concur with those of Cox (1984), as cited earlier.

The Arabo-Indian haemoglobin S haplotype is found in the oases in western Arabia and among tribal peoples in India (Nagel & Fleming, 1992). The percentage of Hb AS carriers is believed to be about 30% in tribal people. In the Nilgiri Hills of Tamil Nadu, the frequency of Hb AS was above 37% and even reached 47% among older children (Ramasamy *et al.*, 1997); this abnormally high frequency could be due to an epidemic early in the century selecting against normal haemoglobin, although this remains to be confirmed.

The relationship between α-thalassaemia (Modiano *et al.*, 1991) and malaria remains to be proven. This type of haemoglobinopathy seems to be less common in tribal peoples.

A total absence of Duffy-negative subjects is observed among the Naga people of the oriental extremity of India (Kar *et al.*, 1992).

G6PD deficiency (Kar *et al.*, 1992) is more frequent among the indigenous population than among Hindus in Andhra Pradesh, and, in Sri Lanka, it is more common in the Singhalese population than in Tamil people. Among the Gonds of the Madhya Pradesh, a corollary was established between G6PD deficiency and malaria (Thakur & Verma, 1992). Despite an abundant literature, the relationships between these factors are still poorly defined and there are more hypotheses than proven facts.

Epidemic malaria

Malaria epidemics are an integral part of the history of the Indian Subcontinent (Bouma, 1995). They were cyclical before the first malaria control programmes were launched in the 1950's. Epidemics were caused by climatic variations that affected both parasite transmission efficiency and the development of immunity (Macdonald, 1953). Variations in life expectancy, anthropophilic behaviour and vector density were other important factors (Onori & Grab, 1980). Changes in vectors' distribution ranges may also have been a result of climatic variations (Zulueta, 1987).

Epidemic malaria ravaged two large zones: the Punjab in Pakistan and neighbouring Indian States, as well as Sri Lanka. In the first, they were triggered by heavy rainfall and, in the second, by a lack of rain.

The first well-studied epidemic occurred in Punjab in 1908. Prior to partition, the Punjab Region included the States of Haryana, Himachal Pradesh and part of Uttar Pradesh in India, as well as that of Punjab in Pakistan. The malaria epidemic led to 300,000 deaths (Christophers, 1911). Other less dramatic epidemics occurred up until 1940 (Yacob & Swaroop, 1944, 1945) but the introduction of DDT indoor spraying in 1958 lead to the temporary end of such outbreaks.

After the recrudescence of malaria (Mathur et al., 1992), a serious epidemic broke out in the semi-desert part of Rajasthan in 1994, killing 4,000 people. The epidemic was triggered by very heavy rainfall after a dry period; its victims were people whose immunity had waned and who succumbed to cerebral malaria (Kochar et al., 1997) (although, according to the WHO [1994], mortality was actually far below the reported figures). All of these epidemics are associated with excess precipitation (often related to the ENSO) during the monsoon following an extended dry period in the Punjab. Ten of the sixteen epidemics that ravaged this region occurred in years following an El Niño episode, and the other six occurred in La Niña years (also characterised by heavy rainfall) (Bouma & Van der Kaay, 1994; Bouma, 1995).

It should be noted that the development of irrigation in the valleys of the Indus and its tributaries has changed anopheline breeding cycles thereby reducing the risk of epidemic malaria and increasing the risk of endemic disease.

In Sri Lanka, epidemics occur in the "dry" zones in the north and east of the country, and in years with low levels of precipitation. Rivers stop flowing and their beds become scattered with residual pools providing ideal conditions for the development of *An. culicifacies* E. Nine out of sixteen epidemics at the start of the century occurred during dry El Niño years (Bouma & Van der Kaay, 1994). The construction of dams, notably at Victoria, cut down flow rates and attenuated the epidemics (Wijesundera, 1988). Not all epidemics seem to be linked to climate. In Sri Lanka after indoor spraying operations had been discontinued, an epidemic in 1964 led to several million infections although there were practically no deaths as only *P. vivax* was involved.

The epidemic of 1967 in the Punjab which affected 790,000 people followed flooding and was probably amplified by the development of *An. culicifacies* resistance to DDT. In 1967, the untreated city of Karachi, Pakistan, experienced an epidemic that affected 400,000 people which Farid (1974) attributed to a massive influx of refugees.

Preventing epidemics—the keystone of malaria control—depends on understanding the underlying factors which cause such epidemics so that the risks can be accurately evaluated; this is why we have chosen to go into the Indo-Pakistani Subregion in such detail.

Tribal malaria

The problem of malaria in ethnic minorities in the Oriental Region was discussed earlier. In India, the tribal people are indigenous groups that persisted following invasion by Indo-Europeans. This invasion resulted in considerable mixing of the populations, particularly in the south of the country. These native peoples practice animism or Christianity and are caste-less. They often live in extremely poor conditions, do not participate in the economic life of the country and have no social protection.

Perry (1914), in the Jeypore Hills of Orissa, and Russel & Jacob (1942) in the Nilgiris Hills of Tamil Nadu, have already drawn attention to the high endemicity of malaria in tribal peoples living in the hilly regions where *An. fluviatilis* sp. S is the vector. The above-mentioned north-eastern States, where the vectors are *An. minimus s.l.* and *An. dirus* sp. D, now called *An. baimai*, are inhabited by indigenous tribal minorities.

There was no particular focus on tribal malaria during the eradication period when uniform strategies were implemented but, since recrudescence of malaria, this form of the disease has attracted special attention. Now, tribal malaria accounts for more than 30% of all cases in India, and this in just 12% of the population.

The District of Koraput in Orissa is home to only 0.36% of the population of India but sees 2-3% of all cases of malaria and 6-9% of cases of pernicious disease, i.e. 300,000 cases with 80 deaths per annum (Rajagopalan et al., 1990); 66% of the children were suffering from malaria (Das et al., 1989). Venkat Rao (1949) contrasted the hyper-endemic plateau home of *An. fluviatilis* (sp. S) with the hypo-endemic or healthy plateau, where *An. annularis* and *An. philippinensis* dominate: 70% of infections were symptomless providing a reservoir of *P. falciparum* malaria. Viswanathan (1951) had reintroduced the notion of the immunity-conditioned pyrogenic threshold. Perry (1914) had long before pointed out that, in Orissa, the immunity of indigenous people confers some degree of "resistance" to the disease. With the expansion of irrigation, *An. annularis* has become an efficient vector of malaria in this State (Dash et al., 1982). Among the Gonds of Madhya Pradesh, Singh et al. (1998) had noted the absence of malaria mortality and the fact that only one abortion occurred in a group of ninety-six *P. falciparum*-infected pregnant women.

Since 1942, the situation in the Nilgiris has been described by Russel & Jacob; they proposed an altitude-based stratification with a **hyper-endemic zone** between 300 and 1,200 m, the limit of the *An. fluviatilis* S vector; these experts did not take the ethnic aspect into account. Tribal malaria has often been rightly associated with the jungle where *An. fluviatilis* S is one of the vectors. In certain regions of the Madhya Pradesh, however, *An. culicifacies s.l.* can play the primary role.

The access of tribal people to proper medical care is limited with few health care facilities and, in any case, a reticent attitude to modern medicine. Little mention is made of the problem of how these people are received in health facilities run by Hindus, whose culture is totally different.

Urban malaria

The majority of cities in Southeast Asia that were never treated during the eradication programs are in fact malaria-free. The exception comes from the Indian Subcontinent where urban malaria has been documented since the beginning of the century. The problem has been associated with the water supply, especially its storage in wells or tanks which provide highly propitious environments for the propagation of *An. stephensi*.

This anopheline, the levels of which are generally stable throughout the year, has a sporozoite rate close to 1% (Das *et al.*, 1979). In Salem, Tamil Nadu, the highly abundant *An. subpictus* (a freshwater species) is also found in wells although it has never been found infected (Batra *et al.*, 1979b).

Urban malaria has been reported in most Deccan cities (Madras, Madurai, Salem, Bangalore, etc.) as well as in Calcutta and Delhi. It tends to prevail in the city even where it is not present in the surrounding countryside, making it a rather case.

The exception of Pondicherry should be noted where urban malaria is not present as the larvae of *An. stephensi* are parasitised by the *Nosema algerae* fungus (Menon & Rajagopalan, 1979). In the neighbouring village of Salem, where the larvae are not parasitised, the prevalence of malaria is significant.

The conclusions to be drawn from the comprehensive literature on the topic are nearly unanimous.

Malaria in different countries

As Nepal, Bangladesh and north-eastern India were discussed under the Indo-Chinese Subregion, India (to the west of Brahmaputra), Pakistan, Afghanistan (to the east of the Hindu Kush), Sri Lanka and the Maldives will be considered in the Indo-Pakistani Subregion.

Prior to the Second World War, there were an estimated 75 million cases of malaria per annum in the Empire territory which included Pakistan, Bangladesh and Sri Lanka as well as India; this territory had less than 400 million inhabitants. All older statistics must thus be reviewed in the light of both the population boom (India alone had 1 billion inhabitants in 2000) and the redrawn borders.

India

The statistics of India's National Malaria Eradication Programme (NMEP) currently provide only aggregate data from which it is impossible to resolve the north-eastern States from the rest of India. After its launch in 1958, the program was restructured into a Control Program in 1975 at the request by the WHO's 14th Expert Committee (1974) after their review of antimalarial strategies. Insecticide treatment was then undertaken only where it was justified for epidemiological and/or strategic reasons.

Table V shows the number of cases declared by the NMEP. The smallest number of cases was declared in 1961 at which time it was believed that eradication was on the right track. 1971 marked a resurgence of transmission as a result of *An. culicifacies s.l.* and *An. stephensi* developing resistance to DDT. 1976 was marked by a genuine post-eradication epidemic following the termination or reduction of insecticide treatments. The incidence curve then began to decline again with the application of modern control measures (*Table V*).

It should be noted that even in 1961, transmission was never completely stopped in zones inhabited by indigenous peoples where *An. fluviatilis* S was the vector (Rao, 1962, personal communication). The information provided at that time by the NMEP concerned the number of declared cases, with priority given to eradication dynamics, i.e. a target of zero incidence. During the massive resurgence of transmission in 1976 however, persistent foci exploded highlighting the importance of tribal malaria, particularly in the jungle. In the Madhya Pradesh, the incidence of malaria was five times greater in jungle villages than in villages on roads outside the jungle (Singh *et al.*, 1996) (*Figure 28*).

One of the major factors which led to the recrudescence of 1971 was the development of resistance in *An. stephensi* and *An. culicifacies s.l.* In the latter complex however, the zoophilic species B is more resistant than the anthropophilic species, which minimised the epidemiological impact of resistance.

A bitter polemic developed regarding the causes of resistance in India. For Sharma & Mehrotra (1983), it was a consequence of widespread DDT use by the public health authorities whereas experience in Turkey, West Africa and Central America was rather in favour of selection by the destruction of larval habitats as a result of agricultural

Table V. Cases of malaria in India from 1961 to 1986. The peak of 1976 marks the end of the eradication program (according to India's NMEP).	
1961	49,000 cases
1965	100,000 cases
1971	1,300,000 cases
1976	6,160,000 cases
1982	2,160,000 cases
1986	1,765,000 cases

insecticide treatment (Chapin & Wasserstrom, 1981), particularly on cotton crops. Regardless of the cause of resistance, it nevertheless compromises the efficacy of indoor spraying strategies.

It has to be underlined that indoor spraying with DDT eradicated *Phlebotomus argentipes* from houses, leading to the near disappearance of kala-azar. In 1977, the disease reappeared with 70,000 cases in the State of Bihar, one of the most affected; cutaneous forms of *Leishmania* had persisted in lesions and, after a period of ten years, these re-launched the disease.

Malaria returned to India after 1972. The first signs were detected in 1973 and key indicators continued to rise, reaching extremely high values in 1976 with more than 6 million cases. In Tamil Nadu (Dutta *et al.*, 1979), the discontinuation of spraying operations and the development of irrigation systems were considered to be responsible for this re-emergence (Hyma & Ramesh, 1980); the same pattern was seen in the Gujarat District (Dutt *et al.*, 1980). Malaria has since become more or less endemic in a large part of the country.

India thus remains an active malaria zone. Endemicity increased in many States and, as in the past, epidemics exploded after eradication efforts (mainly based upon Indoor Residual Spraying – IRS) were discontinued in 1975. In 1984, the Gujarat District and the western part of India were devastated by a terrible epidemic. The more recent epidemics of 1988 and 1994 in Rajasthan were described earlier.

In 1986, the government created a malaria stratification committee to plan control measures. The country was divided into seven strata (*Figure 29*):
- south India with a low epidemic potential, except with regard to urban malaria;
- the centre-west (Maharashtra, Gujarat, Madhya Pradesh, eastern Rajasthan) with many endemic foci;
- the west, along the Pakistani border (western Rajasthan) with moderate to high epidemic potential;
- the north, as far as the foothills of the Himalayas (Punjab, Haryana, Uttar Pradesh) with limited epidemic potential; Jammu and Kashmir are considered to be malaria-free;
- the north, between the previous zone to the west and Bengal to the east (Bihar, Bengal) with very high potential;
- the centre-east (west Bengal, Orissa, north of Andhra Pradesh and west of Madhya Pradesh) with a high potential;
- the north-east (Assam, tribal areas, Sikkim) with very strong receptivity, if not hyper-endemic.

These divisions were inspired by old Indian malaria maps which had been updated on the basis of developments in the country (Singh *et al.*, 1990). However, the experts consider that the decentralisation of malaria control operations should be mapped in terms of primary health care units. The proposed district-based stratification took into account topography, rainfall, vectors, Annual Parasite

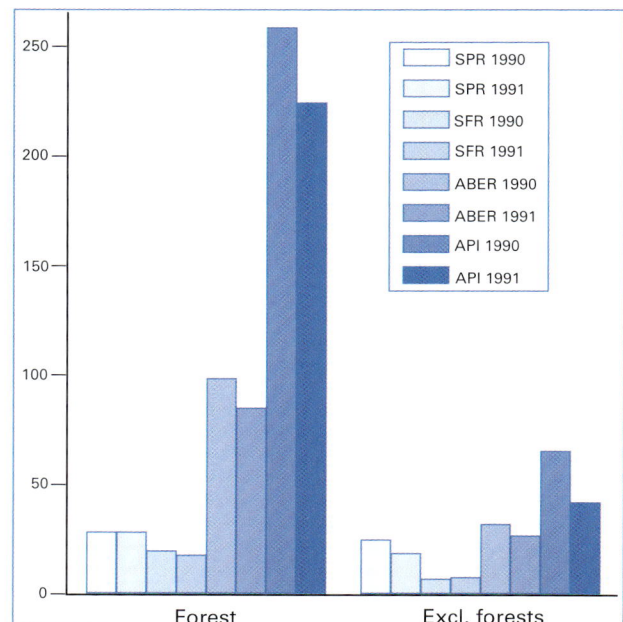

Figure 28. Epidemiology of malaria in cities in and around jungle areas in Madhya Pradesh, India: 1990-1991 (adapted from Singh et al., 1996).
SPR: Slide Positivity Rate;
SFR: Slide falciparum Rate;
ABER: Annual Blood Examination Rate;
API: Annual Parasite Incidence.

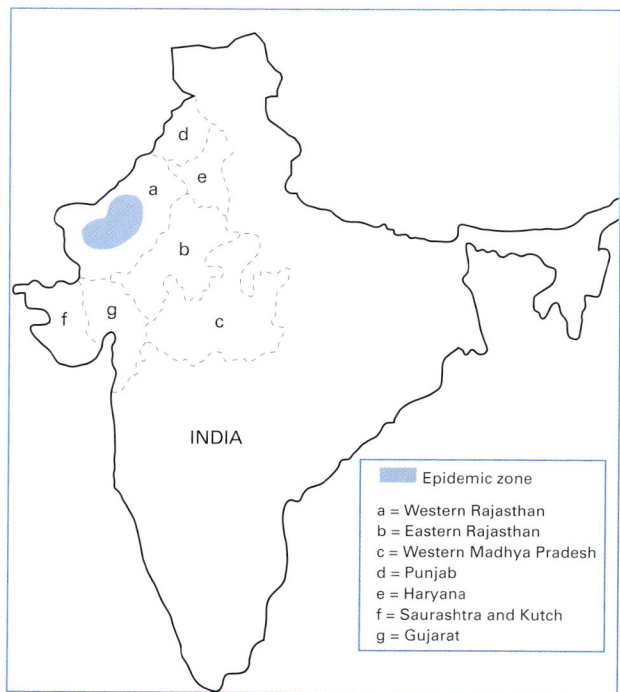

Figure 29. The malaria epidemic of 1994 in Rajasthan, India (adapted from Bouma & Van der Kaay, 1994).

Incidence (API) for five years, epidemic potential (the highest API over a five-year period) and vulnerability. Each factor is assigned a coefficient from 1 to 10 and the sum for the six factors is used to rank districts according to the local seriousness of the malaria problem with a view to deciding what needs to be done in terms of control measures. It appears that the model was successfully tested in the State of Karnataka.

Transmission follows the monsoon rains from July to October, but *P. vivax* is transmitted by *An. culicifacies s.l.* in the springtime throughout the country (Vaid *et al.*, 1974).

The "jungle phenomenon" appears in all regions where this type of vegetation thrives.

Pakistan

Pakistan is divided into four provinces: Punjab, Sindh, North-West Frontier Province (NWFP) and Balochistan.

Table VI. Cases of malaria in Pakistan from 1984 to 1986.			
	1984	1985	1986
Number of slides examined	2,840,000	2,730,000	2,890,000
Number of positive slides	65,000	60,000	90,000
Number of *P. falciparum*	1,725	20,296	29,538

Table VII. Percentage of positive slides.			
Province	1985	1986	1987
Punjab	2.13	2.49	1.49
Sindh	3.06	3.60	3.67
NWFP	3.53	5.80	3.68
Balochistan	2.36	2.19	2.48

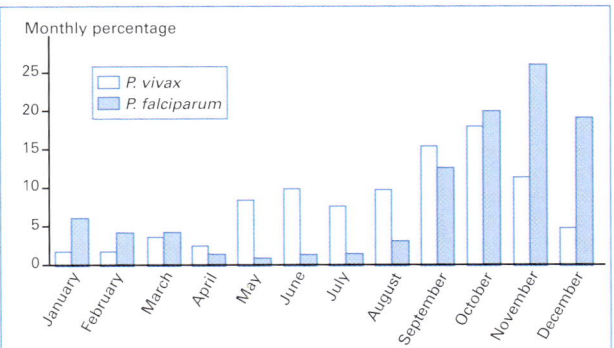

Figure 30. Monthly percentages of P. falciparum *and* P. vivax *in north-eastern Pakistan (adapted from Bouma* et al., *1996).*

In 1960, prior to eradication efforts, 3.7 million cases were reported with 37,000 deaths. The situation from 1984 to 1986 according to Farid (1987) is shown in *Table VI*.

Between 1960 and 1984, the number of cases dropped considerably due to large scale operations of IRS, with DDT but, in 1985, *P. falciparum* numbers began to increase again. This is the major change which has taken place over the last few years. According to the WHO (1990a), the number of cases dropped from 90,000 to 50,000 between 1996 and 1998. The percentage of positive slides per province is indicated in *Table VII*.

The very high rate of positive results in the NWFP in 1986 apparently corresponds to the increase of *P. falciparum*.

In pre-eradication surveys conducted in 1960 (Mashaal, 1962, *in* Farid, 1974), four types of zones were defined on the basis of data collected from a sample of 693 villages:
- malaria-free: 6.3%,
- hypo-endemic: 28.8%,
- meso-endemic: 53%,
- hyperendemic: 12%.

The overall percentage of parasites was 11.4%, half of which corresponded to *P. vivax*.

Transmission is at its peak from July to October although it can extend into November. *P. vivax* numbers begin to drop off in April or May while *P. falciparum* is predominantly a summer species (Strickland *et al.*, 1987). Relapsing *P. vivax* malaria occurs primarily in March and April (*Figure 30*).

The prevalence of malaria varies enormously from place to place within the same region. The highest figures are found in the plain of the Indus River and the valleys of the Punjab (the region of the five rivers) where PRs are two to five times higher in children than they are in adults—reflecting the existence of acquired immunity (Strickland *et al.*, 1987). Bouma (1995) reproduced two maps of malaria: the first, produced by Christophers (1927), includes Pakistan and North West India; the second, published by Jaffar Brothers (*Figure 31*), is used by malaria control managers. Both of these maps show malaria-free zones and endemic zones (which often correspond to irrigated areas) which were the starting points for explosive epidemics. Comparison of the two maps shows shrinkage of the malaria-free zones in the north and along the border with Afghanistan, which is consistent with the increase in temperature (Bouma, 1995). Furthermore, the epidemic zones have disappeared although they may return since the discontinuation of indoor spraying operations.

The vectors in the NWFP are *An. fluviatilis* S and *An. pulcherrimus, An. superpictus* in the mountainous regions of the north-west, *An. culicifacies* A and *An. stephensi* in the flood plains.

Reisen and his team have conducted a great deal of research into the possibilities of genetic control. They have primarily focused on population dynamics and the behaviour of the two vectors rather than on epidemiology.

Biodiversity of Malaria in the World

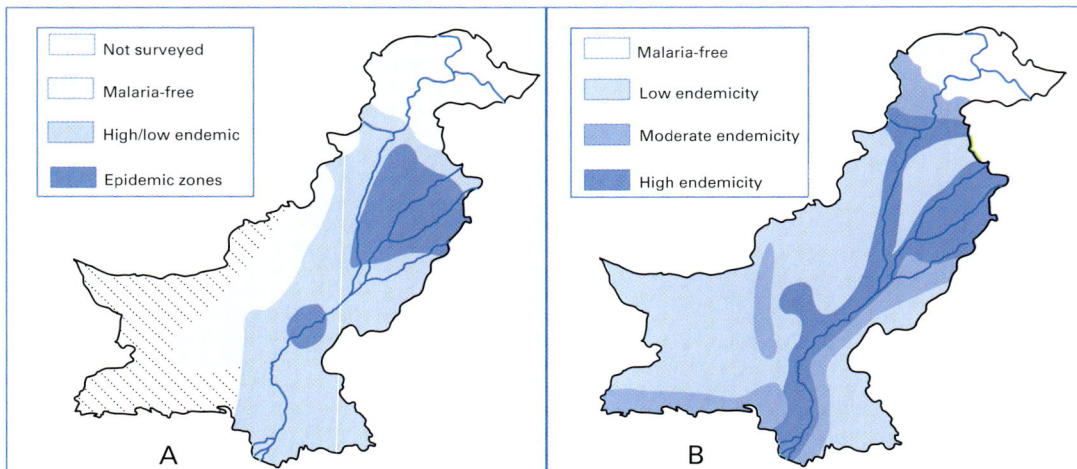

Figure 31. Changes in malaria in Pakistan between 1927 and 1991.
A. Malaria in 1922 (adapted from Christophers in Bouma, 1995).
B. Malaria in 1991 (adapted from Jaffar in Bouma, 1995).

Afghanistan

Only the part to the east of the Hindu Kush will be dealt with in this chapter; the country as a whole will be addressed in the context of the western Asia Subregion of the Palaearctic Region. The Hindu Kush Mountains, a southern extension of the Pamir, splits Afghanistan along a line running from the northeast to the south-west; in the north and in the centre, its peaks exceed 4,000 m, while its slopes flatten out towards the south. For many biogeographers including Rao (1984), this mountain chain marks the limit of the Oriental Region, though numerous Palaearctic species cross this limit to the east and Indo-Pakistani species extend westwards as far as the Arabic Peninsula.

In the part that we are interested in, the vectors are essentially *An. culicifacies s.l.* and *An. stephensi* in the south-east (Rao, 1951), *An. superpictus* and *An. fluviatilis s.l.* in the higher areas. *An. superpictus* was the only vector in Kabul, owing to its altitude (Iyengar, 1954).

Maps of the entire country are relatively old, dating back to the late 1950's when the first eradication operations were being commenced (Dhir & Rahim, 1957). Concerning the south-east specifically, malaria morbidity was particularly high in the Districts of Laghman, Kunar and Jalahabad (Rao, 1951). In 1985, 228,000 cases were reported in Kunar district alone (in the east) (WHO, 1990a). In 1986 in the south-east, Delfini (1987) observed increased incidence in a *P. vivax* epidemic involving 400,000 people, and this was accompanied by a growth in the number of *P. falciparum* cases.

In 1985, in the south in Kandahar and Helmand Provinces, the incidence was 12-18‰, with an increase of *P. falciparum* (WHO, 1990a).

There has been no reliable information from Afghanistan since 1988. NGOs operating near the Pakistani border have indicated, however, that the incidence of *P. falciparum* has become very high as a result of a breakdown in health care logistics and the exclusion of malaria control organisations (Hoffmann, personal communication). The disease spread throughout the region from foci in Afghanistan and Tajikistan was recently the seat of major related epidemics (WHO, 1999b).

Sri Lanka (*Figure 32*)

Malaria was confirmed in Sri Lanka as early as the 16th century (Edrisinghe, 1988). According to various

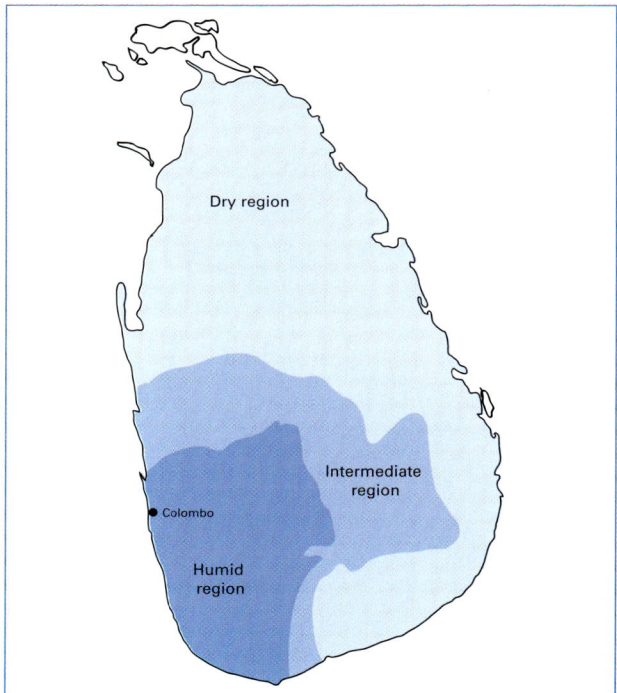

Figure 32. Rainfall and malaria in Sri Lanka (adapted from Dewit et al., 1994).

historians, it was introduced along with its vector *An. culicifacies s.l.* in the 13th century and was responsible for annihilation of the Rajatara civilisation (Murphey, 1957). These hypotheses, based on the "debilitating effect" of malaria are to be treated with great caution. The first documented scientific information was collected by the British army: from 1799 to 1804, an epidemic decimated the 65th Grenadier Guards Regiment during its march into the interior and the survivors had to fall back to healthier coastal areas. Those living in the interior were heavily affected.

In 1852, development of the coffee industry led to the importation of large numbers of Indian labourers. In 1867, the newly created Civil Medical Department noted very high prevalence among railway builders and in 1894, the administration recorded very high mortality from fever, thus pointing to the presence of *P. falciparum*.

Beginning in the early 20th century, epidemics began to arrive at an alarming pace: 1906, 1911, 1914, 1919, 1923, 1928-1929, 1934-1935, 1939-1940, 1943, 1945-1946 (Dewit *et al.*, 1994; Edrisinghe, 1988; Macdonald, 1957). In 1934-1935, malaria killed 80,000 people over a seven-month period (Pearson, 1935). In 1947, 1,350,500 cases were reported. In 1954, 37,400 cases were reported. It was at this time that indoor spraying-based eradication operations were begun, initially using DDT and later, once resistance to this insecticide had appeared, malathion.

In 1962, it was thought that malaria had been eradicated and indoor spraying operations were suspended. In 1964, the first "post-eradication" epidemic occurred, resulting in several million cases. Luckily *P. vivax* was to blame and the number of deaths was limited.

In 1994-1995, Amerasinghe *et al.* (1999) reported small epidemics attributable to *P. falciparum* (50% of the cases); in 1999, these authors estimated the annual number of cases between 150,000 and 400,000 of *P. falciparum*.

An. culicifacies B was considered to be the only vector for a long time (Subbarao *et al.*, 1988). At present, it appears that the vast majority of the transmission is caused by another species of the complex, *An. culicifacies* E, which is believed to invest Sri Lanka and southern India (Kar *et al.*, 1999); this species is both anthropophilic and endophilic. The sporozoite rate was 1.9% for *P. falciparum* and 0.44% for *P. vivax* (Dewit *et al.*, 1994).

Circumsporozoite antigen has been detected in various species that are not usually considered to be vectors, although a role for *An. subpictus* in irrigated areas has been confirmed by demonstration of the presence of sporozoites (Amerasinghe *et al.*, 1992).

Maldives

This 287 km^2 archipelago is made up of 1,190 flat, coral islands, of which 202 are inhabited: the population is roughly 300,000. A large part of its resources are derived from the tourist industry that exerts itself to protect visitors from malaria. Only *P. vivax* had been identified in the archipelago, with very low incidence. Only 1,106 cases were reported in 1975 and this had decreased to 53 by 1980 (WHO, 1983); in 1988, malaria appeared to have been eradicated (Sloof, 1988). Two anophelines, *An. tessellatus* and *An. subpictus,* were reported in the Maldives (Iyengar *et al.,* 1953). Infected specimens of the former were discovered by Covell (1944) but this species appears to have disappeared from the islands since 1980. *An. subpictus* was thus considered to be the only vector (Rao, 1984), although all transmission now appears to have disappeared. The Maldives have become a paradise for sun-and-sea-seeking tourists.

Palaearctic Region

Borders and subdivisions

The Palaearctic Region is the largest of the biogeographical regions, extending from the European shores of the North Atlantic to the eastern coasts of Siberia, and from the Hoggar and the Sahara to the Spitzbergen in the glacial Arctic Ocean. It covers a wide variety of climates from the polar ice caps to the deserts of the Sahara and Central Asia, across temperate forests and the idyllic conditions of the Mediterranean (*Figure 1*).

Different experts divide up this region in different ways. No distinction is necessary between a European Subregion and a Siberian one since Europe is really an outcrop of Asia; the Ural Mountains do not constitute a biogeographical barrier between the two. The change is clearer between the countries to the west and to the east of the Yenisey although there is no clear-cut demarcation.

Should the Mediterranean Subregion include continental France? Based on the distribution of anopheline species, only Corsica should be included in this subregion. The status of Middle Eastern countries—Saudi Arabia, Iran, Iraq, Afghanistan and the Central Asian Republics—is debatable. Although Mediterranean vectors (*Anopheles sacharovi*, *An. subpictus*) are dominant, other species more typical of the Indian Subcontinent (*An. culicifacies s.l.*, *An. stephensi*, *An. fluviatilis s.l.*) play a very important role on the coasts of the Persian Gulf and the Sea of Oman. Some experts distinguish a Touranian Subregion but we prefer the term "Arabo-Persian".

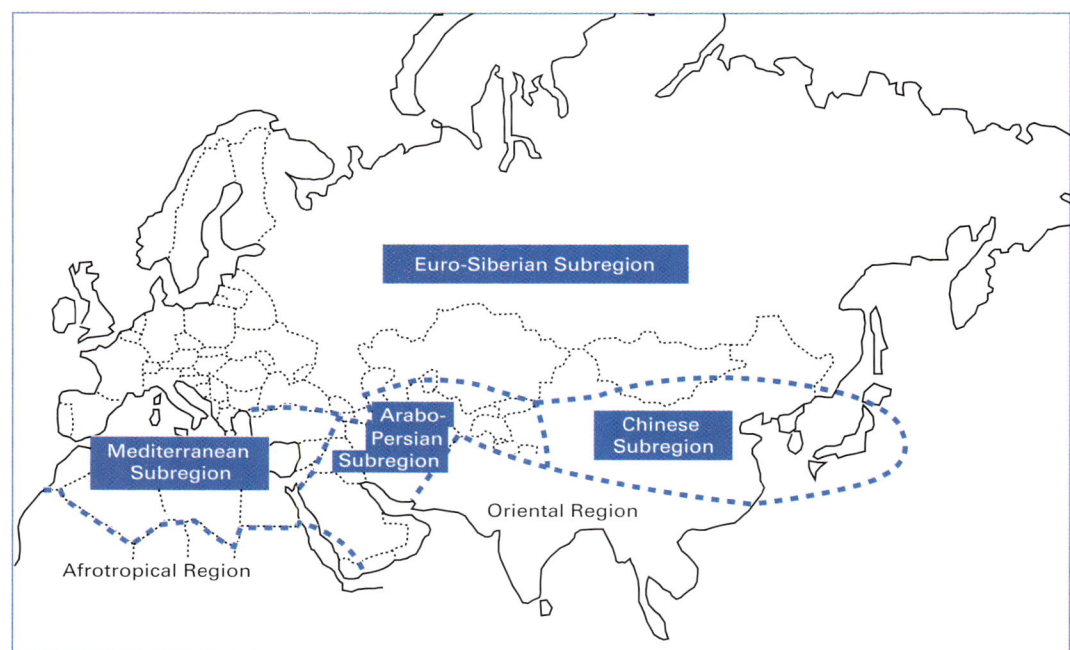

Figure 1. The Palaearctic Region.

Finally, for this classification of malaria epidemiology, we have chosen to use Macdonald's (1957) "Chinese Subregion" in preference to a "Manchu Subregion" since the former extends down as far as the 25th parallel.

These considerations lead to a classification system which includes:
- the Euro-Siberian Subregion: all of Europe including the British Isles and the Mediterranean islands. Although the peninsulas and islands of southern Europe (southern Spain, Italy and the Balkans) and the islands of France (Corsica), Italy (Sardinia, Sicily), and Greece (Crete) all enjoy a Mediterranean climate and support Mediterranean-type vectors, they are classified within the Euro-Siberian Subregion as a result of their economic and political status;
- the Mediterranean Subregion: Turkey, the Caucasian Republics, Syria, Lebanon, Israel, Jordan, Egypt, Libya, Tunisia, Algeria (to the southern Hoggar Region) and Morocco. In the southern Sahara, the frontier with the Afrotropical Region is located between the Mediterranean Hoggar Region in Algeria and the Afrotropical Aïr in Niger;
- the Arabo-Persian Subregion: Saudi Arabia, Yemen, Kuwait, the United Arab Emirates, Oman, Bahrain, Iraq, Iran, Afghanistan, Turkmenistan, Tajikistan, and China (Xin Kiang);
- the Chinese Subregion: Korea, China north of the 25th parallel, Japan, and the eastern tip of Russia (Maritime Province).

These divisions are not absolute and significant overlap occurs between each subregion and its neighbours.

General characteristics

Without going into all the geographical, economic and epidemiological details in depth, a brief analysis reveals some salient points.

Diverse climates and flora

From north to south, a series of different climates and types of fauna mark the transition between the arctic north and the subtropical south; going from west to east, the influence of the Atlantic Ocean steadily wanes.

A polar climate gives way to warmer weather further south, then the Mediterranean climate and finally a subtropical climate. In parallel, the arctic tundra gives way to coniferous forest—the taiga—which is succeeded by various types of mixed, then deciduous forests. The flora of the Mediterranean (where there is very little rainfall in the summer months) gives way to steppe and xerophilic species, and ultimately to the extremely sparse vegetation of the Sahara, and the deserts of Arabia and Central Asia.

As one moves eastwards, precipitation levels drop, the climate becomes more "continental": seasonal and diurnal temperature differences rise (to over 80 °C in Yakutia).

The amount of cultivated land increases as one moves southwards and also nearer the sea in the Euro-Siberian Region. In the Mediterranean Region and Central Asia, aridity limits agriculture along the peripheral areas of the deserts. In the Far East, China, Korea and Japan profit from the influence of the Pacific Ocean and are among the most fertile countries in the world.

Extensive mountain ranges in this subregion—the Alps, the Carpathians, the Caucasus, the Altai Mountains and the vast plateaux of the Hindu Kush, Tibet and Occidental China—have a highland fauna and flora, relics of post-glacial conditions.

To summarise, the Palaearctic Region is characterised by highly diverse climates, fauna, and land usage practices.

Highly variable population densities and levels of economic growth

Seventy-five sovereign States comprise the Palaearctic Region, including forty-six in Europe, twenty-four in Asia and five in Africa (*Table I*). The Russian Federation, a large part of the territory of which is in Asia, is included with the European countries as is Turkey, despite being more part of Asia. Russia remains the largest country in the world with 17,075,000 km² of surface area; while some tiny principalities (Monaco, Andorra, San Marino, Liechtenstein, Luxembourg) maintain their independence by providing tax havens where financial dealings are the only economic activity.

The break-up of the Soviet Union resulted in the creation of fifteen new sovereign republics with the former Yugoslavia accounting for five or six (depending on the status accorded to Kosovo). This would not be of any relevance to this book if it were not for the fact that independence has been accompanied by deteriorating health care organisation and the return of malaria in at least three countries where it had previously been eradicated (Armenia, Azerbaijan, Tajikistan).

The first Neolithic civilisations developed in the fertile crescent of Mesopotamia and in the Nile Valley although evidence of contemporaneous population centres has been found in Ténéré in Niger as well as in India and China. Thriving centres grew up around the Mediterranean Rim long before Western Europe became the global centre of industrial civilisation (only recently surrendering this position to the United States and the Far East). Colonisation had a tremendous impact in India, Indochina and Indonesia. Two recent phenomena have had major impact: firstly the oil boom in the Persian Gulf since 1930, and secondly, the collapse of the Soviet Union and the economic hardship in the various, newly created republics.

Over the last two centuries, industrial development has been accompanied by steady improvement in standards of living and housing, particularly in Western Europe. Simultaneously, scientific progress has helped the development of better public health and sanitation

Biodiversity of Malaria in the World

Table I. Countries of the Palaearctic Region (Wikipedia, 2006).

Region	Country	Size (km²)	Population (million)	Density (inhab/km²)	Country	Size (km²)	Population (million)	Density (inhab/km²)
Western Europe	Andorra	468	0.077	158	Liechtenstein	160	0.035	204
	Austria	84,000	8.1	98	Luxembourg	2,600	0.44	171
	Belgium	30,500	10.5	342	Monaco	2	0.33	16,500
	France	675,000	64	109	Netherlands	41,500	16.3	393
	Germany	357,000	82.5	235	Portugal	92,000	10.6	114
	Great Britain	244,000	59.9	244	Spain	505,000	44.7	79
	Ireland	84,000	5.7	53	Switzerland	41,300	7.5	178
	Italy	301,000	58.1	195	Saint-Marin	61	0.029	448
Scandinavia	Denmark	43,000	5.4	124	Iceland	103,000	0.29	2.8
	Greenland	2,188,000	0.056	0,2	Norway	325,000	4.6	14.2
	Finland	337,000	5.3	16,6	Sweden	450,000	9.1	22
Eastern Europe and the Balkans	Albania	29,000	3.6	113	Macedonia	25,700	2	79
	Bosnia-Herzegov.	51,000	4.2	72	Poland	313,000	38.6	124
	Bulgaria	110,000	8.0	75	Romania	237,500	22.3	94
	Croatia	56,500	4.5	80	Serbia-Montenegro	102,200	10.8	106
	Czech Republic	79,000	10.3	130	Slovakia	49,000	5.4	111
	Hungary	93,000	10.1	110	Slovenia	20,200	2.0	95
Former USSR	Armenia	29,800	3.3	112	Lithuania	65,200	3.4	57
	Azerbaijan	86,000	7.8	91	Moldavia	33,700	4.4	128
	Belarus	208,000	10.3	49.7	Russian Federation	17,075,000	142	8.7
	Estonia	45,000	1.3	38.8	Tajikistan	143,100	7.2	50
	Georgia	67,000	4.7	64	Turkmenistan	488,100	4.7	10
	Kazakhstan	2,717,300	16.7	6.1	Ukraine	603,700	46.7	87.8
	Kirghizstan	198,500	5.1	25.6	Uzbekistan	447,400	26.9	60
	Latvia	64,500	2.3	39				
Eastern Mediterranean	Cyprus	9,500	0.78	83	Lebanon	10,400	3.8	358
	Greece	132,000	11.2	82	Syria	185,000	19	93
	Israel	20,770	7.1	290	Turkey	780,000	74.7	85.3
	Jordan	92,300	5.2	70	West Bank		2.5	424
North Africa	Algeria	2,381,700	33	12,6	Malta	316	0.39	1,249
	Egypt	1,001,000	79	66	Morocco	450,000	33.42	74.4
	Libya	1,759,500	5.7	3	Tunisia	163,600	10	63.8
Arabo-Persian zone	Afghanistan	647,500	31	43	Oman	309,500	2.9	11.2
	Bahrain	707	0.6	826	Qatar	11,000	0.77	69
	Iran	1,648,000	68.7	40	Saudi Arabia	2,150,000	27	9.4
	Iraq	435,000	24	53	United Arab Emir.	83,000	3.9	26
	Kuwait	17,800	2.0	101	Yemen	527,000	21.5	40
Far East	China	9,600,000	1,316	134	North Korea	120,500	23.1	193
	Japan	377,800	127.5	335	South Korea	99,600	48.8	467
	Mongolia	1,565,000	2.6	1.7	Taiwan	35,900	21.9	610

practices. As in many other fields, malaria and malaria control have benefited from the enormous medical progress of recent years—which has resulted in an increase in life expectancy beyond 75 years of age.

Propitious conditions for malaria control

In the 5th century BC, Hippocrates made a clear link between "fever" and splenomegaly, and marshlands. He recommended that villages be built far from such "unhealthy" places. In the 12th century, the kings of Spain banned rice cultivation because of the risk of fever. These empirical observations did not have much impact on the malaria that ravaged populations from southern Finland to the Sahara, and from Yakutia in Siberia to Iran. In the cold regions, *P. vivax* was the primary malaria parasite, although *P. falciparum* may have been present in the Balkans (having since been eradicated there) (Bruce-Chwatt & Zulueta, 1980) and the high malaria mortality rates reported last century in the Dombes Region in France do not appear to be compatible with the idea that *P. vivax* was the only parasite involved.

In continental France, as in many Western European countries, malaria spontaneously disappeared before 1945. In Mediterranean countries, the extensive use of quinine and the drainage of wetlands (e.g. of the Pontine marshes in Italy and the Mitidja marshlands in Algeria) reduced the incidence of malaria, but the key step was implementation of indoor spraying operations. Finally in the early 1950s, malaria had been eliminated in France (Corsica), Italy and Japan. In Europe, it was finally "eradicated" in 1976, in the USSR and South Korea in 1979, in Tunisia, Syria, Lebanon and Israel in 1985, and in Morocco in 2000.

In North Africa, the disease (*P. vivax*) is only seen at a handful of foci in Algeria, Libya, Egypt and Morocco. In Iran and Iraq, it has regressed considerably and its incidence (almost exclusively *P. vivax*) is well below 10‰. The only real residual problem is found in Turkey where the disease's impact is limited by efficient treatment. For the last twenty years, Afghanistan has been at war and the current situation *vis-à-vis* malaria is very poorly understood; according to local NGOs, the frequency of *P. falciparum* has increased considerably.

In China, only *P. vivax* is present north of the 25th parallel (Zhou-Zu Jie, 1981) whereas *P. falciparum* is found to the south of that line; this part of the Chinese territory is assigned to the Oriental Region.

Over the last decade, the pendulum has swung somewhat: autochthonous malaria has reappeared in Armenia, Azerbaijan, Tajikistan, and in South and North Korea. Vigilance is warranted and it remains to be seen how the various new States will respond to the changing epidemiological situation.

In 1950, most if not all countries in the Palaearctic Region had the resources necessary to undertake malaria control operations and the disease has since been eradicated in many of them. Current conditions throughout the region could be considered as being highly propitious, in a number of ways:
- climatic factors: the climate is temperate or cold in more the half of the Palaearctic Region, with transmission only occurring during a short season at particular conducive sites. *P. falciparum* is only found in certain specific regions or in susceptible population groups;
- from the 19th century to the early 20th century, malaria regressed spontaneously with improvements in standards of living, housing and environment;
- malaria control measures within a context of sustainable development with, in parallel, efficient treatment of patients (both autochthonous and imported disease). While medical coverage is still very unequal, it generally covers malaria. Furthermore, the health authorities have or have had sufficient resources to implement vector control operations when necessary.

What does the future hold for Eurasian malaria?

Global warming is a major "ecological" concern for humanity. Among the threatened consequences is an increase in the incidence of various communicable diseases, and malaria in particular. According to mathematical models, Global Warming could extend the altitudinal and latitudinal limits of malaria. These forecasts are based solely on temperature and do not take account of other important determinants of malaria. Currently experts are not unduly worried about deterioration of the situation in the short term and the risk of malaria at the polar circle should not worry us (Mouchet & Manguin, 1999) (*see the Chapter entitled* "The Role of Humans in the Dispersal of Malaria and its Vectors").

In the current ecological context, given the low vector capacity of local *Anopheles* species coupled with the very low prevalence of gametocyte carriers, renewed transmission is highly unlikely. Even if active foci reappeared as a result of rising temperatures, the means would be available to treat all patients in a timely manner and control transmission. Europe is therefore not at high risk. In addition, anophelines of the Maculipennis Complex are not ideal hosts for the *P. falciparum* of Africa and Asia. The re-emergence that occurred in Armenia, Azerbaijan and Tajikistan (WHO, 1999b) took place against a background of social breakdown (even armed conflict) and the collapse of health care infrastructure. Such events warrant vigilance in all "eradicated" regions, but should not lead to pessimism.

Parasites

Three *Plasmodium* species are present in the Palaearctic Region: *P. vivax*, *P. falciparum*, and *P. malariae*. The fourth species, *P. ovale*, has never been reported and if it does exist there, it must be very rare or undiagnosed.

Frequency of the various parasite species

The arrival of *P. falciparum* in Italy, the Balkans and maybe Asia Minor is a phenomenon that occurred in the first or second century BC. In the first century AD, Celsus (1935 translation) described tertian fever. Prior to the Second World War, 40% *P. falciparum* was recorded in Greece (Livadas & Belios, 1948), more than 50% in Yugoslavia (Simic, 1956), 50% in Turkey (Hussamedin, 1930), and more than 50% in both Italy (Hackett, 1944a) and Corsica (Sergent *et al.*, 1921). In all these regions, two vectors were found, namely *An. labranchiae* and/or *An. sacharovi*. Very high frequencies of *P. falciparum* were also noted in southeastern Afghanistan, southern Iran, and Saudi Arabia where oriental vectors were responsible for transmission, as well as in the Sahara and in Saudi Arabia where *An. sergentii* was encountered. In Yemen, which belongs to the Afrotropical Region, *P. falciparum* was very much predominant (> 80%).

On the contrary, throughout all of continental Europe and Siberia, *P. vivax* was the dominant species, at least according to the available information. However, throughout history, mention has been made of numerous epidemics of fevers accompanied by high mortality rates which are difficult to attribute to *P. vivax*, a species which rarely causes fatal disease. The deadliest epidemic of modern European history occurred in the USSR between 1922 and 1936, resulting in more than 9,000,000 cases in 1935. Many of these cases were attributed to *P. falciparum* on the basis of laboratory results, and this in a place where the average temperature was below 18 °C (in the Volga Basin and central Russia as far as Archangel), so vectors would not in theory be able to transmit this parasite. Transmission might be favoured by the length of the summer day in these latitudes, but up to what temperature? It has also been suggested that European strains of *P. falciparum*—since eradicated—might be able to develop at lower temperatures (< 17°C) in local, receptive vectors. For the moment, the adaptation of *P. falciparum* to temperate zones, as suggested by Bruce-Chwatt & Zulueta (1980), remains to be proven. Anophelines of the Maculipennis Group do not currently transmit African strains of *P. falciparum* (Zulueta *et al.*, 1975).

Generally speaking, the frequency of *P. falciparum* used to be 1-2% outside the ranges of *An. labranchiae* and *An. sacharovi*, e.g. in continental France, cases of *P. falciparum* were very rare according to Sautet (1944), although they exceeded 50% in Corsica where *An. labranchiae* and *An. sacharovi* were present. In Portugal, in rice-growing areas where *An. atroparvus* was the vector, Cambournac (1942) reported 10% *P. falciparum*. Outside the USSR, there were very few major epidemics in Europe throughout the 20th century, since the development of microscopic diagnosis.

P. malariae was a rare parasite, although it may persist for several years. After the First World War, malaria contracted by soldiers on the Eastern Front persisted many years after their return, creating the legend of an endless disease. In Macedonia, the frequency of *P. malariae* is estimated at 18-22%, compared with 40% for *P. falciparum* and 27% for *P. vivax*. In Morocco, Guy (1963) had reported 15-18% *P. malariae*.

Plasmodium vivax "hibernation"

The propagation of *P. falciparum* is continuous, meaning that, once transmission has ceased, it generally disappears within six months. On the other hand, owing to its physiology, some strains of *P. vivax* can remain in the body in the latent hypnozoite form, to reactivate weeks or months later. Throughout most of the Palaearctic Region, "relapsing malaria" due to *P. vivax* used to occur in winter and spring (i.e. outside the transmission period) while pernicious malaria due to *P. falciparum* tended to arise during and after the transmission periods, either in early summer after the spring rains or the melting of snow, or in September-October after the summer rains.

Two distinct processes of hibernation—or rather of parasite perpetuation—are possible depending on whether the *Anopheles* species in question undergoes total diapause (e.g. *An. messae*) or partial diapause (e.g. *An. atroparvus*).

Plasmodium vivax hibernation in the northern regions

An. messae females begin hibernation in September or October. They do so without having taken a blood meal but engorged with nectar which they use to create a fat reserve to provide them with energy until spring. They are not carrying sporozoites and only females from the springtime generations can get infected and transmit *Plasmodium*. It is thus humans infected in the autumn and who remain latently infected until spring who are the source of the parasite to infect the vector and sustain the cycle of transmission. This process has been described in Finland and Russia (Hernberg & Tuomela, 1948; Lysenko *et al.*, 1977; Renkonen, 1944; Shute *et al.*, 1977), and also in Korea where the vector is *An. sinensis* (Paik *et al.*, 1988). The validity of defining a distinct taxon, *P. vivax hibernans*, is contested by many experts.

Gonotrophic dissociation in winter

A certain number of *Anopheles* species (*An. atroparvus*, *An. maculipennis*, *An. sacharovi*, *An. labranchiae*, and *An. superpictus*) do not undergo complete winter diapause. They continue to feed although their ovaries do not fully mature. This phenomenon is referred to as gonotrophic dissociation and corresponds to a kind of semi-hibernation (*see the Chapter entitled* "Increase Knowledge about Malaria and Development of Control Measures"). The rare blood meals taken during this period allow *P. vivax* to develop, either prior to the start of hibernation or during the hibernation period when the mosquitoes are resting inside houses. Wintertime domestic malaria was described in The Netherlands by Swellengrebel & De Buck (1938), a classic piece of work in the study of malaria.

Anophelines that hibernate will lay eggs at the end of hibernation. Only the females that result from this "waking-up" batch of eggs can get infected and perpetuate the transmission cycle (Beklemishev, 1944).

In the Middle East, gonotrophic dissociation has been observed in *An. sacharovi* and *An. maculipennis* in Iraq, as well as in *An. superpictus* in Iran and Afghanistan. In Morocco, Guy (1959) has also described gonotrophic dissociation in *An. labranchiae* (or *An. sicaulti*) although the epidemiological significance of this phenomenon is uncertain.

In Morocco, Iran and Iraq, the winter is shorter than it is in The Netherlands and the effects on transmission are less significant. In the Camargue Region of southern France, gonotrophic dissociation is common in *An. atroparvus* hibernating in sheep sheds and stables but, since malaria has been eradicated there, one can only speculate as to the importance of this pattern *vis-à-vis* malaria transmission.

There is a semi-hibernation gradient from the North Sea to Iran in *An. atroparvus*, *An. labranchiae*, *An. sacharovi*, and *An. superpictus*; depending on the winter temperature, female gonotrophic activity stops or slows down. The impact of this phenomenon—seen in most of the countries of the region—on parasite transmission has not generally been quantified.

In China, Yang (1996) showed that the incubation period is longer if the number of parasites inoculated is small (one hundred sporozoites per bite). When many parasites are inoculated—ten bites or ten thousand sporozoites—the incubation period is short. In the mid-range (e.g. an inoculum of 1,000 parasites), the incubation period may be either long or short. This might explain why small inocula at the end of the transmission season give rise to very long incubation periods, with no symptoms (which are in any case usually mild) for several months.

Haemoglobinopathies

At Al Quateef in eastern Saudi Arabia, the Arabo-Indian haplotype of the gene which causes sickle-cell anaemia (HbS), has been observed at frequencies of between 0.149 and 0.001 (El-Hazmi *et al.*, 1996); the percentage of AS carriers was 7.4% and that of SS was 1.06%. In Bahrain, this gene correlates with G6PD deficiencies (Mohammad *et al.*, 1998); this correlation could be explained by the historical presence of endemic *P. falciparum* malaria in the region.

Relationships between malaria and various types of haemoglobinopathy have already been discussed in the Introductory Part (*see the Chapter entitled* "Increase Knowledge about Malaria and Development of Control Measures"). The relationship between malaria and thalassaemia in the Mediterranean Basin and the Far East has always been and still is a controversial subject (although one of purely historical interest since the disappearance of malaria from the Mediterranean Region).

Vectors

The anopheline fauna of the Palaearctic Region is dominated by the Maculipennis Complex, now called the Maculipennis Subgroup (Harbach, 2004) which includes nine species of the *Anopheles* subgenus. In this region there are also two other species that belong to the *Cellia* Subgenus, *An. sergentii*, a desert anopheline, and *An. superpictus* of the eastern Mediterranean and the Iranian Plateaux. The Hyrcanus Group (*Anopheles* subgenus) dominates in China and Japan. A certain number of often-mentioned secondary vectors are of minimal or no importance. At the edges of the Palaearctic Region, species of Indo-Pakistani origin are important in the Arabo-Persian area while the Afrotropical species *An. arabiensis* is found in south-western Saudi Arabia and the Yemen (which come under the Afrotropical Region).

Maculipennis Subgroup

Hackett *et al.* (1934) and Hackett & Barber (1935) proposed a classification system for *An. maculipennis* subspecies based on egg morphology. It was only after the Second World War that cytogenetic methods could be used to fine-tune the taxonomy and define a number of new species.

In 1978, White proposed a classification system that integrated the existing data. Thirteen forms (including four in North America which are not dealt with here) are considered as distinct species; synonymous forms are shown in *Table II*.

In a list of anopheline species throughout the world, Harbach (2004) presented nine species within the Maculipennis Subgroup including *An. atroparvus*, *An.*

Table II. *Anopheles maculipennis* **Complex in the Old World.**

Species	Synonyms
An. atroparvus Van Thiel, 1927	*An. fallax* Roubaud, 1934 ; *An. cambournaci* Roubaud & Treillard, 1936
An. beklemishevi Stegnii & Kabanova, 1976	
An. labranchiae Falleroni, 1926	
An. maculipennis Meigen, 1818	*An. basilii* Falleroni, 1932 ; *An. typicus* Hackett, 1934
An. martinius Shingarev, 1926	*An. relictus* Shingare, 1928 ; *An. elutris* Martini, 1931
An. melanoon Hackett, 1934	*An. subalpinus* Hackett & Lewis, 1935
An. messae Swellengrebel & De Buck, 1933	*An. lewisi* Ludlow, 1920 ; *An. selengensis* Ludlow, 1920 ; *An. alexandraeschingarevi* Shingarev, 1928
An. sacharovi Favr, 1902	*An. elutus* Edwards, 1921
An. sicaulti Roubaud, 1935	

daciae, *An. labranchiae*, *An. maculipennis*, *An. martinius*, *An. melanoon*, *An. messeae*, *An. persiensis*, and *An. sacharovi*. A tenth species has recently been described, *An. artemievi* from Kyrgyzstan, that may play a role in malaria transmission in the Fergana area (Gordeev *et al.*, 2005). Even though it is not of crucial importance since it is not a malaria vector, *An. subalpinus* is now synonymous with *An. melanoon* (Linton *et al.*, 2002).

Anopheles sacharovi and Anopheles martinius

These two species which can only be distinguished on the basis of karyotype, have clearly defined ranges of distribution (*Figure 2*).

An. sacharovi extends from Corsica and Italy to the Caspian Sea and western Iran. It appears to have been eradicated in Cyprus (Zulueta & Chang, 1967).

An. martinius covers Turkmenistan, Uzbekistan, Tajikistan, Kazakhstan, Kyrgyzstan, northern Iran and Afghanistan, as well as the Chinese Province of Xinjiang.

Following indoor spraying operations, *An. sacharovi* disappeared from certain countries, notably Romania and Cyprus where changes in farming practice contributed to its elimination. It had disappeared from Israel, only to return in 1971 (Ben-Dov, 1971).

As with all species in the subgroup, its larval habitats have not been very well defined in ecological terms. It is found in sunny pools of stagnant water with dense aquatic vegetation particularly propitious sites are residual pools near slow-flowing rivers such as the Jordan in the Middle East. In Turkey (the European part), it thrives in rice paddies (Postiglione *et al.*, 1973). *An. sacharovi* is relatively tolerant of salt, which explains its predilection for coastal regions. It is also abundant on the alkaline soils of Macedonia and Montenegro.

Little to no information is available about the larval habitats of *An. martinius* which have not yet been separated from those of *An. sacharovi* (if there are any significant differences between the two).

Generally speaking, the behaviour of *An. sacharovi* is anthropophilic and endophilic in Turkey (Clarke, 1982), Iraq (Abul-Hab, 1958), Iran (Etherington & Sellick, 1956, 1961) and, in fact, throughout its entire range. However, as with all species in the complex, it is an opportunistic mosquito that does not shun livestock or animal shelters if they are readily available.

The hibernation of *An. sacharovi* is incomplete (*see above*), lasting from December to March or April. In Greece, Iraq (Abul-Hab, 1956), Turkey (Clarke, 1982) and Azerbaijan (Artemiev, 1980), it hibernates in homes and stables; it feeds intermittently during the winter (Clarke, 1982) although its ovaries do not develop. In the springtime (usually in April), the females come out of semi-hibernation, their ovaries develop and they lay eggs; the first larvae appear in April or May and the females of the new generation begin to fly in May.

In Central Asia where the climate is cooler, *An. martinius* undergoes full hibernation with fat bodies detectable in all specimens (Artemiev, 1980). In Afghanistan, hibernation of this species appears to be partial.

An. sacharovi was the main vector in the Eastern Mediterranean Region and the Near East prior to insecticide treatment. Sporozoite rates of 1.4% were recorded in Greece (Barber & Rice, 1935), 3.8% in Iraq (Abul-Hab, 1958), and 1-2% in Iran (Motabar *et al.*, 1975).

The current data do not show why malaria has returned to Armenia and Azerbaijan where the vector is *An. sacharovi*.

In Central Asia, *An. martinius*, an essentially zoophilic species, does not appear to transmit human malaria (Artemiev, 1980).

Anopheles labranchiae and Anopheles sicaulti

While White (1978) rehabilitated the Moroccan species *An. sicaulti* and separated it from *An. labranchiae* of Algeria and Italy on the basis of its egg ornamentation, Zulueta *et al.* (1983) put these two species together with *An. sicaulti* being a local variant of *An. labranchiae*. The

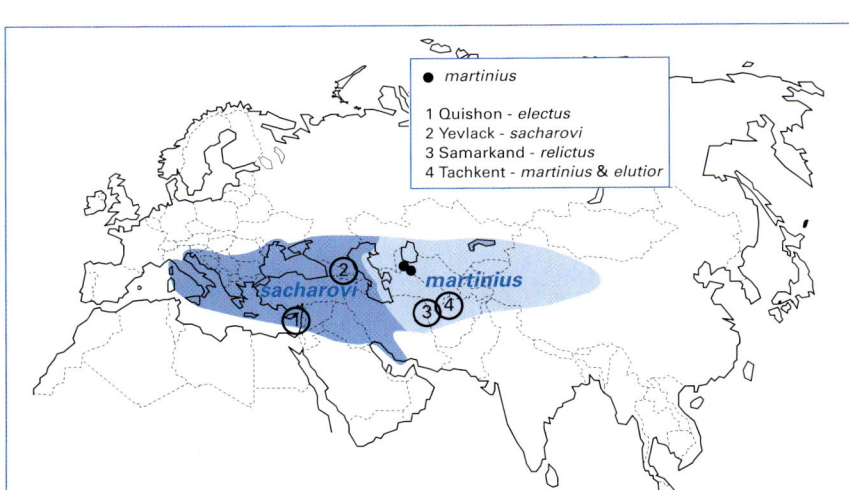

Figure 2.
Distribution of An. sacharovi and An. martinius (adapted from White, 1978).

geographic distribution of *An. labranchiae s.s.* covers Corsica, peninsular Italy and the Italian islands, as well as Algeria, Tunisia and western Libya (around Tripoli) (Macdonald, 1982) to the north of the 200 mm isohyet (around Laghouat) which forms the limit of the desert (*Figure 3*). *An. labranchiae* was eliminated from southern Spain in the 1950s (Blazquez & Zulueta, 1980). In Italy, the density of *An. labranchiae* dropped considerably following drainage of the marshes and pollution of the environment (Coluzzi, 1980). The species is quite abundant in the rice-growing regions which remain under close surveillance (Bettini *et al.*, 1978).

The larval habitats of this species are found in sunny springs, clear water deposits with buttercups and pondweeds; in Morocco, such deposits are referred to as "anopheline ponds" (Guy, 1959). In Algeria, larval habitats extend from the coast to the Djurdjura Mountains (Collignon, 1959). The residual pools formed near intermittently flowing streams are highly productive larval habitats as are the many small hillside dams found throughout North Africa (Bouchité *et al.*, 1991). The larvae are not very tolerant of organic or mineral pollution (Coluzzi, 1980) although they can tolerate a saline concentration of 2-3 g/l in Tunisia (Bouchité *et al.*, 1991).

In Morocco, *An. labranchiae* is zoophilic—67% in homes and 95% in stables—although it still bites humans even if it prefers animals (Guy & Holstein, 1968). Similar behaviour was observed in Algeria (Senevet & Andarelli, 1956).

During the active summer period, the daily life expectancy of *An. labranchiae* in sites that had not been treated with insecticide for over twenty years in Tunisia was 0.9 in July and 0.95 in September (Bouchité *et al.*, 1991). This implies a life expectancy greater than twenty days in at least 10% individuals, i.e. longer than the sporogonic cycle.

This potential danger posed by the summertime longevity of *An. labranchiae* was mitigated by its low density, which would account for the current absence of autochthonous malaria in Tunisia.

As with the above-mentioned *An. sacharovi*, the hibernation of *An. sicaulti* and *An. labranchiae* was incomplete. In Morocco, only 3-7% of "hibernating" females of the former species in the coastal region had a demonstrable fat body compared with 10-50% inland. As far as the latter species is concerned, 23% of the supposedly hibernating females were parous and therefore were or had been sexually active. In Sicily, a large number of them remained gonoactive although they did not lay eggs in winter. The first larvae were found only in April and the females of the new generation appeared in May (D'Alessandro *et al.*, 1971).

The difference in vector potential between the two sibling species—if there is any difference—was not measured. Information about the sporozoite rate of *An. labranchiae* is rare: the only data is that of Boyd (1949) who reported a sporozoite rate of 1.6% in Italy prior to eradication.

Anopheles atroparvus

An. atroparvus is a European species *par excellence* which occupies the entire continent from Spain to a line running from Lithuania to the Azov Sea and Iran. To the north, it reaches the coasts of Sweden, Denmark and England. To the south, the south-eastern portion of Spain, the Italian Peninsula and islands and the Balkans are excluded, but it has reappeared on the northern coasts of the Black Sea (White, 1978) (*Figure 3*). It is a species of the coastal

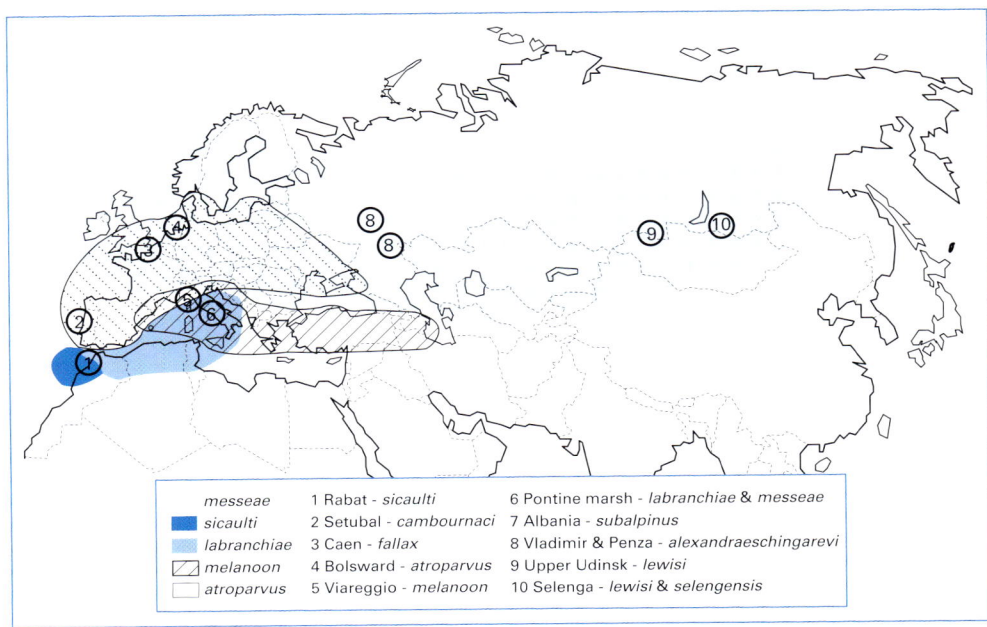

Figure 3.
The species of the An. maculipennis Complex in Eurasia and North Africa (*adapted from* White, 1978).

regions that tolerates saltwater (Bruce-Chwatt & Zulueta, 1980). In The Netherlands, when the NaCl concentration is 8-10‰, the *An. atroparvus/An. messae* ratio is 98/2 whereas in freshwater, it is 10/90 (Swellengrebel & De Buck, 1938). Although this species is considered to be anthropophilic, it also bites animals and this could be exploited for zooprophylaxis.

In southern France, *An. atroparvus* is found together with *An. melanoon* and *An. maculipennis*, and the populations of these three species (which are difficult to distinguish in the field) can become quite dense in animal shelters (Rioux et al., 1958).

In the early 19th century up to the Second World War, *An. atroparvus* was the major malaria vector in Western Europe, particularly in The Netherlands.

Anopheles maculipennis

This species is distributed through Europe from northern Spain to Russia, in the Caucasian Republics, as well as in Turkey, northern Syria, Iraq and Iran (*Figure 4*).

In Turkey, it is found up to an altitude of 2,300 m, inland, while *An. sacharovi* and *An. melanoon* tend to inhabit the coasts; *An. maculipennis* is very abundant in the rice-growing regions of European Turkey (Thrace), around Edirne (Postiglione et al., 1973).

It is one of the most abundant species in Macedonia and Serbia (Adamovic, 1981). In Iran, it is found south of the Caspian Sea, north-west of the Iranian Plateau, and in the Zagros Mountains (Motabar et al., 1975) from where it significantly extends into northern Iraq. It is not found in Sardinia, Crete or Cyprus.

An. maculipennis bites at nightfall then rests in homes and animal shelters (in which it also hibernates in Yugoslavia and Iran). Hibernation is incomplete in the Danube Plain (Adamovic, 1981), but it is associated with complete blockage of ovary development in Iran (Motabar et al., 1975).

Prior to the eradication of malaria, *An. maculipennis* was a major vector in Daghestan in Russia, Georgia, Armenia and the mountains of Azerbaijan (Artemiev, 1980). It is still not known whether or not this anopheline has been involved in the recent resumption of transmission in Armenia and Azerbaijan.

In Iraq, *An. maculipennis* was considered to be the vector in mountainous regions above 900 m (Al Tikrity, 1964). In Iran, before indoor DDT spraying operations, its sporozoite rate was 0.33%, and this was associated with PRS of 70% in adults and 19% in children (Motabar et al., 1975). If this species still has a role in the epidemiology of malaria, it remains a very modest one.

Anopheles messae and Anopheles beklemishevi

An. messae is one of the anopheline species with the most extensive distribution; from the Pyrénées and the British Isles in the west, to 130° east (in Siberia); and from the 65th northern parallel to the south of France, northern Italy, southern Macedonia, the Transcaucasian Republics, Iran and Central Asia, the provinces of Xinjiang and Manchuria in China, and Mongolia (*Figure 3*).

An. beklemishevi (*Figure 4*), which belongs to the *An. quadrimaculatus* Subgroup (Harbach 2004), can be distinguished from *An. messae* and *An. maculipennis* by karyotype analysis. It lives alongside *An. messae* although its range of distribution appears limited to 50° north (White, 1978). Highly zoophilic, it hibernates (full diapause) in outdoor shelters (Artemiev, 1980).

Despite low vector efficiency (as a result of its zoophily), *An. messae* appears to have played an important role in the spread of malaria throughout continental Eurasia, although this picture might be exaggerated as a result of failure to distinguish this species from *An. maculipennis*. In Siberia, *An. messae* was a vector all the way to Yakutia (Lysenko & Kondrashin, 1999). This is one of Macdonald's (1957) examples of transmission in the arctic.

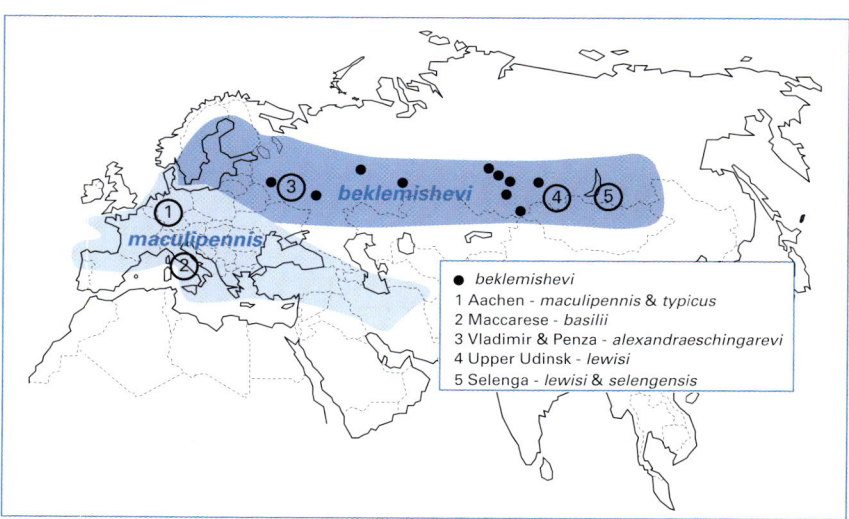

Figure 4. An. maculipennis *and* An. beklemishevi *in Eurasia (adapted from White, 1978).*

The only places where *An. messae* is believed to be a current vector are the Xinjiang and Heilongjiang Provinces in China (Tang-Lin-Hua *et al.*, 1991; Zhou Zu Jie, 1981).

An. beklemishevi is not currently involved in the transmission of malaria; in fact, it was not even described until 1976, by which date malaria had been eradicated from the USSR.

Anopheles melanoon

Neither White (1978) nor Russian experts (Artemiev, 1980) made any distinction between *An. melanoon* and *An. subalpinus* (*Figure 3*).

In France, Rioux *et al.* (1958) perpetuated the name *An. subalpinus*, but Linton *et al.* (2002) defined *An. subalpinus* as being synonymous with *An. melanoon* which is now integrated in Harbach's list (2004). *An. melanoon* does not transmit malaria.

Anopheles daciae and *Anopheles persiensis*

Recently described using molecular markers, *An. daciae* (Nicolescu *et al.*, 2004) and *An. persiensis* (Sedaghat *et al.*, 2003) belong to the Maculipennis Subgroup (Harbach, 2004). The former species has been found in the Black Sea coastal Region and plains adjacent to the Danube River in southern Romania, but its distribution might be wider in Eastern Europe and the Balkan States. *An. daciae* could be responsible for malaria transmission that is currently attributed to *An. messae*. The other species, *An. persiensis*, has been collected in the northern Caspian Sea littoral provinces of Gilan and Mazandaran where it seems to be responsible for malaria transmission otherwise attributed to *An. maculipennis*.

Compatibility of different plasmodia with the various members of the Maculipennis Subgroup

This is an important issue in the context of re-emergent and imported malaria.

Generally speaking, all types of *P. vivax* can be transmitted by species of the *An. maculipennis* Subgroup.

An. atroparvus and *An. labranchiae* are not compatible with the *P. falciparum* of western and eastern Africa (Zulueta *et al.*, 1975), although *An. labranchiae* can become infected with the *P. falciparum* found in Italy and Corsica.

An. atroparvus and *An. messae* of Russia are refractory to African and Asian *P. falciparum*, although in Africa *P. falciparum* could infect *An. melanoon*. The results of most experiments with *An. sacharovi* were negative, although sporozoites were produced in five cases (Daskova & Rasnicyn, 1982).

Anopheles sergentii (Theobald 1907)

Considered as the anopheline of North Africa, as well as being found in most oases, it occurs from Mauritania to Saudi Arabia and southern Pakistan (*Figure 5*). In North Africa, it is found in most oases (Ramsdale & Zulueta, 1983). It thrives in places with moderate rainfall (Guy & Holstein, 1968) from the coast to the Hoggar and Tassili N'Ajjer. However, it has never been found in the Afrotropical Saharan Aïr Massif in Niger (Julvez *et al.*, 1998) or from Tibesti in Chad (Rioux, 1961). In Libya, it has been found in oases of the Fezzan Region (Gramiccia, 1953) and in Egypt, in the Fayoum Region, the Nubian Desert, the Nile River Delta (Gad, 1956) and the Sinai (El Said *et al.*, 1986). Specimens have been collected at oases in Syria, Saudi Arabia and Iraq, as well as along the southern coast of Iran and in Pakistan (Zahar, 1990).

The larvae need clear, well-oxygenated water with abundant aquatic vegetation. In the oases, they are confined to the small canals that irrigate crops grown under date palms.

Outside of the desert, the larvae can be found in clear streams and hillside dams in North Africa. In these biotopes however, they are never very dense, possibly owing to competition from *An. labranchiae*.

In Egypt, Farid (1940) observed a sporozoite rate of 2.7% during an epidemic in the Nile River Delta and one of 0.85% in the Fayoum Region (El Said *et al.*, 1986). In Jordan, a single specimen out of seventy collected in a cave was found to be infected (Farid, 1954).

The seeding of oases with the larva-eating fish, *Gambusia affinis*, gave promising results in the course of vector control operations at both Timimoun in Algeria (Maruto & Fellahi, 1969) and El Thor in Egypt.

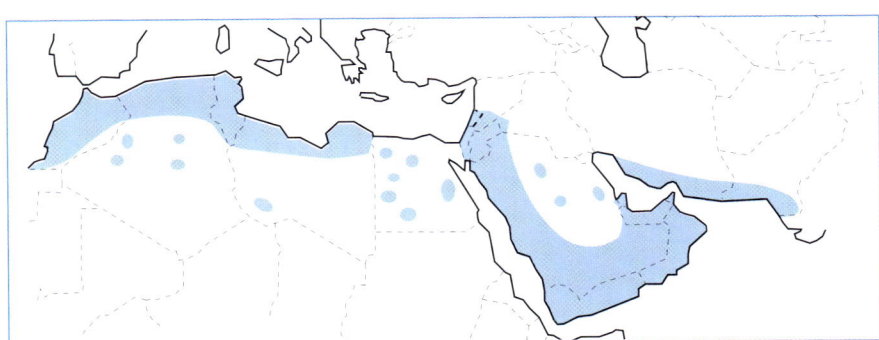

Figure 5.
Distribution of An. sergentii (adapted from Zahar, 1990).

Anopheles superpictus *(Grassi 1899)*

This species extends from Corsica and the Italian Peninsula to the borders of China (Zahar, 1990) *(Figure 6)*. It has also been reported in south-western Spain and Tunisia. In Iraq, it ranges from altitudes of 300 to 1,500 m (Pringle, 1954) and, in Afghanistan, it is found at altitudes of over 2,200 m around Kabul (Iyengar, 1954). Its density has dropped in the north-eastern part of Afghanistan as a result of the development of rice paddies that favoured the rival species, *An. pulcherrimus* and *An. hyrcanus* (Onori *et al.*, 1975).

An. superpictus is one of the main vectors of *P. vivax* malaria in the Eastern Mediterranean and the Middle East. In Israel, Kliger (1930) reported a sporozoite rate of 1.5%. In Iraq, two sporozoite carriers were seen in 27 specimens (Macan, 1950). In Iran, SIs of 0.65-4.5% were reported on the plateau (during an epidemic) and one of 0.9% in the caves (Motabar *et al.*, 1975). In Afghanistan, the sporozoite rate throughout the country was 0.08-0.15% (Dhir & Rahim, 1957); in Kabul, it was 0.39% (Iyengar, 1954) and 0.4% in Laghman (Rao, 1951). The majority of this information dates back to before 1955.

An. superpictus thrives in running water and on irrigated land, notably in Iraq (Macan, 1950). It was particularly abundant in late summer in the Caucasus when the rivers began to dry up, leaving residual pools (Artemiev, 1980).

The annual cycle is marked by a slowing-down during the winter months (October to April) which does not seem to completely interrupt development (Abul-Hab, 1967). In Syria, where it hibernates inside homes, it becomes active again in March or April (Abdel Malek, 1958).

An. superpictus was considered to be endophilic in Kabul, Afghanistan (Iyengar, 1954). In Iran, however, following indoor DDT spraying operations in the Zagros, it appeared to have become exophilic and was resting in caves (Zahar, 1974); owing to this "avoidance" behaviour, it was able to continue to maintain low-level transmission.

Hyrcanus Group

The taxonomy of this group is particularly complex, with seventeen distinct species and two subgroups (Harbach, 2004). Only four of the species are considered to be potential vectors.

The name *An. hyrcanus* Pallas 1717 is currently reserved for the Palaearctic species which extends from France to China through the Mediterranean Basin and Central Asia. Otherwise, in addition to twenty or so non-anthropophilic species, *An. sinensis* Wiedemann 1820, *An. lesteri* (synonymous with *An. anthropophagus* Xu & Feng 1981), *An. liangshanensis* (synonymous with *An. kunmingensis* Ding & Wang 1985), and *An. nimpe* (Nguyen *et al.*, 2000) are found in the Palaearctic Chinese Subregion and the Oriental Region.

Anopheles hyrcanus

The distribution of this species is quite vast, ranging from the south of France to Afghanistan. It is generally considered to be neither endophilic nor anthropophilic (Macan, 1950) and therefore, not a vector. The only exception is the Kunduz Region of north-east Afghanistan near Tajikistan where it was shown to be transmitting *P. vivax* in a rice-growing area (Anufrieva *et al.*, 1977; Onori *et al.*, 1975; Ward, 1972b). Muir (1966) and Anufrieva *et al.* (1977) were able to infect this anopheline experimentally with *P. vivax*. It is difficult, however, to imagine that it is a vector only in one very small area while it ranges over half of the Palaearctic Region. The presence of a closely related but different form cannot be excluded.

Anopheles sinensis and Anopheles lesteri

Long considered to be a subspecies of *An. hyrcanus*, *An. sinensis* only gained species status in 1953 (Reid, 1953). Its distribution is vast, ranging from eastern Siberia to Sumatra in Indonesia, and from Assam in India to the west as far as Japan in the east (Beales, 1984). In such a diversity of climates—from the cold temperate zone down to the equator—it is not certain that the term *An. sinensis* covers

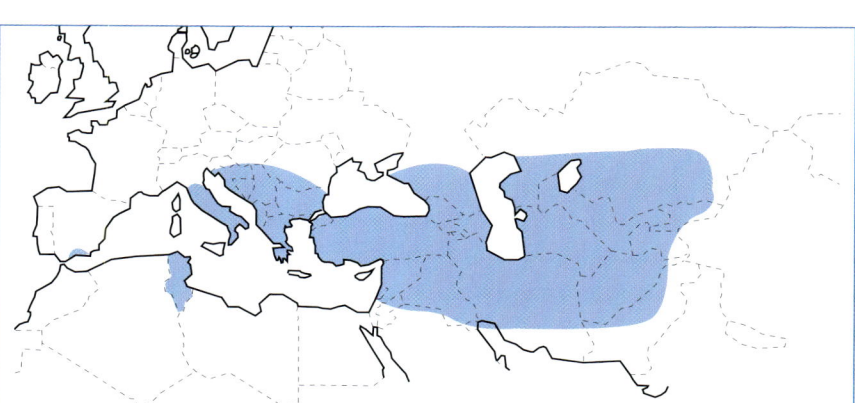

Figure 6.
Distribution of An. superpictus (adapted from Zahar, 1990).

a single species. We will be discussing only the populations of the Chinese Subregion that are involved in the transmission of malaria since the role of populations found in Indochina and Indonesia is still controversial.

An. anthropophagus has recently be synonymized with *An. lesteri* (Wilkerson *et al.*, 2003). Initially described as a subspecies, *An. lesteri anthropophagus*, by Xu & Feng (1975), it was accorded the status of distinct species in 1981, but the subsequent molecular data suggest a single species. *An. lesteri* ranges from 32° north in China down to a point level with the southern Chinese border in Japan. Its presence in Vietnam is restricted to the northern coastal area (Phan, 1998). Throughout its entire range of distribution, *An. lesteri* is sympatric with *An. sinensis* although it occupies only part of the latter's territory.

These two species can be differentiated on the basis of egg morphology (Beales, 1984); the dorsal part of the *An. sinensis* egg is light in colour whereas that of *An. lesteri* has a black band—which is unbroken in the spring generations and discontinuous in the autumn populations (Otsuru & Ohmori, 1960).

Both species are found on rice-growing land in China and Japan, although *An. sinensis* develops in the irrigated part of the rice paddy (which is often rich in fertilizer) while *An. lesteri* is found in the clearer water of irrigation ditches (Ho *et al.*, 1962).

The annual development cycle of both species varies with climate. Up to the 25th parallel, their activities slow down in winter, a phenomenon which could be seen as a diapause. In Japan and Korea, *An. sinensis* hibernates in late September to re-emerge in April or May (Otsuru & Ohmori, 1960; Chen *et al.*, 1967). The females in diapause disperse as early as September and ovary development begins in February; in March, the females group together in animal shelters and begin their summer activity. The hibernation period is shorter in southern China with year-round development in Canton (Ho Kwei-Ming *et al.*, 1965).

The hibernation of *An. lesteri* is exceptional among anophelines. It spends winter in the egg stage, to hatch in the spring (Ho *et al.*, 1962). This form of hibernation does not rule out the possibility that development is arrested in hibernating females. Hibernation habits tend to follow the same climatic variations as *An. sinensis*.

An. sinensis density peaks in July in Korea and northern and central China (Chen *et al.*, 1967). In southern China, the peaks come in July and October, the latter being the more dangerous (Ho Kwei-Ming *et al.*, 1965). According to the same experts, *An. lesteri* peaks between September and November in southern China.

Generally speaking, *An. sinensis* is zoophilic and rests in animal shelters while *An. lesteri* is anthropophilic and rests in homes, although this can only be considered as a tendency. *An. sinensis* feeds mainly in early evening, before 8 pm, after which the number of bites drops off. In contrast, *An. lesteri* feeds mainly between 11 pm and 4 am (Ho *et al.*, 1962), as most efficient vectors do. In Korea, Japan and China to the north of the Yangtze, *An. sinensis* is, or was, the only vector of malaria (more or less exclusively *P. vivax*). Malaria disappeared from Japan in 1949. It also disappeared from Korea, but it has recently reappeared (Feighner *et al.*, 1998) both in the South and North Korea. South of the Yangtze, *An. sinensis* and *An. lesteri* both participate in transmission. In 1960, in Anhwei Province, Ho *et al.* (1962) observed sporozoite rates of 0.5%, 0.7% and 1% for *An. lesteri*, while all dissections of *An. sinensis* gave negative results. In the Henan Region (Huang & Lin, 1986), *An. lesteri* was the vector of *P. falciparum* during an epidemic in which this parasite accounted for 79% of the clinical cases. In the Sichuan Region, during a *P. vivax* epidemic, the sporozoite rate of *An. lesteri* was 0.37% (Liu *et al.*, 1986). In the Jiangxi Region, a sporozoite rate of 0.7% was recorded among *An. sinensis* (Beales, 1984).

An. lesteri is a much more efficient vector than *An. sinensis* where both species are sympatric. In addition, *An. lesteri* can transmit *P. falciparum*. This difference between the two species was not taken into account in the older data. In a previous chapter, we discussed the role of another species of the Hyrcanus Group, *An. kunmingensis*, synonymous with *An. liangshanensis* (Ma *et al.*, 2000) in the provinces of southern China which are part of the Oriental Region.

Secondary and localised vectors

Outside Tropical Africa, *An. pharoensis* Theobald 1901 occurs in Egypt, the coasts of Israel, Saudi Arabia, and Yemen. The species is abundant in rice paddies and is considered to be salt-tolerant (0.5-5 g NaCl/litre).

It can be carried on the wind over distances of over 20 km and wind-borne dispersion from Egypt in 1959 resulted in 21 cases of malaria in the Gaza Strip, 70 km away (Saliternik, 1960).

Barber & Rice (1937) reported a sporozoite rate of 0.33% in Egypt, with a figure of 1.4% having been reported in the course of an epidemic (Madwar, 1936). The only recent reference is from Fayoum where a sporozoite rate of 0.36% was observed in *An. pharoensis* (El Saïd *et al.*, 1986).

An. claviger Meigen 1804 extends from Morocco to Iran; its twin species, *An. petragnani* Del Vecchio, both belonging to the Claviger Complex (Coluzzi *et al.*, 1965), does not extend beyond Italy to the east. Historically implicated in the transmission of malaria in Cyprus, Lebanon and Palestine, *An. claviger* has been blamed for malaria in Jerusalem and Tripoli in Lebanon, where it was found developing in water tanks. It is also reported in the upper valleys of the Pamir Region in Tajikistan. It is suspected of being the vector of *P. vivax* at an altitude of 2,000 m in the Moroccan Atlas (Langeron, 1938).

An. pulcherrimus Theobald, a relatively inefficient vector, occupies Central Asia to the south of the Aral Sea, Afghanistan, Iran, northern Iraq, Syria, Turkey, Azerbaijan and the eastern Arabian Coast.

The species *An. plumbeus* develops in tree cavities and adapts to numerous types of niche, particularly old tyres, near which it represents a genuine nuisance (Karch, 1997). It is suspected of being involved in two recent cases of imported *P. falciparum* malaria in Germany (Kruger *et al.*, 2001) although this remains to be confirmed.

An. multicolor Cambouliu 1902 is a desert species, ranging from Morocco to Pakistan. It is often considered as a vector in the absence of other species, although its role has never been demonstrated. Nevertheless, it can be experimentally infected.

An. dthali Patton 1905 is an anopheline found in dry regions from Mauritania to Pakistan. It has been designated as a vector in Iran in the province of Bandar Abbas, but only on the basis of circumstantial evidence and the absence of other species (Manouchehri *et al.*, 1972). Beside Iran, it has not been included in the list of vectors in its range of distribution.

An. paltrinierii Shidrawi and Gillies 1987 is briefly mentioned because it may have an epidemiological role in Oman, where it was reported.

An. pattoni Christophers was believed to be a vector in China (Macdonald, 1957), but this is no longer discussed; the identification was most probably erroneous.

Oriental and Afrotropical vectors in the Palaearctic Region

Certain species were discussed in depth in the chapters dedicated to vectors found in the Oriental Region. Given the definition retained of the Palaearctic Region, what follows is a reminder of the range of distribution of the species that have crossed regional boundaries.

An. fluviatilis (mainly species T) occupies Afghanistan, Iran, the southern portion of the Central Asian Republics, Iraq, eastern Saudi Arabia, the United Arab Emirates, Oman and southern Yemen (*see Figure 18*, page 204).

An. culicifacies (species A apparently) occupies southern Afghanistan and Iran, the United Arab Emirates, Oman and southern Yemen (Socotra Island) although it makes an incursion into the Afrotropical Region in Eritrea (*see Figure 20*, page 205).

An. stephensi is also an Indo-Pakistani species whose area of distribution extends into the southern parts of Afghanistan, Iran and Iraq, eastern Saudi Arabia, the United Arab Emirates and Oman (*see Figure 21*, page 206).

The Afrotropical species, *An. arabiensis*, extends into western Saudi Arabia and Yemen (*see Figure 12*, page 254) and its range coincides with the highest prevalence of malaria anywhere in the Arabian Peninsula and even the Palaearctic Region.

Euro-Siberian Subregion

Climatic changes and the history of malaria

During the Würm glaciation, Northern Europe, north-western Siberia, the Carpathians, the Alps and the Pyrénées were covered by an ice cap surrounded by tundra permafrost. The ice began to thaw twelve thousand years ago and "modern man" began moving northward as the climate became less hostile.

In southern Europe, around 10,000 BC, the average temperature was 9 °C. In these conditions, only *P. vivax* could possibly be transmitted, and that only in the extreme southern part of the continent for a short period during the year. Climatic conditions precluded the transmission of *P. falciparum*; in addition, the very low densities of human populations and limited exchanges at this epoch were unfavourable to such a "short-lived" parasite.

Around 8,000 BC, the temperature was at least equal to that of today.

The Neolithic Revolution which began around 7,000 BC and led to the stabilisation of people in permanent settlements, created foci of malaria infection within which the parasite could be locally transmitted (Fenner, 1970) (*see the Chapter on* "Man Facing Malaria") resulting in the disease becoming endemic.

In the 5th century BC, Hippocrates described benign tertian fever (*P. vivax*) and quartan fever (*P. malariae*). Malignant tertian malaria (caused by *P. falciparum*) was described by Celsus in the first century BC (*in* Jones, 1908) but it was not until the second century AD that malaria became a major public health problem on the shores of the Mediterranean Sea.

To what can this change for the worse be attributed? It appears that the environment was considerably modified in Asia Minor, Greece and Italy (Butzer, 1972) by deforestation and soil erosion linked to intensive cultivation of the coastal regions. These changes would have promoted the establishment of *An. labranchiae* (originally from North Africa) in Italy, Sicily, Sardinia and Corsica, and the establishment of *An. sacharovi* (originally from inland Asia) in Greece and the Balkans. These two vectors are much more efficient than the continental species of the Maculipennis Group, notably *An. atroparvus*, *An. messae* and *An. maculipennis*. Competition between these "imported" species and the continental species would explain the coastal distribution of *An. labranchiae* and *An. sacharovi* (Grmek, 1994). Their tolerance of salt water, however, is not restricted to this area of their distribution. This explanation of the invasion of Mediterranean Europe by these two vectors remains hypothetical (as do so many questions about the Greco-Roman era) and quite doubtful to our point of view.

The continental species of the Maculipennis Group are refractory to *P. falciparum* strains from the Afrotropical Region and Southeast Asia (Zulueta *et al.*, 1975). There is extensive proof of *P. falciparum* transmission by *An. atroparvus* in Portugal and Spain (Cambournac, 1942; Pittaluga, 1903), and by *An. messae* in Russia (Hackett, 1944). Certain strains of *P. falciparum* must therefore have adapted to European anophelines (Bruce-Chwatt & Zulueta, 1980). Taking their hypotheses a step further, both authors flt that, after "eradication" in 1976, the European populations of *P. falciparum* disappeared. Currently, only imported strains, which cannot be transmitted by European anophelines, are encountered in Europe.

Paradoxically, military history tells us a great deal about malaria. Hannibal considered Italy a "healthy" country during the Punic Wars; Alexander the Great crossed the Middle East without problem even if some authors believe that he died of malaria. Only in the early Middle Ages did the disease begin to take a serious toll on soldiers. Many garrisons were wiped out and many sieges had to be lifted, although it is difficult to be sure of the etiology of the infectious agents implicated in so-called fevers until reliable data begin to become available in the 19th century. The French expeditionary corps lost 450 men at Navarin in 1827, and in 1916 during the First World War, the allied expeditionary corps suffered very heavy losses in Turkey.

Military history is just one of our sources of information about the increase in the prevalence of malaria in Europe since the start of our era. It reached its peak in the 18th century. This situation continued through to the middle of the 20th century in Russia and countries of the former Soviet Union where the polar circle was reached at Archangel and Yakutia in Siberia (Macdonald, 1957). This change was independent of climate, e.g. the 17th century, the "Little Ice Age" was the coldest of modern history with the pack ice extending down as far as Scotland and yet it was during this period that the prevalence of malaria peaked in England (Reiter, 2000).

In their review of malaria in Europe, Bruce-Chwatt & Zulueta (1980) often painted a very dark picture with malaria causing hundreds of thousands of deaths, although they were careful to point out that diagnosis remained highly error-prone until the discovery of the parasite by Laveran in 1880. Before this time, all fevers were considered to be due to malaria, including typhoid fever which was very widespread until quite recently.

It is nevertheless curious that such high mortality rates should be attributed to malaria in countries where the majority of infections involved the benign species, *P. vivax*.

Malaria has certainly played an important role in history, as already discussed in relation to the minorities of Southeast Asia, but blaming the disease for the downfall first of Greece and later the Roman Empire (Ross, 1906) may be taking the hypothesis a bit too far.

Control and eradication of malaria

Malaria spontaneously began to decline in Europe from the middle of the 19th century (earlier in some places). This cannot be attributed to the climate because the temperature increased by 0.6 °C between 1850 and 1940, which would rather be expected to favour spread of the disease. This may put the catastrophic forecasts relative to global warming in context. As of the beginning of the 19th century standards of living and conditions in general were improving in Europe. Wesenberg-Lund (1921) credited the disappearance of malaria in Denmark to changes in animal husbandry methods: the construction of stables and pig sties concentrated *Anopheles*, notably *An. atroparvus*, in animal shelters which are more attractive than homes, so humans were no longer being bitten as often by these mosquitoes. The separation of humans from cattle was considered one of the essential factors in lowering the prevalence of malaria.

Until 1940, malaria remained very active in Italy and Corsica (where it was transmitted by *An. labranchiae*) as well as in the Balkans (*An. sacharovi*). Prevention campaigns in Italy—mainly based on vector control strategies accompanied by quinine distribution—resulted in a 70% decrease in malaria in Italy. Similar campaigns were conducted in Albania, Greece and elsewhere. In all these countries, however, as well as in the foci of Corsica, Portugal, The Netherlands and the former USSR, the disease was not eliminated until control measures based on the indoor spraying of long-acting insecticides were implemented. The last cases were reported in Macedonia (in Yugoslavia) in 1976 and in the former USSR in 1979. In Spain, malaria was eliminated without any specific control measures (Najera, 2001) prior to 1950 although one autochthonous *P. ovale* case was reported in 2001 (Cuadros *et al.*, 2002). In Italy, one *P. vivax* case was linked to a parasite imported from India (Baldari *et al.*, 1998).

Corsica in France was endemic for malaria before 1953 and from 1965 to 1971 during which period a few cases were reported (Ambroise-Thomas *et al.*, 1972; Sautet & Quilici, 1971) although these did not lead to the establishment of endemic disease. However, 35 years later, one case of an autochthonous *P. vivax* infection was reported in August 2006 in Porto, southern Corsica (Armengaud *et al.*, 2006). These cases demonstrate the importance of epidemiological surveillance on the island. The same is true of the many cases either imported by travellers coming back from tropical regions or caused by infected anophelines brought in by planes from endemic areas, a phenomenon referred to as airport malaria (Giacomini *et al.*, 1995).

In Italy, *An. labranchiae* is probably not particularly susceptible to infection by imported *P. falciparum* and the number of gametocyte carriers is very low during the transmission season. The malariogenic potential is thus currently very low and the risks of re-emergence are negligible in most European countries (Romi *et al.*, 2001).

Biodiversity of Malaria in the World

It is too early to define the details of the re-emergences observed in 1999 in Armenia and Azerbaijan, and the causes for this phenomenon. This first reversal of the eradication process warrants great vigilance on the part of the health authorities.

In Europe, malaria never reached the levels witnessed in tropical countries and particularly in Africa but, in the late 19th and early 20th centuries, several tens of millions of *P. vivax* cases per annum in Europe seems a reasonable estimate. While malaria is considered to be eradicated from Europe today, the process required a considerable effort from all countries concerned. Comparing the number of cases reported in the various countries at the start of the century with data gathered during eradication campaign allows us to measure the progress made and understand the real danger that malaria posed on this continent in the relatively recent past (*Table III*).

Mediterranean peninsulas and islands

For historical reasons, we have chosen to include the Mediterranean Peninsulas with continental Europe, although they really constitute part of the Mediterranean Subregion.

The lands covered are Greece, Cyprus, the Balkan Coast and the Black Sea, peninsular Italy, Sicily, Sardinia, Corsica

Table III. Disappearance of malaria from Europe (information gathered by Bruce-Chwatt & Zulueta, 1980).

With indoor spraying			Spontaneous disappearance		
Country	Year	Number of cases	Country	Last case	Number of cases
Albania	1938	16,420	Austria	Around 1946	+ war cases
	1968	Eradicated	Czech Republic + Slovakia	Around 1850	+ war cases 1944-1946
Bulgaria	1946	144,000			
	1946	Eradicated	France (exc. Corsica)	1950	
Greece	1931	1-2 millions	Germany	1938	+ war cases 1944-1946
	1974	Eradicated			
Cyprus	1946	(coastal -) 40% prevalence	Belgium	1938	+ war cases 1940-1945
	1956	Eradicated			
Romania	1948	333,198	Denmark	1921	
	1968	Eradicated	Sweden	1927	
Yugoslavia	1937	240,210	Finland	1945	
	1975	Last case in Europe (Macedonia)	Spain	1962	
France (Corsica)	1921	Prevalence 40%	Great Britain	1926	0 case
	1954	Eradication followed by re-emergence then disappearance		1952	0 case (disappearance)
Italy	1905	323,500	Poland	1956	
	1953	9			
	1962	No more native cases			
Hungary	1948	3,600			
	1966	Eradicated			
Netherlands	1946	15,640			
	1960	Eradicated			
Portugal	1938	45,500			
	1959	Eradicated			
Former USSR	1938	5,014,431			
	1956	13,038			
	1973	211			
	1979	Eradicated			

in France and the extreme southern tip of Spain (there was never any malaria in Crete or the Greek Islands in the Aegean Sea). These regions all host highly efficient vectors, *An. labranchiae* to the west and *An. sacharovi* to the east of Italy (Butzer, 1972; Jones, 1908). The two species are in competition with continental species belonging to the Maculipennis Group, a process in which they are at a disadvantage thus explaining their predominantly coastal range (Grmek, 1994). The relative tolerance of the two Mediterranean species to brackish water explains why malaria is concentrated in coastal regions. Corsica and Sardinia are exceptions as, due to the absence of the other species of the Maculipennis Group, *An. labranchiae* occupies all the territory of these islands (Zulueta, 1990). The vector incriminated in the small outbreak in the Murcia Region of Spain was also *An. labranchiae*.

In all places where these species were present, malaria remained prevalent with periodic epidemics until the end of the Second World War. Indoor spraying with DDT eradicated malaria. Anti-larval operations undertaken prior to 1940, particularly in Italy, as well as widespread quinine distribution, had certainly reduced the number of patients, although the disease was still endemic in 1945. This situation differs fundamentally from that of continental Europe where malaria started to regress spontaneously in the 19th century and had completely disappeared by 1940 (e.g. mainland France).

A small digression should be made to mention the significant vector role played by *An. superpictus* in the Balkans.

In Greece, in 1935, transmission rates were high with a sporozoite rate of 1.3% in *An. sacharovi* and 0.9% in *An. superpictus* (Barber & Rice, 1935). The number of cases varied from one to two million per annum from 1930 to 1940, resulting in malaria mortality of 74 for 100,000 inhabitants. As soon as DDT indoor spraying became widespread, the number of cases dropped below 1,000 in 1951 and to 10 in 1970. The eradication campaign was completed in 1974 (Belios, 1933; Bruce-Chwatt & Zulueta, 1980; Livadas & Belios, 1948).

In Cyprus, PR readings reached 40% in the coastal villages in 1946. Ten years later, eradication had been achieved (Zulueta & Chang, 1967) with the complete disappearance of *An. sacharovi*, the only instance of vector eradication in the Mediterranean.

In Bulgaria, malaria dropped from 144,600 cases in 1948 to 3 cases by 1960; in Romania, from 338,198 cases in 1948 to 24 cases in 1962 (Bilbie *et al.*, 1978; Ciuca, 1956); and, in Yugoslavia (prior to partition), from 240,000 cases in 1938 to under 100 cases in 1960 (most of which were in Macedonia) (Simic, 1956).

In the western Mediterranean Basin, the situation was as critical as in the east. In Corsica, the only part of France that hosts *An. labranchiae*, the prevalence of malaria was 40% on the eastern coast (Sergent *et al.*, 1921). After the Second World War, malaria had been practically eradicated as early as 1949 with no more cases by 1953 (Jaujou, 1954). However since then, a few autochthonous cases have been reported (22 in all) in 1965, again in 1971, and one in 2006.

In Italy, malaria developed steadily as of the beginning of the Christian era. Alaric, after the sack of Rome, died from fever. In 455, the Vandals had to leave Rome after they had sacked it. Several popes died from fever within one year of consecration. Throughout the Middle Ages, Germanic people contracted malaria in Italy. The Roman countryside together with Sicily and Sardinia were the most malaria-ridden. Control measures (particularly drainage operations) were implemented and quinine distributed as soon as the parasite responsible was identified and the mode of transmission defined. Between 1887 and 1947, the number of cases was reduced from 323,000 to 13,750 (down to 9 by 1953). The mortality rate attributed to malaria dropped from 21,000 to 4 deaths per annum. As early as 1945, indoor spraying operations with DDT became commonplace. Biocca (1946) proposed a stratification system that differentiated hyperendemic* regions (Sardinia, Sicily, Calabria, and the countryside around Rome), meso-endemic regions (the "boot" south of the latitude of the island of Elba, Latium, Abbruzes, Pouilles, Campania), hypoendemic regions (Po Valley, Tuscany, the Marches, the Adriatic Coast, Venetia) and malaria-free regions (North and Umbria).

Contrary to initial hopes, it proved impossible to eliminate *An. labranchiae* from Sardinia, although malaria was eradicated anyway (Zulueta, 1990). The old concept of anophelism without malaria regained its significance.

In southern Spain, *An. labranchiae* had disappeared from the Murcia Region even before the DDT spraying operations began (Gil Collado, 1935, 1937).

Owing to their climatic, ecological and epidemiological conditions, the "Mediterranean Peninsulas" can be considered as transition zones between the subtropical regions and the temperate regions of Eurasia. The mild winter temperature does not trigger true anopheline diapause even though their development is slowed down during the cold season. Most importantly however, these regions used to be legendarily "unhealthy" because of the presence of the efficient vectors, *An. labranchiae* and *An. sacharovi*, both of which are able to transmit *P. falciparum*.

---

* The terms "hyper-endemic" and "meso-endemic" correspond to levels of endemicity lower than the corresponding terms in Africa.

Western, Central and Northern Europe

We have grouped all European countries together, apart from those of Eastern Europe and the Mediterranean Peninsulas. These all have one feature in common, namely a spontaneous decline in malaria in the 19th and 20th centuries. The treatment of homes was necessary to obtain eradication in only certain very limited foci in the Netherlands, Portugal and Hungary. This decline in malaria is generally considered to have been a result of improvements in rural housing, standards of living, hygiene and diet.

P. vivax was by far the most common species, accounting for 90% of all cases. *P. falciparum* was frequent in the rice-growing areas of Portugal (Cambournac, 1942) and Spain (Pittaluga, 1903), although rare in the south of France (Sautet, 1944); sporadic cases were reported in the Netherlands, Germany and Central Europe. Currently, the importation of parasites from tropical countries, particularly *P. falciparum*, is a risk for all European countries (Muentener et al., 1999), although a resurgence of local transmission is extremely improbable. *P. malariae* infection was particularly common in soldiers returning from Turkey and the Balkans in 1916.

The vectors all belong to the Maculipennis Group. The majority of the group's species could only be identified as of 1935, often after the malaria focus had disappeared. The halophilic species, *An. atroparvus*, is confined to coastal regions and eggs found in such a region can be identified on the basis of morphology. *An. atroparvus* survives the cold season in a state of semi-hibernation as described above. The females can infect humans in their homes with sporozoites derived from gametocytes either ingested before entering hibernation or from the infected human living in the house. This type of winter transmission has been described in the Netherlands (Swellengrebel, 1950; Swellengrebel & de Buck, 1938) and Germany in western Friesland (Rodenwaldt & Jusatz, 1956; Weyer, 1933).

Separating the respective roles of *An. messae* and *An. maculipennis* is more difficult given that both species are currently found in many places from which malaria disappeared more than fifty years ago. Brumpt and Dao Van Ty (1942) thought that it was impossible to prove retrospectively either species' role in the foci of Sologne and Dombes in France, where both are present (Pichot & Deruaz, 1981).

At the beginning of the 20th century, *An. atroparvus* was the main vector of malaria in Europe (outside the Mediterranean Peninsulas). The malaria centres of Denmark, the Swedish Coast, Germany and in particular the Netherlands (where transmission continued through the winter as mentioned above) were the most "productive" in Europe. Springtime cases were attributable to strains of *P. vivax* with a long incubation period, most often inoculated the previous autumn. In summertime, patients fell ill soon after the infection event (Swellengrebel, 1950).

Hirsch (1883) considered The Netherlands to be the most endemic country in Europe with a mortality rate of 2.6 ‰ in Zeeland. Fifteen thousand cases were recorded in 1946; the disease disappeared in 1947 following the implementation of DDT indoor spraying. In France, the marshlands along the Atlantic and Mediterranean Coasts and particularly the Camargue Region had a reputation of being unhealthy (Sautet, 1944). In Portugal and Spain, where *An. atroparvus* was the only vector, rice-growing appears to have enhanced the spread of malaria (Cambournac, 1942). Rice-growing, which had been introduced by the Arabs around the 12th century, was prohibited by the Catholic Kings in the 14th century as a public health measure (Rico Avello, 1947). Although endemic disease had been nearly eradicated by 1936, a new outbreak (168 cases) broke out in the southern part of the country following the Civil War, giving rise to 253,000 cases in 1941 and 426,000 cases in 1943. The endemic area reached the Castille Mountains, which would prove, in retrospect, that *An. atroparvus* is not necessarily confined to coastal regions. Malaria disappeared in 1962 without any specific control operations after treatment centres had been set up and the socio-economic conditions had improved (Pletsch, 1965). In Portugal, the last autochthonous cases (*P. vivax* and *P. falciparum*) were observed in 1961 (Cambournac, 1978), although more than 550 imported cases were reported in 1972.

In England, Reiter (2000) painted an apocalyptic portrait of malaria which was referred to as "ague" in the south-western part of the country in the 18th century. In 1887, 112,000 cases were reported with high mortality due to anaemia and malnutrition, but can we be sure that the epidemic was really due to malaria?

It would be difficult to attribute the foci of the Danube Delta in Romania and Moldavia (Bilbie et al., 1978; Ciuca, 1956) to *An. atroparvus* alone as it lived there together with *An. sacharovi*, a far more efficient vector.

Beyond the coastal regions, more or less severe epidemics of malaria broke out in all countries from the 15th century to the 19th century. Starting in the middle of the 20th century, these epidemics spontaneously receded for the reasons already discussed. Malaria resurfaced at the end of World War I and then again after World War II following migrations and troop movements. These modern malaria outbreaks, particularly those in the Balkans, are characterised by the high percentage (up to 30%) of *P. falciparum* (Bruce-Chwatt & Zulueta, 1980). Historic foci had been reported in Silesia and Saxony in Germany (Hirsch, 1883), in the Flanders, Sologne, Dombes and Alsace Regions in France (Callot & Rochedieu-Assenmacher, 1953; Marchoux, 1927) and in north-eastern Hungary (Lörincz, 1937). *An. messae* was designated as the vector although a role for *An. maculipennis* cannot be discounted. In the Balkans, the situation outside *An. sacharovi* zones was variable from one country to another. In Serbia, *An. messae* was implicated in Voivonia and *An. superpictus* in Kosovo. The latter species was also implicated in Albania, Greece and Bulgaria. *An. maculipennis* was a major vector in Macedonia and in the mountains of Romania, while *An. messae* maintained a significant role in the rice paddies of the Danube Plain. Now, where malaria has been eradicated, retracing the disease's epidemiology in Europe is a theoretical endeavour—even if one only tries to review the last one-hundred years. Bruce-Chwatt & Zulueta (1980) have produced an excellent review of malaria in Europe which serves as reference work.

Eastern Europe and Siberia

This section includes the former Republics of the USSR, excluding the Caucasian and Central Asian Republics, i.e. the Russian Federation, Moldavia, Ukraine, Belarus, Lithuania, Latvia, Estonia, as well as Finland. It is important to note that the anopheline fauna of the Russian Provinces of the Far East are related to the Chinese fauna but, given the low incidence of malaria in this geographic region, this point will not be discussed further. The regions north of the Caucasus (Dagestan) are similar to that of the Caucasian Republics.

The climates are continental, temperate, cold, and can even be considered polar at certain northern latitudes. In the summer, the long day means that the *P. vivax* cycle can be completed even far north, e.g. at Archangel and Yakutia (Lysenko & Kondrashin, 1999) or even in the lower parts of the Gulf of Botnia where the average temperature is below 15°C in July (Renkonen, 1944). "Polar" malaria in Yakutia (*Table IV*), the example given by Macdonald (1957), is the most northern form of the disease reported so far.

P. vivax hibernans transmission in the cold regions of Finland and Russia was described above. The same "hibernation" process has been observed in Korea in American servicemen (Paik *et al.*, 1988) who had been infected by *An. sinensis*. It should be noted that the incubation period is longer as further north as temperature decreases: 10% of long incubations found in Astrakhan on the shores of the Caspian Sea, 40° north, compared with 80% in Arkhangelsk, 64° north (Lysenko & Kondrashin, 1999).

P. falciparum was very frequent and associated with high mortality in epidemics between 1920 and 1936, particularly in Ukraine, the Volga Basin and the Ural Mountains. Sporadic cases were reported all the way to Archangel (Moschkovsky & Rashina, 1951). Asymptomatic cases were reported by Sergiev & Yakuscheva (1956). This parasite disappeared following eradication operations which began in 1950.

Just a few cases of *P. malariae* have been reported in Moldavia, Ukraine and the Volga Plain.

An. messae is the most widely distributed vector, spanning the entire Euro-Siberian Region apart from the Polar Regions and the Far East (Beklemishev, 1944; Chesnova, 1974). This anopheline, although predominantly zoophilic, was considered the most important in the epidemics of 1920-1940. Exceptional circumstances had to be fulfilled for this anopheline to acquire this level of epidemiological importance. As *An. beklemishevi* has been described since its eradication in 1976, it is impossible to determine the role that it might play. *An. maculipennis* is limited to Ukraine and southern Russia, where it is sympatric with *An. messae*, although no differences between the two species' vector roles have been established. *An. atroparvus* remains a coastal species of Ukraine, Russia and Moldavia. *An. sacharovi* was considered to be an excellent vector in Moldavia, Ukraine and in southern Russian up to the 50th parallel in the valley of the Volga River.

Intermittent fevers were reported in Eastern Europe from the middle of the 15th century on. Epidemics were reported in Saint-Petersburg, Kazan and Odessa (Bruce-Chwatt & Zulueta, 1980). German colonists were decimated by malaria in Astrakhan (Hirsch, 1883).

Table IV. Cases of malaria in Yakutia from 1924 to 1959 (adapted from Lysenko & Kondrashin, 1999).

Year	Number of cases	Year	Number of cases	Year	Number of cases
1924	1,312	1935	16,328	1950	3,825
1925	1,181	1940	5,822	1951	1,355
1926	819	1941	5,501	1952	976
1927	1,004	1942	3,766	1953	1,141
1928	421	1943	3,476	1954	679
1929	860	1944	2,332	1955	1,749
1930	1,504	1945	1,930	1956	1,263
1931	2,161	1946	2,664	1957	734
1933	5,032	1947	3,361	1958	468
1933	12,758	1948	2,084	1959	88

Biodiversity of Malaria in the World

In 1674, quinquina bark was mentioned as a substitute for garlic… and by 1848, the army was using quinine.

As of 1824, epidemics spread among soldiers in western Siberia, Ukraine and on the banks of the Black Sea (2,500 deaths out of 10,000 men) and these are among the few records of malaria during this era.

In 1903, Favr performed the first comprehensive study of malaria in the Russian Empire. The incidence was 2-8 ‰ in the north, rising to 330 ‰ on the banks of the Black Sea and 228 ‰ in Astrakhan. The map compiled by Moschkovsky & Rashina (1951) stratifies malaria by region. Favr initially estimated 1,250,000 cases in 1882, 3,200,000 cases in 1895, and then approximately 3,000,000 cases annually until 1914.

The major event for the USSR was the post-Revolution pandemic between 1922 and 1938 (*Table V*). Hackett (*in* Boyd, 1949) considered this outbreak as the biggest epidemic in modern times, with more than 600,000 deaths. It reached its peak in 1934 with 9.5 million cases. The reasons behind this unprecedented epidemic in Europe are not very clear but certain factors have been singled out, including poor, disorganised health care, a lack of drugs, and the massive slaughter of livestock which would have driven normally zoophilic mosquitoes to feed on humans.

Lysenko & Kondrashin (1999) published a map representing the incidence of malaria (the number of cases per 10,000 people) in 1934 when the pandemic was at its peak (*Figure 7*). Incidences above 2,000 per 10,000 inhabitants were reported in Ukraine, southern Russian, the Volga Basin, south-western Siberia and Transcaucasia; north of the 50th parallel, between the Ob and Yenissey Rivers, the incidence varied between 1,000 and 2,000 per 10,000, and it was 500 to 1,000 per 10,000 in Ukraine and southern Siberia (west of the Yenissey); in eastern Russia, the Astrakhan Region, and south-eastern Siberia, the incidence dropped down to between 500 and 100 per 10,000, and in the Far East, the incidence was less than 100 per 10,000.

This pandemic was particularly severe in the more temperate regions although the cold regions were not spared, e.g. in the Republic of Yakutia in eastern Siberia, between 50° and 60° north, the number of cases of malaria jumped from 421 in 1928 to 16,328 in 1935, dropping back down to 3,825 in 1950 and then to 468 in 1958 (Lysenko & Kondrashin, 1999) (*Table V*).

These authors compiled a table summarising the number of cases in the USSR from 1900 to 1956. There were between 3 and 3.5 million cases in the Soviet Union between 1900 and 1915. Beginning in 1923, the figures jump up to 9,871,919 cases in 1925, before falling back to 3 million in 1930-1931. The epidemic re-emerged with around 9 million cases in 1934-1935, then slowly began to decline from 1936 to 1949. By 1950, fewer than one million cases were being reported. Eradication was considered complete in 1975 throughout all of the Republics.

Caucasian Republics

Throughout Russian history, malaria epidemics have regularly broken out among troops stationed in the Caucasus, with very high mortality rates.

The independent republics of Georgia, Armenia and Azerbaijan, as well as that of Dagestan in the Russian Federation, are home to a highly efficient vector, *An. sacharovi*; other species belonging to the Maculipennis

Table V. Number of cases of malaria and incidence of cases from 1900 to 1956 in the Soviet Union (adapted from Lysenko & Kondrashin, 1999).

Year	Number of cases	Incidence* per 10,000 inhab.	Year	Number of cases	Incidence* per 10,000 inhab.	Year	Number of cases	Incidence* per 10,000 inhab.
1900	3,417,678	256	1930	2,700,105	171	1940	3,176,527	171
1905	3,021,321	208	1931	3,159,453	194	1946	3,364,502	–
1910	3,633,656	229	1932	4,415,324	270	1947	2,820,712	–
1915	2,611,119	185	1933	6,503,827	389	1948	2,296,568	–
1920	508,157	100	1934	9,477,007	552	1949	1,663,536	–
1921	1,226,274	153	1935	9,024,909	523	1950	781,329	43
1922	2,094,275	268	1936	6,503,109	378	1951	351,178	19
1923	5,668,074	424	1937	6,328,889	375	1952	183,603	9.5
1924	5,867,828	445	1938	5,108,431	301	1956	115,869	6.1
1925	9,871,919	388	1939	3,769,056	221			

* In the USSR, the incidence was often evaluated as the number of cases per 10,000 inhabitants while in the majority of countries, it is estimated as the number of cases per 1,000 inhabitants

Palaearctic Region

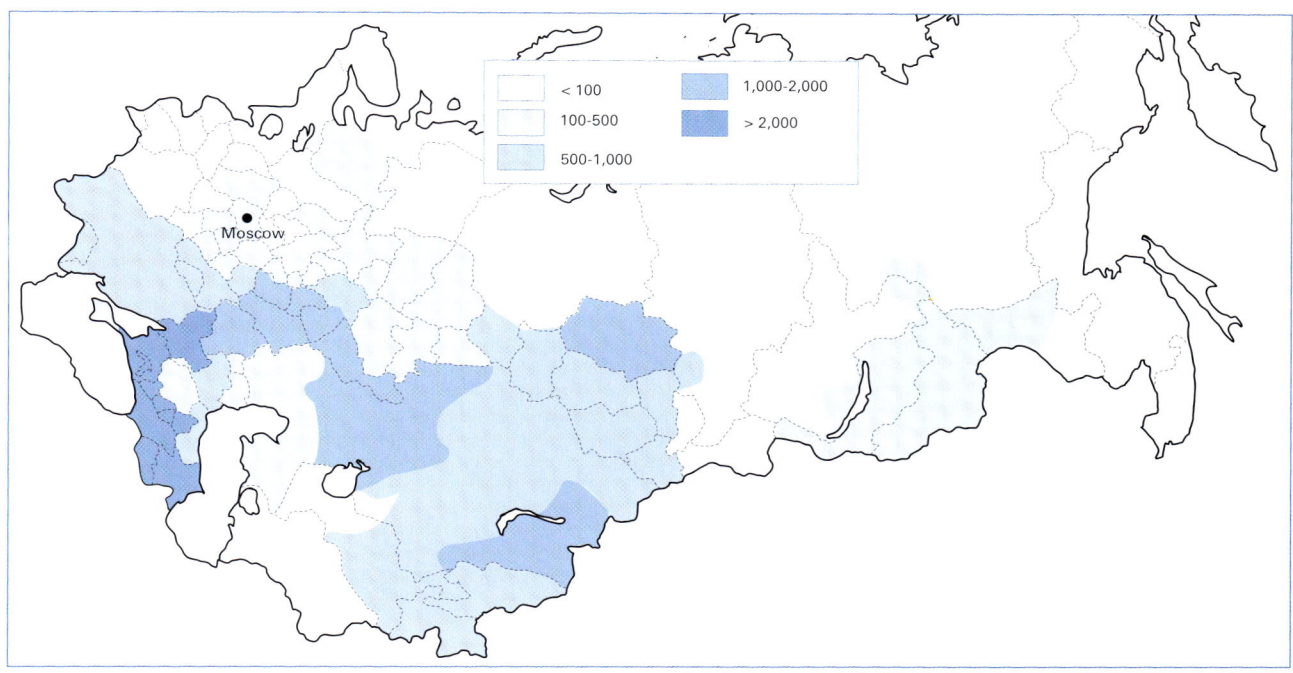

Figure 7. Incidence of malaria (per 10,000 inhabitants) in the USSR in 1934 (highest during the epidemic) (adapted from Lysenko & Kondrashin, 1999).

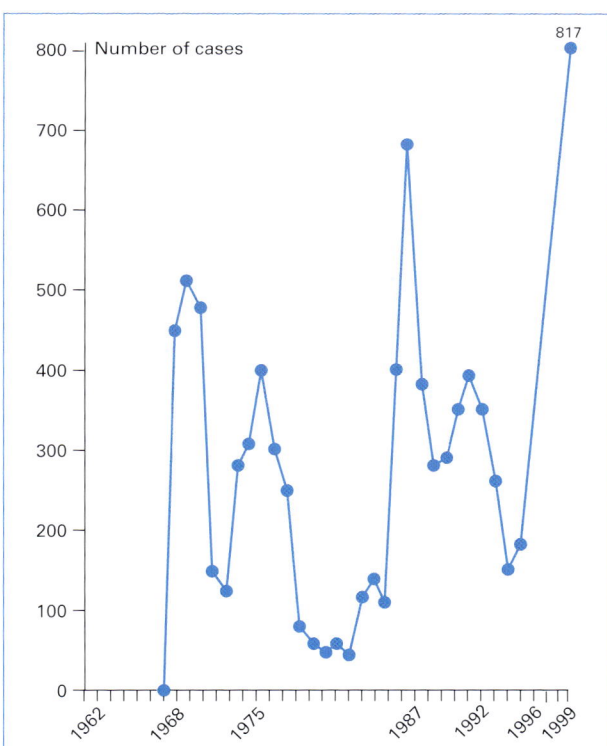

Figure 8. Re-emergence of malaria in Armenia (adapted from Lysenko & Kondrashin, 1999).

group, *An. messae* (which reaches the southern limit of its range of distribution) and *An. maculipennis*, are far less anthropophilic. *An. superpictus* can be found at altitudes of 500 m.

P. vivax was the dominant parasite, but *P. falciparum* was common until 1940 as shown by the high mortality rate; this parasite seems to have been eradicated in the late 1960s. *P. malariae* represented less than 10% of cases.

The Caucasian Republics have always been considered the most malarious areas of the Russian Empire (which later became the Soviet Union). In 1911, Moschkovsky & Rashina (1951) reported incidences of over 100‰ in Georgia, and between 50‰ and 100‰ in Azerbaijan, Armenia and Dagestan. Lysenko & Kondrashin (1999) reported incidences above 200‰ in 1934 during the great pandemic. Owing to rigorous prevention measures, eradication was achieved between 1970 and 1975.

Malaria then resurfaced in the Caucasus in 1990. In Armenia, 140 and 817 autochthonous cases were reported in 1996 and 1997 respectively, after an alert in 1969 which affected 500 people (*Figure 8*).

In Azerbaijan, Lysenko & Kondrashin (1999) followed incidence dynamics from 1936 to 1997. The annual number of cases exceeded 200,000 in 1936; there were no more than 100,000 cases reported in 1950 and this dropped to below 100 in 1960, then to less than 20 in 1990. Starting in 1991, the number of malaria cases skyrocketed, reaching 13,146 cases by 1996 (WHO, 1999b) (*Figure 9*).

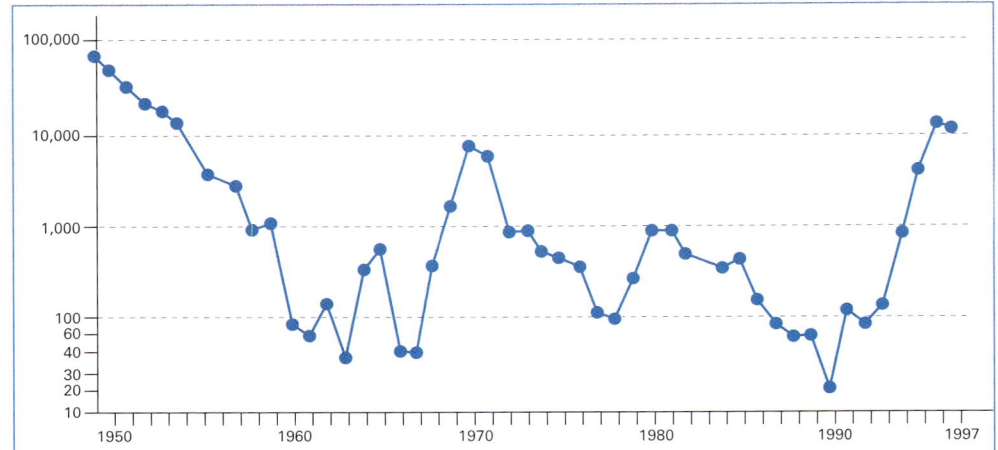

Figure 9.
Cases of malaria in Azerbaijan from 1950 to 1997 (adapted from Lysenko & Kondrashin, 1999).

According to recent unconfirmed reports (Sabatinelli, 2002), *An. sacharovi* and, to a lesser extent *An. superpictus* were responsible, as might be expected.

It appears that Georgia and Dagestan are not as yet affected.

The return of malaria in an "eradicated" region is a warning to countries located in temperate regions which, since 1960, have forgotten that malaria can wreak havok. In many countries, the degradation of social, economic and health care structures could result in its return.

Mediterranean Subregion

In the geographic sense, the Mediterranean Subregion includes all the countries bordering the Mediterranean Sea with similar climatic and ecological characteristics.

The Mediterranean Subregion section will thus include the countries of North Africa, i.e. Morocco, Algeria, Tunisia, Libya, and Egypt, with those of the Near East (to revive a slightly outmoded geographic entity), i.e. Israel, Lebanon, Syria, Jordan, and Turkey. The region extends over more than 7,000,000 km² with a population exceeding 270 million people (*Table I*).

Climate and the history of malaria

It is considered that the limit between the Mediterranean Subregion with its winter rains and the Afrotropical Region with its summer rains is located somewhere between Adrar (Mauritania), Hoggar, Tassili N'Ajjer (Algeria) and Fezzan (Libya) to the north, and, Tagant (Mauritania), Adrar des Iforas (Mali), Aïr (Niger) and Tibesti (Chad) to the south; the first group is therefore part of the Mediterranean Subregion, and the second part of the Afrotropical Region. This climatic partition affects the fauna, both invertebrates, such as *Anopheles* mosquitoes, and vertebrates.

All the countries of the Mediterranean Subregion (except Turkey) have a coastline bordered by a desert: in Algeria, the desert begins in Laghouat (at the 200 mm isohyet) and occupies three quarters of the country; in Tunisia and Morocco, the desert part occupies less than half the country. In Libya and Egypt, green vegetation grows only along a thin coastal area although in Egypt, the Nile River Valley constitutes a kind of "oasis". Israel, Syria and Jordan are backed by the Middle-Eastern deserts, whose origins are essentially identical to those of the Sahara.

Thus, in each country, there is a distinction between the coastal regions and the arid hinterland. Inland, xerophilic or oasis ecological conditions favour certain vectors (notably *An. sergentii*), and contrast with those of the coastal regions where the 400-800 mm of rainfall in the winter months favour vectors of the *An. maculipennis* Group (*An. labranchiae* and *An. sacharovi*); year-round oasis malaria contrasts with malaria associated with the wet season. The coastal vegetation has changed considerably over the past two thousand years. In Numidia (west of Algeria and east of Morocco), extremely dense forest blocked the advance of Roman legions; in Lebanon, the cedar forest provided wood for the Egyptian navy; the Syrtes (Cyrenaica) was Rome's granary. Intensive farming operations had already resulted in deforestation in Asia Minor (Turkey) during the Greek era. Extensive efforts are currently being made to restore an environment compromised by the pressure of massive population growth, e.g. in Egypt, mud constructions are prohibited as they destroy topsoil.

The disease today and control measures

Greek, Roman and later Arab physicians were familiar with intermittent fevers. The disease was endemic in Algeria in particular. It was at Constantine in 1880 that Laveran discovered the malaria parasite. In the late 19th century, drainage operations were undertaken by the French administration. Throughout the Mediterranean Region, clean-up measures were complemented by the distribution of quinine. Malaria had regressed significantly by the end of the Second World War when indoor spraying operations with long-acting insecticides were undertaken.

As of 1946, prevention programs based on DDT spraying were being launched in most of the countries and these were transformed into eradication programs around 1960.

At present, malaria has been eradicated in Tunisia, Libya, Israel, Lebanon and Jordan. The number of autochthonous cases has been considerably reduced, below a few hundred in Algeria, Egypt and Syria (WHO, 1999a). Only Turkey poses a malaria problem, the importance of which must not be exaggerated since only *P. vivax* is involved.

The majority of current cases are of imported *P. falciparum* malaria and this problem is easily managed by local health structures.

The Maghreb

Characteristics

The three countries of the Maghreb have a Mediterranean coastline that stretches nearly 2 000 km, backed by a system of parallel mountain ranges, the Tellian Atlas bordering the Mediterranean Sea and the Saharan Atlas further south.

These two mountain ranges delineate an area of moderately high plateaux (1,000 m) with steppe-like vegetation, interspersed with forests on the higher and wetter elevations. The coastal plain consists of a series of fertile alluvial basins; the plateaux extend roughly 300 km from Algiers in the north to Laghouat in the south. Beyond the Saharan Atlas, the vast Sahara Desert extends 1,700 km from Laghouat to In-Guezzam at the border of Niger.

To the west, the mountain ranges curve southward in Morocco, demarcating the three Atlas lines. A vast plain extends from the base of the mountain range, along the coastline of Morocco. South of Oued Draa, the Sahara joins its Algerian counterpart.

Rainfall decreases from north to south with the 200 mm isohyet marking the beginning of the Sahara Desert.

An initial stratification emerges, separating those regions with a Mediterranean climate in the north from the Saharan Regions to the south. In the former regions, the vector is *An. labranchiae* in Algeria, Tunisia and Morocco (published as *An. sicaulti*). In the Sahara, *An. sergentii* is the vector in oases. This series of climates and botanic facies provides a degree of geographical uniformity to the three countries.

During more than a century of French colonisation, agricultural land was reclaimed for the cultivation of cash crops by draining wetlands, such as the Mitidja Plain in Algeria; this led to the regression of malaria. Population growth in Algeria (five-fold increase since 1830) reversed trends in agricultural production in favour of food crops designed to ensure self-sufficiency.

Marshy zones were transformed into irrigated land. Only Morocco's coastal lagoons remain to shelter migrating birds but it is going to be difficult to preserve these ecological showcases against pollution with the kinds of nitrates, heavy metals and pesticides that are used in intensive farming. Owing to its demography and agriculture, North Africa is undergoing a dramatic ecological transformation. Furthermore, the many new hillside dams create ideal larval habitats for *An. labranchiae* and *An. sergentii* (Bouchité, 1991), although this has not yet been associated with the transmission of malaria.

In the early 20th century, 75% of the North Africa population lived in endemic zones. At present, the number of cases remains in the single digits (or a few hundred at the very most), which gives a measure of the progress made against malaria in this century.

For roughly twenty years, the countries of Maghreb were worried—unjustifiably in the final analysis—about the risk of *An. gambiae* being introduced as a result of trade across the Sahara.

Morocco

A more extensive stratification of Morocco proposed by Guy (1963) defines five zones:
- the Mediterranean zone which extends across the north of the country and the Riff Mountain range. This zone was the least endemic in Morocco in 1963. Three-hundred-and-eighty-nine cases were reported in 1960 as opposed to 166 cases in 1961, in a rural population of 1,131,500. In Tanger Province, there were only 19 cases among 22,500 rural inhabitants. The vector—as throughout the north and centre of Morocco—was *An. labranchiae*, synonymous with *An. sicaulti*;
- the Atlantic coastal zone, bordered by marshes and lagoons, is undergoing extensive agricultural development from Tetouan to Agadir. The zone is propitious for *An. labranchiae*. Transmission occurred in August, and then in October and November. In 1960, there was a sudden increase in the number of cases following heavy spring rains. Seven-hundred-and-fourteen cases were reported in 1960 but only 508 in 1961, for a rural population of 1,958,580;
- the continental plain zone is the most populated region of Morocco, extending beyond the coastal plain up to the Atlas Mountains. There were 3,379 cases reported in 1960 and 2,253 in 1962 for a rural population of 3,139,000. The vector was *An. labranchiae*. Moving towards the interior of the country, the incidence rose and the outbreak was delayed;
- the mountainous zone was endemic until 1963, although the limiting altitude for *Anopheles*, particularly that of *An. labranchiae*, was not clearly established. *An. hispaniola*, which is synonymous with *An. cinereus* (Ribeiro *et al.*, 1980), was very abundant. Only 1,615 cases were declared in 1960 and 1,164 cases in 1961 for a rural population of 1,041,000. High altitude epidemics (above 2,000 m) were reported by Langeron (1938) in the Grand Atlas and Anti-Atlas where *An. claviger* was suspected of being the vector;

- in the pre-Saharan zone, the Agadir coastal area should be distinguished from the interior (Ouarzazate, Ksar el Souq) where *An. sergentii* vector seems to predominate, although information about this region is not precise. There were 900 cases reported in 1961 and 711 cases in 1962 for a rural population of 1,212,000.

Until 1959, diagnosis was based on purely clinical evidence but thereafter, statistics based on parasitological examinations became available, allowing Guy (1963) to compile a first reliable review of the situation. From before, there was a great deal of entomological data available but little epidemiological information, especially considering that malaria was endemic throughout the whole of Morocco. Malaria control was based on drainage and quinine distribution (Houel & Donadille, 1953).

In all districts included in 1963 (Guy, 1963), *P. vivax* accounted for 55-70% of all positive slides compared to 14-28% for *P. falciparum* and 15-18% for *P. malariae*. By 1978, there was no more autochthonous *P. falciparum* or *P. malariae* malaria and only *P. vivax* persisted. However, the number of imported cases of *P. falciparum* malaria continued to grow. The statistics of the last thirty years do not always define whether the cases are autochthonous or imported, leading to confusion.

Data collected by Ben Mansour (1972), Naji *et al.* (1985) (on imported malaria) and by Zahar (1990) show a steady regression of malaria.

Between 1970 and 1971, a generalised rise in the incidence of malaria was recorded following a very rainy spring—from 0.48% positive slides to 0.91%:
- 1982: 62 cases reported,
- 1983: 75 cases reported,
- 1984: 318 cases reported,
- 1985: 714 cases, including imported cases.

In 1987, there were 658 autochthonous cases (all attributable to *P. vivax*) as compared to more than 600 imported cases (mostly due to *P. falciparum*). A very high percentage of these were seen in adults.

In 2000 and 2001, no autochthonous cases were declared in Morocco.

The two main vectors (Guy & Holstein, 1968) are *An. labranchiae* (syn. *An. sicaulti*) in the north and centre, and *An. sergentii* which colonises nearly all of Morocco although it is believed that this species only acts as a vector in the southern pre-Saharan desert; only one infected specimen of *An. hispaniola*, an essentially zoophilic species, has ever been found (Andarelli, 1960) and whether or not it can transmit malaria remains to be proven (despite the species' high density). *An. claviger* is frequent in the mountainous zones although its role has not been demonstrated in North Africa, except for Langeron's very old reference (1938) concerning the High Atlas.

Algeria

Algeria has a long-standing tradition of malaria control based on the drainage of stagnant water, particularly in the coastal region, and since 1936, this has been coupled with the widespread use of larvivorous fish (*Gambusia affinis*) and the distribution of prophylactic drugs (*in* Boyd, 1949). Malaria had regressed considerably prior to 1945 and the incidence of the disease collapsed as soon as eradication measures were implemented.

In 1973, out of 15 million inhabitants (as opposed to 27.5 million in 1997 and 33 million in 2006), 6.5 million were being protected by indoor DDT spraying operations; out of 292,250 slides examined, only 53 were positive (all *P. vivax*). In the unprotected part, more than 3,000 cases were reported. In 1987, only 63 cases including 11 autochthonous cases due to *P. vivax*, were declared throughout the entire country. Most of these cases occurred in the northern Sahara and transmission was due to *An. labranchiae*. This situation continued until 2001.

In the Sahara, epidemics have been recorded since the late 1920's. Following the Djanet epidemic in 1928-1929 (Brousses, 1930), Le Gaonach (1939) reported an epidemic in Hoggar in 1934, followed by one at Doury in 1959. In 1968, Lefèvre-Witier reported an epidemic among the nomads of the Tassili N'Ajjer, while the Djanet Oasis was protected. In 1969, Maturo & Fellahi described the Timimoun epidemic.

All of these epidemics have a common denominator, i.e. a high frequency of *P. falciparum* (up to 90%). It cannot be affirmed that these parasites had come from the Afrotropical Region. Benzerroug & Janssens (1985) showed that, of the 410 cases in the Sahara, 46% were autochthonous compared with 47% imported of which 90% were caused by *P. falciparum* from Mali. However, *An. sergentii*, the main vector (Holstein *et al.*, 1970)—and often the only one—was perfectly able to transmit all strains of *P. falciparum*, while, in northern Algeria, *An. labranchiae* did not readily transmit this parasite of African origin (Zulueta *et al.*, 1975).

Serological studies conducted in 1991 (Benzerroug *et al.*, 1991) confirmed the extinction of the majority of foci, notably in Ouargla and Adrar.

The feared invasion of southern Algeria by *An. gambiae s.l.* has not yet happened and, for Ramsdale & Zulueta (1983), the probability of such an event is very low. In fact, the risk of introduction into Algeria was greater between 1945 and 1960 when the aircraft of the Zinder and Gao lines to Algiers, which made stops at all the oases along the route, were never treated with insecticide. Despite this, *An. gambiae* was never detected in any Algerian oasis (Mouchet, personal observations).

Malaria is now no longer a public heath priority in Algeria and the vast majority of cases are imported.

Tunisia

Since it was founded, the Pasteur Institute of Tunisia has been dedicated to control malaria. In a report compiled in 1909, Husson claimed high malaria indices through the whole country: 20% of schizont carriers among those with splenomegaly in Mendja Kheredine, 80% of people with splenomegaly and 30% carrying schizonts in Souk el Arba, Beja and Ghardimaou, and 20-50% of schizont carriers with splenomegaly at Cap Bon. Malaria control operations were based on drainage and the distribution of quinine with the primary objective being to protect the European colonialists.

It appears that these measures were efficient since, by the time of the pre-eradication survey of 1957, malaria indices had dropped considerably although the entire country was still considered to be at risk (Wernsdorfer, 1973). The vectors were *An. labranchiae* (exclusively *P. vivax*) in the north and *An. sergentii* (both exclusively *P. vivax* and *P. falciparum*) in the south. The eradication program was a great success with malaria having been almost eradicated by the 1970's. Indoor spraying operations were then replaced by the application of larvicide (notably Abate® at 75 ml/ha) in the Cap Bon Region and in the south where *An. sergentii* was well controlled.

In 1976, Ambroise-Thomas *et al.* demonstrated the almost complete disappearance of malaria in a large-scale serological analysis. Chadli *et al.* (1986) reported the last case in Jendoube (*P. vivax*). From 1978 to 1985, only 68 cases of malaria—all imported—were reported in Tunisia. A few cases of transfusional malaria with *P. malariae* were also observed.

Currently, *An. labranchiae* thrives and is able to reach an epidemiologically dangerous age (Bouchité *et al.*, 1991) in the north of the country without there being any sign of resumed transmission. The risk cannot be ignored however, particularly with the multiplication of small hillside dams which offer this anopheline productive larval habitats.

Libya and Egypt

These two countries consist of a vast desert bordered by a narrow swath of coastal land. The Nile traverses Egypt and virtually all life is concentrated along its banks. It enters the Mediterranean Sea at a vast delta whose vegetation contrasts with the aridity of the surrounding desert.

An. labranchiae is limited to a narrow coastal region to the west of Tripoli.

An. sergentii can be found wherever water is present from Fezzan to the Sinai, as well as in the Fayoum depression and on the eastern edges of the Nile Delta. Its sporozoite rate was 2.7% (Farid, 1940) and it was considered to be responsible for the Fezzan epidemic in Libya (Shalaby, 1972).

An. multicolor is very common, particularly in southern Libya. It was considered to be a vector at Fezzan based on circumstantial epidemiological evidence (Lo Monaco Croce, 1931) although its role was never proven.

An. pharoensis is represented in the Nile Delta by a population that is very similar to that in West Africa, particularly from Senegal. With its mixed feeding behaviour (Zahar, 1974), the species was considered a major vector by Barber & Rice (1937), although its sporozoite rate was consistently low, of the order of 0.33% (1,500 dissections). Furthermore, it rarely reached an epidemiologically dangerous age.

The Gambiae Complex, notably *An. arabiensis*, hangs over the region like Damocles' sword. It was reported by Lodato (1935) in Fezzan (Edri and Ubari), but not by Vermeil (1953); various experts considered that this report was mistaken although it is also possible that it temporarily invaded southern Fezzan and did not remain.

In Egypt, the invasion of *An. gambiae s.l.* from 1942 to 1945 was well documented (Shousha, 1948). The larvae passed the winter in sunny pools of stagnant water left by the receding waters of the Nile, and the species was active throughout the year. *An. gambiae* was eliminated by anti-larval measures (Paris Green) complemented by pyrethroid spraying to kill the adult mosquitoes.

Since 1970, Lake Nasser has been closely monitored; *An. gambiae s.l.* does not extend beyond Dal which is 150 km south of the Sudanese border (Gillies, 1972). Before the dam was built, it was found all the way to the Wadi Halfa area on the border between Egypt and Sudan (Lewis, 1944). These experts consider that the risk of invasion is real, especially through the passive transport of anophelines.

In Libya, in the Fezzan, the first cases of malaria were observed by Nachtigal and these were followed by epidemics in Kufra in 1933 (Lodato *in* Gebreel, 1982); the parasite prevalence was 80% among children and 8% among women. In 1953, an epidemic broke out in Edri and Ubari (Vermeil, 1953), and in 1964 at Ghat and Bardkat (Zahar, 1974); the second endemic zone was north-west of Tripoli at the Tunisian border where, in 1933, one third of the population had malaria (Gebreel, 1982).

In 1974, Kadiki & Ashraf traced the history of malaria in Libya; in 1950, the PR was 3%; in 1959, following control operations, the rate had dropped to 0.39%, only to rise again to 2% in 1969 as a result of the construction of irrigation systems.

Based on a sero-epidemiological study conducted in 1985, Gebreel *et al.* considered eradication measures had been successful; in 1978, only 46 cases were reported and all these were imported.

The incidence of malaria in Libya has always been very moderate. In 1974, Kadiki & Ashraf considered that only 150,000 out of the 2 million inhabitants were exposed to the disease.

In a retrospective study conducted in Egypt, Halawani & Shawarby (1957) found that malaria had slowly regressed from 1917 to 1947, except for the epidemic brought about by *An. gambiae* in Upper Egypt from 1942 to 1945. Generally speaking, malaria was always more prevalent in Lower Egypt (6.3%) than in Upper Egypt (3.9%).

The first control operations based on larvicidal DDT application were conducted in the Dakhla Oasis from 1946 to 1948 (Gad, 1956). Prevalence dropped from 13-0.3%

and *An. sergentii* disappeared only to return in 1951. In the Siwa Oasis, prevention programs relied on indoor spraying operations with DDT; prevalence dropped from 14.4-0.18% for *P. falciparum* and *P. malariae*; *P. vivax* completely disappeared. These operations were combined with prophylactic drug distribution campaigns.

In 1960, following indoor spraying operations with long-acting insecticides, parasite numbers dropped by 20%. According to Zahar *et al.* (1966), in 1962, there were 45,600 cases as opposed to 95,000 in 1953.

An. pharoensis began showing resistance to DDT in 1965. Following a test with malathion in Kaith el Sheik (Shawarby *et al.*, 1967a), the number of cases dropped to two (*P. vivax*) in 1966 and no cases were reported in the resistance zone in 1967.

Throughout the country, a total of 1,900 cases were reported in 1969, then 2,300 cases in 1972. Only 423 cases were reported in 1982. There were only 63 cases in 1986, including 19 cases of imported *P. falciparum* malaria. The annual number has since remained very low with most cases concentrated around Fayoum (Zahar, 1990).

The rare cases observed along the western edge of the Sinai (two *P. vivax*, one *P. falciparum*) may be attributed to wind-borne *An. pharoensis* crossing the Suez Canal (Zahar, 1990).

Eastern Mediterranean countries

This small region with a rich historical background includes four countries, namely from north to south, Syria, Lebanon, Israel and the east Bank of the Jordan.

The Jordan River and further south the Dead Sea mark the frontier with the Kingdom of Jordan.

There is a strong contrast between the coastal plains, the river valleys and the arid mountain ranges which further east give place to the desert.

Malaria, endemic in the four countries, was controlled and even eradicated as a result of the effective medical structures and international aid.

An. sacharovi, which nearly disappeared in Israel, is still a vector in eastern Syria. *An. sergentii* was the vector in oases and the Jordan Valley. *An. claviger*, found in cisterns, was vector in Alep (Muir & Keilany, 1972) and Jerusalem (Saliternik, 1978); two specimens out of 20 dissections were positive; this is the only record of this species having been found infected. Mention should also be made of the wind-borne incursions of *An. pharoensis* from Egypt in the Gaza Strip (Garrett Jones, 1957; Saliternik, 1960).

In **Jordan**, at El Gurm in the Jordan Valley, despite a PR of 55% in the population, no vectors were found in homes or in Bedouin tents during the day. However, *An. sergentii* was abundant during the day in the neighbouring caves and in rock cracks. Infected specimens were found in the caves (Farid, 1956; Saliternik, 1967), which demonstrated the inefficiency of indoor DDT spraying. Anti-larval treatments with temephos were then undertaken to solve the problem. These observations were classics of malaria epidemiology.

In **Israel**, the malaria control campaign began in 1918 while Palestine was under the British mandate; operations were based on drainage and the use of larvivorous fish. DDT indoor spraying operations began in 1948 at which time, 1,178 new cases per annum were reported; in 1959, only 16 cases were reported and eradication was achieved in 1962 (Saliternik, 1978). Numerous cases of imported malaria continued to be reported and even airport malaria was observed in Lodz.

In **Lebanon**, Gramiccia (1953) (*Figure 10*) assessed the endemicity of the disease: the PR was 6% in the northern coastal region; in the hills, it was only 1-3% although, in the Oronte it reached 11% while the disease was frankly endemic in the Bekaa Valley. This information is now only of historical value. The eradication program launched in 1956 resulted in complete curtailment of the exophilic transmission by *An. sergentii* in the Jordan Valley; as a result of eradication measures, no new cases were reported after 1970. Numerous imported cases continued to be reported, despite efforts to monitor roads and airports. In 1975, 281 imported cases (92 *P. falciparum* and 189 *P. vivax*) were reported (*in* Zahar, 1990).

Syria is the only Near East country where malaria has not been eradicated; transmission due to *An. superpictus*

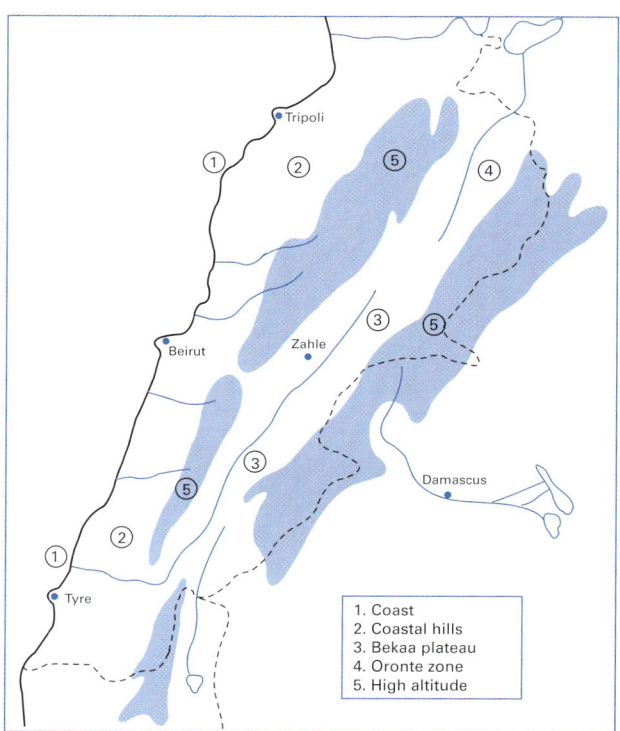

Figure 10. Distribution of malaria in Lebanon according to altitude (adapted from Gramiccia, 1953).

continued in the north-west of the country (Abdel Malek, 1958; Zulueta, 1966 in Zahar, 1974) and *An. sacharovi* continued to transmit the disease near the border with Iraq and Turkey. Exophilic transmission was observed among people who sleep outdoors in the summer. The number of cases has dropped considerably over the last five years and only 6 cases were declared in 2000; a drought in the north-eastern part of the country may have contributed to the near-eradication of malaria (Karch, personal communication).

Turkey

Turkey, with 75 million inhabitants distributed over 780,000 km^2, is the largest and most populated country of the eastern Mediterranean Region. It is flanked on the north and south by two mountain ranges which encircle the Anatolian Plateau. The climate is continental with cold winters. The coastal plains of the north, the west (including the European portion of the country) and the south, all have a gentler, Mediterranean climate.

The anopheline fauna is represented first and foremost by *An. sacharovi*, the main vector which is found throughout the country apart from in the mountains above 1,800 m. *An. superpictus* is particularly abundant in the east up to an altitude of 1,200 m, and this species also plays a significant role. Although mentioned, *An. maculipennis*, *An. melanoon* (syn. *An. subalpinus*) and *An. hyrcanus* are of much lesser importance (Postiglione *et al.*, 1973).

The first epidemics reported in Turkey—at least in western literature—were those of the Dardanelles during the First World War (1914-1918). It is believed that Allies lost more than 100,000 men to disease and German troops, although less severely affected, also suffered heavy losses. It should be pointed out, however, that malaria hit local people just as hard, with 75% of children infected (Bruce-Chwatt & Zulueta, 1980).

The systematic study of malaria based on Spleen and Parasite Rates began in 1925 (Hussamedin, 1930) (*Figure 11*). The disease was found throughout the entire country but was concentrated along the coasts of the Black Sea (Sansum), the Sea of Marmara (Bursa), the Aegean Sea (Manisa, Aydin), and the Mediterranean Sea (from Antalya to Adana), as well as on the Anatolian Plateau (Ankara, Konya). Prevalence varied from focus to focus and from year to year, although it was generally higher in the spring than the autumn (apart from in certain years of unusual rainfall in which this pattern could be reversed). At Bursa in 1926, the prevalence reached 32% (PR) in the spring, to drop down to 7% by the autumn; in Ankara, these values were 24% and 11%, respectively. The highest rates were recorded in 1926. It should be noted that there was little difference in PR between children and adults. The dominant parasite was *P. vivax*, the frequency of which exceeded 90% on the Anatolian Plateau (Konya). *P. falciparum* was omnipresent, exceeding 50% in Bursa and Adana.

Eradication operations were undertaken in 1960 (Ramsdale & Hass, 1978). After two years of malaria control campaigns, only 1,063 cases of *P. vivax* and 19 cases of *P. falciparum* were reported in 1963. The latter species rapidly disappeared. In 1968, malaria had been almost eradicated and, in 1973, only 248 cases were reported in the Adana Region, all attributable to *P. vivax*.

In 1976, the situation suddenly worsened with 88,388 cases in the Churakova and Amikova Regions. The number of cases reached 101,000 the following year before dropping back down to 29,000 cases in 1980. The epidemic then increased to 67,000 cases in 1983, and 55,000 cases in 1984. This second resurgence of transmission was not limited to the Adana Region and it spread to Edirne (in Europe), Izmir, Konya and particularly the Upper Euphrates Region where 21,000 cases were reported in 1983. In 1984, 84,300 cases were declared. The number of cases then dropped to only 34,450 in 1992 (WHO, 1999b). Zahar (1990) analysed the causes of this sustained re-emergence of malaria. The resistance of *An. sacharovi* to DDT, exacerbated by the use of agricultural pesticides, meant that malathion (considered to be inefficient) had to be used. Later, pirimiphos-methyl was used. Moreover, local people were reticent about having their houses sprayed. Decisive

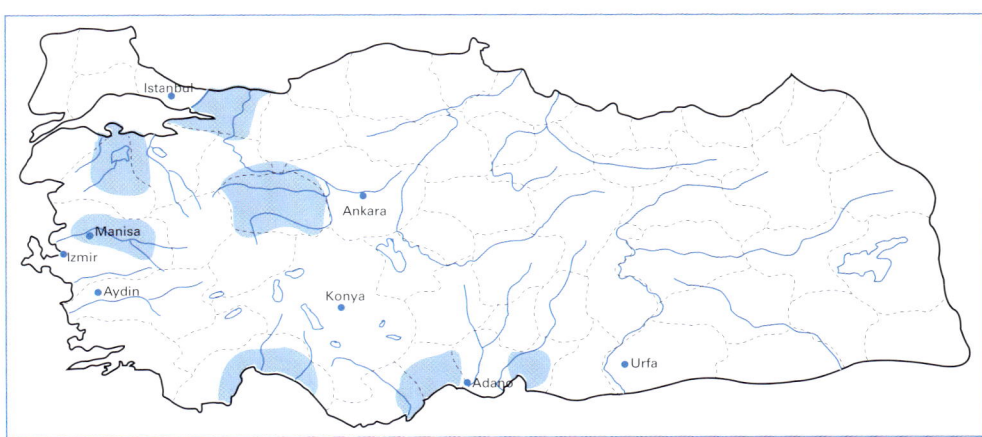

Figure 11.
Malaria in Turkey in 1930 (adapted from Hussamedin, 1930).

results were never attained in anti-larval operations based on the use of the larvivorous fish, *Gambusia affinis*, and the repeated use of *Bacillus thuringiensis* entailed logistical and economic difficulties. The results of these integrated control operations were never truly evaluated (Clarke, 1982) and the administrative and technical modalities employed have been questioned since malaria control policy changes were adopted (Ramsdale & Haas, 1978). Every year, the problem is amplified by the arrival of more than one million seasonal workers in farming areas, although these workers are monitored and treated in the same way as the rest of the population.

In 2000, malaria was still present in Turkey on the eve of its entry into the European Union, and prevention measures are at best only cutting down its prevalence. The idea of eradication has been replaced by the public health notion of maintaining the prevalence of the disease at a tolerable level.

It is not clear whether or not the integration of malaria control organisations within primary health care systems would improve the situation; the opposite is more likely.

In order to plan malaria control, the country was divided into five risk-based strata with a view to defining the measures to be taken in each region:
- stratum 1a, south: Adana, Haçay, the epicentre of epidemic malaria, to be treated in priority;
- stratum 1b, south-east: Anatolia, Syrian and Iraqi borders, to be treated;
- stratum 2, west and European Turkey: moderate risk, surveillance system and action;
- stratum 3, centre and north: very low risk;
- stratum 4, no risk.

The example of Turkey, a country with considerable technical resources, clearly illustrates the difficulties faced when it comes to eradicating focal malaria, even in the temperate zone.

Arabo-Persian Subregion

Limits and characteristics

This area is a transition zone between the Oriental Region to the east, the Mediterranean Subregion to the west, the Euro-Siberian Subregion to the north, and the Afrotropical Region to the south-west. We have considered it as a subregion of the Palaearctic Region, while Macdonald (1957) associated it with the Indo-Pakistani Region to form the Indo-Iranian malaria Region.

From the geographic standpoint, the Arabo-Persian Subregion includes four areas:
- the Arabian Peninsula,
- the plain of Mesopotamia,
- the Irano-Afghani Plateaux, and
- the plains of Central Asia with their extension into Xinjiang Province in China.

The Arabian Peninsula includes Saudi Arabia, Yemen, Bahrain, the United Arab Emirates, Qatar, Oman and Kuwait.

The Mesopotamian Plain is occupied by Iraq. It is overhung by the Irano-Afghan Plateau which covers the north-east of Iraq (Iraqi Kurdistan), Iran and Afghanistan.

Central Asia includes the former republics of the Soviet Union: Turkmenistan, Kazakhstan, Uzbekistan, Tajikistan and Kyrgyzstan. It extends to the east into Xinjiang Province in China (formerly eastern Turkestan).

Geography

The Arabian Peninsula separated from Africa during the Tertiary era. The pronounced relief of Yemen (3,000 m) and south-western Saudi Arabia forms a ridge along the Red Sea. The climate is subtropical with hot summers (the average temperature in July is above 30 °C) and winters with average January temperatures above 20 °C in the southern part of the peninsula. Precipitation ranges between 100 and 300 mm in the mountainous regions in the west, although it is less than 100 mm in the barren centre and east. A few temporary rivers make their way to the sea with difficulty, although the majority dry up somewhere in the sands. Life is thus concentrated in the oases. Except for Yemen and Oman, all the countries of Arabia live off the rich petroleum resources of the region. Saudi Arabia holds 24% of the world's petroleum reserves and its GNP exceeds 10,000 dollars per capita per annum.

The Mesopotamian Plain, occupied by the Tigris and Euphrates River Valleys between Arabia and the Iranian Mountains, represents a major part of Iraq (which also includes the mountains of Kurdistan to the north-east). The climate is subtropical with average July temperatures above 30 °C, more temperate winters with temperatures ranging from 10 to 20 °C in the south, and from 0 to 10 °C in the north (where frost occurs at higher altitudes). Precipitation in the south is below 300 mm but reaches 600 mm in the north-east. Nicknamed the "Fertile Crescent", Mesopotamia has been the home to several civilisations since the Neolithic era. The presence of two major rivers has enabled irrigation to develop since the third millennium BC. Agriculture was for a long time Iraq's source of wealth, and the discovery of oil fields in the north and south has since made it a very coveted prize indeed.

The Irano-Afghan Plateaux consist of a series of closed basins ranging from 200 to 1,000 m in altitude. They are surrounded by two major mountain systems: to the west, the massif of Iranian Azerbaijan and of Kurdistan that extends south-east along the Persian Gulf and Gulf of Oman into the Zagros Mountains (which exceed 4,000 m) and north into the Elburz Mountain range (5,601 m) which runs along the Caspian Sea and then the Turkmenistan border; to the east is the Hindu Kush (above 4,300 m) which rises in the Pamir Plateau in Tajikistan and goes on to divide Afghanistan along a north-east/south-west diagonal. In Iran, the plains are bordered to the south by the Caspian Sea, the north-east corner of the Persian Gulf and along the Gulf of Oman. Rainfall is generally less than 300 mm per annum, except along the Caspian Coast and in the Hindu Kush.

Most of the rivers on the plateaux feed lakes, often brackish, which form in the basins. The climate is subtropical with very hot summers (average July temperatures of over 30 °C); winters are mild in the south (average January temperatures range from 10 to 20 °C), but very cold in northern Iran where average January temperatures range between 0 and 10 °C (with minima as low as –30 °C).

The vegetation is steppe-like and supports only small livestock and camels, the traditional livelihood of millions of nomads. Crop-growing is highly dependent on irrigation which is practised wherever possible. In north-eastern Afghanistan, at altitudes of between 500 and 700 m, rice-growing (in the Kunduz Region) has developed a significant place in the economy. Infrastructure has been drastically disrupted during the twenty years that the country has been at war, particularly health care systems.

Central Asia (former-USSR) is the extension, to the south, of the vast Siberian Plain. The drainage system consists of the Amu-Daria and Syr-Daria Basins which supply, or rather supplied, the Aral Sea, after having drained the water from the Tian-Chan Mountains and the Ob Basin which joins the Arctic glacial area. The climate is continental with massive variations from season to season (hot summers followed by –20 °C in winter) and between day and night (very cold nights and very hot days in the summer). Rainfall is less than 300 mm per annum and, in many places, less than 100 mm. Vegetation is steppe-like or barren; it feeds a few herds of camels, goats and especially sheep (notably the Karakul breed used to make "Astrakhan"). Farming is highly dependant on irrigation for cotton and rice production. The extensive use of fertilizer and the pumping of river water have led to massive pollution. The situation has become very dangerous in terms of public health: in the Aral Sea, the last vestiges of life are slowly disappearing and the fish farmed there are no longer fit for consumption. Man has caused an ecological catastrophe.

Climate and vegetation in the Chinese Province of Xinjiang are very similar to those in the rest of Central Asia.

All the countries of the subregion have or used to have the resources to implement malaria control programs (either on their own initiative or with the assistance of international organisations). Data on the number of declared malaria cases throughout the Arabo-Persian Subregion between 1982 and 1997 were published in 1999 in the WHO's Weekly Epidemiological Record (Table VI).

Arabian Peninsular

The roughly three million km^2 of the Arabian Peninsula are covered by the desert where rainfall is less than 200 mm per annum. Apart from desert oases, life is concentrated in mountains to the west, along the Red Sea and in the Yemen where rainfall exceeds 500 mm per annum. Malaria is very unevenly distributed, mainly along rivers and in oases.

Saudi Arabia (*Figure 12*) is divided into five provinces: the north, west, south, centre and east, to which the zone of the Islamic Holy Land must be added. These administrative divisions correspond to relatively "homogenous" regions in terms of ecology and epidemiology.

In the eastern province, malaria was localised in the oases (Daggy, 1959), where the main vector was and still is *An. stephensi*, a species which is salt-tolerant and thrives in irrigation systems. Anopheline density showed two peaks, one in the spring and another in the autumn. In autumn,

Table VI. Arabo-Persian Subregion. Cases of malaria (‰ inhabitants) 1982-1997 (WHO).

Year	1982	1983	1984	1985	1986	1987	1988	1989	1990	1991	1992	1993	1994	1995	1996	1997
Yemen	28	11	4.5	4.3	4.2	8	9.8	11.7	11.3	12.7	29.2	39.4	37.2	–	416	1,394
Oman	30	34	16.5	16.9	16.7	15.5	24.6	17.8	32.7	19.3	14.8	10.8	7.2	1.8	1.2	1
S. Arabia	15	17	11	16	12	17	9.8	6.5	15	10	19	18	10	18	21	20.6
U.A. Emirates	6.2	4.8	3.5	2.7	3	2.7	3	2.8	3.5	3.4	3.6	3.7	3.3	2.9	0.1	0.1
Iraq	3.2	2.4	3.3	42	2.9	3.7	6.8	3.4	3.9	7.1	5.5	41	96	96	58	14
Iran	42.8	45.9	30.8	26.3	26.3	38.4	53.3	59	77.4	96	76	64	51	67.5	563	38.6
Afghanistan	110	118	155	277	277	428	378	257	317	297	–	–	–	–	305	–
Tajikistan	0.3	0.5	0.5	0.5	0.4	0.3	0.3	0.2	0.2	0.3	0.4	0.6	2.4	6.1	16.5	30.1

Kuwait, Qatar and Bahrain declared no cases although it is known that malaria used to be endemic in Bahrain.
Turkmenistan, Uzbekistan, Kirghizstan, Kazakhstan declared no cases, although there were a few new cases (autochthonous) in Turkmenistan.
Xinjiang Province is included with China.

malaria was hyperendemic with a PR of 85%: with 35% *P. falciparum*, 27.4% *P. vivax* and 14% *P. malariae*. In 1950, malaria was responsible for 8.5% of deaths at the hospital of the Arabian American Company (ARAMCO). The use of DDT (2 g/m^2) provided effective control from 1948 to 1953, until resistance began to appear. It was then replaced by dieldrin, to which *An. stephensi* also became resistant. Larvicides, notably temephos, were then used. *An. stephensi* appears to have been eliminated in the 1960's.

The northern province, along the Iraqi border, was host to just one vector, *An. superpictus*. The incidence of malaria was very low and the disease was quickly eradicated.

There was very little malaria in the barren central province.

The western province of Hedjaz along the Red Sea, which contains the Islamic Holy Lands (Mecca), was known for its malaria epidemics, e.g. that in Djeddah described by Buxton (1944). In 1949, an epidemic extended through October and November with 1,550 cases. In 1955, an epidemic caused by *An. arabiensis* was reported 250 km north of Mecca. This endophilic anopheline had a sporozoite rate of 3.5%. In 1957, *An. arabiensis* disappeared and was replaced by *An. sergentii* which was the usual vector in the province (Zahar & Dabbagh, 1959), while *An. arabiensis* was limited to the south of the 22nd parallel.

In wet years, *An. arabiensis* returned after the rains in October-November (Farid, 1987; Zahar, 1974). In 1958, another epidemic was recorded in a neighbouring untreated region, Djeddah, the arrival point and logistical health care centre for pilgrims.

In 1959, a major epidemic with 65% *P. falciparum* raised the PR of infants to 80% (Mashaal, 1959). Following this epidemic, *An. arabiensis* was eliminated from the region (Zahar & Dabbagh, 1959). The problem of the nomadic people continued as tent spraying operations were never very efficient.

The southern province, north of Yemen, was known as the most endemic place in Saudi Arabia. In the Gizan Region, on the coast (Tihama) which housed 500,000 inhabitants and was a centre for high-technology agricultural development, malaria was hypo- to meso-endemic, and even hyperendemic in certain spots (WHO, 1999a). In Mohayed, 136,600 inhabitants were afflicted in 1980 and indoor spraying operations were transferred to the public health services. Although prevalence was 0.6% in 1982, an epidemic occurred with a PR of 24%. At Lith, a similar phenomenon was recorded with a PR of 10%.

The epidemic of 1954 was remarkable. It took place on the eastern face of the coastal range where conditions are generally more arid. This was due to heavy rains followed by flooding; the PR reached 43% in children. These epidemics were caused by *An. arabiensis* aided by *An. sergentii* (in lesser numbers).

The southern desert is practically uninhabited.

Yemen was reunified only in 1989 and WHO provided separate statistics for the north and south up to this time.

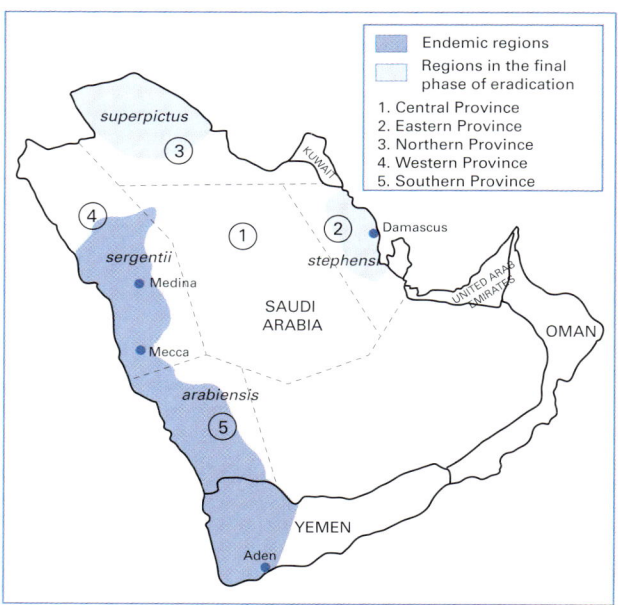

Figure 12. Malaria in Saudi Arabia and Yemen in 1959 (adapted from Zahar, 1959).

From the biogeographical perspective, this country belongs to the Afrotropical Region. The main vector is *An. arabiensis*, found infected in Taiz (Mount, 1953); *An. sergentii* and *An. culicifacies* are less important (Delfini, 1985). Kouznetsov (1976) proposed dividing the country into four natural regions:

- the coastal plain (Tihama), from 0 to 200 m in altitude, where highly irregular rainfall resulted in a highly unstable, focalised malaria, with prevalence ranging from hypo- to hyperendemicity at different foci, depending on local rainfall and the runoff water from the mountains. The prevalence dropped in dry years and rose in wet years. The vectors were *An. arabiensis, An. culicifacies* (possibly), and *An. dthali*;
- the foothills and low mountains, from 200 to 2,000 m, which receive from 800 to 1,200 mm of rain. In the Taiz Region (Thuriaux, 1971), malaria was hypo- or meso-endemic with PRs of 17% and 8% among children less than and over 10 years of age, respectively; malaria was responsible for 5% of admissions at the hospital in Taiz. Peak of malaria transmission was in April and May;
- the central plateau, between 2,000 and 4,000 m, receives no more than 500 mm of rain per annum. *An. sergentii* maintains very low-level endemicity punctuated by epidemics caused by *An. arabiensis*, as was the case in 1946 and 1967;
- on the arid slopes that border the plateau to the east and north and extend to the Arabian Desert, malaria is not endemic although abnormally heavy rainfall can lead to epidemic outbreaks.

In what used to be known as southern Yemen, the city of Aden (500,000 inhabitants) was not endemic although a prevalence of 20% was recorded in the territory on its northern border, towards the mountains, specifically in Abyan (Colbourne & Smith, 1964). Following Afridi (1984), Delfini (1986) confirmed the presence of malaria throughout the entire region of Aden, except in the city itself, the desert and the mountains. In Hadramaut, with a population of only 50,000 (of which 20% are nomads), malaria extended into the desert.

In the island of Socotra, Farid (1988) recorded 3,200 positive cases after examining 40,000 slides; the vector was *An. culicifacies* species A.

In 1996 and 1997, the *WHO's Weekly Epidemiological Record* (1999a) (*Table VI*) reported a sudden increase in the number of cases of malaria in Yemen, which rose from 37,000 cases in 1994 to 416,246 in 1996, and to 1,394,497 in 1997. For a long time in Yemen, diagnosis was based solely on clinical criteria. Numbers based on microscopic diagnosis—insufficient in both quantity and quality—were far from reality. WHO reported epidemics in 1996 and 1998, and a peak of 2.8 million cases in 1999 due to the serious deterioration of surveillance measures. In 2001, the malaria situation greatly improved with the RBM (Roll Back Malaria) control programme which focused on high-risk areas of Yemen. Since 2002, malaria cases have dropped to 200,000 cases anually (WHO, 2005).

In the **Sultanate of Oman**, the first detailed studies of malaria (Farid *et al.*, 1973) showed the scale of this public health problem. The disease was quite different depending on the regions; meso-, or even hyperendemic in the coastal zones of the north-east (Batinah), only hypo-endemic in the oases, and negligible in the desert of Dhofar (south-west). All age groups were affected; adults had little or no immunity and 30% of them experienced at least one paroxysm per annum. Transmission continued throughout the year apart from the very hot months (April and May); the main vectors were *An. culicifacies* along the coast, *An. stephensi* in the hills, and *An. sergentii* and *An. paltrinierii* in the oases and Dhofar (Shidrawi, 1987). Vector numbers were directly dependent on the availability of larval habitats which in turn depended on rainfall and/or irrigation.

Delfini (1987) proposed to divide the country into five ecological zones:
- the north-eastern coast, around the economic growth centre of Batinah, was the country's most malaria-stricken region. Irrigation was a major contributor to the expansion of the vector *An. culicifacies* A; Muir (1988) proposed draining all irrigation channels once a week;
- the foothill region where the vectors were *An. culicifacies* A, *An sergentii* and *An. paltrinierii*; the latter species, first described in the neighbouring Emirates, appears to transmit malaria in the vicinity of streams (wadi) (Shidrawi, 1982). In the Dahira Region, Farid *et al.* (1973) had observed an overall PR of 27.9% with 27% *P. falciparum*;
- the oases, to the south of the coastal zone, where the main vectors were *An. stephensi* and *An. sergentii*. Larvicidal assays were undertaken in this area;
- in Dhofar, a large desert area to the south-west, there is little potential for malaria. *An. stephensi* was reported around Salalah, although further studies are required, notably concerning the role played by watering holes and underground water systems created by the Bedouins;
- the islands of the Persian Gulf were mentioned by Delfini (1987) without any particular comments.

According to WHO statistics (1999a), the various operations in malaria control have considerably reduced the incidence of the disease. The number of cases, which ranged from 33,000 in 1983 to 16,000 in 1993, suddenly dropped to just 7,000 in 1994, then to 1,800 in 1995, and 1,020 by 1997 (WHO, 1999a), without any explanation given for the decrease. In 1990 (WHO, 1990a), a survey of protected zones identified very low PR values of 1.1% on the coast, 1.4% in the hilly areas and 0.7% in the oases.

Farid (1987) considered that the number of cases declared based on microscopic diagnoses (25,000 per annum) was underestimated; 200,000 cases per annum was a more realistic value.

However, transmission has decreased significantly since the implementation of widespread anti-larval operations and the reorganisation of monitoring modalities in 1991. According to WHO, only 603 autochthonous cases were observed in 1996, 129 in 1997, and 114 in 1998 (Beljaev, personal communication), which is very close to eradication. On the other hand, the number of imported cases continues to rise: 662 in 1996, 897 in 1997 and 979 in 1998.

Concerning the **United Arab Emirates**, there is little information about malaria in the western mountainous zones, near the border with Oman.

The report by Farid (1987) mentioned that 300,000 people were exposed to the risk of malaria out of a population of 1,300,000 habitants (in 1987, but 2,300,000 in 2000). Out of 70,000 slides, 3,070 were positive, including 669 for *P. falciparum*. To the east of Abu Dhabi, *An. culicifacies* was the most important vector, while *An. stephensi* was the main vector in the west. Malaria control by indoor spraying operations with DDT and dieldrin had to be subsequently abandoned due to the resistance of two vectors, *An. culicifacies* and *An. stephensi*. Larvicide operations were thereafter based on Abate®.

The number of autochthonous cases, which hovered around 3,000 per annum from 1984 to 1994, dropped from 139 to 4 in 1996, 2 in 1997 and zero in 1998 (WHO-EMRO). The number of imported cases also dropped significantly once neighbouring Oman implemented malaria control operations.

The Island of **Bahrain** was considered endemic until 1980 (Afridi & Majid, 1938; Anjawi, 1983; Delfini, 1977). Since 1982, Bahrain no longer appears on the list of endemic countries, although the number of imported cases (232 in 1976) remains high due to massive immigration (Oddo &

Payne, 1982), as in all the oil-producing countries of the Persian Gulf.

The vector was the ever-present *An. stephensi*, which exhibits two peak periods in April-June and September-December.

In 1959, Anjawi observed an increase in the number of cases which reached 50‰. In 1976, following major earth-moving operations and the importation of Asian labour, Delfini (1977) reported a small epidemic of 35 autochthonous cases.

Malaria control measures based on indoor spraying operations (DDT then organophosphates) encountered problems with a population that was hostile and generally against other people coming into the house. Street fogging was then adopted, although this was probably totally ineffective. Larvicide operations were also undertaken with Abate®. The dissemination of the larva-eating fish, *Aphanius dispar*, appears not to have been successful although malaria seems to have disappeared from Bahrain.

While **Kuwait** and **Qatar** have never been endemic, it would appear that *An. stephensi* is present there. Imported malaria, however, is a serious problem throughout all the oil-producing countries. Prophylactic drugs (600 mg chloroquine + 45 mg pyrimethamine) were administered to all immigrants until the late 1980's. Now Malarone® is the most widely used prophylatic drug.

Mesopotamian plain and the plateaux of Iran and Afghanistan

From an ecological standpoint, separating the Mesopotamian Plain from plateaux of Iran and Afghanistan is legitimate but, in order to present the epidemiological information—that remains very unequal from one country to the next—the following three countries are dealt with separately: Iraq, Iran and Afghanistan.

Iraq

Iraq (*Figure 13*) has been the subject of various classification attempts, be they ecological (Christophers & Shortt, 1921; Ossi, 1969; Pringle, 1954), or political. From the standpoint of malaria and its transmission, it is reasonable to divide the country into three "regions", as did Pringle (1954):
- the north (Kurdistan), a mountainous region set within the Iranian Plateaux, was the seat of a meso- and even hyperendemic malaria (with SRs generally greater than 50%) (Pringle, 1954). Transmission took place from May to November (Macan, 1950) and was attributed to *An. sacharovi*, *An. superpictus* and *An. maculipennis* locally. It was considered to be the most endemic region of Iraq. Pringle (1954) had qualified malaria there as "stable" in order to establish a contrast between the epidemics of the alluvial zones. Variable precipitation—both rain and snow, mostly falling during the winter months—feeds numerous rivers, and results in fluctuations in the incidence of malaria the following summer. All anophelines show some form of interruption of their development during the winter, considered as a diapause;
- the alluvial plains of the Tigris and Euphrates were characterised by malaria that was incorrectly designated as epidemic, transmitted in June-July, then in October-November, after the scorching summer period, by *An. stephensi* and *An. superpictus* in the northern part of these plains. The focus of *An. sacharovi* along the Chatt Al-Arab was eliminated in the early 1980's. On the basis of health centre records, it may be that there was a relationship between the volume of water being carried in the Tigris and the Euphrates, and the incidence of malaria. In 1926, both rivers reached a cumulative flow rate of 84.5 billion m^3 as opposed to 38 billion in 1925; the percentages of malaria cases (as a function of all consultations) were 27% and 8% respectively. In 1946, however, the cumulative flow rate of the rivers was 101 billion m^3, although no "epidemic" was reported. Irrigation systems have a direct impact on the production of *An. stephensi* and constitute the second factor involved in the genesis of epidemics;
- from the endemicity standpoint, the steppes which border the alluvial plain offer an intermediate situation which varies considerably from one village to the next (Pringle, 1954); the vectors are *An. sacharovi* and *An. superpictus*; *An. stephensi* is rare in areas without irrigation. There was a nearly equal number of cases attributable to *P. vivax*

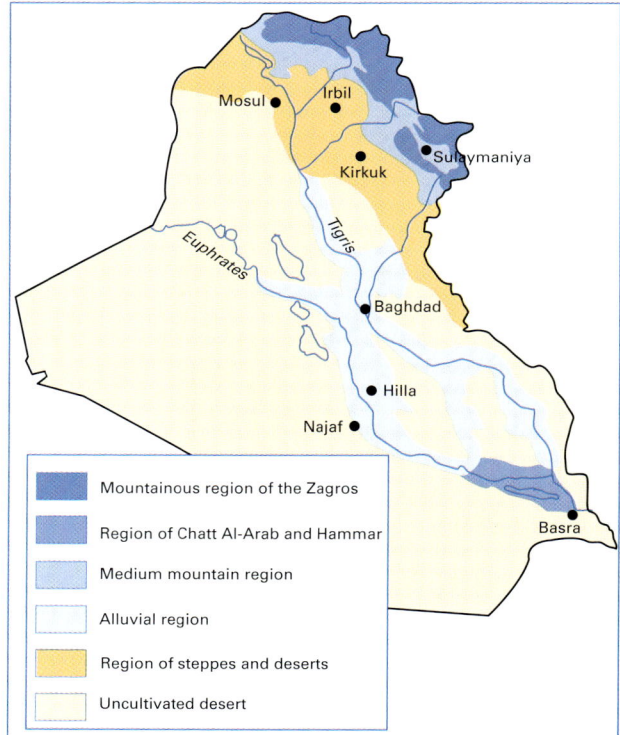

Figure 13. Stratification of malaria in Iraq (adapted from Pringle, 1954).

and *P. falciparum*, although the latter quickly dropped as soon as indoor spraying operations were implemented. No further mention was made of *P. malariae*, originally reported by Covell (*in* Pringle, 1954) in Kirkuk.

The implementation of prevention programs from 1954 to 1957 rapidly resulted in regression of the disease. In 1970 (Ossi, 1969, 1977), only a few foci persisted, primarily in the north, causing 15,000-20,000 cases per annum. In 1978 (Ossi, 1986), transmission was interrupted in the south, but persisted at a few locations in the north where only four cases of *P. falciparum* were reported. Out of 1,800,000 slides examined, only 3,000 were still positive. Malaria had nearly been eradicated as was confirmed by a serological study (Shihab *et al.*, 1987).

In 1987, *P. falciparum* no longer existed in Iraq (Farid, 1987; WHO, 1999a) and the majority of cases were imported. There was a major outbreak from 1993 to 1996, resulting in 96,700 cases in 1995 following the Gulf War. In 1997, numbers began to drop again, reaching 14,006 cases in 1997 (WHO, 1999a) (*Table VII*).

Iran

The first reports of malaria from Iran date back to 1921 and 1941, along the border with Azerbaijan and south of the Caspian Sea (Amdizadeh, 1941; Latisheve, 1921), as well as in the oil-rich region of Khuzestan (Lindberg, 1936); the reports were based on sampling operations. The first overview of the malaria situation was provided by Gilmour in 1925 in a report published by the League of Nations. He noted that 60% of the population of 12 million inhabitants were living in highly endemic areas where malaria caused 4-5 million clinical episodes per annum. Malaria was responsible for 30-40% of deaths. One-third of the Health Ministry budget was allocated to the purchase of quinine. These first steps in the field of the study of malaria in Iran were reported by Motabar *et al.* (1975) and Manouchehri *et al.* (1992).

The use of organic chloride insecticides to control malaria spurred the Malaria Institute to produce a map of endemic areas in 1949 (updated in 1962, and then again in 1971) in order to show the progress made in eradicating the disease (Motabar *et al.*, 1975) (*Figure 14*).

Based on these documents, the preceding experts attempted to produce a stratification ahead of time, taking into account the role of the various vectors in the analysis. The following zones were distinguished:
- hyperendemic zones: along the border with Azerbaijan (the Araxe Valley), the Caspian Sea (with a Mediterranean climate) and the border with Turkmenistan. The vectors were *An. maculipennis* and mainly *An. sacharovi*. The western face of the Zagros, Fars Regions of the south along the Persian Gulf and the Sea of Oman as well as south-eastern Baluchistan, were also classified as hyperendemic. Besides *An. superpictus*, the vectors were *An. sacharovi* in the western mountains, *An. fluviatilis*, *An. stephensi* and *An. culicifacies* species A throughout all southern regions;
- meso-endemic zones surrounding the hyperendemic belt in the interior; the vectors were primarily *An. superpictus*, *An. stephensi* and *An. culicifacies* in the south;

Table VII. Cases of malaria in Iraq from 1982 to 1998 (*Relevé Épidémiologique Hebdomadaire*, 1990).							
1982	1983	1984	1985	1986	1987	1988	1989
3,300	2,400	3,340	4,770	2,953	3,724	6,830	3,420
1990	1991	1992	1993	1994	1995	1996	1997
3,924	7,105	5,534	41,071	96,368	96,738	58,345	14,006

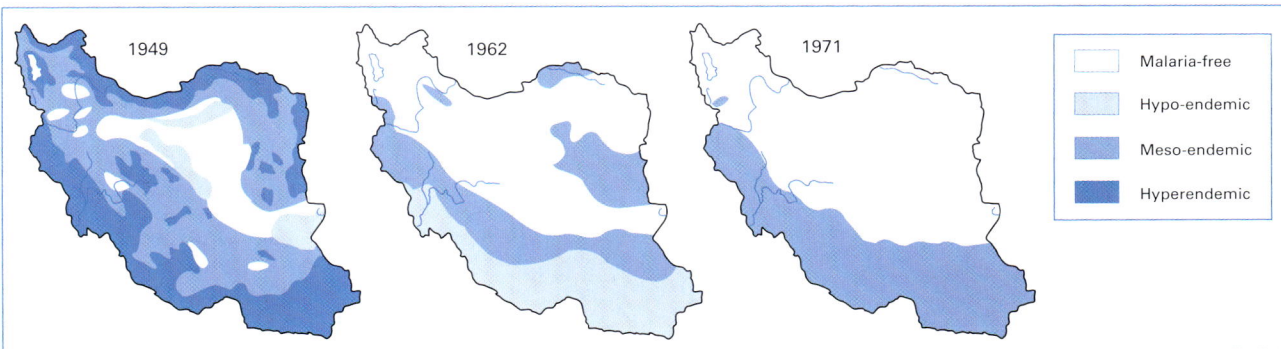

Figure 14. Decline of malaria in Iran from 1949 to 1971 (adapted from Motabar et al., 1992).

- hypo-endemic zones, limited in extent although somewhat broader to the east;
- malaria-free zones in the desert regions of the central Iranian Plateau.

Control measures were an immediate success. After three years, in 1953, prevalence had dropped to 0.75% and malaria had disappeared throughout most of the country; on the 1962 map (*Figure 14*), the hyperendemic zones were eliminated, notably those where *An. sacharovi* and *An. maculipennis* were the vectors; in 1971 (*Figure 14*), the result remained steady and only the meso-endemic foci in the south-west and south remained (Motabar *et al.*, 1975). These results were confirmed by a serological study conducted by Edrissian *et al.* (1976); *P. falciparum* had nearly disappeared and only *P. vivax* persisted (owing to its very long winter incubation period, as in Russia).

The final eradication phases were complicated by the acquisition of multiple insecticide resistance by the vectors, the exophilic behaviour of some of them, and population movements, particularly those of the nomad peoples. *An. stephensi*s resistance to both DDT and dieldrin necessitated the use of more expensive organophosphate compounds and shorter-acting products (malathion and fenitrothion). The exophilic behaviour of *An. superpictus*, which rested in caves during the day, continued to maintain transmission levels in Khorassan (north-east); at least one infected specimen of this anopheline was found in caves (Charles, 1960). In the south of the country, after *An. stephensi* had disappeared, the exophilic and exophagic behaviour of *An. fluviatilis* was a problem as the population continued to sleep outdoors during the hot months.

The nomadic lifestyle which takes shepherds from Zagros into southern Fars is still considered an obstacle to malaria control and treatment (Motabar *et al.*, 1975).

In 1987, after having reviewed the problems related to malaria control treatment operations in Iran, Zaïm compiled an inventory of the current situation. In the north (Zagros and plateau), 35 million people were in the maintenance phase. Out of 1,024,727 slides, only 5,246 were positive (roughly 0.5%). These can be broken down as follows: 95% *P. vivax*, 3% *P. falciparum* and 1% *P. malariae*. In the south, where malaria control was still in the attack phase, 20,400 out of 1,600,000 slides were positive (1.4%) with 83% *P. vivax* and 16% *P. falciparum*.

Since 1982, the number of declared cases has fluctuated from a minimum of 26,363 cases in 1985 to 96,310 cases in 1991 before dropping back down to 38,680 cases by 1997 (WHO, 1999a). The increase between 1988 and 1994 may be attributed to the influx of Afghani refugees fleeing the war.

If there is still any malaria in Iran, it cannot be considered as a major public health problem. In fact, since 1975, imported cases far outnumber autochthonous cases (Manouchehri *et al.*, 1992) (*Table VIII*).

Table VIII. Results of studies dealing with cases of malaria in two endemic zones in Iran (1975-1990) (*in* Manouchehri *et al.*, 1992).

	Region north of Zagros (number of cases)					Southern and south-western Iran (number of cases)				
Year	Autochthonous	Introduced	Imported	Relapses	Unknown	Autochthonous	Introduced	Imported	Relapses	Unknown
1975	932	54	1,652	232	19	842	191	742	746	34
1976	343	385	2,888	572	76	585	201	841	670	23
1977	61	68	3,088	470	24	624	15	1,061	741	25
1978	31	45	1,396	121	3	556	19	793	614	22
1979	211	5	591	65	2	510	59	469	381	10
1980	87	31	884	130	8	1,478	48	527	626	48
1981	37	28	917	156	12	1,153	49	607	927	124
1982	123	53	2,287	190	9	1,343	69	660	724	107
1983	38	169	3,440	103	12	1,091	46	918	815	52
1984	44	33	3,715	164	32	605	106	921	451	49
1985	244	36	4,563	142	15	481	24	1,341	509	25
1986	378	41	4,279	317	4	267	69	929	237	23
1987	428	43	4,706	174	9	273	24	999	123	28
1988	574	69	3,125	160	19	172	36	213	85	15
1989	256	21	3,665	284	24	133	16	165	73	7
1990	83	99	3,654	225	14	158	14	157	48	9

Afghanistan

Afghanistan, as far as the eastern part of the Hindu Kush is concerned, has already been addressed under the Oriental Region, so it is impossible to avoid some degree of redundancy here.

According to Dhir & Rahim (1957), two of the twelve million inhabitants were living in endemic zones which are spread around four regions (*Figure 15*):

- the eastern region, already discussed (*see the Chapter on the* "Oriental Region"), where the vectors of oriental origin, *An. stephensi, An. culicifacies s.l., An. fluviatilis s.l.* and *An. superpictus*, maintained meso- or hyperendemic transmission with an increasing proportion of *P. falciparum* (which is believed to have reached 50%);
- the north-east region, between 200 and 500 m in altitude, where *An. hyrcanus* and *An. pulcherrimus* were vectors of a malaria that was refractory to indoor spraying in the neighbouring rice-growing valleys of Tajikistan; the parasite was exclusively *P. vivax*. Beyond the Kunduz Basin, the vector was *An. superpictus*;
- the steppe-like plateaux, at an altitude of 500 to 2,000 m, are a seat of meso- or hypoendemic malaria, transmitted by *An. superpictus*; *P. vivax* represented more than 95% of infections;
- the southern basins, at an altitude of 200 to 1,000 m with generally halophilic steppe or desert vegetation, where malaria is meso- or hypoendemic and transmitted by a wide variety of different vectors, namely the Palaearctic species *An. superpictus* and *An. stephensi*, as well as *An. culicifacies s.l.* and *An. fluviatilis s.l.* of oriental origin. While *P. vivax* was the main parasite, an increase in *P. falciparum* has been reported since 1988. Generally speaking, malaria was localised in the cultivated valleys.

The Kunduz Region in the north-east, very similar to neighbouring Tajikistan from a geographic standpoint, has been extensively studied since 1970 (Onori *et al.*, 1975) as indoor spraying operations proved to be ineffective there. The region featured four distinct types of landscape: the rice paddies in the valleys, irrigated zones, mountain valleys and foothill regions (Polevoy *et al.*, 1975). *An. hyrcanus* (identical to the Western European forms) and *An. pulcherrimus* were considered to be relatively inefficient vectors because they are highly zoophilic. The first species was no longer biting in the zone treated with DDT although it continued to enter untreated homes; it was very exophilic, however, as it rested outdoors. The second species, while continuing to bite indoors (endophagy), rested outdoors (exophily). This "refractory" behaviour of the second species led to continued transmission in spite of indoor spraying. Beginning in the 1980's, larvivorous fish were widely used in places where the only plasmodia species was *P. vivax*.

Throughout the whole of Afghanistan, anopheline sporozoite rates were very low: 0.4% in *An. culicifacies s.l.*, and from under 0.1% to 0.4% in *An. superpictus* (Dhir & Rahim, 1957).

The tragic events that have taken place in Afghanistan since 1980 have caused disorganisation in health services. Also, there are many problems with the statistics available (WHO). In 1987, Delfini questioned their reliability; he felt that 428,128 cases must be an underestimate and suggested two million as a more plausible figure. Since 1992, the situation does not appear to have improved; indeed, it has probably deteriorated. Reports were not issued from 1992 to 1995, nor in 1997 and the number of cases announced in 1996 remains to be confirmed (WHO, 1999a).

For example, in the north-eastern region, out of 46 villages with 42,000 inhabitants, the incidence varied from 232‰ to 674‰ (Kouchasov, 1985, unpublished WHO document). High morbidity levels were observed in Kunar where the percentage of *P. falciparum* was greater than 30% (Hoffman, personal communication). For the time being, we have to make do with such fragmentary information.

Central Asia

This section includes the Asian republics of the former Soviet Union and the autonomous territory of Xinjiang, in China, all of which represent a land mass of 4 million km² between the 36th and 47th north parallels and between the Caspian Sea to the west and the plateaux of China to the east. The climate throughout all these regions is an extreme continental one with very cold winters and hot summers (at least during the daytime). The lack of precipitation, less than 300 mm, precludes the growth of steppe or even desert vegetation. Life concentrates around high-altitude, glacier-fed rivers which are exploited (and sometimes over-exploited) for the purposes of irrigation.

The republics of Turkmenistan, Uzbekistan, Tajikistan, Kazakhstan and Kyrgyzstan, an area which used to be

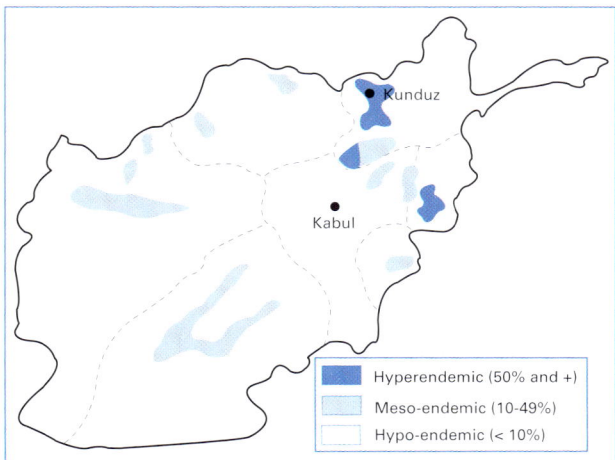

Figure 15. Malaria in Afghanistan in 1957 (adapted from Dhir & Rahim, 1957).

called Russian Turkestan prior to the Russian Revolution, form the southern extension of the large Siberian plain which abuts the Iranian Plateaux, the Hindu Kush, the Pamir and Tian-Chan. These landforms, reaching altitudes of 7,000 m in the Pamir and Tian-Chan, offer a stark contrast with the plains to the north and west. The autonomous territory of Xinjiang in China (known in the past as Chinese Turkestan) is a region of mountains, plateaux and scattered basins at altitudes below 500 m which communicate extensively with Kazakhstan, *via* the Gate of Dzungaria, a former silk route, and which are drained *via* the Ili Valley which joins China to Lake Balkhash.

The anopheline fauna is typically Palaearctic. The species *An. martinius*—very similar to *An. sacharovi* although not a vector of malaria—occupies the entire region, and *An. messae* is confined to north of the 40th parallel. Both species are indicated in Xinjiang on White's maps (1978), although Zhou Zu-Jie (1981) only mentions the second species as being a vector in China. *An. maculipennis s.s.* appears only in southern Turkmenistan. *An. superpictus* is mentioned in the five Republics while *An. pulcherrimus* and *An. fluviatilis s.l.* are found south of the Aral Sea (Zahar, 1990). Finally, owing to similarities in landscape, *An. hyrcanus* must be included with the vectors (Polevoy *et al.*, 1975) of the upper Amu-Daria Basin, as well as *An. claviger* in the valleys of the Pamir Mountains in Tajikistan.

Malaria was considered to be endemic in Central Asia. Favr (1903 *in* Bruce-Chwatt & Zulueta, 1980) reported incidences of 36.4‰ on the Syr-Daria and 25.3‰ in Samarkand.

On the map of Lysenko & Kondrashin (1999) produced in 1934 at the peak of the great malaria pandemic, indices of 100-200‰ are shown in eastern Kazakhstan and Kyrgyzstan, of 50-100 ‰ in Tajikistan, Uzbekistan and northern Kazakhstan, and of 10-50 ‰ in Turkmenistan.

These two authors traced the dynamics of malaria in Tajikistan (*Figure 16*). In this country, the number of cases was around 100,000 per annum from 1934 to 1950; from 1955 to 1960, the number of cases dropped below 100 during the eradication period, an objective which was reached in 1975. Starting in 1991, following the abandonment of control operations as a result of civil war, the incidence "skyrocketed" to 120,000 in 1996, even more than in 1934, before dropping back down to 30,000 in 1997 (WHO, 1999a). This epidemic is very closely related to the epidemic which occurred in the Kunduz Region in north-eastern Afghanistan. The landscape is very similar in both regions (Polevoy *et al.*, 1975), although it appears that in Tajikistan, the vector responsible for the epidemic wave was *An. superpictus* (Kondrashin, personal communication).

Still within the same country, *P. falciparum* returned (16% *P. falciparum* and 84% *P. vivax*) to a region from which it had been eliminated in 1960 (Pitt *et al.*, 1998). It appears as though the monitoring reports underestimated the

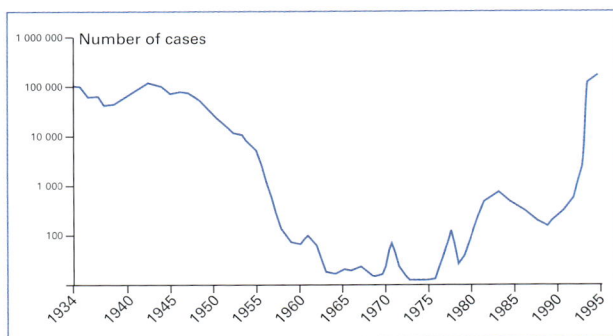

Figure 16. Cases of malaria in Tajikistan from 1934 to 1995 (adapted from Lysenko & Kondrashin, 1999).

prevalence values. Within the district of Boktus with a population of 15,000 people, 499 of the 700 slides examined were positive.

In Turkmenistan, the 104 cases reported in the district of Kuscha were imported by soldiers returning from Afghanistan (WHO, 1999a).

A few isolated cases were reported in the various Republics. Almost all of these cases were imported (Nemirovskaia *et al.*, 1975).

In the Xinjiang Province of China, Zhou Zu-Jie (1985) reported seasonal epidemics of *P. vivax*, occasionally associated with *P. falciparum*, in the Ili Valley where the PR reached 5%. *An. messae* was the only vector mentioned.

Chinese Subregion

Borders

The Chinese Subregion occupies the eastern part of the Palaearctic Region. It includes China to the east of Tibet and north of the 25th north parallel; to the south of this line, the Chinese territory is included in the Oriental Region. The high parts of Tibet and Qinghai are outside the endemic zone, although their fauna resembles that of the Chinese Subregion. The autonomous territory of Xinjiang, in the western part of the country, can be assimilated to Central Asia. Besides China, Japan (except the Ryukyu Islands with oriental affinities), the Republic of Korea (ROK) (South Korea), the Democratic People's Republic of Korea (North Korea), and the maritime province of Russia belong to this Chinese Subregion where *An. sinensis* is the dominant anopheline species. The rest of Siberia is included in the Euro-Siberian Subregion.

Malaria has not been reported in Mongolia, the fauna of which shares much with that of eastern Siberia.

The territory of this subregion represents approximately 2 million km² with a total population of about 1.7 billion people. The Chinese part accounts for nearly 80% of this population.

Our biogeographical, ecological and epidemiological approach has led us to divide China into three entities: Xinjiang to the west, part of the Palaearctic Region (Arabo-Persian Subregion); China south of the 23rd parallel, part of the Oriental Region; and central and northern China (Palaearctic Region, Chinese Subregion).

General characteristics

The first descriptions of malaria in China date back roughly 3,500 years and the disease has marked the country throughout its history although there have always been enormous differences from region to region.

To the west, the mountains of Tibet, Sichuan and Qinghai, then the deserts of Mongolia, isolate the Chinese Subregion. The most common parasite was *P. vivax* which could be found beyond the Amour River. *P. falciparum* levels have been significantly reduced and it is close to elimination in Central China; it was probably never very common in northern China, Korea or Japan. *P. malariae* never represented more than 1-2% of the cases in southern China.

Malaria was eliminated in Japan at the end of the Second World War and in South Korea in the 1960's, although it reappeared in that country in 1994.

China

Stratification

Ho (1965), Zhou Zu-Jie (1981) and later Tang Lin-Hua *et al.* (1991) proposed dividing China into five regions, based on climatic differences and the epidemiological characteristics of malaria—corresponding to the distribution of the various vector species (*Table IX*): this epidemiological division will lead us into some redundancy since, in biogeographical terms, China is split between three different regions or subregions. Nevertheless, we have chosen to present here an overview of malaria throughout this massive territory:

- from north to south, malaria can be stratified into longitudinal zones which follow the isotherms south of the 25th parallel to the borders of Indochina. The vectors in this tropical region are *An. minimus s.l.* and *An. dirus s.l.*, *An. minimus* (formerly species A) and species C of the Minimus Complex are present in this area sometimes in sympatry, with species C found up to 32.5°N. They are both responsible for malaria transmission (Chen *et al.*, 2002). Within the seven species of the Dirus Complex, only two occur in southern China, *An. dirus* (species A) and *An. baimaii* (species D) which are very efficient malaria vectors (Sallum *et al.*, 2005). Malaria was often associated with jungle and was characterised by hyperendemic foci in broader meso-endemic zones. The dominant parasite, *P. falciparum*, has been in regression ever since effective malaria control measures were implemented;
- a temperate zone extends from the 25th to the 33rd north parallel, limited by the Sichuan Mountains to the west. The dominant vector is *An. anthropophagus* (former *An. lesteri* Baisas) which is highly anthropophilic, and twenty times more effective as a vector than the secondary species, *An. sinensis* (Liu *et al.*, 1986). In rice-growing areas, the larvae of *An. lesteri* (syn. *An. anthropophagus*) are generally found in irrigation ditches while those of *An. sinensis* tend to be concentrated on the irrigated land itself. Transmission lasts six to eight months in the year. Malaria used to be meso- or hypoendemic with seasonal epidemic outbreaks. *P. falciparum* was responsible for more than 20% of paroxysms in Henan (Huang & Lin, 1986; Huang, 1987);
- only one single vector, *An. sinensis*, appears north of the 33rd parallel; this species is zoophilic and relatively inefficient as a vector. However, the disease has often reached epidemic proportions, as in 1960 with 10 million cases in northern China (Zhang *et al.*, 1998). In this region, *P. vivax* is practically the only parasite and it is only transmitted during three months out of the year. To the west, this region is limited by the mountains of

Table IX. A few characteristics of the transmission of malaria in China.			
Region	Transmission period	*Plasmodium* species	Vectors
South of the 25th parallel	9-12 months 6-8 months	*P. vivax* *P. falciparum* *P. malariae*	*An. minimus** *An. dirus** *An. candidiensis* *An. sinensis*
From the 25th to the 33rd parallel	6-8 months	*P. vivax* *P. falciparum* *P. malariae*	*An. sinensis** *An. lesteri**** *An. candidiensis*
North of the 33rd parallel	3-6 months	*P. vivax*	*An. sinensis**
West (Xinjiang)	3-5 months	*P. vivax*	*An. messae***
North-west of the 33rd parallel	Non endemic		
* Main species, ** Mainly localised species, *** *An. lesteri*: synonym with *An. anthropophagus*			

Qinghai and Gansu Provinces, as well as the deserts of Mongolia;
- the malaria-free regions are essentially the mountains to the west of Sichuan and Gansu Provinces, as well as Qinghai, Tibet and south-west Xinjiang. The deserts of Mongolia are also considered as non-endemic. These autonomous regions or provinces are home to only 7.9% of the population;
- the lower regions of Xinjiang Province which open onto the plains of Central Asia were discussed above.

Changes in the malaria situation

Prior to the Second World War, a deadly epidemic broke out in the valley of the Yang-Tse-Kiang following flooding in 1931. This epidemic touched 60% of the 28 million inhabitants (Zhang et al., 1998). In 1933, an epidemic in Yunnan resulted in the deaths of 33,000 people (Huang & Lin, 1986), although these figures are confusing since, in Yunnan, malaria was considered to be stable.

In 1949-1950, Zhou Zu-Jie (1985) reported 3.5 million cases per annum, associated with 6.46% morbidity and 1% mortality. Zhang et al. (1998) collected data on malaria between 1950 and 1980. In 1950, the disease was endemic in 80% of counties. In 1955, 6.97 million cases were reported but by 1958, the incidence had dropped by 50%. In 1960, a *P. vivax* epidemic devastated the entire hypoendemic region south of Beijing with 10 million cases. In 1970, during the Cultural Revolution, malaria control operations were interrupted and the number of cases increased to 24 million.

In 1978, after the departure of the "Gang of Four" (extensively discussed by epidemiologists), control operations were resumed by the provincial anti-epidemic services within the primary health care system (*Figure 17*).

Between 1980 and 1990, the number of cases dropped from 3.3 million to 117,000; the incidence went from 0.33-0.1% but the corresponding mortality rate did not follow the same curve, dropping only from 65 to 35 (a negligible figure in the light of the size of China). This decline in malaria mortality resulted from priority being given to the treatment of the most severe forms and the use of the Qinghaosu.

The latest statistics published by WHO (1999a) confirm the overall efficiency of malaria control in China.

The number of cases recorded dropped from 204,100 in 1982 to 86,000 in 1990 and 26,816 in 1997.

In 1999, no cases of malaria were reported in the northern provinces, and the overall incidence was less than 0.1‰. *P. falciparum* no longer thrives in the south, with just a few isolated cases in the centre accounting for just 8.9% of all confirmed cases.

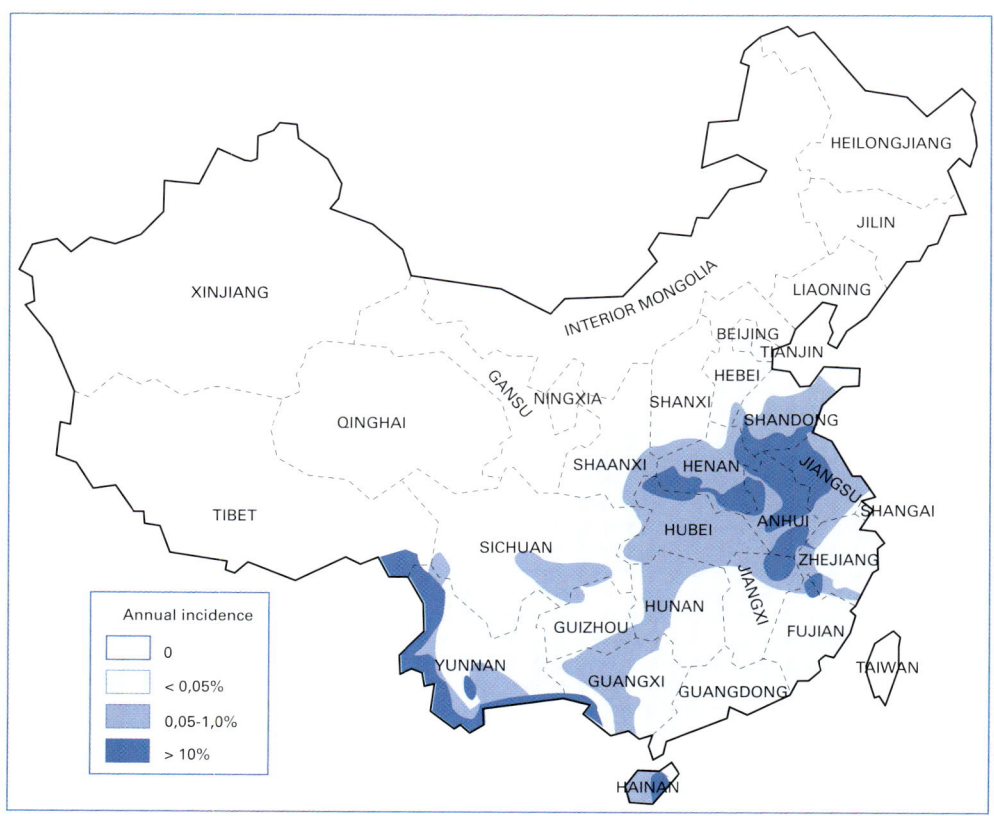

Figure 17. Malaria annual incidence in China in 1979 (after the Cultural Revolution) (adapted from Zhou Zu Jie, 1981).

The health authorities are being remarkably effective at reducing residual foci and managing imported cases (which could lead to reintroduction of the disease), e.g. in Guangdong Province, a small epidemic among seasonal labourers led to *P. vivax* infection of 21% of the district's population: all were immediately treated and malaria control operations were implemented (Zhang, 1986).

This is probably one of the best results reported in the last twenty-five years.

Korea

Malaria was first reported in Korea in 1913. *P. vivax* was involved and was the only parasite that has ever been described in this country (Paik *et al.*, 1988). The parasite has an exceptionally long incubation period (Shute *et al.*, 1977) and subjects who had been infected in late summer or autumn did not experience any paroxysm until the following spring (which we know because the disease cannot possibly be transmitted during the winter months). These observations, made on Japanese soldiers, are consistent with others made in Finland and Russia where the parasite was named *P. vivax hibernans* (Garnham *et al.*, 1975; Renkonen, 1944): from 1931 to 1939, numerous cases were reported prior to April even though *Anopheles* was not yet active.

From 1922 to 1930, the number of cases dropped significantly due to improved living conditions (Païk *et al.*, 1988). However, the incidence was still above 50‰ in the forest-covered mountains of eastern South Korea.

Following partition of the country, 19,500 cases were reported in 1968 in South Korea (WHO, 1983) but, once indoor spraying operations were initiated, malaria was eliminated.

Statistics regarding North Korea have never been submitted to WHO and the country remains terra incognita.

The only vector reported to date is *An. sinensis*; sporozoite rates of 0.006% were reported by Chow (1970) and Chen *et al.* (1967). The vector potential of this zoophilic species is very low and, although in regions where there is very little livestock *An. sinensis* frequently bites humans, no appreciable transmission has ever been recorded (Chen *et al.*, 1967).

The transmission season is short, lasting only three to four months. The female mosquitoes hibernate in animal shelters and may feed without their ovaries developing (Whang, 1961).

In 1993, a re-emergence of malaria was reported in South Korea along the demilitarised border zone (Feighner *et al.*, 1998). The number of cases continued to grow exponentially, signalling an epidemic process: one case in 1993 (Chai *et al.*, 1994), 24 cases in 1994, 107 cases in 1995, 356 cases in 1996 and 1,724 cases in 1997.

It would have been surprising if the epidemic wave along the demilitarised border zone had not had any effect in North Korea. In fact, the six provinces in the south of the country were stricken by a very serious epidemic. In 1998, 2,100 cases of *P. vivax* were reported in Kaesong, South Hwanghae and Kangwon Provinces. In 1999, the epidemic was estimated at 100,000 cases, including 900 cases reported in the capital Pyongyang (Kondrashin, as reported at Roll Back Malaria, WHO, Geneva, February 2000); 39% of the cases (including relapses) appeared during the first semester, 29% in July, 21% in August and 11% in September. Microscopic diagnosis was performed in only 30% of cases. Most cases (about 90%) involved adults between the ages of 20 and 45, with an equal distribution between males and females. *An. sinensis* was the only anopheline concerned.

It thus appears that the epidemics in both countries are part of a parallel process. The reasons why malaria re-emerged twenty-five years after eradication remain very obscure. The introduction of parasite carriers is the theory proposed by the North Korean authorities, although this does not make much sense in the light of the country's political isolation. It is, however, certain that poor heath care provision and malnutrition may well have played a role.

Japan

Malaria, endemic in Japan until 1945, disappeared at the end of the Second World War. The only parasite was *P. vivax* which was transmitted by *An. sinensis* (Chow, 1970).

It appears as though the last epidemic outbreak occurred in 1946 when troops were returning from the various fronts (Sawada, 1949); more than 460,000 cases of "imported" malaria were diagnosed.

In Ryukyu, *An. saperoi* was considered a vector after the war. *An. minimus* E is a species of the Minimus Complex recently described in this archipelago (Somboon *et al.*, 2001). This species is not incriminated as malaria vector since it occurs in a malaria-free area.

An. lesteri also was reported in Japan (Otsuru & Ohmori, 1960).

Far-eastern Russia

An. sinensis has been reported in eastern Siberia where it seems to substitute for species of the Maculipennis Group, notably *An. messae* and *An. beklemishevi*.

According to the 1934 map of malaria in the USSR (*in* Lysenko & Kondrashin, 1999), the incidence of malaria in the Far East was very low, below 100 per 10,000 inhabitants. Eradication was achieved there as early as 1958.

American Regions

In this book, the two American Regions—the Nearctic Region (North America down to the Isthmus of Tehuantepec in Mexico) and the Neotropical Region (the Caribbean Islands, Central America south of the Isthmus of Tehuantepec, and South America)—are addressed together. Considering the entire American continent together thus allows us to take the overall distribution of each vector into account, particularly those found in both regions, such as *Anopheles pseudopunctipennis* which ranges from Texas to Argentina. This grouping is all the more pertinent given that malaria is now only a memory in North America.

The total land mass (*Figure 1*) is 39,863,000 km^2 and the current population is 884 million (*Table I*). Malaria was a major cause of mortality until 1943; in Central America and southern Mexico, the number of deaths by malaria was between 200 and 500 per 100,000 inhabitants with peaks of up to 1,000. A spectacular decline was recorded following indoor DDT spraying operations. By 1975, the incidence of the disease had declined significantly and eradication had almost been realised in several countries. Since 1975, however, the developing countries of the American continent have had to deal with an increase in the number of cases and a spread in the areas affected (Roberts *et al.*, 1997). This upsurge is primarily due to discontinuation or attenuation of control measures as a result of difficulties associated with the use of DDT. It is in fact difficult or nearly impossible to obtain alternative insecticides that are both as efficient and cheap as DDT (which is now banned in many countries). The movements of rural and mining populations, who live in precarious conditions in which the vectors are difficult to control, are also involved in the reemergence of malaria. The increase in malaria since 1975 has led certain countries and WHO to consider integrating malaria control operations into primary health care systems, the main function of which is patient care. This horizontal approach, in compliance with the Global Control Strategy adopted by the Ministerial Conference on Malaria in Amsterdam (1992), was developed in parallel with or to the detriment of indoor insecticide spraying operations, which are essentially vertical strategies (Brown *et al.*, 1976).

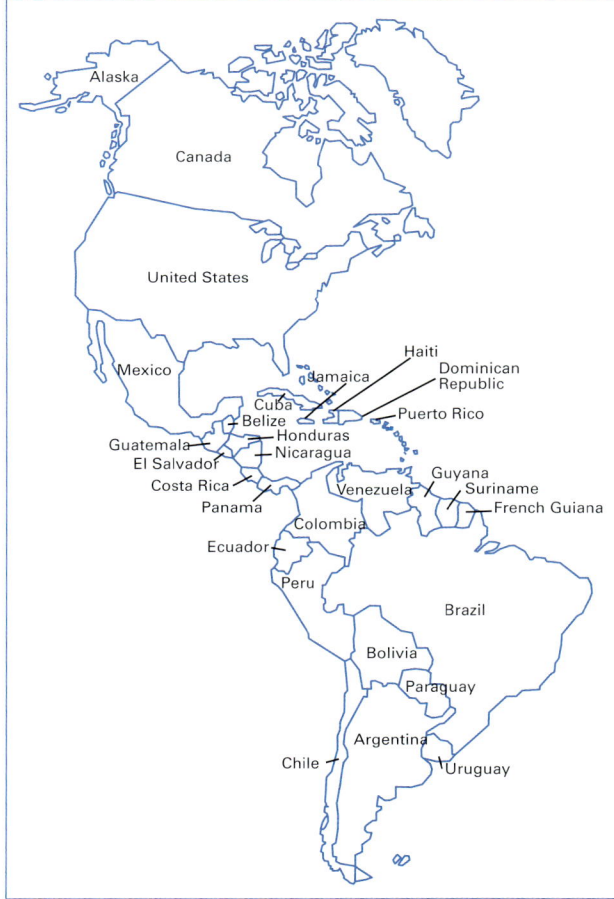

Figure 1. *Countries of the American continent.*

Table I. Countries of the American Continent (Wikipedia, 2006).							
	Size (km²)	Population	Density		Size (km²)	Population	Density
North America	21,306,436	436,200,000	20.5	Mexico	1,967,183	107,000,000	54.4
Canada*	9,976,130	32,200,000	3.2	United States*	9,363,123	297,000,000	34.7
Central America	540,740	39,900,000	73.8	Guatemala	108,900	12,600,000	115.7
Belize	22,900	290,000	12.7	Honduras	112,100	7,200,000	64.2
Costa Rica	50,700	4,200,000	82.8	Nicaragua	148,000	5,600,000	37.8
El Salvador	21,040	6,900,000	327.9	Panama	77,100	3,100,000	40.2
South America	17,782,940	369,600,000	20.8	French Guiana	91,000	170,000	1.9
Argentina	2,766,900	38,600,000	14.0	Guyana	215,000	750,000	3.5
Bolivia	1,088,600	8,900,000	8.2	Paraguay	406,752	5,900,000	14.5
Brazil	8,511,950	184,000,000	21.6	Peru	1,285,200	28,000,000	21.8
Chile*	756,948	16,300,000	21.5	Suriname	163,270	490,000	3.0
Colombia	1,138,900	43,000,000	37.8	Uruguay*	177,500	3,300,000	18.6
Ecuador	270,670	13,400,000	49.5	Venezuela	910,250	26,800,000	29.4
Caribbean	232,681	38,600,000	166.2	Guadeloupe*	1,780	450,000	252.8
Antigua*	442	80,000	176.5	Haiti	27,750	8,500,000	306.3
Bahamas*	13,900	320,000	23.0	Jamaica*	11,425	2,700,000	236.3
Barbados*	431	270,000	626.5	Martinique*	1,100	380,000	345.5
Cayman Islands (GB)*	260	50,000	180.8	Puerto Rico (USA)*	8,897	3,900,000	438.3
Cuba*	110,800	11,300,000	102.0	Saint Lucia*	616	160,000	259.7
Dominica*	751	70,000	91.9	St Kitts & Nevis*	269	50,000	174.7
Dominican Republic	48,400	8,900,000	183.9	St Vincent and the Grenadines*	388	12,000	309.3
Grenada*	344	100,000	290.7	Trinidad and Tobago*	5,128	1,320,000	3.5
				"Americas" Total	39,862,797	884,300,000	22.2

* Countries in which malaria never existed or has been eradicated

Introduction of malaria into the Americas

When and how malaria first came to the American continent remains debatable. In the 1940's, most of authors including Boyd (1949), Gabaldon (*in* Boyd, 1949) and Bruce-Chwatt (1965), thought that human *Plasmodium* had been introduced by Europeans and African slaves in the 16th century. As far as *P. falciparum* is concerned, this hypothesis is still accepted but it is now thought that *P. malariae* and *P. vivax* were probably present in Amerindians prior to the arrival of Christopher Columbus. This hypothesis is supported by two types of evidence, ethnological and parasitological. *P. malariae* and *P. vivax*—and not *P. falciparum*—were first found in groups of highly isolated Peruvian Indians by Sulzer *et al.* (1975). Furthermore, the two simian *Plasmodium* species—*P. brasilianum* in Aotus monkeys and *P. simium* in Saimiri monkeys—are closely related to *P. malariae* and *P. vivax*, respectively; most experts actually believe that they are identical, which would argue in favour of a long history of contact between human and simian parasites which could readily pass from one group of hosts to another. Another hypothesis has it that malaria parasites were introduced by Asian explorers who crossed the Pacific Ocean long before Columbus arrived (Bruce-Chwatt *in* Wernsdorfer & McGregor, 1988). None of these hypotheses have been confirmed.

History, development and distribution of malaria

In 2000, it is difficult to imagine what malaria may have been like between the arrival of the first colonisers and 1940, and to estimate the devastation that it caused among indigenous people, voluntary emigrants and slaves. Here we review what is known about this period which came to an end with the DDT revolution, and then we will track how the disease pattern has changed since to give a picture of the current situation.

From Columbus to DDT

The first cases of malaria or intermittent fever in America are documented in the chronicles of the conquistadors; at least one of Cortez's soldiers succumbed in 1542 although it is not known whether the disease had been imported from Europe or contracted there. In the following years, reports multiplied; soldiers, colonists, governors and clergymen also fell victim and fuelled the literature of the 16th and 17th centuries, not to forget the discovery of the antimalarial activity of the *Cinchona* tree bark, as mentioned earlier (*see the Part entitled* "Malaria, a Vector-Borne Parasitic Disease").

It appears that malaria was most widespread in the Americas between 1850 and 1880, ranging from the banks and coasts of the Saint-Laurence River and British Columbia in Canada, to the 32nd parallel south at Cordoba in Argentina. In terms of altitude, the "highest" case of *P. vivax* malaria was observed at 2,770 m above Cochabamba in Bolivia (Hackett *in* Boyd, 1949; Hackett, 1945).

North America and Mexico
Canada

Prior to 1880, malaria was endemic in British Columbia in the west and along the banks of Lake Ontario and the Saint Laurence River in the east. It began to regress in 1892, finally disappearing in about 1900 (Faust *in* Boyd, 1949).

United States

Essentially rural in the United States and imported by pioneers and slaves, malaria was endemic throughout the territory except in the mountains and deserts. Its incidence reached a peak in 1875. In the east it was transmitted by *An. quadrimaculatus*, and in the west by *An. freeborni*.

The prevalence of the disease appears to have decreased spontaneously following improvements in living conditions from 1890 to 1920. The dominant parasite was *P. vivax*, except in Mississippi and Florida, states with large African American populations, where *P. falciparum* predominated.

There were an estimated 600,000 cases in 1914. The first reports of the number of cases per state were compiled by Von Ezdorf (*in* Faust, 1949) in 1915 and 1916. Mississippi was one of the most endemic states with 154,000 cases, followed by Arkansas with 145,000 cases (8.53% of the population), Louisiana (126,000 cases) and Alabama (85,000 cases or 3.75% of the population). Among the 25 million inhabitants of the eastern States, 13.28% of slides were positive and 4% of the population had clinical malaria. Incidence varied from 17‰ in Alabama to 410‰ in the Mississippi Delta.

In Mississippi, the number of cases dropped considerably following the implementation of control measures, notably the drainage of wetlands and quinine administration. These efforts resulted in a decrease from 159,000 cases in 1916, to 64,800 cases in 1929, and 17,400 cases in 1948 (Faust, 1949). In 1943-1945, malaria disappeared from Mississippi, then from the rest of the United States following the first indoor DDT spraying operations (Gahan & Lindquist, 1945).

The disease began to decline in the early 20th century with the drift of people from malaria-ridden rural areas to the malaria-free cities. This decline can also be attributed to an overall improvement in housing and living conditions, drainage of marshland and better organised health care (notably, readily available quinine) (PASB, 1969). These efforts were enhanced by a malaria control program initiated in 1943 based on indoor DDT spraying and larvicidal treatment (Gahan & Lindquist, 1945). By late 1945, 300,000 homes had been treated. Monitoring operations conducted by the Centers for Disease Control and Prevention (CDC) concluded that malaria had been eradicated in the United States in the 1950's.

Mexico

Prior to 1940, *P. vivax* was the dominant parasite in Mexico. In the north and the highlands, it was transmitted by *An. pseudopunctipennis*; *An. aztecus* and *An. hectoris* were cited as unconfirmed secondary vectors. In the Neotropical South, the vectors were *An. albimanus* and, locally, *An. darlingi*. Malarial mortality was over 990 per 100,000 in the tropical part, only 100-500 per 100,000 in the centre, and very low in the north. In the highly endemic region of Tabasco and Oxoaca in the south, the incidence of cases was greater than 500‰, while in the north it was only 50‰. Throughout Mexico as a whole, the incidence was 200‰ (Faust *in* Boyd, 1949) (*Figure 2*).

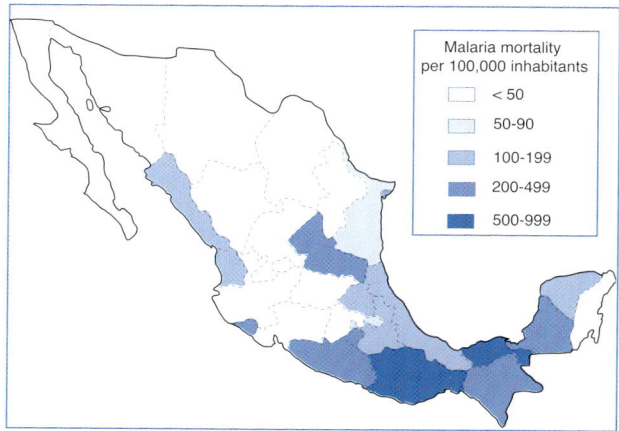

Figure 2. Malarial mortality in Mexico in 1940 (adapted from Boyd, 1949)).

Central America and the Caribbean

Central America

Malaria was endemic in all the Central American countries and evaluating malarial mortality was a priority for all epidemiologists during the first half of the 20th century. In the highly infested region of Peten in Guatemala, malarial mortality reached 1% (*Table II, Figure 3*); there were major differences from country to country and from place to place (and from expert to expert). The main vectors responsible for transmission were *An. albimanus* and *An. pseudopunctipennis*, with contributions from *An. darlingi* in Guatemala, Honduras and Belize, and *An. vestitipennis* in Belize (*Table III*).

The inconsistency of the data, collected mainly by Faust, does not make it possible to draw up a generally coherent picture of malaria in Central America, prior to 1940.

The Caribbean

In 1948, the Caribbean Islands had a population of only 10 million on a land mass amounting to 230,000 km^2. Malaria was meso-endemic with hyperendemic foci in Haiti and the Dominican Republic (on the island of Hispaniola). On most of the other islands, the disease was hypoendemic with generally meso-endemic foci in Jamaica, Puerto Rico, Trinidad and Tobago, and in most of the Lesser Antilles. The Bahamas were spared by the disease and it was encountered only in the form of small coastal foci in Cuba, Saint Croix and Barbados (Gabaldon *in* Boyd, 1949). The negative impact of rice growing was already manifest in Puerto Rico where the malaria mortality rate was 387 per 100,000 in irrigated zones, as opposed to 135 per 100,000 in other villages. The appearance of *An. albimanus* in Barbados in 1927 was one of the first instances of *Anopheles* being introduced by rapid transport.

South America

Gabaldon's review of malaria in South America (*in* Boyd, 1949) remains the best overall interpretation of the disease in the Neotropical Region although it suffers from the uncertainties of the era about the Amazon, an epidemiological

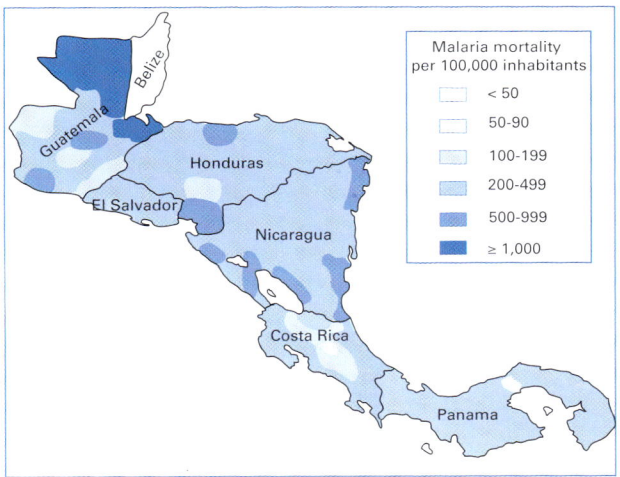

Figure 3. Malarial mortality in Central America in 1940 (adapted from Boyd, 1949).

Table II. Malaria in Central America prior to 1940.				
Country	Malaria mortality (per 100,000 inhab.)	Prevalence	Observations	References
Guatemala	1,000 (Petén) 500 and 100 (Cole)	25%		Faust *in* Boyd, 1949
Belize	14 to 91	50% (rural)		
Honduras	744	42% (1932) 30% (1937-1939)		Faust *in* Boyd, 1949
El Salvador			Incidence : 270‰ San Salvador 440‰ Pacific coast *P. vivax* 26% *P. malariae* 20% *P. falciparum* 27%	Sutter & Zuniga, 1942
Nicaragua	451 (27% of all deaths)	50%	*P. vivax* 79%	
Costa Rica		1%	*P. vivax* 22% *P. malariae* 26% *P. falciparum* 24%	
Panama	88 (total country) 1.2 (canal zone)			

Country	Prevalence		Parasites: F = P. falciparum M = P. malariae V = P. vivax	Vectors	Observations	References cited by Gabaldon in Boyd, 1949
	Parasite rates	Spleen rates				
Bahamas					No malaria	
Cuba		2% of 8,800 exams	F M V	An. albimanus	Malaria limited to the coasts, 201 positive slides out of 42,000 samples	Carret Hill, 1942
Jamaica	8.9% 72% locally	5,9%	F: 90% V: 9%	An. albimanus	No malaria above 800 m, very unequally distributed in brackish zones	Muirhead-Thomson & Mercier, 1949 Faust, 1941
Haiti	46.3% maximum 55%	46%	F: 87% M: 8.9%	An. albimanus	The greatest infection rate of the Caribbean	Paul & Bellerive, 1947
Dominican Republic	16%	8-24%	F: 56% V: 29% M: 11%	An. albimanus	Malaria very irregular depending on the year	Thomen et al., 1943
Puerto Rico	55% in places	23%	F V (depending on the season)	An. albimanus	Particularly in coastal foci	Earle, 1930
Virgin Islands Saint Croix				An. albimanus ?	Low malarial mortality: 18 per 100,000 Epidemic in 1931	Faust, 1941 Show, 1932
Antigua	7%	5-23 %	F: 88% M: 9%	An. albimanus An. aquasalis		Charles, 1943
Martinique	15-20%	6%		An. albimanus An. aquasalis		Montestruc, 1936
Dominica	19.3%	9.8%	F: 67% M: 30%	An. aquasalis		Charles, 1943
Guadeloupe		2-59%		An. aquasalis	Micro-coastal foci	
Saint Lucia		11-39%	F: 56% M: 38%	An. aquasalis		Charles, 1943
Grenada	5.1%		F: 45% V: 43% M: 11%	An. pseudo-punctipennis		Root & Andrews, 1938
Barbados				An. albimanus An. aquasalis	Introduced epidemics	Seager, 1927
Trinidad and Tobago		9.4% (Afro-Americans) 7.2% (Indians)	F: 62% V: 45% M: 5%	An. aquasalis An. bellator	Bromeliad malaria	Downs et al., 1943

Table III. Malaria in the Caribbean in 1940.

* Supply of the synthesis of Gabaldon in Boyd (1949). Many indices are derived from samples from only one part of the island. As malaria had been eradicated in this region (except for Haiti and the Dominican Republic), these figures give only an idea of what the situation may be like in the West Indies

terra incognita at the time. While the main vectors, *An. darlingi*, *An. pseudopunctipennis*, *An. albimanus* and *An. aquasalis* had already been identified, other "secondary" vectors were and still are discussed. Although *P. falciparum* was the most common parasite in African-Americans in Guyana and its neighbours as well as certain parts of Brazil and the coastal regions of Venezuela, Colombia and Ecuador, *P. vivax* remained the most common throughout the rest of the Americas; foci in which *P. malariae* topped 50% had been identified in Peru (Sulzer *et al.*, 1975).

Like all the experts of his day, Gabaldon tried to attribute a periodicity to the disease, proposing a five-to-eight year cycle linked with climatic and/or ecological events; it should be noted that the role of El Niño was not yet well understood. Epidemics, reported pretty much everywhere, were difficult to differentiate from seasonal outbreaks of malaria which, in some years, were exacerbated by particularly heavy rainfall. During certain epidemics, particularly in Venezuela, the mortality rate reached 5.4% (accounting for more deaths than "Spanish Flu"), as opposed to 0.1-0.25% in ordinary years. There was already awareness of the problems associated with irrigation for sugar cane and rice cultivation (Guyana, Peru, Venezuela). Most of these epidemiological differences disappeared as of 1945 when indoor DDT spraying was instigated.

The south-west: Argentina, Bolivia, Chile, Paraguay, Peru

In **Argentina**, two independent types of foci were observed north of the 33rd parallel south: the north-eastern zone, in the Mission Territory, associated with the Chaco Zone (at the confluence of Argentina, Paraguay, Bolivia and Brazil) where the vector was *An. darlingi*; and the zone of the Andes foothills (up to 1,600 m), an extension of the endemic Bolivian Region where the vector was *An. pseudopunctipennis*. The most common parasite species was *P. vivax*.

In the lowland areas of **Bolivia**, the Parasite Rate (PR) was 15% in Tarija, near the Argentine border and the vector appeared to be *An. darlingi*. In the foothills (the Medioplano) and high valleys of the Yungas (above 1,500 m), the vector was *An. pseudopunctipennis* and the parasite *P. vivax*, although there were also extensive *P. malariae* foci.

In **Chile**, malaria was eliminated in 1945 from where it had been localised in the extreme north in the Arica Region along rivers flowing down from the Andes through the Atacama Desert, although the vector *An. pseudopunctipennis* persisted. The only parasite had been *P. vivax*.

In **Paraguay**, a country that remains understudied from the epidemiological perspective, the only suspected vector was *An. darlingi*. According to samples analysed by Gabaldon, the PR was 7.48%.

Along the Pacific Coast of **Peru** and in the valleys of the low Andes, the PR was 10-25%. Highly endemic foci were seen in zones of rice and sugar cane cultivation (Paz Soldan, 1943; Villalobos, 1942). In the Andes, high-altitude epidemics had been reported up to 2,800 m (Hackett, 1945). Almost nothing is known of the Peruvian Amazonia, except that *An. darlingi* is found along the Madre de Dios River (Shannon, 1933).

The northern Andes: Colombia, Ecuador, Venezuela

Ecuador marks the southern limit of *An. albimanus* (which overlaps into northern Peru), which is responsible for meso-endemic disease along the coast with Spleen Rates (SRs) of 48% in rural areas and 17% in Guayaquil. The dominant parasite was *P. falciparum* (62% in the Afro-American population); epidemics due to *An. pseudopunctipennis* have been reported above 700 m and up to an altitude of 2,500 m along the Cordillera; only *P. vivax* and *P. malariae* were involved. Ecuadorian Amazonia was supposedly highly endemic and the vector was *An. darlingi*.

Along the coast of **Colombia** where the vector is *An. albimanus*, SRs of 79% were recorded with *P. falciparum* predominant in Afro-Americans. Elsewhere, the main parasite was *P. vivax* and the vector was *An. darlingi* in Amazonia and at the Venezuelan border; the SR was 45%.

Venezuela is the country that has been most extensively studied in South America. In the sparsely populated south-east (with less than 2 inhabitants per km^2), the SR varied from 10-50%; the vector was *An. darlingi*. It should be noted that this vector does not breed in the acidic waters of forest rivers, so the disease is not endemic along their banks. In the north-west, as one moves away from the coast, *An. albimanus* gives way to *An. darlingi* which is succeeded by *An. pseudopunctipennis* in the Cordillera. In the coastal rice paddies, the SR was greater than 50%, while it was less than 29% in regions of rain-dependent farming. In the Llanos, epidemics due to *An. albimanus* broke out in years of heavy rainfall.

Guyana and its neighbours

In 1943, only three countries in South America were still colonies: Guyana (formerly British Guiana) and Suriname (formerly Dutch Guiana) eventually won their independence, but French Guiana remained a French overseas department.

In these three countries with a total surface area of 469,000 km^2, a more or less deforested coastal band of no more than 90 km in depth bordered an inland plateau covered with virgin forest. The coastal plains were occupied by people from elsewhere, including Europeans, Afro-Americans and Metis (incorrectly referred to as "Creoles"), Indians, Indonesians and Chinese. This area was the only part of the country that was farmed, although the arable zone penetrates inland along the lower parts of the bigger rivers. The few Amerindians in the region lived inland in villages near rivers.

The two vectors were *An. aquasalis* in the brackish waters of the coastal plain, and *An. darlingi* along the inland rivers and the coast, wherever there were freshwater deposits available.

Guyana (formerly British Guiana) is the largest and most populous of the three. SRs ranged from 20-50% in the coastal regions, but exceeded 50% in the Rupununi savannahs (Giglioli, 1949) where malaria prevalence used to be over 37%. *P. vivax* caused 75% of cases along the coasts whereas inland, 53% were due to *P. falciparum*.

SRs of 20-50% were recorded in **Suriname** (formerly Dutch Guiana) (Swellengrebel & Van Der Kuyp, 1940);

rates were higher inland (50-80%) with a high proportion of *P. falciparum*.

In **French Guiana**, the PR was 6% in Cayenne, the healthiest part, and 24% in Saint-Georges on the Oyapock River, and Sinnamary on the coast. *P. falciparum* accounted for 85% of infections, *P. vivax* 15% and *P. malariae* 10% (including mixed infections) (Floch & Lajudie, 1946).

Brazil

Gabaldon divided the largest country of South America (8,512,000 km^2) into five regions:
- the Amazon basin in the north, covered by virgin forest which extends into neighbouring countries; the altitude does not exceed 300 m,
- the north-east,
- the east,
- the south,
- the centre-west.

In his review, Gabaldon (*in* Boyd, 1949) widely cited the unpublished findings of Deane (1946), Causey & Deane (1946), and Pinotti (1946). Only SR seems to have been taken into account, and the overall picture given is very sketchy.

In **Amazonia**, which occupies 41% of the country, the population density is only 0.4 inhabitants per km^2. Along the coasts and the Amazon estuary, the vectors are *An. darlingi* and *An. aquasalis*; *An. albitarsis*, although infected, was considered not to transmit malaria. SRs were between 25% and 50%, lower in the marshy zones of middle Amazon Basin where *An. darlingi* was rare and higher south-east of Belém (50-75%).

In the **north-east**, the States of Maranhão and Piauí had abundant rainfall, while the eastern States of Ceara, Rio Grande do Norte, Paraíba, and Pernambouco (which were invaded by *An. gambiae* in 1938) received only 1,000 mm (or less) of rain per annum. Here, periods of extreme drought were followed by epidemic outbreaks when the rains eventually came. *An. aquasalis* was present throughout all of the coastal regions, while *An. darlingi* was limited to regions with more rainfall; it appears that it was not found in the zone that had been invaded by *An. gambiae*. In the State of Alagoas, where *An. darlingi* was abundant, SRs were 25-50%.

The **eastern region** along the "Planalto" (the central highlands) is bordered by a coastal band dominated by the pervasive presence of *An. darlingi* with *An. aquasalis* along the shore line. The States of Sergipe and Bahia had important malaria transmission at altitudes below 1,000 m; according to Pinotti (1946), the SR was 68%. In the State of Minas Gerais, the SR was only 20-30% and in the States of Espírito Santo and Rio de Janeiro, malaria was apparently localised along certain valleys (Rio Doco) where the SR was 20-50%.

In the **southern region**, the southern part of the "Planalto", rainfall is abundant in the States of Sao Paulo, Paraná, Santa Catarina and Rio Grande do Sul, ranging from 1,500 to 2,000 mm. Besides *An. darlingi*, in the State of Sao Paulo, *An. (K.) cruzii* and *An. (K.) bellator* were also vectors in the coffee plantations where the epiphyte bromeliads thrive in the shade of the tree cover. In the foci, nearly exclusively due to *P. vivax*, SRs were 20-25%; *P. malariae* was common in the State of Santa Catarina.

The **central-western region** represents the "western planalto" of the Paraná Basin, in the States of Goiás and Mato Grosso. *An. darlingi* was present but malaria (all due to *P. vivax*) was rare. A SR of 16% was reported by Pinotti (1946, *in* Gabaldon, 1949) in the La Plata Basin.

This review draws attention to the gaps in our knowledge about the distribution of malaria in the Americas: it tries to give a snapshot of the malaria situation in 1945 but it is incomplete, despite all the efforts of Gabaldon, one of the most important malaria experts of the 1935-1999 period.

The eradication period

Such was the state of malaria in the Americas at the eve of the Second World War when two technological advances turned conventional malaria control methods upside down: indoor spraying methods to kill adult mosquitoes and the discovery of the insecticidal activity of DDT. Weekly spraying of homes with natural pyrethrins had given excellent results in South Africa (1936), then in The Netherlands and Brazil during *An. gambiae* eradication operations (Soper & Wilson, 1943), although the complicated organisation involved and the need for repeated treatment were limitations. Following Müller's discovery of the long-acting insecticidal activity of DDT in 1938 (Müller, 1946), the United States undertook extensive indoor DDT spraying operations. These operations rapidly eliminated the disease in the Mississippi Valley in 1943 (Gahan & Lindquist, 1945). In Guyana (formerly British Guiana) (Giglioli, 1949) and Venezuela (Gabaldon, 1949), this new control strategy was adopted with overwhelming success. Galbadon considered that he had effectively increased the size of his country—meaning its arable surface area—without war; furthermore, widespread coverage of the entire population was a truly **democratic endeavour that benefited all social strata, even the most impoverished people**.

Following these successes, the 14th Pan-American Health Conference, held in 1954 in Santiago, Chile, proposed expanding eradication operations throughout the entire continent. This corresponded to the wishes of most countries in the western hemisphere. The attack phase was implemented between 1956 and 1959 throughout all endemic countries in the Americas.

In 1970, out of 491 million inhabitants, 176 million people were living in at-risk zones, including 119 million in zones that were already in the consolidation phase and 36 million in zones that were still in the attack phase (*Figure 4*); only the insecure zones under guerrilla control in Colombia were not covered, representing only about 0.2 million people. Malaria had been eradicated in the United States, Puerto

Rico and most of the West Indies (except for Haiti and the Dominican Republic). Argentina, Paraguay and Peru were close to eradication. A significant decline in the disease was recorded in Brazil, Suriname, French Guiana, Venezuela, Guatemala, Mexico, Costa Rica, El Salvador and Belize. Malaria persisted in Colombia, Honduras, Nicaragua and Haiti.

In 1969, *P. vivax* was the dominant species by far, although *P. falciparum* persisted in the Guyanas, Brazil, Colombia and Panama as well as Haiti where it was the only parasite present.

In 1969, following difficulties with the international eradication programme, the 2nd meeting of the PAHO Advisory Committee, held in Washington DC, addressed questions of implementation problems and considered postponing targets. However, the eradication objective was maintained after the identification of a certain number of problematic areas in which different strategies would have to be used.

Numerous problems appeared: resistance in *An. albimanus* to DDT and organophosphate insecticides, and drug resistance, initially to chloroquine, followed by resistance to sulfadoxine-pyrimethamine in some places. But the main problem was the mass migration into the Amazon which began in 1970 with the construction of the first roads. This gave access to the gold miners (garimpeiros) and people who settled on cleared forest land. In the Amazon Basin, the population in the States of Roraima, Pará, Amazonas, Rondônia, Acre, Mato Grosso and Goiás (pro-parte) multiplied four to five-fold; immigrants converged from the Andes to the Amazonia in Venezuela (diamond mines), Colombia, Ecuador, Peru and Bolivia (after the metal mines

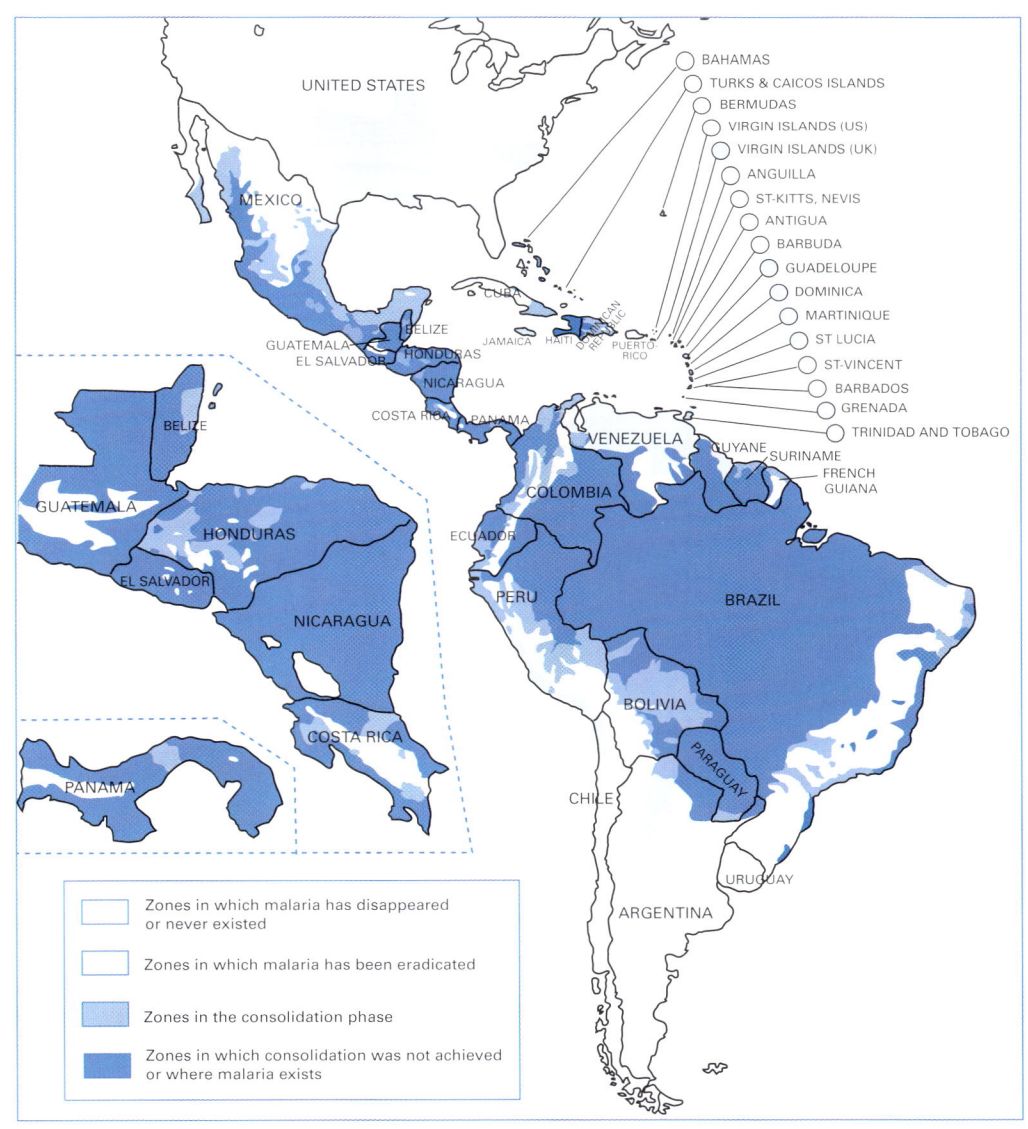

Figure 4.
Eradication of malaria in 1970 (WHO).

of Altiplano shut down). During the early years following their installation, the settlers—who lived in huts often without walls—were heavily exposed to the vectors, and the nearest health care centre was usually far away; these were the main victims of malaria. Many of these immigrants then brought parasites back to their home province or country of origin. Treating the disease in these populations proved difficult and indoor spraying was ineffective in such rudimentary dwellings. According to WHO figures for the period 1962 to 1981 (WHO, 1983) and then, for 1982 to 1997 (WHO, 1999a), the number of malaria cases on the continent rose sharply in 1970 after a spectacular decline; up to 1997, there were about one million cases per annum. This number has dropped from 600,000 to 400,000 in Brazil since 1995 with decreased migration into the Amazon, although this country—together with the Guyanas—remains the main source of malaria in the Neotropical Region.

Implementation of the Global Control Strategy

After the Ministerial Conference on Malaria in Amsterdam (1992), most of countries on the American continent followed a control strategy based on the integration of malaria control operations into the general primary health care services. These specialists had a good understanding of the people and the territory, which should have been of benefit when it came to implementing the new strategy.

Early diagnosis and treatment are the corner-stones of control. However, in remote locations, microscopic diagnosis remains impossible in more than 80% of cases (Najera, 2001). In these conditions, treatment guided by a simple clinical diagnosis is conditioned by the availability and acceptability of drugs.

In addition, most of the countries continue to implement indoor spraying operations in active centres, based on the resistance profiles of local anophelines (e.g. *An. albimanus*). Due to pressure from environmentalists, pyrethroids are often used instead of DDT, even though the latter is approved by WHO.

Difficulties have been encountered in promoting the use of impregnated mosquito nets for reasons of both cost and acceptability.

Current malaria situation

Of the entire population of the Americas, 36% live in regions considered to be at risk vis-à-vis *P. vivax*, *P. falciparum* and, locally, *P. malariae*. *P. vivax*, with its variants (*P. vivax* VK210, VK247 and *vivax-like*), are predominant on the American continent; *P. falciparum* is the dominant parasite in the regions where populations of African origin live (Guyanese mountains, Haiti and the Dominican Republic). Malaria is endemic in twenty-one countries from northern Mexico to southern Argentina, with a continuous zone in the Amazon Basin and Guyanese mountains.

Within the Neotropical Region, malaria increased from 269,000 confirmed cases in 1974 to more than 1.3 million cases in 1995 (PAHO, 1996). In a review covering 1998 to 2004 (PAHO, 2005), the number of malaria cases since 2000 has dropped below one million, stabilizing around 900,000 cases per annum. The highest incidences are in Guyana (460‰), Suriname (340‰) and French Guiana (320‰) (Carme & Venturin, 1999). In Brazil and Central America, the incidence is less than 200‰ and it is about 100‰ in the rest of Tropical America.

Ecological zones

Among the attempts to correlate malarial epidemiology to the natural regions of the Americas, that of Rubio-Palis & Zimmerman (1997) is one of the most useful.

They distinguish five ecological zones defined by their vectors and environmental characteristics. The five main factors taken into account are rainfall, temperature, vegetation, altitude and type of landscape. These five zones comprise the coastal region, the lowland forests, savannah, foothills and the high valleys (*Figure 5, Table IV*).

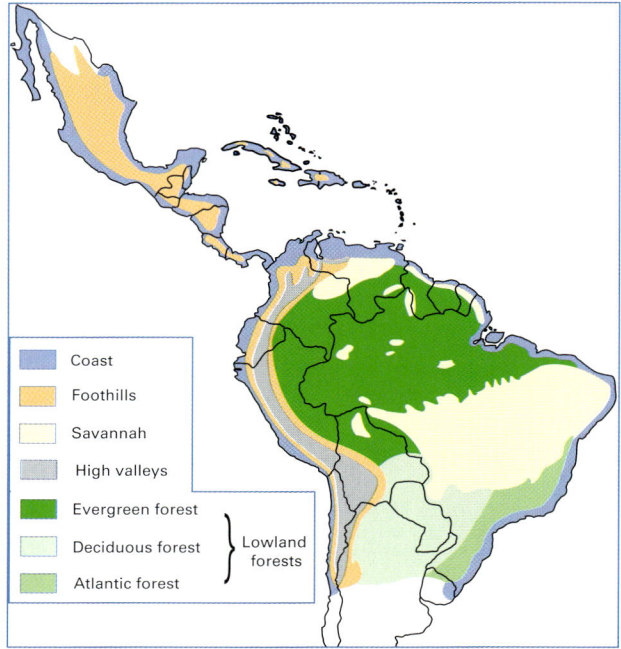

Figure 5. Ecological zones in the Americas (*adapted from Rubio-Palis & Zimmerman, 1997*).

Ecological zones	Characteristics			Vectors	
	Altitude (m)	Annual rainfall (mm)	Average yearly temp. (°C)	Regional	Local and/or secondary
Coast	< 550	> 1,000 (seasonal)	25-27	*An. albimanus*, *An. aquasalis*, *An. darlingi*, *An. pseudopunctipennis*	*An. punctimacula*, *An. albitarsis*, *An. calderoni*, *An. braziliensis*, *An. neivai*, *An. bellator*, *An. cruzii*, *An. homunculus*
Plain forest	100-500	1,500-6,000 (seasonal)	26-28	*An. darlingi*	*An. albitarsis*, *An. nuneztovari*, *An. oswaldoi*, *An. trinkae*, *An. rangeli*, *An. neivai*, *An. bellator*, *An. cruzii*, *An. homunculus*
Savannah	0-1,200	< 100-2,000 (variable, seasonal)	20-27	*An. darlingi*, *An. nuneztovari*	*An. albitarsis*, *An. aquasalis*, *An. braziliensis*
Foothills					
- East Andes	200-1,500	400-4,000 (variable, seasonal)	25-27	*An. nuneztovari*, *An. darlingi*, *An. pseudopunctipennis*	*An. oswaldoi*, *An. trinkae*, *An. rangeli*
- West Andes				*An. albimanus*, *An. pseudopunctipennis*	*An. nuneztovari*, *An. calderoni*
- Mexico, Central America				*An. albimanus*, *An. darlingi*, *An. vestitipennis*, *An. pseudopunctipennis*	*An. gabaldoni*, *An. punctimacula*
- Caribbean				*An. albimanus*	*An. aquasalis*, *An. pseudopunctipennis*
High valleys	1,500-3,200	800-2,000 (variable, seasonal)	variable < 0 (1 month/year)	*An. pseudopunctipennis*	
North America	0-500	< 100-1,000 (variable, seasonal)	20-27	*An. freeborni*, *An. quadrimaculatus*	*An. hermsi*, *An. pseudopunctipennis*, *An. aztecus*, *An. punctipennis*

Table IV. Ecoregions in the Americas and their vectors (Rubio-Palis & Zimmerman, 1997).

Coastal

This ecological zone is represented by the coastal land bordering the Atlantic and Pacific Oceans where the temperature ranges between 25 °C and 27 °C and the humidity between 20% and 70%. Generally speaking, the hot months are from January to March and the period with heavy rainfall is from July to September. Rainfall generally exceeds 1,000 mm. The population is concentrated along the coasts in Central and South America. Two vectors, *An. albimanus* and *An. aquasalis*, are specific to this halophilic environment. The first species ranges from Mexico to Venezuela, just north of Peru and the Greater Antilles (*Figure 5*). It is present at low altitude (under 500 m) and can be found more than 100 km from the ocean. *An. albimanus* is the major malaria vector from southern Mexico to northern Peru and along the Caribbean Coast from Colombia to Venezuela, as well as on the island of Hispaniola (which includes Haiti and the Dominican Republic) (Faran, 1980). The distribution of *An. aquasalis*, a much less efficient vector, somewhat overlaps that of *An. albimanus* as it ranges from Nicaragua to Ecuador (Kroeger *et al.*, 1995) and from northern Colombia to south-eastern Brazil (Forattini, 1962); it is considered a local vector from eastern Venezuela to the coasts of central Brazil and Trinidad and Tobago (Faran, 1980; Forattini, 1962).

Two other major vectors, *An. darlingi* and *An. pseudopunctipennis*, can also transmit malaria along the coasts, although only in certain conditions. The first species requires heavy rainfall (1,500-4,000 mm), high humidity (80-85%), temperature around 26 °C, and the presence of humid tropical forest near the ocean. *An. pseudo-*

punctipennis can transmit *P. vivax* in the coastal plains next to the Chiapas Mountains (Mexico) and the desert coasts, the Lima Valley in Peru and formerly, in the desert valleys of Atacama in Chile.

Wooded lowlands

The lowland forests represent the most extensive of the five ecological zones. They cover the entire fluvial zone of South America, including the Amazon Basin where the altitude does not exceed 500 m. The local vector is *An. darlingi* which essentially transmits *P. vivax*, despite an increase in the prevalence of *P. falciparum* in certain zones, notably the Guyanas (PAHO, 1996) and the Choco tropical rainforest in Colombia.

There are three types of forest in this ecoregion: evergreen rain forest in the Amazon Basin, various forms of deciduous forest, such as the Chaco open woodland (Paraná Basin) and the coastal forest of the Brazilian Medioplano. They have different features including, respectively, an average temperature of 26 °C or 28 °C and rainfall of 2,000 to 4,000 mm over at least a nine-month period or 1,500 to 2,500 mm over five to seven months. These differences define two epidemiological situations: stable malaria* characteristic of evergreen forests; and unstable malaria that is specific to deciduous forests.

In the coastal forests of southern Brazil and Colombia, *Anopheles* of the subgenus *Kerteszia* are something of an ecological and epidemiological curiosity. Their larvae develop in phytotelmata, i.e. water which collects at the bottom of bromeliad leaves in the forest canopy in places with heavy rainfall (4,000-8,000 mm) and high relative humidity (> 90%) (Murillo et al., 1988). The anthropophilic females are active during the daytime (Downs & Pittendrigh *in* Boyd, 1949). *An. (K.) bellator* used to transmit malaria in Trinidad (Downs & Pittendrigh, 1946; Rozeboom & Laird, 1942) and *An. neivai* is a vector on the Colombian Pacific Coast (Astaiza et al., 1988). Not long ago, *An. (K.) bellator, An. (K.) cruzii* and *An. (K.) homunculus* were local vectors of the coastal rain forest in the Brazilian States of Sao Paulo and Santa Catarina where annual rainfall reaches 3,000 mm (Coutinho et al., 1944; Forattini, 1962; Rachou, 1958). Sporozoite rates are often very low in these anophelines and infections tend to be isolated.

Savannah

This ecological zone consists of several zones of various sizes throughout South America. The largest zone is located in the centre of Brazil, while smaller savannahs are found in northern Venezuela and Colombia as well as along the coastal fringe of the Guyanas. Such regions are characterised by grasslands extending from sea level to 1,200 m in altitude. Annual rainfall, spread over a five to seven-month period, amounts to 1,000-2,000 mm and the average temperature fluctuates between 20 °C and 26 °C. The relative humidity varies considerably from season to season, ranging from 10-80%. The major vector is *An. darlingi* (*Table IV*), whose riparian distribution and abundance are highly dependent on annual rainfall, vegetation and topography.

Foothills

The foothills region covers all of inland Central America as well as in the Andean Cordillera (*Figure 5*) which constitutes an interface between the high Andean valleys and the lower inland forests. Altitudes range from 200 to 1,500 m with an average temperature of 25°C to 27°C. In these regions, malaria varies from hyperendemic in Mexico to meso-endemic from Venezuela to Bolivia. Seasonal transmission is mainly of *P. vivax* although cases of *P. malariae* have been reported at 1,000 m in the Rio Erné Valley (Peru), as well as cases of *P. falciparum* associated with the presence of *An. darlingi* at lower altitudes. The vectors primarily tend to be zoophilic, exophagic and exophilic, except for *An. darlingi* (Zimmerman, 1992). Anopheline populations overlap and various epidemiological situations abut each other, resulting in the designation of three distinct subregions, namely East of the Andes, West of the Andes and Mexico-Central America, and the Caribbean Islands.

East of the Andes

This subregion covers the Andes foothills from Venezuela to Argentina (*Figure 5*). The altitude limits are somewhat unclear and it is often difficult to separate this region from the high Andean valleys with which it is continuous. In Bolivia, for example, the "Sierrelas", which border the Amazonian plain between 500 and 1,000 m, continue into the Alto Beni (800-1,500 m) and then into the Yungas, (1,000-3,000 m). The vectors are *An. pseudopunctipennis* at higher altitudes and *An. darlingi* at lower ones (*Table IV*). The role of *An. nuneztovari* was proven in Venezuela and Colombia (Rubio-Palis et al., 1992), although it did not appear in the other Andean countries. *P. vivax* is the dominant parasite.

West of the Andes

The countries concerned span from Venezuela to Peru. *An. albimanus* is the main vector from north-eastern Colombia to northern Peru (*Table IV*), while at higher altitudes, *An. pseudopunctipennis* is the major vector, particularly in Ecuador and Peru.

---

* American authors use the word "stable" to mean something more like "perennial" as opposed to Macdonald (1957) when he spoke about West Africa or Sri Lanka (*refer to the Part* "Malaria, a Vector-Borne Parasitic Disease").

Mexico, Central America and the Caribbean islands

The two main vectors are *An. albimanus* and *An. pseudopunctipennis* and, locally, *An. vestitipennis* and *An. darlingi* (*Table IV*).

High valleys

These high valleys extend along the Cordillera of the Andes from Colombia to Argentina (*Figure 5*). *P. vivax* malaria is transmitted seasonally by *An. pseudopunctipennis* (*Table IV*) at altitudes up to 2,800 m in Bolivia (Gorham *et al.*, 1973; Hackett, 1945). However, the often-violent winds at high altitudes can cause sudden drops in temperature which slows down the development of this anopheline. It is often the only vector species at altitudes of over 600 m. Rainfall is variable, ranging from 800 to 2,000 mm, and the temperature drops below zero at least once a month (*Table IV*). The distribution of *An. pseudopunctipennis* and the epidemiology of malaria can vary from one valley to another as a function of climatic conditions, with epidemics common in years with a mild winter followed by a summer with only moderate rainfall (Hackett, 1945).

North America

Two historical malaria foci existed, one to the east in the Mississippi River Valley where *An. quadrimaculatus* was the vector, and the other in California with *An. freeborni* and *An. hermsi*.

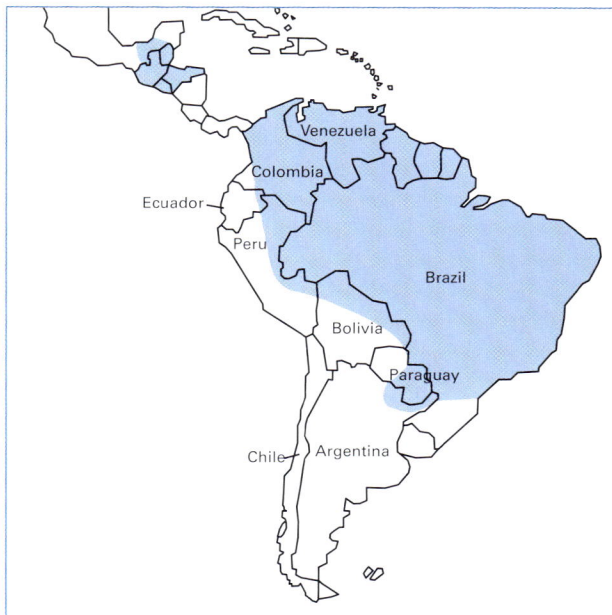

Figure 6. *Distribution of* An. darlingi.

Anopheline vectors

The genus *Anopheles* includes six subgenera, three of which are of major importance in the Americas (Harbach, 2004). One of these three, *Nyssorhynchus*, includes 33 species, all from the American continent. Some of them are major vectors of malaria in the Neotropical zone, including *An. darlingi*, *An. albimanus*, *An. aquasalis*, and *An. nuneztovari*. Another of these subgenera, *Anopheles*, includes 189 species worldwide among which are neotropical vectors such as *An. pseudopunctipennis*, *An. vestitipennis* and the North American species of the *An. maculipennis* Complex (*Table V*). The third important subgenus represented in the Americas is *Kerteszia*, which is associated with bromeliads. There are two additional small subgenera with neotropical species only, *Lophopodomyia* (6 species) and *Stethomyia* (5 species), but they are of no epidemiological interest (Harbach, 2004).

Regional vectors

Anopheles darlingi

This is by far the most efficient vector in the Neotropical Region owing to its anthropophilic, endophagic and often endophilic behaviour. This species has early biting activity with a peak at 9 p.m. in Belize (Achee *et al.*, 2006) and between 7 p.m. and 9 p.m. in the Bolivian Amazon (Harris *et al.*, 2006), although a second smaller peak before sunrise was also noticed in Belize. This riparian species covers a vast, low-altitude (under 450 m) part of South America (from northern Argentina to Venezuela), including the entire Amazon Basin and part of Central America (from Honduras to southern Mexico) (*Figures 6 and 7*). It has the particular feature of a discontinuous distribution as it does not occur in Panama, Costa Rica or Nicaragua. Larval habitats are localised in slightly shaded, slow-flowing rivers and streams or the freshwater lakes into which they flow. The larvae (which are difficult to sample because they are not gregarious) are found in floating clusters of plant debris (Manguin *et al.*, 1996a). This species is capable of flying considerable distances—up to 7 km—to find a host and feed, and a recent study showed that this species has a much higher biting rate (278 times) in areas that have undergone deforestation (Vittor *et al.*, 2006). People living along rivers run a high risk of contracting malaria. A study of the genetics of *An. darlingi* populations in South and Central America illustrates a remarkable degree of genetic homogeneity throughout the entire range of distribution (Manguin *et al.*, 1999a). It is thus not a complex of species and controlling it should be approached on the grand scale, meaning throughout the entire Neotropical zone apart from the high Andean valleys (Manguin *et al.*, 1999b). In Central America, the populations of *An. darlingi* appear to have originated from South America and arrived in the relatively recent past. Insecticide-based control strategies against *An. darlingi* are still successful here as the species does not appear to have developed resistance to DDT as it has in Colombia (Suarez *et al.*, 1990).

Biodiversity of Malaria in the World

Table V. Vectors in the Americas (adapted from Darsie & Ward, 1981 ; Lounibos et al., 1998 ; Rubio-Palis & Zimmerman, 1997 ; Wilkerson et al., 1990).

Anopheline species	Positive			Country										
	Glands	CSP Pf	CSP Pv	North America	Mexico	Caribbean	Central America	Venezuela	Colombia-Ecuador	Peru	Bolivia	Brazil	Guyanas	Southern Cone
Subgenus *Anopheles*														
quadrimaculatus	+		+	+	+									
hermsi			+	+										
freeborni			+	+	+									
vestitipennis	+	+				+		+						
gabaldoni			VK210					+						
pseudopunctipennis		?	+	+	+	+	+	+	+	+	+			+ Argentina
Subgenus *Nyssorhynchus*														
darlingi	+	+	+		+		+	+	+	+	+	+	+	+ Argentina, Paraguay
albimanus	+	+	VK210 VK247	+	+	+	+	+	+					
aquasalis	+					+	+	+				+	+ Guyana	
nuneztovari	+	+	+				+ Panama	+	+	+	+	+	+ not infected	
braziliensis								+				+		
oswaldoi	+	+	+				+					+ Amazonia		+
albitarsis	+											+		
marajoara (= *allopha*)	+	+	+				+ Costa Rica Panama					+		
deaneorum	+	+	+									+ Acre		
triannulatus	+	+	+				+					+ Amazonia		
strodei						+	+					+ Amazonia		
benarocchi	+									+				
galvaoi												+		
trinkae		+	+						+	+	+			
Subgenus *Kerteszia*														
cruzii	+		+									+ Sao Paulo		
homunculus	+											+ Sao Paulo		
neivai	+		+			+	+		+					
bellator	+						+					+ Sao Paulo		

Pf : *P. falciparum* ; Pv : *P. vivax* ; CSP : circumsporozoite protein detected

Anopheles albimanus

An. albimanus (*Figures 8 and 9*) is a vector that is associated with lowlands areas (0-400 m in altitude) in Central America, north-western South America and the Caribbean Islands. It has the ability to fly up to 3 km. Its larvae can be found in fresh or brackish water, generally exposed to sunlight (flooded pastures, lakes, ponds, and marshes), and they colonise a wide variety of larval habitats

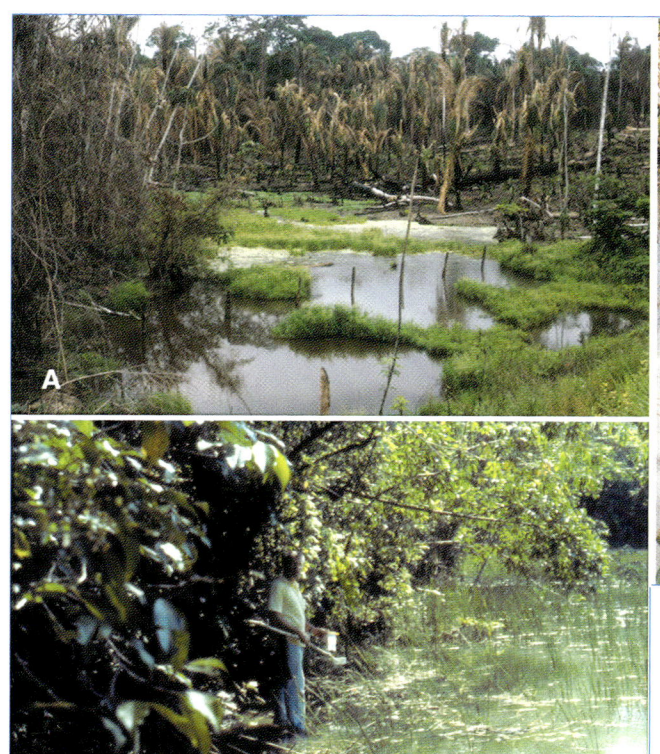

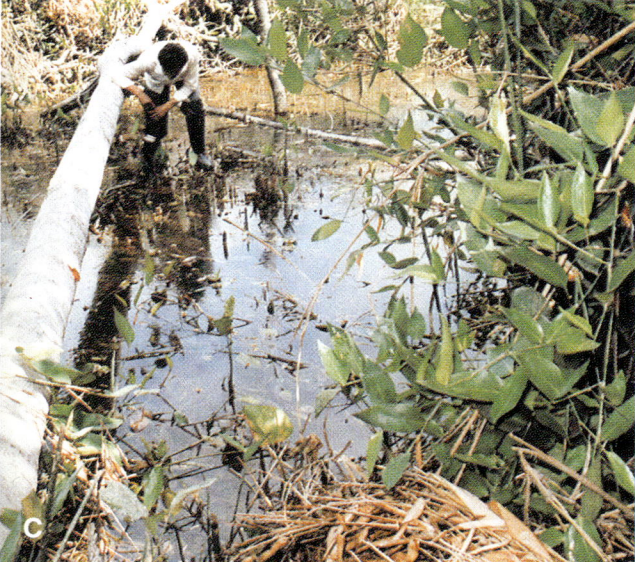

Figure 7. An. darlingi *larval habitats.*
A. *Brazil, Pará State, destroyed forest (photograph by Coosemans).*
B. *Belize (photograph by Manguin).*
C. *Bolivia (photograph by Mouchet in Danis & Mouchet, 1991).*

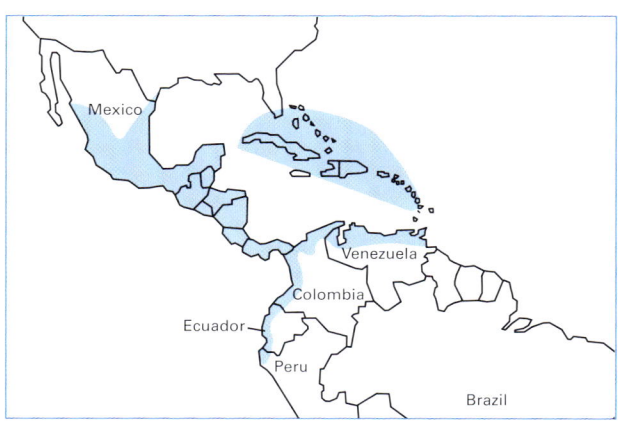

Figure 8. Distribution of An. albimanus.

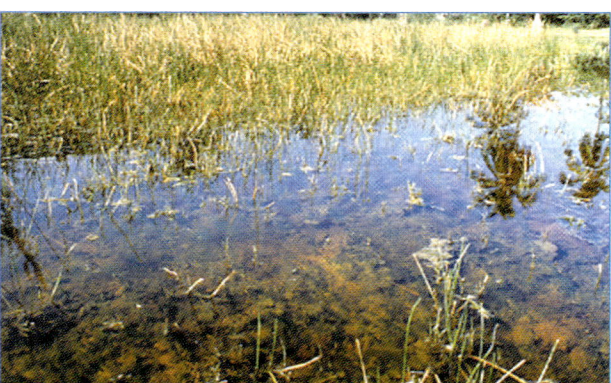

Figure 9. Larval habitat of An. albimanus, *Haiti (photograph by Désenfant in Danis & Mouchet, 1991).*

(streams, ditches, puddles). Its ecology was particularly well studied by Rejmankova *et al.* (1993, 1996) who showed that, in southern Mexico, its larvae prefer flooded pastures containing phytoplankton while in Belize, they prefer permanent marshes with large clusters of floating cyanobacteria mats (blue-green algae) and sparse emergent vegetation such as rushes (*Eleocharis*) and sawgrass (*Cladium*). Its behaviour tends to be exophagic (> 65%) and zoophilic (80-85%), and its vectorial capacity mainly depends on the density of females, particularly at the end of the rainy season. Dieldrin resistance appeared in 1965, followed by resistance to DDT, carbamates and organophosphates in the 1970's (Ayad & Georghiou, 1975; Davidson & Sawyer, 1975; Georghiou, 1972), and to pyrethroids since 1998 (Brogdon *et al.*, 1999; Penilla *et al.*, 1998). A recent study by Molina-Cruz *et al.* (2004) showed little genetic variation among populations from Central America but a barrier to gene flow between Central and South American populations seems to occur. Their data also suggest that current continental populations may have originated from the Caribbean.

Anopheles aquasalis

An. aquasalis also covers the coastal fringe of southern Central America, eastern South America and the Caribbean Islands (*Figure 10*), penetrating 8-10 km upriver due to its long flight capability (8 km). Its larvae generally develop in brackish water (lagoons, canals, rice paddies and swamps), and sometimes freshwater. Its vector role depends on its density and specific behaviour patterns (which vary from place to place). It is zoophilic, exophagic and exophilic on the Amazonian coast and in south-eastern Brazil, although it has been defined as anthropophilic and endophilic in north-eastern Brazil. It can become a vector of malaria when its density is high and there are no domestic animals, its usual food source. In Guyana, the mechanisation of rice farming resulted in the disappearance of buffalos which used to be the main sources of blood for this *Anopheles* species which then switched to humans resulting in an increase in the incidence of malaria (Giglioli, 1951). In Trinidad, an epidemic of *P. vivax* transmitted by *An. aquasalis* was reported in 1990-1991 (Chadee & Kitron, 1999). While the vector capacity of this species remains ten times less than that of *An. darlingi*, it is or used to be the vector along the Brazilian coast (Deane, 1986). In French Guiana, despite very high densities along the coast, it is not associated with malaria transmission (Silvain, 1979).

Anopheles nuneztovari

An. nuneztovari is a low-altitude (under 500 m) species which ranges from eastern Panama in the north, down to the Amazon Basin in South America (Faran, 1980) (*Figure 11*). Its immature stages cluster in floating or emerging vegetation in freshwater along generally sunny river banks, ponds and streams. Its behaviour varies according to its geographical location. It can be either a highly anthropophilic (80%), exophilic vector, as it is in Venezuela, Colombia and Peru (*in* Gabaldon 1981; Hayes *et al.*, 1987; Rubio-Palis *et al.*, 1992), or it is zoophilic and only considered as a secondary vector, not really involved in transmission, as is the case everywhere else it is found, notably in Suriname (Brokopondo Dam) and Brazil (Panday, 1977; Silva-Vasconcelos *et al.*, 2002; Tadei *et al.*, 1998; Tadei & Dutary Thatcher, 2000). A search for *P. falciparum*, *P. vivax* and *P. malariae* circumsporozoite antigens in this species in Brazil (in the Amazonian States) did not suggest that it transmits malaria—and human cases of the disease are always found in zones infested by *An. darlingi* (Tadei *et al.*, 1998; Tadei & Dutary Thatcher, 2000). *An. nuneztovari* numbers are high during and at the end of the rainy season and it tends to bite at nightfall, from 6 to 9 p.m. (Silva-Vasconcelos *et al.*, 2002; Tadei *et al.*, 1998). Differences in vector capacity, observed from one region to another, have raised suspicions as to the existence

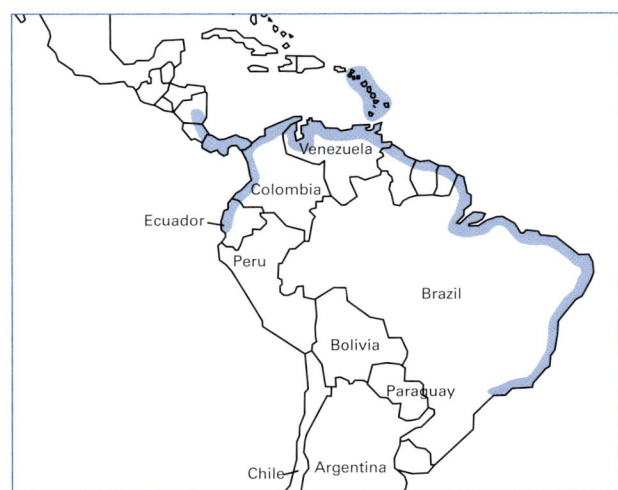

Figure 10. *Distribution of* An. aquasalis.

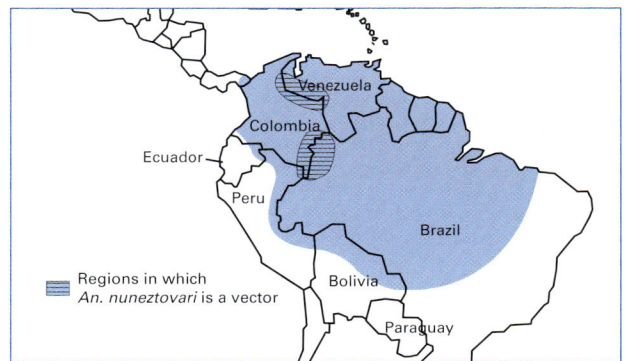

Figure 11. *Distribution of* An. nuneztovari.

of a species complex. At least two cryptic species have been differentiated on the basis of various criteria: behavioural (Elliott, 1972; Renjifo & Zulueta, 1952), cytogenetic (Conn *et al.*, 1993; Kitzmiller *et al.*, 1973), egg ultrastructure (Linley *et al.*, 1996), the morphology of the male genitalia (Hribar, 1994), isozyme analysis (Scarpassa *et al.*, 1999; Scarpassa & Tadei, 2000) and molecular approaches (Fritz *et al.*, 1994; Onyabe & Conn, 1999). One corresponds to the populations of *An. nuneztovari* of Venezuela and Colombia, and the other is found in the Brazilian Amazon. The low degree of genetic divergence between these cryptic species suggests recent speciation (Onyabe & Conn, 1999; Scarpassa *et al.*, 1999).

Anopheles pseudopunctipennis

An. pseudopunctipennis is a major vector from Mexico to northern Argentina. Its vast geographic distribution (*Figures 12 and 13*) extends from the southern United

American Regions

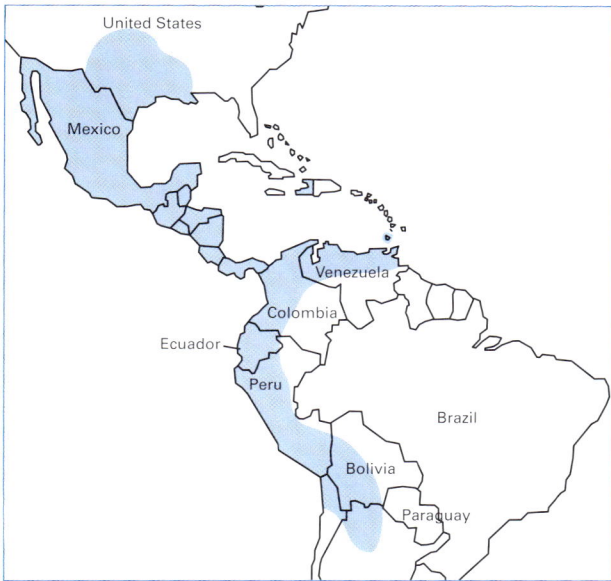

Figure 12. Distribution of An. pseudopunctipennis.

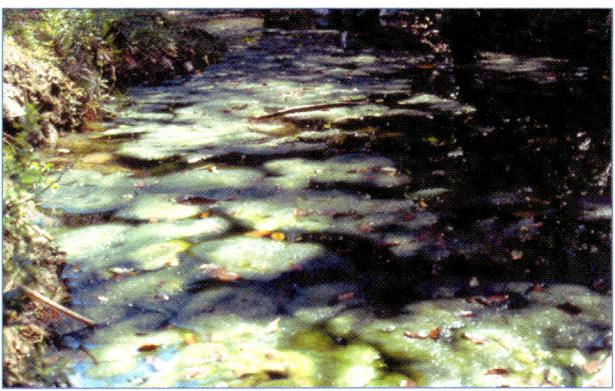

Figure 13. An. pseudopunctipennis *larval habitats, Island of Grenada (photograph by Manguin).*

States (Kansas, Texas) (Darsie & Ward, 1981) to northern Argentina and Chile. In the east, it colonises certain islands of the Caribbean, including Haiti (Molez *et al.*, 1987) and Grenada where the species was described by Theobald (1901). Its larvae develop in pools of water left by receding rivers or streams, well exposed to sunlight and colonised by green filamentous algae such as *Spirogyra* (Manguin *et al.*, 1996b). Its highest densities are seen during the dry season. This species, considered as the only vector above 600 m, ranges from sea level to altitudes of up to 3,200 m. The distribution of malaria in the Andes (*P. vivax*, and to a lesser extent *P. malariae*) is thus conditioned by the presence of this vector. Its behaviour is anthropophilic and endophagic (Gabaldon, 1949), although due to its opportunistic behaviour it is often zoophilic, biting different hosts such as sheep, goats, donkeys (Lardeux *et al.*, 2007)

Three geographically separated groups of *An. pseudopunctipennis* (Central America, South America and Belize, and the island of Grenada) have been defined, based on an extensive isozyme analysis (Manguin *et al.*, 1995). The isolation of the population on Grenada Island does not allow any gene flow with the population from the continent which is now considered to be a separate species (Coetzee *et al.*, 1999).

Anopheles vestitipennis

An. vestitipennis ranges from southern Mexico and Central America to northern South America, Cuba, the Dominican Republic and Puerto Rico. Its larval habitats are shallow, very shady swamps, in either a forest setting or in areas covered by high, dense herbaceous vegetation (Rejmankova *et al.*, 1998). A recent study showed that this species is associated with *Typha* cover and marshes around farmland (Grieco *et al.*, 2006). Although this species is present throughout the year, its density peaks during the rainy season (Arredondo-Jimenez *et al.*, 1996). It is endophagic and endophilic, and both anthropophilic and zoophilic subpopulations have been found in southern Mexico (Ulloa *et al.*, 2005). In Belize, it is most aggressive after sunset (6.45-9.45 p.m.) and usually leaves the house between 11.45 p.m. and 4.45 a.m. (Grieco *et al.*, 2000). It has been identified as being infected by *P. falciparum* and *P. vivax* VK210 in Chiapas, Mexico (Loyola *et al.*, 1991) and Belize (Achee *et al.*, 2000); it is an efficient vector (Roberts *et al.*, 1993) in both these countries. This anopheline remains susceptible to insecticides and is efficiently repelled: indoor spraying operations reduced the number of female *An. vestitipennis* inside huts by 66% with deltamethrin and 97% with DDT (Grieco *et al.*, 2000).

Maculipennis Group

In the Americas, this group, which is also found in the Palaearctic Region, includes thirteen species (Porter & Collins, 1996).

The neotropical species are included in two subgroups. The first subgroup consists of four species, *An. freeborni s.s.* which covers the entire western part of the United States and south-western Canada (British Columbia) (Darsie & Ward, 1981), *An. hermsi* in California, *An. earlei* and *An. occidentalis*. The two former species are efficient vectors that transmit *P. vivax* (Porter & Collins, 1990) and more recently, in 1986 and 1988, *An. hermsi* was determined to be responsible for epidemics or rather introduced cases of *P. vivax* infection in San Diego, California (Barr & Guptavanij, 1988; Turley *et al.*, 1986).

The second subgroup includes five neotropical species, *An. diluvialis, An. inundatus, An. maverlius, An. quadrimaculatus* and *An. smaragdinus* (Kaiser *et al.*, 1988; Narang *et al.*, 1989; Reinert *et al.*, 1997), which occupy the United States east of the Rocky Mountains and south-eastern Canada (Quebec and Ontario) (Darsie & Ward, 1981). Prior to 1945, it was the main vector of malaria in the United States. It was apparently responsible for transmitting *P. falciparum* among *P. vivax*-resistant African-Americans.

An. aztecus is no longer considered to be a vector in Mexico.

Local vectors

All the species belonging to the *Kerteszia* Subgenus are found in the Neotropical Region and they are distinguished by the uniqueness of their larval habitats which are in epiphytic bromeliads. It is comprised of twelve species among which are *An. bambusicolus, An. bellator, An. boliviensis, An. cruzii, An. homunculus, An. laneanus* and *An. neivai*. The idea that certain vectors of malaria (*An. cruzii*) might have a specific association with bromeliads was first advanced in the State of Sao Paulo, Brazil (Lutz, 1903). Since then, malaria transmitted by such species has been described in Trinidad with *An. bellator* and *An. homunculus* (Downs & Pittendrigh, 1946), in Colombia with *An. neivai* (Astaiza *et al.*, 1988) and in Brazil with *An. bellator, An. cruzii* and *An. homunculus* (Coutinho *et al.*, 1944; Forattini, 1962; Rachou, 1958). Sporozoites were detected in salivary glands (Downs & Pittendrigh, *in* Boyd, 1949) once in 2,150 dissections of *An. bellator* in Trinidad (Rozeboom & Laird, 1942), and once in 700 dissections of *An. cruzii* in Brazil (Corrêa & Renato, 1943). These vectors can be highly anthropophilic, endophilic and endophagic (Forattini *et al.*, 1999). *An. bellator* and *An. homunculus* were blamed for a *P. malariae* epidemic in Trinidad in 1994-1995 (Chadee & Kitron, 1999).

Many species of the *Nyssorhynchus* Subgenus have been considered local or secondary vectors, often based on the detection of circumsporozoite protein or circumstantial evidence.

After the reclassification of the Albitarsis Group, it appeared that *An. deaneorum* was an important vector in the States of Rondônia and Acre in western Brazil (Branquinha *et al.*, 1996; Rosa-Freitas, 1989). *An. marajoara* (also known as *An. allopha*) plays a significant role in the deforested zones of the State of Amapa in Brazil (Conn *et al.*, 2002). Other reports of *An. albitarsis s.l.* lack precise information.

An. triannulatus, An. strodei and *An. oswaldoi* are often mentioned as being infected in the Amazon and sometimes in Central America.

An. trinkae was considered to be one of the most important species along the eastern foothills of the Peruvian Andes (Hayes *et al.*, 1987).

A few species, including *An. braziliensis, An. mediopunctatus, An. rangeli, An. forattinii* and *An. galvaoi*, are occasionally found infected. Although it is suspected throughout Central America of being a vector, the role of *An. punctimacula* has never been proven.

The question of secondary or local vectors in South America is far from being solved; many only have an incidental role and have little or no impact on the transmission of malaria (*Table V*).

Parasites

Three *Plasmodium* species prevail on the American continent (listed here in decreasing order of frequency): *P. vivax, P. falciparum* and *P. malariae*.

The study of circumsporozoite proteins has allowed several variants to be differentiated among *P. vivax* (Rosenberg *et al.*, 1989), such as VK210 and VK247. *P. vivax-like*, which appears to be identical to *P. simiovale*, a parasite found in the macaques of Sri Lanka, has also been detected in Brazil in humans (Qari *et al.*, 1993a, 1993b). The extent of the genetic isolation of these variants and their epidemiological role is currently being studied. In addition, several authors have confirmed that *P. simium* (found in Saimiri monkeys) is exactly the same species as *P. vivax* (in humans).

If the distribution of these three variants of *P. vivax* is global, a recent study mentions two subspecies referred to as Old and New World, each having a distinct geographic distribution. The American subspecies has been provisionally named *P. vivax collins* (Li *et al.*, 2001).

P. falciparum, despite its significant polymorphism, is still considered to be a monotypical species.

It seems now to be accepted that human *P. malariae* is exactly the same species as *P. brasilianum* in Aotus monkeys. This parasite is rare in humans, except among Amerindian tribes where it seems to constitute a zoonosis and its level reaches 10%. It should be remembered that *P. malariae* was found in more than 50% of members of a group of Peruvian Amerindians (Sulzer *et al.* 1975).

Epidemiology

In 1995, 1.3 million cases of malaria were reported in the thirty-seven countries of the American continent. Five years later, the situation has not substantially changed with nearly 1.15 million cases in 2000 (PAHO, 2001). However, since then malaria morbidity has decreased by 23% with 882,361 cases reported in 2004 (PAHO, 2005). Approximately 57% of the population lives in the twenty-one countries where transmission occurs and where control programs are in place. Eleven of these countries are in South America: Argentina, Bolivia, Brazil, Colombia, Ecuador, Guyana, French Guiana, Paraguay, Peru, Suriname, and Venezuela. The other ten countries are in Central America: Belize, Costa Rica, El Salvador, Guatemala, Honduras, Nicaragua and Panama, and in the Dominican Republic, Haiti and Mexico. Within these twenty-one countries, approximately 293 million people live in zones at risk.

The level of malaria risk is determined in the following manner:
- high risk: over 10 cases per 1,000 inhabitants,
- moderate risk: between 1 and 10 cases per 1,000 inhabitants,
- low risk: under 1 case per 1,000 inhabitants.

In 2004, 96.5% of the 882,361 cases reported in the Americas occurred in the following ten countries:
- the vast majority were in Brazil: 52.6%,
- followed by Colombia: 13.25%,
- Peru: 10.62%
- Venezuela: 5.29%,
- Guatemala: 3.53%,
- Guyana: 3.27%,
- Ecuador: 3.26%,
- Honduras: 1.78%,
- Bolivia: 1.69%,
- Haiti: 1.22%.

These countries account for most of the 1.15 million cases reported in 2000.

Of the 514 million people who live in these twenty-one endemic countries, 260 million people (50.6%) live in risk zones and 87 million (17%) are spread throughout the nine countries that form the Amazonian Basin. This population is itself spread between regions where the epidemiological risk is high (16.4%), moderate (16.4%) or low (67.2%).

The other subregion includes the seven countries of Central America plus Mexico for a current population of 147 million people among which 27 million people are living in at-risk zones. In 7 million blood smears examined in 2004, 64,666 cases were detected. The distribution of the number of cases per country is as follows:
- Guatemala: 31,127 cases (48.1%),
- Honduras: 15,689 cases (24.3 %),
- Nicaragua: 6,897 cases (10.7 %),
- Panama: 5,095 cases (7.9%),
- Mexico: 3,400 cases (5.3%),
- Costa Rica: 1,289 cases (2%),
- Belize: 1,057 cases (1.6%),
- El Salvador: 112 cases (0.2%).

These figures show that Guatemala, Honduras, Nicaragua and Panama account for 91% of the cases in this subregion.

In South America, with the exception of the Amazonian Basin, malaria is also endemic in Argentina and Paraguay with 9.7% and 57.9% of the respective populations living in zones where there is a risk of transmission. In Argentina, 3.5 million people are exposed to a moderate or low risk, while in Paraguay, of the 3.2 million people exposed, 1.3 million live in high-risk zones. In 2000, of 7,949 blood smears examined in Argentina, 440 were positive compared to 115 cases in 2004. In Paraguay, the situation has further improved with 6,853 cases confirmed from the 97,026 blood smears analysed in 2004 for 694 cases in 2004 (PAHO, 2005).

In 2000, the twenty-one countries reported that approximately 86 million people were living in regions where they were at high or moderate risk of contracting malaria, representing an increase of 9 million over the 77 million reported in 1999. Nearly 94% of the 1.14 million cases of malaria were detected in zones of high and moderate risk. The API (Annual Parasite Incidence) in these regions was approximately 12.36 cases per 1,000 inhabitants in 2000 and dropped to 7.6 in 2004 (PAHO, 2005). This figure is below that of 1999 which was 13.61 cases per 1,000.

P. vivax is the dominant parasite on the American continent. In zones where the risk is considered to be high or moderate, it was responsible for 73.7% of the cases in 1999 and 73.2% in 2004, as compared to 82.2% in 2000. The large majority of cases attributed to *P. falciparum* (26% in 2004) are found in populations with a significant proportion of African-Americans in the Guyanas, Haiti and along the coasts of Venezuela, Colombia and Ecuador.

In Mexico and Central America, the approximate proportion of each of the three *Plasmodium* species can be broken down to 97% for *P. vivax*, 2.9% for *P. falciparum* and 0.1% for *P. malariae*. In South America, the balance between *P. vivax* and *P. falciparum* varies, while *P. malariae* remains very rare (or absent). In Brazil, the dominant species is *P. vivax* and the proportion of cases due to this parasite rose from 75.5% in 1997 to 81.4% in 2000. In Argentina and Paraguay, *P. vivax* is responsible for all cases of malaria. On the other hand, in Guyana, French Guiana and Suriname, *P. falciparum* is the dominant species responsible for 65.5% of cases in 2000 (PAHO, 2001), while *P. vivax* mainly infects Amerindians.

Since 1996, the availability of a good range of first-line antimalarial drugs has significantly improved. Cases of chloroquine resistance had already been reported several decades before and it appears that increased consumption of antimalarial drugs might well have accelerated the selection of resistance strains.

In 1993, national budgets and funding from other sources exceeded $185.4 million. Since that time, the budget has been continually cut back, down to $85.7 million in 1996 and only $10.7 million in 2003 and $12.5 million in 2004 (PAHO, 2005). However, finances remained relatively constant until 2002 at nearly $80 million per year and lately a substantial increase was made through contributed funds and loans that raised the total budget for malaria control programs to $172.5 million in 2004 (PAHO, 2005). The Roll Back Malaria (RBM) initiative was launched in 2000, and contributions and loans increased the available funds by 15% in this region, with an average budget of $0.57 per person living in the endemic region (PAHO, 2001).

Country by country

North America

Malaria is endemic only in Mexico, although anophelines such as *An. freeborni*, *An. hermsi* and *An. quadrimaculatus* are present and often abundant in North America.

United States

Since the eradication of malaria from the United States in the 1950s, nearly all cases of malaria there have been contracted during visits abroad or imported by immigrants. However, between 1957 and 1994, 74 cases of locally transmitted malaria were reported in twenty-one States (Zucker, 1996), including three in the northern United States (Oregon, New York and New Hampshire). Of the various *Plasmodium* species identified, the vast majority were *P. vivax* (80% of cases), followed by *P. malariae* (8%) and *P. falciparum* (7%); the other 5% could not be identified. Of these 74 cases, 56 represented isolated transmission events, 77% of which involved a single patient, 16% two patients and 7% three or more individuals being infected. Occasionally, these local cases can occur when a *Plasmodium*-infected human happens to be in the same place as a potential vector. The most severe epidemics occurred in 1986 and in 1988 in San Diego County (California), where, respectively, 27 and 30 cases of *P. vivax* malaria were transmitted locally by *An. hermsi* (Barr & Guptavanij, 1988; Turley *et al.*, 1986). These micro-epidemics generally occur in rural areas (89%), although episodes of undetermined origin have been reported in densely populated semi-urban zones, e.g. a 1993 case of *P. falciparum* malaria in New York (Layton *et al.*, 1993; Layton, 1996) and two autochthonous *P. vivax* cases in Maryland and Virginia in 2002 and in Florida in 2003 (CDC, 2002, 2004).

Canada

No autochthonous case has been reported in the last fifty years.

Mexico

Malaria is endemic throughout nearly all of Mexico, with a high proportion of *P. vivax* (98%) and only 2% *P. falciparum*; *P. malariae* is sporadic (Rodriguez *et al.*, 2000). The parasites are the VK 210 and VK 247 polymorphic variants of *P. vivax*. The first is essentially coastal in distribution and it is often found in the same places as *An. albimanus*; the second is more broadly distributed and is associated with *An. pseudopunctipennis*. A transmission-blocking immune factor has been detected in the coastal populations (Ramsey *et al.*, 1996), the activity of which is mainly manifest in relapses. Primary cases were associated with a 92% chance of infection as opposed to one of 4% for relapses. This poorly understood factor should be taken into account when evaluating parasite reservoirs.

Mexico encountered difficulties in stopping transmission throughout the eradication period. *An. aztecus* and *An. quadrimaculatus* were initially suspected of maintaining exophilic transmission but Bruce-Chwatt (1961) refuted this. On the southern Pacific coast, transmission due to *An. pseudopunctipennis* persisted in villages although satisfactory results were obtained in isolated homes: the repellent effect of DDT was thus suspected as being the cause of failure (Zulueta & Garrett-Jones, 1965). Chiapas was classified as a difficult zone. Furthermore, in Oaxaca, the openness of the dwellings played a major role in facilitating transmission. Various treatments were tried, including the carbamate insecticide Bendiocarb®. Pyrethroids were eventually chosen, notably lambdacyhalothrin which is still in use.

The main vectors are *An. albimanus* on the coastline and low altitude marshland, and *An. pseudopunctipennis* inland; the latter is the major vector in the highlands where it is helping the VK 247 variant of *P. vivax* to spread (Fernandez-Salas *et al.*, 1994). Other vectors can also participate at the local level, e.g. *An. quadrimaculatus* in the northern part of the country, *An. vestitipennis* (Loyola *et al.*, 1991) in Chiapas (the Lacandon forest where this species has a sporozoite rate/CSP of 0.47%), and *An. darlingi* in the south-eastern region (Loyola *et al.*, 1991; Manguin *et al.*, 1996a).

The zones at risk in the coastal region of Chiapas have been classified according to *An. albimanus* density, and on the basis of the surface area of the larval habitats in marshes and swampy pastures. The use of remote sensing, particularly satellite imaging coupled with a geographic information system (GIS), has enabled zones with high vector densities to be identified. The habitats of *An. albimanus* and *An. pseudopunctipennis* have been studied using satellite images with a view to developing a model to predict the densities of these two species in Chiapas, and to identify villages with a particularly high risk of malaria justifying targeted insecticide treatment (Beck *et al.*, 1994, 1997; Pope *et al.*, 1994; Rejmankova *et al.*, 1998; Roberts *et al.*, 1991; Savage *et al.*, 1990).

In Mexico, this strategy reduced the incidence of malaria. After a peak of 133,700 cases in 1985, it then dropped to 7,300 cases in 2000 and 3,400 cases in 2004 (PAHO, 2005). This significant reduction in incidence is attributed to the reinforcement of epidemiological stratification, sustained control policies based on indoor spraying with DDT or pyrethroid (lambdacyhalothrin), and the early treatment of patients.

Central America

Malaria in Central America over the last twenty years is summarised in *Table VI*, which shows the annual number of cases. These data are a reminder that most diagnoses (over 80%) are based on purely clinical criteria, so there is the possibility of a significant margin of error (perhaps over 50%).

Table VI. Changes in the annual number of cases in the seven countries of Central America from 1982 to 2000 (PAHO, 1994, 1996, 2001).

Country	1982	1988	1995	2000
Belize	3,868	2,725	9,413	1,486
Costa Rica	110	1,016	4,515	1,879
El Salvador	86,202	9,095	3,362	753
Guatemala	77,375	52,561	24,178	48,213
Honduras	57,482	29,737	59,446	34,736
Nicaragua	15,601	33,047	69,444	20,381
Panama	334	1,000	730	1,036

Following a difficult period prior to 1980, only El Salvador has witnessed a constant decrease in the number of cases from 1982 to 2004. In Nicaragua, from 1983 to 1985, during the guerrilla war, the number of cases of malaria increased as a result of disruption of health services (Garfield et al., 1987), but subsequent macro-economic structural readjustments had more negative impact on malaria control than the war had (Garfield, 1999). The instability of the economic situation led several countries to change their methods of control and/or evaluation. A lack of information prevents us from providing explanations for the differences that occur from one year or one period to another, e.g. in 1995 when all of the figures increased (except for in Guatemala and Panama). It would be particularly interesting to know the impact of political changes. It should also be noted that, the Global Control Strategy (devised at the Amsterdam Ministerial Conference on Malaria) was adopted as soon as 1993 (WHO, 1992a).

It is difficult to know if fluctuations in the number of cases from one year or period to another accurately reflect epidemiological changes or simply changes in the notification system—or even new control strategies.

Guatemala

The incidence of malaria has dropped considerably in Guatemala, decreasing by a factor of 3.8 between 1982 (77,375 cases) and 1996 (20,268 cases). Since that time, this trend has begun to reverse with twice as many cases documented in 2000 than were in 1995. In 2000, 53,311 cases were reported, an increase of 18% in just one year, although the number of cases dropped since then to 31,127 cases in 2004. The pathogenic agents are *P. vivax* (98% of cases) and *P. falciparum* (2%) (PAHO, 2005). The three main vectors are *An. albimanus*, *An. pseudopunctipennis* and *An. vestitipennis*. Defined as a local vector, *An. darlingi* has also been collected along the various river systems (Kumm et al., 1943; Manguin et al., 1996a). Transmission is exacerbated by environmental conditions that favour vector and parasite development, as well as by migration, inadequate control measures, a lack of local participation, and limited heath education. In order to enhance efficacy and motivate local people, volunteer workers "*medicators*" were recruited to administer drugs and take blood samples within the framework of epidemiological monitoring operations (Ruebush-Trenton et al., 1994). The National Malaria Control Program in Guatemala has received support from similar institutions in Belize, El Salvador and Mexico.

Belize

In the 1980's, the number of cases of malaria ranged between 2,700 and 4,500 per annum and then, in the 1990's, the incidence of the disease rose to nearly 10,000 cases in 1994 in a population of just 200,000. This increase can be attributed to the lack of funds for control measures. After the resumption of indoor DDT spraying operations in 1995, the number of cases of malaria dropped by 85% from 9,413 in 1995 to 1,486 in 2000. Since then, the number of cases had remained constant around 1,000 cases per year (1,057 in 2004). *P. falciparum* infection was eliminated in 1972, but it reappeared in 1978 and spread rapidly so that this parasite was implicated in 13.8% of all infections in 1983. Since then, the proportion of *P. falciparum* has dropped considerably (1.3% in 2000 and 0.5% in 2004) (PAHO, 2001, 2005) with the two *P. vivax* strains, VK210 and VK247, accounting for the rest (Achee et al., 2000). There are four main vectors of malaria in Belize: *An. darlingi*, *An. albimanus*, *An. vestitipennis* (Achee et al., 2000) and *An. pseudopunctipennis* (Roberts et al., 1993).

An. darlingi and *An. pseudopunctipennis* are riparian species: the larvae of the former develop along rivers and those of the latter in residual ponds rich in filamentous algae in the dry season; the larvae of *An. albimanus* occupy ponds with clusters of floating cyanobacteria mats (Rejmankova et al., 1993).

The gathering of reliable entomological, epidemiological, environmental and spatial information has made targeted, effective control possible in villages where there is a high malarial risk (Roberts et al., 1999, 2002b).

Honduras

Since 1975, the prevalence of malaria in Honduras has fluctuated between 14,000 and 75,000 cases per annum with 15,689 cases reported in 2004 (PAHO, 2005). A 32% drop in the number of cases was reported in 2000, although a large part of this could be attributed to the 30% reduction in the number of microscopic examinations compared with 1999. Since 1985, the proportion of *P. falciparum* has varied from 1-5%, the rest being *P. vivax*. This country has experienced major ecological upheavals over the last three decades. As a result of overgrazing and intensive sugarcane and cotton farming, the southern part of the country (Choluteca) has become hot and parched, underlying a decrease in *Anopheles* numbers and a 75% decrease in the incidence of malaria. The population has migrated northward and cleared the north-eastern rain forest where the number of cases of malaria has increased significantly (Almendares *et al.*, 1993).

In other respects, an epidemic in January 1997 linked to environmental changes resulted in a significant increase in *P. falciparum* malaria in the north of the country (Colon); the percentage of slides positive for this parasite was 21% (79% *P. vivax*) (Palmer *et al.*, 1998).

Immigration from adjacent countries represents an important risk factor which is difficult to control.

The major vectors are *An. darlingi*, *An. albimanus*, *An. pseudopunctipennis* and *An. vestitipennis*.

Diagnostic field tests using dipsticks (OptiMAL®) are also used to differentiate *P. vivax* and *P. falciparum* (Palmer *et al.*, 1998).

El Salvador

Since 1980, the incidence of malaria has dropped considerably in El Salvador, from a peak of 95,835 cases to 86,202 in 1982, then 9,095 in 1988, 3,362 in 1995, 745 in 2000, and 112 in 2004 in a current population of 6.9 million, i.e. a drop of 99.9% in twenty four years. Malaria control activities—focused in hyperendemic zones which account for 80% of the country's infections—have extensively contributed to this drastic reduction. They are based on reinforcement of epidemiological and entomological monitoring (insecticide treatments and the elimination of larval habitats) as well as diagnosis and immediate treatment of suspect cases. The main vectors are *An. albimanus* and *An. pseudo-punctipennis*; a few specimens of *An. darlingi* have also been documented (Manguin *et al.*, 1996a). This country has the lowest incidence of malaria of all the Central American countries.

El Salvador has become famous for insecticide resistance—first to DDT, then organic phosphates and finally carbamates (propoxur)—which appeared on the coastal plain where cotton is grown intensively with up to thirty insecticide treatments per year. In 1973, *An. albimanus* was found to be resistant to all of the products used for indoor spraying (Mason & Hobbs, 1978). These studies focused attention on how agricultural pesticides can induce resistance in vectors (Georghiou, 1982; Mouchet, 1988). Resistance was not the only problem encountered in El Salvador. The rudimentary housing of seasonal labourers—simple huts open to the four winds—promoted transmission (Rachou *et al.*, 1966) by *An. albimanus* which bites at nightfall. Unlike those in the coastal zones, the anophelines found in the hills where coffee beans are cultivated (particularly *An. pseudopunctipennis*), were susceptible to insecticides.

Nicaragua

Malaria was transmitted in rural zones around large cities from May to December. Owing to the highly-motivated participation of communities and enhanced monitoring during the Sandinista period from 1983 to 1987, there was a 62% decline in malaria in zones not affected by the war although incidence apparently increased in the theatre of operations (Garfield *et al.*, 1987). After the war, there was widespread relaxation of control measures due to cuts in health care service budgets as a result of economic hardship. Slide samples were no longer taken regularly and some nurses and/or volunteer workers demanded money for the drugs (Garfield, 1999).

Since this period, Nicaragua has witnessed two significant increases in the last twenty years with a peak of 46,000 cases in 1989 and nearly 70,000 in 1995. The trend has since begun to reverse with just 23,878 cases reported in 2000 in a total population of 4.6 million. Since then, the number of cases dropped to 6,897 in 2004 for a population of 5.5 million (PAHO, 2005). A reduction of 38.2% in *P. vivax* infections and one of 24.3% in *P. falciparum* infections were recorded in Nicaragua; the former accounts for 94% of cases (PAHO, 2001). Monitoring operations in *P. falciparum* zones were significantly hindered by regional social conflicts which created logistical difficulties that cut down access to health services and exacerbated the lack of human and financial resources.

The two main vectors are *An. albimanus* and *An. pseudopunctipennis* (Heinemann & Belkin, 1977a).

Costa Rica

Costa Rica has the lowest incidence of malaria in Central America. Transmission was nearly interrupted in 1975 (Warren *et al.*, 1975). A serological survey conducted in villages along the Pacific coast, the region at highest risk, concluded that prevalence was more or less zero in under-15 year-olds.

There were only a few hundred cases of malaria in the 1980's but the incidence started to climb back up, reaching a peak of 6,951 cases in 1992. The trend has since reversed with the incidence dropping 73% over the last eight years to just 1,879 documented cases in 2000 (PAHO, 2001) and around 1,000 cases since that date (1,289 cases in 2004) (PAHO, 2005). The incidence of malaria remains one of the lowest in the region. Laboratory diagnosis and hospital treatment are available throughout the country in the decentralised laboratories and health centres.

The two main vectors are *An. albimanus* and *An. pseudopunctipennis* (Heinemann & Belkin, 1977a).

Panama

For more than twenty years, the incidence of malaria in Panama has fluctuated significantly, from a minimum of 125 cases in 1984 through more than 1,000 cases (1986-1988, 1991 and 2000) to a peak of 5,095 cases in 2004 for a current population of 3.1 million. This represents a huge increase (500%) over the last four years ranking this country in fourth place (instead of seventh in 2000) with nearly 8% (*vs* 0.8% in 2000) of all malaria cases reported in Central America (PAHO, 2005). After having achieved a significant reduction in the incidence of malaria since 1991, the country has focused its efforts on its Amerindian populations. Cultural factors and difficulties related to the accessibility of health care centres impede the efficiency of the Panamanian National Malaria Control Program. The proportions of *P. vivax* and *P. falciparum* appear rather variable, ranging from 77.5-98% *versus* 12.5-2%, although there is no evidence of an increase in the relative frequency of *P. falciparum*. The main vectors are *An. albimanus* and *An. pseudopunctipennis* (Heinemann & Belkin, 1977a).

Caribbean islands

Most of the Caribbean Islands were probably infected as a result of the trade in slaves from West Africa, although the disease has steadily disappeared among many members of this population. In the other islands, eradication programs were effective in eliminating the disease, particularly in Martinique and Guadeloupe between 1952 and 1955, in Grenada, Cariacou and Saint Lucia in 1962, in Trinidad and Tobago in 1965, in Dominica and Jamaica in 1966, in Puerto Rico and the Virgin Islands (United States) in 1970, and in Cuba in 1973 (Haworth *in* Wernsdorfer & McGregor, 1988). Malaria is only endemic in Haiti and the Dominican Republic.

Haiti and the Dominican Republic

Hispaniola, the first land of the New World discovered by Christopher Columbus, is shared between two countries. The Republic of Haiti occupies the western third of the island, while the Dominican Republic occupies the eastern two-thirds. These are the only two countries of the Caribbean in which malaria is still endemic. The percentage of *P. falciparum* reaches 99%, with occasional cases due to *P. malariae* and *P. vivax*. The main vector is *An. albimanus*; *An. pseudopunctipennis* is very localised.

Despite the lack of reliable official statistics following internal unrest, **Haiti** has witnessed a significant decline in malaria since 1982 when 65,000 cases were declared. The figure of 18,000 cases declared in 1993 appears to be more realistic (WHO, 1999a). *P. falciparum* is almost the only parasite involved and its vector, *An. albimanus*, is most dense in the lower parts of the island which receive heavy rain; the sporozoite rate is always very low (Molez *et al.*, 1998). Another vector, *An. pseudopunctipennis*, is also present on the island although its epidemiological role remains unclear (Molez *et al.*, 1988). Malaria tends to be concentrated in foci. Depending on environmental conditions, villages in which the Slide Positivity Rate (SPR) exceeds 10% can be found next to places where the same parameter is zero (Duverseau *et al.*, 1989; Kachur *et al.*, 1998). In a study conducted in remote health care centres in 1995, the average SPR was 4%, varying from 5.5% among adults to 0.16% among children between the ages of 1 and 5, indicating the near-total absence of immunity among the adults. Of the forty-one health care units surveyed, six had an SPR of over 10%, five had an SPR between 5% and 10%, eight between 0.1% and 5%, and twenty-two had no infected patients at all. It should be stressed that the SPR is not representative of the general population, but only of those attending health care centres (entailing some degree of over-estimation). Haiti's political difficulties have interfered with malaria control activities. Although epidemiological monitoring is very limited, the number of reported cases in 2000 was 16,897, decreasing to 10,802 cases in 2004; morbidity and mortality data are incomplete (PAHO, 2005). However, the very dark projections issued in 1995 by a USAID team do not appear to have become reality and malaria seems to have stabilised at one of the lowest levels since 1945.

In the **Dominican Republic**, malaria is confined to the western border with Haiti. Almost all cases are due to *P. falciparum* which supports the idea that the disease was introduced here *via* Haiti. The vector is *An. albimanus*. Epidemic foci have been controlled since 1985 and the incidence has been oscillating between 356 cases in 1990 and 1,808 cases in 1995; in 2000, 1,233 cases were reported and 2,355 in 2004 (PAHO, 2005). These relatively low figures compared to its neighbouring country are due to improved monitoring, stratification and targeted intervention in affected zones as well as the close monitoring of cases imported by travellers coming from Haiti.

Cuba, Jamaica, Puerto Rico, the Lesser Antilles, Grenada, Trinidad and Tobago

These various islands are home to anophelines that can transmit malaria but, since no human *Plasmodium* species are present, transmission no longer occurs. Nevertheless, importation means that there is a risk of the disease returning. *An. albimanus* can be found in most of the islands of the Greater Antilles, including Puerto Rico, Cuba, Jamaica, Hispaniola, and the islands of the northern arch of the Lesser Antilles including Martinique and Dominica. In the southern islands of the Lesser Antilles, *An. aquasalis* has been reported in Dominica, Guadeloupe and Trinidad.

In **Jamaica**, the vector used to be *An. albimanus* which is particularly dense along the island's southern coast in the brackish coastal marshes where PRs of 72% used to be seen before insecticide spraying operations were initiated (Muirhead-Thomson & Mercier, 1952a, b). In Afro-American people, the predominant parasite was *P. falciparum*.

In **Grenada**, *An. pseudopunctipennis* and *An. aquasalis* are an integral part of the anopheline fauna (Manguin *et al.*, 1993).

The island of **Trinidad** was highly endemic with 18,000 cases in 1949; following eradication operations, only eleven cases were reported in 1960. Transmission was attributed to *An. aquasalis* in the coastal zones and *An. bellator* in inland areas and plantations where this vector develops in bromeliads (*see above*) (Faust *in* Boyd, 1949). Population movements between the coast and inland plantations maintained the flow of malaria. As *An. bellator* was not affected by the control measures, prophylactic drugs were administered as a complementary eradication measure. An epidemic of *P. vivax* broke out in 1992, twenty-five years after eradication had been achieved. The nine cases were attributed to the infection of *An. aquasalis* by a patient who had come from Venezuela (Chadee *et al.*, 1992).

In **Martinique**, Montestruc (1936) identified malaria around Lamentin Bayet and more sporadically to the east (Le Robert) and south (Sainte-Anne). The PR was 14% at Lamentin and 15% at Rivière Salée; all three plasmodial species were present there. In 1955, he distributed prophylactic quinine. The first indoor spraying operations were undertaken as early as 1951-1952. The only vector appeared to be *An. aquasalis* and malaria disappeared.

According to Léger (1932), the PR was between 5% and 20% in **Guadeloupe** and malaria was increasing; four foci had been identified by Languillon (*in* Aldighieri, 1953) who had produced a malaria map in 1951, before the control campaign had begun. Prophylactic quinine treatment was undertaken. The vectors were *An. albimanus* and *An. aquasalis* in Guadeloupe and Marie-Galante, although the disease was not endemic on Saint Barthelemy. Malaria control operations based on DDT were launched in homes and the neighbouring larval habitats. Malaria disappeared between 1952 and 1955. A so-called indigenous case, declared in Guadeloupe, appears to have been imported in 1999, probably from Haiti.

In **Cuba**, in 1940, a SR study (Carr & Hill, 1942) showed low-prevalence malaria with a maximum of 16% in Camaguey Province; only nine of the 134 communities had a SR greater than 20%. The low incidence of malaria was due to the porosity of the soil, which precludes the formation of larval habitats. In places where malaria was not endemic, seasonal outbreaks (false epidemics) and epidemics occurred at regular intervals. They were originally anthropogenic and the vector was *An. albimanus*. Malaria had disappeared from Cuba by 1963 after repeated DDT spraying operations.

In **Puerto Rico**, from 1939 to 1943 malarial mortality ranged from 60-120 per 100,000 inhabitants. Eradication operations began in the 1950s, after a series of indoor DDT spraying operations.

South America

A division of the countries of South America based on political and linguistic criteria has been proposed, making distinction between the:
- **Andean countries**, the territory of which includes part of the Andean Cordillera. The northern countries—Venezuela, Colombia, Ecuador and Peru—have a maritime coast (Atlantic for the first two and Pacific for the last two) and an Amazonian continental border; the southern countries, often referred to as the Southern Cone, include land-locked Bolivia and Paraguay, Chile on the Pacific coast, and Argentina and Uruguay on the Atlantic coast. All of these countries are Spanish-speaking;
- **Guyana** and its neighbours: these territories are or were under European control; the official languages are English, Dutch and French. They are populated by Afro-Americans or Indian or Indonesian immigrants, alongside a sparse Amerindian population. They stand out from the other American countries by virtue of their very high incidence of malaria in general with a high proportion of *P. falciparum* malaria;
- **Amazonia**: this area covers a large part of Brazil, which is the Portuguese-speaking centre of South America, and extends substantially into the adjacent Andean countries.

The Andes

Venezuela

Venezuela was the first American country to extend malaria control measures (indoor DDT spraying) to cover the entire population. After remarkable initial success, it became evident that transmission had not been completely interrupted and the disease still persists today in certain foci in the north-west, north-east and Amazonia. Since the 1980's, the number of cases rose from about 4,000 to a peak of 47,000 in 1990, before stabilising at around 20,000 cases in 1998, 1999 and 2001. Since then, the number increased progressively to 26,049 cases in 2000, reaching 46,655 cases in 2004 (PAHO, 2005).

In the foci in the north, *P. vivax* is involved in more than 90% of the cases, while *P. falciparum* can reach 50% and *P. malariae* 1% in the southern territories. In the Amazonian zone in the southern part of the country, where the major vector is *An. darlingi* (Gabaldon, 1965), the prevalences of *P. vivax* and *P. falciparum* are equal.

The anopheline fauna is particularly varied in Venezuela; *An. albimanus* is found in all coastal and subcoastal regions, *An. aquasalis* is located along the north-eastern coast, *An. pseudopunctipennis* in the Andes foothills (where malaria has often disappeared) and *An. darlingi* in the Amazonian South along rivers with low acidity levels. *An. nuneztovari*, a confirmed vector in north-western Venezuela, maintained a focus which was refractory to control operations, possibly together with *An. oswaldoi*. Out of 60,000 anophelines tested for *P. vivax* CSP, six specimens were positive (0.019%). The Entomological Inoculation Rate (EIR) was 10 infective bites/person/year (Rubio-Palis *et al.*, 1992). The zone was populated with settlers who cleared the forest and lived in rudimentary shelters open to the elements in which spraying was not effective. *An. nuneztovari* was biting in homes or outdoors but did not rest there, which would explain its failure to respond to insecticide treatment (Gabaldon *et al.*, 1963; Scorza *et al.*, 1976). The parasite in the zone was *P. vivax*.

After a twenty-year absence, malaria returned to the north-east of the country at the base of the coastal chain between May and December 1985 (Barrera *et al.*, 1999). The vector was *An. aquasalis*. Following the heavy rains caused by La Niña in 1988, malaria increased by 36% (Bouma & Dye, 1997); control efforts remained ineffective.

In Bolivar Province, the discovery of diamond reserves created an influx of gemstone hunters; a malaria epidemic with a high percentage of *P. falciparum* exploded in this highly mobile population whose housing was very basic (Berti *et al.*, 1998). The vector was *An. darlingi*.

There are 37,900 Amerindians in Venezuelan Amazonia, 9,000 of which belong to the Yanomani ethnic group whose villages range from the Sierra Parima to the Brazilian border. Over the last few years, ethnologists, biologists and, to a lesser extent, epidemiologists have studied these peoples. Their traditional territories have been invaded by gold diggers, particularly Brazilians who, according to Médecins Sans Frontières (MSF), are thus risking their lives. *P. vivax* is present in most of villages and relapsing forms are perpetuating the disease (although this is not a necessary condition for persistence). *P. falciparum* outbreaks have been due to importation of the parasite by people from elsewhere (Laserson *et al.*, 1999a). Malaria has affected the Yanomani for more than a century, having been originally introduced by the gold diggers; the vector is *An. darlingi* although other secondary vectors may be involved.

During an epidemic among the Yanomani in November 1994, two isolates of *P. falciparum* exhibited the same merozoite surface proteins (msp) allele frequencies, suggesting that a single genotype of *P. falciparum* was involved and that it remained constant during the outbreak (Laserson *et al.*, 1999b).

Over 90% of Yanomani people show signs of sideropenia (Perez, 1998). Hyperactive splenomegaly is frequent with acute haemolytic forms of the disease, probably due to auto-immune responses. While 44% of subjects had splenomegaly, only 3% were found to be carrying the parasite (Torrès *et al.*, 2000).

In 1999, in the eastern part of Guyana, 51% of strains were susceptible to chloroquine, S.P. (sulfadoxine, pyrimethamine) and 80% to Fansidar®. There was only resistance to the former drug (6%) (Caraballo &Rodriguez-Acosta, 1999).

Field testing of the quantitative buffy coat (QBC) test showed that this method was more sensitive than thick smear testing when it comes to detecting parasites, although it did not differentiate *P. vivax* from *P. falciparum* (Bosch *et al.*, 1996).

The ENSO (El Niño Southern Oscillation) must be taken into account when deciding how to prevent epidemics. In northern South America, this phenomenon has resulted in periods of drought during El Niño, followed the next year by excess rainfall, particularly during La Niña. The phenomenon is cyclical, although irregular. The alternation of drought during El Niño and heavy rainfall during La Niña may be associated with a 36% increase in malaria mortality. ENSOs can be predicted from temperature changes at the surface of the ocean (SSTs: sea surface temperatures) (Bouma & Dye, 1997), if the meteorologists are right (*see the Part entitled* "Spatiotemporal Dynamics of Malaria").

Colombia

Since the end of the Second World War, Colombia has been through a period of insecurity associated with a bitter guerrilla war and, more recently, drug trafficking. All official functions are affected, including malaria control measures. This has been compounded by many factors, including the anarchic colonisation of new territories, the continual movement of labour in search of often illegal employment, and the inaccessibility of malarial foci, all of which compromise the efficiency of health care operations in rural zones.

The annual number of cases remains at more than 100,000, and even 206,195 in 2001 and 221,834 in 2003 (116,872 cases in 2004) (in 1991, 1992, 1995, 1997) in a current population of 43 million (PAHO, 2005). Official figures are under-estimated since certain regions fail to submit declarations. Malaria is present throughout the country, except for in the mountains.

P. vivax, the most widespread species in the valleys west of the Andes, is responsible for 65-70% of all cases, *P. falciparum* is responsible for 25-30%, particularly along the Pacific coast and in the southern jungle; the role of *P. malariae* is anecdotal. As a result of migration and environmental changes, small epidemics broke out in 2000 in zones considered to be of only moderate risk; these were attributed to *P. falciparum* .

Furthermore, it was noted that the incidence of malaria rises by approximately 17% during El Niño years and 35% the following year. Understanding and predicting the El Niño phenomenon may be of help in preventing malaria outbreaks, as discussed above.

The vectors are *An. albimanus*, locally *An. aquasalis* along the coast, *An. neivai* in the forest along the Pacific coast, *An. pseudopunctipennis* on the Andean relief, *An. nuneztovari* in the eastern part of the country and *An. darlingi* in the Amazonian Region.

Until recently, urban malaria was not considered a problem in the American Regions. In Buenaventura, the main port on the Pacific Coast, the number of cases increased from 576 in 1987 to 3,296 in 1991 (Olano *et al.*, 1997); it is transmitted by *An. albimanus* which represents 90% of captures in homes; its parous rate is only 55%; the density of this species in and around houses peaks between 6 p.m. and 8 p.m. It finds abundant larval habitats in mining pits and fish/shrimp farm basins.

In the city, based on a sample of 1,380 subjects, the overall prevalence was 4.4% although this parameter tended to decrease with age; 93% of the cases were contracted in the city itself with the rest contracted in the course of forestry work in the surrounding area. The incidence varied from 1‰ to 3‰ throughout the city, but it was five to six times higher in the suburbs than it was in the centre. On the other hand, the API in the rural zones was 60‰ to 100‰ (Mendez *et al.*, 2000). This pattern is very similar to that seen in African cities where species of the *An. gambiae* Complex are the vectors.

On the Pacific Coast, in the forest regions (the Chocó Region), *An. neivai*—a member of the bromeliad-dependent *Kerteszia* family—is an important vector. The young females of this mosquito species bite in the evening between 6 p.m. and 7 p.m. and the older females are active from 5.30 a.m. to 6.30 a.m., either indoors or outdoors (Astaiza *et al.*, 1988). The female has a very long life expectancy, with 1.5% of them showing traces of ten egg-laying cycles (an exceptionally high number). In the village of Charambira (near Chocó), where malaria was transmitted year-round, 4,720 *An. neivai* were collected for just 5 *An. albimanus*. CSP testing showed eight *P. falciparum* infections and one *P. vivax* infection (Carvajal *et al.*, 1989).

In a village with high levels of malaria (Zubaletas), 20% of slides were positive with 73% *P. falciparum* and 27% *P. vivax*, although only eight subjects were showing symptoms (Gautret *et al.*, 1995).

A negative correlation between rainfall and malaria was established in a region of low transmission and unstable malaria. Of the 319 subjects examined, 8 were carrying parasites; 6 of these had no symptoms and the symptoms that were seen were very mild (due to premunition, according to the authors) (Gonzales *et al.*, 1997). Serological testing revealed a history of exposure to *P. falciparum* in 90% of cases. The vector was *An. neivai* which accounted for more than 60% of the local anophelines. During the month of greatest transmission, the EIR was four infective bites/person/month (Gonzales *et al.*, 1997).

In Amazonas, at Arica on the Putamayo near the Peruvian frontier, 8% of febrile subjects tested positive for malaria; the prevalence was relatively low among coca farmers (27% positive). *An. darlingi* was not detected and the only possible vector was *An. oswaldoi*. There were 76% *P. vivax* as opposed to 24% *P. falciparum* (Perez *et al.*, 1999). Malaria was considered to be unstable but, in a neighbouring city, Tarapaca, transmission was year-round (Perez *et al.*, 1999).

The desire to improve and automate diagnosis, a preoccupation in all American countries, has led to a comparison of three methods: thick smear (reference technique), QBC (Quantitative Buffy Coat Analysis) and PCR (Polymerase Chain Reaction). *P. falciparum* prevalence was 5.8% using the thick smear, 7.3% by QBC and 21.8% by PCR. This last method is certainly the most sensitive and it can detect very low-level parasitaemia (Carrasquilla *et al.*, 2000) although its clinical significance is open to debate.

Ecuador

According to statistics published in 2005 by PAHO, Ecuador is the South American country (outside of the Guyanas) where the incidence of malaria is the highest with 50% of the population living in endemic regions. Malaria extends over three eco-geographic zones:

- the Pacific coast, where the vector is *An. albimanus* and its preferred larval habitats are shrimp farm basins along the coast;
- the Amazonian plain to the east of the Andes, where the vector is *An. darlingi*;
- the slopes of the Andes and the south of the valley within the range where *An. pseudopunctipennis* transmits *P. vivax* (Reyes, 1992).

Autochthonous malaria is rare in the higher-altitude Andean Provinces, and neither *Anopheles* nor malaria are found in the Galapagos Islands.

The number of notified cases has fluctuated considerably since 1982: 14,633 in 1982, 78,599 in 1984, 23,274 in 1989, 71,670 in 1990, 11,882 in 1996, 104,528 in 2000 and 28,730 cases in 2004 (WHO, 1999a; PAHO, 2001, 2005). Such variations correspond to bias in the reporting rather than actual changes in incidence.

Deterioration of the malaria situation was attributed to political instability and the resultant disorganisation of health care services. Environmental changes with intense deforestation may also have played a role, as well as climatic changes (although the information remains imprecise). For example, from September 1982 to July 1983, El Niño led to abnormally high precipitation that supposedly resulted in an increase in the number of cases from 14,000 to 51,000. Furthermore, epidemics were recorded in zones that had hitherto been free of malaria, with a gradual increase in the number of cases and the geographical spread of infections attributed to *P. falciparum*.

It should be remembered that it was at Loja in the Andes that, in the 17th century, the first European was treated with *Cinchona* bark administered by a local traditional doctor (Riofrio, personal communication).

Peru

In 1944, Peru declared 95,000 cases of malaria; in 1965, after the eradication programme was initiated, the number dropped to 1,500; in 1988, at the lowest level, 641 cases were declared, all due to *P. falciparum*. Beginning in 1991, the trend reversed and 140 cases of *P. falciparum* were reported; in 1998, the disease culminated at 247,229 cases. In the Amazonian department of Lloreto alone, 128,269 cases, including 54,280 cases due to *P. falciparum* were reported; these cases resulted in 85 deaths (Guarda *et al.*, 1999). This spectacular increase was initially due to a decrease in indoor spraying operations after DDT was banned (after regular application until 1990); it was replaced with pyrethroid but operations were reduced. Interference with surface waters (for irrigated rice growing) and the clearing of the Amazonian forest—coupled with extensive immigration—may also have been instrumental. In 2004, the number stabilized at 93,581 cases—nearly the level reported 60 years ago before the eradication programme was implemented. This represents 10.62% of all malaria cases reported in the Americas, ranking Peru in third place after Brazil (52.6%) and Colombia (13.25%)

out of the twenty-one countries where transmission occurs (PAHO, 2005).

Faced with this situation, Peru implemented extensive control operations in application of the Global Control Strategy. Diagnosis was improved and 95% of the cases were confirmed microscopically or by "ParaSight-F dipstick" tests in difficult situations (Forney et al., 2001). *P. vivax* malaria was treated with chloroquine and primaquine, and uncomplicated *P. falciparum* disease was treated with Fansidar® and primaquine; drugs were administered to 94.5% and 92.8% of patients, respectively. The most serious cases were treated with quinine or a combination of artesunate (or a derivative) and mefloquine. These measures resulted in a 58% drop in malarial mortality, a 69% decrease in the number of *P. falciparum* cases, and a decrease of over 50% in the number of cases of *P. vivax* malaria.

Malaria is very unequally distributed in Peru as a result of differences in altitude, climate and anopheline fauna. On the Pacific coast, north of the 8th south parallel, malaria is transmitted by *An. albimanus* (as in Colombia and Ecuador). South of this, there is less rainfall and a desert zone follows the coast down to the 30th south parallel in Chile. This desert, one of the most arid in the world, is created by the cold Humboldt Current flowing up from Antarctica and along the South American coast. It prevents all precipitation below 600 m in altitude. The only surface water is from streams flowing down from the Andes which create oases along their path. These oases are the home of *An. pseudopunctipennis* that transmits *P. vivax* from the slopes of the Andes to the ocean.

On the slopes of the Peruvian Andes, *An. pseudopunctipennis* had been found at altitudes of up to 3,200 m (Hackett, 1945), although malaria does not appear to go above 2,600 m; the only parasite is *P. vivax*. On the eastern slopes of the Andes, below 1,000 m, infected *An. nuneztovari* has been found in the Junin Region.

The main source of malarial infection remains the Amazonian Region which covers 50% of the country's territory. Lloreto Province alone represents 25% of the country's total surface area, although only 3.4% of the population lives there (about 820,000 inhabitants). The incidence in this province, in 1997, was two cases per person per year (Roper et al., 2000). Sixty percent of the cases were among men (hunters, fishermen, farmers) as opposed to 40% among the more house-bound women. The disease is hyperendemic but local people do not appear to be protected in any way. From 1994 to 1998, malarial mortality varied from 1.3 to 1.8 per 1,000 inhabitants. The seasonality of malaria is dictated by the water-level in the level of the rivers which peaks at the end of the rainy season (January to July), e.g. in Padre Cocha, the level of the Rio Nonay varies by 10 m between the highest and lowest levels.

The vectors are *An. darlingi*, which accounts for 90% of all anophelines around Iquitos, *An. benarrochi* (part of the Strodei Subgroup) in the west of Lloreto Province, and *An. triannulatus* in the east. In the region of Junin, on the last foothills of the Andes in the Amazonian forest, *An. trinkae* sporozoites have been found in dissections, not only of well known vectors such as *An. nuneztovari* and *An. pseudopunctipennis*, but also of *An. trinkaae, An. oswaldoi, An. rangeli* and a species related to *An. fluminensis* (*An. sp. nr. fluminensis* of the *Arribalzagia* series) (Hayes et al., 1987).

Finally, there is a hyperendemic *P. malariae* focus in south-eastern Peru among Amerindians who are isolated from the Campas Group; here the prevalence of this parasite is 63% (Sulzer et al., 1975); monkeys in the surroundings were found to be carrying *P. brasilianum* which was at that time considered as distinct from *P. malariae*.

Bolivia

This large country of more than one million km² has a population of only 8.9 million, one of the lowest population densities (7.3 inhabitants/km²) in South America. Set within the western Cordillera of the western Andes, Bolivia is landlocked.

Distinction is made between three altitude-defined ecological zones, ranging from 200 m to more than 5,000 m:
- the Altiplano is the highest plateau of between 3,500 to 4,500 m in altitude, bounded on the east and west by the Occidental and Oriental Cordilleras which rise to altitudes of over 5,000 m. The northern part of the plateau is occupied by Lake Titicaca and the south by "salars", more or less dried out salt lakes. This region is the historical centre of the country and is home to nearly two-thirds of the population (who are Hispanics, Aymara and Quechua with variable degrees of intermixing). Silver, tin, platinum and tungsten mining provided a large part of the region's resources. In the 17th century, San Luis de Potosi was one of the largest cities in the world. The gradual closure of the mines which began in 1970 resulted in an exodus of the population to lower-lying areas where the migrants encountered tropical diseases, notably malaria and leishmaniasis, which did not exist in the highlands;
- the foothills (500-1,200 m) and the upper Andean valleys (1,200-3,000 m), the only ways into the massif, form an intermediate stratum characterised by a remarkable diversity of fauna and flora, the inventory of which is far from complete. This zone is marked by the contrast between the talwegs where *An. pseudopunctipennis* thrives during the dry season, and the coca-covered slopes;
- the plain between 500 and 200 m is dominated by the Amazonian forest in the north (in the departments of Pando and Beni) and its exceptionally rich fauna and flora. In the south in the upper Paraná basin, the landscape is more contrasted and most of the vegetation is typical of the savannah. Marshland and savannahs, periodically flooded, cover large portions of the departments of Santa

Cruz and Tarija. The main vector, otherwise only found in the south-east, is *An. darlingi*.

In 1955 (Villaroel, personal communication, 1999), malaria flourished in the plains, foothills and upper Andean valleys up to 2,700 m in altitude. In Cochabamba, at 2,600 m, severe epidemics of *P. falciparum* malaria erupted in 1930, 1936, 1941 and 1946. In the "warm" valleys, between 1,000 and 2,500 m, in the Yungas of La Paz and Iquiziti, Chiapare, the Mizqué Valley, and the Rio Chico, the high infant mortality was responsible for the depopulation of this formerly booming area (Moscoso Carrasco, 1963). Malaria morbidity was 820‰ and mortality was 35 per 100,000. The vectors involved were *An. darlingi*, below 500 m and *An. pseudopunctipennis* above.

In 1956-1957, during the pre-eradication period, surveys conducted throughout the country covering a total of more than 25,000 subjects estimated the prevalence of malaria at 6%. For Bolivia as a whole, the balance between the different parasites is 65% *P. vivax*, 23% *P. falciparum*, and 12% *P. malariae* (Moscoso Carrasco, 1963). *P. falciparum* was confined to the Amazonian basin, although it was also reported in Cochabamba; *P. vivax* occupied the entire endemic area, particularly sites at higher altitudes.

From 1963 to 1975, morbidity dropped to 1 or 2 cases per 1,000 inhabitants; these residual cases were due to settling on new lands with changes in the country's economy (from one based on mining to one based on agriculture). Since that time, the number of cases has appeared to stabilise between 10,000 and 2,000, depending on the efficacy of control operations (Villaroel, personal communication).

In 1990, a small epidemic of *P. vivax* occurred in Arque near Cochabamba at an altitude of 2,700 m, attributed to an imported case. In 1992, while the country was supposedly protected, in eight villages around Camiri (in the department of Santa Cruz), PRs were 1.59% during the dry season and 25% at the end of the rainy season; the only parasite was *P. vivax* (Cancrini *et al.*, 1992). In 1997 and 1999, many *P. vivax* infections were detected in Pazuela, in the Yungas of Inquiziti at 1,800 m (Villaroel, personal communication). These examples show how vulnerable to malaria are the Andean valleys.

After eradication plans were implemented in the 1960s, malaria disappeared from the Yungas and considerably diminished in the lower plains. After 1982, with a decline in indoor spraying operations and colonisation of the lowland areas, the incidence of malaria continued to climb until 1997 (WHO, 1999a). In the last three years, the number of confirmed cases has dropped considerably and the Annual Parasite Incidence (API) dropped from 74,350 cases in 1998 to 31,469 cases in 2000 and 14,910 cases in 2004 (PAHO, 2005). The number of notified cases dropped by 80% after the Global Control Strategy was implemented; indoor spraying operations are still being conducted in high-risk foci.

The Southern Cone

This term refers to the geographic region composed of the southernmost countries of South America: Chile, Argentina, Paraguay and Uruguay (and occasionally Bolivia).

Chile

Chile marks the southern limit of malaria west of the Andes; the endemic zone was limited to the Arica Region, not extending below the 19th south parallel, along the border with Peru. In the region of the Atacama Desert, *An. pseudopunctipennis* can only breed on the banks of rivers flowing down from the Andes, particularly the Rio Lluta and Rio Azapa which form oases along their journey to the ocean (Manguin *et al.*, 1996b). Malaria control, which included prophylaxis and treatment (quinine) as well as anti-larval measures, began in 1937. Ever since it became available, DDT has been used and autochthonous malaria was definitively eradicated in the early 1950's (Reyes, 1999). However imported cases occur with 24 reported during the 1945-1988 period. Between 1980 and 2001, 66 cases were recorded with 5 deaths (8.8%). The entomological surveillance system is focusing its efforts in foci where the only vector is *An. pseudopunctipennis* (Schenone *et al.*, 2002).

Argentina

Argentina is the southern limit of malaria east of the Andes, at the level of Cordoba on the 32nd south parallel. It should be noted that west of the Andes, the limit of malaria in Chile is far higher.

Malaria was endemic in the north-west (in the Salta and Jujuy Provinces), extensions of the Bolivian foci of Tarija and in the north-east (Missiones). In the latter region, malaria reappeared due to the return of *An. darlingi*. Bolivian migrants are believed to be implicated in this return in the northern provinces, although this remains contentious. *An. pseudopunctipennis* is the most abundant species encountered in the Yungas de Salta, but *An. argyritarsis*, *An. nuneztovari*, *An. rangeli* and *An. strodei* were also collected (Juri *et al.*, 2005).

In a country in which many consider malaria to have been "eradicated", the number of cases—mainly due to *P. vivax*—remained very low with a maximum of 2,000 cases in 1986 and 1996, followed by a significant drop to 500-600 cases since 1997 and less than 250 cases since 2001 (115 cases in 2004) (PAHO, 2005). In 2000, of the 484 documented cases, 80% were imported (PAHO, 2001).

Owing to its position at the latitudinal (Cordoba) and altitudinal limits of malaria, Argentina is very concerned by the possible impact of climatic changes on the distribution and abundance of vectors, and thus on malaria. Models were formulated in 1993 (Burgos *et al.*, 1994a) but, by 2002, there was no evidence that they had been verified or that they were in the progress of being verified.

Paraguay

In contrast, malaria is endemic throughout the whole of Paraguay, a landlocked country. Approximately

3.05 million people (51.7% of the population) live in zones considered to be at some degree of risk. The most affected populations are the Guarani who do not have access to health care services. There are less than 1,000 cases per year (694 cases in 2004), except for an outbreak of 9,947 cases in 1999, all due to *P. vivax*. *An. darlingi* is the only vector reported. This country is essentially a transition zone between the Andean countries (Bolivia and Argentina) and Brazil.

Uruguay

Uruguay is not considered endemic and all cases reported there were imported.

Guyana and its neighbours

The Guyanas, which include Guyana* (formerly British Guiana), Suriname (formerly Dutch Guiana) and French Guiana (a French overseas department), are the three countries of the American continent where malaria incidences are the highest, greater than 500‰ in Guyana and 700‰ in the Oyapock Basin in French Guiana (*Table VII*).

Geographically speaking, these three countries are located within the Guyana Shield which corresponds to a subcropping of the Precambrian basement of the ancient supercontinent of Gondwana, similar to the Goyas Shield in Brazil; it contrasts with the Amazonian basin of recent alluvial origin. This "ancient" land, for the most part covered in forest, possesses flora and fauna of remarkable biodiversity. The major vector, *An. darlingi*, is omnipresent along rivers and in the wooded areas of the coastal plain. In the brackish waters along the coast, *An. aquasalis* is a relatively weak vector, despite the enormous densities that it can attain. *An. nuneztovari*, present everywhere and extremely abundant in dam reservoirs (e.g. the Brokopondo Dam in Suriname) is not a vector in this part of South America (Panday, 1977).

The population is concentrated along coastal strips, while the inland territories are nearly empty. The population consists of:
- Amerindians, minorities, concentrated (or pushed back) inland, along rivers and in a few coastal enclaves;
- Afro-Americans, descendants of slaves, who are concentrated near the coast and along the lower courses of rivers (where the plantations are located). They have either returned to their tribal customs, particularly the Boni in French Guiana and the Djukas along the Maroni River in Suriname as well as in French Guiana (also referred to as the "Black Maroons"), or have settled in the coastal regions, often mixing with the Caucasians to form a population that is incorrectly referred to as "Creole";
- Asians, Indians and Indonesians, brought to Guyana and Suriname as labour in the late 18th and the 19th centuries;
- a few recent migrations, such as the Hmongs from Laos, who have settled in French Guiana. They have retained the health care logistics of their former colonisers, particularly *vis-à-vis* malaria control operations.

This "melting pot" aspect is reflected in the parasite distribution; *P. falciparum* is the dominant parasite among African-Americans and the only one along the Maroni River whereas *P. vivax* is more common in Amerindians and immigrants of Asian origin.

Guyana

Formerly British Guiana, Guyana*, a member of the Commonwealth, is the largest country of the Guyanas and the most populous (750,000 inhabitants in 2006 compared to 70,000 in 1970) (*Table I*). People of Indian origin and the Afro-Americans dispute power there. For the most part, these two groups live in the coastal regions which concentrate 90% of the population in just 18% of the territory. The inland areas are sparsely populated; thick jungle and broad forest cover most of the territory.

In 1945, when the country was under British administration, this territory was one of the first to implement malaria control operations, the success of which was rapid and highly publicised; malaria and its vector, *An. darlingi*, disappeared from the coastal regions as early as 1951 (Giglioli, 1951). However, in 1963, a small epidemic appeared around Georgetown; the vector was *An. aquasalis* (Lobel *et al.*, 1977). It had been negligible not long beforehand but the disappearance of its preferred host, the buffalo (resulting from the mechanisation of rice

Table VII. Changes in the number of cases of malaria in the Guyanas from 1963 to 2000.									
Country	1963	1968	1973	1978	1983	1988	1993	1995	2000
Guyana	476	61	42	927	2,102	35,470	33,172	59,311	24,018
Suriname	716	1,555	1,948	876	1,943	2,691	4,704	6,606	12,321
French Guiana	70	50	484	266	1,051	3,188	3,974	4,711	3,416

* Depending on the author, the term Guiana or Guyana is used to designate the former British Guiana. Since 1970, the official term is "Cooperative Republic of Guyana" (Anonymous, 1999 ; *État du Monde*, 2000).

farming operations) drove it towards more anthropophilic behaviour (Giglioli, 1963).

Transmission never stopped among the Amerindians in the sparsely populated inland savannahs of Rupununi. The exophilic *An. darlingi* was the vector in the open houses (which are, moreover, difficult to treat with insecticide). In addition, in regions of heavy rainfall in the west, *An. bellator*, a bromeliad anopheline, was believed to be responsible for small foci (Charles, 1959).

In 1977, a sero-epidemiological study based on two surveys, conducted one year apart, showed the absence of transmission; malaria had disappeared inland following elimination of the coastal foci (Lobel *et al.*, 1977).

Beginning in 1980, malaria initially reappeared with cases of *P. vivax* along the coast, transmitted by *An. darlingi* in a region that had been malaria-free for more than twenty years (Rambajan, 1984); this was followed by the return of *P. falciparum* malaria in force (Rambajan, 1994). The API jumped from 260‰ in 1986 to 776‰ in 1991 and then to over 1,000‰ by the end of the decade. The number of cases increased from 927 in 1978 to 3,200 in 1980, then jumped to 7,900 in 1985, to 16,388 the following year and to 35,470 in 1988. This increase in malaria continued until 1995 with 59,311 cases after which the number of cases dropped to 24,018 in 2000 with a slight increase at 28,866 cases in 2004 (PAHO, 2001, 2005). Chloroquine resistance which was brought in from Brazil by migrants does not explain why the situation degraded so rapidly and so dramatically. Cutbacks in control operations bear a large part of the blame.

Two parasites, *P. falciparum* and *P. vivax*, are responsible for all malaria infections. Until 1985, the proportions of *P. vivax* were greater (70%) than those of *P. falciparum* (30%) but, from 1986 to the present, the similar numbers of cases have been attributed to each parasite and now, there are even reports of *P. malariae* infection although rare.

Suriname

Since 1980, Suriname, formerly Dutch Guiana, has experienced a long period of political and social instability. Dispensaries along the Maroni River have been periodically closed and local people—mainly Djukas—had to go to French Guiana for treatment. All health care statistics from this country should be interpreted with caution.

The main vector is *An. darlingi* (Hudson, 1984; Rozendaal, 1987, 1990), which is abundant along all the rivers; along the banks of the Maroni, it represented 85% of the anophelines, while in the inland forest region along small streams, it represented only 20%—as opposed to 63% *An. nuneztovari* and a small number of *An. oswaldoi*. Following the construction of the Brokopondo Dam, *An. nuneztovari*, present throughout the country, was considered a vector, as it was the only species present during a 1976 epidemic of *P. falciparum* malaria in Amerindians (Panday, 1977, 1980). However, the role of this species has not been confirmed, and neither have the roles of *An. aquasalis* on the coast or *An. oswaldoi* in the forest been confirmed (Panday, 1980).

Between 1985 and 1990, the number of cases was about 1,600; in 1996, it rose to 18,800 and 17,074 in 2001 and dropped to around 13,000 in 1999, 2000 and 2002 and at 8,021 cases in 2004 (PAHO, 2001, 2005). The civil wars that ravaged the country for more than ten years facilitate neither control operations nor the establishment of health care statistics, which have thus become very unreliable. *P. falciparum* is by far the most dominant parasite, particularly among the Djukas, an Afro-American group: this parasite accounts for 72% (1996) to 99% (1992 and 1993) of infections. Severe outbreaks of malaria were recorded in 1978-1980 among the Djukas on the Maroni River; these were classified as epidemics—perhaps wrongly (Rozendaal, 1992).

The percentage of *P. vivax*, which particularly affects forest-dwelling Amerindians and those of Asian origin along the coast (Rozendaal, 1987), is no higher than 20%. *P. malariae* is poorly represented (< 6%).

French Guiana

This is the only French overseas department in which malaria is endemic and where it persists despite an operational malaria control programme and the treatment of all cases, measures which account for the exceptionally low mortality rate: out of the 4,000-odd cases declared each year, only two deaths were reported in 1986 and 1989, and there were less than five deaths per year from 1991 to 2001. In 1986 the two documented deaths were both of marginal people who had refused treatment. In 1997, Hommel *et al.* traced 71 severe cases over the last fifteen years, many of which were imported from Haiti. Moreover, local physicians feel that these figures are very high.

French Guiana still has a very low population density of just 1.8 inhabitants/km^2 even though immigration has doubled the population over the last fifteen years. Eighty percent of the population is concentrated in the narrow coastal region. The Amerindian population, although on the increase, still only numbers 5,000 people living along the Oyapock River on the Brazilian border, along the Litani (upper Maroni) on the Suriname border, and in a few coastal cities. The "Black Maroons" (Boni and Djukas), having fled slavery, resumed a semi-tribal life along the Maroni River. The highly mixed "Creole" population concentrated in the coastal zone although recent immigration by people from Suriname, Haiti, Brazil, Laos (Hmongs) and mainland France has created a cosmopolitan society, particularly around the centres of Cayenne and Kourou.

As throughout all the Guyanas, two ecoregions predominate; broad expanses of virgin evergreen forest with many rivers and, to the east of this, the densely populated coastal band of mangrove, more or less marshy savannah, and man-made habitats. Despite a few ranches in the coastal savannahs, agriculture is limited to food crops for home consumption.

In the late 1950s, malaria was thought to have been eradicated in Guyana (Floch & Lajudie, 1946) following indoor DDT spraying operations. The efficacy of these programmes remains questionable, as the homes of the Amerindian populations do not have walls.

The annual distribution of malaria is very discontinuous. In 1989, three types of foci were designated in Guyana (Mouchet *et al.*, 1989):
- the Amerindian foci along the Oyapock on the Brazilian border, and along the Litani (upper Maroni) on the Suriname border; the annual incidence ranged from 300 to 900 per thousand, depending on village and region, e.g. there were 1.5 paroxysms per person per year around Saint-George. Generally speaking *P. falciparum* accounted for 65% of cases and *P. vivax* for 35%;
- the foci of the Maroni, at Maripasoula and downstream, populated by "Black Maroons" (Boni and Djukas), where the only parasite was *P. falciparum*; the continuous movements of people to and from Suriname across the river made it impossible to calculate the true incidence; the parasite prevalence was 3% (according to a single survey);
- the coastal foci, previously meso-endemic, have disappeared (Floch & Lajudie, 1946) except for the island of Cayenne where transmission persists, particularly among Haitian and Brazilian migrants. In 1987, a small outbreak due to *P. vivax* occurred in a Laotian Hmong village, affecting a third of the population (Mouchet *et al.*, 1989).

The only vector is *An. darlingi* (Pajot *et al.*, 1977). In the coastal halophilic zone, *An. aquasalis* is very abundant and represents a serious menace for man, although its low life expectancy prevents it from being considered a vector (Silvain & Pajot, 1981). *An. (K.) neivai* was suspected of transmission in an Amerindian village, although without conclusive proof (Pajot *et al.*, 1978).

For spraying operations, DDT—to which bedbugs were resistant—was replaced by pyrethroid. The Bonis along the Maroni had a difficult time accepting spraying operations in their rudimentary homes, and in Amerindian houses, there were no walls to be sprayed.

Between 1991 and 2001, the number of cases stabilised between 3,000 and 3,800 with a peak at 5,307 in 1999 (3,037 cases in 2004) (PAHO, 2005). The percentage of *P. vivax* dropped from 51-19% and *P. falciparum* became the dominant parasite.

P. brasilianum was detected (by microscopic examination and PCR assays) in monkeys, namely *Alouatta seniculus*, *Saguinus midas*, *Pithecia pithecia* and *Ateles paniscus*. Blood examinations and PCR results indicated positive rates of 5.6% and 11%, respectively. *P. malariae* is rare in humans (under 5%) and the transmission of simian parasites to man can only occur at a very low rate, if it occurs at all (Fondeur *et al.*, 2000).

Brazil - Amazonia

In all, 99.7% of the malaria cases in Brazil occur in the Amazonian Region and 74% of cases are concentrated in just three of the nine states (Rondônia, Mato Grosso and Pará) (*Figure 14*). The annual number of cases has oscillated between 400,000 and more than 600,000 since 1985 (*Table VIII*), due to *P. vivax* (80%), *P. falciparum* (20%), and sporadically *P. malariae* (0.1%). The malaria situation in Brazil is very heterogeneous and influenced by many factors that we will attempt to identify below.

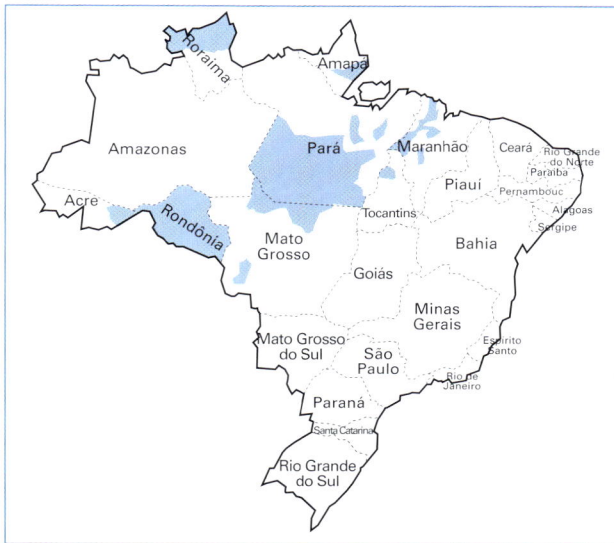

Figure 14. Brazilian Regions with high malaria transmission rates in 1985 (adpated from Marquès, 1987).

Table VIII. Number of cases of malaria in the Amazon Legal Region in 1983 (Marquès, 1986).

Administrative unit	Number of cases	Proportion of autochthonous cases (%)
Rondônia	168,690	96
Mato Grosso	128,832	63
Parà	113,649	76
Maranhão	37,889	48
Roraima	15,830	96
Amazonas	11,198	63
Acre	10,120	70
Amapá	7,460	98
Tocantins	6,928	39
Rest of Brazil	14,859	7
Total in 1983	515,455	

Biodiversity of Malaria in the World

Migrations and recent epidemiological changes

In 1940, the number of cases of malaria in Brazil was estimated at 4-5 million for a population of 55 million—about 10%. Following implementation of the eradication program, the number of cases continually dropped and, in 1970, only 54,600 cases were documented (WHO, 1988); outside Amazonia, the disease appeared to have been eradicated (SUCAM, 1970). With the opening of the roads through the Amazon beginning in 1975 and the development of cleared forest as well as the search for gold, malaria started to gain ground with 614,430 cases reported in 1990. Since then, the number of cases dropped to 392,000 in 1997 (WHO, 1999a). It should be stressed that, since 1995, settlement on cleared forest land slowed considerably following economic setbacks.

During the 1980-1995 period, 99% of the cases were contracted in the "Amazon Legal Region" (made up of the States of Amazonas, Rondônia, Acre, Pará, Roraima, Amapá, Mato Grosso and, pro parte, Maranhão and Goiás). In 1984, 41% of the cases occurred in new farming regions in Rondônia State and 35% in the Pará gold mines (Tauil, 1986). The focal distribution of the cases should be stressed. Of the 483 municipalities concerned, 78 (i.e. 17%) hosted 81% of the cases.

In Pará State, the gold mines of São Félix do Xingu declared 3,000 cases of the 112,000 notified in the whole State. In Rondônia State, the Ariquemes project accounted for 34% of all cases (although designation as a hyperendemic focus was somewhat overdone with a prevalence of under 25%) (Marquès, 1986).

Malaria affected the miners very little as their employers provided chloroquine or other antimalarial drugs. Farmers, however, being very poor and often isolated, had very variable access to health care and were heavily exposed during clearing and harvesting operations. Malaria never inhibited migration and its impact on this social and economic phenomenon was limited. Upon their return home, migrants spread the parasites that they were carrying (Marquès, 1987). Of the 14,000 cases observed outside Amazonia in 1985, 13,000 originated there. Secondary transmission foci could even be formed (twenty-six foci in six States in 1985) (*Figure 15*).

Malaria and Amerindians

There is little information about the Indian forest tribes. Four ethnic groups were studied in the north of Amazonas State. The incidence of malaria was very low there and the average parasitaemia was just 0.2%. The four groups (Arana, Parakana, Asurini and Metuktine) had high antisporozoite antibody levels (90% of the Asurini and all Metuktine adults). More than 50% of the monkeys were *P. brasilianum* positive; in the villages, these monkeys are treated as pets and may represent parasite reservoirs. Of the 755 specimens of *An. darlingi* taken in the camps, three tested positive for *P. brasilianum-P. malariae* and one for *P. falciparum* (Arruda *et al.*, 1989). In 1993, an epidemic was declared in the Vale de Javari reserve in the extreme west of Amazonas State; among its population of 3,000, the incidence was 98.9 per 1,000. In 1994, the prevalence climbed from 4.5% to 25%. Only *P. falciparum* was involved, and it may have been introduced by prospectors (Sampaio *et al.*, 1996).

In the villages along the Rio Machado in Rondônia State where most inhabitants are indigenous, Alves *et al.* (2002) detected a very high proportion of asymptomatic carriers (by PCR and by microscopic examination): 49.5% were carrying *P. vivax* and 10% *P. falciparum*. For the migrants, these carriers are permanent sources of re-infection.

The Yanomani group of the Sierra Parima, whose territory is located in both Brazil and Venezuela, has already been mentioned in the section on Venezuela. At Boa Vista Hospital, at the "Casa del Indio", malaria was considered the most common disease accounting for 15 out of 495 patients in 1987, 65 in 1988 and 74 in 1989; 23% of patients with a severe form died. Most of the patients were living near gold mines (Pithan *et al.*, 1991). According to Veeken (1993), it was the arrival of the miners that posed the most serious risk in this ethnic group, despite all the medical support provided by MSF.

Primate malaria

Primate malaria takes on particular importance in South America, particularly in Brazil, since two species, *P. brasilianum* and *P. simium*, are transmissible to man. The first is related to *P. malariae* and, for many authors, it is the same species (that they designate *P. brasilianum-P. malariae*). The other case of similarity concerns *P. simium* and *P. vivax*; this is less common and whether or not the two are exactly the same is sometimes disputed (Deane *et al.*, 1966).

In the subcoastal forests of Sao Paulo State, simian malaria is enzootic among certain primate species, particularly howler monkeys (*Alouatta fusca*), 60% of which were infected in Cantareira State Park. The capuchins (*Cebus apella*), marmosets (*Callithris anita*) and the masked titi *Callicebus personatus* are also infected. The vector was *An. cruzii* with a sporozoite rate of 2% (in the absence of humans). These acrodendrophilic anophelines (living in the tree canopy) have frequent exchanges with the ground and can transmit parasites from monkey to man. *P. brasilianum* is the most frequent, although *P. simium* is also present (Deane *et al.*, 1966). In the coastal forests—now often reduced to shrub vegetation—of the States of Espirito Santo, Santa Catarina and Rio Grande do Sul, simian malaria is also found in howler monkeys. The presence of homes in the area results in human infections. As the vectors (particularly *An. cruzii*) attack primarily at dawn, people try to stay out of the woods at this time (Deane *et al.*, 1984).

In northern Amazonia and Rondônia, the squirrel monkey *Saimiri ustus* and spider monkey *Ateles paniscus* are infected by *P. simium* (up to 8%). The vectors belong to subgroups *Nyssorhynchus* with *An. nuneztovari*, *An. oswaldoi* and *An. triannulatus*, on the one hand, and

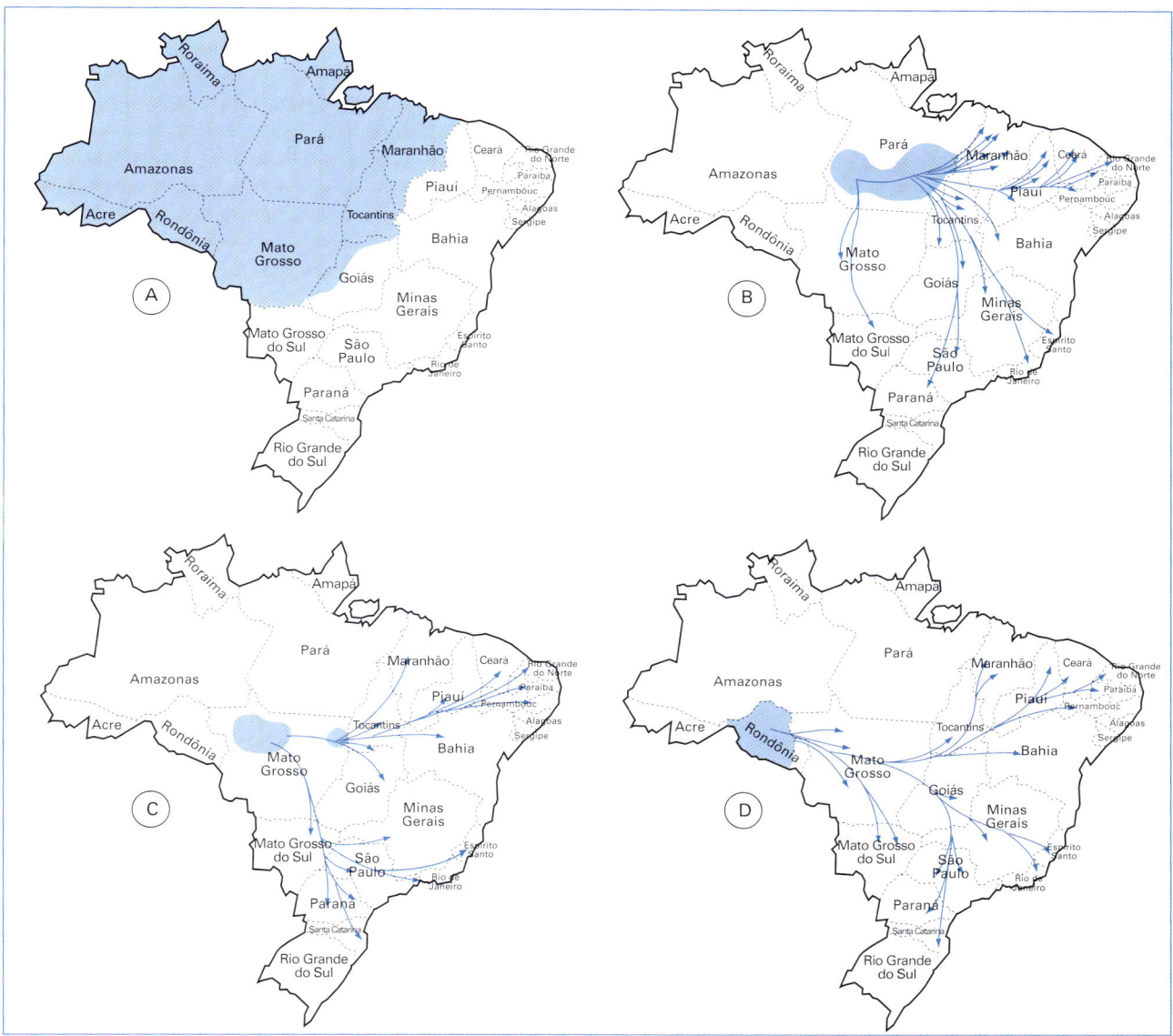

Figure 15. Migrations in Brazil between 1980 and 1995.
A. Amazonia versus the rest of Brazil. **B.** Migrations in Pará State.
C. Migrations in the Mato Grosso. **D.** Migrations in the Rondônia.

Anopheles, belonging to the *Arribalzagia* series, with *An. shannoni* and three twin species, *An. mediopunctatus, An. forattinii* and *An. costai*, on the other (Sallum *et al.*, 1999; Wilkerson & Sallum, 1999). The main human vector, *An. darlingi*, is rarely found in the forest and in consequence, is probably not very involved (Lourenço de Oliveira & Luz, 1996; Lourenço de Oliveira & Deane, 1995).

In Santa Catarina State, *P. simium* has been observed in both primates (particularly howler monkeys) and the *Kerteszia* anophelines (Deane *et al.*, 1966).

The attractiveness of monkeys for *Anopheles* depends on their body weight and the size of the resting area (which conditions the intensity of the odour in the vicinity) (Davies *et al.*, 1991)

Regional epidemiology

The malaria map has been significantly changed by control operations (which started in 1950) and migration (from 1970 to 1995). Currently, 90% of the cases occur in the Amazon Legal Region or originate there. However, the different States of this super-region (which covers half the surface area of Brazil) are concerned in different ways.

Rondônia State, measuring 238,512 km^2, has received the greatest amount of immigrants with its population having multiplied ten-fold between 1970 and 1992; 66% of its population are immigrants. In the 1980's, more than half of all malaria cases declared in Brazil were from here. Since 1990, migration has stabilised, but in 1992, the incidence of malaria was still high at 111‰ (Camargo *et al.*, 1994, 1996, 1999).

Prior to 1970, the population was concentrated in small, highly sedentary, isolated groups living along the rivers from fishing, gathering and a little cultivation. On the Rio Madeira, a study of people living in Portachuelo showed that malaria was a major influence with an API of 292‰—three times that in Rondônia as a whole. The dominant parasite was *P. vivax* (66%). The population, essentially comprised of subjects borne there, exhibited a certain level of immunity. The highest prevalence was observed among children of under 16 years of age (1.9%), and more particularly in new born babies (6.8%). Transmission was perennial and the malaria was stable*. Transmission was mediated by *An. darlingi* in or around homes, although contributions from other, more exophilic species are not ruled out. These villages represent permanent sources of infection for the migrants (Camargo *et al.*, 1999).

In the agricultural settlement zones along major roads, malaria was hypo-endemic and unstable, with annual seasonal outbreaks (wrongly referred to as "epidemics") during the dry season transmitted by *An. darlingi*. During the first three years after settling, the new arrivals lived in temporary shelters where they were very exposed to *Anopheles*. This pioneer malaria mainly concerned men (70-85%) working outdoors. The annual incidence was 130 to 140‰, and prevalence increased with age: 1.5% among children less than 1 year of age compared with 6.5% among adults of 16-40. In addition to *An. darlingi*, exophilic vectors such as *An. oswaldoi* or *An. triannulatus* may also have been involved (Camargo *et al.*, 1996).

Following this pioneer phase, those who decided to remain in the area settled either in isolated farms or in and around villages. In Candeiras, a small city of 7,000 inhabitants about 20 km from Porto Velho, "imported" cases were superimposed on the indigenous cases. All cases seen in the city in subjects who had spent the previous fifteen days in a rural zone were considered to be imported. Around the villages, the forest had given way to pastures and crop fields. Ordinary cases were treated at the local clinic while serious cases were referred to a hospital.

These three examples summarise most of the situations encountered in Rondônia (Camargo *et al.*, 1999). Migration began to wane in 1991 and malaria, originally rural, took on a "village" or even urban aspect, with a whole variety of different situations. Around Ariquemes, a city with a population of 102,000 that is an important food processing centre, radiating urban-type malaria is seen with the transmission rate rising as one moves from the centre out. *An. darlingi* was the main vector during the dry season.

In Rondônia State, malaria was most commonly asymptomatic, particularly that due to *P. vivax*. Among 190 infected subjects, 133 (70%) did not have any fever. On the contrary, fever was observed among 22 (3%) of the 689 uninfected subjects (McGreevy *et al.*, 1989).

Six species were incriminated based on salivary gland dissections and/or circumsporozoite antibody assays (Oliveira-Ferreira *et al.*, 1990, 1992a). Of the 13,000 anopheles tested, CSP was detected in 61 specimens (0.47%): 41 (67%) *P. falciparum* and 20 (33%) *P. vivax*. There were 47 *An. darlingi*, 5 *An. triannulatus*, 4 *An. albitarsis* (identified as *An. allopha*), 2 *An. braziliensis*, 2 *An. strodei* and 1 *An. oswaldoi*. *An. darlingi* was the only species present at sites where transmission had been confirmed and it was, consequently, considered to be the main vector.

Anaemia (as measured by haematocrit) was studied in the village of Candeiras. Of the 1,086 subjects examined, 23% were anaemic, 70% of these being babies of 6-12 months, 38% children (1-6) and 41% pregnant women. Of the ten subjects with malaria, eight were anaemic (Cardoso *et al.*, 1992).

Acre State is located north-west of Rondônia in the extreme west of Brazil. Despite its modest surface area (153,150 km^2), it declared 3.2% of the cases in Brazil, even more than Mato Grosso State which is nearly six times larger (906,800 km^2) (Tauil, 1986).

The apparently primordial role of *An. oswaldoi* and *An. deaneorum* in certain parts of the State has sparked interest (Branquinho *et al.*, 1996). These two species were the most highly represented in captures: 2,610 individuals for the first, 361 for the second as opposed to 24 *An. darlingi*. In one of the three locations prospected, the infection rate of *An. oswaldoi* by *P. falciparum* was 3.4%, by *P. vivax* 2.26%, by *P. vivax* VK-247 1.22 % and by *P. malariae* 0.42%. The infection rate of *An. deaneorum* was 2.7% for *P. falciparum*, 0.55% for *P. vivax* and 0.82% for *P. vivax* VK-247. It should be remembered that *An. deaneorum* which belongs to the Albitarsis Group was first described in Acre State (Rosa-Freitas, 1989).

For the first time, antibodies to the circumsporozoite protein of *P. vivax-like/P. simiovale* were detected in the vectors *An. oswaldoi* and *An. deaneorum* (Marrelli *et al.*, 1998).

In 1985, **Pará State**, with a surface area of 1,253,000 km^2, accounted for 35% of all cases of malaria in Brazil—largely in the gold mining region of São Félix do Xingu with

---

* The term "stable" is the equivalent of perennial (Camargo *et al.*, 1999).

31,000 of the 120,000 cases in the State as a whole (Marquès, 1986). The miners were a very mobile population that took parasites to the neighbouring States. This malaria did not have significant economic importance as the febrile subjects were immediately treated with chloroquine or sulfadoxine-pyrimethamine, either by nurses, their employers or on their own initiative.

Upon leaving Pará, the miners headed to the north-eastern States and Minas Gerais State, while the farmers from Roraima tended to exchange with States to the south.

The southern half of Pará State is considered a region with a level of high transmission (Marquès, 1986) owing to mining activities and the presence of settlements (*Figure 16*).

In 1985, the prevalence of *P. falciparum* was 16% and that of *P. vivax* 20% (Arruda *et al.*, 1986). Out of 9,046 anophelines tested, *P. falciparum* circumsporozoite antibody was present in 2.7-4.2% of *An. darlingi* specimens and a small number of *An. oswaldoi*; the *P. vivax* antibody was present in *An. darlingi*, *An. triannulatus*, *An. nuneztovari* and *An. albitarsis* (mentioned under one of its synonyms, *An. allopha*), at percentages ranging from 0.9-12%.

In **Amazonas**, a vast State with a surface area of 1,577,800 km^2, the prevalence continued to decline from 1970 to 1980, except in Manaus and along the roads through the Amazon, particularly those between Manaus and Boa Vista and Manaus and Porto Velho, along which settlements had been established. Fifty-six percent of the patients hospitalised in Manaus came from this area (Ferraroni & Hayes, 1979). Men aged 30 to 45 were the most frequently infected (> 70%) with 32 infections (6.7%) identified in 480 examinations (Dixon *et al.*, 1979).

Cases of urban malaria are rare in the Americas. In Manaus, which was malaria-free up to 1975, autochthonous cases began to appear in 1988 with the return of *An. darlingi*. Since that time, the number of cases has continued to climb (Roberts *et al.*, 2002c). Malaria is currently present throughout the year with an upsurge during the hot and rainy months between July and October.

Roraima State, with a surface area of 225,116 km^2, was considered as a high transmission risk after development of the area around Boa Vista (Marquès, 1986) and uncontrolled mine prospecting operations. The impact on the Yanomani peoples was discussed above. The population in this State, the northernmost of Brazil, had doubled from 1980 to 1985. The incidence of malaria was extremely variable from one community to another, depending on the make-up of the population and food industry activities. However, no correlation was apparent between population growth and the incidence of malaria (Chaves & Rodrigues, 2000).

Amapá State, measuring 143,453 km^2, is a high transmission zone, at least around the city of Macapá, owing to local agricultural and mining activities (Marquès, 1986). *An. marajoara* is a good vector in deforested zones. A study along the Matapi River showed that *An. darlingi* has the highest human blood indices followed by *An. nuneztovari*, *An. triannulatus* and *An. intermedius* which were relatively zoophilic, also feeding on pigs and bovine (Zimmerman *et al.*, 2006).

The **Mato Grosso**, with a surface area of 906,800 km^2, took second place (*Table VIII*) in the list of malaria-stricken States with 128,832 cases (Marquès, 1986). The search for gold, particularly in the Colider Region, resulted in significant mixing of populations; only 63% of the cases were autochthonous. In a gold diggers' camp, twenty of the ninety-eight subjects examined were positive, although fourteen were asymptomatic (Andrade *et al.*, 1995).

Goiás and **Tocantin States**, located at the boundary of the Amazon Region (with surface areas of 341,289 km^2 and 278,420 km^2, respectively) had declared less than 7,000 cases, only 39% of which were autochthonous (Marquès, 1986). Statistics on deaths due to *P. falciparum* from 1981 to 1993 showed that 46% of cases involved those of between 20 and 50 years of age: 35% were farmers and 14% miners. The rate of malaria morbidity was 0.24‰, the rate of malaria mortality was 0.005‰ and the lethality rate was 2.3‰ (Pineli *et al.*, 1997).

Maranhão State, with a surface area of 333,365 km^2 only part of which is in the Amazon Region, had declared 37,300 cases in 1985, which put it in fourth place in terms of the number of cases of malaria. This was one of the first States where the wave of migration was felt in the 1970's.

Ever since 1985, throughout the settlement period, the number of cases continued to grow until 1991 when it reached 614,431 cases (WHO, 1999a). Since the readjustment of malaria control policies in 1993, the number of cases has continued to drop; early diagnosis of cases and immediate treatment have proved to be very effective in zones where indoor spraying operations were unsuccessful (Gusmao, 2002). However, in 1999 and 2000, 635,646 and 613,241 cases were reported respectively

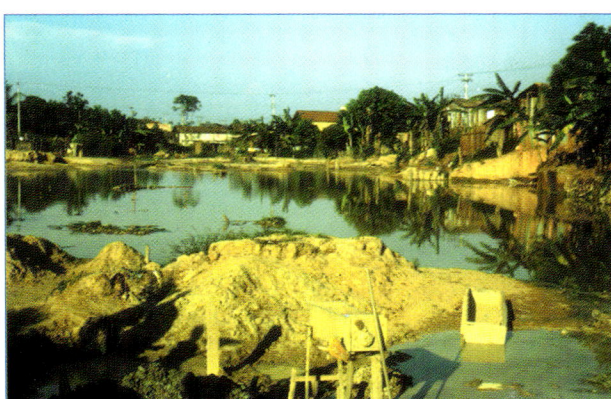

Figure 16. Mining operation, Brazil, Pará (photograph by Coosemans).

(PAHO, 2005). Since then, the annual number of cases has been fluctuating between 348,259 in 2002 and 463,792 in 2004.

Outside of Amazonia, high urban immigration appears to have caused a malaria epidemic in Camacari in **Bahia State** (Souza *et al.*, 1988). This is one of the rare instances of urban malaria in the Americas (together with Manaus and in Colombia). In **Minas Gerais State**, incidences were very low between 1980 and 1992, from 0.08 to 0.27‰ with a maximum of 0.25‰ in 1985. Cases imported from Amazonia represent 93% of the total and only 10 cases were autochthonous; 87% of the patients were men, including 26% gold diggers. *P. vivax* was the parasite in 75% of cases; 26 infectious foci emerged, which resulted in 471 autochthonous cases. In **Pernambouc State**, migrants returning from Amazonia reintroduced malaria and approximately 100 cases were declared (Menelau *et al.*, 1981).

Malaria due to the bromeliad anophelines of the Kerteszia Group has become a feature of coastal Atlantic forests, especially in Sao Paulo State where this very peculiar environment is protected. One of the species, *An. cruzii*, is always responsible for sporadic benign cases (2% of all cases in the State), with a low *P. vivax* parasitaemia. Out of the 2,000 *An. cruzii* specimens, 0.17% were positive for *P. vivax* circumsporozoite antibodies, and 0.08% for the VK-247 variant. The low infectivity of the vectors was compensated for by their large number and aggressiveness (Branquinho *et al.*, 1997). The role of another *Kerteszia*, *An. bellator*, is still debated, although its markedly endophilic, endophagic behaviour exacerbates its epidemiological role (Forattini *et al.*, 1999). The core of the problem is the importation of cases (95%) from the mines and agricultural development areas of Amazonia; it primarily affects men (80%) from 24 to 40 years of age with *P. vivax* the parasite in 60-70% of cases. The mortality in *P. falciparum* cases is 6.6% and malaria mortality reaches 5‰ for all patients taken together (Wanderley *et al.*, 1994), e.g. in the city of Campinas, of the 2,780 cases documented from 1980 to 1995, 95% of the infections came from Amazonia; there were only 5 local cases as well as a few cases due to blood transfusion (5), drug use (3) and congenital malaria (1) (Alves *et al.*, 2000).

Secondary foci became established on the Sao Paolo Plateau where the vector was *An. darlingi*. In the Mato Grosso do Sul, along Paraguay's northern border, no autochthonous case of malaria has been reported since 1990 (Matsumoto *et al.*, 1998) but the return of migrants warrants close monitoring in places where *An. darlingi* is abundant. In Paraná State, the density of *An. darlingi* has increased considerably following the construction of the Itaipu Dam; this has been accompanied by an increase in the incidence of malaria, essentially *P. vivax* malaria (Consolim *et al.*, 1991). Along the border with Argentina and Paraguay, the return of *An. darlingi* is assumed to have been the reason for the increase in malaria on the Argentinean side (Casa & Isabel, 1992).

Conclusions on malaria in the Americas

Comparing the endemicity of malaria in 1945 (prior to eradication) and 2004 shows how drastically the disease has declined, despite the persistence of endemic foci in the Guyanas (primarily due to *P. falciparum*), Central America (*P. vivax*), Amazonia and, to a lesser extent, the Andean countries (Colombia, Peru, Ecuador, and Bolivia). Adoption of the Global Control Strategy in 1993 seems to have led to a decrease in the incidence in certain countries, such as Brazil, while many experts believe that the discontinuation of spraying operations is responsible for the revival of other foci (Roberts *et al.*, 2002b).

There are practically no more hyperendemic foci in the region and mortality due to malaria is very low since the routine treatment of suspect cases became widespread. Political instability as in Colombia, Ecuador and Suriname still constitutes a major malaria risk factor.

If eradication was not achieved in the Americas, malaria as a public health problem has nevertheless been substantially attenuated throughout the region and the future looks optimistic.

Spatiotemporal Dynamics of Malaria

Climate, humans and malaria from a global point of view

Malaria dynamics across the planet have been conditioned by two series of events:
- climatic changes, especially in the last 15,000 years;
- the appearance of modern humans (*Homo sapiens sapiens*) some 100,000 years ago and their remarkable evolution (Coppens & Picq, 2001). Ever since the Neolithic revolution which occurred between 9,000 and 8,000 BC, humans have been remodelling the surface of the planet for the purposes of arable farming and animal husbandry, and have come together to form settlements of ever-increasing size—to the point that today 60% of the world's population live in an urban setting.

In contrast to the slow pace of climate change, demographic patterns evolve in an exponential fashion so that today overcrowding is one of humanity's great problems.

Technological changes, notably since the beginning of the Industrial Revolution, have induced changes in the very air we live in with gaseous emissions—carbon dioxide generated as a result of the burning of fossil fuels, methane, steam and nitrogen oxide—contributing to the "greenhouse effect". In decades to come, the temperature of the planet is expected to rise by between 1.5 °C and 6 °C; for the first time, climate is being influenced by human activities.

Malaria, a vector-borne parasitic disease, has to be reviewed in the context of this evolving spiral. The malaria species which infect humans are closely related to those of African apes and there is no evidence that hosts and parasites did not evolve in parallel in Africa until the hominid lineage* split off from the ancestor of modern chimpanzee six to eight million years ago. Thereafter, the parasites evolved separately when bipedal hominids descended from the trees to adopt a savannah life style. Savannah anophelines—the *An. funestus* Group and members of the *An. gambiae* Complex—which are not found in the woody environment then took over the role of transmitting *Plasmodium* to humans; thereafter, ecologically segregated hominids and apes continued to evolve apart together with their parasites. These hypotheses are largely speculative with the earliest traces of *P. falciparum* DNA having been detected in mummies from Ancient Egypt, dating from no earlier than the third millennium BC (Miller *et al.*, 1994).

Passage of the parasite into the mosquito represents the weak link in the epidemiological chain, this step being highly susceptible to climatic and environmental factors. In consequence, the "history" of malaria cannot be dissociated from that of its vectors which will be the key parameter if global warming is going to have any effect on this disease.

Although climatic factors are very important, they are not the only variables that affect malaria. Anthropogenic modification of the environment, changes in vegetation, modifications of the water network, changing cultivation techniques, new livestock-raising methods, etc.—all can affect the mode and intensity of transmission.

Today, humans travel extensively using conveyances that allow them to transfer parasites and vectors between

---

* In general, the hominids are considered to consist of Australopithecines and the various types of *Homo* which gave way to one another over the two to three millenia preceding the appearance of the human, *Homo sapiens sapiens*. The pongids—chimpanzees, orang-utans and gorillas—which separated from the hominids between seven and ten million years ago maintained stayed in woodlands.

different places anywhere in the world within a time frame of less than forty-eight hours. The outcome is usually a dead-end in terms of transmission but the risk always exists.

At the end of the Würm glaciation period around 8,500 BC, the Mediterranean Basin was already conducive to the transmission of malaria. According to most experts, the Neolithic Revolution began in about 9,000 BC, as of which time the development of arable farming and livestock raising began to lead to the abandoning of the nomadic life style and the establishment of permanent settlements. The major town of Jericho was believed to exist in 7,000 BC. Settlements have played a major role in the establishment of endemic and epidemic malaria (as well as of other transmissible diseases in all likelihood). Communal living promotes the fast, continuous transfer of pathogenic microorganisms between human beings, notably *Plasmodium*. Moreover, sunny fields provide a propitious terrain for the development of vectors, at least in Africa and the Mediterranean Basin (Fenner, 1970).

In the 5th century BC, Hippocrates described the pathology of intermittent fevers, i.e. benign tertian fever (due to *P. vivax*) and quartan fever (caused by *P. malariae*). Pernicious malaria due to *P. falciparum* did not apparently make any appearance in the Mediterranean Basin until between the 3rd century BC and the beginning of the Christian era; the deadly effects of this form of fever were described by Celsus in Rome. As of the 3rd century AD, sanitary conditions were seriously deteriorating in the most important city in the western world.

Such fevers were not confined to the Mediterranean world but ravaged throughout Europe and North America. In tropical lands, especially Africa, the history of fever cannot be dissociated from that of exploration and discovery: Europeans could only colonise vast swathes of the globe once the prophylactic and curative properties of quinine (or rather of the bark of the Andean *Cinchona* tree) had been discovered.

It was not until the end of the 19th century that the etiologic agent of "fever" was isolated (Laveran, 1880) and the fact that it was vector-borne elucidated (*see the Part on* "Malaria, a Vector-Borne Parasitic Disease"). For two-and-a-half millennia, the causes of "intermittent fever" remained shrouded in mystery.

Malaria determinants

The determinants which affect malaria include all those which are involved in transmission of the parasite as well as those which determine the expression of the disease.

Whatever the classification system used, most factors are interdependent, e.g. vector distribution (a biogeographical criterion) is affected by environmental changes, and the ability of *Anopheles* to thrive at higher altitudes (a biological determinant) depends on the quality of the habitat and the presence of livestock. It is impossible to isolate each and every determinant: a global appreciation is essential if all the many and various factors which condition the expression of malaria are to be taken into account.

The major factors have been classified as follows:
- intrinsic biological factors related to the parasite and its cycle;
- transmission factors related to the parasite's behaviour inside the mosquito;
- biogeographical factors which rule the distribution of vectors (and possibly of the parasites);
- climatic factors: variations in temperature and precipitation;
- environmental factors: changes in vegetation, manipulation of surface water, urbanisation, and cultivation and livestock-raising methods;
- human factors : ethnic, demographic and occupational factors, and migration;
- operational factors: malaria control operations and/or their discontinuation.

Climate and Malaria

Direct impact of temperature and rainfall on malaria

Wherever there is *Anopheles* capable of transmitting malaria, the rate of transmission will depend on the number of times each subject is bitten and the proportion of infected mosquitoes. The resultant of these two factors corresponds to the Entomological Inoculation Rate (EIR) which corresponds to h_e in the equation of Ross; $h_e = ma.s$ (in which s is the sporozoite rate, and ma is the number of times each subject is bitten every 24 hours) (*see the Part on* "Malaria, a Vector-Borne Parasitic Disease").

The **number of times** a subject is **bitten** depends on the **productivity of larval habitats** given that without water, anophelines cannot reproduce. The **number of habitats** depends on geographical phenomena which determine whether or not streams and stagnant water pools are present. The **productivity of larval habitats** depends on **rainfall**, **water flow** and the **accumulation of pools** of any size and origin. Drought, be it seasonal or prolonged, dries up larval habitats but the **seasonal interruption of flow** can induce the **formation of residual pools** of great epidemiological importance.

Anopheline infectivity is the other major parameter of the transmission which depends on the length of the **sporogonic cycle** which varies according to the local temperature. Between the lower limits of 15 °C for *P. vivax* and 18-19 °C for *P. falciparum*, and an upper limit of 35 °C, the optimal temperatures are 22 °C for *P. vivax* and 25 °C for *P. falciparum*. Below this optimal temperature, the length of the cycle increases and the proportion of insects reaching the epidemiologically dangerous age diminishes together with the efficiency of transmission. In contrast, it increases when the temperature rises above the transmission threshold. The effect of temperature on the anopheline infection rate was modelled by Macdonald (1957), a system which has been used by forecasters to predict an increase in transmission rate resulting from global warming (*see the Part on* "Malaria, a Vector-Borne Parasitic Disease").

Temperature is subject to microclimatic fluctuations. One of the most common variations is the higher temperatures indoors during the night and at high altitudes: differentials of 3-5°C between the inside of the house and outdoors are common in the mountains of eastern Africa (Meyus *et al.*, 1962) and on the plateaux of Madagascar (Mouchet *et al.*, 1997). The presence of animals inside homes compounds this effect. In Holland, *Anopheles* used to be able to survive through the winter inside houses, meaning that malaria transmission continued despite the cold weather (Swellengrebel & Buck, 1938).

In any epidemiological review or short- or medium-term projection of malaria incidence, reference must always be made to temperature and rainfall, the two most important climatic factors that determine the rate of malaria transmission.

Malaria since the Quaternary Period

Appearance of humans and of the pathogenic malaria complex

The Quaternary Period only lasted two to three million years, a mere instant in the 4.5 billion-year lifetime of our planet, although an important evolutionary event occurred in this short time frame, namely the appearance of hominids; major meteorological perturbations also gave rise to ice ages.

Although the oldest known hominid or near-hominid species is dated 6-7 million years ago (nicknamed Toumaï), it is believed that the first hominids appeared four million years ago with the australopithecines followed by *Homo habilis, Homo ergaster, Homo erectus*, and ultimately *Homo sapiens sapiens* who most likely developed in East Africa before spreading out over the planet. Traces of *Homo erectus* have been found in China, and traces of the pithecanthropines in Java. In Europe, Neanderthals—the last descendants of earlier hominids—disappeared between 7,000 and 4,000 years ago, according to the fossil record, having been supplanted by modern humans which first appeared in East Africa between 100,000 and 50,000 years ago, i.e. relatively recently. After a period in the Middle East, *Homo sapiens* expanded remarkably rapidly compared with other hominids. Forty thousand years ago, before the Würm glaciation, he was already living in southern Europe; traces found in the Cro-Magnon caves in France date this occupation. By 30,000 years ago, he had reached Australia and 5,000 years later, he could cross the Bering Straits by virtue of the glaciation-related drop in sea-level. Cro-Magnon men may have replaced the Neanderthals or may have interbred with them, a controversial question that may well be resolved in the near future using the techniques of molecular biology.

Based on what we know about the ecology of malaria parasites and their vectors, modern man must have evolved in a malaria-ridden African environment, given that the climate has changed little in East Africa over the last 30,000 years and the same species of *Anopheles* (the *An. gambiae* Complex and the *An. funestus* Group) have always been present. After the phase that modern man seems to have passed in the Middle East, his progress brought him into very diverse climates—temperate or tropical, sometimes conducive to malaria transmission, sometimes not.

In the following paragraphs, we will address first the ice ages and their consequences in the Holarctic Region and then general changes in tropical zones before dealing with the current situation, including the possible effects of global warming and major meteorological disturbances.

Glaciation events and post-glacial periods in Holarctic Regions

The Quaternary Period was marked by a series of ice ages, each lasting about 100,000 years, with intermediate periods lasting 10-20,000 years. Since the end of the Würm glaciation about 10,000 years ago, the planet has been going through an interglacial period (Gribbin, 1989) (*Figure 1*).

The four best-characterised ice ages, the story of which is told in the Alps, are named in chronological order starting with the earliest: Guntz, Mindel, Riss and Würm. These coincide with moraines found in North America with the Wisconsin strata corresponding to the Würm glaciation. According to the results of both the CLIMAP (Climate Long-range Investigation Mapping and Prediction) programme and tests on ice cores sampled in Antarctica and Greenland, it would seem that ice ages were simultaneous in both hemispheres.

In the 1940's, Milutin Milankovitch provided a cosmological explanation for the ice ages by showing that

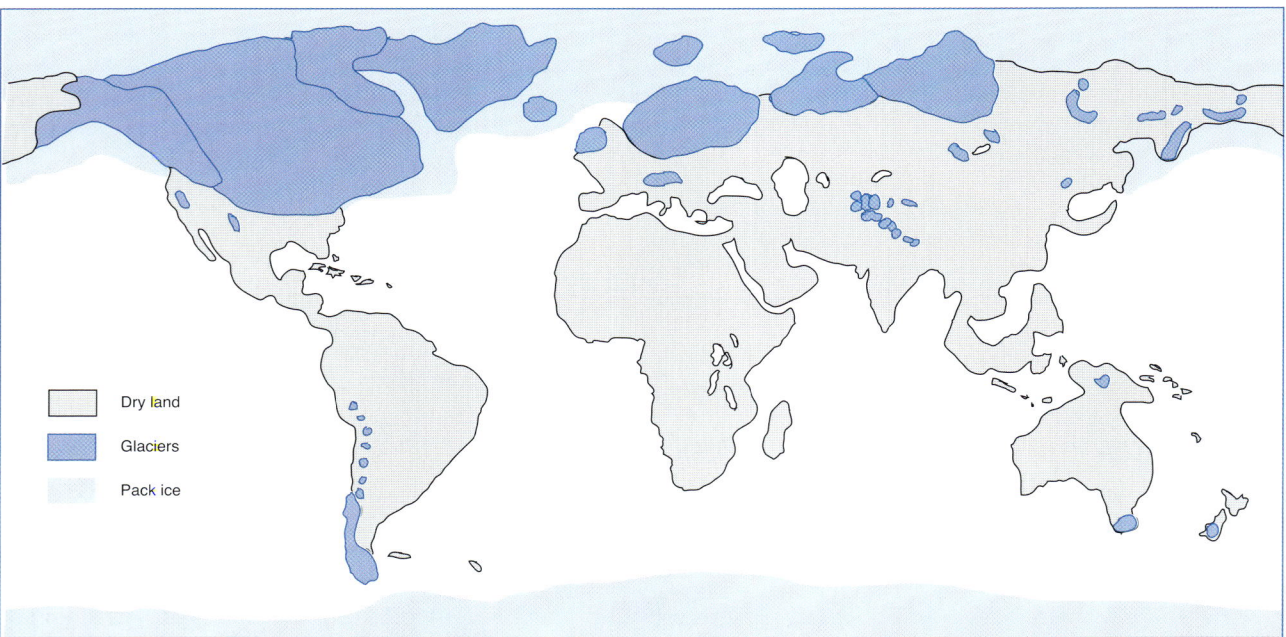

Figure 1. Glaciation of Würm.

Climate and Malaria

the amount of heat incident on the earth depends on three factors: the periodic variation in the "eccentricity" of the earth's orbit around the Sun (100,000 years); the change in the angle of the Earth's axis *vis-à-vis* the plane of the ecliptic (21,000 years); and variation in the obliquity parameter between the polar axis and a perpendicular to the plane of the ecliptic (40,000 years). Nevertheless, the astronomical account fails to provide any explanation for the rapid temperature changes which can occur over a single century or even in a matter of decades, as observed in ice core samples from Greenland (Dansgaard & Oeschger, 1989).

The ice ages were accompanied by changes in the atmospheric carbon dioxide concentration as can be measured in ice core samples. The concentration was lowest about 20,000 years ago and peaked during the Würm glaciation (of the order of 200 ppm). It began to rise in about 16,000 BC when the ice caps began to melt, eventually stabilising around 10,000 years ago. It then remained fairly constant (at about 275 ppm) until the Industrial Revolution in the middle of the 19th century. Since that time, it has been steadily rising to reach the current level of about 367 ppm, a 30% increase, and model-based predictions for the 21st century forecast considerable rises—to 540-970 ppm by 2100 according to the third Assessment Report of Working Group I (Scientific Bases) of the Intergovernmental Panel on Climate Change (IPCC) at the beginning of 2001.

Glaciation resulted in a drop in the sea-level corresponding to 120 metres 20,000 years ago all around the coastline of the ancient continent. This opened up passages between Asia and America, between the islands of Indonesia, the Philippines, and the western Pacific Ocean, and—closer to home—between the British islands and the European continent. This was the last great biogeographical remodelling event before the hand of man came into the picture (*Table I*).

Recent climatic changes in the Palaearctic Region

During the Würm glaciation, the temperature in Eurasia was 6-7 °C lower than it is now and only the southern regions were habitable.

As of 8,300 BC, temperatures approached current values (Dansgaard & Tauber, 1969) and most of the continent was ice-free.

Table I. Climate and malaria in Europe.			
Dates	**Glaciation, interglacial periods and humans**	**Temperature**	**Malaria**
60,000 BC	Riss glaciation, Neanderthals		
30,000 to 10,000 BC	Würm Glaciation appearance of modern humans Cro-magnon sea level: -120 m	8-10 °C lower than now	
10,000 to 8,000 BC	End of the Würm glaciation	Current temperatures	
8,000 to 6,000 BC	Post-glacial optimum	+ 2°C	
800 to 300 BC	Hellenic period	1-2°C cooler than now	Hippocrate describes *P. vivax* and *P. malariae* in Greece
300 BC to 500 AD	End of the classical period. Great invasions	Current temperatures	Appearance of *P. falciparum*. Worsening of malaria in Southern Europe
1,000 to 1,500 AD	Middle Ages	Warming	Malaria throughout the European Continent
1,500 to 1,700 AD	Renaissance	Little ice age. Lowest temperatures of the Christian Era	Zenith of malaria in continental Europe
1,700 to 1,850 AD	Industrial Revolution	Glaciers retract. Temperatures rising	Beginning of the spontaneous regression of malaria
1,850 to 1,950 AD	Industrial Era	Temperature stable, tending to rise	Malaria regressing apart from in the Mediterranean peninsulars
1,945 to 1,985 AD		Same trend	Malaria eradication in 1985
1,985 to 2,002 AD		Temperature rising over recent decades; global warming	No effect on malaria, already eradicated. Re-emergence events are not related to climate

Biodiversity of Malaria in the World

From 8,000 to 6,000 BC, the post-glacial optimum entailed a temperature (Dansgaard *et al.*, 1993) two degrees higher than now, evidence of a certain degree of climatic instability (Planton, 1999). After stabilising around the beginning of the Christian era, another climatic optimum occurred from 750 to 1,250 AD with considerable warming between the 11th and 12th centuries. Then, the small Ice Age occurred in the 16th and 17th centuries (Lamb, 1995), probably the coldest period since the end of the last real Ice Age, marked by the expansion of glaciers and ice caps: Inuit people even reached Scotland! Beginning in the mid-18th century, the climate was a little cooler than now (by about one degree) but there were considerable fluctuations. The glaciers (e.g. in the Alps) did not really begin to retract until 1850. As of that time, accurate data—from large-coverage measurement networks—make it possible to follow mean temperature changes to the present day. Over the last 140 years, the temperature has risen by 0.6 ± 0.2 °C, with particularly steep rises from 1910-1945 and since 1975 (Third IPCC Assessment Report). In the northern hemisphere, it is likely that the last decade was the hottest of the century, with the highest temperatures recorded since the beginning of accurate records (i.e. 1861) in 1998.

As of 8,000 years ago, climatic conditions in the Mediterranean Region, the Middle East and western European coastal zones were conducive to the transmission of malaria.

In the 5th century BC, the malaria described by Hippocrates in Greece was a mild disease likely caused by *P. vivax* or *P. malariae*. By the 2nd century AD, the situation had deteriorated in Rome where Celsus (translated 1935) described malignant tertian fever (likely *P. falciparum*). Historians of science (Grmek, 1994) believe that this deterioration was not due to climate change but to the introduction of new, more efficient vectors in the form of *An. labranchiae* in Italy and *An. sacharovi* in the Balkans. There is no concrete evidence that these two vectors were ever imported other than the arrival of *P. falciparum* and the spread of malaria, the incidence of which remained high in both regions until the end of the 19th century.

In the 17th century Ice Age—the most dramatic meteorological event of the Christian era—no decrease was observed in the incidence of malaria in Western Europe; in fact, "ague" was at its zenith in southern England at this time (Reiter, 2000).

However, as of the middle of the 18th century, malaria began spontaneously to regress—despite the rising temperature. This paradox is explained by improvements in standards of living and conditions, notably the removal of livestock from dwellings. This spontaneous regression continued until the disappearance of the disease in 1945 from all parts of the region apart from the Mediterranean peninsulars and the Soviet Union which saw the most savage pandemic in its history between 1929 and 1936 (which was not a result of climatic phenomena) (Lysenko & Kondrashin, 1999).

Recent climatic changes in the tropics

In contrast to the Holarctic Regions and the southernmost latitudes, **temperatures are conducive to the development of *Plasmodium* in all tropical regions**.

The Ice Ages which affected the middle and high latitudes had only limited effects in the high lands of Africa where glaciers covered 800 km^2 in East Africa (Ethiopia, Mounts Elgon and Kilimanjaro, Kenya, etc.) 15,000 years ago. Today, only 10 km^2 is ice-bound (Hastenrath, 1984) and this is shrinking rapidly. In the Andes and the Himalayas, glaciers are similarly receding (although all these are found well above the altitude at which malaria is transmitted).

At the peak of Würm glaciation, the level of the great Rift Lakes was relatively low and drainage was endoreic. With the subsequent warming, their levels rose, peaking between 10,000 and 8,000 BC (Butzer *et al.*, 1972).

Study of what has happened in the Sahara (in the broadest sense) over the last twenty millennia has revealed a whole series of alternating dry and wet periods. Palaeo-climatologists are beginning to get a better understanding of the chronology of these events but there are a number of special cases (the Atlantic coast, mountain massifs, river basins) which account for diverse climatic behaviour patterns in different regions and the absence of any overall synchronisation in wet and dry periods across this vast region (up until the last two millennia).

A prolonged arid period culminating around 18,000 BC—contemporary with the Würm glaciation—seems to have lasted up to the end of the Pleistocene (Ogolian period, Rognon, 1989). Temperatures must have been 3-4 °C lower than now and it was very windy. Sand drifts blocked great rivers like the Senegal and the Niger.

Towards the beginning of the Holocene (11,000 years ago in Mauritania, 9,000 years ago in Arabia), the region became wetter with rainfall spread throughout the year, and temperatures were lower than now (by about two degrees). Abundant traces bear witness to the density of human settlements in certain places and a Neolithic civilisation grew up around the banks of the Saharan Lakes that existed at that time. Many taxa with a Sudanese origin invaded the Sahelo-Sudanese Region, at least to the south of a line joining Aïr, Teneré and Tibesti. All the conditions for tropical malaria were fulfilled in places like Teneré in Niger. This was the period of the green Sahara, probably consisting of a mosaic of zones, some unconducive to life (e.g. regs, wind-polished gravel) and other more propitious savannah zones inhabited by large herbivorous animals (elephants, giraffes) as represented in contemporary cave paintings. After a minor dry phase between 7,500 and 6,500 BC, cattle-raising became common during a relatively wet phase characterised by a change in rainfall patterns (heavy rainfall with a long dry season) and temperatures higher than those of today. In Mauritania, the Nouakchott Lakes formed during a later localised wet phase (5,000-2,500 BC). However, as of 4,000-3,500 BC, creeping desertification began at certain points in the Sahara, eventually to create a **barrier between the Afrotropical Region and the Mediterranean**.

This barrier has separated and is still separating North Africa from the Afrotropical Region in many ways: in terms of flora, fauna and peoples as well as the epidemiology of malaria (which is generally stable and hyper- or holo-endemic south of the Sahara, and unstable and meso-endemic, hypo-endemic or epidemic to the north of it). *P. falciparum* dominates to the south (accounting for 80-95% of all cases), whereas *P. vivax* is or was the most common species in North Africa and Egypt. From the malaria point of view, there are two Africas: sub-Saharan Africa and Africa to the north of the desert—as is reflected in the biogeographical distinction made between the Palaearctic Region and the Afrotropical Region.

After the Saharan separation, Africa continued to cycle through dry and wet periods as reflected in the varying level of Lake Chad and, in the last century, as shown by measurements. From the 13th century on, we have the Arab chronicles, oral traditions and historical investigations on cultural practices (Olivry & Chastanet, 1986).

The evidence points to massive floods in the Chad Basin in the 17th century, and profound droughts in around 1680 and 1750 (Nicholson, 1980, 1981). Since the beginning of the 20th century, we have accurate measurements of rainfall and flow rates. For the Sahelian Region—one of the most closely studied—three dry periods have been identified (in 1913, 1940 and from 1970 to 1998) and two especially wet ones (1925-1935 and 1950-1965) (Mahé & Olivry, 1991). In the basin of the Senegal and the Middle Niger, 20% less rain fell in 1980-1990 than in 1951-1960. Further south, although the Guinean zone is wetter, severe droughts struck in 1972-1973 and 1983-1984. The surface area of Lake Chad shrunk from 23,000 km² in 1963 to just 2,000 km² in 1988. In general, sub-Saharan Africa has suffered the most dramatic reduction in precipitation anywhere in the world in the last thirty years (Hulme, 1999).

This has been reflected in the anopheline fauna and malaria transmission. One of the most important vectors, *An. funestus*, has disappeared from the Sahelian zone, and densities of *An. arabiensis* have significantly decreased. In consequence, malaria indicators have dropped by 60-80%, as has malaria incidence in northern Senegal and Niger (Faye *et al.*, 1995a; Mouchet *et al.*, 1996) (*Figure 2, Table II*).

West Africa and the Sahara serve as models to study the effects of climatic fluctuations on malaria. However, all tropical zones saw successive periods of dry and wet weather up until the 16th century, and this was reflected in the prevalence and incidence of malaria (apart from South America where there was no *P. falciparum* malaria before the 16th century).

In Southeast Asia and China, the chronicles are peppered with stories of famines following dry years and epidemics in wet years. Most of the tropical world has been affected by malaria but not to the same extent as tropical Africa in terms of either coverage or intensity. For example, in Southeast Asia, the disease, which is concentrated in the forests, has receded with deforestation and the development of rice-growing on the plains (*see the Chapter on the "Oriental Region"*).

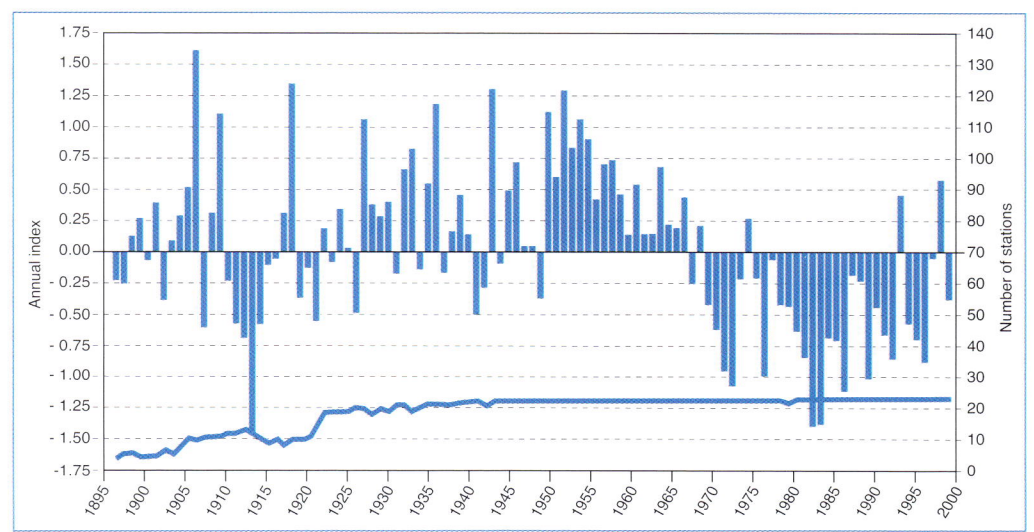

Figure 2.
Variation in a measure of rainfall in the Sahel (*top*) and the number of reporting stations (*bottom line*) (*adapted from* L'Hôte et al., 2002).

Biodiversity of Malaria in the World

Table II. Changes in the Saharan climate between 30,000 BC and 2,000 AD.

Geological period	Dates	Ecology	Sea-level	Country	Authors
Pleistocene	30,000 to 21,000 BC	Arid		Arabia	
	18,000 BC (max. Würm)		– 100 m	Gabon	Delibrius
	19,000 to 12,000 BC	Arid	– 120 m	Mauritania	Descamps
	11,000 to 8,000 BC	Humid		Mauritania	Descamps
Holocene	9,000 to 5,000 BC	Sahara green	Close to current level	Arabia - Ténéré	Mahé & Olivry, 1991
	7,500 to 6,500 BC	Short dry period			Maley, 1981
	5,000 to 2,500 BC	Humid period (Nouakchott lakes)		Mauritania (localised)	Nicholson, 1980
	4,000 to 3,500 BC	Beginning of desertification			
	2,500 BC	Saharan desertification to the present day			
Recent climatic events in the Saharo-Sahelian and Sahelo-Sudanese areas	5th-12th centuries	More humid than now	+10-20 cm	Sahel	Olivry & Chastanet, 1986
	13th century	Aridity of the Sahel			Mahé & Olivry, 1991
	14th-15th centuries	Improved weather			
	17th-18th centuries	Sahelian aridity and Sudanese humidity		Sahel and Sudanese zones	Nicholson, 1981
	19th century	Humid optimum		Sahel	
	20th century 1913, 1954 and 1968-2000	Dry periods		Sahel-Sudan	Olivry, 1993 Hulme, 1999 Sircoulon, 1990 IPCC, 2001
	1925-1935 and 1950-1968	Humid periods		Sahel-Sudan	

Global warming

The greenhouse effect induced by the gaseous envelope of the lower layers of the atmosphere is of itself a blessing since it maintains the earth's surface at a mean temperature of 15 °C (rather than –18 °C if there were no such effect). It is known that most of the solar energy received at the surface of the earth is delivered in the form of short-wavelength radiation. Part of this energy is reflected back in the form of long-wavelength infrared radiation which is absorbed by certain atmospheric molecules (notably carbon dioxide, methane, nitrous oxide and water vapour). The concept of Global Warming due to increased concentrations of greenhouse gases in the atmosphere goes back over one-hundred years (Svante Arrhenius in 1896). The hypothesis that the greenhouse effect may be potentiated by the burning of fossil fuels, deforestation and modern farming practices emerged in the 1930's (Houghton, 1995), and it was supported by evidence of the 30% increase in atmospheric carbon dioxide levels since 1850, a steady rise which has been followed by the Mauna Loa weather station in Hawaii since 1958. According to the Third Assessment Report of the IPCC, the current level is the highest in 420,000 years and in just 150 years, the concentration of methane has risen from 750-1,750 ppm, and that of nitrous oxide from 270-310 ppm.

The mean annual temperature of the planet has risen by 0.6 ± 0.2 °C in the last one-hundred years which can be divided into four distinct phases:
- moderate fluctuations between 1860 and 1910,
- a rise of 0.4 °C between 1910 and 1945,
- a significant drop between 1945 and 1975 (– 0.2 °C),
- followed since 1976 by a rise which gained pace in the last decade.

The drop observed over thirty years while CO_2 levels were continuing to rise lent support to the astronomical cycling theory of Milankovitch (1940) who predicted another ice age. This explained why most scientists at the First Global Climate Conference held at Geneva in 1979 believed that a period of cooling was coming. At the Second Conference just ten years later, the general opinion had reversed. Nevertheless, the first Assessment Report of the IPCC (published in 1992) remained cautious as to the confidence accorded to the results of climate modelling: a range of different scenarios resulted in predictions of temperature rises ranging from 1 °C to 3.5 °C by 2100.

In 1995, the Group's Second Assessment Report pointed more firmly to the probability of global warming and the results of the different model systems used were more consistent.

At the beginning of 2001, after a decade in which the seven hottest years recorded since 1861 had been seen, the IPCC's Third Assessment Report was far more affirmative as to the reality of global warming, predicting a rise of 1.5-6 °C by 2100, on the basis of simulations produced using far more robust models. Moreover, the causality of human activity was generally agreed upon.

The Report included the statement that "On average, between 1950 and 1993, night-time daily minimum air temperatures over land increased by about 0.2 °C per decade. This is about twice the rate of increase in daytime daily maximum air temperatures (0.1 °C per decade)".

The mean sea-level rose by 10-20 centimetres during the 20th century.

It is very likely that precipitation increased by a factor of 0.5-1% per decade during the 20th century in the middle and high latitudes of the northern hemisphere, and by 0.2-0.3% on land in the equatorial regions (between 10° north and 10° south). However, there is no evidence of increased rainfall in the Tropics over the last few decades and it is likely that the amount of rain in the continents between 10° and 30° north has been falling at a rate of 0.3% per decade.

No systematic changes have been detected in the southern hemisphere and the data are insufficient to allow any conclusions about rainfall on the oceans.

Ever since the issue of global warming became current, various groups of scientists—in particular epidemiologists—have been predicting the expansion of malaria to higher altitudes and greater latitudes on the basis of Macdonald's model, or others that similarly emphasise the importance of temperature.

Loevinshon (1994) reported the effect of global warming in Rwanda in a simple correlation between temperature variations over eight years and the numbers of hospitalised patients. This perhaps ignored the fact that the factors that determine the incidence of malaria are many, complex and continually changing.

In 2000, in a colloquium organised in Lausanne to discuss the factors that determine the incidence of malaria, it was concluded that global warming had not yet had any impact on the prevalence or incidence of malaria. Neither altitudinal nor latitudinal limits had changed in Africa, Asia or South America. Similar conclusions have been drawn by Mouchet & Manguin (1999) and, more recently by Hay et al. (2002a, 2002b).

The situation must nevertheless be very closely monitored, especially if higher temperatures are accompanied by increased rainfall.

This possibility will be addressed in the following paragraphs.

El Niño, La Niña and the ENSO

Many scientists have tried to discern periodic patterns in climatic variations and the outbreak of epidemics in order to make predictions. Sergent (1932) detected a twenty-year rhythm in malaria epidemics in Algeria but subsequent observations have not confirmed this hypothesis. Similarly, other experts believed that rainfall in West Africa was following a thirty-year cycle and predicted abundant rainfall towards the mid-1980's—in fact, the opposite was seen in the Sahel.

Climate works like a pendulum swinging to the alternating rhythms of cool and warm seasons in temperate zones, and dry and wet seasons in the tropics. Human life styles adapted to these patterns. However, sometimes the machinery is thrown out of equilibrium. The equatorial Pacific Ocean and the massive volume of air over it march to a different rhythm, upsetting the flora and fauna and, in consequence, the lives of the human beings who depend on that ecology. This far-reaching climatic event, the El Niño Southern Oscillation (ENSO) which arises irregularly, corresponds to westward air movements from the equatorial Pacific Region. Its magnitude is measured by the Southern Oscillation Index (SOI), the difference in pressure at Darwin in Australia and Tahiti. Because the Southern Oscillation is fairly closely linked to the El Niño phenomenon, the term El Niño Southern Oscillation is used to describe the phenomenon which combines the warming of the seas with the atmospheric shifts of air masses over the equatorial Pacific.

As soon as the mechanisms which trigger this phenomenon are first observed, a fairly accurate prediction can be made on how it will evolve and its impact. Models can be used to forecast several months of weather in the regions usually most affected, permitting appropriate action before devastating repercussions occur (including flooding and famine). However, such forecasts have limitations because no ENSO is ever exactly comparable to the previous one.

The El Niño phenomenon was named by fishermen in South America who had four hundreds of years noticed that, from time to time, the water along the equatorial coast was unusually warm as Christmas was approaching (el Niño referring to the Christ Child). The waters remained warm for months provoking a drastic drop in the numbers of fish caught (due to the absence of the key nutritional elements which depend on the cold waters of the Humbolt Current).

It was not until the 20th century that we began—through the work of Walker & de Bjerknes and later with data collected by international monitoring systems like TOGA (Tropical Ocean and Global Atmosphere)—to understand that this phenomenon involved the entire equatorial Pacific Ocean and that it had repercussions all over the planet (Voituriez & Jacques, 1999).

• In "normal" conditions, a vast zone of low pressure over Indonesia leads to heavy rainfall there, while a zone of high pressure extends over the eastern Pacific. The winds blow from east to west, pushing the warmer surface waters towards the centre of the Ocean and inducing the upwelling of colder water along the South American coastline where conditions are arid, precisely due to the presence of the cold Humbolt Current (*Figure 3*).

• In an El Niño (hot episode) year, the winds blow less strongly (or even change direction and blow the other way), and the above-mentioned zones of high and low pressure at the edges of the equatorial Pacific are inverted. Warm waters build up along the South American Pacific coastline bringing heavier-than-normal rainfall there, while in Indonesia and Australia, there is drought. These phenomena are also usually accompanied by failure of the Monsoon in India and Sri Lanka, and East Africa is deluged with abnormally heavy rain while the south of the continent experiences severe drought.

• La Niña—a cold episode—corresponds to the accentuation of normal conditions, i.e. the temperature of the surface water of the eastern Pacific is well below the normal. This explains why an El Niño episode is not necessarily followed by a La Niña one (which is therefore less frequent). In the La Niña situation, the winds blow more strongly leading to a more pronounced upwelling effect and the accumulation of hot water in the western Pacific. This results in heavy rainfall in India (the Monsoon) and southern Africa, and more or less normal rainfall in East Africa. Along the South American coastline, the cold ocean waters promote the subsidence of bodies of cold air and aridity predominates.

• The ENSO cycle has a periodicity of two to seven years with a mean of four; the true El Niño usually lasts 12-18 months but there is major variation from one episode to the next.

Since 1950, there were strong El Niño episodes in 1951-1952, 1965-1966, 1972-1973, followed by a stepped up rhythm in the 1980's and 1990's with episodes in 1982-1983, 1986-1987, 1991-1992, 1994-1995 and 1997-1998. In just fifteen years, the two most severe El Niño episodes of the century (1982-1983 and 1997-1998) were recorded and this period was also marked by practically continuous El Niño conditions between 1991 and 1995; this period featured three La Niña years (1984-1985, 1988-1989 and 1995-1996).

Global climatic effects of the El Niño (a hot episode)

The most deeply affected places are around the tropical Pacific Rim although the climate is modulated over much of the planet.

• During the winter months (October to March) in the northern hemisphere, El Niño causes heavy rainfall on the coasts of Peru and Ecuador, in southern Brazil, the south-eastern United States, the central Pacific and East Africa (from Somalia to Tanzania). In contrast, there is severe drought in Indonesia, the Philippines, New Guinea, northern Australia, north-eastern Brazil, and from Mozambique to South Africa. Higher-than-normal temperatures are seen in the maritime provinces of Canada, Alaska, Korea and Japan.

• During the summer months (April to September) in the northern hemisphere, heavy rainfall occurs in the central Pacific and the western United States while drought reigns in Indonesia, eastern Australia and, to a lesser extent Central America, Colombia and Venezuela as well as much of southern India and Sri Lanka.

An El Niño year is usually followed by a La Niña episode. In the Indian sub-continent therefore, drought is often followed by excessive rainfall (Bouma, 1995). However, the timing and intensity of La Niña episodes are not always understood.

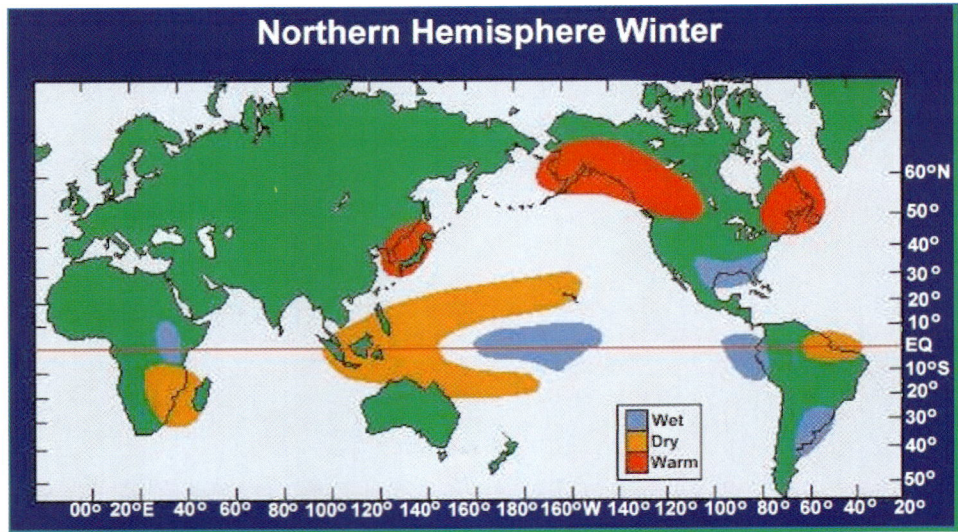

Figure 3. El Niño effects on temperature and precipitation (hhtp://nsipp.gsfc.nasa.gov/enso/primer/images/primer7.jpg)

Regional effects: the Sahel

It is not always easy to see a direct relationship between El Niño or La Niña episodes in the equatorial Pacific and rainfall in West Africa—the links can seem weak and some of the observations are contradictory (Janicot, 2000). Two periods can be singled out over the last fifty years. Between 1954 and 1973—a relatively wet period in the Sahel but progressing towards a drier phase—fluctuations in rainfall can be linked to surface water temperatures in the tropical Atlantic. But between 1970 and 1989—a period marked by persistent drought in the Sahel—this influence waned and certain inverse correlations begin to appear vis-à-vis the situation in the eastern Pacific. Since 1975, indicators have been steadily dropping in the Atlantic and significantly rising in the Pacific.

Regional effects: southern Africa

It has long been recognised that there exists a relationship between rainfall in southern Africa and the El Niño phenomenon. The impact is greatest in the middle of summer (January to March) in the south-east of the continent, although hot episodes are not always accompanied by reduced rainfall and the correlations do not seem to be stable over time. Ocean surface temperature (OST) plays a central role but a change is observed in abnormal temperature patterns in association with the droughts at the end of the 1960's. Up until this time, droughts in the south were linked to negative OST abnormalities in the Indian and Atlantic Oceans whereas, since 1970, it is hotter OST abnormalities in the east and central Pacific Ocean, the tropical Indian Ocean and the equatorial Atlantic Ocean which are involved (Trzaska, 2000).

The exceptional El Niño of 1997-1998

The global climate was profoundly marked by the exceptional development of this hot ENSO episode (WMO, 1998 and 1999; Ropelewski, 1999) which caused damage and loss of life on a massive scale (The El Niño Episode of 1997-1998: a scientific and technical review by the Special El Niño Inter-institutional Group, 1999). The Compendium of Climate Variability estimates that, in Africa alone, the episode led to 13,325 deaths, that the associated morbidity touched 107,300 people, and that 10 million people were displaced or otherwise adversely affected by the disastrous consequences of this phenomenon (although all these figures are of course compromised by the fragmentary nature and incompleteness of the underlying data).

Meteorological experts were closely monitoring the rapidly rising temperature of surface waters in the equatorial Pacific at the end of 1996 and the beginning of 1997 and it soon became clear that an exceptional hot episode was on its way. This El Niño really took off in March or April 1997 and grew rapidly over the following two months: during the last six months of the year, it was more intense than the episode of 1982-1983 with equatorial water temperatures off the South American coast being at least 5°C higher than normal between May and December. The effects continued to be felt through June and July of the next year, while surface water temperatures were plunging in the centre of the equatorial Pacific and a moderate La Niña phenomenon was developing. This extreme episode had a substantial impact on the mean global temperature, exacerbating the general trend towards warming. In 1997, the mean temperature was 0.43 °C higher than the terrestrial mean temperature recorded over the period 1961-1990; and the difference rose to 0.57 °C in 1998, the hottest year of the century.

Although no effect of global warming on malaria incidence has been observed yet, the ENSO is known to have had major epidemiological consequences—and often dramatic ones—as discussed throughout the Part on the "Epidemiological Biogeography of Malaria". In Pakistan, Bouma (1995) observed that prior to 1945 (when indoor spraying begun), most of the epidemics in the Indus Valley occurred during wet periods (probably due to La Niña) following dry El Niño years. On the other hand, in Sri Lanka, epidemics were seen in dry El Niño years because the local vector, *An. culicifacies* species E was able to develop in water residual pools generated when rivers stopped flowing. The cessation of vector control measures can result in epidemics.

In Vietnam (Shapira, 2002), the 1997 drought caused by El Niño decimated crops and drove farmers into the jungle for food where they were exposed to malaria infection by *An. minimus*, thereby creating a dangerous situation. At the same time, forest fires caused an ecological catastrophe.

In East Africa, the 1997-1998 ENSO episode caused catastrophic flooding and led to a devastating malaria epidemic in southern Somalia and Ethiopia as well as north-eastern Kenya, the effects of which were felt as far away as Uganda (*see the Part on* "Epidemiological Biogeography of Malaria").

In southern Africa, many of the epidemics that were common before the widespread implementation of vector control measures seem to have been related to El Niño.

Climate and other factors that affect malaria

The study of variations in the incidence of malaria linked to climate changes over the course of human history is a fascinating subject but, most importantly, it shows how plastic the situation is. It is all the more difficult to predict how the incidence of the disease will be affected by global warming since, above and beyond meteorological phenomena, it is vital to take into account ongoing anthropogenic modifications of the environment as well as human efforts to combat the disease.

Anthropogenic Changes of the Environment and Malaria

Different stages of demographic and technological development

As discussed above, **modern humans** (*Homo sapiens sapiens*) appeared on earth relatively recently, sometime between 50,000 and 100,000 years ago.

Human beings—hunter-gatherers integrated into their ecosystems as either predators or herbivores—were sparse; it is estimated that there were no more than 250,000 on the planet at the end of the Würm Ice Age 10,000 years ago (Lutz, 2002).

The Neolithic Revolution occurred between 10,000 and 7,000 years ago, when hunter-gatherers began to overcome the restrictions of their natural environment by cultivating food plants and domesticating certain types of animal. To protect themselves against their enemies (often other groups of humans) and enhance their productivity, they banded together in organised settlements near their fields. The first towns grew up in Mesopotamia about 7,000 years ago.

The role played by the concentration of people in the installation and spread of malaria has already been discussed (Fenner, 1970).

From the Neolithic Revolution on, the human population of the planet has steadily expanded. The figure of one billion was reached by 1750 and two-hundred-and-fifty years later, in 2000, the threshold of six billion was passed; the population of the world had more than doubled between 1950 and 2000.

The scientific and industrial revolutions

By the end of the 18th century, humans had explored most of the surface of the planet; in 1850, geographical knowledge was sufficient to warrant the conclusion that malaria was present wherever the conditions were conducive for transmission (Hackett *in* Boyd, 1949). This date marks the high (or low) point of the disease's geographical coverage.

The succession of scientific discoveries which marked the end of the 19th and beginning of the 20th centuries led to major improvements in sanitary practices and medicine, entailing a substantial reduction in infant mortality and increased life expectancy, both of which contributed to exponential population growth.

Less technologically developed countries were the last to benefit from such improvements in public health, and the imbalance between rich and poor countries is still enormous. The story of malaria and malaria control is an instance: after a period of regression between 1960 and 1975, the disease has increased in the years since, largely due to economic problems.

Population growth and technological progress have had significant impact on the environment. More land has had to be turned over to arable farming to feed a growing population, and increased productivity has in turn promoted population growth. New fields have been created at the expense of primary natural land by the clearance of trees, the conversion of natural grasslands, the drainage of marshes, slash and burn cultivation etc.

Water requirements for arable farming have led to modification of waterways across the planet, with the construction of dams and/or reservoirs to supply irrigated land. Irrigation was first developed four thousand years ago in the so-called Fertile Crescent, and it has since been massively expanded all over the Earth, notably with the creation of rice paddies, rice being the staple diet of one-third of all human beings.

The appropriation of arable land has been accompanied by improvements in farming practices and in the crops themselves. The Green Revolution of the 1960's in combination with progress in the field of genetics provided farmers with new, highly productive varieties. The development and distribution of genetically modified organisms (GMO) is a controversial topic in both philosophical and scientific terms. The new varieties are often susceptible to pests and many have nutritional requirements which are quite different from those of the indigenous plants, necessitating the use of pesticides and fertilisers which pollute the environment and may threaten the health of humans and animals. Nitrates are making water undrinkable, not only in the industrialised countries but also in some parts of the southern hemisphere where intensive agriculture is practised. Uncontrolled large scale use of pesticides in agriculture is selecting for insects that are resistant to DDT, pyrethroids and other insecticides, thereby compromising control efforts, including those targeting *Anopheles* in some countries (Corbel *et al.*, 2007; Asidi *et al.*, 2005; Weill *et al.*, 2003).

There are lively debates about the pros and cons of intensive animal husbandry—not to mention cloning—but this is beyond the scope of this book.

Finally, urban development, the whole scale of which underwent a massive change in the last century, is modifying the geographical distribution of human beings, concentrating them in agglomerations of ever-increasing size. Already, more than half the world's population lives in cities.

It seems likely that there have been more environmental changes in the last fifty or one-hundred years than since the beginning of humanity. The main factors which affect the epidemiology of malaria are:
- the modification of vegetation;
- interference with surface water;
- changing farming methods and agrochemical pollution;
- galloping urbanisation.

Changes in vegetation

Deforestation

Forests and forest-dwellers

The move from the dark, highly compartmentalised and three-dimensional forest environment to the wide-open, sunny and two-dimensional world of the savannah or steppe represents a major ecological change. For anophelines, this underlies the segregation of forest and savannah species which have completely different larval habitats, e.g. the contrast between members of the *An. dirus* Complex in Southeast Asia which rarely leave the jungle, and sun-loving *An. gambiae s.l.* in Africa which does not breed in the shade of trees.

But forests are encroached upon by villages, fields and roads, which allows sun-loving species like *An. gambiae s.s.* in Africa to thrive in villages in the forest zone. Similarly, species associated with the forest (members of the *An. dirus* and *An. minimus* Complexes) can be found in villages far from the actual forest. When talking about forest anophelines or malaria as defined in Southeast Asia or Africa, it is important to stipulate whether the place in question is in the true forest or simply wooded.

For a long time, the forest was home to only sparsely distributed populations of hunter-gatherers who were well integrated into their environment, e.g. the Pygmies of Central Africa, Amerindians in the Amazon, the Oran Asli of Malaysia, Dayaks in Borneo, and the indigenous peoples of the Philippines and New Guinea.

Later, tribal people expelled by the Indo-Europeans in India (the tribal peoples) or by various invaders in China and Southeast Asia (the so-called ethnic minorities) fled into the forest, a difficult, uncovetted environment that provides a natural refuge. In such relatively hostile environments, many such peoples are obliged to carry out slash-and-burn agriculture, a practice which is inefficient and ecologically disastrous.

In Southeast Asia, inhabitants of the forest and its edges were and still are at high risk of contracting malaria because of the presence of efficient vectors such as *An. minimus s.l.* and *An. dirus s.l.* in Indochina, and *An. fluviatilis* S in India (*see the Chapter on the* "Oriental Region"). Many experts (Perry, 1914) have proposed that the presence of vectors prevents incursions by non-immune intruders. In Thailand (Somboon *et al.*, 1998), the incidence of malaria among villagers who spend part of the year in crop huts around the edges of the forest is far higher than among those who spend all their time in the forest village itself.

In the central African forest in Cameroon, the prevalence of malaria drops with the degree of isolation of the village and the number of man-made larval habitats (along footpaths, in ruts on roads, at mining sites, etc.) suitable for the development of *An. gambiae s.s.* ("Forest" form). It has been said that malaria is linked to human activities that create sunny larval habitats (Livadas *et al.*, 1958).

Among Pygmies who live inside or at the edges of the forest, vectors used to be rare and the prevalence of malaria was very low in Cameroon (Languillon *et al.*, 1955), in the Central African Republic (Carnevale, personal observation), and in the Ituri forest of the Congo (Schwetz *et al.*, 1934).

In the Amazon, malaria (essentially due to *P. vivax*) did not pose a major problem among Amerindians, most of whom lived on the banks of the river (*see the Chapter on the* "American Regions").

Exploitation of forest

In the second half of the 20th century and at an accelerated pace in the last twenty-five years, the forest has become a highly lucrative resource for wood to be used in the construction and paper-making industries, as well as for its potential as farming land. How it is exploited in Asia and South America has evolved, from the selective felling of only the most valuable trees in the 1950's to indiscriminate clearance by 2000.

In Asia, lumberjacking is generally a temporary activity practised by migrant workers from the cities or the over-populated plains. These "seasonal" workers from malaria-free zones have no immunity at all and often fall victim to the disease when they come into direct contact with vectors. In response to the adverse ecological impact of deforestation, most countries in the region have imposed restrictions. In Vietnam, Cambodia and Thailand, jungle work used to be considered as being at the root of most cases of severe malaria transmitted by *An. dirus s.l.*, a forest mosquito.

In Africa, most woodcutters come and stay in endemic zones and are solidly immunologically protected.

Up until 1975 in the Amazon, the population was very sparsely distributed, Amerindians and the inhabitants of a few commercial and administrative centres were, for the most part, located along rivers. After the construction of transamazonian roads through the forest, there were massive migrations to make the most of these "new lands", a movement which was supported by government subsidies (*see the Chapter on the* "American Regions"). Millions of people participated in the felling of the forest, especially in the western States (Rondônia, Pará, Roraima, Acre) which are referred to as "legal Amazonia". This migration continued until 1991 when doubts began to surface about the viability and sustainability of the new colonies and the subsidies expired. Clearance was focused along the major roads and involved two distinct phases: a pioneer phase during which migrants lived in open huts with only the most rudimentary health care services, followed by the construction of more permanent dwellings within estates and villages with improved sanitation and health coverage.

Malaria was most serious during the pioneer phase. Clearance created ideal conditions for vectors, notably *An. darlingi* in streams with floating debris. Once the new population had stabilised somewhat, the number of cases began to drop and, even more importantly, patient care improved. Between 1980 and 1990, almost 90% of malaria cases in Brazil were notified in Amazonia. In addition, infected migrants re-migrated to other places (Marques, 1986, 1987).

Similar population displacements into the Amazon Basin were seen in Bolivia, Peru and Colombia. The problems of Amazonian malaria were discussed in the Chapter on the "American Regions".

Destruction of the forest

Complete levelling is the end point of the destruction of the forest ecosystem. As villages grow and the fields surrounding them spread, the site loses its forest character.

In West and Central Africa, the forest has given way to post-forest facies, comprising patches of woodlands in vast expanses of savannah, the latter constantly expanding with exploitation of the local environment. The proliferation of *An. gambiae s.s.* (and *An. funestus* in some places) leads to the establishment of generalised holo-endemic malaria with the number of infective bites rising to 300-1,000 per person per annum and transmission all the year long (Carnevale, 1979; Trape & Zoulani, 1987a).

In Southeast Asia, the term "forest malaria" is used to describe the epidemiological entity seen in the forest setting, taking into account its exploitation. The situation is currently evolving with intensive forest exploitation, e.g. its levelling in Thailand and Vietnam. In contrast, rubber plantations have created neo-forest facies in which *An. dirus s.l.* develops. In the aftermath of this deforestation, the kinds of measures that were recommended by Phan (1991) and McArthur (1947)—designed to control *An. dirus s.l.* around villages in cleared forest land—now seem irrelevant. In levelled areas, species of the Maculatus Complex (*An. maculatus, An. pseudowillmori, An. sawadwongporni*) have been confirmed as vectors in Thailand (Harbach *et al.*, 1987b).

Damaged herbaceous strata

Forest is not the only threatened setting. In the savannah, regular bush fires result in leaching of the top soil leading, in the most extreme case, to ecological desertification. Madagascar's other name, the "Red Island", derives from the stripping of the top soil which has rendered much of the High Plateaux unfarmable; these days, life is focused around rice paddies in the valleys.

Two recent phenomena deserve special notice: over-grazing in dry regions and the draining of wetlands.

Over-grazing of dry pastureland

In the arid zones south of the Sahara and Kalahari Deserts, the traditional activity is livestock raising. The boring of wells has made it possible to increase herd sizes, sometimes beyond what the region's ecology can support. During droughts, starving animals gather around wells and pack the surrounding ground down with their hooves. When the rains eventually arrive, the water soaks in more slowly, leaving puddles which provide ideal larval habitats for *An. arabiensis*; related outbreaks of malaria among unprotected or inadequately immune populations were recorded in 1988 in Botswana and the Sahel, and then again in Botswana in 1997 (Samba, 1997).

Draining wetlands

In the mountains of Central Africa (Rwanda, Burundi, Uganda, Kenya), the valley bottoms used to be home to vast stands of papyrus. These plants secrete an essential oil which forms a film over the water surface which impedes the development of mosquito larvae (McCrae, 1975). The only anophelines found in these high lands (1,500-2,000 m) were *An. chrystii, An. cinereus* and *An. marshalli* which did not transmit malaria.

After 1945, to reclaim this land, the papyrus was destroyed, and the valley bottoms drained to create basins and fields for fish farms and food crops. These depressions were then invaded by malaria vectors, first *An. funestus* (Jadin & Fain,

1949) and more recently *An. gambiae s.s.* (Mouchet *et al.*, 1998; White, 1972). The latter species is confined to villages close to the valley bottom but its vectorial capacity is remarkably high.

Mention was made above of the disappearance of *An. funestus* following the drought in West Africa. This occurred in two phases in the Niayes in Senegal (Faye *et al.*, 1995a). At the height of the drought, the anophelines (notably *An. funestus*) disappeared; to make the most of the persistent humidity in the depressions, local farmers pulled up the aquatic vegetation and planted food crops. In subsequent rainy periods, without the shelter afforded by the reed stands, *An. funestus* never came back (although it did in irrigated areas).

In Bangladesh, marshlands in which the local malarial vector *An. philippinensis* (or *An. nivipes*) develops, were converted into rice paddies which are suitable for the development of *An. aconitus* (Elias *et al.*, 1983; Maheswary *et al.*, 1992); whether or not this species transmits malaria in this area is not yet known.

There is now a popular movement to protect wetlands: it is important to be careful that such well-intentioned actions to preserve the environment do not have any negative effects on vector-borne diseases.

Interference with surface water

Bore holes

In dry places, modern technology makes it possible to dig deep wells reaching all the way down to fossil freshwater pools. These vary in volume but none are of infinite capacity. This brings freshwater into regions where hitherto the mineral content of the surface water precluded the development of freshwater species, e.g. in the Republic of Djibouti between 1905 and 1975, there was no indigenous malaria because conditions were hostile for anophelines of the *An. gambiae* Complex (Courtois & Mouchet, 1970); after 1975 however, malaria became endemic throughout the territory with the proliferation of *An. arabiensis* in many water pools and even in relatively shallow bore holes (Rodhain *et al.*, 1977). The reasons for this change are not really known but the influx of fresh well water may have been involved in the invasion of a desert region by this vector

The drilling of deep wells in Fezzan, Libya has not yet had any epidemiological impact, the most common anopheline being *An. multicolor* which does not transmit malaria.

Cisterns and wells

In some places where the ground is particularly permeable to water, like in Grande Comore, there are few surface water places and, therefore, there is little if any malaria. Widespread cistern construction in the 1920's led to the installation of *An. gambiae s.s.*, which caused a terrible malaria epidemic from 1920 to 1923 (Raynal, 1928). Since then, malaria remained meso- or hyperendemic throughout the island even though, with an effective water supply system having been constructed, many of the cisterns are now disaffected (Blanchy *et al.*, 1987, 1999).

In Somalia, half-buried cisterns (Haud Tanks) in the northern provinces are used by *An. arabiensis* (Alio *et al.*, 1985; Choumara, 1961). Basins which catch rain water in homes in the arid south of Madagascar were suspected of providing larval habitats for *An. arabiensis* and these structures have been replaced by larger-capacity, communal reservoirs which are less favourable for anopheline development.

Wells are only propitious for *Anopheles* if they are shallow and exposed to the sun (at least, according to most of the studies on this subject). In Indian towns, especially in the south, wells—along with domestic water tanks and cisterns—provide larval habitats for *An. stephensi* and *An. subpictus*; the former causes urban malaria. In northern Vietnam, larvae of *An. minimus s.s.* develop in domestic cisterns which is quite unusual for this running water mosquito, and in Myanmar, *An. dirus s.l.* has been found in city cisterns (*see the Chapter on the* "Oriental Region").

Interestingly, *An. culicifacies* A is found in cisterns in Assab in the Eritrean desert, the only place in Africa where this Asian anopheline is found.

Dams and watering basins

Small earth dams for village use have been constructed all over the world, especially in dry regions where they provide water reserves for local people, livestock and, possibly, watering plants. In North Africa, high densities of *An. labranchiae* in these dams have not yet caused the re-emergence of malaria in either Tunisia (Bouchité *et al.*, 1991) or Morocco where the disease has greatly decreased.

In West Africa, ground around wells which has been packed down by the hooves of animals provides ideal larval habitats for members of the *An. gambiae* Complex, and the same is probably true throughout most of the Afrotropical Region, notably in Swaziland (Mouchet, 1987) where wells provide the water used on sugar cane plantations. However, since the incidence of malaria is already very high in these endemic regions, this factor has no particular impact on the disease.

In urban settings such as Pikine in Senegal (Vercruysse & Janclos, 1981), Ouagadougou in Burkina Faso (Rossi *et al.*, 1986), Niamey in Niger (Julvez *et al.*, 1997a), and Bouaké in Ivory Coast (Tia *et al.*, 2006), watering holes for gardens provide sites for the larval habitats and dispersion of urban anophelines.

When it comes to big dams which retain huge volumes of water, only the edges where the level varies with the season, provide larval habitats for *Anopheles*. In different ecological zones in Africa, *An. arabiensis* and/or *An. gambiae s.s.* breed there; *An. funestus* is confined to places with abundant standing vegetation, e.g. reed beds. Apart from Lake Nasser in Egypt and Sudan, most of the great dams of the Afrotropical Region are found in places where malaria is stable (the Kariba Dam on the Zambesi, the Volta Lake in Ghana, the Senna Dam in Sudan) so their presence does not affect the prevalence of the disease. Many of the studies which have been carried out lack both clear results and solid conclusions.

In Brazil and Surinam, it was expected that *An. darlingi* would take hold once waters built up behind the Tucuaru and Brokopondo Dams; in fact, it was *An. nuneztovari* which developed, apparently without any epidemiological consequences (Panday, 1977).

In Turkey, the proliferation of *An. sacharovi* around dams on the Euphrates probably played a role in the re-emergence of malaria (Clarke, 1984; Mather & That, 1984).

In the Indochina and Malaysia Peninsular, no significant vectors are found around dams. In South India, the situation is less clear: species of the *An. culicifacies* Complex seem to develop in the agricultural lands of Tamil Nadu. In Vietnam and Laos, dam construction has not had any direct effects but it has forced the displacement of villages closer to the highly endemic forest, resulting in a high malarial toll. In the Vientiane Province in Laos, such displacements have had significant health repercussions (Pholsena, 2001, personal communication).

Irrigation ditches and irrigated land

Most treatises on the subject have addressed the anopheline faunas of irrigation ditches and irrigated land together. On the High Plateaux of Madagascar, it was believed that *An. funestus* mainly developed in irrigation ditches rather than in the actual rice paddies until Marrama (1999) convincingly proved the contrary, i.e. that this vector actually develops on the irrigated land itself.

In the Southern Chinese province of Guangdong, *An. anthropophagus* (synonymy with *An. lesteri*), an efficient, anthropophilic vector, mainly develops in the ditches whereas *An. sinensis*, a poor, zoophilic vector, is found in the actual paddies (Li Zu Zi, 1992, personal communication).

In Java in Indonesia, *An. aconitus* colonises both types of water habitats but prefers stagnant, obstructed channels (Sundararaman *et al.*, 1957). The same is true of *An. gambiae s.s.* in West Africa (Robert *et al.*, 1988b), and probably for many other species, the ecology of which has not yet been thoroughly studied.

Rice paddies

Rice paddies account for most of the irrigated land in the tropics, and their surface area is growing in response to increased food needs. This intensive, high-yield crop requires heavy labour—which is amply available in the southern hemisphere.

Ecological conditions in a rice paddy evolve with the growth of the crop, from the nursery stage through planting out, seeding, growth, maturation, harvesting and fallowing (Marrama *et al.*, 1999). During the first three stages, the flooded, sun-exposed rice paddy is propitious for sun-loving species whereas shade-loving species which seek standing vegetation prefer the next three; conditions in the fallowing stage are intermediate between the two. In consequence, different species are successively favoured, the details depending on the biogeographical region, altitude, salinity and cultivation methods. The health risk represented by rice paddies will depend on the exact species that develop there as well as the local epidemiological conditions and history.

In Southeast Asia—in the Indochina, Malaysia and the Philippines—, the incidence of malaria is not linked with rice paddies. The major vectors—the *An. minimus* and *An. flavirostris* Complexes which develop in slow running water, and the *An. dirus* and *An. balabacensis* Complexes which prefer pools at the edges of the forest—do not like irrigated surfaces. This is why the "healthy" rice-growing plains are contrasted with the malaria-ridden forest (*see the Chapter on the* "Oriental Region"). Of course, many anopheline species breed in rice fields, including *An. culicifacies* B, *An. sinensis, An. subpictus, An. tessellatus*, but these are predominantly zoophilic and are therefore not infected. A few exceptions warrant mention, notably an epidemic due to *P. vivax* being transmitted by *An. subpictus* in the Red River Delta in Vietnam, as well as a few cases of the same origin in the Mekong Delta (Phan, 1998). Cases reported in Laos close to rice paddies inside a forest zone might well have been due to forest species as well as the vector suspected at the time, *An. nivipes* (Kobayashi *et al.*, 2000). In Indonesia, Sumatra, Java and Bali, *An. aconitus* is considered as the most widespread vector, mainly spreading *P. vivax; An. sundaicus* which develops in brackish water (i.e. not irrigation water), transmits *P. falciparum* more efficiently.

In China and Korea, *P. vivax* malaria transmitted by *An. sinensis* in rice paddies used to extend up as far as Amour. After its eradication from Korea, it re-emerged in both North and South Korea (Feighner *et al.*, 1998; Kondrashin, 2000) although the reasons are not fully understood.

South of the 32nd parallel in China, *An. sinensis* and *An. anthropophagus* (synonymy with *An. lesteri*) transmit only *P. vivax*. Periodically interrupted irrigation in rice paddies, where human fertiliser is used, has been considered to control mosquitoes (Lu Bao Lin, 1984) but this does not seem to have gone beyond the experimental phase.

In India, *An. culicifacies* A seems to be well installed in development projects in Tamil Nadu.

In north-eastern Afghanistan (around Kunduz), the creation of rice paddies has been blamed for malaria. The two vectors, *An. hyrcanus* and *An. pulcherrimus*, are both only moderately efficient but they are completely exophilic and difficult to control (Anufrieva *et al.*, 1977; Onori *et al.*,

1975) by means of indoor spraying; while larvivorous fish do not seem to have been very effective either.

In Turkey, *An. sacharovi* proliferates on all irrigated land, both in the European part and the Asian part of the country, particularly in the agricultural development regions of Adana and the Higher Euphrates, projects which are considered to have been responsible for the massive come back of malaria in Turkey.

In Spain, rice-growing was banned by the Catholic Kings in the 17th century because it was associated with fever (Najera, 1999).

Prior to 1940 in Portugal, the proliferation of *An. atroparvus* in rice paddies coupled with a worsening malaria situation led the authorities to try intermittent irrigation (Hill & Cambournac, 1941). In France, there is no malaria in the rice paddies of the Camargue where the main anopheline is *An. hyrcanus*.

In the Afrotropical Region, anophelines of the *An. gambiae* Complex, *An. funestus* and *An. pharoensis*, are the most important vectors found in rice fields.

On brackish land in the Senegal River Delta, species belonging to the Gambiae Complex were always found (*An. arabiensis*) but only at low densities. In contrast, *An. pharoensis* numbers were very high; although they were positive for CSP, the transmission rate was low, as in neighbouring regions (Faye *et al.*, 1995c).

In the Kou Valley in Burkina Faso, the "Mopti" form of *An. gambiae s.s.* is more or less the only vector. This mosquito seems like an efficient vector in laboratory conditions and is associated, in the Niger loop, with meso- or hypo-endemic malaria. In the above-mentioned Kou Region, transmission rates were seven times lower than in villages of rainy season cultivation in which the vector was the "Savanna" cytotype of *An. gambiae s.s.* Nevertheless, malaria was holo-endemic and stable, as throughout the entire Sudanese Region.

The rice paddy vector was *An. arabiensis* in the valley of the Logone and the Benoué in northern Cameroon (Robert *et al.*, 1985), on the Kenyan Plateau, at Kisumu (Highton *et al.*, 1979) and in the Rusizi Valley in Burundi (Coosemans, 1985); in the first two, where malaria was already holo-endemic, neither its prevalence nor its incidence changed, but in the hypo-endemic Rusizi Region, the introduction of rice-growing triggered a sharp increase in the disease's incidence—in contrast to the low endemicity seen in the rest of the valley where crops were grown only during the rainy season (Coosemans, 1985).

In the Sudanese part of Ivory Coast where malaria is stable and holo-endemic, rice-growing has not fundamentally changed the prevalence or incidence of the disease which is transmitted by the "Savanna" form of *An. gambiae s.s.* (Carnevale *et al.*, 1999).

Compared with the continent, a quite different picture is seen in Madagascar: on the plateaux, the introduction of irrigation for rice-growing caused endemic malaria in regions that had been considered as "healthy" up until 1860 (the date of the first high-altitude epidemic). The vector is *An. funestus*; the zoophilic *An. arabiensis* plays no more than an accessory role. At medium altitudes (800-900 m) around Lake Alaotra and along the west coast—both regions of intensive rice growing—*An. arabiensis* seems to play a more important part (Laventure *et al.*, 1995).

In the Americas, although rice growing is becoming more common, it nevertheless remains limited in scope. In Guyana, *An. aquasalis*—which is zoophilic and a very inefficient vector—dominated the rice fields created by immigrants from India. It is possible that the situation changed with the mechanisation of cultivation, which entailed the banishment of buffaloes driving *An. aquasalis* towards more anthropophilic habits, although this information is probably out of date (Giglioli, 1964) and needs re-investigation. In the Peruvian Amazon (Iquitos), rice-growing resulted in an increase in *An. darlingi* densities.

This review of the place of rice paddies in malarial epidemiology shows the extreme diversity of outcomes, highlighting the problem of trying to make generalisations about different parts of the world (or even different regions).

Cultivation and animal husbandry

Arable farming

The change to modern cultivation methods has had little direct effect on malaria. The effects on rice paddy anophelines of intermittent or interrupted irrigation were discussed above.

However, farming is using ever-increasing amounts of fertiliser and pesticides to enhance yields and protect crops against pests. This is the price to be paid for growing higher-yield (and often more fastidious) varieties. Pesticides used in the growing of cotton and, to a lesser extent, of rice, have been involved in the selection of most of the strains of *Anopheles* that are resistant to DDT, pyrethroids, organic phosphates and carbamates (Corbel *et al.*, 2007). It is believed that the selection pressure is expressed on larvae developing in ruts in the ground or along the edges of cotton fields. Selection is constant in these fields which are treated up to thirty times a year (in the rainy season). This is the mechanism believed to underlie the resistance of *An. gambiae s.s.* in West Africa, *An. culicifacies* A in the Middle East, *An. sachavori* in Greece and Turkey, and *An. albimanus* in Central America (Georghiou, 1982; Ramsdale *et al.*, 1980; Subbarao, 1988; Tia *et al.*, 2006).

DDT resistance can be mediated enzymatically—through oxidase activities—or physiologically by means of the modification of a sodium channel so that the pesticide can no longer reach the insect's nervous centres where it is active, a mechanism which is dependent on the *kdr* (knock-down resistance) gene. The same gene also confers pyrethroid resistance (which can similarly be also mediated enzymatically by oxidases).

In West Africa, pyrethroid-resistant *An. gambiae s.s.* have been found in regions where this family of insecticides had never been used for the purposes of public health (Elissa *et al.*, 1994); this is the case of a *kdr* cross-resistance to DDT and pyrethroids due to leucine-phenylalanine substitution at position 1014 of the voltage-gated sodium channel (Chandre *et al.*, 1999).

In East Africa, a similar *kdr* cross-resistance to DDT/pyrethroids was found in Kenyan *An. gambiae* populations with an alternative substitution (leucine to serine) at the same position 1014 (Ranson *et al.*, 2000).

In South Africa and Mozambique, the pyrethroid resistance of *An. funestus* is mediated by elevated levels of oxidases conferring also cross-resistance to the carbamate insecticide propoxur (Brooke *et al.*, 2001). However, the resistant populations are still susceptible to DDT. The lack of cross-resistance between pyrethroids and DDT suggests that a *kdr*-type target site resistance mechanism has not been selected (Casimiro *et al.*, 2006). These observations draw attention to how important it is to define the resistance mechanism in order to establish control measures which will be both effective and will inhibit the development of further resistance.

Mechanisms underlying resistance to organophosphate insecticides have been extensively described in *An. albimanus* in Central America (Georghiou, 1982; Penilla *et al.*, 1998). In Sudan, *An. arabiensis* resistance to malathion is due to a decarboxyesterase which acts on the pesticide's side-chains.

Resistance to dieldrin appeared soon after the first use of the product in West Africa, first in *An. gambiae*, then *An. funestus*, and later in most anopheline species; this led to the complete abandonment of this excellent insecticide. It does not seem to have been generated as a result of agricultural use but rather as a direct effect of public health measures (Hamon & Garrett-Jones, 1963; WHO, 1981a). There is cross-resistance between dieldrin and the more recently developed fipronil.

Two stories illustrate the role played by farming in the development of resistance:
- in Turkey, *An. hyrcanus*, a non-vector species which does not enter houses, is as resistant to DDT as the anthropophilic, endophilic *An. sachavori*; both these species develop in rice paddies and around cotton plantations;
- inversely, in Thailand where the whole country has been covered by indoor DDT spraying operations for the last thirty years, *An. minimus s.l.* (a running water mosquito) and *An. dirus s.l.* (a forest mosquito) are still susceptible to the insecticide. No cotton is grown in Thailand and, by virtue of their ecological and behavioural characteristics, neither species ever comes into direct contact with agricultural insecticides (Mouchet, 1988).

Throughout the history of "eradication", the local development of resistance (especially to DDT) was accompanied by the recrudescence of malaria. The effects of the various instances of resistance need to be evaluated and weighed up because they have not always led to the complete cessation of treatment operations. In this context, it is important to remember that, in addition to its direct toxic effects, DDT also acts as a repellent. Much has been written about the avoidance of treated surfaces and the rapid flight from treated houses (be it before or after feeding). A long time ago, Zulueta (1959) observed that, despite resistance, DDT was still an effective way of controlling malaria. More recently, Roberts *et al.* (2002b) came to the same conclusion which led to re-evaluation of this product in malaria control.

In India and Salvador, Chapin & Wasserstrom (1981) claimed that the increased use of pesticides in the context of the Green Revolution had exacerbated resistance, leading to a dramatic return of malaria. Sharma & Mehrotra (1983) eventually concluded that the rise in malarial incidence was due to the discontinuation of spraying operations at the end of the eradication programme—and nothing to do with the Green Revolution or anopheline insecticide resistance.

Over the last thirty years, vector resistance has become a media topic. It is a real issue of great concern for malaria control but it is important not to let this become an excuse for abandoning measures to target vectors.

Livestock raising

Where malaria is concerned, livestock—in particular cattle and horses—play an ambivalent role. On the one hand, they can maintain high anopheline densities by providing food for them but on the other hand, they may attract mosquitoes away from human beings. The balance between these two sides will depend on the feeding preferences of the local anopheline species or forms, environmental conditions and the epidemiological context.

Distinction can be made between:
- anthropophilic species and forms which feed almost exclusively on humans, such as *An. gambiae s.s.* ("Forest" form) in the Cameroon forest where there are neither cattle nor horses (because of the presence of tsetse flies). In Indochina, *An. minimus* mainly bites humans despite the presence of animals as does *An. darlingi* in South America, at least up until the development of extensive animal husbandry. Because their behaviour takes them into houses, these highly efficient malarial vectors have proved very vulnerable to indoor spraying in Cameroon (Livadas *et al.*, 1958), in the Indochina (Phan, 1998; Vien *et al.*, 1992) and in the Amazon (Roberts *et al.*, 2002b), in all of which cases, control measures have seen remarkable success with eradication not far from being achieved;
- amphophilic species and forms, that is those which feed indiscriminately on both humans and animals (according

to Roubaud's expression), with high vectorial capacity, have been studied in the wet African savannah. Their response to insecticide treatment has been considered one of the main causes for continued transmission in spite of house spraying. Since they do not have to enter houses to maintain their biological cycle, anopheline densities remain high immediately following treatment, and later they are able to enter the houses as the activity of the insecticide on the walls begins to wane (Cavalié & Mouchet, 1962). This is the case with *An. gambiae s.s.* and *An. arabiensis* in the West African savannahs (Carnevale & Mouchet, 1990);

- mainly zoophilic species—poor vectors because of their preference for animals—have been used for the purposes of prevention: interposing livestock between the larval habitats and human dwellings attracts mosquitoes away from human hosts. This type of zooprophylaxis has been used in Europe against species belonging to the *An. maculipennis* Group but its efficacy has never been evaluated.

Living together with or close to more zoophilic species has been considered a factor which favours transmission. In Madagascar, it was thought that stabling livestock on the ground floor of dwellings (as protection against theft) amplified the 1986 epidemic in places where *An. arabiensis* was practically the only vector (Mouchet *et al.*, 1997).

In Europe, improved living conditions, and the separation of stabling facilities, were considered as essential factors underlying the spontaneous disappearance of malaria on the continent (Bruce-Chwatt & Zulueta, 1980).

The sudden disappearance of livestock can alter the behaviour of anophelines which are then obliged to feed on human beings, thereby potentiating their vectorial capacity. After 1921 in the Soviet Union, famine drove the people to consume all their livestock and species like *An. messae* (normally a very inefficient vector) were transmitting malaria as far up as the Arctic Circle (cases of *P. falciparum* malaria were recorded at Archangel). It seems clear that the decimation of livestock was a key element in the great pandemic that ravaged this country up until 1935, causing nine million cases of malaria per annum (Bruce-Chwatt & Zulueta, 1980; Lysenko & Kondrashin, 1999).

It is important to remain cautious about changes in vector feeding preferences and their epidemiological impact because the extent to which samples collected in the course of surveys are representative of the various anopheline populations as a whole is often uncertain.

Habitat, Urbanisation and Professional Activities

Habitat

Habitat and dwellings

By the 5th century BC, Hippocrates was already advising that villages to be constructed far from marshland, to prevent fever and splenomegaly. This advice was followed to a variable extent in Europe where members of the Maculipennis Group depend on the presence of stagnant water habitats. As far as we know, the choice of where to settle was conditioned as much by the desire to avoid being bitten by mosquitoes as the need to avoid fever, the link between *Anopheles* and malaria not being established until the end of the 19th century (Ross, 1897).

In many parts of the world, malaria-ridden zones are associated with taboos, e.g. in the malaria-free Bafoussam Region of Cameroon at an altitude of 1,200-1,500 m, it used to be taboo to spend the night in the lower Noun Valley (500 m) where malaria was indeed hyperendemic (Mouchet & Gariou, 1960); and in South China, spending the night in the "dragon-infested" forest was believed to be dangerous; the forest was also infested with the malarial vectors *An. minimus* and *An. dirus*. Whether or not all such taboos are indeed associated with "fever" is always uncertain—they could well have other origins.

In South Africa, the Boers associated the presence of the "fever tree" (*Acacia xantholacca*) with malaria. In Europe, the existence of "unhealthy" places was recognised in Italy (the Pontine Marshes, Sardinia), France (Dombes, Camargue, the east coast of Corsica, the marshes of the Vendée), Holland (the Zeeland Polders), Germany (western Freesia), Greece, Albania, etc. People continued living in these malarial foci—where life expectancy seems to have been very low—until the 19th century, defenceless but unable to move to a healthier place. Malaria was simply part of daily life.

In holo-endemic regions of Africa, malaria is a component of the environment. Every inhabitant is permanently infected from the day they are born to the day they die, and survival depends on acquired immunity. The risk can be considered as omnipresent and permanent in places where malaria is stable (Mouchet & Carnevale, 1998).

Many people do not choose their habitat. It is often imposed on them by invasion—so they have had to adapt to life in places where they can get by. This is so with the tribal peoples of India, and the ethnic minorities of China, Indochina and Indonesia. Driven up into the mountains or other hostile habitats, they experience a far higher prevalence of malaria than the majority population but they resist the disease far better. It has long been said that malaria "protected" these people against the incursions of their neighbours (Perry, 1914) although this is a somewhat simplistic view.

Many farmers in Africa, Southeast Asia, and Central and South America have secondary dwellings near their fields, usually rudimentary huts designed to afford basic protection against bad weather. These are often located in dangerous, high-transmission zones, e.g. in Thailand (Somboon *et al.*, 1998) and Vietnam (Marchand *et al.*, 1997) as well as many other places. Huts of "farmers' malaria" are often difficult to monitor and pose a problem for control operations, as has been seen in many programmes, e.g. in Cameroon (Livadas *et al.*, 1958) and Burkina Faso (Choumara *et al.*, 1959).

In Irian Jaya (now called Western New Guinea), Indonesia, Javanese immigrants coming from a place where the prevalence of malaria is low fall victim to severe malaria but, within two years, they have acquired a solid immunity to the local parasites, showing that humans can adapt rapidly to a new environment (Baird *et al.*, 1999).

Building houses

Dwellings are designed and constructed according to materials available: thatch, wood, clay, stone, corrugated iron, etc. With increasing levels of development, simple wall-less shelters—such as Amerindian dwellings in the Amazon and crop huts in Southeast Asia—are replaced with enclosed buildings, perhaps with more than one room, coated walls, a separate kitchen, and removed from stabling facilities. Solidly constructed houses with roofs made of corrugated iron or tiles are becoming more and more common in the southern hemisphere.

No building is ever truly mosquito-proof, even houses with air-conditioning and insect screens over all the openings (which are difficult to maintain). Personally, I have never seen a genuinely mosquito-proof house in over fifty years in endemic zones (Mouchet, personal observation). However, the risk of occupants being bitten does depend on the construction of the dwellings although no correlation has ever been established between level of exposure and the incidence of malaria among the occupants; in practice, the degree of correlation varies a great deal, being more dependent on the distance between the dwelling and the larval habitats than on structural considerations.

Anopheles can find larval habitats inside houses. In Mauritius, *An. arabiensis* develops in accumulations of rain water on the terraced roofs (Gopaul & Konfortion, 1988). The role of cisterns, wells and other types of reservoir inside homes has already been discussed in detail, mainly in the context of urban malaria in India.

The building of mud huts necessitates the creation of holes which are among the most productive larval habitats for members of the Gambiae Complex throughout the whole Afrotropical Region. The same type of hole is created when materials are extracted to construct roads and tracks. When towns are being built, e.g. Brazzaville, excavation work leads to major outbreaks of malaria; such outbreaks are often misleadingly referred to as urban malaria although the situation returns to normal once the construction work is over (Trape & Zoulani, 1987b). In Madagascar, it has been suggested that the massive construction works undertaken to build religious edifices in the middle of the 19th century led to a massive rise in the numbers of *Anopheles* at the same time as infected workers were brought onto the Plateaux from the malaria-infested west coast (Raison, 1984), leading to the introduction of malaria in 1879 into areas which had hitherto been free of the disease. Without detracting from the significance of this coincidence of circumstances, it is nevertheless important to bear in mind that this first epidemic was also associated with the introduction of irrigated rice-growing, and that the timing of the outbreaks is more consistent with the vector having been *An. funestus* which is almost exclusively associated with rice paddies (Laventure *et al.*, 1996), rather than *An. arabiensis*, the species which is more likely to develop on construction sites.

Urbanisation

Urban development is a major social phenomenon which has followed the population growth of the 20th century. While population growth as a whole was 3% in the southern hemisphere, the growth rate in towns was 6% (and reached 9% in some African countries). This was not associated with an decrease in the rural population (which has remained fairly stable). More than half of humanity already lives in towns containing more than 5,000 inhabitants; various projections are predicting that the percentage will reach 70% by the year 2020 (Lutz, 2002).

Different experts define towns in different ways, using variously architectural, economic or sociological criteria. In this book, we will first address anopheline ecology in the urban setting and repercussions thereof on the transmission of malaria. The importation of parasites by immigrants from rural areas is but a side issue since transmission will only be sustained if potential vectors are present *in situ*.

A town is located within the territory of an ecosystem defined by a specific fauna, flora and environment, in other words a certain biogeographical setting. A great part of this territory is occupied by man-made structures—housing, storage facilities, roads and tracks, sewers, etc. The primary fauna of the ecosystem, including *Anopheles*, is more or less assimilated into the urban matrix, depending on its nature. As a general rule, *Anopheles* numbers decline as one moves from the suburbs towards the centre of town, as the density of infrastructure increases and clean surface waters are replaced by polluted waste water, the latter being unsuitable to anopheline larvae. In parallel, a specific fauna becomes established within and around buildings—quite distinct from that in surrounding rural areas.

Distinctions are therefore made between urban malaria, urbanised malaria and malaria-free agglomerations.

Urban malaria

The term urban malaria was first used in the early 20th century by Christophers (1931) who was working in Madras, in a classic study of Indian malaria epidemiology. The subject was taken up by many scientists in various Indian cities, including Salem, Bangalore, Calcutta and Bombay (*see the Chapter on the* "Oriental Region"). The parasite is transmitted by *An. stephensi* which develops in water deposits and cisterns inside houses and sometimes, in wells. It is often accompanied by *An. subpictus* which does not seem to transmit malaria (or at least, not efficiently) (Das *et al.*, 1979).

To date, strictly urban malaria has only been seen in South India. The most remarkable feature of this epidemiological entity is the **absence of malaria from surrounding rural areas**.

Urbanised malaria

We use this term to describe malaria transmitted in an urban setting by anophelines that are also found in the surrounding, malaria-infested rural environment. It is different from the above-described urban malaria in that there is continuity between the rural and urban settings.

In the Afrotropical Region, urbanised malaria is usually transmitted by species belonging to the *An. gambiae* Complex, namely *An. arabiensis* in dry places and *An. gambiae s.s.* in wetter and forest regions, thus following the general distribution of these species, although there is the interesting exception of *An. arabiensis* being found in towns of the Nigerian forest, notably Benin City (Coluzzi *et al.*, 1979).

Vector numbers again drop going from the outskirts towards the centre and the number of bites falls as the density of the urban matrix increases. At Bobo-Dioulasso in Burkina Faso, the number of infective bites delivered by *An. gambiae s.s.* per person per year was 350 in outlying villages, 4.6 in the suburbs and 0.4 in the middle of town (Robert *et al.*, 1986). The prevalence of malaria of 65-90% in the countryside dropped to 21-48% in the town centre (Gazin *et al.*, 1987). In the Congo, the same radial pattern *vis-à-vis* vector numbers and malarial prevalence has been documented in Brazzaville (Trape & Zoulani, 1987c). At Cotonou—which has grown up on an offshore bank—transmission was intense throughout the entire city (Chippaux *et al.*, 1991a).

A second centre for the urban anophelines dispersion is constituted by water pools found within the town's limits. The density of *Anopheles* decreases in Niamey with distance from the River Niger and permanent watering pools (Julvez *et al.*, 1997a), and at Ouagadougou in Burkina Faso, with the distance from reservoirs (Sabatinelli *et al.*, 1986b). At Pikine in the dry part of Senegal, watering pools constitute dispersion points for malaria infection (Trape *et al.*, 1992; Vercruysse & Jancloes, 1981).

In town, the number of possible larval habitats is lower than in the countryside because of the presence of buildings and water pollution. But ever-increasing numbers of towns are expanding to absorb surrounding villages, between which household gardens are set up, even small rice paddies as in Bouaké in Ivory Coast. Where exactly the town finishes can become very vague—and the prevalence of malaria in the outskirts can approach that in the surrounding countryside (Dossou-Yovo *et al.*, 1998a).

Unusually, *An. funestus*—a species not considered at all as urban—is found in the suburbs of Yaoundé (Manga *et al.*, 1997b).

In Brazil, Manaus is encroaching further and further into the jungle (or rather what remains of the jungle), and *An. darlingi* is now found in the suburbs.

At Buenaventura on the Pacific Coast of Colombia, the disease was transmitted by *An. albimanus*, but only in the suburbs (*see the Chapter on the* "American Regions").

At Gurgaon in North India, a few *An. culicifacies* have been found in the suburbs, breeding in natural sites; *An. stephensi* was found in the same place but this species was developing in man-made cisterns and wells (*see the Chapter on the* "Oriental Region").

In towns, the sheer density of the population means that the risk—associated with a finite number of *Anopheles* larval habitats—is shared between a greater number of individuals (each of whom is bitten less often), so the personal risk is reduced.

Malaria-free towns

There is no malaria in many towns located in endemic areas. In the Indochina, in Malaysia, Indonesia and the Philippines, towns were considered to be healthy and were not treated during the eradication period. The same was true in the Mediterranean Basin, the Middle East and the Americas. The anophelines there, although often abundant, were not vectors, e.g. *An. subpictus* at Jakarta in Indonesia, *An. aquasalis* in Cayenne in French Guiana, and *An. vagus* in the cities of North India. In the **urban setting**, it is important **not to confuse the presence of *Anopheles*** (or other culicines) **with that of malaria**.

Although the risk of malaria in towns should not be understated, the problem should not be exaggerated either, given the reduced incidence there as well as the easy access to treatment. Endemic malaria remains essentially a rural problem.

Excavation work

Excavation work is not exclusively involved in the construction of buildings; it is also undertaken in the contexts of road-building and mining.

Roads require materials taken from holes which remain along the constructed road and provide suitable larval habitats for mosquitoes, initially without any vegetation and later with standing plants. On the island of Mayotte in the Indian Ocean, *An. gambiae s.s.* larval habitats created along newly-built roads triggered the re-emergence of malaria in 1981 (Julvez *et al.*, 1987).

Ruts along tracks in the Cameroon forest provide important larval habitats for *An. gambiae s.s.*—sometimes the only ones they use (Livadas *et al.*, 1958); simply reworking a track can eliminate *Anopheles* from villages in the vicinity.

The opening up of new roads across the Amazon has been blamed for the recrudescence of malaria in the area; in point of fact, deforestation and the establishment of settlements along the road were probably more often responsible than the construction work itself.

Gold and gemstone mines use huge volumes of water to wash the precious ore or stones. In and around mines in Africa, this creates a plethora of highly productive larval habitats for anophelines of the *An. gambiae* Complex. In a gold-diggers' camp in the heart of the Cameroon forest near Batouri, there can be several thousand *An. gambiae* per hut, which is exceptional in the forest environment (Mouchet, personal observation). At Kanungu in the Ugandan mountains where illegal gold-digging is practised, local people used to work at night-time, thereby directly exposing themselves outside to anophelines that were breeding in the ore extraction pits. This occurred at the altitude limit of transmission and people who stayed inside at night were hardly ever infected.

In Brazil, *An. darlingi* develops in the immense pits that are dug by gold-hunting garimpeiros in several Amazonian States, especially Pará. Miners sleeping in the most rudimentary shelters are heavily exposed but the owners or managers of mines administer chloroquine (or other prophylactic drugs) at the first sign of malaria, so the disease does not usually have serious consequences.

In the jungle in the Southeast Asian mountains, gemstone hunters from town fall victim to severe malaria. Excavation work is not the problem here with transmission mediated by *An. dirus s.l.* and *An. minimus s.l.*, which are abundant throughout the dense forest cover.

The Role of Humans in the Dispersal of Malaria and its Vectors

Humans are found in all habitable parts of the planet, but each anopheline species is only found over a defined geographic region. We are fairly knowledgeable about the geographic distribution of each species, even each different form. The range is the result of an evolutionary process of adaptation to environmental factors—some of which we do not understand. By changing local ecology, man has sometimes affected anopheline distribution although he has not altered the major patterns. Nevertheless, he has sometimes transported species far from their place of origin to places where they have found conditions conducive to sustained development.

These are the two themes, the spread of parasites and the introduction of vectors by human beings, which constitute the basis of this chapter, with special emphasis on the epidemiological consequences that are the fundamental subject of this book.

Spread of the parasites and the disease

Great historical migration events

Population displacements at the dawn of humanity

Ever since their appearance on earth, human beings have continually expanded their territory. *Homo erectus* left its African birthplace and arrived in China and Indonesia although it later disappeared from those places, as Neanderthals later disappeared from Europe, western Asia and North Africa.

Homo sapiens sapiens—modern man—first appeared at most 100,000 years ago, during the Upper Pleistocene, almost certainly in East Africa (Coppens & Picq, 2001).

The new arrival was soon occupying all available spaces. There are traces of his passage in the Fertile Crescent in the Middle East, from where he spread across Europe to the west, and into Asia to the east and thence to America via the Behring Straits and Australia by way of the Sunda Islands.

This gradual occupation of the planet involved successive migrations over relatively small distances (given the limited means of transport at man's disposal).

Beginning with the Neolithic revolution in the prehistoric period, more or less structured groups migrated further to flee enemies or natural catastrophes (e.g. earthquakes, volcanoes, drought or locusts) or in the search for new lands (which were often already occupied). We can only speculate about malaria in this period but this revolution would certainly have created more favourable conditions for the establishment of the disease which could then have been spread by migrants from original foci. This does not rule out the possibility that parasites were already present in small groups of hunter-gatherers.

Successive migrations have occurred throughout five or six thousand years of our history. Without attempting a comprehensive list, we will address certain events that might have helped determine the geography of malaria up until 1850 (Hackett, 1949).

Migrations in the Afrotropical Region

East and South Africa were occupied by the Koi-San or San peoples (Bochimans, Hottentots and their relatives), traces of which are believed to have been found at Oldoway in Tanzania. These were not of Melano-African origin and their descendants (numbering about 50,000) are found in the Kalahari Desert and its surroundings in Namibia, Botswana and the Republic of South Africa, as well as in small groups in Tanzania (the Hamza); these people carry the Duffy+ antigen and are susceptible to all human malaria parasites.

The territories of the Koi-san shrunk with expansion of the Bantus and other Melano-African peoples coming from either Bar el Ghazal or the Bénoué (in Nigeria and Cameroon) according to different experts (Cornevin, 1963). They steadily spread through eastern and southern Africa—more *via* a process of gradual expansion than by means of organised invasions, although some groups such as the Zulu might have been warriors. It is believed that the Digoya reached the Transvaal in the 16th century, the Zulu reached Natal in about 1670, and the Herero reached Namibia around 1700. The Kikuyu were already in Kenya by about 1550 but the Gulf of Guinea was not reached until the end of the 18th century. All these dates are approximate, and are often contested by linguists. What is of relevance to malaria is the genetic status of these Bantus who, like all Melano-Africans, do not have the Duffy antigen and are therefore refractory to infection by *P. vivax*. In addition, when they grow up and live with hyper- or holo-endemic malaria, they seem to be remarkably well adapted to *P. falciparum*, surviving in the presence of this potentially deadly parasite as shown by the high proportion (over 90%) of symptomless carriers. In such regions, these people constitute important "parasite reservoirs". Bantus are associated with stable malaria in the Afrotropical Region. It is interesting to wonder whether their genetic make-up might not have given them some advantage over the Koi-San, although it has to be borne in mind that, being able to work iron, they already had some degree of technological superiority. The Bantu migrations constitute one of the major events in the last two thousand years of history in Africa.

The Pygmies are people of small stature of diverse ethnic origins who live in the equatorial forest and surrounding lands. It seems that they are the descendants of a large number of groups who used to live on savannah land (Tikar in Cameroon); in this context, the myth of dwarf peoples is present in many cultures. None of the Pygmy groups that have been studied possess the Duffy antigen, so they are refractory to *P. vivax* infection like Melano-Africans. Differential malarial prevalences, such as those documented in Cameroon (Languillon *et al.*, 1956) and in the Central African Republic, are due to differences in their forest habitats which dictate the extent to which they are exposed to vectors. African Pygmies are unrelated to peoples of small stature found in the Andaman Islands, Borneo and the Philippines.

The populations of West Africa and the Upper Nile region have been substantially modified by migrations although this has not affected the epidemiology of malaria in these places where the disease is stable and holo-endemic.

It seems likely that malaria would have restricted Moroccan expansion south of the Sahara as well as the activities of Yemenites on the Ethiopian High Lands, although historians prefer to focus on wars and political aspects rather than questions of epidemiology. Nevertheless, these mostly immunologically naïve people would not have been able to escape malaria when they were expanding into endemic zones.

Migrations in Southeast Asia

In India, Indo-Europeans—who call themselves Aryans—came from the Iranian and Afghani Plateaux in the second millennium BC, and introduced Hinduism and the caste system. They intermixed with the aboriginal people (especially in the southern Deccan), but excluded all who failed to accept their social and religious system. The many animist "tribal" groups of the Deccan, Madya Pradesh and north-eastern States lost their social status and were relegated to deep poverty. It is these people who are today malaria's main victims although they are significantly more resistant to the disease than the Hindu majority. The same pattern is seen in Nepal. Many of these marginalised people are conducting a guerrilla war in the north-eastern States of India.

In the 10th century, Burmese and Thai people chased out of China by the Mongols descended on the plains of Myanmar (former Burma), Thailand and Laos, pushing out—often without a fight—Shang, Karen, Meo, Li and Lao-Teung peoples. The Vietnamese (Khins), originally from the plain of the Red River, gradually conquered the whole of Vietnam. All over ethnic minorities were pushed back into malaria-infested jungle areas as the so-called ethnic majorities—the Burmese, the Thais and Lao-Thais, and the Khin, occupied the fertile, malaria-free plains. On the island of Hainan in China, the same separation is seen between the Han (i.e. the Chinese) in the healthy rice paddies of the north, and the Li in the malaria-ridden mountains in the south. This partition between rich (and often over-populated) plains and malaria-infested highlands dominates the epidemiology of malaria in Southeast Asia.

In addition to the above-mentioned instances, the same pattern is seen in Cambodia, Malaysia, Borneo and the Philippines although in these places, some ethnic groups have almost disappeared.

These disparities are the final outcome of various migration processes—both peaceful and bloody—which have created a mosaic of high-risk and healthy areas.

Arrival of Europeans and the slaves in the Americas

The arrival of Europeans in America and the importation of slaves from Africa is the beginning of a migratory process uninterrupted to this day. Many experts think that the pre-Colombian peoples did not know malaria (Boyd, 1930) although others believe that *P. malariae* and possibly *P. vivax* were already present before the arrival of the Spanish, especially in Peru where hyperendemic foci of *P. malariae* persist in the absence of *P. falciparum* (Sulzer *et al.*, 1975). But everyone agrees that *P. falciparum* arrived in the Americas as a result of the slave trade (Gabaldon, 1949a).

Recent and ongoing migration events

Reasons for population shifts

Migrations can be classified on the basis of:
- duration, i.e. whether they are temporary, seasonal or permanent;
- distance: within the same region or country, to a foreign country, transcontinental;
- reasons: a search for arable land or work, tourism, pilgrimages (Kondrashin & Orlov, 1985).

Whatever the classification system used, dichotomies cannot be avoided, e.g. work may be sought close to home or in a foreign country, possibly on a seasonal basis or the stay may last a matter of years. Rather than trying to apply some rigid system, we will review some of the most common migratory scenarios.

Rural exodus

Today's most widespread migration is from the countryside to town. The concentration of people in urban agglomerations has led to the phenomenon of urban malaria (as discussed in the preceding chapter). The new arrivals often maintain close links with their villages of origin and congregate in specific neighbourhoods. Within a limited urban space, a mosaic of different epidemiological pictures can be seen, depending on the topography and geography of the different neighbourhoods and differential vector densities; this has been studied in depth in Brazzaville (Trape & Zoulani, 1987c), Khartoum (El Sayed *et al.*, 2000) and Kinshasa (Coene, 1993; Mulumba *et al.*, 1994).

Quest for arable land

In response to population growth, finding fresh arable land has become a priority for many communities. In Southeast Asia, clearing the surrounding jungle is often one of the only options for minority people. In the Andes, especially in Bolivia, closure of the metal mines pushed Aymara and Quetchua people onto the Andean foothills and into the Amazon Basin. These people, who did not change country, maintain close links with their villages of origin on the Altiplano. In Brazil, it is farmers from the northeast and southeast who are felling the Amazon jungle, and the same phenomenon is happening in Peru and Colombia. In Burkina Faso in Africa, the peaceful Mossi people are clearing the rest of the country and Ivory Coast. In Cameroon, the Bamiléké in the western mountains have made exploited most of the west of the country. In Indonesia, Javanese people are settling in Western New Guinea, Kalimantan and Sulawesi.

The new arrivals may settle permanently on the new land or just work it for a few years. Temporary occupation can have disastrous environmental impact with destroyed vegetation not necessarily ever coming back (as is the case with the Mossi in Ivory Coast). More and more countries are trying to control migration in the context of organised development projects with integrated health care and financial aid, e.g. the Indonesian Transmigration Programme in Western New Guinea (former Irian Jaya). Many rice-growing development projects arose in West Africa. The settlement of Hmongs from Laos in French Guiana was successful as they have found their place in society within just twenty-five years.

A comprehensive list of migrations in search of arable or grazing land would be extremely long. We have chosen to highlight a few examples which have had obvious epidemiological repercussions. In Brazil, resettlement programmes have triggered a resurgence of malaria which, up until then, had been on the way to eradication. In Ivory Coast where malaria is stable and holo-endemic, the epidemiological situation of migrants has not changed compared to local ethnies. In Western New Guinea, the incidence of malaria is far higher in Javanese immigrants than it is in the indigenous population.

Refugees and people who have been displaced within their own country of birth

In 1994, it was estimated that 20 million refugees were living outside of their own country and 25 million had been displaced within their own country, a total of 45 million people, i.e. 6‰ of the world's population.

Distinction is often made between **economic refugees** fleeing from natural catastrophes (drought, flooding, etc.) who tend to return in their country of origin, and **political refugees** who have been forced out of their country or region by oppression, in the broadest sense of the word; the latter include many **political prisoners** who are often being kept in very harsh conditions—a kind of suspended death sentence.

Most refugees have been grouped together in camps, either in their country or in a neighbouring one. Many are assisted by international non-governmental organisations and/or charities that help them survive and usually provide very basic medical care, particularly antimalaria drugs (Luxemburger *et al.*, 1996).

Economic refugees usually return home once the climatic abnormality has passed, e.g. once the floods have receded. But prolonged drought—like the one that has been affecting the Sahel since 1973—can have irreversible consequences: in Niger, a significant proportion of the Tuaregs—who lost their livestock which is their livelihood—have settled around the capital Niamey where they are homeless and unemployed.

Political refugees are condemned to exile for as long as the relevant political situation persists. In Cambodia, most of the refugees who had fled to camps on the Thai border returned home after the defeat of the Khmer Rouge but many Karen people from the Thai-Burmese border region were still living in refugee camps in Thailand in 1999, since there had been no political settlement.

After the genocide of the Tutsi in Rwanda, people who were believed to be responsible for the tragedy fled to camps in the Democratic Republic of Congo, and their future remains precarious.

Refugees are completely dependent on political events and/or climatic conditions. The ever-changing situation is closely monitored by United Nations institutions UNHCR which can give details on the current problems.

Malaria is not necessarily a major problem for refugees who have usually fairly good access to antimalarial drugs in the camps.

Temporary, seasonal and long-term migrants

This section deals with all who move to improve their economic situation by finding work—be it temporary or permanent and close or far from their place of origin, they are called "economic migrants".

Nomads who move with their herds seeking new pastures now represent an archaic social system. Although they are still numerous on the southern and northern reaches of the Sahara, in Somalia and Iran as well as, to a lesser extent, in Afghanistan and Pakistan, they are tending to settle down. These permanent migrants are somewhat difficult to classify although their movements are clearly undertaken for economic reasons. These people are often exposed to epidemic malaria and their isolation complicates treatment. Malaria control among nomads has been the subject of numerous studies, particularly in Iran (Manouchehri *et al.*, 1992).

Workers from developing countries settle for highly variable stays in foreign countries, especially in Europe, the Persian Gulf and North America. This constitutes a mass migration involving many tens of millions of people. Many of these "immigrant workers" maintain close links with their home country and send money back to keep their families going, although they are increasingly tending to seek to settle permanently in their new home where living standards are higher. The influx of labour—which is essential for industrialised societies—is usually organised by the destination country.

Temporary agricultural labourers (working on rice farms, tea and rubber plantations) constitute large populations in countries of the South, e.g. between the Adana and Upper Euphrates Regions of Turkey, there are more than a million seasonal workers. These labourers are often poorly paid, poorly accommodated and without adequate medical protection. They tend to be all the poorer since they are sending part of their wages back home to look after the family. Most seasonal workers remain in their country of birth or seek work in neighbouring countries. In Turkey, they represent most of the victims of malaria, as is the case in India, although there the authorities remain more discreet.

Forestry—practised on an individual basis or by companies—is a high-malaria-risk enterprise in Southeast Asia, in Malaysia and Indonesia (*see the Chapter on the* "Oriental Region").

The mining of gemstones in Southeast Asia and South America, diamonds in Africa and South America, and gold in the Americas and Africa, is poorly supervised with individuals working alone or alongside company employees, depending on the methods used. These are rootless people seeking immediate profit—often without hope of success. They are highly exposed to malaria.

Fishing is often seasonal and usually the prerogative of particular ethnic groups such as the Bozo in the Niger loop. Auxiliary activities include drying and selling. In a dam lake located in a place where malaria had disappeared thirty years beforehand in Zimbabwe, night time poaching led to a localised epidemic among young adults (Mouchet, personal observation, *see the Chapter on the* "Afrotropical Region"). In the Amazonian Basin, fishing is a community activity to produce food for immediate consumption and its epidemiological impact is minimal.

Hunting and poaching are killing off big game animals which are now only found in national parks and reserves in large parts of Africa, Asia and even America; this does not have any direct epidemiological impact but safari tourism, especially to Kruger National Park in South Africa, gives rise to thousands of cases of malaria every year (*see the Chapter on the* "Afrotropical Region").

Travellers

Since Ulysses took twenty years to get back to Ithaca, the duration of most voyages has considerably shortened. Sailing is now only a recreational activity and the salt caravans of Taoudenni (Mali) and Bilma (Niger) are well on the way to becoming relics of the past. Almost all boats are used for cargo while road and air transport are shrinking distances to the extent that a parasite or a vector can cross the globe in less than 48 hours.

Travelling may be for reasons of work, religion (pilgrimage) or pleasure (tourism). The boom in intercontinental travel has given rise to a new speciality, travel medicine. This discipline assumes a preventive mission, informing travellers about the health risks in the country to be visited and advising prophylactic modalities. It also aims to inform the authorities in the destination country and at home about how to treat diseases that tourists might contract.

Risks associated with migration

Migration is associated with two types of risk—that run by the migrants themselves and that incurred in the host country.

Risks to the migrants

The degree of risk will depend on origin and destination.

For those from malaria-free places

Most foreign aid workers and tourists come from industrialised countries in the northern hemisphere (North America, Europe, northern Asia) or the far south (Australia, New Zealand, countries of the South American Cone) and are a high-risk group *par excellence*; these are the primary target of travel medicine. The risk run varies enormously according to whether the traveller is heading for a town or the countryside, how he or she will be living, and where he or she will be staying.

The consequences when mountain-dwellers descend from a malaria-free environment onto infested plains have been well documented in Ethiopia (Gebre Mariam, 1988; Teklehaimamot, 1994) and in the Andean foothills (in Bolivia, Peru and Colombia). These population movements are usually staggered and do not trigger sudden epidemics, e.g. during the steady emigration of Bamiléké people from western Cameroon to the holo-endemic south-western part of the country, they never seemed more vulnerable than the indigenous population.

In contrast, massive, sudden population shifts—be they organised or not—have often led to epidemics as occurred during the emigration of Javanese people to Irian Jaya (now called Western New Guinea) and Borneo in Indonesia (Baird et al., 1993), and the moves of mountain-dwellers down into the Awash Valley and Gambella Region in Ethiopia (Kloos, 1990; Gebre Mariam, 1988).

The malaria risk associated with resettlement programmes based in endemic zones will be all the greater if the settlers come from malaria-free places (Roundy, 1985), be it in Asia, Africa or the Americas (e.g. Brazil).

More insidious is the risk run by people from malaria-free enclaves within endemic zones who move to a place where the disease is highly endemic; this scenario has been seen over many years in the Indochina, and malaria has been known among seasonal tea pickers in Darjeeling, India, for sixty years (Gilroy, 1939).

For those from malaria-endemic places

When moving into a malaria-free area, the immigrants are free of any risk of malaria. Most infections—symptomatic or not—resolve spontaneously.

In endemic regions, immunologic status varies significantly with the transmission rate. If the migrant comes from a region where the epidemiological picture resembles that at the destination, the risk is not affected. If however, he comes from somewhere where the transmission rate is lower, he may experience attacks (the severity of which will depend on the differential in transmission rate).

Malaria in refugees

Refugees—whether their displacement was for economic or political reasons—are highly exposed to all sorts of health problem, especially in poor countries. In Africa, mortality is far higher than average among refugees: in the special cases of displaced populations in northern Ethiopia in 1985 and southern Sudan in 1988, the differential was more than sixty-fold (Toole & Waldman, 1990, 1997). Mortality rates more than 100-fold higher have been recorded in Rwandan refugees in the Democratic Republic of Congo in 1995, although these figures need to be confirmed. The most diseases in these people are malnutrition, diarrhoea, measles, HIV, respiratory infections and malaria.

Most of the information available is fragmented and should be considered as no more than indicative.

In a camp in north-western Tanzania containing 22,000 refugees from the relatively malaria-free mountains of Burundi, weekly malarial mortality averaged 10-20 people, with a peak of 37 in one week (Crowe, 1997).

Starting in 1969, many refugees from Ethiopia and Eritrea fled to camps in the Gedaref Region in north-eastern Sudan, where they founded families. The incidence of malaria there was 80‰, the same as in the local people living around the camps (Lienhardt et al., 1990). After a very difficult period, the refugees changed their life style and the incidence dropped.

A new wave of refugees arriving from Tigre in 1985 was exposed to the same dangers as those who had arrived in 1969 and 1974, and they experienced a mortality rate of 0.89‰ per day, in which malaria played a significant role (Shears et al., 1987) with an incidence of 112‰ in under-5 year-olds, and 84‰ in those of 14 and over.

Afghani refugees in Pakistan were shown to have been infected on arrival (as opposed to having brought the parasites with them) (Suleman, 1988); they even seemed to have become infected faster than local people because they were being bitten more often by anophelines. The parasite balance was 70% *P. vivax* versus 30% *P. falciparum* (Rowland et al., 1997).

Camps on the border between Cambodia and Thailand sheltered 216,000-248,000 refugees between 1983 and 1985. The incidence of malaria ranged from 37‰ in camps on the plains to 562‰ in the mountains and bushlands with low rainfall, and 2,073‰ in mountainous jungle with abundant rivers. These incidences were directly proportional to vector density, i.e. of *An. minimus s.l.* and especially *An. dirus s.l.* The API (the percentage of positive slides) was 359-116‰ (depending on age) inside camps compared with just 5-6‰ in Thailand as a whole.

On the frontier between Thailand and Myanmar there are long-standing refugee camps for Karen people where well-organised medical services coupled with effective vector control measures rapidly reduced the incidence of malaria (Shanks et al., 1990).

Epidemiological dangers for the host country

If there are no competent vectors in the destination country, i.e. if the country is not receptive, no chain of transmission will be established but cases may nevertheless be imported, either in migrants or in travellers coming back home. Malaria is now a significant health problem even in developed countries (a subject which is addressed in a separate chapter).

In countries where malaria has been eradicated but which are still receptive (with vectors present), imported cases may be seen but, in addition, transmission may also recommence.

Introduced malaria usually only affects the victim and a few people in the immediate vicinity, especially if control measures are rapidly implemented. This is the case with the 22 cases of *P. vivax* malaria documented in Corsica in 1961 and 1971 (Ambroise-Thomas *et al*., 1972; Sautet & Quilici, 1971) as well as in California where 28 cases of *P. vivax* malaria were caused by introduction of the parasite by Mexican workers. The vector of this mini-epidemic was *An. hermsi* (of the *An. maculipennis* Group) (Maldonado *et al*., 1990). Other cases of *P. vivax* malaria—apparently introduced—have been reported in both New Jersey and Texas in the United States (Zucker, 1996); the suspected vector was *An. quadrimaculatus*. The cases of malaria seen in New York in 1993 are believed to have been introduced although, since there does not seem to have been any vector present, these may correspond to airport malaria (Layton *et al*., 1995). On the other hand, a case of *P. vivax* malaria at Maremma in Italy (Baldari *et al*., 1998) could be considered as having been introduced. On the island of La Réunion, introduced cases are seen every year (Julvez *et al*., 1982), although real transmission is never resumed because the capacity of the vector, *An. arabiensis*, is so low.

To date, there is no documented instance in which introduced cases—or more generally, the introduction of parasites by migrants—have caused genuine **re-emergence of malaria** which could only happen if **parasite introduction** were coupled with **increased transmission potential**, i.e. an increase in the number of competent vectors where the parasites have been introduced. The most common current reason for an increase in vector numbers is the cessation of control measures, as happened in Swaziland (Fontaine, 1987; Mouchet, 1987) where the interruption of DDT spraying was followed by a major outbreak of malaria. In this case, the arrival of immigrants from Mozambique only represented a spatially contained epi-phenomenon of very dubious epidemiological significance (Packard, 1986). After the collapse of the Soviet Union, malaria re-emerged in the Republics of Armenia, Azerbaijan and Tajikistan and this was simultaneous with massive population displacements and major social unrest as well as the complete discontinuation of vector control operations and profound disruption of health services. The importance of migration in such re-emergence events can only be assessed on a case-by-case basis.

Imported malaria

Background

The term "**imported malaria**" is used to describe cases of the disease that are contracted in an endemic area but diagnosed in a non-endemic one (WHO, 1964). It is quite distinct from "**introduced malaria**" which can lead to local transmission.

There are barely 10,000 cases of imported malaria annually (according to official figures) but it nevertheless constitutes a public health problem in both developed countries and countries where malaria is well on the way to being eradicated. Imported malaria is often severe because the victim is usually immunologically naïve: death is always possible, which is why diagnosis is urgent, even if it is difficult on the basis of the symptoms alone.

Impact on public health

Most cases of imported malaria involve either people from non-endemic regions coming home after a stay in an endemic place, or emigrants originate from an endemic zone returning to their non-endemic place of residence after a trip home.

Muentener *et al*. (1999) recently produced a review of imported malaria between 1985 and 1995, a summary of which is presented in *Table I*.

A total of about 100,000 cases were recorded over this period, i.e. about 10,000 per annum. With 2,200 cases per annum (and a maximum of 2,350 in 1991), the United Kingdom was the most affected "host" country, followed by France (1,270), the United States (1,050), Germany (980) and Australia (760).

Despite annual 10% increases in air travel, the number of cases of imported malaria did not rise between 1989 (when the number peaked) and 1995 (although this year's figures were lowered due to a delay in United States notifications). This is evidence of the efficacy of travel medicine centres and services *vis-à-vis* the information of travellers about prevention. It seems that the development of multi-drug resistance in many parts of the world has not had any direct impact on imported malaria. Given that the numbers of air travellers have increased dramatically, it can even be said that imported malaria has decreased, especially since it used to be under-estimated to a greater extent than it is today.

Marginal cases

Although they are not classified among the industrialised countries, the petroleum-exporting countries of the Persian Gulf and the Middle East attract many labourers from poorer countries, often on a temporary basis.

In Bahrain, Kuwait, Qatar and the United Arab Emirates, since 1995 all cases were imported, e.g. 534 cases in Kuwait in 1984 and 234 in Bahrain in 1998. In the Emirates, 2,164 cases were imported and 40 were autochthonous in 1994; most of the emigrants came from the Sultanate of Oman. In 1998, after the implementation of an eradication programme in Oman, the number of imported cases fell to just 6 (compared with 2 autochthonous cases) (Beljaev, 2002).

In Iraq in 1984, at which time malaria was close to eradication, 3,346 cases of imported malaria were notified, most of them due to *P. vivax*; these occurred in natives of Southeast Asia working in oil fields (Shibab *et al*., 1987).

In northern and eastern Iran from 1986 to 1991, there were more cases imported from Afghanistan, Pakistan and Bangladesh than there were indigenous cases (respectively 3,500 and 2,800 (Manouchehri *et al*., 1992).

Biodiversity of Malaria in the World

Table I. Number of cases of malaria imported into industrialised countries (1985-1995).

	1985	1986	1987	1988	1989	1990	1991	1992	1993	1994	1995	Number of cases per annum	Total number of cases
Europe													
Austria	82	92	52	83	98	112	111	58	89	75	80	85	932
Belgium	208	298	258	271	272	264	314	249	320	423	304	289	3,181
Czechoslovakia	9	11	20	26	28	7	8	7	8	n/a	n/a	14	124
Denmark	128	178	138	142	125	114	110	110	113	136	175	134	1,469
Finland	30	28	19	n/a	52	46	33	39	31	49	31	36	358
France	631	1,125	1,143	1,664	1,863	1,491	1,165	905	769	824	1,167	1,159	12,747
Germany	591	1,137	794	1,030	1,143	976	900	773	732	830	941	895	9,847
Greece	34	39	47	52	48	28	45	29	35	27	24	37	408
Ireland	22	21	28	30	23	12	11	15	9	12	9	17	192
Italy	178	191	287	350	468	521	471	499	688	782	743	471	5,178
Luxembourg	7	3	5	n/a	8	7	5	1	4	6	6	5	52
Malta	4	5	2	2	10	3	5	0	4	2	6	4	43
Netherlands	137	167	153	259	244	248	272	179	223	236	312	221	2,430
Norway	53	68	47	53	52	60	71	36	76	73	80	61	669
Poland	15	14	16	21	22	21	16	17	27	18	20	19	207
Portugal	62	95	119	113	161	129	108	61	49	67	n/a	96	964
Romania	10	8	13	n/a	5	9	11	19	21	20	30	15	146
Spain	112	179	166	176	118	161	159	154	171	268	263	175	1,927
Sweden	140	147	155	172	180	205	149	124	143	160	161	158	1,736
Switzerland	200	196	192	322	340	295	322	261	285	310	289	274	3,012
United Kingdom	2,212	2,309	1,816	1,674	1,987	2,096	2,332	1,629	1,922	1,887	2,055	1,993	21,919
(Former) USSR	1,918	1,686	1,323	1,580	1,145	356	254	188	293	485	548	889	9,776
Yugoslavia	57	75	64	53	46	23	18	10	20	n/a	n/a	41	366
Total	6,840	8,072	6,857	8,073	8,438	7,184	6,890	5,363	6,032	6,690	7,244		77,683
Other parts of the world													
Australia	421	696	574	601	770	874	939	743	670	710	610	692	7,608
Canada	314	436	515	307	284	417	674	407	n/a	637	447	444	4,438
Japan	53	50	40	48	49	49	52	49	51	64	n/a	51	505
New Zealand	n/a	n/a	n/a	n/a	27	32	39	29	58	34	41	37	260
United States of America	1,045	1,091	932	1,023	1,102	1,098	1,046	910	1,275	1,014	n/a	1,054	10,536
Total	1,833	2,273	2,061	1,979	2,232	2,470	2,750	2,138	2,537	1,822	1,288		23,338

n/a: information not available

In Saudi Arabia, although imported malaria was considered a serious problem, it was not possible to obtain reliable figures.

From 1981 to 1989, 7,683 cases of *P. vivax* malaria were imported into the USSR by soldiers returning from Afghanistan (Sergiev *et al.*, 1992). From 1991 on, during the collapse of the Soviet Union, the return of soldiers from Afghanistan and population movements that followed the granting of independence to various former republics led to marked increases in the numbers of imported cases in the new Republics of the Caucasus and Central Asia as well as in the Russian Federation. These led to outbreaks of introduced malaria which were easily brought under control (or disappeared spontaneously) in Georgia, the Russian Federation, Turkmenistan, Uzbekistan, Kirghizstan and Kazakhstan. However, the same processes led to genuine epidemics in Armenia, Azerbaijan and Tajikistan (Sabatinelli, 2001).

In Brazil from 1978 to 1990, many people settled in Amazonia (especially in the States of Rondônia and Pará). Many settlements, in which living conditions were very basic, constituted foci of re-emergent malaria. And the settlers maintained close links with their home states which were in turn contaminated when they returned home (Marquès *et al.*, 1999).

"Wartime malaria" which swept through the Balkans between 1916 and 1918 and then through Central and Eastern Europe from 1944 to 1946 has been well documented (Bruce-Chwatt & Zulueta, 1980). In Japan in 1945 and 1946, many soldiers returning from the Pacific combat zones brought malaria parasites back with them, causing a genuine epidemic which struck 460,000 people (Sawada, 1949).

Between 500 and 1,000 sailors contract malaria every year and treatment at sea can pose problems. This number is seriously under-estimated because shipping companies whose boats are registered under a flag of convenience are not subject to the obligatory notification process (Tomaszunas, 1998).

Seriousness of imported malaria

More than 50% of imported malaria cases are due to *P. falciparum*, the most virulent species which can cause death. This percentage can reach 84% in France where there are more exchanges with sub-Saharan Africa.

In Europe, 1.10% of cases result in death, from 3.9% in Germany to 0.7% in Great Britain (two countries where the percentage of *P. falciparum* is similar but the reasons for this disparity are unclear).

The diagnosis of malaria does not represent a problem but the disease has to be considered. Given the scarcity of the condition in developed countries, tests for *Plasmodium* are not systematically ordered in a patient with a fever.

Any patient with prolonged, unexplained fever should be closely questioned ("Have you been to the Tropics?" "Do you live near an airport?") to help the physician to decide whether or not to order the appropriate tests which is the only way of definitively characterising malaria. Thrombocytopaenia is a common alarm signal. Any delay in diagnosis and treatment could entail serious complications and possibly lead to death (Giacomini *et al.*, 1997).

Travel medicine institutions—with back-up from many hospital departments—are making great efforts to inform travellers about the risk in different countries, and inform them about the right prophylactic drugs to take in the light of the specific parasite resistance profiles they are likely to encounter where they are going.

However, the failure to comply with prophylactic prescriptions or the use of drugs that are not matched to local epidemiological conditions remain responsible for most cases.

In Kenya, an attempt was made to estimate the malaria risk by assaying antibodies directed against circumsporozoite antigens. Such antigens were detected in 6-49% of the tourists who had visited the country but were not showing any symptoms of malaria (Selinek *et al.*, 1996). These results are preliminary because, in non-immune subjects, the details of the relationship between the sporozoite inoculation rate and the appearance of plasmodia in the blood have not been established; the epidemiological significance of these antibodies is not therefore clear.

Anthropogenic vector spread

Although the experts have had a great deal to say about the role of population displacements in the spread of malaria and plasmodia through the world, they have been far more discreet about the introduction and fate of their vectors (Longstreith & Kondrashin, 2002). This is a complex topic on which controlled scientific data are often lacking.

Before any animal can establish itself in a new region, it must overcome a series of obstacles related to transport and in the case of *Anopheles* its acclimatisation to its new environment.

Introduction of Anopheles

Anopheles can be introduced as a result of active migration, or it can hitch a ride (passive spread) in a boat, an airplane, a train or a truck.

Active spread

This essentially corresponds to wind-borne migration. This mode of spread has been suspected in a number of cases but without any proof other than circumstantial evidence. In 1868, La Réunion was probably invaded by *An. gambiae* blown over from Mauritius by a tropical storm. The presumed landing point in the north-east of the island is 250 km as the crow flies from Mauritius, on the opposite side of the island to Saint-Paul and the port where boats arrive (Julvez *et al.*, 1990) which is in favour of the proposed hypothesis.

In Niger in 1990, it has been proposed that the oasis of Bilma (Develoux *et al.*, 1994)—more than 500 km north of the nearest water pools in the Sahel—was invaded by anophelines borne on monsoon winds from the south-west as the tropical front was rising. Such seasonal migration is not ruled out for anophelines of the *An. gambiae* Complex and could explain why these mosquitoes occasionally appear in oases in the southern Sahara (e.g. Tagant in Mauritania and Largeau in Chad).

Passive spread

Anopheles does not usually reproduce on boats—the female mosquito that gets off is the same individual as the one that got on. Although it can live for a month, the survival time on a boat cannot be expected to be more than a week to ten days.

In the days of sailing when sea voyages were long, no example of *Anopheles* having been imported was ever recorded. It was suggested that the merchants who criss-crossed the Mediterranean between the 5th and 2nd centuries BC may have brought *An. sachavori* into Greece and *An. labranchiae* into Italy, which would explain the appearance of *P. falciparum* as described by Celsus in the 1st century AD, although there is no concrete evidence for this plausible hypothesis.

The arrival of maritime steam technology considerably shortened voyages. In 1864, the commissioning of a steamship line which cut the crossing time between Tamatave in Madagascar and Port Louis from 45 to just 5 days, was followed in 1866 by the appearance of *An. gambiae* and probably *An. funestus* which brought malaria transmission to Mauritius which had hitherto been reputed for being healthy (Julvez *et al.*, 1990). The introduction of *An. gambiae* into Brazil at the end of 1929 has been blamed on the *avisos rapides* which took mail between Dakar and Natal (Soper & Wilson, 1943). Navigation up and down the Nile (which was particularly intense during the war) spread *An. gambiae* in the Nile Valley in Upper Egypt.

Trucks and the train coming from Diré Daoua brought *An. arabiensis* to the Republic of Djibouti, which was believed to be free of indigenous malaria until 1975 when this anopheline became established on a permanent basis. In Ethiopia, *An. arabiensis* was regularly brought into the lower neighbourhoods of Addis Ababa in trains and trucks (Ovazza & Neri, 1955), and in South Africa, trucks continuously took vectors up onto the Transvaal Plateaux (de Meillon & Gear, 1939).

But today, it is the airplane which represents the most efficient means of spreading *Anopheles*. The first controlled research into the role of aircraft was carried out in 1933 and 1934 by Symes (1935) in Kenya, at Kisumu and Nairobi. Of 77 planes (mostly "Hannibal" belonging to Imperial Airways) checked at Kisumu, 33 contained mosquitoes, including 38 *An. funestus* and 24 *An. gambiae*; in Nairobi, 6 *An. funestus* and 4 *An. gambiae* were collected from 65 planes. Most of the infested planes had come from Juba in southern Sudan or Entebbe in Uganda. In 1968, five *An. gambiae* were collected from the 28 airplanes examined (Highton & Van Someren, 1970). After the eradication of *An. gambiae* from Brazil, aircraft coming from Africa were monitored in the context of re-invasion surveillance operations between 1942 and 1945: from a total of 1,060 planes, 352 *An. gambiae* were collected (Mendonça & Cerqueira, 1947).

Over the last thirty years, very few articles on anopheline capture experiments in airplanes have been published, although *An. subpictus* was found in Tokyo on planes coming from Thailand (Ogata *et al.*, 1974). It is true that looking for *Anopheles* in huge cargo planes is difficult and moreover requires official approval, which is not always easy to get—and all for a very meagre harvest. On the other hand, multiply resistant *Culex quinquefasciatus* are often found. In mosquito hunts carried out in response to the increasing problem of airport malaria, *An. gambiae s.s* was found in a number of big cargo planes arriving at Paris Roissy-Charles-de-Gaulle Airport from West Africa (Karch *et al.*, 2001), suggesting that this anopheline is often being introduced into European airports.

Vector acclimatisation and establishment

Few of the many animal species that are introduced into a new place find climatic and ecological conditions conducive to their sustainable installation.

For *Anopheles*, the first obstacle to overcome is finding larval habitats of suitable dimensions, sun exposure, vegetation, organic content, and salt and mineral content which are devoid of pathogens, predators and competitors. In 1942 in Egypt, *An. gambiae* found a highly conducive habitat in the marshes left after recession of the Nile floods (Shousha, 1948). In Mauritius, deforestation for sugar cane plantations promoted the expansion of *An. gambiae* (Julvez *et al.*, 1993).

Failure is probably more common than success but it leaves no trace.

A distinction can be made between:
- **sustained establishment** with ongoing maintenance of the species, e.g. *An. arabiensis* in Mauritius and La Réunion. This category also covers the establishment of *An. gambiae* in Brazil and Egypt, and *An. funestus* in Mauritius although in these cases, the mosquitoes were eliminated by specific antilarval measures coupled with pyrethroid spraying; it may be that these species were not fully adapted because they could be eliminated with relative ease. In La Réunion and Mauritius in contrast, *An. arabiensis* has persisted for decades despite sustained control, including indoor DDT spraying campaigns;
- **seasonal establishment** lasting a matter of days or weeks in oases where the species disappears as suddenly as it appears. At Faya-Largeau in Chad, large numbers of *An.*

gambiae were found by Rioux *et al.* (1961) but it had disappeared by the time Taufflies & Saugrain performed their survey of the same location the next year. Mention has already been made of the Bilma Oasis in Niger (Develoux *et al.*, 1994). These cases warranted in-depth study given the danger of spread of members of the *An. gambiae* Complex into Algeria *via* the roads across the Sahara (Benzerroug & Janssens, 1985; Julvez *et al.*, 1997b); however, there is no reason to exaggerate the risk because, between 1945 and 1958, airplanes from Bamako and Zinder regularly landed at the oases and, despite no insecticide treatment during this period, *An. gambiae* was never introduced in a sustained way into the oases of the central Sahara;

- **accidental introduction**, meaning the introduction in airplanes, or any other vehicle, of vectors that fail to find conditions favourable to their reproduction at the end of their journey. Their stay is therefore self-limiting but in the meantime, they can feed on humans and inoculate them with parasites they might be carrying. This category includes airport malaria;
- the **introduction of an insecticide-resistant strain of a vector** into a place where the species was hitherto susceptible to the insecticide in question; this is related to the importation of a novel vector into a place in which it is perfectly adapted.

Epidemiological consequences of vector importation

In all the documented cases, vector importation has had serious—and sometimes catastrophic—consequences. In 1865, neither the island of Mauritius nor the neighbouring Rodrigues were home to any anophelines. The arrival of *An. gambiae* and, in certain spots *An. funestus* led to an epidemic which eventually killed 25% of the population of the capital Port-Louis. In April 1866 alone, 6,224 of the 87,000 inhabitants died. In 1868 on the island of La Réunion, the arrival of *Anopheles* triggered a massive epidemic (although its scale might have been exaggerated) (Julvez *et al.*, 1990).

In Brazil, *An. gambiae* was confined to the Natal Region until 1929 when it began to spread, first to the State of Rio Grande del Norte and then Ceara. The resultant epidemic peaked in 1938 and has been reviewed by Soper & Wilson (1943). In the worst-affected parts of Rio Grande del Norte, there were 48,000-51,000 cases in the 43,700 inhabitants, with 5,290 deaths according to contemporary estimates. In 1938 in the State of Ceara, 80% of the rural population had malaria according to Chagas (*in* Soper & Wilson, 1943). In July 1938 in the Jagouribe Valley alone, there were 60,000 cases and 8,000 deaths. With the implementation of a well-conceived control programme, *An. gambiae* had been eliminated from Brazil by November 1940.

In southern Egypt in 1942, at the height of the War, an epidemic of *P. falciparum* malaria broke out at Abou Simbel and Ballana. Over 80% of the population of Abou Simbel was affected, and 60% of that of Ballana. In these villages in May, the mortality rate rose from 2 in 1941 to 34 in 1942. The epidemic was soon attributed to *An. gambiae s.l.* (almost certainly *An. arabiensis*) which had never hitherto been seen north of the Second Cataract. This *Anopheles* rapidly spread to Edfou and Assouan (by July 10), to Luxor and Gerga (August), and to Assiout (November) where it reached the township of Montfalour—referred to as the El Alamein of *An. gambiae* by Shousha (1948). It seems to have made a few incursions into the delta in September but did not become established there. At Assiout, it persisted through three winters even though the temperature dropped to 6-10 °C at night. The number of cases of malaria in 1942 was estimated at 63,000 and in 1943 at 72,000, with 6,300 and 3,800 deaths respectively; in 1944, there were 32,800 cases and 1,789 deaths. In March 1945, *An. gambiae* was chased out of Egypt and the epidemic died down (Shousha, 1948).

Since then, no anopheline invasion has been reported, possibly because, since 1950, improved vector control measures have made large-scale invasion less likely to happen.

Airport malaria

Earliest cases

Towards the end of the 1960's in Western Europe (particularly in France), cases of indigenous malaria were seen in people who had never visited an endemic area. The parasite concerned was *P. falciparum* which was supposed to have been eliminated over fifty years before. Moreover, the research of Zulueta *et al.* (1975) had shown that "European" anophelines (notably *An. atroparvus*) were not conducive to the development of this species. These autochthonous cases excited a great deal of interest. It was deduced that the "Breton" cases reported in 1969 by Doby & Guigen (1981) had probably been contracted around the airport of Bourget. Subsequently in 1970, three cases were reported in Zurich (WHO, 1978). In 1976, several cases occurred in or around the Paris airports (Auvergnat *et al.*, 1979; Bentata-Pessayre *et al.*, 1978; Gentilini *et al.*, 1978; Gentilini & Danis, 1982). No evidence was found of local transmission, neither by autochthonous anophelines nor by imported species (Cassaigne *et al.*, 1980). But it became ever more probable that these cases of malaria had been transmitted by anophelines which had arrived on airplanes.

In 1984, Giacomini *et al.* introduced the term "airport malaria" to define the situation in which the disease is transmitted in a malaria-free place by *Anopheles* imported from an endemic region. This is quite distinct from introduced malaria which is transmitted by autochthonous *Anopheles*.

Scale of the problem

Since the first description of airport malaria around Le Bourget in 1969 (Doby & Guigen, 1981), a total of 78 cases have been described in Western Europe, including 28 in France, 18 in Belgium, 12 in Switzerland, 9 in Great Britain, 5 in Italy, 3 in Luxembourg, 2 in Germany and 1 in Spain. Since 1995 (Giacomini et al.), no comprehensive list has been compiled on airport malaria cases and one or two cases are somewhat doubtful.

Almost all these cases are due to P. falciparum. It is not yet possible to define the geographic origin of this parasite. It is responsible for severe malaria, especially since the diagnosis of this very rare form of the disease—which is not always evident from the results of routine tests (e.g. blood tests)—is often delayed. The interview does not reveal any recent foreign travel but the patient living near or working in an airport may incite the doctor to order a microscopic blood examination in the case of prolonged, unexplained fever (Giacomini et al., 1997); similarly, primary plasmodial infection often causes thrombocytopaenia. The global lethality rate of airport malaria is particularly high: 16.9% according to Isaacson (1989) and 26% according to Danis et al. (1996).

P. vivax has only been seen twice, at Maremma in Italy (Baldari et al., 1998) and at Rosny near Paris (Saliou et al., 1978). In neither case can the possibility of introduced malaria be ruled out.

A single case of P. malariae malaria was reported in Zurich in Switzerland (WHO, 1978). Mixed P. falciparum-P. vivax infection was seen in two different patients admitted into the same hospital department at the same time in France.

One patient, who had been treated and cured of an attack of P. falciparum malaria, subsequently presented an attack due to P. malariae (Lusina et al., 2000).

In the United States, three cases of P. falciparum malaria occurred in the Borough of Queens in New York. Layton et al. (1995) suggested that the disease had been transmitted autochthonously by An. quadrimaculatus but this hypothesis was never backed up by capture evidence; there is nothing to suggest that these were not cases of airport malaria (which has never been reported in America).

It is important to note that here, only severe cases that involved admission into hospital are addressed (Giacomini et al., 1995); no information is available on the number of benign cases.

Given the rarity of airport malaria, it is not a serious public health problem but its lethality rate is very high and it represents a local danger. However, the development of new air travel routes from Africa suggests that the relative risks identified will continue to increase and, based on climate suitability methods, it will be important to optimise Anopheles-specific disinfection and control efforts (Tatem et al., 2006).

Infection pathways

Danis et al. (1996) distinguished between five different infection pathways: inside the airplane; inside the airport; around the airport; far from the airport; and from baggage.

Inside airplanes

This has been observed in Great Britain in two groups of passengers travelling from London to Rome in different flights, one of which had come from Addis Ababa (where there are no anophelines!) (Smeaton et al., 1984; Weir et al., 1984). Two other cases occurred in passengers travelling from Johannesburg to London via a stop-over in Abidjan. The passengers had not left the plane but the doors had been left open in the middle of the night (Colon et al., 1990; Oswald & Lawrence, 1990). Another case involves a passenger who had got off the plane for a stretch at Banjul in Gambia. To date, infection inside the plane is a British speciality although other such cases may have been classified as simple imported malaria.

Inside the airport and associated buildings

This category accounts for most cases of airport malaria. Victims include people who were working on the runway, baggage handlers, postal service employees who had opened containers and security staff. Given this range, it seems that vectors must be flying around the airport. One case even involved a musician who had come to welcome a Head of State—in the middle of winter (Saliou et al., 1978).

Infection of those living near the airport

Almost the same number of cases has been reported in those living within four kilometres of an airport (as long as the population density is low between the airport and the house). Four cases—a mini-epidemic—were described near Cointrin, the airport of Geneva in Switzerland (Bouvier et al., 1990).

Infection further away

The distance of four kilometres was set arbitrarily on the basis of observations. Other cases suggest that the anophelines had been transported by car, particularly those of airport workers. At Villeparisis, six kilometres from the airport, two subjects living 300 m from one another developed malaria (and one of them subsequently died). Neither had been anywhere near the airport but both their houses were surrounded by those of airport workers, some night-shift workers (Giacomini et al., 1995). Two similar cases occurred in an airport personnel estate near Geneva. In England, near Gatwick Airport in Sussex, Curtis & White (1984) attributed the infection of a publican whose pub was located ten kilometres from the airport as well as that of a motorcyclist crossing the village to a single mosquito; still, it is rare that an anopheline bites a moving target in a strong head wind!

Baggage handling

In Italy, two infections—one at Asti (Rizzo *et al.*, 1989) and the other at Brescia (Castelli *et al.*, 1994)—were attributed to baggage coming from an endemic zone having been brought into the house (which was far from the nearest international airport). One of these cases occurred in wintertime (February). A less clear-cut case was reported in France (Guillet *et al.*, 1998). When one thinks about how tightly packed suitcases usually are, it is difficult to imagine that a fragile anopheline could survive there although chests might be more propitious: indeed two cases involving chests brought back from Vietnam have been documented in France (Mouchet, personal observation).

Sources of infection

It is not yet possible to define the geographic origin of *P. falciparum*, even using DNA analysis (Eldin de Pecoulas *et al.*, 1996). Only two *An. gambiae* have ever been found in aircraft coming from tropical Africa to France. More research in European airports would be required to measure the infectivity of imported anophelines. In the absence of any direct evidence, we are obliged to speculate as to the sources of airport anophelines.

Most of the cases have occurred in France, Belgium and Switzerland, three countries which have close relationships with countries of West and Central Africa where more than 80% of the population is infected by *P. falciparum*, especially children; in contrast, there is hardly any *P. vivax* anywhere on the continent. In France, all the cases involved Roissy Airport where most of the flights from sub-Saharan Africa arrive. Before Roissy opened, two cases had been reported at Bourget which, at the time, was the hub for African flights. No case has ever been linked to Orly airport which does not serve sub-Saharan Africa.

Most international airports in Asia, America and Oceania are located in zones where *P. falciparum* has either never existed or from which it has been eliminated, e.g. Hanoi, Ho Chi Minh City, Bangkok, Delhi, Bombay, Madras, São Paulo, Rio de Janeiro and Lima, to mention just a few airports in the Tropics with regular flights to Western Europe.

In contrast, all the airports of West Africa are considered to be a risk. Guillet *et al.* (1998) were able to collect *An. arabiensis* and/or *An. gambiae* near or inside airplanes at night in Dakar (Senegal), Abidjan (Ivory Coast), Cotonou (Bénin) and Douala (Cameroon), which are very likely embarkation sites (especially given that two passengers were infected after just a stop-over in Abidjan). During the rainy season (which corresponds to the European summer), all parts of the Afrotropical Region are at risk. Guillet *et al.* (1998) attempted to compile a (non-exhaustive) list of high-risk airports in West and Central Africa. At and south of the Equator, the change of seasons affects when anopheline numbers peak, but the airports of Libreville (Gabon), Brazzaville (Congo), Luanda (Angola) and Kinshasa (Democratic Republic of Congo) must all be considered as being at risk throughout the year. In East and South Africa, high altitude airports—Nairobi (Kenya), Addis-Ababa (Ethiopia) and Harare (Zimbabwe)—are at lower risk and malaria is not endemic in Johannesburg (South Africa). In the northern hemisphere, Khartoum (Sudan), Entebbe (Uganda) and Djibouti are at risk during the summer (though a small risk in the last case). From the southern hemisphere—Mombasa (Kenya), Dar ès Salam (Tanzania), Lusaka (Zambia), Antananarivo (Madagascar) and Moroni (Comoros)—anophelines could be imported in winter but they would be unlikely to survive long in the cold European winter.

Outside of Africa, Port-au-Prince (Haiti) is in a transmission zone. In Oceania, Honiara (Solomon Islands) and Port Moresby (Papua-New Guinea) are not directly linked to Europe and represent only a risk to Australia, especially since many of the flights concerned involve small airplanes crossing between non-international airports. Vanuatu is linked to New Caledonia, and there are regular flights between Fiji and Australia.

These lists are by no means exhaustive. It would be fairly easy to compile a list of all the airports where there is a real risk of embarking infected *Anopheles*, but this would only be of use if it were possible to compile a complementary list of other vectors that are transported in airplanes, notably *An. aegypti*. Such malaria risk estimates have been compiled for African mosquito air transportation (Tatem *et al.*, 2006).

Distribution of cases

How cases are distributed does not seem to be governed by any law. Five cases were documented in the United Kingdom in 1983, five in Brussels in 1986, seven at Roissy in 1994 and another four there in 1998, and five in Geneva, Switzerland in 1989 (that Bouvier *et al.* [1990] defined as a "mini-epidemic").

There does not seem to be any correlation between the incidence of cases and July temperature figures. The summers of 1983 and 1994 were particularly hot whereas those of 1974, 1978 and 1980 were cool. In 1983, when there were five cases in Great Britain and one in Belgium, no other cases were seen anywhere else in Europe. The summer of 1994 was hot everywhere; seven cases were seen at Roissy but none anywhere else. During the "cool" summers of 1974 and 1980, no case was reported anywhere, although there were two cases in Holland during the "cool" summer of 1978. There were five cases in Brussels in 1986 when temperatures were perfectly average. In 1989, summer was hot in Geneva and four cases were notified; this summer was relatively cool in Great Britain. Although there is a little evidence that the risk may be higher in hot years than in cool years, no statistically significant conclusions can be drawn (Giacomini *et al.*, 1995; Guillet *et al.*, 1998).

Nor does the geographical distribution of cases follow any rule. Apart from the "mini-epidemic" in Geneva (Bouvier *et al.*, 1990), most of the other incidents correspond to isolated cases. Double cases have been seen in passengers on a flight between London and Rome, soldiers on duty at Zurich airport, brothers in Brussels, a mother and daughter in Luxembourg, neighbours at Villeparisis, and two other cases near Roissy Airport; this is indicative of transmission by a single mosquito as had previously been suggested by Curtis & White (1984) in a double case near Gatwick airport.

These cases can be explained in terms of the biology of *Anopheles*. Most take a blood meal and then digest the ingested blood over a period of two or three days, during which time their eggs mature; after laying, the female is ready to bite again. This so-called gonotrophic cycle is sometimes upset and the mosquito does not take a full meal. Most of these disturbed individuals then seek a second host to finish feeding. This type of interrupted feeding is seen in 5-8% of individuals according to Boreham (1975). If the mosquito is carrying sporozoites, it can infect two people in one interrupted meal (Kulkarni & Panda, 1984). The probability of double infection has been investigated by means of PCR analysis of *P. falciparum* isolates from the two subjects—who lived 300 m apart— infected on the same day at Villeparisis (Eldin de Pecoulas *et al.*, 1996): the two strains were found to be identical.

Uncertainties of airport malaria

Studying airport malaria is of cognitive value since each case poses a special problem with respect to the time and place of infection as well as the candidate vector. Any results are uncertain and it is important to bear the possibility of error in mind.

It has been shown in various experiments that anophelines, in particular *An. gambiae* from Africa, can be transported in all types of airplane, either in the cabin, the hold or even in the wheel housings. These insects may also be transported in chests although it is less likely in tightly packed suitcases (with the insects all killed in our experiments to investigate this possibility).

Guillet *et al.* (1998) showed that *An. gambiae* could be embarked in aircraft heading from west Africa to Europe. It is only in September 2000 that a "tropical" anopheline (*An. gambiae*) was found in an Air France Airbus arriving at Roissy-Charles-de-Gaulle Airport (Karch *et al.*, 2001). *An. gambiae* was also collected in Kenya (Highton & Van Someren, 1970) and Brazil (Mendonça & Cerqueira, 1947) in small aircraft (in which finding mosquitoes was relatively easy). In larger airplanes, manual searching is more difficult—and light traps do not work for many anopheline species (including *An. gambiae*).

The distribution of cases still poses a problem. Evidence of the infection of two (at least) subjects by a single mosquito sheds some light on the subject but does not resolve the entire problem. There remains the possibility of more than one infected anopheline having been brought in on one or more aircraft arriving from the same place.

Airport malaria therefore remains a very stimulating subject for epidemiologists.

Finally, the only certainty we had on the transport of mosquitoes was the capture of *An. gambiae* inside an Airbus at Roissy and a capture of another one in the corridor of Roissy airport five years ago (Karch *et al.*, 2001)

Malaria Control

History of Control Policies

Control measures before the Second World War

The earliest evidence of a preoccupation with malaria control dates back to Hippocrates who recommended that villages should be built near rivers but far from marshlands as a way of avoiding fever. The first active treatment for fever was based on *Cinchona* bark from which quinine was eventually extracted by Pelletier and Caventou in 1820. The efficacy of this compound made it the drug of choice for curing fever and protecting both residents and travellers. On the other side of the planet, qinghaosu has been in use in China for over 2,000 years.

The idea of unhealthy places—for the most part, associated with intermittent fever—has been a key factor determining population distribution throughout history. European marshlands were traditionally under-populated and the few people that lived there were often sick. Intercontinental exploration and voyages revealed the planetary scale of the problem. The mangrove-fringed coast of West Africa, the first part of the greater world that Europeans came into contact with, was particularly unhealthy and the survival of crews depended on taking cinchona (and later quinine), and sleeping offshore on the boat. Carlson (1984) has reviewed how early European colonialists were decimated by fever.

At the end of the 19th century, isolation of the etiologic agent of the disease and discovery of how it was transmitted (*see the Chapter on the* "Increase Knowledge about Malaria and Development of Control Measures") completely changed the medical community's attitude to malaria. Now, not only was there a curative and prophylactic drug available (quinine), but also the parasite could be identified and its vector eliminated.

As early as 1887, measures directed at suppressing the vector—*Anopheles*—came to be considered the bedrock of malaria control when it comes to planned public health operations. The soundness of this strategy was demonstrated by Gorgas (1915) in Panama. The Rockefeller Foundation, as represented by Hackett, considered treatment as belonging to the medical field rather than coming into the domain of public health operations: malaria control meant preventing infection by abolishing transmission (Hackett *et al.*, 1938).

Arguments between the advocates of direct medical intervention and those of disease prevention have been an almost constant feature of the debate ever since and, until recently, it was underlying in all health policies.

National and international malaria policies have been influenced by various different "schools": the Italian, the English, the Dutch and the American as well as those associated with international institutions such as the League of Nations from 1920 to 1939 and, after 1948, the WHO. The history of policy has been marked by a series of far-reaching changes in which everything that had hitherto been considered sacred was abandoned, e.g. the replacement in 1992 of the **Global Eradication Programme** with the **Global Strategy for Malaria Control**.

The 125-year history of malaria control has been reviewed by Najera (2001) with copious details on the strategies of the operations conducted at various times.

Italian strategy

The Law of December 23, 1900 regularised the production and sale of quinine. The drug was made available free of charge in malaria-ridden regions and to travellers. Provincial inspectors ensured compliance with the Law in line with the guidelines of the **League of Nations Health Commission** (as of 1920). During the same period, clean-up operations ("*picola bonifica*") were undertaken in villages, the use of **mosquito nets** was encouraged, zooprophylaxis was instigated, and **larval control**

measures were implemented based on the release of the fish, *Gambusia affinis*, or the **spread of Paris Green** or **mineral oil** on larval habitats.

The number of deaths due to malaria dropped from 70 per 100,000 inhabitants in 1897 down to under 5 in 1915; after a climb back up to about 30 during the Great War, it had fallen back down to about 1 by 1939 (Benn, 1947 *in* Najera, 2001) (*Figure 1*).

Mussolini-era propaganda claimed that organised clean-up operations had transformed the Pontine Marshes into a granary but priority was still accorded to a strategy based on the treatment of isolated cases with the stockpiling of drugs to prepare for possible future epidemics.

Larval control in the Americas

In Central America, the success of Gorgas led to a dogmatic position (even though there was confusion between the killing of *Aedes aegypti* and *Anopheles*): blanket larval control will prevent the transmission of malaria. According to Hackett *et al.* (1988), the incidence of malaria depended directly on anopheline density and reducing the number of bites would reduce the incidence of the disease.

But in parallel to the success in **Panama**, control measures in the Tropics met with failure, e.g. operations directed against *Anopheles melas* in Sierra Leone (Ross, 1911) and the Mian Mir project in India from 1902 to 1904 (Bynum, 1994).

Adult control by indoor pyrethrin spraying

The rationale underlying the weekly pyrethrin spraying operations in South Africa organised by Swellengrebel *et al.* (1931) was that, given that they are only active during the night, **anophelines must necessarily enter houses** to find their blood meal and then to be killed. The same type of treatment was performed in Brazil and Egypt to eliminate *An. gambiae*, as well as in Panama and Holland.

Return to drugs

The Europeans were not convinced by the results in America, and Hackett (1937) proposed that methods used successfully in the New World would not be effective in Europe.

Under the influence of Koch (*in* Najera, 2001), the Germans based their attempts to control malaria in their colonies of New Guinea and Tanganyika on treating declared cases and **prophylactic quinine distribution**.

During the 1916 epidemic on the Eastern Front, troops were successfully protected by prophylactic drugs (Sergent & Sergent, 1932).

Watson in Malaysia (1928) and then Swellengrebel (*in* Takken *et al.*, 1990) in Indonesia proposed adapting measures to the relevant vector, an approach referred to as species sanitation which was successfully implemented against *An. sundaicus* in Java.

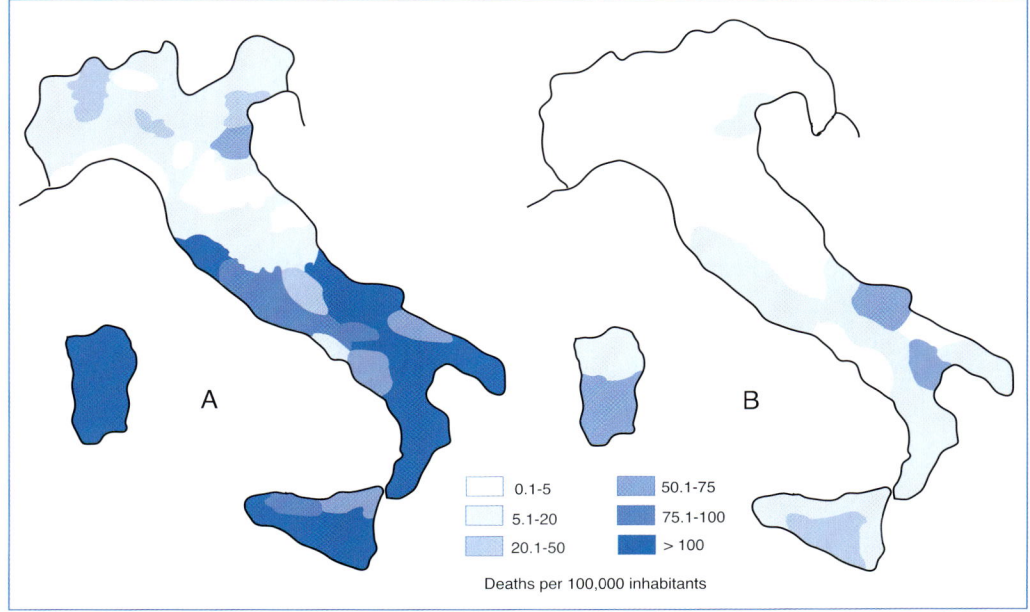

Figure 1. Decline of malaria in Italy. Malarial mortality per 100,000 inhabitants in 1887-1889 (**A**) and 1920-1930 (**B**) (in Najera, 2001).

Deaths per 100,000 inhabitants

Disappearance of malaria from Europe

During the 19th century and at the beginning of the 20th century, malaria was on the decline throughout Europe, ultimately disappearing from the major part of the continent. Hardly any part of Italy was endemic by 1940 (*Figure 1*), but the disease persisted in the Balkans, in a focus in Holland and, most importantly, in the USSR where 2 million cases were recorded in 1941 (*Figure 2*) at the end of the great epidemic which followed the Bolshevik Revolution.

World Eradication Programme

DDT and the hope of eradication

Muller's discovery of the insecticidal activity of **DDT** in 1939 revolutionised malaria control (Muller, 1946, 1955). The sustained action of the new compound as well as its low cost and ease of use meant that treatment could be repeated every six-to-twelve months.

After the first trials in the **Mississippi Valley** in 1943 (Gahan & Lindquist, 1945), indoor spraying methods spread throughout the **United States**, **Venezuela** and **British Guiana**, and then through the Mediterranean Basin, **India** and the Middle East, with apparently miraculous results (*see the Chapter on the* "Increase Knowledge about Malaria and Development of Control Measures").

Launch of the Eradication Programme

In 1954, ten years after the first trials, the 14th Panamerican Health Conference held at Santiago in Chile proposed eradicating malaria from the American continent. A programme sponsored by UNICEF and the Regional Office was launched in Central America.

In the same year, the 2nd Asian Conference held at Baguio in the Philippines also opted for the objective of eradication.

In 1955 in **Mexico**, the 8th World Health Assembly decided that the WHO ought to encourage eradication and authorised the Director-General to create a special fund for the eradication of malaria and launch a **Global Eradication Programme**. This resolution was adopted by 46 votes for with two votes against and six abstentions; Liberia opposed the resolution and France and the United Kingdom expressed reservations. Russel (*in* Najera, 2001) countered these objections by pointing out that, in reality, an eradication strategy was already underway. **Macdonald's mathematical model** (1957) provided a scientific support to the Programme which carried significant weight in the decisions of many of the countries.

In 1957, the 6th Expert Committee defined **eradication as the complete blockage of malaria transmission and elimination of the parasite reservoir within a defined time frame, by means of a campaign conducted effectively enough to preclude resurgence of the disease once operations are terminated**. The various operational phases and how long each would take were scheduled (*see the Chapter on the* "Increase Knowledge about Malaria and Development of Control Measures").

The Committee recognised that Africa presented special problems, notably the behaviour of *An. gambiae*, the length of the transmission season, the omnipresence of malaria, extremely high transmission rates, poor transportation, and administrative deficiencies. It was decided to postpone the

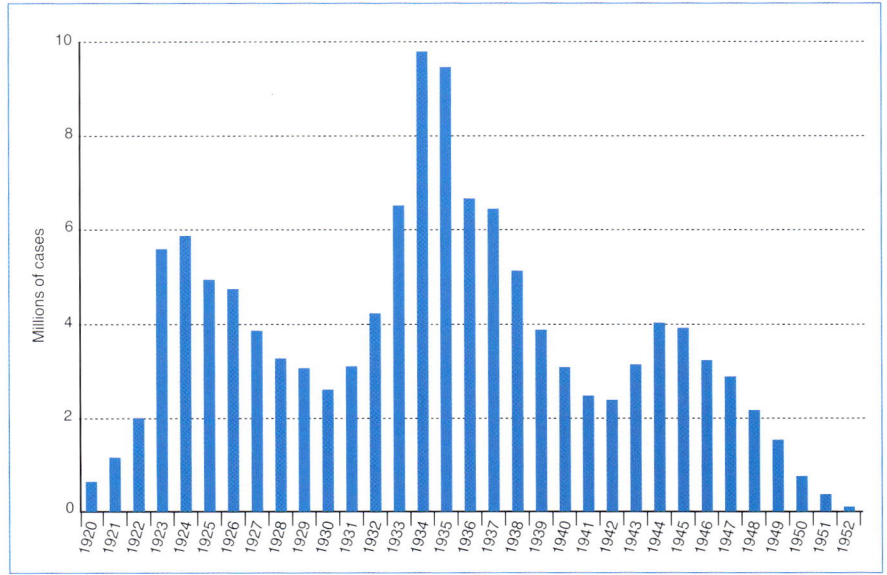

Figure 2.
Malaria incidence in the former Soviet Union from 1920 to 1952 (almost eradicated) (adapted from Sergiev & Duhanina in Najera, 2001).

objective of eradication in Africa and instead, to create pilot zones representative of the various African Regions.

Rapid drops in prevalence in treated regions meant that new indicators had to be devised to follow malaria on the way to eradication.

Eradication problems

From the start of the Programme, anopheline resistance to insecticides was a source of worry—especially since alternative products (like **malathion**) had their own disadvantages. Multiple resistance in Central America fostered a great deal of research but never really presented a serious obstacle to control.

In 1960, **chloroquine-resistant parasites** first emerged in Colombia and Thailand.

Problems soon arose associated with exploitation of the jungle and "crop huts" in Asia, as well as with various border disputes and armed conflicts, making it necessary to define **special zones** (Zulueta & Garrett-Jones, 1965).

But the most serious problem was the **inability** of indoor DDT spraying to **block transmission** in the **West African savannah** (Burkina Faso, Nigeria and northern Cameroon). Without a solution to this problem, eradication—in the strictest sense of the word—would never be possible. There were doubts about the results obtained between 1960 and 1965 but nobody who had actually worked in the areas concerned was in any doubt at all that transmission was proceeding exactly as before despite all the control measures (Cavalié & Mouchet, 1961) To investigate this, WHO established the scientifically robust Garki Study Project in northern Nigeria. It was only twenty years later that WHO recognised that transmission would never be blocked (Molineaux & Gramiccia, 1980).

From 1960 on, more and more National Eradication Departments were experiencing technical, financial and logistic difficulties. The inadequacy of monitoring instruments became evident and the numbers of voluntary workers (who were usually unpaid) collapsed.

End of the programme: lessons learned

At the 1963 Congress of Tropical medicine and Malaria in Tehran, Gabaldon—one of the godfathers of eradication—recognised that even in his own country, Venezuela, there were parts where eradication was not technically possible; other speakers described problems in other countries, especially in Africa. A motion passed at the Congress asked **WHO to review its malaria control policy**.

In 1969, the 22nd World Health Assembly acknowledged the failure but eradication remained the ultimate objective until 1972 when, at a meeting in Brazzaville, countries which could no longer subscribe to the eradication objective opted for a control strategy.

Over the following years, eradication programmes were steadily abandoned in favour of control policies.

Obviously, the eradication strategy never reached its objective but it nevertheless brought massive public health benefit by decreasing the incidence and mortality of the disease, and shrinking the fraction of the planet's surface ravaged by malaria; medical services were also brought for the first time to remote areas and hitherto neglected populations. The programme certainly does not deserve the opprobrium showered on it by the advocates of horizontal structures, notably primary health care provision systems.

Revision of the Global Malaria Control Strategy in 1992

Problems with the switch from eradication to control

Starting in 1969, the switch from eradication caused a great deal of upset in public health institutions which found it difficult to define targets once control had been ratified as a strategy in 1978 by the 31st World Health Assembly.

When spraying operations were stopped, epidemics broke out in Sri Lanka, India, Pakistan, Sudan, Swaziland, Madagascar, and Turkey. In India, more than a million cases per annum were seen between 1995 and 1998, and attack-phase measures had to be resumed. Similarly in Madagascar, nearly 100,000 people were dying from malaria every year from 1992 to 1995. Outside of Africa, the number of cases notified doubled between 1970 and 1985, and the proportion due to *Plasmodium falciparum* rose from 15% to 38%; the seven countries declaring the most cases were India (66% of cases, mostly occurring in the Tribes), Brazil (97% in the Amazon), Sri Lanka, Afghanistan, the Philippines and Vietnam. Nevertheless, 90% of all cases and deaths were still in tropical Africa.

Amsterdam Conference (1992) and the Revised Global Malaria Control Strategy

Following the Ministerial Conference in Amsterdam in November 1992, a Revised Global Malaria Control Strategy was formulated which was subsequently reviewed by United Nations Economic and Social Council and adopted, first by the General Assembly in 1994 and later at the 33rd Session of the Africa Unit Organisation in 1997.

The goal of this WHO Global Strategy was to prevent mortality and reduce morbidity and social and economic losses, through the progressive improvement and strengthening of local and national capabilities.

Four basic technical elements of the strategy were:
- early diagnosis and prompt treatment;

- implementation of selective and sustainable preventive measures, including vector control;
- the prevention, detection and containment of epidemics in their early satges;
- to reassess regularly a country's malaria situation, in particular the ecological, social and economic determinants of the disease.

Conclusion

Table I illustrates the time taken to reach a decision when strategy is changed: twelve years before opting for eradication; fourteen years to decide to abandon the objective of eradication; thirteen years before a control policy was defined.

The prevarications which followed the death throes of the eradication strategy confused many countries deprived of guidance on malaria control. This largely explains why the number of cases doubled (at least) between 1970 and 1985.

The policy of primary health care adopted after Alma-Ata in 1978 was a shock in all countries which were being protected by vertical antimalarial operations. Such policies have not meshed well with the Global Control Strategy.

The Programme proposed in 1992 constitutes a good framework for the development of malaria control strategies, well-conceived in both epidemiological and socio-economic terms. Implementation is up to the countries.

Effective control operations will depend on a number of factors:
- the manifestation of political will at all governmental and administrative levels;
- recognition of the variability in both malaria epidemiology and socio-economic conditions in different countries, i.e. stratification of zones of action and the tailoring of control methods;
- the community should be the favoured partners in control, and the strategy should be firmly rooted in primary health care structures which are, by definition, decentralised (although this is no more than wishful thinking in many countries);
- when it comes to preventive measures, sustainability should take priority over ephemeral success, however spectacular. Although the word sustainable is in fashion at the moment, its meaning is vague. How long does sustainable last? It is important not to use a lack of sustainability as an excuse for doing nothing;
- research is a stated objective of the strategy but targets need to be specified; over the last twenty-five years, the direct contribution of research to malaria control has been at best moderate.

The Global Strategy is far from authoritarian, true methods and drugs are largely dictated by local circumstances. The drugs selected will depend on local parasite susceptibility profiles; vector control may include time-limited indoor spraying at selected sites, insecticide-treated mosquito nets and, possibly, larval control, provided that it is

Table I. Malaria control 1880-2002.

Period	Year	Methods and strategies
Before 1943 Control measures focused 　in North America 　and the Mediterranean Basin	From 1820 From 1890 1930 1934	Curative and prophylactic treatment using quinine Larvicidal treatment Targeted clean-up Pyrethrin used against adult mosquitoes
From 1943 to 1955 Expansion of adult insect control Duration 12 years	1943 1944 1955	Indoor DDT spraying (Gahan & Lindquist, 1943) United States Indoor DDT spraying, Venezuela, Guyana Indoor DDT spraying, Mediterranean Basin, South America, Southeast Asia, India, Middle East
From 1955 to 1969 Global Eradication Programme Duration 14 years	1955 to 1969	Beginning of the eradication policy Implementation of eradication measures Exclusion of Africa
Laborious implementation 　of control strategies Duration 13 years	1969 1972 1978	End of the official eradication policy Review of control strategies. Brazzaville Conference Alma-Alta Conference. SSP policy and abandonment of vertical programmes Abandonment of spraying programmes leading to the recrudescence of malaria (with the number of cases doubling between 1970 and 1985) Return to attack phases
Application of the 1992 Strategy Duration 10 years to present	1992 to 2002	Amsterdam Conference, 1992 Global Malaria Control Strategy Roll Back Malaria - Reactivation of the Control Strategy

sustainable. Since laboratory diagnosis is impossible in 90% of cases, clinical or even presumptive diagnosis is often the only option.

Finally, the incidence of malaria has always been related to economic development throughout history: if the former has often conditioned the latter, the inverse is also true in some cases.

Given that many countries have serious financial difficulties, it is legitimate to ask the most affluent countries to provide international or bilateral aid.

The targets and methods proposed in the Roll Back Malaria program are summarised in *Figure 3*. This initiative focuses on implementing the strategy defined at Amsterdam in 1992 by setting up collaborative projects and partnerships.

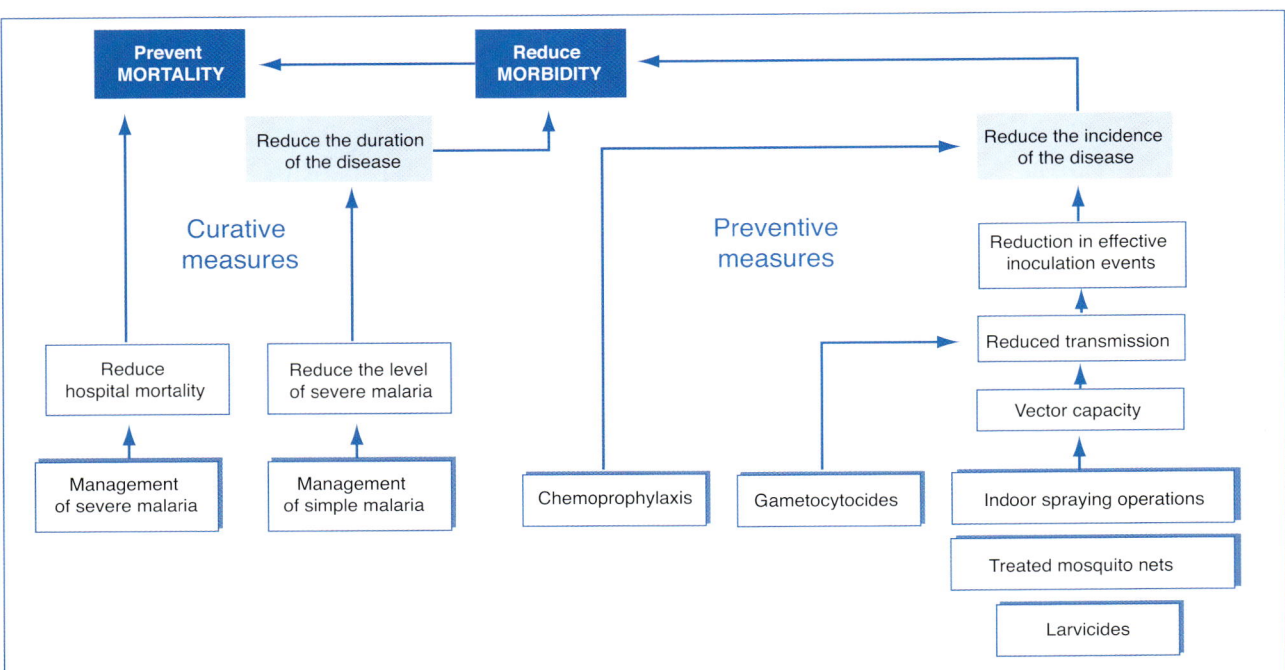

Figure 3. Goals, mid-points and actions in malaria control (from Coosemans).

Patient Care and Malaria Diagnosis

Patient care—a term which covers both diagnosis and treatment—is the cornerstone of malaria control in the Global Strategy. The process is divided into three phases:
- realisation that the patient is sick by the mother or another family member, then presentation of the patient at health care facility. In the absence of this, on the first signs, usually fever, many families are reduced to "caring" for the patient with drugs available from a pharmacy or dispensary—or very often, from the local general store or a travelling peddler; consulting a traditional practitioner does not always preclude such self-medication;
- establishment of a diagnosis, initially on clinical criteria and subsequently—if the centre has the resources for blood examination or rapid diagnosis—on a parasitological basis; 90% of diagnoses are purely clinical—and more than half of these are wrong (Baudon *et al.*, 1984);
- drug prescription and, if necessary, hospitalisation of the patient. In principle, health care and drugs should be free or at least affordable although this is not always the case, which is one reason why so many patients resort to self-medication. The high cost of modern drugs, especially the artemisinin derivatives, means that many patients are denied access to the most effective treatment, although such drugs are spreading through even the poorest countries (e.g. the Comoros);
- if a patient is not responding to treatment, parasitological examination should be performed before the therapeutic strategy is changed;
- severe malaria requires immediate treatment which can only be effectively administered in a specially equipped medical facility.

Treatment is not a new thing, on the contrary, it was being practised with qinghaosu more than 2,000 years ago and with *Cinchona* bark in the 17th century, long before the discovery of *Plasmodium*. But, since the launch of the Global Malaria Control Strategy in 1992, it is supposed to be available to all subjects living in endemic areas. It is therefore important to inform and educate whole populations, notably mothers and all categories of care provider, both professional and voluntary. This education—perhaps more aptly described as training—should cover the earliest signs of a malarial paroxysm, how patients can be treated, and what care providers should do when confronted with severe malaria.

Clinical diagnosis

Attitudes of mothers and family members

It is usually the mother who is the first to become aware that a child is sick. Fever—measured using a thermometer or simply by hand—accompanied by sweating and shivering are the first suggestive symptoms although they are not always seen. There may also be headache, loss of appetite, nausea, vomiting, diarrhoea and, in babies, convulsions, but all of these may be mild and short-lived at the beginning, and can be missed.

When confronted with these alarm signals, the family should consult a health care facility. However, they often buy drugs directly or go to see a traditional practitioner, thereby delaying effective treatment. Chloroquine—along with bottled beer—is one of the few modern consumer products to have reached the most isolated villages in West and Central Africa. The availability of this drug made presumptive treatment possible throughout most of Africa but the spread of resistance—not only to chloroquine but also to sulfadoxine-pyrimethamine—and the resultant increasing incidence of therapeutic failure is seriously compromising self-medication. Moreover, if treatment is not effective, a mild attack can develop into severe disease.

Attitudes of local health care workers

How the patient and his or her family is received at the health care centre is a sensitive topic. Most care providers are highly motivated and competent but absenteeism, lack of drugs or their sale at too high a price are among the problems that have undermined the reputation of some facilities.

That said, it is important to remember that the non-specificity of the clinical symptoms of a malaria attack makes clinical diagnosis difficult. Even a temperature of over 38 °C—the most common symptom—is not always present. Differential diagnosis *vis-à-vis* arbovirus infection (dengue, sandfly fever), nascent visceral leishmaniasis and even tuberculosis or brucellosis is not possible at the average health care centre, save for well-characterised epidemics (e.g. measles or meningitis).

Parasitological diagnosis

The roles of parasitological diagnosis are to:
- support the clinical observations and confirm (or rule out) the diagnosis of malaria;
- investigate the reasons for failure to respond to treatment;
- confirm cases of severe malaria;
- detect simple attacks in places where transmission is relatively rare.

Parasites can be detected in thick or thin blood smears, both of which methods are described in the first part of this book (*see the Chapter on* "Epidemiological Basis").

In places where malaria is stable, 60-80% of children carry parasites in their blood, therefore the simple detection of parasites is not enough to confirm the diagnosis of a malaria attack. Only if the parasite density is above the so-called "pyrogenic threshold" (3,000-15,000 parasites per µl, depending on the locality and age) and the patient is febrile can a firm diagnosis be made (*see the Chapter on* "Epidemiological Basis"). In regions of stable malaria, it is essential to differenciate asymptomatic carriers from those suffering a malaria crisis, requiring immediate treatment.

Modern diagnostic methods

These methods were described above (*see the Chapter on* "Epidemiological Basis") but new ones are constantly being developed and it can be hoped that, in the near future, detecting malaria will be a simple process which does not require a meticulous—and error-prone—microscopic examination.

Many laboratories in developed countries are capable of concentrating parasitized red blood cells by centrifugation and staining them with acridine orange (the QBC Malaria Test®), but this system requires an ultraviolet read-out system.

The Parasight F Test®, the ICT Malaria Pf Test®, the Now® ICT Malaria Pf/Pv test and Paracheck Pf® all detect plasmodial antigens and are available as strip tests (RDT = Rapid Detection Test).

The Opti Mal Test® is based on the detection of plasmodial lactate dehydrogenase.

Some of these tests have recently been used in large-scale surveys, notably in Burundi. In highly endemic areas, plasmodial antigens persist in asymptomatic carriers, reducing the value of this approach for diagnosis although it makes diagnosing the disease easy in returning travellers.

Simple attacks

Table I lists the main symptoms of malaria together with accompanying signs.

Severe paroxysms

If untreated, severe malaria attacks or paroxysms usually result in death. Specific malaria mortality is due to such paroxysms (often following the deterioration of a simple case) but malaria is also associated with considerable indirect mortality—which often counts for more deaths than the specific mortality. Almost all severe paroxysms are due to *P. falciparum*. WHO (2001a) has republished an easy-to-use handbook containing basic information on diagnosing and treating malaria (*Table II*).

A severe paroxysm constitutes a medical emergency with the death of the patient likely to ensue within days or even hours unless treatment is rapidly administered.

The first four syndromes described—all associated with a very high *P. falciparum* parasitaemia—are the most commonly encountered.

Cerebral malaria is the most common complication. Coma can be evaluated in adults and older children using the Glasgow Scale (*Table III*), or with the Paediatric Blantyre Scale (*Table IV*) in very young children who have not yet learned to talk. If the comatose state is prolonged, irreversible sequelae are seen in more than 10% of children (but less than 5% of adults). Convulsions are far more common in children than they are in adults.

Anaemia with a haematocrit reading of below 20% is usually only seen in young children or primigravidae. The risk of severe malaria in the third trimester of pregnancy is between two and ten times higher in the immunologically naïve than in semi-immune mothers-to-be.

Impaired kidney function with hypouresis and high blood creatinine levels may warrant peritoneal dialysis although few health centres in the developing world are capable of administering this form of treatment. Instead, isotonic infusion has been recommended.

The WHO Handbook (Geneva, 2001a) gives recommendations as to what to do when confronted with each of the syndromes associated with severe malaria.

Patient Care and Malaria Diagnosis

Table I. Symptoms of the simple malaria attack.

The symptoms of the simple malaria attack are often misleading, being variable according to immune status and the *Plasmodium* species involved. They may be differently interpreted by the mother of a febrile child, a doctor or health care worker (with or without laboratory back-up)

Simple, primary attack in a "naïve" non immune person (a young child, a visitor)
- Short-lived fever
- Gastrointestinal problems (nausea, vomiting). Respiratory symptoms are common and particularly misleading

Symptoms more intense with *P. falciparum*, milder with *P. vivax*, *P. ovale* and *P. malariae*

Simple malaria in a partially immune subject
- Malaria attack:
  - sustained fever (a few days)
  - asthenia
  - splenomegaly
  - anaemia/pallor
- Simple attack: a triad of symptoms rarely complete for *P. falciparum*
  - **shivering** and headache
  - **hot**, fever with splenomegaly
  - **sweating**, end of the attack
- Possible concomitant symptoms, often associated with a poor prognosis:
  - convulsions
  - digestive problems (vomiting, diarrhoea)
  - respiratory problems
  - anaemia, pallor
  - nascent jaundice
  - nascent neurological problems (*P. falciparum*)

At any point, an attack of *P. falciparum* malaria may progress to a severe form, possibly leading to death

Table II. Syndromes associated with a serious paroxysm (adapted from WHO, Geneva, 2001).

Syndrome	Symptoms
Cerebral malaria	Coma, convulsions, motor deficit
Anaemia	Haematocrit often lower than 20%
Kidney failure	Oliguria, elevated creatinine
Hypoglycaemia	After quinine treatment: hyperinsulinaemia
Electrolyte imbalance	Urine sodium concentration below 20 mml/l
Pulmonary oedema	Complication during or after treatment (50% fatality)
Circulatory collapse	Low body temperature, often associated with infection
Bleeding and intravascular coagulation problems	Bleeding from the gums, epistaxis, generalised bleeding, thrombocytopaenia
Hyperpyrexia	Generally associated with convulsions
Hyperparasitaemia	Parasite density over 5%, severe anaemia
Blackwater fever	In subjects with G6PD on primaquine. Role of quinine?

Table III. Glasgow Scale for progressive coma.		
		Score
Eyes open	Spontaneously	4
	In response to a voice	3
	In response to a painful stimulus	2
	No response	1
Verbal response	Normal	5
	Confused	4
	Inappropriate word usage	3
	Incomprehensible sounds	2
	None	1
Motor response	Execution of orders	6
	Localisation of painful stimulus	5
	Flexion in response to pain: return normal	4
	return abnormal	3
	Extension in response to pain	2
	None	1

Table IV. Paediatric scale for progressive coma.		
		Score
Motor response	Localisation of painful stimulus	2
	Retraction of member in response to pain	1
	Response non-specific or absent	0
Verbal response	Appropriate	2
	Inappropriate or mumbling	1
	None	0
Eye movements	Orientated (following the mother's face)	1
	Disorientated	0

Drug and Treatment Policies

National drug policies

Most countries have a national drug policy which covers malaria drugs. Once first-line, second-line and sometimes even third-line drugs have been defined, stocks are distributed around health centres and community-based facilities. Above and beyond the official, public-sector outlets and private-sector pharmacies, large volumes of drugs are also sold at dispensaries or by general stores and travelling peddlers. National drug regulation institutions are often dysfunctional and many poor-quality or dangerous drugs are available on the black market, e.g. drugs containing less than the stipulated dose or even no active substance at all. In Africa and Southeast Asia, such parallel distribution short-circuits health centres which often run out of medicine. The products available to members of the community are not always those that are recommended by the health authorities (usually in accordance with WHO guidelines).

Choice of drugs

The selection of first-line and second-line drugs is conditioned by various considerations, some of them mutually contradictory:
- efficacy must be the primordial criterion: the drug should cure the patient with a minimum of adverse effects;
- the susceptibility of the parasite to the compound in question; drug resistance restricts the use of many drugs, notably chloroquine and sulfadoxine-pyrimethamine (*Table I*).
- cost is a major factor for health authorities. In 2004, a course of chloroquine costs 0.07 € whereas artemether-lumefantrin can be as much as 2.5 € (and even then, only if it is obtained from WHO); a course of halofantrin costs 4.20 €;
- acceptability is an important parameter, especially when it comes to drugs with known side effects. Mefloquine on its own or in combinations is rejected in Cambodia because it is known to induce vomiting and chloroquine used to be unpopular in Africa because people with very high parasite loads may experience pruritus. Serious adverse reactions remain rare or very rare, e.g. eye problems with chloroquine, liver problems with amodiaquine, and heart problems with halofantrin; however, they contribute to poor compliance and therapeutic failure.

Changing national policies: monotherapy or multiple drugs?

Changing national policy—even as simple a switch as that from chloroquine to sulfadoxine-pyrimethamine as first-line drug—is complicated and difficult to implement. Many African countries still distribute first-line chloroquine despite significant local resistance to this drug.

Until recently, **monotherapy** has been the rule: chloroquine or sulfadoxine-pyrimethamine for first-line treatment with quinine in the event of non-response or for severe paroxysms (NB: the combination of sulfadoxine and pyrimethamine, two active substances which block different stages of the folic acid synthetic pathway, is considered as monotherapy).

Combination therapy involves combining at least two schizont-active compounds with distinct mechanisms of action and different biochemical targets, with a view to enhancing efficacy and preventing the development of resistance to each of the active substances. It is likely that, in the near future, the need for multiple therapy to deal with multi-drug resistant parasites will increase. Combination therapy is ten times more expensive than

Table Ia. Drug resistance and changes in first-line medicinal products (WHO/CD/RBM 2001-33).

Country	Resistance	First-line drug (2001 recommendation)	Second-line drug
Botswana	Chloroquine (1984)	Sulfadoxine-pyrimethamine	Quinine
Kenya	Chloroquine (1979) Sulfadoxine-pyrimethamine (1998)	Sulfadoxine-pyrimethamine	Amodiaquine
Ethiopia	Chloroquine (1979) Sulfadoxine-pyrimethamine (1998)	Chloroquine + sulfadoxine-pyrimethamine *P. vivax*: chloroquine	Quinine
Ghana	Chloroquine (1987) Sulfadoxine-pyrimethamine	Chloroquine	Sulfadoxine-pyrimethamine
Malawi	Chloroquine (1984)	Sulfadoxine-pyrimethamine	Quinine
Mali	Chloroquine Sulfadoxine-pyrimethamine	Chloroquine	Sulfadoxine-pyrimethamine
Tanzania	Chloroquine (1978) Sulfadoxine-pyrimethamine (1982)	Sulfadoxine-pyrimethamine	Amodiaquine
South Africa		Sulfadoxine-pyrimethamine	Quinine
Uganda		Chloroquine + sulfadoxine-pyrimethamine	Quinine
Zambia	Chloroquine (1978)	Sulfadoxine-pyrimethamine	
Papua New Guinea	Chloroquine (1976) Amodiaquine (1987) Quinine Sulfadoxine-pyrimethamine *P. vivax* resistant to chloroquine	Chloroquine + sulfadoxine-pyrimethamine (adults) Amodiaquine + sulfadoxine-pyrimethamine (children) *P. vivax* : chloroquine + primaquine	Artesunate + sulfadoxine-pyrimethamine
Salomon	Chloroquine (1980) Sulfadoxine-pyrimethamine (1995)	Chloroquine + sulfadoxine-pyrimethamine *P. vivax* : chloroquine + primaquine	Quinine
Vanuatu	Chloroquine (1987) Sulfadoxine-pyrimethamine (1991)	Chloroquine + sulfadoxine-pyrimethamine *P. vivax* : chloroquine	Quinine
Afghanistan	Chloroquine	Chloroquine	Sulfadoxine-pyrimethamine
Bangladesh	Chloroquine (1970) Sulfadoxine-pyrimethamine (1985)	Chloroquine + primaquine	Quinine + sulfadoxine-pyrimethamine
Cambodia	Chloroquine (1960) Sulfadoxine-pyrimethamine (1965) Mefloquine (1995)	Chloroquine (limited regions) Artesunate + mefloquine	Quinine + tetracycline
India	Chloroquine (1987) Sulfadoxine-pyrimethamine (1982) *P. vivax* resistant to chloroquine	Chloroquine + primaquine *P. vivax* : chloroquine	Sulfadoxine-pyrimethamine + primaquine
Malaysia	Chloroquine Sulfadoxine-pyrimethamine *P. vivax*: chloroquine	Chloroquine	Sulfadoxine-pyrimethamine
Myanmar (Burma)	Chloroquine Sulfadoxine-pyrimethamine Mefloquine Quinine	Chloroquine or sulfadoxine-pyrimethamine + primaquine	Mefloquine + primaquine Quinine + primaquine
Thailand	Chloroquine Sulfadoxine-pyrimethamine Mefloquine Quinine	Mefloquine + primaquine Mefloquine + artesunate + primaquine on the frontiers *P. vivax* : chloroquine	Quinine + tetracycline
Vietnam	Chloroquine Sulfadoxine-pyrimethamine Mefloquine	Chloroquine (north) Artemether or artesunate (south-center) *P. vivax* : chloroquine + primaquine	Artesunate + mefloquine
Yemen	Chloroquine	Chloroquine	Sulfadoxine-pyrimethamine

Drug and Treatment Policies

Table Ib. Drug resistance and changes in first-line medicinal products (WHO/CD/RBM 2001-33).

Country	Resistance	First-line drug (2001 recommendation)	Second-line drug
Brazil	Chloroquine (1961) *P. vivax*: chloroquine Sulfadoxine-pyrimethamine (1972) Mefloquine (1996)	Quinine + tetracycline	Mefloquine
Colombia	Chloroquine (1958) Sulfadoxine-pyrimethamine (1985)	Amodiaquine + primaquine + sulfadoxine-pyrimethamine	Sulfadoxine-pyrimethamine
Guyana	Chloroquine (1987) Sulfadoxine-pyrimethamine (1982) *P. vivax*: chloroquine	Quinine + clindomycine	Sulfadoxine-pyrimethamine
French Guiana	Chloroquine (1990)	Artemether + lumefanthrin	
Peru	Chloroquine (1987) Sulfadoxine-pyrimethamine (1997)	Sulfadoxine-pyrimethamine + artesunate (Pacific coast) Mefloquine + artesunate (Amazonia)	Sulfadoxine-pyrimethamine
Venezuela	Chloroquine (1960) Sulfadoxine-pyrimethamine (1978)	Chloroquine + primaquine	Quinine + doxycycline

chloroquine, and even more if it includes an artemisinin derivative*.

Africa—where 90% of cases of malaria occur—will only be able to meet this challenge with international or bilateral aid. Otherwise, local health care services will be unable to cope.

Therapeutic arsenal

WHO (2001) has compiled a list of malaria drugs together with usual dosages, presentations, contraindications and resistance details. This list is summarised in *Table II* (agents used in monotherapy) and *Table III* (combination therapy).

Drugs used in monotherapy

For over fifty years, **chloroquine** (CQ, a 4-aminoquinoline) was ideal for both the treatment of simple attacks and for prophylaxis. However, its usefulness is steadily waning with the spread of resistance.

Amodiaquine (AQ, another 4-aminoquinoline) is not used for prophylaxis because it can occasionally cause liver and blood problems. Resistance is common but usually low-level, not leading to non-response. This drug was recommended for first-line treatment in many countries (e.g. Kenya and Tanzania) where chloroquine resistance is common.

Sulfadoxine-pyrimethamine (SP) is the most commonly proposed alternative when chloroquine resistance is common, although resistance to this combination—which from the beginning was associated with therapeutic failure—appeared almost immediately after that to chloroquine and the switch has not brought any sustained benefit (Ogutu *et al.*, 2000).

Despite some very demarcated foci of resistance in Thailand and Vietnam, **mefloquine** (ME) is in widespread use in Asia against multi-resistant strains. It is often combined with an artemisinin derivative to improve the efficacy of the treatment. Side effects are quite common with mefloquine, including neuropsychiatric impairment, nausea and vomiting. This drug can only be taken orally.

Halofantrin was developed for the treatment of resistant strains and is often reserved as a stand-by for immunologically naïve travellers to high-risk places. It is expensive (over 4 € per course, i.e. 130 times the price of chloroquine) and its heart toxicity necessitates close monitoring. It is only taken orally to treat simple attacks.

Quinine (Q) is the oldest of the antimalarial drugs and still has a place in the treatment of severe disease and multi-drug resistant infections. It is quickly cleared from the body which means that it has to be taken regularly; however, this is also the reason why it has remained active for so long: the parasite does not have enough time to acquire high-level resistance.

---

* Derivatives of Qinghaosu (notably artemisinin and artesunate) or semi-synthetic compounds based on the same active substances (e.g. artemeter).

Table II. Drugs used on their own.		
Drug	**Dosage**	**Side effects and contraindications**
Chloroquine	25 mg/kg for 3 days	Sometime pruritus, visual perturbation following prolonged overdose
Amodiaquine	30 mg/kg for 3 days	Not recommended for prophylactic treatment (hepatitis, agranulocytosis)
Sulfadoxine-pyrimethamine	150 mg + 75 mg/kg in 3 installments over one day (adults)	Rare dermatitis
Quinine	24 mg/kg/day in 3 doses, for 3, 7 or 10 days	Reversible side effects (acusia, heart rate)
Mefloquine	25 mg/kg in single dose in 3 installments	Nausea, vomiting, dizziness Neuropsychological problems possible
Halofantrine	24 mg/kg in 1 day in 3 installments at 6-hour intervals	Avoid in patients with heart disease
Pyronaridine		Under development in China
Artemether	4 mg/kg on D1, 2 mg/kg from D2-5	Few side effects
Artemisinin	20 mg/kg on D1, 10 mg/kg from D2-6	Few side effects
Artesunate	4 mg/kg on D1, 12 mg/kg from D2-6	Few side effects
Primaquine	0,25 mg/kg from D1-14	Gametocytocide. Radical treatment for *P. vivax* Not recommended in subjects with G6PD

Pyronaridine is only used in China.

Primaquine (PQ, a 8-aminoquinoline) is the drug most often used against hepatic forms and gametocytes. It is used to prevent relapsing *P. vivax* malaria This product is not suitable for G6PD-deficient subjects (i.e. over 30% of the population in some countries).

Qinghaosu derivatives—artesunate (ASU), artemisinin and artemether (ATM)—are extracted from a species of wormwood (*Artemisia annua*). They are effective, fast-acting and very safe. Because they have a very short biological half-life, they are usually used in combination therapy in which they cut down the length of the course of treatment and prevent the development of resistance. Recent studies sponsored by WHO showed the efficacy of combinations of artesunate with amodiaquine (Adjuick *et al.*, 2002) and sulfadoxine-pyrimethamine (Von Seidlein *et al.*, 2000).

Combination therapy

The most commonly used drug combinations are:
- chloroquine + sulfadoxine-pyrimethamine: no advantage over monotherapy since resistance usually involves both drugs; this combination is now mistrusted and rarely prescribed;
- amodiaquine + sulfadoxine-pyrimethamine: no obvious advantage over amodiaquine on its own; rarely prescribed;
- mefloquine + sulfadoxine-pyrimethamine: exerts a strong selection pressure on parasites and is therefore associated with a high probability of acquired resistance (Watkins & Mosobo, 1993); no longer in production;
- quinine + tetracycline or quinine + doxycycline are used where quinine resistance is low;
- chloroquine + proguanil: until recently one of the most commonly used combinations for prophylaxis in Africa (Savarine®) but failure is not rare;
- atovaquone-proguanil (Malarone®): used for both prophylaxis and cure; highly effective against chloroquine and mefloquine-resistant strains; acts on asexual hepatic forms; very expensive;
- chlorproguanil-dapsone: used against multi-drug resistant parasites;
- artesunate + chloroquine: of little use in places where chloroquine resistance is common;
- artesunate + amodiaquine: useful where chloroquine resistance is moderate;
- artesunate + sulfadoxine-pyrimethamine: efficacy limited in East Africa where sulfadoxine-pyrimethamine resistance is common; useful in West Africa;
- artesunate + mefloquine: first-line treatment in many parts of Southeast Asia; mefloquine's side effects have led to this combination being discouraged in Africa;
- artemether-lumefantrin (Coartem®): very effective and safe; not recommended for pregnant women;
- artesunate + chlorproguanil + dapsone: made available in Africa in 2003 after very promising field trials.

Drug and Treatment Policies

Table III. Combination therapy for *P. falciparum* and *P. vivax* (adapted from WHO, 2001).		
Drugs	**Dosage and course**	**Comments***
Associations without an artemisinin derivative		
Chloroquine + sulfadoxine-pyrimethamine		No demonstrated benefit over sulfadoxine-pyrimethamine
Amodiaquine + sulfadoxine-pyrimethamine		Risk of amodiaquine toxicity not excluded. Advantage?
Quinine + tetracycline	8 mg quinine + 250 mg tetracycline 4 times a day/8 days	For strains that are not very sensitive to quinine
Quinine + doxycycline	8 mg quinine + 100 mg doxycycline a day/8 days	For strains that are not very sensitive to quinine
Chloroquine + proguanil	1 g chloroquine + 400mg proguanil	Used for prophylaxis (tourists, servicemen, etc.)
Atovaquone + proguanil	1 g atovaquone + 400 mg proguanil	Prophylaxis. Avoid in subjects with kidney failure. The best prophylactic drug
Chlorproguanil + dapsone		Treatment of resistant strains
Combinations with an artemisinin derivative		
Artesunate + chloroquine		Does not induce resistance to chloroquine or amodiaquine
Artesunate + amodiaquine		
Artesunate + mefloquine		Used for first-line treatment in Thailand. Nausea, vomiting, neuropsychiatric problems possible
Artemether + lumefantrine	4 tab. at the beginning then 4 tab. after 8 hours. Then twice a day for 2 days	Apparently good outcomes. Better tolerated than artesunate + mefloquine
Chlorproguanil-dapsone + artesunate	Rapid and effective	Available in Africa in 2003
Products far along in the development process		
Pyronaridine + artesunate		In China
Piperaquine-dihydro-artemisinine-trimetoprime	3-5 days course	Very promising
Artecom + primaquine		Trials in China, Vietnam, Cambodia, Peru
Artemether + benflumentol (CGP56695)		Very effective, promising combination
* Unless specifically mentioned, combination therapy does not present problems of resistance		

New drugs in development

- pyronaridine + artesunate developed in Korea;
- piperaquine + dihydro-artemisinin + trimethoprim; a 3-5 day course of treatment;
- artecom + primaquine: trials in China and Vietnam;
- artemether + benflumentol (CGP 56695): one of the most effective combinations—apparently without side effects. For the treatment of simple attacks in adults and children, even due to multi-drug resistant strains;
- naphthtoquine + dihydro-artemisinin: under development but the toxicological testing is still in the early stages.

The Walter Reed Institute is experimenting with 8-aminoquinolines, namely tafenoquine (a primaquine analogue, WR 138.605) and guanyhydrazone (WR 182.393) for the radical cure of *P. vivax* malaria.

Trioxaquine (Meunier, Toulouse) is a conjugate of 4-aminoquinoline and trioxane.

Ferroquine (SSR 97-19371) (Sanofi-Brocard-Lille) is a 4-aminoquinoline.

Fosmidocyne (Jonaa Pharma, Germany) is an antibiotic that blocks parasite isoprenoside synthesis. In trials in Gabon, it has been administered together with clindamycin and artesunate.

Less advanced, active research is underway into the synthesis of artemisinin-related compounds (Hoffmann Laroche and the University of Nebraska), and active substances (e.g. T16) that inhibit parasite membrane protein binding and phospholipid metabolism (Vial, University of Montpellier G25).

Counterfeit drugs and inappropriate products

No discussion of the topic of antimalaria treatment can ignore counterfeit drugs which are increasingly common in countries where intellectual and industrial property rights are not effectively protected. The most common trick is under-dosing the active substance, or even omitting it; the packaging and the capsules or tablets look exactly like the true version. Forgers usually carry on with impunity, in particular in the African and Asian marketplaces.

Often due to the ignorance of distributors rather than deliberate dishonesty, patients (many of whom are illiterate or insufficiently aware) are given drugs which are devoid of activity against *Plasmodium*. A survey conducted in Cambodia by McDonald & Lek Sandi (personal communication) indicated that only 30% of the drugs sold as anti-malarials by general stores and travelling peddlers were actually intended for the indication; 30% of patients were being given Vitamin C.

Attention has already been drawn to the importance of educating everyone involved in malaria control. Distribution circuits can easily be improved, even in rural settings, as long as the tradesmen are of good faith, although it cannot be denied that genuinely cynical counterfeit drug distribution networks exist. Forging needs to be combated by reinforcing regulatory and monitoring systems, and by raising awareness.

Resistance to malaria drugs

What induces resistance

Chloroquine used to be ideal for treatment by virtue of its efficacy and low cost, and for prophylaxis by virtue of its lack of toxicity.

Unfortunately, the simultaneous emergence of chloroquine resistance in Latin America and Southeast Asia in the 1960's followed by its spread is now restricting its usefulness (D'Alessandro & Buttiens, 2001; Wéry & Coosemans, 1980). In Africa, the first chloroquine-resistant strains made their appearance towards the end of the 1970's in Kenya and Tanzania.

An increase in the level of chloroquine resistance in a given place is almost always accompanied by a significant increase in malaria mortality (Trape *et al.*, 1998). Switching from chloroquine to another first-line antimalarial (e.g. sulfadoxine-pyrimethamine or mefloquine) may resolve the problem temporarily but only until resistance to the new drug appears.

Resistance is not an all-or-nothing phenomenon and its degree is highly variable. The development of resistance depends on multiple interactions (D'Alessandro, 1998). Naturally-occurring *P. falciparum* populations are genetically heterogeneous mixtures which respond in different ways to different drugs. The efficacy of any drug will depend on its concentration, the intrinsic susceptibility of the parasite, and the length of time the parasite is exposed to an active concentration of the drug. A small fraction of the original parasite load may survive a course of treatment and can be eliminated by immune mechanisms. However, the infection will persist if too many parasites survive, either because they have some degree of resistance to the drug or if the concentration of the drug has been allowed to fall below a critical threshold; this is why under-dosed drugs tend to select for resistant parasites.

The propagation of resistant strains is exacerbated by the fact that sulfadoxine-pyrimethamine induces rapid over-production of gametocytes (Robert *et al.*, 2000). Drugs with a long half-life have the advantage that they can be taken as a single dose (notably sulfadoxine-pyrimethamine and mefloquine) but these exert a major selection pressure (Hasting *et al.*, 2000). Artemisinin and its derivatives have very short half-lives, which makes them particularly valuable for combination therapy together with a product with a long half-life (e.g. mefloquine, piperaquine or lumefantrin), which cuts down the chance of resistance developing. Moreover, artemisinins drastically reduce the production of gametocytes which might have an impact on transmission.

Monitoring resistance

Monitoring for new forms of resistance is an essential part of any national malaria control programme. Different types of test exist.

In vivo tests

Testing *in vivo* means estimating the parasite's response in a patient treated with a fixed dose of the medicinal product under investigation (taking into account variable responsiveness). This gives an overall estimate of resistance but with a possible interference of the immune mechanisms In addition to susceptible (S), three different levels of resistance are recognised (RI, RII and RIII) (WHO, 1973). RI is defined as reduction of the parasite load below the microscopic detection limit for at least two of the first seven days of treatment but with recrudescence within two to four weeks. With RII, the parasitaemia drops substantially but never below the microscopic detection limit, and with RIII, it drops little if at all. In places where transmission rates are high, it is difficult to distinguish between recrudescence and new infection but these days, PCR genotyping can be used to this end (Magesa *et al.*, 2001).

In 1996, WHO changed the protocol to put more emphasis on therapeutic outcomes. A new fourteen-day test involves clinical and parasitological monitoring as well as measurements of haematocrit and temperature: this makes it possible to distinguish between a satisfactory clinical response and early or delayed therapeutic failure (WHO, 1996b). However, because of inconsistencies in inclusion criteria, care standards and the interpretation of results, it is not always possible to compare different studies. Following changes in resistance over time and in different places is often very problematic.

In vitro tests

Culture-based assays measure the degree to which schizogony is inhibited in the presence of increasing concentrations of the drug being tested. This excludes some of the confounding factors to which *in vivo* tests are prone, namely host immunity and drug bioavailability. But not all strains grow well *in vitro* and this could lead to selection-related distortion although, as a rule, *in vivo* and *in vitro* tests give concordant results. This type of testing requires highly competent laboratory technicians.

Molecular methods

Mutations—even point mutations—in the genome of the resistant parasite can be detected using molecular biology techniques. Various mutations have been linked with resistance to sulfadoxine-pyrimethamine and it is the number of such mutations accumulated in the genome that determines the degree of resistance (Plowe *et al.*, 1997). Chloroquine resistance is partially due to a mutation in the *pfcrt* gene which leads to decreased build-up of chloroquine in the parasite's digestive vacuole. This type of resistance can be reversed by the administration of verapamil. The same gene is implicated in resistance to other antimalarial drugs (quinine, mefloquine and artemisinin) but strangely, not to amodiaquine (Sidhu *et al.*, 2002). The methods of molecular biology can be used in the field to measure drug resistance (Djimde *et al.*, 2001).

Distribution of resistance (Table IV)

Chloroquine resistance is spreading in all parts of Southeast Asia, Africa and Latin America, not only in *P. falciparum* but also, in the last five years, in *P. vivax* in Papua New Guinea and India. In some countries like Cambodia, *P. falciparum* is still susceptible in some provinces of the interior whereas it is extremely resistant in frontier areas where there is a great deal of population exchange and large quantities of malaria drugs are consumed (i.e. the selection pressure is high). Over-aggressive or too-frequent courses of treatment (e.g. in refugee camps or among private-sector company employees) as well as under-dosed self-medication products can foster drug resistance.

The spread of resistance to sulfadoxine-pyrimethamine seems to be following that to chloroquine, albeit somewhat later.

Mefloquine resistance is seen in only a few places in Southeast Asia and is very rare in South America.

Reports of reduced susceptibility to quinine require confirmation.

Resistance to chloroquine and sulfadoxine-pyrimethamine has led some countries to change the first-line drug they recommend, although the advantage associated with the switch has not always been observed (*Table I*). Switching from monotherapy to a combination is, at this time, the only strategy envisaged to counter resistance.

Treatment

Whether it concerns a simple attack, an attack with complications, or a severe paroxysm, the following factors need to be taken into account when prescribing a drug:
- the species of *Plasmodium* and its—or their—susceptibility to the usual drugs;
- the patient's general condition and age, any intercurrent diseases, pregnancy, certain genetic conditions (haemoglobinopathy, G6PD-deficiency) and recent or concomitant courses of other drugs. Oral forms cannot be prescribed to a patient who is vomiting or in a coma;
- treating a simple attack in a remote facility or at home should prevent deterioration to a potentially life-threatening paroxysm. The outcome will depend on the rapid accessibility to acceptable and affordable drugs (*Table IV*).

		Table IV. Treating a simple attack.	
Susceptible parasites	**Parasites resistant to chloroquine or sulfadoxine-pyrimethamine**	**Parasites resistant to chloroquine and sulfadoxine-pyrimethamine**	
		Monotherapy	**Combination therapy**
All products acceptable Chloroquine Amodiaquine Sulfadoxine-pyrimethamine	Chloroquine resistance: give sulfadoxine-pyrimethamine Resistance to sulfadoxine-pyrimethamine: give chloroquine	Amodiaquine if susceptible Mefloquine Halofantrine	Chlorproguanil-dapsone Chlorproguanil-dapsone + artesunate Artemether + lumefantrine Artesunate + mefloquine (SE Asia) Artesunate + amodiaquine

A severe paroxysm is a life-threatening emergency which requires immediate care in a hospital setting, preferably with intensive care facilities. Any delay to treatment may put the patient's life in danger. In addition to the parasitic infection, it is important to manage all the complications which may be associated with malaria (detailed in the preceding chapter).

The WHO handbook (2001a) on managing malaria gives advice for all the stages of care and treatment.

Quinine solutions are available: Quinmax containing 125 mg of alkaloid per ml; and Quinoform containing 219 mg of quinine base per ml. The loading dose is 17 mg/kg over 4 hours followed by maintenance treatment of 8 mg/kg every 8 hours, either infused over 4 hours or administered continuously. Subsequently, quinine is to be orally administered as soon as possible, and continued for 7 days. If it is suspected that the susceptibility of the parasite to quinine may be diminished, doxycycline or clindamycin should be added.

In Asia, quinine is increasingly being replaced by qinghaosu derivatives (artesunate, artemisinin, artemether), often together with mefloquine to ensure sustained antiplasmodial activity. Dosages of the various drugs are presented in *Tables II and III*.

Chemoprophylaxis

Definition and mass trials

Malaria chemoprophylaxis could be defined as regularly taking a medicinal product to protect against the onset and development of malaria disease. Until 1940, this was characterised by quinine distribution in Italy, North Africa and the United States, countries in which the disease was either prevented or treated. From the beginning of the century, taking quinine was a ritual act for expatriates living in malaria-ridden places. As early as 1789 during an epidemic in Mexico, Masdewall was advising anyone who had to stay in the affected area to chew *Cinchona* bark (*in* Najera, 2001). Sailors visiting African ports were also accustomed to consuming a decoction of *Cinchona* bark in wine.

After 1945, the widespread availability of chloroquine—a compound that is cheap, highly effective when administered in a single dose and which does not cause major side effects—made generalised prophylaxis possible.

But the results of trials in pilot zones in Africa—in Burkina Faso (Choumara *et al.*, 1959) and Cameroon (Cavalié & Mouchet, 1962)—soon proved disappointing. Although at first, 100% of the local people participated in the distribution of chloroquine + pyrimethamine on a monthly basis, participation soon dropped below 50%, then below 30%. People who were not experiencing any direct effects of the disease failed to procure the drugs—only those who actually had symptoms took them, effectively boiling down to presumptive treatment. In Madagascar, child prophylaxis at "nivaquinisation" centres continued until 1975 but in effect, ever since the 1960's, these centres had been functioning as no more than dispensaries with a clientele almost exclusively of people that were already sick.

The spread of *P. falciparum* chloroquine resistance as of 1962, the principal prophylactic drug, spoiled this preventive option which was replaced by indoor spraying methods using remanent insecticides (DDT and malathion).

After 1975, in the context of the various reviews of strategy, chemoprophylaxis was reinstated as a possible means of "controlling" malaria. However, the lessons of the past showed that it was neither reasonable nor possible to attempt to treat entire populations, especially in highly endemic zones.

According to the 1992 Global Strategy, chemoprophylaxis was to be reserved for:
- pregnant women;
- travellers (spending less than three months in an endemic area);
- immunologically naïve people staying in an endemic region.

For the high-risk group of under-2 year-olds, prophylaxis was rejected in the light of the practically insurmountable difficulties associated with implementation. In addition, some experts believed that chemoprophylaxis might inhibit the acquisition of immunity and installation of the state of premunition although this has never been demonstrated. This philosophy is currently being re-evaluated and children are being intermittently treated in some places.

Prophylaxis for pregnant women

Rationale

Malaria is more common in pregnant than in non-pregnant women. Both the prevalence and the severity of the symptoms depend on the woman's immune status prior to pregnancy which, in turn, will depend on the local transmission rate (Mutabingwa, 1994): in parts of tropical Africa where malaria is stable, the disease causes fewer problems—for both mother and child—than in places where it is unstable.

It is important to point up the difference between women pregnant for the first time and those who have already had children:

- malaria is more common in the former than in the latter (Meuris *et al.*, 1993);
- the infected babies of the former weigh less than the infected babies of the latter (McGregor, 1984);
- and the women's haematocrit readings are lower.

Even so, although first-time mothers are at higher risk, all pregnant women need to be protected against malaria.

When protecting pregnant women was first recommended in the context of malaria control strategies, chemoprophylaxis was based on the continuous administration of chloroquine; however, with the spread of resistance to this drug, it became necessary to resort to other compounds at different dosages and this in the absence of any proof that any other drug or combination was devoid of toxicity for mother and/or child. Moreover, the known teratogenic activity of many drugs restricts the number of options available for the treatment of this high-risk group.

Intermittent Preventive Treatment (IPT)

A Cochrane review of malaria prevention in pregnant women compared the efficacy of:
- a series of different medicinal products, namely chloroquine, sulfadoxine-pyrimethamine, mefloquine and dapsone-pyrimethamine;
- different prophylactic protocols: weekly, twice-weekly and monthly dosing.

Intermittent treatment was a promising option in that its efficacy may be comparable to that of continuous chemoprophylaxis. The first study was conducted in Malawi: a protocol based on two doses of sulfadoxine-pyrimethamine (one administered during the second trimester of pregnancy and the other at the beginning of the third trimester) was compared either with another one with a single dose of sulfadoxine-pyrimethamine or with a full chloroquine treatment followed by weekly doses of the same drug. The double dose of sulfadoxine-pyrimethamine gave significantly better results in terms of peripheral and placental parasite loads as well as mean birth weight and the number of hypotrophic (under 2.5 kg) babies (Schulz *et al.*, 1994).

Another trial in Malawi showed significantly higher mean birth weight and a significant decrease in the number of low birth-weight babies after two or three doses of sulfadoxine-pyrimethamine as opposed to just one; the number of doses of sulfadoxine-pyrimethamine had no effect on placental or peripheral parasitaemia, or on haemoglobin concentration (Verhoeff *et al.*, 1998). Two studies conducted in Kenya compared intermittent treatment with sulfadoxine-pyrimethamine to placebo and the conventional management regimen: one of these showed that intermittent sulfadoxine-pyrimethamine treatment was associated with a significant reduction in the incidence of severe anaemia (Shulman *et al.*, 1999); and the other showed a positive effect in terms of mean birth weight and the proportion of hypotrophic babies (Parise *et al.*, 1998).

Intermittent sulfadoxine-pyrimethamine treatment is therefore effective when it comes to preventing some of the adverse consequences of malaria in pregnant women. However, this drug is contraindicated before the sixteenth week of gestation because of the possibility of teratogenic activity (Philipps-Howard & Wood, 1996).

In Malawi where intermittent treatment was introduced in 1993, only one-third of women delivering at the central Blantyre Hospital had taken both recommended doses, evidence of the difficulties associated with compliance (Rogerson *et al.*, 2000).

In HIV-positive women, intermittent treatment does not seem to be enough to confer adequate protection although the effective dosage regimen has not yet been defined (Verhoeff *et al.*, 1999).

Most studies have shown a significant reduction in parasitaemia and a significant increase in haematocrit, especially in first babies (Greenwood *et al.*, 1984), but no study has included enough subjects to demonstrate any effect on perinatal or neonatal mortality. It can be concluded that the administration of an effective antimalarial prophylactic drug protects against complication during pregnancy and has positive effects on the new-born babies (Gulmezoglu & Garner, 1999).

Insecticide-treated mosquito nets in the protection of pregnant women

Treated mosquito nets (*see the Chapter on the* "Prevention by Means of Vector Control") represent an alternative way of controlling malaria during pregnancy (D'Alessandro *et al.*, 1995) although there is not enough evidence to make it possible to draw any firm conclusions about efficacy (for both treated and untreated nets) (Gulmezoglu & Garner, 1999).

The National Treated Mosquito Net Programme in Gambia yielded positive results but only in first-time mothers during the transmission season.

Mean birth weight was significantly higher in first-time mothers from villages where the mosquito nets had been treated with insecticide; in parallel, the number of premature births was lower as was the prevalence of parasitaemia in the mothers in the third week (D'Alessandro *et al.*, 1996). A Kenyan study confirmed the beneficial effects of treated mosquito nets for pregnant women and new-born babies in an endemic region (Gamble *et al.*, 2007; Lengeler, 2004)).

Protection is warranted in all pregnant women from endemic and epidemic areas but first-time mothers are a priority target—and this is the most difficult group to reach: the mean age of 651 first-time mothers-to-be in Gambia was just 17, and most were illiterate farmers. Although most of the women had attended at least one prenatal consultation (the mean number being four), only a very small number had been given any prophylactic drugs. Most had received iron supplementation and folic acid but this had had little effect on mean haematocrit and 18% suffer from anaemia (haemoglobin ≤ 8) after 32 weeks of gestation.

Conclusions: the future

In places where chloroquine resistance is a problem, intermittent treatment based on two doses of sulfadoxine-pyrimethamine is an useful option although when resistance to this medicine develops quickly (as happened in southern and East Africa), a therapeutic alternative needs to be sought.

Prophylaxis for travellers

Prophylaxis concerns all travellers—whatever the reason for the journey—as long as the stay in the endemic zone is not to exceed three months. In France, Travellers' Health Centres which can be consulted on the Internet give advice about the risk in different places and the appropriate precautions to take, including the drugs to take during and after the trip. A variety of factors needs to be taken into account.

Destination

Malarial prophylaxis relies on drugs that are active against *Plasmodium*, especially *P. falciparum*. In April 1999, the French-Language Infectious Disease Society's 12th Consensus Conference on Anti-Infectious Therapy (Anonymous, 1999d) divided the world into four different groups of countries on the basis of resistance to chloroquine, sulfadoxine-pyrimethamine and (less frequently) mefloquine and quinine:
- **Group 0**: no malaria;
- **Group 1**: *P. vivax* present but no *P. falciparum* or, if the latter is present, it is susceptible to chloroquine;
- **Group 2**: moderate drug resistance (an imprecise term);
- **Group 3**: highly resistant *P. falciparum*, possibly to multiple drugs. These are the countries that obviously pose the greatest problem in terms of prophylaxis and include almost all of tropical Africa, the Amazon Basin, Guyana and its neighbours in South America, the borders of Cambodia, Laos, Myanmar, Thailand, China (Yunnan and Haïnan) and Bangladesh, Irian Jaya (now called Western New Guinea) in Indonesia, and Papua New Guinea.

Other factors which determine prophylactic strategy

The risk run by a traveller will depend on the habitats being visited (urban or rural) and the quality of the accommodations (air-conditioning, mosquito nets, insecticide coils and diffusers, etc.). In the air-conditioned hotels of Asia and Latin America, the risk of infection is close to zero but in rural Africa (where mosquito nets are often in bad condition), there is a major and daily risk.

Risk depends on local epidemiology and the traveller's surroundings but these factors can be difficult to assess for travellers' advice institutions, e.g. a tourist passing eight days in Phnom-Penh and Siam Reap (Angkor Wat) runs hardly any risk of contracting malaria whereas someone who spends one night in the Cardamone Mountains will be highly exposed to multi-drug resistant Plasmodium, even though they are both visiting Cambodia.

People who have emigrated to the developed world often fall sick with malaria after returning to their adoptive country following a trip home to see the family.

People who are taking medications for hypertension, heart disease or diabetes as well as those with neurological disease and the immunodeficient ought to check the compatibility of the prophylactic antimalarial prescribed. Serious adverse reactions have been seen with mefloquine in people with neurological problems, and with halofantrin in people with heart disease. Travellers should seek advice from their general practitioner.

Travellers' Centres can usually provide advice about the recommended drugs and dosages. "Tips" should always be treated with caution, especially those from other tourists. Anyone who suffers from some specific condition or deficiency should seek advice from their general practitioner before travelling.

For the more conscious, travelling with a course of curative treatment on hand may be a viable option: medical personnel often opt for this strategy.

Prophylaxis

Table I summarises the prophylactic protocols recommended for the various country groups; dosages for children are shown although as a general rule, travelling to malaria-ridden places with very young children is not to be recommended.

The information in this Table is strictly provisional and it may be changed at any point as a result of the appearance of new resistance patterns or if new drugs become available.

In general, prophylactic drugs (especially mefloquine) should not be taken for a period of more than three months.

After returning home, the traveller should continue taking the drug for four more weeks to preclude attacks. In France, 85% of attacks occur within two weeks of coming home (Danis & Legros, 2002); only 2% are seen after two months or more.

A three month course of atovaquone + proguanil costs, in 2004, 350 €, compared with just 65 € for doxycycline or chloroquine.

Country	Adults		Children	
	Product	Posology	Product	Posology
Group 1	Chloroquine	100 mg/day	Chloroquine	< 2-5 kg: 12,5 mg/day 9-17 kg: 25 mg/day 17-33 kg: 50 mg/day 33-45 kg: 75 mg/day
Group 2	Chloroquine + proguanil (Savarine®)	100 mg chloroquine + 200 mg proguanil a day	Chloroquine + proguanil	Not suitable for children weighing under 50 kg
Group 3 Strong resistance or multiple drug resistance	Mefloquine	250 mg/week	Mefloquine	<15 kg: do not use 15-20 kg: 50 mg/week 20-30 kg: 100 mg/week 30-45 kg: 200 mg/week
	Atovaquone + proguanil (Malarone®)	250 mg atovaquone, 100 mg proguanil a day	Atovaquone + proguanil	Not established for < 40 kg
	Doxycycline		Doxycyline	

Table I. Prophylaxis for travellers.

Prophylaxis for non-immune inhabitants

How to protect non-immune people living long-term in a malaria-infested place is a much-discussed problem. Active protection is often recommended, at least immediately after their arrival although to date, there are few real examples of this type of mass prophylaxis ever having been implemented, e.g. in south-western Ethiopia, land was prepared to receive immigrants from the malaria-free plateaux but, apart from the installation of health care centres and early treatment programmes, little was done by way of prophylaxis, even though protecting the immigrants had been recommended in a WHO consultant's report.

The Indonesian Transmigration Programme was associated with a very high incidence of malaria among Javanese immigrants to Western New Guinea. The victims were treated but no prophylactic measures seem to have been implemented for new arrivals.

The case of foreign aid workers is somewhat different since these people generally have substantial financial resources and support as well as a better understanding of the disease and its treatment. For a long time, taking 100 mg of chloroquine a day ensured complete security for any expatriate living in the Tropics but, with the spread of resistance, this drug is steadily losing its prophylactic efficacy.

Today, most expatriates opt for keeping a stand-by course of curative treatment on hand. On the first suggestive symptoms, they go to a clinic to confirm the diagnosis and, if necessary, start taking the drugs. A clinical diagnosis—often the only diagnosis possible in a rural setting—warrants drugs that are easy to use and safe, e.g. atovaquone + proguanil (Malarone®) and artemether + lumefantrine (Coartem®) are often used. Many people residing in remote areas keep stocks of drugs chosen according to local resistance patterns—this is particularly necessary where local clinics are likely to run out of drugs. In the final analysis, this strategy often amounts to a form of self-medication.

Members of the armed services are usually closely monitored and given prophylactic or fast-acting curative drugs chosen according to the epidemiological picture and local resistance profiles.

Prevention by Means of Control Vector

Objectives

Prevention is one of the four cornerstones of the Global Malaria Control Strategy and one of the approaches recommended by the Roll Back Malaria Programme. In the absence of any effective vaccine, prevention depends on the distribution and use of prophylactic drugs (an approach compromised by resistance) and vector control.

The Global Malaria Control Strategy emphasises that preventive operations must be selective and sustainable. But operations must always be adapted to the local epidemiology and the behaviour of the vectors involved—which means having an in-depth understanding of how the disease is being transmitted in the targeted place.

The goal of vector control is to reduce transmission so that the incidence of malaria is actually reduced. Each stage of anopheline development could be a potential target as discussed by Coosemans & Carnevale (1995) and summarised in *Figure 1*.

According to the methods being considered and the vector species involved in malaria transmission, one or other of the targets—or a number of them—will be focused upon.

Depending on social considerations, the resources available and the state of local public health institutions, vector control may be personal or community-based. In the latter case, a mass effect on transmission—which is often the key to success—is superimposed on the beneficial effects of the actions of individuals and families.

Targets

The first step is to identify the vector concerned, i.e. the anopheline species. Mosquitoes found inside houses and/or biting humans can be sampled in three ways:

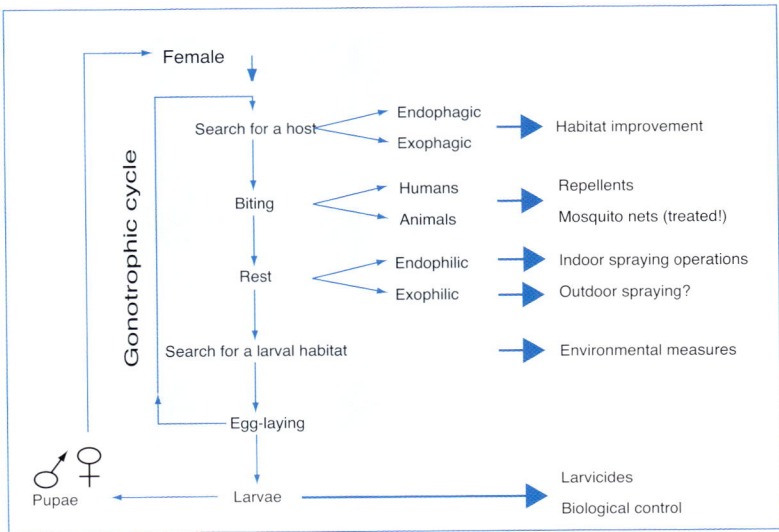

Figure 1.
Targets in vector control at various stages of the gonotrophic cycle (adapted from Coosemans & Carnevale, 1995).

- "indoor resting population" (IRP) = anophelines resting on the walls of a house can be collected using a simple haemolysis tube (*Figure 2A*) or some kind of "suction" system especially designed for mosquito collection;
- IRP can be caught after spraying with pyrethrum, a sheet spread out on the floor can be used to collect all the insects killed (*Figure 2B*);
- biting insects can be captured when biting—either on humans (*Figures 2C and 2D*) or on an animal, most often on cattle (*Figure 2E*).

Specimens collected in this way are in good condition and can therefore be reliably identified and dissected (dry specimens cannot be dissected) and, if necessary, tested for insecticide resistance. Identification can be made using

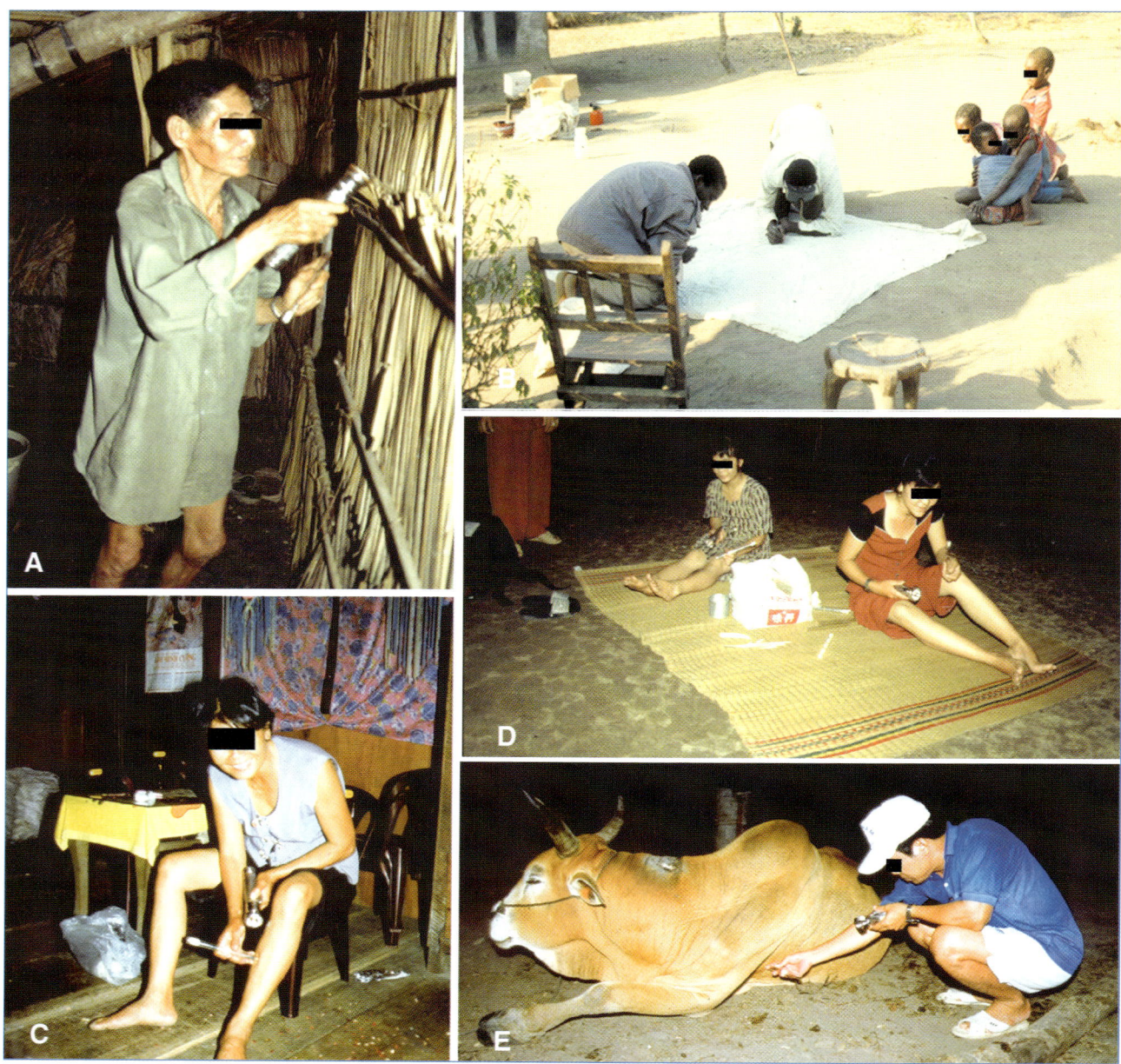

Figure 2. Anopheles *trapping.* **A.** *Manual sampling inside a house in Vietnam (photograph by Coosemans).* **B.** *Collection after pyrethrin spraying in Burundi (photograph by Coosemans).* **C.** *Capture on a human subject inside a house (photograph by Coosemans).* **D.** *Capture on a human subject outside in Vietnam (photograph by Coosemans).* **E.** *Capture on animals in Vietnam (photograph by Coosemans).*

morphological characteristics and cytogenetic or molecular assays (which can be done with dry specimens). Infection rates can be measured on fresh (salivary glands) or dried (CSP ELISA tests) specimens. Blood meal sources can be analysed by transferring stomach contents to filter paper (*see the Part on* "Malaria, a Vector-Borne Parasitic Disease").

Window traps (*Figure 3*) sample anophelines leaving or entering the house. Light traps can be used as an alternative to night-biting collections (Davies *et al.*, 1995), but results are not always consistent, and or of limited ecological significance (Carnevale & Le Pont, 1973; Le Goff *et al.*, 1993). However, light traps are now more and more used due to ethical problems with biting collections.

Morphological identification of the vector species is up to the entomologist who will use the keys available for the various parts of the world. Computerised inventories (Brunhes *et al.*, 1999) are available in CD-ROM form for the Afrotropical Region, as well as the Southeast Asian Region with the interactive key for the mosquitoes of the Malesiana fauna (White *et al.*, 2004). On a national level, other computerised systems have also been developed, especially in India, Iran, North America, etc.

At the community level, identification boils down to distinguishing non-biting "mosquito-like" insects (e.g. chironomids or crane flies) from blood feeding culicids. Many village-dwellers can be easily taught to distinguish *Anopheles* from *Culex* and *Aedes*, although all are still considered as an unwanted nuisance.

Distinguishing between sibling species of a complex involves other methods that can be based on cytogenetics, isozyme analysis and molecular techniques, which can only be performed in adequately equipped laboratories with well trained human resources.

Knowledge of the larval biotopes is basic to any larval control strategy which aims at more than simply cleaning up around the living area. It is hardly ever possible to define all the larval habitats (apart from in special places like in the desert), which is why larva control is only attempted in particular circumstances.

The ecology of the adult *Anopheles* centres on the house which represents an obligatory point of passage for endophagic mosquitoes when seeking a host: this is why indoor spraying is such an effective strategy. However, operations must be carried out at the right time of year (before anopheline density is at its peak) using products taking into account safety and environmental considerations, and the susceptibility of the vector.

Without getting bogged down in these introductory remarks, it is clear that the entomologist's contribution is essential to defining the geography and timing of vector control operations, and advising governmental or community authorities on which products and methods are the most suitable.

Personal measures

Personal protection measures—mosquito nets (treated or not), insect repellents, insecticide diffusers and bombs, etc.—are as relevant to permanent residents as they are to travellers.

Treated mosquito nets and protective screens (Coosemans & Guillet, 1999)

Avoiding mosquito bites is a natural reflex and the use of mosquito nets dates back to the earliest antiquity, in Egypt on the banks of the Nile (Bruce-Chwatt, 1980).

In theory, when a net is used correctly and kept in good condition, it protects the sleeper throughout the night. However, they are often poorly hung and/or torn, in which case they may tend to concentrate the mosquitoes rather than protect the user.

Mosquito nets are hung from the ceiling or from frames made of metal or wood. They may be completely closed (with the fabric tucked under the mattress) or they may have an access slit. The latter type is in widespread use in Africa but if the two strips of fabric do not overlap enough, the mosquito can get in; entomologists often find well blood fed anophelines inside such nets in the morning.

These problems are resolved if the net is impregnated with an insecticide, usually a pyrethroid which has a repellent, as well as a lethal effect (*Figures 4A and 5*).

The products used belong to the pyrethroid family (*Table I*) that are safe for humans (deltamethrin, lambdacyhalothrin, cypermethrin, cyfluthrin, permethrin and etofenprox being the most commonly used). Most of the products remain active for six to twelve months after which retreatment will be necessary; retreatment must also be done after 3 washes of the net. Unfortunately, many families either do not know that retreatment is necessary or they cannot or do not want to perform the operation. To avoid the problem of re-impregnation of nets, Long Lasting insecticidal Nets (LN)

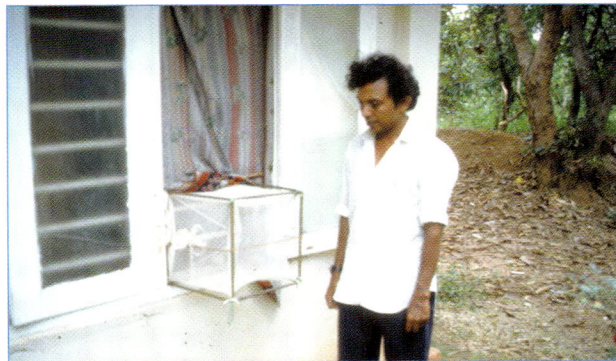

Figure 3. Window trap to harvest anophelines leaving a house in Sri Lanka (photograph by Coosemans).

are now more widely used by the control programmes. These nets are factory-treated with insecticide either incorporated into or coated around fibres. They resist multiple washes and remain active throughout the net's lifetime (3 to 4 years for polyester nets, 4 to 5 years for polyethylene ones). Three long lasting nets have been so far recommended by WHO: one polyethylene net blended with permethrin (Olyset®, 1,000 mg/m²),and two polyester nets coated with deltamethrin (PermaNet®, 50 mg/m²) or α-cypermethrin (Interceptor®, 200 mg/m²).

Using a mosquito net is routine where bites are common, whatever the local risk of malaria, e.g. in tropical cities where *Culex quinquefasciatus* is abundant but *Anopheles* less so.

The treatment of mosquito nets has been described in detailed by Coosemans & Carnevale (1995):
- calculate the net's surface area which is usually between 10 m² for those of less than 1.65 m in height and 20 m² for double nets and for tall people);
- measure the volume of fluid (water or diluted insecticide) needed to saturate the net (usually 0.7-1.0 l per net);
- calculate the quantity of insecticide formulation needed using the equation $C = (S \times D)/(F \times A)$
    C: the amount of formulated insecticide needed per litre water expressed in g or ml,
    S: surface area of the mosquito net in m²,
    D: treatment dosage in grams of active ingredient per m²,

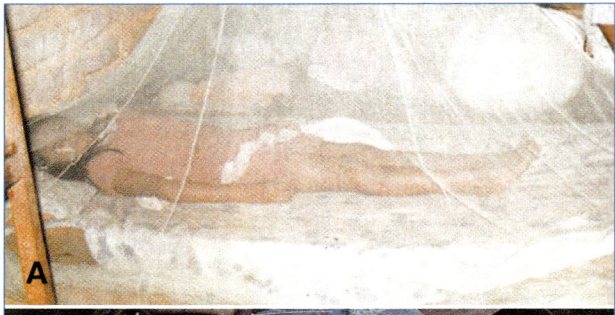
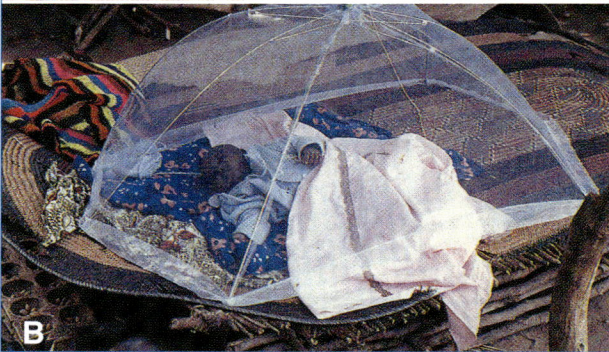

Figure 4. A. Using a treated mosquito net in Guajaramerin, Bolivia (photograph by Mouchet in Danis & Mouchet, 1991. B. Baby under a bell-shaped net (photograph by Mouchet in Danis & Mouchet, 1991).

Table I. Insecticides recommended for indoor spraying and/or the treatment of mosquito nets.										
Compound	Class[1]	IS[2]	ITN[2]	Dosage[3]	Toxicity (mg/kg)		Toxicity category[4]		Remanence on a wall	Remanence on an ITN
					Oral	Dermatological	Compound	Formulation		
DDT	OC	+		2 g/m²	113	200/500	II	III	6 months	
Malathion	OP	+		2 g/m²	1,370-2,100	4,000	III	III	2/3 months	
Fenitrothion	OP	+		2 g/m²	500	3,500	II	III	3/6 months	
Pirimophos-methyl	OP	+		1/2 g/m²	2,000	> 4,500	III	III	2/3 months	
Bendiocarb	C	+		0.1/0.4 g/m²	40-126	> 560	II		2/6 months	
Propoxur	C	+		1/2 g/m²	95	> 2,400	II	III	3/6 months	
Alpha cypermethrin	P	+	+	20/30 mg/m²	72	> 2,000	II	III	3/6 months	6-12 months
Cyfluthrin	P	+	+	25/50 mg/m²	250	> 5,000	II	III	3/6 months	6-12 months
Deltamethrin	P	+	+	10/25 mg/m²	128	2,940	II	III	3/6 months	6-12 months
Lambdacyhalothrin	P	+	+	20/30 mg/m²	79	632	II	III	3/6 months	6-12 months
Bifenthrin	P	+		20/40 mg/m²	54	700	II	III	3/6 months	6-12 months
Permethrin	P		+	500 mg/m²	540	2,690	III	III	2/3 months	6-12 months
Ethofenprox	NP	+		300 mg/m²	> 10,000	> 2,100	III	III	3/6 months	

1. Class: OC = organochlorine; OP = organophosphate; C = carbamate; P = pyrethroid; NP = neopyrethroid
2. IS = indoor spraying; ITN = impregnated treated nets
3. OC, OP and C dosages are expressed in g/m²; P and NP dosages are expressed in mg/m²
4. Insecticides are classified according to toxicity below (*Table II*)

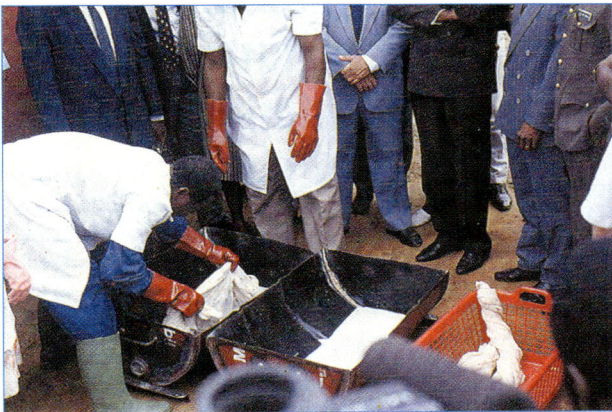

Figure 5. Mosquito net impregnation in a village (photograph by Mouchet, 1991).

F: proportion of active ingredient of the formulated insecticide (NB: 0.025 rather than 2.5%),
A: amount of water absorbed per mosquito net (in l).
E.g. for an 11.5 m² net to be impregnated with deltamethrin, 2.5% SC at a dose of 15 mg of active ingredient per m², 6.9 ml of the insecticide formulation will be needed. For one litre of ready-to-use solution, 6.9 ml/0.84 l = 8.21 ml of the insecticide formulation will be needed.
It will be possible to treat 143 mosquito nets with one litre of deltamethrin SC 25 (suspended concentrate);

- the calculated amount of the product formulation is mixed with water and the mosquito nets immersed therein. Then, they are spread out on a non-absorbent surface to dry out.

In places where mosquito nets are not commonly used and the nuisance is relatively low (fewer than 10 bites per night), a full-scale "marketing" operation will be necessary, based on health education and making local people aware of the efficacy of mosquito nets in the prevention of malaria.

Prices vary enormously from one country to another (between $3.5 to $15 in 2007). The installation of production facilities in developing countries is tending to bring the price down: a mosquito net can be obtained for $3-4 (depending on size) plus $0.5 for transport costs. But cost remains a problem for people living at or below the poverty threshold. When mosquito nets are handed out free of charge, care must be taken to check that they are not being resold. Special low prices or monthly payment schemes have also been suggested (Coosemans & Guillet, 1999). With free or highly subsidised insecticide treated net distribution through antenatal care services, routine immunisation programmes, and measles vaccination campaigns, coverage of vulnerable groups, e.g. pregnant women and children, has considerably improved in many countries.

People's adherence to net usage depends on the degree of satisfaction they feel, particularly regarding their sleeping comfort and general inconvenience.

In principle, efficacy is guaranteed as long as the net is used correctly and sleeping patterns remain unchanged; people who go to bed very late after an evening of watching the village television may be exposed to anophelines which bite at the beginning of the night, e.g. *An. baimaii* (former *An. dirus* D) in Myanmar. Moreover, some species (e.g. *An. farauti*) may be able to change their behaviour and begin biting earlier in the evening before people go to bed, although this observation requires confirmation.

Treated curtains

Whether or not treated curtains are effective remains controversial since it depends on how they are used. Remarkable results have been observed in Burkina Faso where hanging permethrin impregnated curtains around the house substantially cut transmission down (Pietra *et al.*, 1991; Procacci *et al.*, 1991), whereas, on the Madagascan plateaux, treated curtains on windows and doors had no tangible effect (Rabarison *et al.*, 1995; Mouchet, personal observation, 1995).

Protecting living quarters

Stopping mosquitoes from getting into houses has been widely recommended since the beginning of the last century. Solid construction techniques and maintenance of the screens covering windows, porches and verandas are essential to keeping a house "mosquito proof". Air conditioning is to some extent replacing metallic and plastic screens but such means of protection remain the preserve of the rich. The great majority of dwellings—especially in the Tropics—are not and cannot be fitted with any type of protective screen: there is a considerable disparity between the reality in the rural, tropical habitat and the advice of some experts which is often impracticable.

Domestic spraying of insecticide and repellents

Such measures are implemented for personal comfort against flying insects (mosquitoes, flies, sandflies, and chironomids) and even crawling ones (bed bugs, cockroaches, fleas, etc.). Preventing malaria is not usually the major concern even though such measures may contribute to attenuating malaria transmission.

Repellent products

Since time immemorial, smoke has been used to chase mosquitoes away with some types of wood (e.g. margosa) considered as particularly effective.

Locally applied plant extracts stop mosquito bites, including lemon grass which is very popular although its effect lasts barely an hour. Palm oil affords 4-6 hours of protection against *Simulium* in Benin although it has an unpleasant smell (Mouchet, personal observation).

Chemical repellents—especially **N,N-diethyl-3-methylbenzamide (DEET)**—in lotion, cream or cosmetic mixture forms act for 4-6 hours (depending on how much the user is sweating). The addition of silicone prolongs the duration of protection to about 12 hours, i.e. the whole night (Mehr *et al.*, 1985). Topical products do not induce adverse reactions in adults but DEET should not be regularly used on the skin of young children (< 30 months) so the product should be applied to their clothing. In India, using **N,N-diethylphenylacetamide** has been suggested; it is as effective as DEET but cheaper. Now the products with 35/35 or KBR 3023 (Icaridin) are often recommended instead of DEET for toxicological reasons and Icaridin is performing as well as DEET. However, according to some experts, Icaridine based-products should not be used for more than one month on a continual basis.

Except in high risk situations, skin repellents cannot be used in children before 30 months of age.

Repellent products—whatever their type—have only a limited role in the prevention of malaria in endemic regions because they are rarely used all the time and malaria vectors bite during the night, although they are of great use against day-biting mosquitoes such as *Aedes* and in the prevention of diseases they transmit (dengue, Chikungunya, etc.)

Repellent soaps containing 20% DEET and 0.5% permethrin have been developed for use by the subject before going to bed (Yap, 1986). There are no recent articles on this topic but the associated discomfort seems to present a major disadvantage. Treated items of **clothing impregnated** with 1.25 g/m² permethrin have been used in places where *Culex* biting was intolerable. In the Arctic, **very loose-knit** polyester and cotton vests treated with 10-15 g/m² DEET are used, sometimes with added permethrin (Schreck *et al.*, 1979). Barnard's WHO document (2000c) gives a list of repellent products that can be used to treat clothing (e.g. 1 g/m² permethrin).

Transmitters which emit sound waves to repel female mosquitoes are not effective and some companies have been fined for misleading advertising (Curtis, 1970).

Domestic insecticide products

These are of two types: solids that vaporise when heated (mosquito coils, thermal bricks) and aerosols.

Spray guns (e.g. Fly-tox which has already been available for one hundred years) used to contain natural pyrethrins dissolved in kerosene. Since cheaper pyrethroids were developed, a mixture of 0.1% bioallethrin and 0.5% permethrin in a mixture of equal volumes of kerosene and white spirit has been used.

A more modern presentation is the **aerosol** which is as popular in the developing countries as it is in developed countries. The active products are fast-acting pyrethroids with a strong knock-down effect, (e.g. kadethrin, resmethrin and esbiothrin) mixed with piperonyl butoxide (synergizer). Some companies sell aerosols for flying insects as described above, and others for crawling insects which include in addition a stable pyrethroid (cyfluthrin or deltamethrin) or a carbamate (propoxur). Since the ozone layer-damaging chlorofluorocarbons (CFCs) were banned, the propellents used are non-inflammable hydrofluorocarbons (HFCs) or, more commonly, highly inflammable propane or butane.

Mosquito coils (*Figure 6*) are used in all poor countries where there is often no electrical supply (Chadwick, 1975). The market is supplied by many manufacturers and lots of different presentations are available; efficacy varies enormously. Originally, the coils contained pyrethrin or pyrethrum but they are now usually based on allethrin (0.2-0.3%) and/or transallethrin (0.10-0.15%). Inferior, relatively ineffective products were sold containing γ HCH. The moulded vehicle is commonly a mixture of starch and coconut husk flour, sometimes supplemented with a fungicide, although many different sorts of vehicle are used in different places. The coil is designed to burn slowly for 6-8 hours, supported on a wire holder to prevent fires (Rozendaal, 1997).

In India, jute fibres impregnated with insecticide (1 mg/kg esbiothrin) hung from the ceiling burn for 10-12 hours (Sharma *et al.*, 1989).

Small portable devices containing coils can be used outside in places with many mosquitoes, especially at night (rubber plantation workers, miners) (Rozendaal, 1997).

Dichlorvos dispensers are highly effective in confined spaces but they can induce health problems in young children and the elderly and they have been withdrawn from the market.

In houses with a main electricity supply **insecticide vaporizing mats** can be used with good effect at night although in some towns, *Culex quinquefasciatus* is very resistant to pyrethroids. These mats consist of rectangular blocks of compressed paper (35 x 22 x 2 mm) impregnated with a fast-acting pyrethroid such as allethrin, esbiothrin or esbiol. They are placed on an electric plate at 145-160°C which safely induces sublimation of the active substance (Chadwick & Lord, 1977).

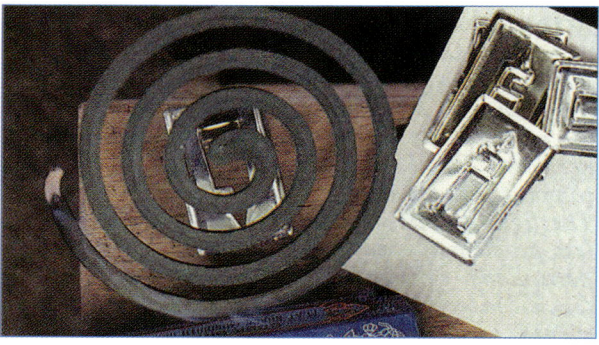

Figure 6. Mosquito coils, the most popular domestic insecticide/repellent modality in developing countries (photograph by Mouchet, 1991).

Electric vaporisers are sometimes used to evaporate a pyrethroid solution, a system which precludes the need to change the brick every day since one bottle lasts a month (Coosemans & Guillet, 1994).

WHO (Geneva, 1998) has produced a guideline for domestic products including their specifications since the products available in developing countries are often not in line with the minimum standards (CTO/WHOPES/IC/98.3).

Clearance of larval habitats around the house

Cleaning up the area around dwellings has been considered a panacea in primary health care systems. Removing small larval sites (used containers, water deposits, hollows in trees, old tyres) may reduce the density of *Stegomyia* (*Ae. aegypti, Ae. albopictus, Ae. polynesiensis*) which transmit arboviruses and filariasis; and in India, draining and clearing the vegetation from the small swamps which surround all the houses in Kerala can reduce the number of *Mansonia* which carries *Brugia*.

But in general, anophelines avoid polluted domestic water deposits and clearing up around the house rarely has any great effect on malaria vectors which prefer more open bodies of clean water.

Systematic treatment with larvivorous fish will be addressed later on.

Chemical treatment (temephos) and biological control (*Bacillus thuringiensis* H 14) in water deposits are rarely used alone but often account for a component of structured programmes directed against *Ae. aegypti*—more rarely against *Anopheles* (although these modalities are being used against *An. stephensi* in India).

Nothing can be said against operations designed to clean up around dwellings although the effect on malaria will be minimal.

Community-based preventive measures

Methods

A critical level of coverage in terms of houses or people needs to be attained if any mass effect is expected to benefit those who are not directly protected.

From 1945 to 1975—both before and during the eradication period—indoor residual spraying (IRS) operations with long-acting insecticides constituted the basis of malaria control. This lost its preeminent role in the course of several revisions of control strategy. However, in the Global Strategy of 1992, IRS plays an important role for selective control of transmission in some zones and for limited periods.

After some degree of reluctance in the 1980's, insecticide treated mosquito nets are now considered as a sustainable means of protection specially with the recently developed Long Lasting Nets, applicable to large cross sections of the population. Their efficacy has been epidemiologically demonstrated. Although coverage of vulnerable groups, e.g. young children and pregnant women, should still be prioritised, it will deliver limited protection and equity to these groups. Large reductions of the malaria burden, including in children, can only be achieved by a broader population coverage with these nets (Gerry *et al.*, 2007).

Larva control—be it physical, chemical, bacteriological, biological or environmental—is now only recommended in special situations, notably in oases and against urban malaria.

The possibility of genetic control, notably using transgenic mosquitoes, has attracted enormous amounts of funding and stimulated a great deal of research but practical applications are decades away, at least.

Indoor spraying with long-acting insecticides

Vector behaviour in response to indoor spraying

Houses act as mosquito traps in which the residents are the bait. After biting and feeding, the anopheline—now more than quadrupled in weight—rests close by, i.e. on the house wall to digest the blood and maturation of ovaries. It may either remain inside the house (endophilic behaviour) or leave (exophilic behaviour). If the walls have been treated with a toxic product, the insect is killed inside the house and the parasite transmission cycle is curtailed.

There are exceptions to this basic outline.

Some anopheline species or strains spend very little time on an interior wall after a blood meal, leaving the house very soon after. Such exophilic behaviour is facilitated if the house has only makeshift walls or none at all. This is true for members of the *An. dirus* Complex in the jungles of Southeast Asia. After the endophilic vector *An. minimus* s.l. had disappeared, *An. dirus* s.l. continued transmitting malaria in rudimentary crop huts ("forest malaria").

In newly colonised areas of the Amazon in western Brazil, many immigrants living in shacks with hardly any walls were infected, notably by *An. darlingi* against which indoor spraying was completely ineffective.

On the other hand, in the dry Senegalese Sahel where people sleep outside and there is no other shade, anophelines (*An. arabiensis, An. gambiae* s.s.) take refuge inside houses during the daytime; thus an exophagic anopheline behaves endophilically.

An. sergentii has been reported as behaving in the same way in the Jordan Valley where it feeds on Bedouin people while they are watering their camels and then, in the daytime, rests in caves.

Much has been written about the impact of exophilic behaviour on the efficacy of insecticide treatment but what is important to remember is that, after biting, most anophelines pass at least one hour inside the house during concentration of the blood meal. They are therefore very likely to come into contact with any long-acting insecticide to be confronted with both the toxic and excitatory/repellent effects of the product.

Insecticide toxicity and excito-repellent effects

The excito-repellent effect of some insecticides (DDT, pyrethroid and some carbamates) makes anophelines quickly leave treated surfaces (induced exophily) that they have settled on before receiving lethal dose of insecticide. This excito-repellent effect may also reduce the entry rate (deterrence) and blood feeding of mosquitoes. The excito-repellent effect of DDT on some species has clearly been assessed, e.g. in northern Cameroon, it was two times more important with *An. gambiae s.l.* than with *An. funestus* (Mouchet *et al.*, 1961). This excito-repellent activity was exactly the same at every DDT concentration (1%, 2% and 4%). In contrast, insecticide toxicity waned rapidly after treatment—by over 50% in two and a half months—so an ever-increasing proportion were quitting the treated house alive.

This pattern meant that anopheline densities remained high, especially if alternative hosts were available in the form of livestock. Malaria continued to be transmitted at a high rate with over 35% of children infected during the transmission season (Cavalié & Mouchet, 1962). By 1965, it was becoming clear that it was not going to be possible to block transmission using DDT or other available insecticides in the humid, holo-endemic savannahs of West Africa although some experts were not convinced of the truth of this until the results of the Garki Project came out (Molineaux & Gramiccia, 1980).

An even more important excito-repellent effect was shown by pyrethroids, with their faster-acting and knock-down effect which practically corresponds to lethality since, while on the ground, mosquitoes are eaten by scavengers such as ants and spiders. Propoxur also has excitatory and repellent activities.

In places where malaria is hypo-endemic such as KwaZulu-Natal in RSA, the same phenomena are seen but the irritant effect combined with the more or less effective toxicity of DDT has been sufficient to prevent contact between humans and vectors, even when the mosquito exhibits low-level resistance (Roberts *et al.*, 2002b; Zulueta, 1959).

The excito-repellent effect of deposits of insecticide or sublethal concentration, as well as house improvements can induce exophilic behaviour, thereby reducing the mosquito's life expectancy to the point that they no longer act as vectors. This is why malaria has not returned to La Réunion (Girod *et al.*, 1999) despite the continued presence of *An. arabiensis*.

During the eradication period, in-depth studies were conducted to estimate how insecticides are absorbed onto walls. Bamboo, wood, palm leaves and thatch do not absorb the insecticide which is subsequently lost through mechanical abrasion. The extent to which deposited insecticide is absorbed by mud bricks depends on their humidity content. Alkaline surfaces (e.g. lime plaster) break insecticides down as do the high temperatures of corrugated iron roofs.

Current trends

Since 1970, indoor residual spraying has become less widespread. In 1964, 15 million houses were treated in the Americas whereas, by 1997, the figure was just 1.6 million, and a similar reduction was seen in Asia. This strategic change results from the adoption of the Global Strategy in 1992. To this, we should add, in the Americas, the shift of cases to the Amazon, where house spraying was abandoned because of the rudimentary nature of the dwellings.

In Southeast Asia, Vietnam, China and Cambodia, there is a trend towards replacing indoor spraying with treated mosquito nets.

Under pressure from environmentalists, DDT has been banned in many countries and replaced by pyrethroids. However, DDT is still accepted by WHO for indoor spraying only and it was used in Madagascar to tackle the epidemic in 1988 (Mouchet *et al.*, 1997), and to control pyrethroid-resistant *An. funestus* in South Africa (Maharaj *et al.*, 2005).

Today, indoor spraying is still recommended to **prevent** an epidemic once the warning signs have been seen, e.g. excessive rainfall, higher-than-normal minimum temperatures and influxes of immunologically naïve immigrants. Indoor spraying is also recommended to **control epidemics** if it can be done before the peak of transmission (Protopopoff *et al.*, 2007). It also remains the basis for **protecting high-risk, non-immune groups**, e.g. temporary workers, servicemen and refugees.

In places where very high seasonal transmission occurs, the **peak incidence** can be brought down by well-targeted spraying operations (Coosemans, 1987).

Finally, some development projects are sufficiently well funded to guarantee permanent protection of the inhabitants by indoor spraying.

Formerly indoor spraying mainly relied on special units of the Ministries of Health, but nowadays public health authorities want control operations to be decentralised, if possible with the help of community-based collaborators. However, this requires considerable effort in training and follow up to assure the quality of the treatments.

The problem of wall-less shelters is currently unresolved and new strategies need to be found.

In indoor spraying programmes, misgivings on the part of local people often have to be overcome such as:
- the need to clear the house and to accept visible deposits of wettable powder on furniture and walls, especially in richer homes;
- odour of the product, especially malathion, which is refused at Mohéli in the Comoros;

- the resistance of bedbugs to DDT, which led to the abandonment of houses in Maroni in Guyana and on the Madagascan Plateaux;
- the weariness on the part of people who will not let teams into their houses. Problems related to the cost, availability, storage and distribution of insecticides have to be dealt with by health services or community-based institutions.

Insecticide: choice, safety, poisoning

The choice of an insecticide and its formulation must be based on its biological effectiveness, the susceptibility of the vectors, the method of application, its safety to humans and its toxicity for the environment (WHO, 2006).

All insecticides are to some degree toxic to humans, but for those used in public health the acute toxic doses to humans are far higher than those required for killing insects. The hazard is inherent in the compound and the risk of a hazardous chemical depends on the amount and route of exposure of users and applicators. Handling of pesticides in Public Health should give particular attention to:
- the residents in treated homes, especially children who might be directly exposed to products running down walls or dropping on the ground;
- the spray team members who must wear appropriate clothing despite the temperature in tropical regions and must be well trained about handling and using insecticides and cleaning the spray pumps after the work, etc.;
- the environment and any food stocks.

The toxicity of insecticides is measured following either oral or dermal administration and expressed in terms of their lethal dose (LD50) in rats, i.e. the dose in mg per kg body weight which kills 50% of a significantly-sized population of animals. A list of products has been drawn up on the basis of their differential toxicity.

Rather than the toxicity of the product, what the health authorities are interested in is the toxicity of the formulation. The formulations recommended by the WHO/WHOPES for indoor spraying operations belong to Class III and are based on technical products belonging to Class II or III.

Table I lists the dozen-odd products currently recommended for indoor spraying operations with their toxicities.

Depending on which compound is used, the operatives (responsible for mixing and spraying) must be provided with special equipment (face-masks, gloves, boots, overalls). In those who are using organophosphates or carbamates, cholinesterase levels should be monitored; a colorimetric test based on whole blood can be used to detect elevated cholinesterase activity with possibly a confirmatory spectrophotometric assay.

DDT has rarely been responsible for acute accidental poisoning. Pyrethroids are very safe although they sometimes cause local, reversible paraesthesia. Most acute and chronic poisoning events are caused by the organophosphates and carbamates, both of which inhibit cholinesterase and can be absorbed passively while the victim is resting. Poisoning demands specific treatment with atropine and oximes for organophosphates, only atropine for carbamates. Whatever the product, any contaminated clothing should be removed and the subject's airways should be kept open; it may be necessary to pump the stomach, wash the skin to remove any residual product, and administer specific drugs (atropine, oximes, diapruzam) before the patient is taken to hospital.

A single person should be able to lift the insecticide container (usually made of metal but sometimes cardboard) which should be resistant to shocks and humidity. The product is often contained in a water-proof plastic bag inside the outer packaging. Many companies supply single-dose sachets containing the correct amount of product for one pump-load; sometimes, the sachet is made of a water-soluble substance which means that the mixer never has to touch the product. The name of the product and its toxicity should be displayed and well labelled on the outside of the container (*Figure 7*) which should be stored away from extreme conditions and theft. After use, the container should be washed, stored and, if possible, recycled. Residual product is not considered as a source of pollution but, following switches in strategy, decommissioned product should be destroyed according to WHO recommendations. High-temperature incineration, chemical destruction or burying are approved methods although burning in the air can be dangerous. FAO and WHO (1996) have published a guide on destruction of unneeded pesticides.

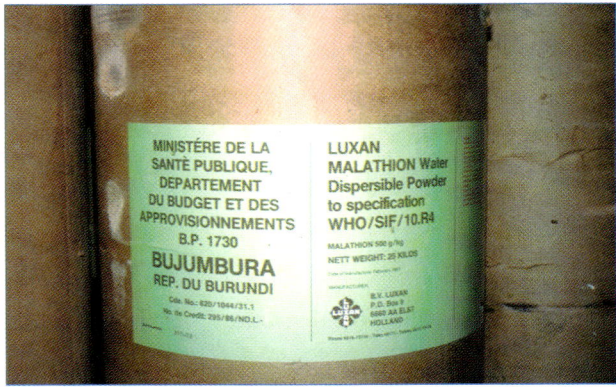

Figure 7. *Storage and labelling of malathion (photograph by Coosemans).*

Application

Logistics

If indoor spraying operations are to be successful, they need to cover a large surface of the houses (the whole surface or the lower portion only) within a given perimeter. Incomplete coverage is a source of gaps. This is a **collective initiative** designed to **protect the entire community**.

Indoor spraying was the basis of the eradication strategy between the 1950's and 1970's and operations were performed through vertical, hierarchical structures. Such structures were gradually abolished with the establishment of decentralised, primary health care systems which depend on community participation. In period during which the new structures were being set up, the quality of operations deteriorated: the operatives were often poorly trained staff and the operations sometimes conducted at the wrong time of year. Moreover, population growth meant that the geographical survey data were obsolete; geographical distribution of the households should be regularly updated. Remote sensing methods can here be useful (Booman *et al.*, 2000; Roberts *et al.*, 1991). Finally, local people began to tire of the repeated invasion of their homes.

There are few models of decentralised spraying operations, although mention could be made of those in Burundi which were supervised at the municipal level and conducted by local people provided with the appropriate training. Technical directives and supervision at the national level seem indispensable to ensuring efficiency and efficacy, and maintaining a motivated work force. The role of NGOs is particularly important, e.g. *Médecins Sans Frontières* (MSF) in Burundi. Operatives must be fully trained, adequately equipped, and provided with a way of reaching even the most remote settlements with regular monitoring.

One major stumbling block for indoor spraying is sustainability. It is always difficult to estimate how long a programme will last and recent history shows that those advocating treatment programmes have often been mistaken. However, it is clear that many programmes supported by time-limited funding have met with failure. It is moreover important that the programme has been accepted by local people if it is to receive their support. Effective targeting of treatments—both temporal and spatial—can enhance sustainability.

Such constraints are a major reason for the waning of indoor spraying operations.

Formulations, specifications, dosages, cycles

The formulation to be used will depend on the types of surface to be treated and the wishes of the inhabitants.

Wettable powders are the most commonly used products: powdered 75% DDT was the mainstay of eradication. Such products contain an active substance mixed with an inert powder (e.g. bentonite) supplemented with a wetting agent (Triton X100) and a dispersing agent (for DDT). Pyrethroids can be diluted much more and the wettable powders usually contain only 5% (sometimes up to 20%) of active ingredient. Liquid products like malathion are pre-adsorbed onto an inert substrate before the addition of wetting and dispersing agents; malathion is supplied as a 50% wettable powder.

Wettable powders leave stains on walls and furniture and this is seen as increasingly unacceptable as social status rises. Moreover, some organophosphates, including malathion, have an unpleasant smell which is unpopular, whatever the insecticide activity.

Emulsifiable concentrates (EC) are suspensions of an active substance in an organic solvent (often the highly inflammable kerosene) supplemented with an emulsifier. After dilution in water, these products do not usually stain surfaces. This type of suspended concentrate presentation containing 2.5% active substance is common for pyrethroids—both for the spraying of walls and the treatment of mosquito nets. Generally EC are not used for impregnation of nets.

Flowable **suspended concentrates** consist of insecticide particles with a wetting agent diluted in water to generate an aqueous solution: these are not inflammable and leave no residue on surfaces.

Microencapsulated suspensions release the insecticide slowly thereby increasing the exposure of the target insect.

The most commonly used **dosages** are listed in *Table I*, expressed in g/m^2 for DDT, organophosphates and carbamates, and in mg/m^2 for the pyrethroids.

DDT needs to be applied every six months, and the other products every three months. In places with a humid tropical or equatorial climate, operations have to be repeated twice a year for DDT, and three or four times a year for the other products. In places with a harsh winter or a marked dry season, DDT needs only to be applied once a year although twice a year may be necessary for the other products. In regions, where malaria has a focal distribution spatial targeting of the indoor spraying can be recommended (Carter *et al.*, 2000). In African highland, spraying rounds can be limited to valley floors where more than 90 % of transmission occurs, leaving the tops untreated.

Most of these products were patented more than 25 years ago and are no longer under licence. Hence they can be produced by anyone, which brings problems in quality control. In the course of the tender process, it is important to check the product's purity, its active substance content, and the quality of the formulation (suspensibility, wettability), e.g. in Pakistan, a batch of malathion (which is itself of low toxicity) containing a high concentration of iso-malathion (the concentration of which is usually below 0.5%) caused five deaths and hundreds of poisonings among spraying operatives (Baker *et al.*, 1978). All insecticides used in public health initiatives must be in line with the most recent WHO specifications (http://www.who.int/whopes).

WHO (WHOPES) can help national authorities to choose a suitable source and WHO Regional Offices can help them obtain high-quality products.

Method of application and auxiliary equipment*

Before treatment starts, all perishable products and foodstuffs must be collected together at a point inside or, preferably, outside the house (*Figure 8*).

The dilution factor necessary for the suspensions should be calculated according to the concentration of active ingredient in the formulation and the amount to be applied (*Figure 9*), given that using a standard, pre-pressurised sprayer, one litre of suspension is enough to treat a surface area of 25 m² **.

Pre-pressurised sprayers—which have not significantly changed in forty years—are usually used (*Figure 10*). These consist of a 10-litre cylindrical tank unit made of galvanised steel with a hermetically sealed (rubber gaskets) cover. The upper part is perforated by a pump, a pressure gauge, and a rubber tube connected to a spray lance.

After the tank has been filled with 8 l of suspension, an internal pressure of 380 kg PA is generated using the hand pump and monitored at the pressure gauge (*Figure 11*). The high pressure drives suspension into the tube at the base of the tank and thence into the external rubber tube.

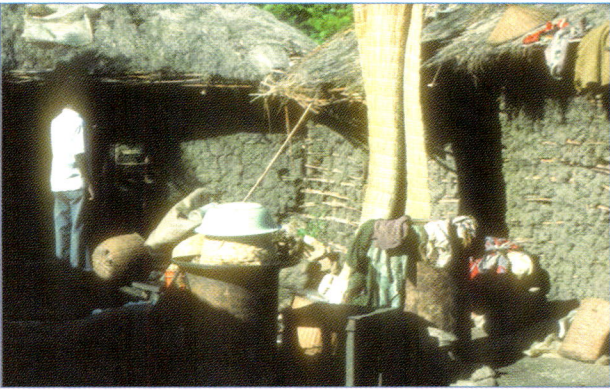

Figure 8. Indoor spraying in Burundi. Emptying of the house (photograph by Coosemans).

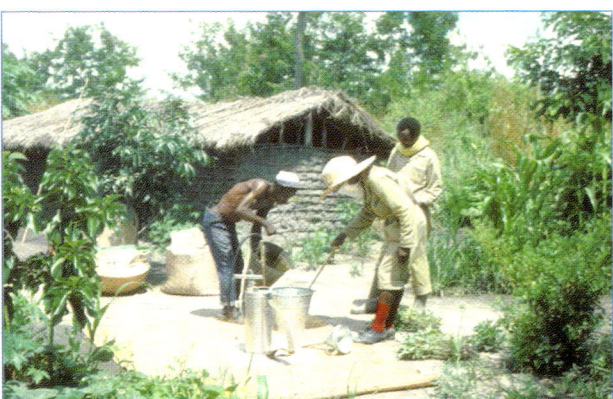

Figure 9. Indoor spraying in Burundi. Making up the insecticide mixture (photograph by Coosemans).

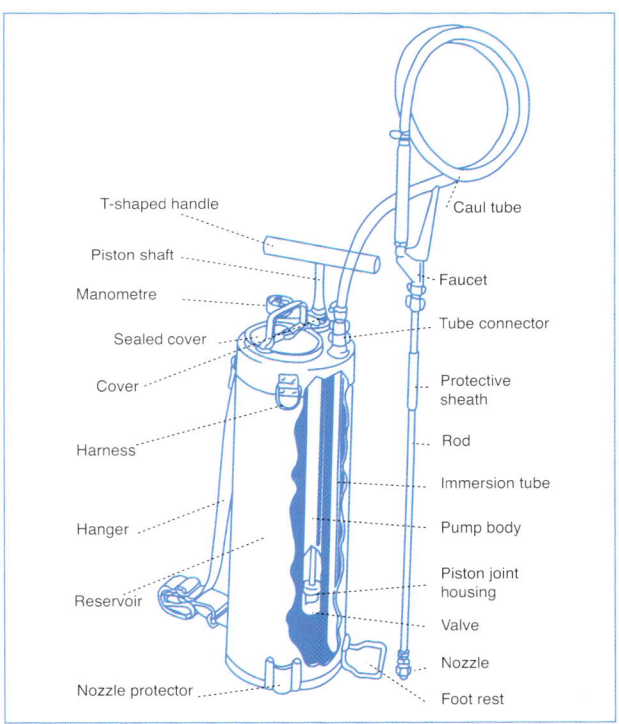

Figure 10. Section through a pre-pressurised spraying tank (adapted from Rozendaal, 1997).

---

* The key issues associated with long-lasting indoor spraying have been addressed by WHO in Geneva (2000c). See also Najera & Zaïm (2001).

** To make up suspensions of the desired dilution, use equation X: $25xy/C$ (*in* Rozendaal, 1997)
x: weight of formulation per litre; C: concentration of the active product; y: application dosage (g/m²)
For 75% DDT powder to be used at 2 g/m², $X = 25 \times 2 = 66.6$ g/l, i.e. 533 g for a pump load of 8 l. Dosed sachets containing the correct amount of powder for 8 l of suspension can be pre-prepared. For 2.5% deltamethrin microencapsulated suspension to be used at 0.025 g/m², 40 g of microencapsulated suspension will be needed for 8 l.

Biodiversity of Malaria in the World

Using the control valve, the spray operative can now open and close the flow as desired. As the tank empties and the internal pressure drops (to below 170 kg PA), it is necessary to pump again to restore the pressure. The most fragile part of the device is the spray nozzle: if this gets blocked, it has to be gently cleared and if it is corroded (some of the products are corrosive), it must be changed.

Standing 45 cm away from the wall, the operative sprays a 75 cm-wide strip moving from top to bottom then moves laterally one step still spraying to treat from bottom to top and so on till the whole wall is treated (*Figure 12*); for a three metre-high wall, each strip should be sprayed in 6.7 seconds. In one day, a single person can treat 8-10 houses, each with an interior surface area of 200 m² (*Figure 13*).

Treating the tents of nomads and refugees

Treating the tents of nomads, notably in Iran, has always posed a problem in malaria control programmes because of their mobility. Wettable powders do not remain active for very long on fabrics and hides that are frequently folded up, and emulsifiable DDT concentrates do not seem to last any longer than six weeks (even shorter if the tents are moved in the meantime) (Motabar, 1974). The continuous movements of nomads compromise the efficacy of treatment.

The last three decades have seen a massive increase in the number of refugees in the world, fleeing warfare, political persecution and climatic events (drought and famine): it is believed that there are currently 20 million displaced people. Most are living in camps set up by the United Nations High Commission for Refugees or NGOs. They are provided with a minimum of resources—food and medicine—although this does not prevent high mortality rates on arrival due to diarrhoea and lung disease, especially among the young. Blanket malaria treatment is practised on any subject with suspected fever. In camps located in malaria-endemic areas, tents are systematically treated (Najera, 1996). In camps near Goma in the RD Congo, shelters covered by the classical UN plastic sheeting were treated with 25 mg/m² deltamethrin (Carnevale, personal communication).

The best product for treating nets seems to be permethrin (500 mg/m²) which has a broad safety margin. Good outcomes have been obtained in Afghan refugee camps in Pakistan (Hewitt *et al.*, 1995) with the prevalence of *P. falciparum* dropping from 46% to 13% in the refugee children while it was rising in local Pakistani children (Bouma *et al.*, 1996).

Tarpaulins and plastic sheets designed for the construction of shelters can be impregnated directly with 25 mg/m² deltamethrin.

The current trend is to integrate refugees into local populations.

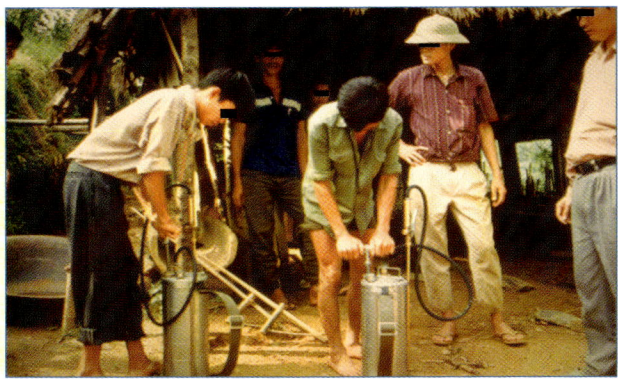

Figure 11. Indoor spraying in Vietnam. Pressurising the pumps (photograph by Coosemans).

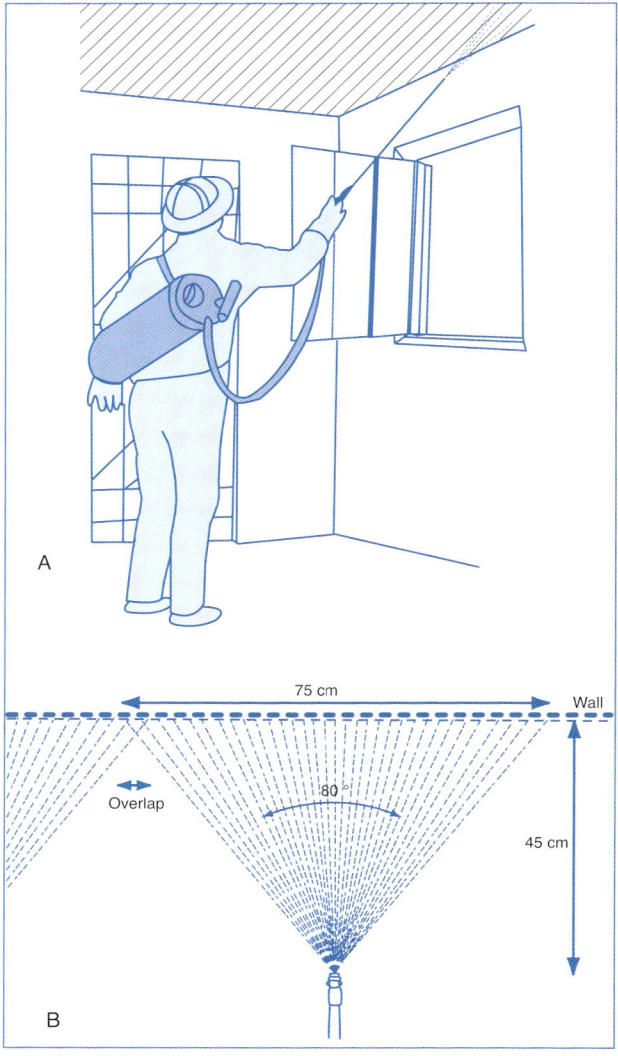

Figure 12. **A.** Correct position when spraying a wall. **B.** Insecticide jet (adapted from Rozendaal, 1997).

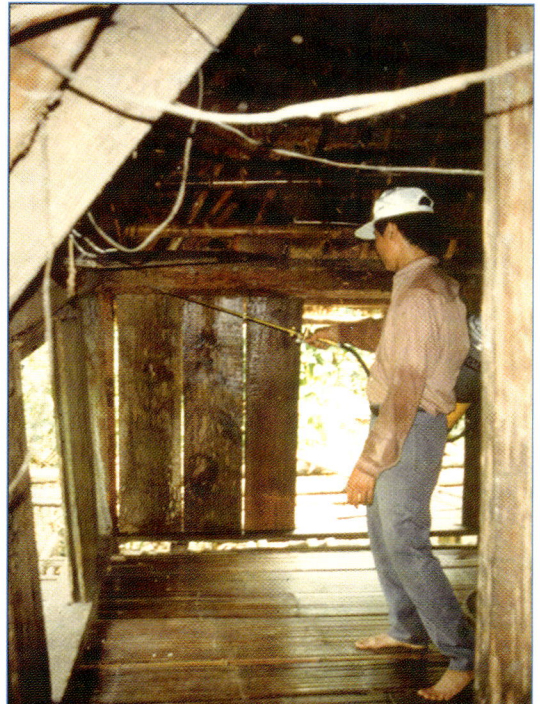

Figure 13. Indoor spraying, Vietnam. Spraying a wall (photograph by Coosemans).

Indoor low volume insecticide spraying

This is an alternative to indoor spraying with long-acting insecticide. To date, it has only been used in Mexico against *An. pseudopunctipennis* (Arredondo-Jimenez *et al.*, 1998).

The insecticide—bendiocarb—was dispensed using a mist blower, a back-pack device driven by a two-stroke motor. The dose dispensed by these devices is estimated at 20 ml/m^3. A house can be treated quickly (in just 30% of the time needed for conventional indoor spraying), so labour as well as insecticide costs are reduced; the global reduction of the cost is of 43%. The residual activity inside the house is almost as long, although mist blower equipment is more expensive and requires well trained personnel.

Community-based protection using treated nets

Key points on the treatment and efficacy of mosquito nets—a highly effective means of personal protection—were addressed above. During the Second World War, DDT-treated canvas sheets were used to protect soldiers although when the Chinese tried the same strategy in the 1960's, they apparently had little success (Li Zu Zi, personal communication). Only with the development of the highly effective pyrethroids in the 1980's (Darriet, 1991) did mass protection of whole communities using this tool (without significant human toxicity) become feasible (Carnevale *et al.*, 1988; Lengeler, 1998).

Mass effect

Insecticide-treated nets (ITNs) provide a high degree of protection for those sleeping under them. Mosquitoes attempting to feed come into contact with the insecticidal net surfaces and are either killed or repelled. Where mosquitoes contacting the net are not immediately killed, their survival may be considerably reduced. The protection remains high even where nets have holes in them, or are not tucked in. However, when treated nets are used by a significant proportion of households in a community, there are additional benefits due to what has been termed the mass effect. A high proportion of the host-seeking mosquitoes will risk lethal contact with a treated net. In this way, a mass anti-*Anopheles* effect is added to the toxic and excito-repellent effect of each individual net. This is especially true with deltamethrin or lambdacyalothrin impregnated nets that have a strong and quick acting knock down effect on anophelines that are not knock-down resistant (*kdr*). In this case, the mosquito will spend sometime on the impregnated net and will have no time to fly away as it will quickly be knocked down and killed. The mass effect can be far more significant than the effect of each treated net taken individually. It depends on:
- the proportion of people sleeping under a treated mosquito net;
- sleeping patterns (e.g. if people go to bed late after watching the village television or usual events);
- the behaviour of certain vectors, either natural (*An. albimanus*) or induced exophily (*An. farauti* in former Irian Jaya, Sloof, 1960);
- finally, the area protected; in a zone containing 3,744 inhabitants in the Shenzhen Region of China, the incidence of *P. vivax* malaria dropped from 11.6‰ down to 4.6‰ after the adoption of deltamethrin-treated mosquito nets; when the trial was expanded to cover a total of 32,367 people, the incidence dropped right down to 2.5‰, and after all 236,700 inhabitants of the entire district had been included, the incidence was no more than 1.09‰ (Li Zu Zi *et al.*, 1986). The vectors were *An. sinensis* and *An. lesteri*.

The level of coverage and the extent of the zone covered are the two parameters that determine the efficacy of a treated mosquito net distribution programme instigated as a control measure on a community basis.

Efficacy

Wherever community-based trials of treated mosquito nets have been conducted, positive results have been seen in terms of reduction in the number of bites, transmission levels, parasitaemia (density of parasites) in the blood, incidence rate of the disease, anaemia,, and even overall infant mortality (Lengeler *et al.*, 1996). However, parasite prevalence was not substantially affected in many of the trials in endemic areas.

It is difficult to rank the various insecticides used to impregnate nets (500 mg/m^2 for permethrin and 15-30 mg a.i./m^2 for deltamethrin, lambdacyhalothrin or cyfluthrin) in terms of efficacy; all these products give the hoped-for results.

Of the large number of trials described in the literature, we have singled out few with particularly interesting results (*Table II*). Lengeler (1998) published an exhaustive review, including all the randomised trials and some of the more reliable unrandomised ones.

Fewer bites

The reduction in the number of bites is the parameter which is most important to local people when judging the utility of treated mosquito nets distribution programme, and this is key when it comes to motivating the population and getting them to accept the initiative. In China, in Guangdong Province, the number of *An. sinensis* bites was reduced by 93% and the number of *An. anthropophagus* (now called *An. lesteri*) bites by 76% after the introduction of treated mosquito nets (Li Zu Zi *et al.*, 1986); and in Sichuan Province, the number of bites was reduced by 99% in 1986-1987 (Cheng *et al.*, 1995). In Burkina Faso, the density of *An. gambiae s.s.* was not changed by the introduction of treated mosquito nets but two-thirds of the *An. funestus* population disappeared. In Africa, the mass effect of insecticide treated nets is measured by the biting rate outside a mosquito net, or even better in sentinel houses without nets.

Curtailed transmission

Entomological Inoculation Rates have been estimated in several trials in Africa. After the introduction of mosquito nets, this measure dropped by 78% in Benin (Akogbeto & Nahum, 1996) and by 98% in RD Congo (Karch *et al.*, 1993) while in south-western Kenya a reduction of only 50% was seen (Beach *et al.*, 1993).

In a savannah village of Burkina Faso, the sporozoite rate of *An. gambiae s.s.* dropped by 89%, and that of *An. funestus* by 74% (Carnevale *et al.*, 1988); in Tanzania, it dropped by nearly 90% (*in* Curtis *et al.*, 1990).

Lower incidence

The results presented in *Table II* illustrate the inconsistent effects of treated mosquito nets on malaria in terms of incidence, number of cases, attenuation of high-level parasitaemia and anaemia.

A number of large-scale randomised trials carried out in places with different transmission rates have been subjected to a meta-analysis by Lengeler (1998). In places where malaria is stable, treated mosquito nets cut the number of simple malaria attacks by half (48% compared to controls without any mosquito net at all and 34% compared to controls protected by an untreated mosquito net). A protective effect was also seen in places where people were receiving less than one infective bite per year: (65% and 43% with respect to controls for *P. falciparum*, and 42% and 25% for *P. vivax*).

In a single trial conducted in Kenya (Nevill *et al.*, 1996), the number of severe episodes was reduced by 45%, a particularly revealing observation. Only a moderate impact was seen on the prevalence of *P. falciparum* and *P. vivax*.

Treated mosquito nets have a markedly positive effect on anaemia (packed cell volume).

Reduced mortality

Reducing malaria mortality by 50% is the primary objective of the WHO Roll Back Malaria programme.

More than 90% of malaria deaths occur in Africa and mostly in children of between 6 months and 5 years of age.

Lengeler's analysis (1998) of five African trials showed a decrease in overall infant mortality of 17% in protected children compared with unprotected children, and of 23% compared with children only protected with an untreated net. The number of deaths prevented by the use of a treated mosquito net was 6 per 1,000 children. The trials were carried out in Gambia (D'Alessandro *et al.*, 1995), Kenya (Nevill *et al.*, 1996), Ghana (Binka *et al.*, 1996) and in Burkina Faso (Habluetzel *et al.*, 1997) where the yearly EIR were 1-10 10-30, 100-300, and 300-500 respectively. In the last case, people were being protected using impregnated curtains.

A more recent study carried out in Tanzania (Armstrong-Schellenberg *et al.*, 2001) in the framework of a demographic surveillance programme running since 1997 covering 480,000 people, demonstrated in a more solid manner the beneficial effects of treated mosquito nets on infant mortality: the survival of children of between 1 month and 4 years of age rose by 27%; and in two districts, the nets prevented one death in twenty among the protected children.

Without any doubt at all, treated mosquito nets and—in certain circumstances—impregnated curtains are extremely valuable tools in the fight against overall infant mortality.

Curtains

At the moment, there is no standard form of curtain for impregnation. In Madagascar, treated curtains were hung across windows and doors, whereas in Burkina Faso, special canvas curtains were hung over porches to seal the house at night, so it is difficult to compare the poor results in the former (Rabarison *et al.*, 1995) with the very good results obtained in the latter (Pietra *et al.*, 1991; Procacci *et al.*, 1991). In Kenya, Beach *et al.* (1993) documented a reduction in incidence from 32% to 10%, similar to that seen in Mozambique (Crook *et al.*, 1995) although the type of curtain used was not specified. If curtains are to be used on a large scale, it will be important to define their size and shape as well as how they should be placed. Another parameter to be studied is how quickly the insecticide breaks down under the action of ultraviolet radiation.

In Mali, the impregnation of bed covers seems to reduce the number of *An. gambiae s.s.* bites (Doumbo *et al.*, 1991).

More and more articles deal with treated clothes and overgear, e.g. treated chadors (the long moslem dress) effectively protect sleeping women in Afghanistan (Rowland *et al.*, 1999).

Problems associated with treated nets

Encouraging mosquito net use encounters various problems at the community level.

The degree of **acceptance** will depend on local habits which will itself depend on the degree of resultant inconvenience; it is relatively independent of malaria which

Table II. Efficacy of insecticide-treated mosquito nets.

	Permethrin	Deltamethrin	Lambda-cyhalothrin	Anopheles concerned	Reduction Transmission[1]	Reduction Incidence[2]	Authors
China Guangdong		+		*An. anthropophagus* *An. sinensis*		from 13-1 ‰	Li Zu Zi *et al.*, 1986
China Jiangxi	+	+		*An. sinensis*		–85% of cases	Li Zu Zi *et al.*, 1989
China Sichuan		+		*An. sinensis* and *An. anthropophagus*		close to 0	Cheng *et al.*, 1995
China Hainan		+		*An. dirus*		from 33-1,2‰	Li Zu Zi *et al.*, 1986
India - Orissa			+	*An. fluviatilis*		–50% of cases	Das *et al.*, 1993
Thailand (NO)	+			*An. minimus*		–38% *P. falciparum*	Luxemburger *et al.*, 1994
Malaysia - Sabah			+	*An. balabacensis*		from 400 to 5,5 %	Hii *et al.*, 1993
Salomon	+			*An. farauti*		–50% *P. falciparum*	Kere *et al.*, 1993
Pap.-New-Guinea Madang	+			*An. farauti*		–50% in 1-4 years	Graves *et al.*, 1987
Guatemala	+			*An. albimanus*		from 200-86 ‰	Richards *et al.*, 1993
Colombia Ecuador Peru	+			*An. albimanus*		–40% of cases	Kroeger *et al.*, 1995
Benin		+		*An. gambiae s.s.* *An. melas*	–78%	0.9 in treated nets 1.4 in untreated nets	Akogbeto et Nahum, 1996
Burkina Faso		+		*An. gambiae s.s.*	–94.3%	-59% in child cases	Carnevale *et al.*, 1988
Burundi		+		*An. gambiae*		–42% to –53% of cases	Van Bortel *et al.*, 1996
Gambia	+			*An. gambiae s.s.*	–90%	–63% of cases	Snow *et al.*, 1988a
Guinea-Bissau	+			*An. gambiae s.s.*	–78%		Jaenson *et al.*, 1994
Kenya (Kisumu)	+			*An. gambiae s.s.* *An. arabiensis*	–50%	–49% of cases	Beach *et al.*, 1993
Sierra Leone			+	*An. gambiae s.s.*		N° attacks in children: 0.65 *versus* 1.3 (untreated)	Marbiah *et al.*, 1998
Tanzania	+			*An. gambiae s.s.*		–54% anaemia	Premji *et al.*, 1995
Democratic Republic of Congo		+		*An. gambiae s.s.*	–98%	– 83% high parasitaemias	Karch *et al.*, 1993

1. Transmission evaluated by the reduction in infective bites per person per year
2. Incidence: the authors undertook evaluations based on the reduction in incidence (the drop in the number of clinical cases per 1,000 subjects, e.g. line 1: from 13‰ to 1‰); others just mentioned the lower incidence as a percentage reduction (e.g. line 2: -85%); finally, a few authors measured the reduction in *P. falciparum* or of high-level parasitaemia or even anaemia.

is rarely a direct motive for use. In towns, many people exposed to *Culex quinquefasciatus* regularly sleep under a mosquito net. In contrast, in the Central African forest where the number of bites per night per person is often under ten, there is little interest in this type of protection even though malaria is holo-endemic there. In many regions, health education campaigns have to be conducted before treated mosquito nets are introduced.

The **costs** and distribution methods for treated nets were discussed above.

Treatment is usually carried out by a specially trained unit or personnel who know how to minimise the risk of poisoning. The currently available products mainly the newly developed kits ("do it yourself") all come with safety guarantees for both users and treatment operators.

The need for re-treatment is the main problem associated with treated mosquito nets. This is why the current trend is to supply people with nets impregnated directly during the manufacturing process which remain active throughout the life of the mosquito net ("Long Lasting Insecticide Treated Nets" or "LLIN").

An. gambiae s.s. resistance to pyrethroids, due to the *kdr* mutation, was first detected in Ivory Coast and then noticed throughout most of West Africa (Chandre *et al.*, 1999; Elissa *et al.*, 1993). However, in contrast to what might have been expected, this does not seem to have compromised the protection afforded by treated mosquito nets (Darriet *et al.*, 1998 ; Henry *et al.*, 2005).

Antilarval and environmental measures

From 1890 to 1940, antilarval drainage operations, environmental measures and the use of chemical products (mineral oil, Paris Green) were the basis of vector control. Some degree of success was observed in Italy, the Balkans, Algeria, the United States and India, to mention the best known examples, but despite massive civil engineering efforts, malaria was not eliminated.

As of 1943, success on a global scale was obtained by means of indoor spraying operations with long-acting insecticides, the prototype being DDT, and larva control was demoted to the rank of a historical curiosity.

In 1978, before the end of "Eradication" and the development of primary health care systems, larva control became part of domestic clean-up operations (*see the Chapter on the* "History of Control Policies"). Many biological and bacteriological control methods were proposed together with environmental measures to reduce vector density. Trials were conducted more or less throughout the world without any epidemiological impact (Rafatjah, 1988 *in* Wernsdorfer & McGregor, 1988; WHO, 1983). Everything that had been known since the 1950's (Macdonald, 1957) was forgotten, notably that reducing longevity is far more effective than reducing vector density when it comes to controlling malaria.

The great engineering works carried out to reduce the incidence of malaria in Italy at the beginning of the last century (Pampana, 1937) were replaced by development plans aimed at enhancing agricultural production. In terms of health, these programmes aimed at no more than avoiding environmental changes that would favour increases of vector numbers that might lead to malaria exploding.

Intermittent irrigation as a mean of reducing malaria transmission is only possible where water supply systems are very well organised: it has been attempted in China in regions where human fertiliser is used necessitating regular drying out. Growing the alga azolla—a green fertiliser—which covers the entire water surface should prevent the development of mosquito larvae (Lu Bao Lin, 1984).

Environmental modifications are often only complementary to water management projects, as in the rice-growing regions of Burundi (*Figure 14*).

Integrated operations, undertaken with strong scientific back-up in the Kheda in the State of Gujarat in India (Sharma *et al.*, 1987), did not prove very effective against the "first wave" of malaria due to *An. culicifacies* in 1988: the incidence there was comparable to that in neighbouring States although, without any control, this experiment is difficult to evaluate.

The bacterial insect pathogen *Bacillus thuringiensis* H14 is highly effective against anopheline larvae but its usefulness has been restricted by the brevity of its action—under two days—whatever the agent in which it is resuspended, meaning that large-scale operations are prohibitively expensive: in Madagascar, it was estimated that repeated treatment of rice paddies (the main source of *Anopheles*) with *B. thuringiensis* H14 would cost twenty times as much as one DDT treatment, and success was not guaranteed.

B. sphaericus is not very effective against anopheline larvae. This product used to be recommended for the

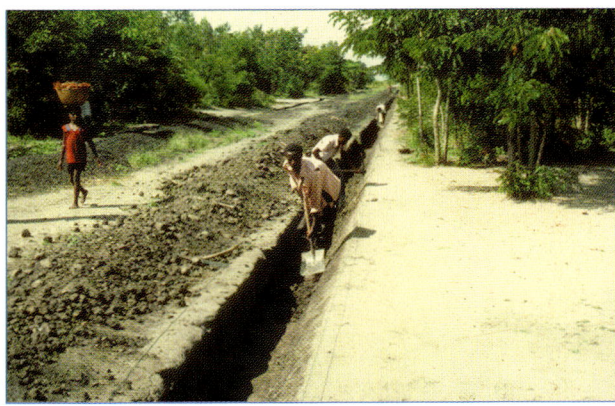

Figure 14. Maintenance of drainage ditches in Burundi (*photograph by Coosemans*).

control of *Culex* but its use has waned since *Culex pipiens* and *C. quinquefasciatus* acquired resistance to this bacterium in many parts of the world.

Many experts have invested enormous hope in larvivorous fish although this hope has proven empty according to others. In some habitats, indigenous fish species are natural regulators of mosquito populations, with a stable balance between prey and predator but, more commonly, mosquito larvae and the relevant fish occupy different biotopes, e.g. in the Camargue in France, an imported fish species, *Gambusia affinis*, has colonised the freshwater channels and *Anopheles* and *Culex* larvae are rare; however, in the residual brackish marshes into which the fish fail to penetrate, *Aedes caspius* thrives and is responsible for something like 5,000 bites per day (between 6 and 9 p.m.). In Madagascar, when the same fish was introduced on the High Plateaux, it thrived in natural water bodies but had little impact on the numbers of *An. funestus* or *An. arabiensis* which develop in rice paddies.

The introduction of larvivorous fish—usually *Gambusia affinis* in clean water and guppies (*Poecilia reticulata*) in polluted water—has been successful in some instances. The volcanic island of Grande Comore emerged relatively recently and does not have much surface water, so *An. gambiae s.s.* can only find larval habitats in mosque bathrooms and domestic water tanks. Many such tanks were constructed in 1920 when the vanilla boom began, and their massive invasion by *Anopheles* led to an epidemic which killed one quarter of the island's population before the current hyperendemic malaria became installed (Blanchy *et al.*, 1999). In a guppy seeding experiment conducted on 120 tanks (supplying 1,200 people), a drop of 45% was obtained in PR (Sabatinelli *et al.*, 1991): this is one of the very few positive results from this type of experiment which were unfortunately not pursued.

In the oasis of Timimoun in the Algerian Sahara, the introduction of *Gambusia affinis* into *An. sergentii* larval habitats brought a small epidemic (70 cases) to an end (Montillier, 1954).

In northern Chile, *An. pseudopunctipennis* develops in a few rivers flowing down from the Andes. Even though, there is no longer autochthonous malaria in this country, this mosquito is being controlled by the presence of *Gambusia affinis* introduced at the beginning of the last century and the use of chemical larvicidal compounds to prevent any reintroduction of malaria from neighbouring countries (Manguin, personal observation).

In northern Somalia, the treatment of water tanks—which provided the only larval habitats available for *An. arabiensis*—with the fish *Oreochromis spilurus* eliminated *Anopheles* and malaria (Alio *et al.*, 1985) although it has been impossible to follow more recent developments because of the political situation in the country.

In water tanks and wells in Assab in Eritrea where *An. culicifacies* thrives, *Aphanius dispar* was introduced on an experimental basis but this does not seem to have ever been followed up. The impact of this species in wells and water bodies in Djibouti where it thrives has not been clearly evaluated. In any case, *An. arabiensis* continues to flourish even in the presence of the fish.

In urban water tanks and reservoirs in India where *An. stephensi* (and also *An. subpictus*) develop, most larvicidal modalities have been investigated (Rajagopalan *et al.*, 1987): temephos gave excellent results. Larvivorous fish and the bacterial insect pathogen *Bacillus thuringiensis* Bt-14 were also tested.

Today, chemical larvicidal compounds are only being used on a large scale in very arid regions where vector densities are low. In the Sultanate of Oman, the generalised control strategy is based on once-weekly temephos treatment of watering holes in wadis and underground channels with substantial success, the incidence of malaria having dropped by over 90% (Beljaev, personal communication).

In Djibouti, temephos treatment of water tanks is still implemented (*Figure 15*).

Resistance to insecticides

Ever since insecticides were first used to protect crops and human health, resistance has been observed (Brown & Pal, 1971). DDT resistance was first documented in 1947, in domestic flies in Sweden; the first resistant anopheline (*An. sachavori*) was observed in Greece in 1953 (Livadas &

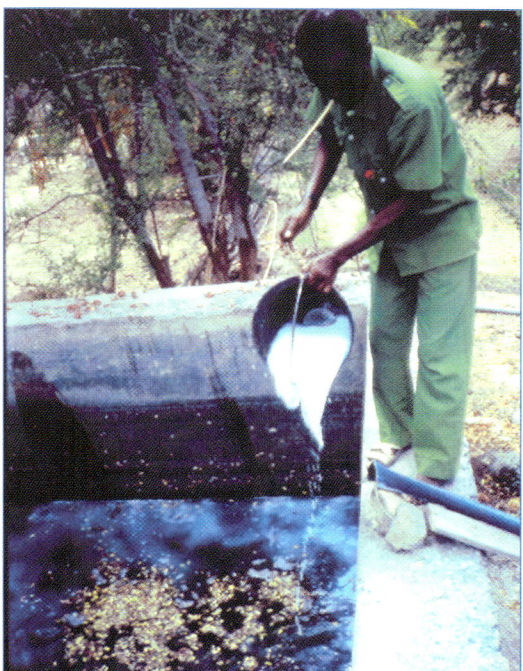

Figure 15. Treating water tanks with temephos to eliminate An. arabiensis *larval habitats in Djibouti (photograph by Carnevale).*

Georgiopoulos, 1953). Since then, many anopheline species have developed resistance to various insecticides, posing a major problem when it comes to malaria control.

Main resistance mechanisms

Insecticide resistance has been defined as the **presence of insects which survive doses of insecticides which would normally kill all the individuals in that population**. This is essentially an empirical definition.

A distinction is made between physiological and behavioural resistance mechanisms.

Behavioural resistance arises when a mosquito has changed from an endophilic and/or anthropophilic behaviour pattern to a more exophilic and/or zoophilic one. This seems to be the simple result of the natural presence of several—often related—species. Some of these disappear as a result of insecticide use and are supplanted by others which are less susceptible to the compounds in question. In South Africa and Swaziland, *An. arabiensis* had disappeared and only the zoophilic, exophilic *An. quadriannulatus* was left; since both species were at the time considered as the same entity, i.e. *An. gambiae s.l.*, it was concluded that it had changed its behaviour and was no longer feeding on humans. The same thing happened in Thailand with the endophilic *An. minimus* (former species A) and the more exophilic and partially zoophilic *An. minimus* C (Ismael *et al.*, 1978). In point of fact, no proven case of behavioural resistance has been documented to date.

In contrast, physiological resistance is an all-too-real phenomenon. This results from the process of genetic mutation which occurs at a very low frequency. Massive insecticide treatment can select for mutants which then supplant the initial, wild-type population.

Such mutations can affect:
- enzymes that inactivate insecticides, including esterases, mono-oxygenases and transferases;
- the insecticide's site of action, e.g. the receptor for gamma-amino-butyric acid (GABA) in the case of dieldrin (Rdl);
- sodium channels, e.g. the *kdr* (knock-down resistance) gene for DDT and pyrethroids;
- acetylcholinesterase for organophosphates and carbamates.

WHO (1986) has developed simple tests which can be carried out in most entomological laboratories to assess the resistance of adult and larvae of anophelines to various insecticides. They have developed simplified protocols and set discriminating concentrations which makes it possible to define whether or not a population of vectors is resistant on the basis of a small number of specimens (minimum 100) (Tables III and IV).

Resistance and control measures

Dieldrin resistance (Rdl) appeared very soon (in 1955 in Nigeria) in *An. gambiae* and spread throughout most of the countries in which this insecticide had been used for public health operations. There is no proof that resistance was selected for by the presence of agricultural insecticide. Dieldrin is long-acting and does not induce an excito-repellent effect, and it was probably the best compound for indoor spraying. However, it is no longer used because of widespread resistance.

Anopheline dieldrin resistance is due to the inhibition of GABA receptors. It is extremely stable with the mutant allele being transmitted through the generations even when the toxin has not been encountered for forty years. In addition, this trait confers cross-resistance to the phenylpyrazoles which have the same mechanism of action; this class was therefore useless even before it had ever been used.

DDT and pyrethroid resistance is due to the *kdr* gene which codes for a voltage gated sodium channel. In *An. gambiae s.s.* in West Africa, up to 90% of individuals may be carrying the *kdr* mutation as a result of ongoing selection pressure exerted by the ever-present insecticide. In Burkina Faso, the first DDT-resistant *Anopheles* appeared in 1967, long after the product had been abandoned for use in public

Table III. Discriminatory doses for detecting resistance in adult *Anopheles*.		
Pesticide	**Concentration %**	**Exposure time (hours)**
DDT	4	1
Malathion	5	1
Fenitrothion	1	2
Permethrin	0.75	1
Deltamethrin	0.025	1

Table IV. Discriminatory doses for *Anopheles* larvae (mg/litre) (ppm)	
Pesticide	**Dose in ppm (24 hours exposure)**
DDT	2.5
Chlorpyrifos	0.025
Temephos	0.25
Fenitrothion	0.05
Fenthion	0.05
Malathion	3.125

health operations in 1959. It seems more than likely that resistance had been selected for by use of the insecticide on cotton crops (Mouchet, 1988). In 1994, pyrethroid resistance was observed in Ivory Coast (Elissa *et al.*, 1994), a hangover from DDT resistance which has exactly the same biochemical mechanism of action. Since then, it has been documented in most of West Africa (Chandre *et al.*, 1999), as well as Cameroon (Etang *et al.*, 2007) and Kenya (Ranson *et al.*, 2000). Resistant *An. sacharovi* carrying the *kdr* gene have been observed in Turkey (Luleyap *et al.*, 2002).

In population of *An. gambiae s.s.* from East Africa (Kenya), a *kdr* mutation different from that found in West Africa has been observed. Both are found at the same locus but, in the East African form, a serine is substituted by a phenylalanine (West Africa form): this mutation confers strong resistance to DDT but lower-level resistance to pyrethroid (Ranson *et al.*, 2000).

Some forms of **DDT resistance** are due to **altered enzyme activities**. Resistance due to a modification of the GST (glutathion S-transferase) gene which enables the mosquito to detoxify the toxic molecule has been seen since 1955. Dehydrochlorinase converts DDT into the less toxic DDE, a type of resistance that has been observed in *An. gambiae s.s.* in Zanzibar, *An. sinensis* in China, and various species in South Asia (including *An. culicifacies*). In Kwazulu-Natal in South Africa, the same type of resistance is apparently seen in *An. arabiensis*.

In South Africa and southern Mozambique, *An. funestus* pyrethroid resistance is due to elevated levels of mixed function oxidases responsible for the detoxification of pyrethroids in resistant mosquitoes. This mechanism is also conferring cross-resistance to the carbamate insecticide propoxur (Brooke *et al.*, 2001) ; the high level of metabolically based pyrethroid resistance has major impact on current malaria control programs (Casimiro *et al.*, 2006) in both countries .

Three types of **organophosphate and carbamate resistance** have been characterised:
- modified acetylcholinesterase so that the insecticide can no longer bind the mutated enzyme, e.g. the multiple resistance of *An. albimanus* to organophosphates in Central America (El Salvador) (Georghiou, 1982) and resistance of *An. gambiae s.s.* to carbosulfan in Ivory Coast (Nguessan *et al.*, 2003);
- a modified oxidase activity which acts on the thiophosphate core of temephos;
- carboxyesterase activities which act on side-chains, e.g. malathion resistance which is not usually associated with cross-resistance to other organophosphates (Davidson, 1982).

Some mosquitoes are also resistant to pathogenic bacteria, e.g. most populations of *Culex pipiens* and *C. quinquefasciatus* are now highly resistant to *B. sphaericus* which produces a single toxin (which has never been very effective against *Anopheles*).

On the other hand, no resistance has ever been documented vis-à-vis *B. thuringiensis* H14; this bacterium produces three toxins, which may explain why resistance fails to develop.

What to do about resistance

First and foremost, it is important to emphasise that the existence of resistance does not necessarily mean that the compound concerned can no longer be used at all for vector control because it may have repellent activity—be it immediate or delayed—above and beyond its lethal effect.

The discovery of pyrethroid resistance in *An. gambiae* in Ivory Coast (Elissa *et al.*, 1993, 1994) provoked a full-scale panic throughout Africa where pyrethroid impregnated mosquito nets constitute the only feasible means of control in the near future. Tests of repellent impregnated nets have been quite positive, even against *An. gambiae kd*-resistant (*kdr*) (N'Guessan *et al.*, 2006). Nevertheless, to date, impregnated mosquito nets are continuing to provide effective protection (Henry *et al.*, 2005). It seems that because resistant individuals are less susceptible to the insecticide's excito-repellent effect, they remain in contact longer with the treated surface, which induces a higher mortality (Darriet *et al.*, 1998).

In the holo-endemic Korhogo Region of Northern Ivory Coast, *kdr* resistance exists at very high level but large scale use of mosquito nets treated with lambdacyhalothrin induced a ten-fold decrease in transmission (Carnevale *et al.*, personal observation) and a major drop in malaria morbidity (56%) among children under 5 years old (Henry *et al.*, 2005).

A number of more or less sophisticated strategies have been proposed to prevent the development of resistance, including rotating insecticides, applying them in a mosaic pattern, using mixtures of different compounds on the same mosquito net, or defining protection zones for high-risk populations (WHO, 1986). Apart from the rotation of larvicidal products in the control of *Simulium* vectors in West Africa, few of these proposals—especially when it comes to adult insects—have ever gone beyond the theoretical stage, given the small number of families of products available, the complicated logistics of application, and drastic restrictions in the choice of of insecticides due to their toxicity.

For instance, only pyrethroid insecticide with a residual effect are safe enough and quick acting when used in impregnated mosquito nets. However, there is cross-resistance between different pyrethroids and resistance to one is usually associated with reduced susceptibility to all the others. The only other long- and fast-acting product suitable is carbosulfan although this compound is fifty times as toxic as most of the pyrethroids and is not ideal for public health usage. Encouraging results were recently obtained by treating nets with a mixture of a non-pyrethroid insecticide (propoxur) and a repellent (DEET).

The replacement of DDT with other compounds as a result of resistance or to avoid irritating environmental activists has seriously compromised most IRS programmes. Whichever product is used, it will not remain active for more than three months on walls and treatment will have to be repeated. Malathion, the only compound which can compete with DDT in terms of cost, is often rejected for indoor spraying because of its unpleasant odour. All the other options, namely the organophosphates (fenitrothion, methyl pyrimiphos), carbamates (propoxur) and pyrethroids (deltamethrin, cyfluthrin, lambdacyhalotrin, etc.) are far more expensive, although pesticide cost is relatively low comparing to the operational costs. In addition, only few developing countries (e.g. South Africa) possess enough resources to conduct spraying operations without any external help.

Detection, Control and Prevention of Epidemics

In places where malaria is transmitted exceptionally, irregularly or rarely, an epidemic may break out at any time. This may apply in mountainous or arid tropical regions as well as in places where malaria control operations have been abandoned. Such epidemics strike people who have little or no immunity against *Plasmodium* and are therefore very susceptible to infection. Similarly, an epidemic may break out in a population that has migrated from a healthy region into a malaria-infested one (Najera *et al.*, 1998).

It is important to make the distinction between epidemics—acyclic phenomena—and annual, seasonal outbreaks which are triggered by rain or some other meteorological event which is to some extent predictable; nevertheless, the two may coincide in a year of particularly heavy rainfall.

Control of epidemics

Detection

The first step—crucial when it comes to an epidemic—is detecting it as early as possible. Few epidemics break out suddenly without a more or less obvious build-up period. In most cases, health institutions are notified by local bodies (or the media!) about an unusual rise in mortality and morbidity due to high fever. The regions affected are often rural and poorly served by the health care system, and responses from the centralised health structures are often slow.

An efficient health monitoring system should nevertheless detect an epidemic in its early stages. Whenever the incidence of fever doubles, an epidemic should be suspected. To evaluate the incidence of fever to this end, it is necessary to have to hand monthly or fortnightly mean variations for the preceding ten years. However, these figures are rarely available and other signs may need to be monitored such as unusually high consumption of malaria drugs, exhaustion of stocks in local dispensaries, high absenteeism from school, etc.

It must be confirmed that the epidemic is indeed one of malaria rather than of relapsing fever, visceral leishmaniasis, an arboviral disease or meningitis. Failure to respond to antimalaria drugs does not rule out the possibility that the epidemic is due to malaria since drug resistance is often a factor underlying the spread of an epidemic. Cases must be confirmed by clinical and parasitologic diagnosis. In this respect, rapid diagnostic testing (RDT) can be a valuable tool (Verlé *et al.*, 1996). The spatial dimensions of the problem (geographical extent, distribution of cases in foci or clusters) and temporal features (daily or weekly incidence, progression) need to be defined as well as target groups (age groups, occupations, social parameters).

Combating epidemics

As soon as an epidemic has been detected, the most urgent needs of the affected population need to be addressed as quickly as possible. **Care of the sick** is certainly the priority but other essential needs cannot be ignored, including food, accommodation, water supplies and clothing, especially if the epidemic has broken out against a background of some natural catastrophe such as a famine or flood. Medical services will have to cope with more than just patients with malaria and immunisation campaigns may be considered (e.g. against measles).

Vector control operations to block transmission may be indicated, depending on the dynamics of the epidemic. In epidemic zones, transmission is usually short-lived (e.g. highland malaria) and there is a lag period between the period of transmission and the peak incidence, so vector control operations—even if they reassure local people—will be quite useless if they are conducted as transmission is on the wane (Protopopoff *et al.*, 2007). Aerial spraying measures (or using motorised ULV units) are often purely for show. The picture may be different if the epidemic is due to the introduction of a new vector, to the migration of non-immune people into places where malaria is stable, or to the cessation of control operations, in which cases well-targeted vector control operations may prove very effective.

Pre-defined emergency plans can enhance the coordination and mobilisation of human and logistical resources thereby ensuring more efficient implementation. The place of the national and international authorities, bilateral agencies and non-governmental institutions will depend on the scale of the epidemic and the capacity of local bodies to deal with the problem effectively and rapidly enough. Such plans are rare and, even when they exist, they often fail to take stock of past experience and earlier mistakes. At-risk zones can be mapped and the detection of epidemics could be improved by strengthening the data gathering and analysis capabilities of the public health authorities.

Given that drug resistance is a major issue when it comes to controlling epidemics (Hay et al., 2002), specific treatment protocols have to be established—and these may be different from those recommended in endemic zones or at other times in the place where the epidemic is occurring. The usual first-line drug (often chloroquine) may be replaced by other drugs (e.g. Coartem®) that may be more expensive but which guarantee efficacy (Etchegorry et al., 2001). In an epidemic, keeping the rate of therapeutic failure as low as possible is essential since the capacity of the local health care system will already be overloaded. Every effort should be made locally to treat severe cases with intramuscular injections of quinine dihydrochloride. Drug prices should be cut and strategic stocks built up to ensure preparedness for an epidemic. The emergency plan should provide for the rapid establishment of an effective drug distribution system. In the most remote villages, it may be profitable to increase the number of treatment points. Education of the population and the targeting of specific messages is a necessary component of any emergency plan, emphasising how to recognise the symptoms of the disease and stipulating first aid measures that can be undertaken at home (Najera et al., 1998). It should be underlined that mass treatment programmes have a relatively low ratio of cost to efficacy.

Prevention

Predicting epidemics?

The period following an epidemic is too rarely studied with a view to analysing the circumstances which led to the outbreak and what could have been done to improve its control—or even how to prevent an outbreak in the future Extremely complex models—which are mainly based on satellite imaging data and weather forecasts (Hay et al., 2001)—are of little use when it comes to predicting epidemics, so systematic monitoring and flexible prevention instruments are to be preferred to a strategy based on highly targeted interventions. Many recent epidemics were not the result of major climate events (like floods or global warming), despite what certain authors have suggested.

The sporogonic cycle and gametogenesis of *P. falciparum* are slower than those of *P. vivax*, so the epidemic waves of the former grow more slowly, even though the ultimate consequences of the two types of epidemic are far from comparable (*in* Najera et al., 1998). In practice, most epidemics—especially those due to *P. falciparum*—break out in endemo-epidemic zones where there is already a parasite reservoir in people who are not immunologically naïve.

The factors which trigger epidemics are many and various but some constant features can be discerned. Most commonly, the number of cases of malaria rises gradually, possibly over several years (although on a seasonal basis). This spiralling rise in the size of the reservoir can explode at any moment under the influence of seasonal factors that promote transmission, e.g. a rise in temperature foreshortening the sporogonic cycle at higher altitudes. Vector populations are also subject to seasonal factors such as rainfall which usually leads to increased anopheline densities (Lindblade et al., 1999) but not always. Particularly heavy rain may flush out larvae from shallow habitats or reduce the temperature in highlands, both resulting in the curtailment of transmission. Other factors can exacerbate the spiralling effect, including ineffective control programmes or the cessation of operations, health care system deficiencies, and therapeutic failure due to resistance to antimalaria drugs (Lindsay & Martens, 1998). War and political instability often cut large populations off from access to health care. It should be noted that sulfadoxine-pyrimethamine treatment induces a spectacular increase in gametogenesis which has been suspected of promoting the spread of resistance as well as enhancing transmission (Hogh et al., 1998); conversely, combination therapy including an artemisinin derivative induces a no less spectacular decrease in gametocyte production (Nosten et al., 2000).

Land development can create conditions which favour vector installation and proliferation; this has been seen when lower-lying enclaves in mountainous regions have been turned over to arable farming and when rice-growing was introduced in the Sahel. In Madagascar highlands, such land developments led to epidemics at the end of the 19th century and throughout the first half of the 20th century (Mouchet et al., 1998). In the 1950's, indoor DDT spraying programmes were shown to be effective in the curtailment of epidemics. It can be said that, in most places where land development has created an epidemic risk, the situation is largely irreversible. Given the agricultural and industrial prerogatives at issue, it is impossible to imagine remodelling these areas purely for reasons of public health.

Nevertheless, well-conceived prevention strategies should aim to block expression of the epidemic risk.

What strategy to adopt?

Prevention is essentially based on indoor spraying operations with residual insecticides and the use of insecticide-impregnated mosquito nets.

The first objective of any prevention programme is to reduce the size of the gametocyte reservoir in order to block transmission. A *P. falciparum* infection may last one year, and *P. vivax* can persist in the body for three years. An effective two-to-three year programme should reduce the human *P. falciparum* reservoir to preclude any sudden resumption of transmission. At the end of this period, the prevalence and incidence of malaria should be assessed before deciding whether or not to continue operations. It is important to remember that such interventions can hit vectors very hard, and a species may even disappear—temporarily like *An. funestus* on the Plateaux of Madagascar or forever like *An. gambiae s.l.* in Brazil and Egypt. This is particularly true for anophelines surviving despite sub-optimal ecological conditions: on the cool African highlands, *An. gambiae* and *An. funestus* are markedly more endophagous and endophilic than at lower altitudes, so indoor spraying and sleeping under mosquito nets are highly effective measures.

Temporal and spatial targeting

A good preventive strategy aims at being effective but also sustainable and easy to implement. In consequence, precise targeting—in both time and space—will reduce the cost of the operation and limit the period during which human resources need to be deployed. The sustainability of operations will depend on political will.

Targeting in time

It is not always easy to interpret seasonal variations in the malaria figures and this is compounded by the fact that it is often impossible to separate cases of malaria from those involving other forms of fever. However, in epidemic zones, transmission can only occur at certain times of the year: summer in temperate regions, the hottest months at altitude, the rainy season in arid zones or the beginning of the dry season where the vector can propagate in pools left behind by the receding flood waters as happens in Sri Lanka. To cut the number of indoor spraying rounds down to a minimum, vector control measures should target the periods of transmission.

Targeting in space

In places at risk of epidemic malaria, anopheline larval habitats are usually well-defined and localised, e.g. in mountain valleys, river-beds and oases. *Anopheles* is at its densest in dwellings close to these larval habitats, so highly selective treatment operations can have a major impact (including possible protection of dwellings further away by virtue of a barrier effect). In this way, operations could be targeted to just 25% of the community. This will involve an in-depth geographical analysis coupled with a meticulous inventory of dwellings and local particularities.

Reflections on different vector control methods

There are two well-adapted ways of controlling malaria vectors, both aimed at the adult mosquito; targeting the larvae presents too many problems.

Indoor spraying with a residual insecticide can be very effective as long as the coverage is adequate: this will depend on the team conducting the operation. If prevention is to be sustainable, it is to be strongly recommended that teams be decentralised and that they operate under the aegis of a community-based authority (a municipal or regional institution). Efficacy will also depend on the anophelines resting habits; at higher altitudes, a given species will tend to be far more endophilic than it is elsewhere because it is so cold outdoors.

Using a treated mosquito net can be an extremely effective means of personal protection although coverage—and therefore collective protection—will depend on compliance, which could be low if the nuisance is not an issue.

Vaccination

Vaccines and fundamental problems associated with the physiology of *Plasmodium*

A vaccine against malaria has been the hope of a generation, ever since it became evident that the goal of eradication would not be achieved. By 1996, it was clear that no single vaccine would suffice, given the diversity of plasmodial species and the polymorphism at all stages of development (Jeffrey, 1966).

To date, most candidate vaccines have been directed against *P. falciparum*, the molecular biology of which we are understanding more and more fully.

Three vaccine targets are being investigated:
- against pre-erythrocytic forms, i.e. sporozoites and hepatic forms, to protect immunologically naïve immigrants and travellers as well as those living in places where malaria is endemic but at low-level. This has been disparaged as a vaccine for tourists and military personnel from rich countries;
- against asexual erythrocytic forms to protect groups at higher risk (young children, pregnant women and immigrants) living in places where malaria is highly endemic. This vaccine which would reduce malaria mortality and morbidity is the one needed in endemic zones, especially in Africa;
- against sporogonic stages to block transmission, an "altruistic" vaccine.

In their review, Richie & Saul (2002) drew attention to two *Plasmodium*-specific properties:
- after an attack or malaria, the parasite persists in the host's body despite immune mechanisms which inhibit its growth: in other words, this **immune response does not protect against new infection**;
- at each stage of its development, the parasite expresses **different antigens** and each of the proteins involved is **highly polymorphic**, thereby potentially limiting the efficacy of a putative vaccine, e.g. one parasite clone contains fifty copies of the gene encoding Pf EMP1, an erythrocyte membrane protein; in the course of chronic infection, **each new wave** of parasites expresses a **new variant** of this surface antigen, so it can continue to proliferate in the presence of antibodies elicited against the previous waves;
- the number of plasmodial proteins—between five and six thousand—offers a wide choice of possible vaccine components (sub-units);
- finally, stock has to be taken of the heterogeneity of the human immune response (histocompatibility groups, genetic traits, different forms of haemoglobin, etc.).

In these circumstances, can an effective vaccine ever be produced? Richie & Saul (2002) believe so, but it is clear from their review that the development process will be long and expensive. Their confidence is inspired by the results of trials.

Immunisation with irradiated sporozoites protects, at least partially, rodents (Nussenzweig *et al.*, 1967), monkeys and humans (Rickman *et al.*, 1979) although it is not known which immune mechanisms mediate this protection (Collins & Contracos, 1972). No single dominant immune response has been identified in immunised subjects, which suggests that protection must result from a whole series of different responses directed against a broad spectrum of different antigens contained in the attenuated vaccine organism, each individual response being of limited efficacy but which sum to generate a protective mechanism (Richie & Saul, 2002).

In addition, it is known that regular infection elicits acquired immunity or "premunition" which protects against the most serious clinical manifestations. If we could mimic this state of premunition by means of a vaccine, we could protect against clinical disease. One research avenue is to elicit antibodies directed against antigens of the erythrocytic stages. Stowers *et al.* (2001) successfully protected *Aotus* monkeys against *P. falciparum* using a merozoite surface protein (MSP1). This type of vaccine would fulfil the requirements of highly endemic areas.

Both types of vaccine have shown protective activity in field trials but they are insufficiently effective and the duration of protection is too short.

Candidate antigens

A whole series of different antigens have been proposed for inclusion in a malaria vaccine (Hoffman *et al.*, 1996; Richie & Saul, 2002):
- on sporozoites in liver cells: neutralising antibodies can be found against antigens expressed on the sporozoite surface, the best-characterised of which is the circumsporozoite protein (CSP);
- on hepatic stages: when T cells recognise plasmodial antigens expressed on the surface of the liver cell, the cell is killed;
- on merozoites: neutralising antibodies directed against merozoite surface proteins 1, 2, 3 and 4 block red cell invasion, and promote parasite phagocytosis and destruction;
- in erythrocytic stages;
- in the mosquito: neutralising antibodies against the PFs 25 parasite antigen block fertilisation.

The preferred approach is now to include combinations of antigens from different physiological systems at all the various stages of development of all three human plasmodial species.

Sequencing the genome of *P. falciparum* should lead to the identification of candidate antigens; the immune responses against hundreds of proteins are currently being evaluated.

Any vaccine will have to meet a dual challenge: on the one hand, it has to be easy to use and cheap; and on the other hand, it should cover all parasite populations with all their diversity and polymorphism.

Vaccine trials

Some forty vaccine trials have been conducted over the last twenty years, most of the vaccines having been directed against sporozoites (with a few against blood forms and just one designed to block transmission).

There have been relatively few field trials. The SPf 66 vaccine consisting of an alum-adsorbed synthetic peptide which targeted blood forms (Patarroyo *et al.*, 1988) proved quite ineffective in Africa (Graves & Gelbrand, 2001) although it had slightly reduced the clinical incidence of the disease in South America.

In a trial in adult males in Gambia, the RTS,S vaccine was found to reduce substantially the level of infection (Bojang *et al.*, 2001). More recently, in a trial in children of Mozambique, the RTS,S vaccine was shown to reduce by half severe malaria episodes (Alonso *et al.*, 2004).

In 5-9 year-old children in Papua-New Guinea, a combination of three surface protein fragments—part of the MSP1 antigen, one polymorphic form of MSP2, and a part of the ring infected erythrocyte surface antigen (RESA)—reduced the parasite load and the frequency of attacks (in those whose parasite load exceeded 1,000 per μl of blood).

Genes for plasmodial antigens carried on DNA plasmids have been shown to be able to induce antibodies in animal models but not yet in humans. This approach is being extensively investigated in the search for a malaria vaccine.

Evaluating the results of a vaccine trial means extremely well-prepared preliminary planning and constitutes a genuine epidemiological exercise. More and more institutions are qualified to test vaccines, at the international level (WHO and TDR), in Europe (European Malaria Vaccine Initiative), in America (Malaria Vaccine Initiative, National Institutes of Health, USAID and US Department of Defence): sites have already been selected for trials in Gambia, Mali, Ghana, Kenya, Mozambique, Tanzania and Papua New Guinea. The only element missing is the vaccine: to date, no candidate has proved adequately immunogenic or has conferred sufficiently long-lived protection.

Until a vaccine is developed

While we are waiting for a vaccine—the targets and protective activity of which are quite unknown—, it is essential to keep up the fight against malaria using the tried and tested instruments of malaria control, i.e. patient care, the targeted protection of high-risk groups, prevention by means of vector control, and preventing and controlling epidemics.

The impact of the disease with one million deaths per annum in Africa makes it vital that we keep our guard up in terms of malaria control operations—which have already been reduced to a minimum—on the pretext that a vaccine is going to be developed in the future.

Immunising against a parasite that is only weakly immunogenic is always going to be a problem and it is by no means sure that sequencing the genomes of *Plasmodium* and *Anopheles* will bring an effective vaccine any closer (Butler, 2002) although the resultant information may help with the development of new medicinal products.

Bibliography

- Abdel-Malek AA. The anopheline mosquitoes in Northern Syria. *Bull Soc Entomol Egypte* 1958 ; 42 : 591-5.
- Abderrazak SB, Oury B, Lal AA, *et al*. *Plasmodium falciparum*: population genetic analysis by multilocus enzyme electrophoresis and other molecular markers. *Exp Parasitol* 1999 ; 92 : 232-8.
- Abdurrahman MB, Edington GM, Narayana TP, Babaoye FA. Pathology of childhood nephrotic syndrome in Northern Nigeria. *Trop Geogr Med* 1981 ; 33 : 269-73.
- Abel L, Cot M, Mulder L, Carnevale P, Feingold J. Segregation analysis detects a major gene controlling malaria blood infection levels in human malaria. *Am J Hum Genet* 1992 ; 50 : 1308-17.
- Abul-Hab JK. Observations on the overwintering of *An. sacharovi* in Suleimaniya Liwa, Northern Iraq. *Bull Endem Dis (Baghdad)* 1956 ; 1 : 298-310.
- Abul-Hab JK. The seasonal occurrence of *An. superpictus* and *An. sacharovi* in Suleimaniya Liwa, Northern Iraq. *Bull Endem Dis (Baghdad)* 1958 ; 2 : 152-5.
- Abul-Hab JK. Resting habits of *Anopheles superpictus* Grassi and *Anopheles sacharovi* Faure in Northern Iraq. *Bull Endem Dis (Baghdad)* 1961 ; 4 : 54-9.
- Abul-Hab JK. Overwintering of *Anopheles superpictus* Grassi in Suleimaniya and Kirkuk Liwas in Northern Iraq. *Bull Soc Entomol Egypte* 1967 ; 51 : 243-50.
- Achee NL, Korves CT, Bangs MJ, *et al*. *Plasmodium vivax* polymorphs and *P. falciparum* circumsporozoite proteins in Anopheles from Belize, Central America. *J Vector Ecol* 2000 ; 25 (2) : 203-11.
- Achee NL, Grieco JP, Rejmankova E, *et al*. Biting patterns and seasonal densities of Anopheles mosquitoes in the Cayo District, Belize, Central America with emphasis on *Anopheles darlingi*. *J Vector Ecol* 2006 ; 31 : 45-57.
- Adam JP, Bailly-Choumara H. Les *Culicidae* et quelques autres diptères hématophages de la République de Guinée. *Bull IFAN* 1964 ; 26 : 900.
- Adamovic ZR. Anopheline population in East Macedonia, Yugoslavia. *Bull Acad Serbe Sci Arts* 1981 ; 75 : 81-91.
- Ademowo OG, Falusi AG, Mewoyeka OO. Prevalence of asymptomatic parasitaemia in an urban and rural community in South Western Nigeria. *Cent Afr J Med* 1995 ; 41 : 18-21.
- Adjuick M, Agnamey P, Babiker A, *et al*. Amodiaquine-artesunate *versus* amodiaquine for uncomplicated *P. falciparum* malaria in African children: a randomised multicentre trial. *Lancet* 2002 ; 359 (9315) : 1365-72.
- Adou-Bryn KD, Kouassi D, Ouhon J, Assoumou A, Kone M. Essai clinique de l'amodiaquine dans la commune d'Attecoube (Abidjan, Côte d'Ivoire). *Bull Soc Pathol Exot* 2000 ; 93 : 115-8.
- Adugna N, Petros B. Determination of the human blood index of some anopheline mosquitoes by using ELISA. *Ethiopian Med J* 1996 ; 34 : 1-10.
- Afari EA, Nakano T, Binka F, Owusu-Agyei S, Asigbee J. Seasonal characteristics of malaria infection in under-five children of a rural community in Southern Ghana. *West Afr J Med* 1993 ; 12 : 39-42.
- Afridi MK. *Review of malaria situation and research activities carried out in the control of malaria in Democratic Yemen* (Jordan, 31 March/ 12 April 1984). OMS EM/WKD.IMP.MAL.CNT.AFR./5.2, 1984.
- Afridi MK, Majid SA. Malaria in Bahrein Islands (Persian Gulf). *J Malaria Inst India* 1938 ; 3 : 427-72.
- Akogbeto M. Étude entomologique sur la transmission du paludisme côtier lagunaire : cas d'un village construit sur un lac d'eau saumâtre. *Ann Soc Belg Med Trop* 1995 ; 75 : 219-27.
- Akogbeto M. Le paludisme côtier lagunaire à Cotonou : données entomologiques. *Cahiers Santé* 2000 ; 10 : 267-75.
- Akogbeto M, Chippaux JP, Coluzzi M. Le paludisme urbain côtier à Cotonou (Bénin). Étude entomologique. *Rev Épidémiol Santé Publique* 1992a ; 40 : 233-9.
- Akogbeto M, Modiano D, Bosman A. Malaria transmission in the lagoon area of Cotonou, Benin. *Parassitologia* 1992b ; 34 : 147-54.
- Akogbeto M, Nahum A, Massougbodji A. Impact des moustiquaires imprégnées d'insecticides sur la morbidité palustre : résultats préliminaires. *Med Trop (Marseille)* 1995 ; 55 : 118-9.
- Akogbeto M, Nahum A. Impact des moustiquaires imprégnées de deltaméthrine sur la transmission de la malaria dans un milieu côtier lagunaire, Bénin. *Bull Soc Pathol Exot* 1996 ; 89 (4) : 291-8.
- Akogbeto M, Romano R. Infectivité d'*An. melas* vis-à-vis du *Plasmodium falciparum* dans le milieu côtier lagunaire du Bénin. *Bull Soc Pathol Exot* 1999 ; 92 : 57-61.
- Alam MT, Das MK, Ansari MA, Sharma YD. Molecular identification of *Anopheles (Cellia) sundaicus* from the Andaman and Nicobar islands of India. *Acta Trop* 2006 ; 97 : 10-8.
- Alcantara AK, Buck RL, Uylangco CV, Cross J. Cerebral malaria at San Lazaro Hospital, Manila Philippines. *Southeast Asian J Trop Med Public Health* 1982 ; 13 : 563-7.
- Aldighieri R. Quelques réflexions, à propos de la chute artificielle du paludisme dans un secteur à haute endémicité palustre en pays tropical (Guadeloupe). *Bull Soc Pathol Exot* 1953 ; 46 : 121-36.
- Ali Halidi M. Paludisme à Mayotte : passé, présent et futur. *Cahiers Santé* 1995 ; 5 : 362-7.
- d'Almeida JJ. *Contribution à la connaissance de l'épidémiologie du paludisme en République Togolaise*. Thèse Université Bordeaux, 1966, n° 524.
- Alio AY, Isaq A, Delfini LF. *Field trial on the impact of Oreochromis spilurus spilurus on malaria transmission in Northern Somalia*. WHO/MAL/85.1017 1985 ; 18 p.
- Allan R, Nam S, Doull L. MERLIN and malaria epidemic in northeast Kenya. *Lancet* 1998 ; 351 : 1966-7.
- Allison AC. Protection afforded by sickle-cell trait against sub-tertian malarial infection. *Br Med J* 1954 ; 6 : 290-4.
- Almendares J, Sierra M, Anderson PK, Epstein PR. Critical regions, a profile of Honduras. *Lancet* 1993 ; 342 : 1400-2.

- Alonso PL, Sacarlal J, Aponte JJ, *et al.* Efficacy of the RTS,S/AS02A vaccine against *Plasmodium falciparum* infection and disease in young African children: randomised controlled trial. *Lancet* 2004 ; 364 (9443) : 1411-20.
- Al Serouri AW, Grantham-McGregor SM, Greenwood B, Costello A. Impact of asymptomatic malaria parasitaemia on cognitive function and school achievement of school children in the Yemen Republic. *Parasitology* 2000 ; 121 : 337-45.
- Al Tikrity AB. The geographical distribution of *Anopheles* species and vectors of malaria in Iraq. *Bull Endem Dis (Baghdad)* 1964 ; 6 : 91-117.
- Alves FP, Durlacher RR, Menezes MJ, Krieger H, Pereira da Silva LH, Camargo FP. High prevalence of asymptomatic *Plasmodium vivax* and *P. falciparum* infections in native Amazonian populations. *Am J Trop Med Hyg* 2002 ; 66 (6) : 641-8.
- Alves MJ, Rangel O, de Souza SS. Malaria in Campinas region, Sao Paulo, Brazil, 1980 to 1994. *Rev Soc Brasil Med Trop* 2000 ; 33 (1) : 53-60.
- Alves W. Malaria parasite rates in Southern Rhodesia: May-Sept. 1956. *Bull World Health Organ* 1958 ; 19 : 69-74.
- Alves W, Blair DM. Malaria control in Southern Rhodesia. *J Trop Med Hyg* 1955 ; 58 : 273-80.
- Ambroise-Thomas P. La réaction d'immunofluorescence dans l'étude séro-immunologique du paludisme. *Bull Organ Mond Santé* 1974 ; 50 : 267-76.
- Ambroise-Thomas P. Diagnostic immunologique du paludisme en pratique individuelle et de masse. *Med Mal Infect* 1981 ; 6bis : 382-7.
- Ambroise-Thomas P, Quilici M, Ranque P. Réapparition du paludisme en Corse. *Bull Soc Pathol Exot* 1972 ; 65 : 533-42.
- Ambroise-Thomas P, Wernsdorfer WH, Grab B, Cullen J, Bertagna P. Étude séro-épidémiologique longitudinale sur le paludisme en Tunisie. *Bull Organ Mond Santé* 1976 ; 54 : 355-67.
- Ambroise-Thomas P, Pinel C, Pelloux H, Picot S. Le diagnostic du paludisme : actualités et perspectives. *Cahiers Santé* 1993 ; 3 : 280-4.
- Amdizadeh G. Recherche sur le paludisme en Iran. *Acta Med Scand* 1941 ; 107 : 579-683.
- Amerasinghe PH, Amerasinghe FP, Wirtz RA, *et al.* Malaria transmission by *Anopheles subpictus* in a new irrigation project in Sri Lanka. *J Med Entomol* 1992 ; 29 : 577-81.
- Amerasinghe PH, Amerasinghe FP, Konradsen F, Fonseca KT, Wirtz RA. Malaria vectors in a traditional dry zone village in Sri Lanka. *Am J Trop Med Hyg* 1999 ; 60 : 421-9.
- de Andrade AL, Martelli CM, Oliveira RM, Arias JR, Zicker F, Pang L. High prevalence of asymptomatic malaria in gold mining areas in Brazil. *Clin Infect Dis* 1995 ; 20 (2) : 475.
- Aniedu I. Dynamics of malaria transmission near two permanent breeding sites in Baringo District, Kenya. *Indian J Med Res* 1997 ; 105 : 206-11.
- Anker M, Black RE, Coldham C, *et al. A standard verbal autopsy method for investigating causes of death in infants and children.* Genève : OMS, 1999.
- Anonyme. *Intercountry Border Meeting in Malaria Control.* Djibouti, octobre 1990.
- Anonyme. Mekong malaria. *Southeast Asian J Trop Med Public Health* 1999a ; 30 (suppl. 4) : 101 p.
- Anonyme. *Comité interinstitutions sur El Niño. L'épisode El Niño 1997-1998 : rétrospective scientifique et technique.* Genève : OMM, UNESCO, PNUE, CIUS, 1999b.
- Anonyme. Prise en charge et prévention du paludisme d'importation à *Plasmodium falciparum*. 12ᵉ conférence de consensus en thérapeutique anti-infectieuse de la Société de Pathologie Infectieuse de Langue Française (SPILF). *Med Mal Infect* 1999c ; 29 (6) : 37-159.
- Anonyme. Conférence de consensus thérapeutique antipaludique, avril 1999. *Med Mal Infect* 1999d ; 29 : 373-9.
- Anonyme. *L'état du monde. Annuaire économique géopolitique mondial, 2000.* Paris : La Découverte & Syros, 2000 : 675 p.
- Antelme F. *Causerie sur la fièvre de Maurice. Extrait du Bulletin de la Société Médicale de l'Ile Maurice.* Port Louis : Nouvelle Imprimerie Dupuy, 1888 : 48 p.
- Antheaume B, Bonnemaison J. *Atlas des îles et États du Pacifique Sud.* Montpellier/Paris : GIP Reclus/Publisud, 1990 : 128 p.
- Anthony RL, Bangs MJ, Hamzah N, Basri H, Purnomo MY, Subianto B. Heightened transmission of stable malaria in an isolated population in the Highlands of Irian Jaya, Indonesia. *Am J Trop Med Hyg* 1992 ; 47 : 346-56.
- Anufrieva VN, Koshelev BA, Markin II. Confirmation of the role of *Anopheles hyrcanus* Pall. and *An. pulcherrimus* Theo. 1902 in the transmission of tertian malaria in the rice-growing areas of North-Eastern Afghanistan. *Medskaya Parazitol* 1977 ; 46 : 414-6.
- Anyanwu GI, Davies DH, Molyneux DH, Phillips A, Milligan PJ. Cuticular hydrocarbon discrimination/variation among strains of the mosquito *Anopheles stephensi*. *Ann Trop Med Parasitol* 1993 ; 87 : 269-75.
- Appawu MA, Baffoe-Wilmot A, Afari EA, Nkrumah FK, Petrarca V. Species composition and inversion polymorphism of *Anopheles gambiae* complex in some sites of Ghana, West Africa. *Acta Tropica* 1994 ; 56 : 15-23.
- Arbani P.R. Malaria control program in Indonesia. *Southeast Asian J Trop Med Public Health* 1992 ; 23 : 29-8.
- Argawal A, Guindo A, Cissoko Y, *et al.* Hemoglobin C associated with protection from severe malaria in the Dogon of Mali, a West African population with a low prevalence of hemoglobin S. *Blood* 2000 ; 96 : 2358-63.
- Ariey F. *Typage moléculaire d'isolats guyanais de Plasmodium falciparum.* Thèse Université Paris VII, 2 Septembre 1996.
- Armengaud A, Legros F, Quatresous I, *et al.* A case of autochthonous *Plasmodium vivax* malaria, Corsica, August 2006. *Eurosurveillance* 2006 ; 11 : 11.
- Armstrong-Schellenberg JR, Abdulla S, Nathan R, *et al.* Effect of large scale social marketing of insecticide-treated nets on child survival in rural Tanzania. *Lancet* 2001 ; 357 : 1241-7.
- Arnot D. Unstable malaria in Sudan: the influence of the dry season. Clone multiplicity of *Plasmodium falciparum* infections in individuals exposed to variable levels of disease transmission. *Trans R Soc Trop Med Hyg* 1998 ; 92 : 580-5.
- Arredondo-Jimenez JI, Rodriguez MH, Brown DN, Loyola EG. Indoor low-volume insecticide spray for the control of *Anopheles albimanus* in Southern Mexico. Village-scale trials of bendiocarb, deltamethrin and cyfluthrin. *J Am Mosq Control Assoc* 1993 ; 9 (2) : 210-20.
- Arredondo-Jimenez JI, Gimnig J, Rodriguez MH, Washino RK. Genetic differences among *Anopheles vestitipennis* subpopulations collected using different methods in Chiapas state, Southern Mexico. *J Am Mosq Control Assoc* 1996 ; 12 (3) : 396-401.
- de Arruda M, Carvalho MB, Nussenzweig RS, Maracic M, Feirreira AW, Cochrane AH. Potential vectors of malaria and their different susceptibility to *P. falciparum* and *P. vivax* in Northern Brazil identified by immunoassay. *Am J Trop Med Hyg* 1986 ; 35 (5) : 873-81.
- de Arruda M, Nardin EH, Nussenzweig RS, Cochrane AH. Sero-epidemiological studies of malaria in Indian tribes and monkeys of the Amazon basin of Brazil. *Am J Trop Med Hyg* 1989 ; 41 (4) : 379-85.
- Artemiev MM. Anopheles mosquito. Main malaria vectors in USSR. *Internat Sc Project Ecolo Safe Methods for Control of Malaria and its vectors.* Collected lectures, Moscow, 1980 ; 2 : 45-71.
- Asidi AN, N'Guessan R, Koffi AA, *et al.* Experimental hut evaluation of bednets treated with an organophosphate (chlorpyrifos-methyl) or a pyrethroid (lambdacyhalothrin) alone and in combination against insecticide-resistant *Anopheles gambiae* and *Culex quinquefasciatus* mosquitoes. *Malar J* 2005 ; 4(1) : 25.
- Asinas CY. Current status of malaria and control activities in the Philippines. *Southeast Asian J Trop Med Public Health* 1992 ; 23 (suppl. 4) : 55-9.
- Asindi AA, Ekanem EE, Ibia EO, Nwangwa MA. Upsurge of malaria-related convulsions in a paediatric emergency room in Nigeria. Consequence of emergence of chloroquine-resistant *P. falciparum*. *Trop Geogr Med* 1993 ; 45 : 110-3.
- Astaiza R, Murillo C, Fajardo P. Biology of *Anopheles (Kerteszia) neivai* H, D, K, 1913 (Diptera: Culicidae) in the Pacific coast of Colombia. II. Fluctuation of the adult population. *Rev Saude Publica* 1988 ; 22 (2) : 101-8.
- Audibert M, Josseran R, Josse R, Adjidji A. Irrigation, schistosomiasis and malaria in the Logone valley, Cameroon. *Am J Trop Med Hyg* 1990 ; 42 : 550-60.
- Auvergnat JC, Massip P, Armengaud M. Actualité du paludisme autochtone à *P. falciparum* : à propos d'une observation. *Rev Med Toulouse* 1979 ; 15 (suppl. 3) : 369.
- Avery JG. A review of the malaria eradication programme in the British Solomon Islands, 1970-72. *Papua New Guinea Med J* 1974 ; 17 : 50-60.
- Ayad H, Georghiou GP. Resistance to the organophosphates and carbamates in *Anopheles albimanus* based on reduced sensitivity of acetylcholinesterase. *J Econ Entomol* 1975 ; 68 (3) : 295-7.
- de Azevedo JF, Gandara AF, Fereira AP. II. Subsidios para o conhecimento da endemia malarica na provincia de Timor. *An Inst Med Trop (Lisb)* 1958a ; 15 : 35-52.
- de Azevedo JF, Gandara AF, Ferreira AP. III - Subsidios para o conhecimento dos mosquitos da tribo Anophelini na provincia de Timor. *An Inst Med Trop (Lisb)* 1958b ; 15 : 53-70.
- Azubuike JC, Izuora GI, Obi GO. Anaemia in non-sickling Nigerian children around Enugu. *Trop Geogr Med* 1977 ; 29 : 365-8.

- Babiker HA. Unstable malaria in Sudan: the influence of the dry season. *P. falciparum* population in the unstable malaria area of Eastern Sudan is stable and genetically complex. *Trans R Soc Trop Med Hyg* 1998 ; 92 : 585-9.
- Babiker HA, Charlwood JD, Smith T, Walliker D. Gene flow and cross-mating in *P. falciparum* in households in a Tanzanian village. *Parasitology* 1995 ; 111 : 433-42.
- Babiker HA, Lines J, Hill WG, Walliker D. Population structure of *P. falciparum* in villages with different malaria endemicity in East Africa. *Am J Trop Med Hyg* 1997 ; 56 : 141-7.
- Babiker HA, Abdel-Mushin AM, Ranford-Cartwrigh LC, Satti G, Walliker D. Characteristics of *Plasmodium falciparum* parasites that survive the lengthy dry season in Eastern Sudan where malaria transmission is markedly seasonal. *Am J Trop Med Hyg* 1998 ; 59 (4) : 582-90.
- Babiker HA, Ranford-Cartwright LC, Walliker D. The epidemiology of multiple *P. falciparum* infections. 3. Genetic structure and dynamics of *P. falciparum* infections in the Kilombero region of Tanzania. *Trans R Soc Trop Med Hyg* 1999 ; 93 : 11-4.
- Babiker HA, Abdel-Mushin AA, Hamad A, Mackinnon MJ, Hill WG, Walliker D. Population dynamics of *P. falciparum* in an unstable area of Eastern Sudan. *Parasitology* 2000 ; 120 : 105-11.
- Bafort JM. *An. marshalli*, a secondary vector of malaria in Africa. *Trans R Soc Trop Med Hyg* 1985 ; 79 : 566-7.
- Baimai V. Population genetics of the malaria vector *Anopheles leucosphyrus* group. *Southeast Asian J Trop Med Public Health* 1988 ; 19 : 667-80.
- Baimai V, Harbach RE, Sukowati S. Cytogenetic evidence for two species within the current concept of the malaria vector *Anopheles leucosphyrus* in Southeast Asia. *J Am Mosq Control Assoc* 1988a ; 4 : 44-50.
- Baimai V, Kijchalao U, Sawadwongporn P, Green C. Geographic distribution and biting behaviour of four species of *An. dirus* complex in Thailand. *Southeast Asian J Trop Med Public Health* 1988b ; 19 : 151-61.
- Baird JK, Basri H, Purnomo MY, *et al.* Resistance to chloroquine by *Plasmodium vivax* in Irian Jaya, Indonesia. *Am J Trop Med Hyg* 1991 ; 44 : 547-52.
- Baird JK, Purnomo MY, Basri H, *et al.* Age-specific prevalence of *P. falciparum* among six populations with limited histories of exposure to endemic malaria. *Am J Trop Med Hyg* 1993 ; 49 : 707-19.
- Baker EL Jr. Warren M, Zack M, *et al.* Epidemic malathion poisoning in Pakistan malaria workers. *Lancet* 1978 ; 8054 : 31-4.
- Bakri G, Noguer A. *Impact of a single DDT spraying application on malaria vector densities and Entomological Inoculation Rate in Togo.* WHO/MAL/77.891, 1977.
- Baldari M, Tamburro A, Sabatinelli G, *et al.* Malaria in Maremma, Italy. *Lancet* 1998 ; 351 : 1246-7.
- Baldet MC, Camara M, Barry AO, *et al.* Étude de la prévalence du paludisme dans 24 villages de Guinée. *Bull Soc Pathol Exot* 2001 ; 94 : 192-4.
- Barat. Étude sur la fièvre épidémique qui a régné en 1869 à l'île de La Réunion. *Arch Med Nav*, 1869 ; 12 : 422-40.
- Barber MA, Olinger. Studies on malaria in Southern Nigeria. *Ann Trop Med Parasitol* 1931 ; 25 : 461-502 .
- Barber MA, Rice JB. Malaria studies in Greece. *Ann Trop Med Parasitol* 1935 ; 29 : 329-48.
- Barber MA, Rice JB. A survey of malaria in Egypt. *Am J Trop Med Hyg* 1937 ; 17 : 413-36.
- Barbie Y, Timbala R. Notes sur le paludisme en République Islamique de Mauritanie. *Med Trop (Marseille)* 1964 ; 24 : 427-36.
- Barnard DR. *Global collaboration for development of pesticides for Public Health: repellent and toxicant for personal protection.* WHO/CDS/WHOPES/GCDPP/200.5 : 49 p.
- Barnish G, Maude GH, Bockarie MJ, Eggelte TA, Greenwood BM. The epidemiology of malaria in Southern Sierra Leone. *Parasitologia* 1993 ; 35 (suppl. 4) : 1-4.
- Barr AR, Guptavanij P. *An. hermsi* n. sp, an unrecognised American species of the *Anopheles maculipennis* group. *Mosq Syst* 1988 ; 20 : 352-6.
- Barrera R, Grillet ME, Rangel Y, Berti J, Ache A. Temporal and spatial patterns of malaria reinfection in Northeastern Venezuela. *Am J Trop Med Hyg* 1999 ; 61 (5) : 784-90.
- Basco LK, Ruggeri C, Le Bras J. *Molécules antipaludiques, mécanismes d'action, mécanismes de résistance et relations structure-activité des schizontocides sanguins.* Paris : Masson, 1994 : 364 p.
- Bashford G, Richens J. Travel to the coast by highlanders and its implication for malaria control. *Papua New Guinea Med J* 1992 ; 35 : 306-7.
- Bassett MT, Taylor P, Bvirakare J, Chiteka F, Govere E. Clinical diagnosis of malaria: can we improve? *J Trop Med Hyg* 1991 ; 94 : 65-9.
- Bassignot T. *Rapport à l'administration sur la fièvre endémo-épidémique qui règne à La Réunion.* Saint-Denis : Lahuppe imprimeur, 1872 : 62 p.
- Bassiouny HK. Bioenvironmental and meteorological factors related to the persistence of malaria in Fayoum Governorate: a retrospective study. *East Mediterr Health* 2001 ; 7 : 895-906.
- Batra CP, Reuben R, Das PK. Studies on day-time resting places of *Anopheles stephensi* in Salem (Tamil Nadu). *Indian J Med Res* 1979a ; 69 : 583-8.
- Batra CP, Reuben R, Das PK. Urban malaria vectors in Salem, Tamil Nadu: biting rates on men and cattle. *Indian J Med Res* 1979b ; 70 (suppl.) : 103-13.
- Batra CP, Reuben R. Breeding of *Anopheles stephensi* in wells and cisterns in Salem, Tamil Nadu. *Indian J Med Res* 1979c ; 70 (suppl.) : 114-22.
- Baudon D, Gazin P, Rea D, *et al.* Épidémiologie clinique : morbidité palustre, mortalité palustre. *Études Médicales* 1984 ; 3 : 135-44.
- Baudon D, Gazin P, Rea D, Carnevale P. A study of malaria morbidity in a rural area of Burkina Faso. *Trans R Soc Trop Med Hyg* 1985 ; 79 : 283-4.
- Baudon D, Carnevale P, Robert V, Peyron F, Sibi Sona L, Gniminou L. Étude épidémiologique du paludisme dans la région de Tillabéri (Nord-Ouest du Niger). *Med Afr Noire* 1986a ; 33 : 281-90.
- Baudon D, Gazin P, Sanou JM, *et al.* Morbidité en milieu rural au Burkina Faso. Étude de 526 accès fébriles. *Med Afr Noire* 1986b ; 33 : 767-76.
- Baudon D, Robert V, Darriet F, Huerre M. Impact de la construction d'un barrage avec retenue d'eau sur la transmission du paludisme. *Bull Soc Pathol Exot* 1986c ; 79 : 123-9.
- Baudon D, Galaup B, Ouedraogo L, Gazin P. Une étude de la morbidité palustre en milieu hospitalier au Burkina Faso, Afrique de l'Ouest. *Med Trop (Marseille)* 1988 ; 48 : 9-13.
- Beach RF, Ruebush TK, Sexton JD, *et al.* Effectiveness of permethrin-impregnated bed nets and curtains for malaria control in a holoendemic area of Western Kenya. *Am J Trop Med Hyg* 1993 ; 49 (3) : 290-300.
- Beale GH, Walliker D. Genetics and biological characterisation of malaria parasite. In : Wernsdorfer WH, McGregor I, eds. *Malaria principles and practice of malariology.* London : Churchill Livingstone, 1988 : 379-409.
- Beales PF. *A review of the taxonomic status of Anopheles sinensis and its bionomics in relation to malaria transmission.* WHO/MAL/84.1007, 1984 : 35 p.
- Beauperthuy LD. Transmission of yellow fever and other diseases by mosquitoes. Gaceta Official de Cumana ; Venezuela ; 1854, ano 4, n° 57. Reproduced by Boyce R. *Mosquito or man.* London : Murray, 1909 : 100-9.
- Beck LR, Rodriguez MH, Dister SW, *et al.* Remote sensing as a landscape epidemiologic tool to identify villages at high risk for malaria transmission. *Am J Trop Med Hyg* 1994 ; 51 (3) : 271-80.
- Beck LR, Rodriguez MH, Dister SW, *et al.* Assessment of a remote sensing-based model for predicting malaria transmission risk in villages of Chiapas, Mexico. *Am J Trop Med Hyg* 1997 ; 56 (1) : 99-106.
- Beebe NW, Foley DH, Cooper RD, Bryan JH, Saul A. DNA probes for the *Anopheles punctulatus* complex. *Am J Trop Med Hyg* 1996 ; 54 : 395-8.
- Beklemishev VN. *The ecology of the malaria mosquito.* Moscow : Medzig, 1944.
- Belios GD. *L'histoire du paludisme en Grèce depuis l'Antiquité jusqu'à la découverte de Laveran.* Paris : Jouvès, 1933.
- Beljaev AE. Determinants of malaria in the Middle East and North Africa. In : Casman E, Dowlatabadi H, eds. *The contextual determinants of malaria.* Washington : Resources for the Future Press, 2002 : 137-66.
- Benasseni R, Gazin P, Carnevale P, Baudon D. Le paludisme urbain à Bobo-Dioulasso, Burkina Faso. 3. Étude de la morbidité palustre. *Cahiers ORSTOM, Entomol Med Parasitol* 1987 ; 25 : 165-70.
- Ben-Dov Y. Note on the occurrence of *Anopheles sacharovi*. *Isr J Entomol* 1971 ; 6 : 313.
- Ben Mansour N. Le paludisme au Maroc en 1972. *Bull Inst Nat Hyg Rabat* 1972 ; 52 : 21-43.
- Bentata-Pessayre M, Schnurmann D, Krivitsky A, Callard P, Delzant G. Paludisme autochtone et foie palustre. *Bull Soc Pathol Exot* 1978 ; 71 : 417-23.
- Benzerroug EH, Janssens PG. La surveillance du paludisme au Sahara algérien. *Bull Soc Pathol Exot* 1985a ; 78 : 859-67.
- Benzerroug EH, Wery M. Séro-épidémiologie du paludisme au niveau d'un foyer résiduel en Algérie : commune de Khemis El Kechua. *Rev Épidémiol Santé Publique* 1985b ; 33 : 276-82.
- Benzerroug EH, Janssens PG, Ambroise-Thomas P. Étude séro-épidémiologique du paludisme au Sahara algérien. *Bull Organ Mond Santé* 1991 ; 69 : 713-23.

- Berger J, Dick JL, Galan P, *et al*. Effect of daily iron supplementation on iron status, cell-mediated immunity and incidence of infections in 6-36 months old Togolese children. *Eur J Clin Nutr* 2000 ; 54 : 29-35.
- Bernard P. Trois ans de lutte antipaludique à Madagascar. *Bull Madg* 1954 ; 96 : 387-458.
- Berti J, Vanegas C, Amarista J, *et al*. Preliminary inventory and biological observations of the anopheline mosquitoes (Diptera: Culicidae) of a mining region of Bolivar State, Venezuela. *Bol Entomol Venezolana* 1998 ; 13 (1) : 17-26.
- Besnard P, Foumane V, Foucher JF, *et al*. Impact of a new parasitologic laboratory for malaria diagnosis on diagnosis and cost of malaria in a company setting: experience from Angola. *Med Trop* 2006 ; 66 : 269-72
- Bespiatov VF, Khromov AS, Chistiakov DA, Zhil'tsov IP. The current malariological situation in the countries of Western Africa. 1. Republic of Guinea. *Med Parazitol (Mosk)* 1992 ; 5-6 : 32-4.
- Bettini S, Gradoni L, Cocchi M, Tamburro A. *Rice culture and Anopheles labranchiae in Central Italy*. WHO/MAL/78.897, 1978 : 6 p.
- Bhat HR. A survey of haematophagous arthropods in Western Himalayas, Sikkim and Hill districts of West Bengal. *Indian J Med Res* 1975 ; 63 : 232-41.
- Bhat HR. A note on *Anopheles dirus* Peyton and Harrison 1979 in India. *Indian J Malariol* 1988 ; 25 : 103-5.
- Biemba G, Dolmans D, Thuma PE, Weiss G, Gordeuk VR. Severe anaemia in Zambian children with *Plasmodium falciparum* malaria. *Trop Med Int Health* 2000 ; 5 : 9-16.
- Biggar RJ, Collins WE, Campbell CC. The serological response to primary malaria infection in urban Ghanaian infants. *Am J Trop Med Hyg* 1980 ; 29 : 720-4.
- Bilbie I, Critescu A, Enescu A, Tacu V, Giurca I, Cristodorescu-Nicolescu G. Up-to-date entomological aspects in the previously endemic areas of malaria in the Danube plain and Dobrudja. *Arch Roum Pathol Exp Microbiol* 1978 ; 37 : 389-97.
- Binka FN, Kubaje A, Adjuik M, *et al*. Impact of permethrin impregnated bednets on child mortality in Kasseina-Nankana district, Ghana. *Trop Med Int Health* 1996 ; 1 : 147-54.
- Binka FN, Indome F, Smith T. Impact of spatial distribution of permethrin impregnated bednets on child mortality in rural Northern Ghana. *Am J Trop Med Hyg* 1998 ; 59 : 80-5.
- Binka FN, Hodgson A, Adjuik M, Smith T. Mortality in a seven-and-a-half-year follow-up of a trial of insecticide-treated mosquito nets in Ghana. *Trans R Soc Trop Med Hyg* 2002 ; 96 : 597-9.
- Bjorkman A, Hedman P, Brohult J, *et al*. Different malaria control activities in an area of Liberia: effect on malariometric parameters. *Ann Trop Med Parasitol* 1985 ; 79 : 239-46.
- Black RH. *Malaria control and research in Netherlands New Guinea CPS - Noumea TP 80*. Noumea : Rap. Commission Pacifique Sud, mars 1958.
- Blanchy S, Benthein F, Sabatinelli G. Épidémiologie du paludisme en République Fédérale Islamique des Comores. *Cahiers ORSTOM, Entomol Med Parasitol* 1987 ; n° spéc. : 45-52.
- Blanchy S, Benthein F, Houmadi A. Morbidité palustre en Grande Comore. *Med Trop (Marseille)* 1990 ; 50 : 209-14.
- Blanchy S, Rakotonjanabelo A, Ranaivoson G, Rajaonarivelo E. Épidémiologie du paludisme sur les hautes terres Malgaches depuis 1878. *Cahiers Santé* 1993 ; 3 : 155-61.
- Blanchy S, Julvez J, Mouchet J. Stratification épidémiologique du paludisme dans l'archipel des Comores. *Bull Soc Pathol Exot* 1999 ; 92 : 177-85.
- Blazquez J, de Zulueta J. The disappearance of *Anopheles labranchiae* from Spain. *Parassitologia* 1980 ; 22 : 161-3.
- Bloland PB, Boriga DA, Ruebush TH, *et al*. Longitudinal cohort study of the epidemiology of malaria infections in an area of intense malaria transmission. II. Descriptive epidemiology of malaria infection and disease among children. *Am J Trop Med Hyg* 1999 ; 60 : 641-8.
- Bockarie MJ, Service MW, Toure YT, Traore S, Barnish G, Greenwood BM. The ecology and behaviour of the forest form of *Anopheles gambiae s.s. Parassitologia* 1993 ; 35 : 5-8.
- Bockarie MJ, Service MW, Barnish G, Maude GH, Greenwood BM. Malaria in a rural area of Sierra Leone. III. Vector ecology and disease transmission. *Ann Trop Med Parasitol* 1994 ; 88 : 251-62 .
- Bockarie MJ, Service MW, Barnish G, Toure YT. Vectorial capacity and entomological inoculation rates of *An. gambiae* in a high rainfall forested area of Southern Sierra Leone. *Trop Med Parasitol* 1995 ; 46 : 164-71.
- Bockarie MJ, Alexander N, Bockarie F, Ibam E, Barnish G, Alpers M. The late biting habit of parous Anopheles mosquitoes and pre-bedtime exposure of humans to infective female mosquitoes. *Trans R Soc Trop Med Hyg* 1996 ; 90 : 23-5.
- Bockarie MJ, Gbakima AA, Barnish G. It all began with Ronald Ross: 100 years of malaria research and control in Sierra Leone (1899-1999). *Ann Trop Med Parasitol* 1999 ; 93 : 213-24.
- Boisier P, Spiegel A. Relation parasitémie-fièvre selon la transmission. *Arch Inst Pasteur Madagascar* 1999 ; 65 : 22-3.
- Bojang KA, Milligan PJ, Pinder M, *et al*. Efficacy of RTS, S/AS02 malaria vaccine against *Plasmodium falciparum* infection in semi-immune adult men in The Gambia: a randomised trial. *Lancet* 2001 ; 358 (9297) : 1927-34.
- Bolton JM. The control of malaria among the Orang Asli in West Malaysia. *Med J Malaysia* 1972 ; 27 : 10-9.
- Bone-Wepster J, Swellengrebel NH. *The anopheline mosquitoes of the Indo-Australian Region*. Amsterdam : De Bussy, 1953 : 504 p.
- Booman M, Durrheim DN, La Grange K, *et al*. Using a geographical information system to plan a malaria control programme in South Africa. *Bull WHO* 2000 ; 78 : 1438-44.
- Boreham PF. Some application of bloodmeal identifications in relation to the epidemiology of vector-borne tropical diseases. *J Trop Med Hyg* 1975 ; 78 : 83-91.
- Borel M. Paludisme en Cochinchine. *Bull Soc Pathol Exot* 1926 ; 19 : 811-5.
- Bosch I, Bracho C, Perez HA. Diagnosis of malaria by acridine orange fluorescent microscopy in an endemic area of Venezuela. *Mem Inst Oswaldo Cruz* 1996 ; 91 (1) : 83-6.
- Bosman A, Modiano D, Voglino MC, *et al*. Malaria transmission in a central area of Futa Djalon (Guinea). *Parassitologia* 1992 ; 34 : 135-42.
- Bottius E, Guanzirolli A, Trape JF, Rogier C, Konate L, Druilhe P. Malaria: even more chronic in nature than previously thought: evidence for sub-patent parasitaemia detectable by PCR. *Trans R Soc Trop Med Hyg* 1996 ; 90 : 15-9.
- Bouchet. *Observations sur les fièvres endémiques de l'Isle de Madagascar*. Curepipe, Mauritius : Carnegy Librairy, manuscrit, 10 août 1770.
- Bouchité B, Kennou MF, Chauvet G. *Éthologie et capacité vectorielle des anophèles de Tunisie*. Rapport Institut Pasteur Tunis, 1991 : 28 p.
- Boudin C, Robert V, Verhave JP, Carnevale P, Ambroise-Thomas P. *Plasmodium falciparum* and *P. malariae* epidemiology in a West African village. *Bull World Health Organ* 1991 ; 69 : 199-205.
- Boudin C, Herrman C, Gouagna C, Mulder B, Bonone R, Tchuinkam T. L'infectivité des porteurs de gamétocytes de *P. falciparum* pour les moustiques vecteurs, un nouveau paramètre épidémiologique. *Bull Liaison OCEAC* 1997 ; 30 (2).
- Bouffard. Géographie médicale : Djibouti. *Ann Hyg Med Col* 1905 ; 8 : 333-75.
- Boulard JC, Chippaux JP, Ayivi B, Akogbeto M, Massougbodji A, Baudon D. Une étude sur la morbidité palustre dans un service hospitalier de pédiatrie au Bénin en 1988 et 1989. *Med Trop (Marseille)* 1990 ; 50 : 315-20.
- Bouma MJ. *Epidemiology and control of malaria in Northern Pakistan*. Leyde : Thèse Université, 1995 : 175 p.
- Bouma MJ, Van der Kaay HJ. Epidemic malaria in India and the El Niño Southern Oscillation. *Lancet* 1994 ; 334 : 1638-9.
- Bouma MJ, Sondorp HE, Van der Kaay HJ. Health and climate changes. *Lancet* 1994 ; 343 : 302.
- Bouma MJ, Van der Kaay HJ. The El Niño Southern Oscillation and the historic malaria epidemics on the Indian subcontinent and Sri Lanka: an early warning system for future epidemics. *Trop Med Int Health* 1996 ; 1 : 86-96.
- Bouma MJ, Dye C, Van der Kaay HJ. *Falciparum* malaria and climate change in the North-West frontier province of Pakistan. *Am J Trop Med Hyg* 1996a ; 55 : 131-7.
- Bouma MJ, Parvez SD, Nesbit R, Winkler AM. Malaria control using permethrin applied to tents of nomadic Afgan refugees in Northern Pakistan. *Bull World Health Organ* 1996b ; 74 (4) : 413-21.
- Bouma MJ, Dye C. Cycles of malaria associated with El Niño in Venezuela. *JAMA* 1997 ; 278 (21) : 1772-4.
- Bouvier M, Pittet D, Starobinski M, Loutan L. Paludisme des aéroports à Genève : une mini-épidémie. *Bull Off Fédéral Santé Publ* 1990 ; 24 : 358-9.
- Bovay GM. *Malaria : l'épopée du paludisme*. Paris : Denoël, 1972 : 314 p.
- Boyd MF. *Malariology*. Philadelphia : WB Saunders, 1949 : 1643 p.
- Brabin L, Brabin BJ, Van der Kaay HJ. High and low spleen rates distinguish two populations of women living under the same malaria endemic conditions in Madang, Papua New Guinea. *Trans R Soc Trop Med Hyg* 1988a ; 82 : 671-6.
- Brabin BJ, Brabin LR, Sapau J, Alpers MP. A longitudinal study of splenomegaly in pregnancy in a malaria endemic area in Papua New Guinea. *Trans R Soc Trop Med Hyg* 1988b ; 82 : 677-81.

- Branquinho MS, Araujo MS, Natal D, *et al*. *Anopheles oswaldoi*, a potential malaria vector in Acre, Brazil. *Trans R Soc Trop Med Hyg* 1996 ; 90 : 233.
- Branquinho MS, Marrelli MT, Curado T, *et al*. Infeccao do *Anopheles (Kerteszia) cruzii* por *P. vivax* e *P. vivax* variante VK 247 nos Municipios de Sao Vicente e Juquitiba, Sao Paulo. *Rev Panam Salud Publica* 1997 ; 2 (3) : 189-93.
- Bransby-Williams WR. House catches of adult *An. gambiae* sp. B in two areas of Zambia. *East Afr Med J* 1979 ; 56 : 557-61.
- Brasseur P, Guigemde R, Diallo S, *et al*. Amodiaquine remains effective for treating uncomplicated malaria in West and Central Africa. *Trans R Soc Trop Med Hyg* 1999 ; 93 : 645-50.
- Breman JG, Campbell CC. Combating severe malaria in African children. *Bull World Health Organ* 1988 ; 66 : 611-20.
- Brewster DR, Kwiatowski D, White N. Neurological sequelae of cerebral malaria in children. *Lancet* 1990 ; 336 : 1039-43.
- Brinkmann U, Brinkmann A. Malaria and health in Africa: the present situation and epidemiological trends. *Trop Med Parasitol* 1991 ; 42 : 204-13.
- Brogdon WG, McAllister JC, Corwin AM, Cordon-Rosales C. Oxidase-based DDT-pyrethroid cross-resistance in Guatemalan *Anopheles albimanus*. *Pest Biochem Physiol* 1999 ; 64 (2) : 101-11.
- Brooke BD, Kloke G, Hunt RH, *et al*. Bioassay and biochemical analyses of insecticide resistance in southern African *Anopheles funestus* (Diptera: Culicidae). *Bull Entomol Res* 2001 ; 91(4) : 265-72.
- Brooker S, Guyatt H, Omumbo J, Shretta R, Drake L, Ouma J. Situation analysis of malaria in school children in Kenya: what can be done? *Parasitol Today* 2000 ; 16 : 183-6.
- Brousses A. Contribution à l'étude du paludisme en région saharienne. Observations recueillies à Djanet au cours de l'épidémie de 1928-1929. *Arch Inst Pasteur Algérie* 1930 ; 8 : 77-85.
- Brown AW, Pal R. *Insecticide resistance in arthropods*. Geneva : World Health Organization, 1971 : Monographie 38.
- Brown KG, Abrahams C, Meyers AM. The nephrotic syndrome in Malawian Blacks. *S Afr Med J* 1977 ; 52 : 275-8.
- Brown V, Issak MA, Rossi M, Barboza P, Paugam A. Epidemic of malaria in North Eastern Kenya. *Lancet* 1998 ; 352 : 1356-7.
- Browne EN, Frimpong E, Sievertsen J, *et al*. Malariometric update for the rain forest and savannah of Ashanti Region in Ghana. *Ann Trop Med Parasitol* 2000 ; 94 : 15-22.
- Bruce-Chwatt LJ. Malaria in Nigeria. *Bull World Health Organ* 1951 ; 4 : 301-27.
- Bruce-Chwatt LJ. Malaria in African infants and children in Southern Nigeria. *Ann Trop Med Parasitol* 1952 ; 46 : 173-200.
- Bruce-Chwatt LJ. A longitudinal survey of natural malaria infection in a groupe of West African adults. *West Afr J Med* 1963 ; August : 141-213.
- Bruce-Chwatt LJ. Paleogenesis and paleo-epidemiology of primate malaria. *Bull World Health Organ* 1965 ; 32 : 363-87.
- Bruce-Chwatt LJ. Resurgence of malaria and its control. *J Trop Med Hyg* 1974 ; 77 : 62-6.
- Bruce-Chwatt LJ. Malaria threat to the Seychelles. *Br Med J* 1976 ; Sept : 754-5.
- Bruce-Chwatt LJ. *Essential malariology*. London : William Heinemann Med Books Ltd, 1980 : 354 p.
- Bruce-Chwatt LJ. History of malaria from prehistory to eradication. In : Wernsdorfer WH, McGregor I, eds. *Malaria*, vol. 1 . Edinburgh : Churchill Livingstone, 1988 : 1-59.
- Bruce-Chwatt LJ, *et al*. *An experimental malaria schema, in a semi-rural holoendemic area of Southern Nigeria*. Inf. Bull n°3, Dept. Med. Service, Nigeria 1955, 30 p.
- Bruce-Chwatt LJ, Archibald HM. *Malaria pilot project in Western Sokoto, Northern Nigeria*. Lisbon : Proceedings 6th International Congress for Tropical Medicine and Malaria, 1958 ; 7 : 347-61.
- Bruce-Chwatt LJ, Draper CC, Konfortion P. Seroepidemiological evidence of eradication of malaria from Mauritius. *Lancet* 1973 ; 2 : 547-51.
- Bruce-Chwatt LJ, Draper CC, Avramidis D, Kazandzoglou O. Seroepidemiological surveillance of disappearing malaria in Greece. *J Trop Med Hyg* 1975 ; 78 : 194-200.
- Bruce-Chwatt LJ, de Zulueta J. *The rise and fall of malaria in Europe*. London : Oxford University Press, 1980 : 240 p.
- Brumpt E. *Précis de parasitologie*. Paris : Masson, 1949 : 2138 p.
- Brumpt E, Dao Van TY. Distribution des biotypes d'*An. maculipennis* en France. *Ann Parasitol Hum Comp* 1942 ; 19 : 69-74.
- Brunhes J. Les moustiques de l'archipel des Comores. I. Inventaire, répartition et description de quatre espèces ou sous-espèces nouvelles. *Cahiers ORSTOM, Entomol Med Parasitol* 1977 ; 15 : 131-52.
- Brunhes J, Le Goff G, Geoffroy B. Afrotropical anopheline mosquitoes. III. Description of three new species: *An. carnevalei* sp. nov, *An. hervyi* sp. nov. and *An. dualaensis* sp. nov. and resurrection of *An. rageaui*. *J Am Mosq Control Assoc* 1999 ; 15 : 552-8.
- Bryan JH. Studies on the *Anopheles punctulatus* complex. Identification by proboscis morphological criteria and by cross-mating experiments. *Trans R Soc Trop Med Hyg* 1973 ; 67 : 64-9.
- Bryan JH. *Anopheles gambiae* and *An. melas* at Brefet, the Gambia, in their role in malaria transmission. *Ann Trop Med Parasitol* 1983 ; 77 : 1-12.
- Bryan JH, Petrarca V, Di Deco MA, Coluzzi M. Adult behaviour of members of the *An. gambiae* complex in the Gambia with special reference to *An. melas* and its chromosomal variants. *Parassitologia* 1987 ; 29 : 221-49.
- Bryan JH, Foley DH, Reardon T, Spark R. How many species are in the *Anopheles punctulata* group? *Ann Trop Med Parasitol* 1990 ; 84 (3) : 295-7.
- Bryskier A, Labro MT. *Paludisme et médicaments*. Paris : Arnette, 1988 : 276 p.
- Buck AA, Anderson RI, Macrae AA. Epidemiology of poly-parasitism. 1. Occurrence, frequency and distribution of multiple infections in rural communities in Chad, Peru, Afghanistan and Zaire. *Tropenmed Parasitol* 1978 ; 29 : 61-70.
- Bullini L, Coluzzi M, Cancrini G, Santolamazza C. Multiple phosphoglucomutase alleles in *Anopheles stephensi*. *Heredity* 1971 ; 26 : 475-9.
- de Burca B, Shah JI. The anophelines mosquitoes of Eritrea and their relation to malaria transmission. *J Malaria Inst India* 1943 ; 5 : 235-45.
- Burgess RW. Comparative susceptibility of *An. gambiae* and *An. melas* to infection by *Plasmodium falciparum* in Liberia, West Africa. *Am J Trop Med Hyg* 1960 ; 9 : 652-5.
- Burgos JJ, Curto de Casas SI, Carcavallo RU, Galindez Giron I. Global climate change influence in the distribution of some pathogenic complexes (malaria and chagas' disease) in Argentina. *Entomol Vect* 1994 ; 1 : 69-78.
- Burkot TR, Dye C, Graves PM. An analysis of some factors determining the sporozoite rates, human blood indexes and biting rates of members of the *Anopheles punctulatus* complex in Papua New Guinea. *Am J Trop Med Hyg* 1989 ; 40 : 229-34.
- Butler D. What difference does a genome make? *Nature* 2002 ; 419 (6906) : 426-8.
- Butzer KW. *Environment and archaeology*, 2nd ed. London : Methuen, 1972.
- Butzer KW, Isaac G, Richardson JL, Washbourn-Kaman C. Radiocarbon dating of East African lake levels. *Science* 1972 ; 175 : 1069-76.
- Buxton PA. Rough notes: Anopheles mosquitoes and malaria in Arabia. *Trans R Soc Trop Med Hyg* 1944 ; 38 : 205-14.
- Bynum WF. An experiment that failed: malaria control at Mian Mir. *Parassitologia* 1994 ; 36 : 107-20.

- Cabrera BD, Ramos OL, Cruz IT. Malaria transmission by *Anopheles litoralis*, a salt-water breeder, in Pangutaran, Sulu, Republic of the Philippines. *Southeast Asian J Trop Med Public Health* 1970 ; 1 : 193-204.
- Cabrera BD, Arambulo PV. Malaria in the Republic of the Philippines. *Acta Tropica* 1977 ; 34 : 265-79.
- Callot J, Rochedieu-Assenmacher V. Le paludisme en Alsace. *Rev Pathol Gen Comp* 1953 ; 53 : 1153-85.
- Camargo LM, Ferreira MU, Krieger H, de Camargo EP, da Silva LP. Unstable hypoendemic malaria in Rondonia (Western Amazon Region, Brazil): epidemic outbreaks and work-associated incidence in an agro-industrial rural settlement. *Am J Trop Med Hyg* 1994 ; 51 : 16-25.
- Camargo LM, dal Colletto GM, Ferreira MU, *et al*. Hypoendemic malaria in Rondonia (Brazil Western Amazon Region): seasonal variation and risk groups in an urban locality. *Am J Trop Med Hyg* 1996 ; 55 : 32-8.
- Camargo LM, Noronha E, Villalobos, *et al*. The epidemiology of malaria in Rondonia (Western Amazon Region, Brazil): study of a riverine population. *Acta Tropica* 1999a ; 72 : 1-11.
- Camargo EP, Alves F. Pereira da Silva LH. Symptomless *Plasmodium vivax* infections in native Amazonians. *Lancet* 1999b ; 353 (9162) : 1415-6.
- Cambournac FJ. *Sôbre a epidemiologia do sezonismo em Portugal*. Lisboa : Soc Indust Tipografia, 1942 : 235 p.
- Cambournac FJ. Sur l'introduction et la transmission du *P. vivax* dans une zone de l'Afrique Occidentale. *Rev Portug Doencas Inf* 1981 ; 4 : 5-8.
- Cambournac FJ, Gandara AF, Pena AJ, Teixera WL. Subsidios para o inquerito malariologico em Angola. *An Inst Med Trop (Lisb)* 1955 ; 12 : 121-52.
- Cambournac FJ, Petrarca V, Coluzzi M. *Anopheles arabiensis* in the Cape Verde Archipelago. *Parassitologia* 1982 ; 24 : 265-7.

- Cambournac FJ, Santa Rita Vieira H, Coutinho MA, Soraes FA, Brito Soares A, Janz GJ. Note sur l'éradication du paludisme de l'île de Santiago (République du Cap Vert). *An Inst Hig Med Trop (Lisb)* 1984 ; 10 : 23-34.
- Cancrini G, Bartoloni A, Guglielmetti P, Roselli M, Pereira L. Malaria parasitological indices in the Cordillera Province, Santa Cruz Department, Bolivia. *Ann Trop Med Parasitol* 1992 ; 86 (3) : 217-23.
- Capellan SC, Delpech M. *Biologie moléculaire et médecine*. Paris : Flammarion, 1993 : 235 p.
- Caraballo A, Rodriguez-Acosta A. Chemotherapy of malaria and resistance to antimalarial drugs in Guyana area Venezuela. *Am J Trop Med Hyg* 1999 ; 61 (1) : 120-4.
- Cardoso MA, Ferreira MU, Camargo LM, Szarfarc SC. Anemia em populaçao de area endemica de malaria, Rondonia, Brasil. *Rev Saude Pub* 1992 ; 26 (3) : 161-6 .
- Carlson DG. *African fever. A study of British science, technology, and politics in West Africa, 1787-1864*. Canton, MA: Science History Publications, 1984 : 101 p.
- Carme B, Guillo du Bodan H, Molez JF, Trape JF. Étude rétrospective sur la mortalité de l'enfant de moins de 5 ans dans une zone rurale de la région de Brazzaville (RP Congo). *Bull Soc Pathol Exot* 1984 ; 77 : 104-14.
- Carme B, Venturin C. Le paludisme dans les Amériques. *Med Trop (Marseille)* 1999 ; 59 : 298-302.
- Carnevale P. Variations saisonnières d'une population d'*Anopheles nili* en République Populaire du Congo. *Cahiers ORSTOM, Entomol Med Parasitol* 1974 ; 12 : 165-74.
- Carnevale P. *Le paludisme dans un village des environs de Brazzaville*. Université Paris Sud : Thèse Doctorat Sciences, 1979 : n° 2175.
- Carnevale P, Le Pont F. Épidémiologie du paludisme humain en république populaire du Congo. II Utilisation des pièges lumineux "CDC" comme moyen d'échantillonnage des populations anophéliennes. *Cahiers ORSTOM, Entomol Med Parasitol* 1973 ; 11 : 263-70.
- Carnevale P, Frezil JL, Bosseno MF, Le Pont F, Lancien J. Étude de l'agressivité d'*An. gambiae* A en fonction de l'âge et du sexe des sujets humains. *Bull Organ Mond Santé* 1978 ; 56 : 147-54.
- Carnevale P, Mouchet J. Le paludisme en zone de transmission continue en Région afrotropicale. *Cahiers ORSTOM, Entomol Med Parasitol* 1980 ; 18 : 162-71.
- Carnevale P, Robert V, Molez JF, Baudon D. Épidémiologie générale : faciès épidémiologiques des paludismes en Afrique Subsaharienne. *Études Méd* 1984 ; 3 : 123-33.
- Carnevale P, Bosseno MF, Zoulani A, Michel R, Molez JF. La dynamique de la transmission du paludisme humain en zone de savane herbeuse et de forêt dégradée des environs nord et sud de Brazzaville (République Populaire du Congo). *Cahiers ORSTOM, Entomol Med Parasitol* 1985 ; 23 : 95-115.
- Carnevale P, Robert V, Boudin C, et al. La lutte contre le paludisme par des moustiquaires imprégnées de pyréthrynoïdes au Burkina Faso. *Bull Soc Pathol Exot* 1988 ; 81 (5) : 832-46.
- Carnevale P, Mouchet J. *The role of livestock in vector borne disease epidemiology in Africa*. WHO/FAO/UNEP. Panel of Experts on Environmental Management for Vector Control. Rome, 10th annual meeting, 3-7 Sept. 1990 : 13 p.
- Carnevale P, Le Goff G, Toto JC, Robert V. *Anopheles nili* as the main vector of human malaria in villages of Southern Cameroon. *Med Vet Entomol* 1992 ; 6, 135-8.
- Carnevale P, Robert V, Le Goff G, et al. Données entomologiques sur le paludisme urbain en Afrique tropicale. *Cahiers Santé* 1993 ; 3 : 239-45.
- Carnevale P, Coosemans M. Some operational aspects of the use of personal protection methods against malaria at individual and community level. *Ann Soc Belg Med Trop* 1995 ; 75 : 81-103.
- Carnevale P, Guillet P, Robert V, et al. Diversity of malaria in ricefield growing areas of the Afrotropical Region. *Parassitologia* 1999 ; 41 : 273-6.
- Carr HP, Hill RB. A malaria survey of Cuba. *Am J Trop Med* 1942 ; 22 : 587-607.
- Carrara G, Petrarca V, Niang M, Coluzzi M. *Anopheles pharoensis* and transmission of *Plasmodium falciparum* in the Senegal river delta, West Africa. *Med Vet Entomol* 1990 ; 4 : 421-4.
- Carrasquilla G, Banguero M, Sanchez P, et al. Epidemiologic tools for malaria surveillance in an urban setting of low endemicity along the Colombian Pacific Coast. *Am J Trop Med Hyg* 2000 ; 62 (1) : 132-7.
- Carter R, Schofield L, Mendis K. HLA effects in malaria: increased parasite-killing immunity or reduced immunopathology? *Parasitol Today* 1992 ; 8 : 41-2 & 57.
- Carter R, Mendis KN, Roberts D. Spatial targeting of interventions against malaria. *Bull World Health Organ* 2000 ; 78 : 1401-11.
- Carteron B, Morvan D, Rodhain F. Le problème de l'endémie de paludisme dans la République de Djibouti. *Med Trop (Marseille)* 1978 ; 38 : 299-304.
- Carvajal H, de Herrera MA, Quintero J, Alzate A, Herrera S. *Anopheles neivai*: a vector of malaria in the Pacific lowlands of Colombia. *Trans R Soc Trop Med Hyg* 1989 ; 83 (5) : 609.
- de Casa C, Isabel S. Malaria reinfestation on the Northern border of Argentina. *Geojournal* 1992 ; 26 (1) : 65-7.
- Casimiro S, Coleman M, Mohloai P, Hemingway J, Sharp B. Insecticide resistance in *Anopheles funestus* (Diptera: Culicidae) from Mozambique. *J Med Entomol* 2006 ; 43 : 267-75.
- Cassaigne R, Bruaire M, Leger N. Paludisme autochtone. Cent ans après Laveran : le paludisme à Paris. I. Les victimes. *Cahiers ORSTOM, Entomol Med Parasitol* 1980 ; 18 : 177-9.
- Castelli F, Cabona MG, Brunori A, Carosi G. Short report: imported mosquito: an uninvited guest. *Am J Trop Med Hyg* 1994 ; 50 : 548-9.
- Cavalie P, Mouchet J. Les campagnes expérimentales d'éradication du paludisme dans le nord de la République du Cameroun. Les vecteurs de l'épidémiologie du paludisme dans le Nord-Cameroun. *Med Trop (Marseille)* 1961 ; 21 : 847-69.
- CDC. Local transmission of *Plasmodium vivax* malaria-Virginia, 2002. *MMWR* 2002 ; 51 : 921-3.
- CDC. Multifocal autochthonous transmission of malaria-Florida, 2003. *MMWR* 2004 ; 53 : 412-3.
- Celli A. *Storia della malaria nell'Agro Romano*. Roma : Academia dei Lineei, 1925.
- Celsus AA. *De medicina* (trad. Spencer WG). London : Loeb Classical Library Heinemann, 1935.
- Chabasse D, Dumon H, Tounkara A, Maiga A, Ranque P. Indices paludométriques chez 938 enfants et adolescents en savane humide au Sud du Mali. *Bull Soc Pathol Exot* 1980 ; 73 : 254-8.
- Chadee DD, Le Maitre A, Tilluckdharry CC. An outbreak of *Plasmodium vivax* malaria in Trinidad, WI. *Ann Trop Med Parasitol* 1992 ; 86 : 583-90.
- Chadee DD, Kitron U. Spatial and temporal patterns of imported malaria cases and local transmission in Trinidad. *Am J Trop Med Hyg* 1999 ; 61 (4) : 513-7.
- Chadli A, Kennou MF, Kooli J. Les campagnes d'éradication du paludisme en Tunisie : historique et situation actuelle. *Arch Inst Pasteur Tunis* 1986 ; 63 : 35-50.
- Chadwick PR. The activity of some pyrethroids, DDT and Lindane in smoke for coils for biting inhibition, knock-down and kill of mosquitoes. *Bull Entomol Res* 1975 ; 65 : 97-107.
- Chand D. Malaria problem in Ethiopia. *Ethiopian Med J* 1965 ; 4 : 27-34.
- Chandler JA, Highton RB. The succession of mosquito species in rice fields in the Kisumu area of Kenya and their possible control. *Bull Entomol Res* 1975 ; 65 : 295-302.
- Chandler JA, Highton RB, Hill MN. Mosquitoes of the Kano plain, Kenya. Part I. Results of indoor collections in irrigated and non-irrigated areas using human bait and light-traps. *J Med Entomol* 1975 ; 12 : 504-10.
- Chandler JA, Highton RB, Hill MN. Mosquitoes of the Kano plain, Kenya. Part II. Results of outdoor collections in irrigated and non-irrigated areas using human and animal bait and light-traps. *J Med Entomol* 1976 ; 13 : 202-7.
- Chandrahas RK, Sharma VP. Malaria epidemic in Shahjahanpur, Uttar Pradesh. *Indian J Malariol* 1983 ; 20 : 163-6.
- Chandrahas RK, Jambulingam P, Sabesan S, Rajagopalan PK. Epidemiological aspects of malaria in Rameswaram Island (Tamil Nadu). *Indian J Med Res* 1984 ; 80 : 37-42.
- Chandramohan D, Setal P, Quigley M. Effect of misclassification of causes of death in verbal autopsy: can it be adjusted? *Int J Epidemiol* 2001 ; 30 : 509-14.
- Chandre F, Darriet F, Manga L, et al. Status for pyrethroid resistance in *Anopheles gambiae* s.l. *Bull World Health Organ : Int J Public Health* 1999 ; 77 : 230-4.
- Chang TL, Watson RB, Chow CY. Notes on the seasonal prevalence of Anopheles mosquitoes in Southern Formosa. *Indian J Malariol* 1950 ; 4 : 281-93.
- Chapin G, Wasserstrom R. Agricultural production and malaria resurgence in Central America and India. *Nature* 1981 ; 293 : 181-5.
- Charles LJ. Observations on *Anopheles (Kerteszia) bellator* D and K in British Guiana. *Am J Trop Med Hyg* 1959, 8 : 160-7.
- Charles LJ. Rapport OMS/MEI/551.12, 1960.
- Charlwood JD, Graves PM, Alpers MP. The ecology of the *Anopheles punctulatus* group of mosquitoes from Papua New Guinea: a review of recent work. *Papua New Guinea Med J* 1986 ; 29 : 19-26.

- Charlwood JD, Bryan JH. A mark-recapture experiment with the filariasis vector *Anopheles punctulatus* in Papua New Guinea. *Ann Trop Med Parasitol* 1987 ; 81 : 429-36.
- Charlwood JD, Graves PM. The effect of permethrin-impregnated bednets on a population of *An. farauti* in coastal Papua New Guinea. *Med Vet Entomol* 1987 ; 1 : 319-27.
- Chauvet G. Répartition et écologie du complexe *An. gambiae* à Madagascar. *Cahiers ORSTOM, Entomol Med Parasitol* 1969 ; 7 : 235-75.
- Chaves SS, Rodrigues LC. An initial examination of the epidemiology of malaria in the state of Roraima in the Brazilian Amazon basin. *Rev Inst Med Trop Sao Paulo* 2000 ; 42 (5) : 269-75.
- Chayabejara S, *et al. Investigation on malaria situation in Zambia.* WHO/AFR/MAL/139/1974a : 40 p.
- Chayabejara S, Sobti SK, Payne D. *Investigation on malaria situation in Malawi.* WHO/AFRO/MAL/137/1974b : 42 p.
- Chayabejara S, Sobti SK, Payne D, Braga F. *Malaria situation in Botswana.* WHO/AFRO/MAL/144/1975 : 28 p.
- Chen YK, Ree HI, Hong HK, Chow CY. *Bionomics and vector efficiency of Anopheles sinensis in Korea.* WHO/MAL/67.633, 1967 : 11 p.
- Chen B, Harbach RE, Butlin RK. Molecular and morphological studies on the *Anopheles minimus* group of mosquitoes in southern China: taxonomic review, distribution and malaria vector status. *Med Vet Entomol* 2002 ; 16 : 253-65.
- Chen B, Butlin RK, Pedro PM, Wang XZ, Harbach RE. Molecular variation, systematics and distribution of the *Anopheles fluviatilis* complex in southern Asia. *Med Vet Entomol* 2006 ; 20 : 33-43.
- Cheng H, Yang W, Kang W, Liu C. Large-scale spraying of bednets to control mosquito vectors and malaria in Sichuan, China. *Bull World Health Organ* 1995 ; 73 (3) : 321-8.
- Cheong WH, Warren M, Omar AH, Mahadevan S. *Anopheles balabacensis balabacensis* identified as vector of simian malaria in Malaysia. *Science* 1965 ; 150 : 1314-5.
- Chesnova LV. *Problems of general entomology.* Moscou : Nauka, 1974.
- Chin W, Contacos PG, Coatney GR, Kimball HR. A naturally acquired quotidian-type malaria in man transferable to monkeys. *Science* 1965 ; 149 : 865.
- Chinery WA. Effects of ecological changes on the malaria vectors *An. funestus* and the *Anopheles gambiae* complex of mosquitoes in Accra, Ghana. *J Trop Med Parasitol* 1984 ; 87 : 75-81.
- Chinery WA. Impact of rapid urbanisation on mosquitoes and their disease transmission potential in Accra, Ghana. *West Afr J Med Sci* 1995 ; 24 : 179-88.
- Chippaux JP, Akogbeto M, Massougbodji A, Adjagba J. Mesure de la parasitémie palustre et évaluation du seuil pathogène en région de forte transmission permanente. In : Robert V, *et al.*, eds. *Le paludisme en Afrique de l'Ouest.* Bondy : ORSTOM, 1991a : 55-65.
- Chippaux JP, Akogbeto M, Massougbodji A. Le paludisme urbain lagunaire : étude de la morbidité palustre dans un dispensaire périphérique de Cotonou (Bénin). In : Robert V, *et al.*, eds. *Le paludisme en Afrique de l'Ouest.* Bondy : ORSTOM, 1991b : 67-75.
- Chippaux JP, Schneider D, Aplogan A, Dyck JL, Berger J. Effets de la supplémentation en fer sur l'infection palustre. *Bull Soc Pathol Exot* 1991c ; 84 : 54-62.
- Chippaux JP, Massougbodji A, Ekoue S, Lanmasso T, Akogbeto M, Aguessi-Ahyi B. Note sur le passage transplacentaire de *P. falciparum* chez les parturientes non fébriles en région holo-endémique. *Bull Soc Pathol Exot* 1991d ; 84 : 458-64.
- Chippaux JP, Massougbodji A, Boulard JC, Akogbeto M. Étude de la morbidité palustre et de la gravité des accès pernicieux chez les porteurs du trait drépanocytaire. *Rev Épidémiol Santé Publique* 1992a ; 40 : 240-5.
- Chippaux JP, Massougbodji A, Castel J, Akogbeto M, Zohoun I, Zohoun T. Parasitémies à *Plasmodium falciparum* ou *P. malariae* chez les porteurs du trait drépanocytaire dans différents biotopes du Bénin. *Rev Épidémiol Santé Publique* 1992b ; 40 : 246-51.
- Chooi CK. Status of malaria vectors in Malaysia. *Southeast Asian J Trop Med Public Health* 1985 ; 16 : 133-8.
- Choudhury DS, Ghosh SK. *Plasmodium falciparum* malaria in Haryana villages and a case report of Aphasia. *Indian J Malariol* 1982 ; 19 : 69-70.
- Choudhury DS, Malhotra MS, Shukla RP, Ghosh SK, Sharma VP. Resurgence of malaria in Gardapur PHC, District Nainital, Uttar Pradesh. *Indian J Malariol* 1983 ; 20 : 49-58.
- Choumara R. Notes sur le paludisme au Somaliland. *Riv Malariol* 1961 ; 40 : 9-34.
- Choumara R, Hamon J, Ricossé J, Bailly H, Adam JP. Le paludisme dans la zone pilote de Bobo-Dioulasso. *Cahiers ORSTOM* 1959 ; 1 : 1-125.
- Chow CY. *The bionomics of two important malaria vectors in China.* Proceedings 4th International Congress for Tropical Medicine and Malaria. Washington, 1948, 1 : 861.
- Chow CY. Bionomics of malaria vectors in the Western Pacific region. *Southeast Asian J Trop Med Public Health* 1970 ; 1 : 40-57.
- Chow CY, Watson RB, Chang TL. Natural infection of Anopheline mosquitoes with malaria parasites in Formosa. *Indian J Malariol* 1950 ; 4 : 295-300.
- Chown M. Satellite monitors Madagascar's shrinking rainforest. *New Scientist* 1990 ; 32 : 32.
- Christophers SR. *Malaria in the Punjab.* Scientific Memoirs by Officers of the Medical and Sanitary Departements of the Government. Calcutta : Superintendent Government Printing, 1911 : New Series n° 46.
- Christophers SR. Malaria map of India. In : Hehir P, Milford H, eds. *Malaria in India.* London : Oxford University Press, 1927.
- Christophers SR. Studies on the anopheline fauna of India. *Rec Mal Surv India* 1931 ; 2 : 305-32.
- Christophers SR. Endemic and epidemic prevalence. In : Boyd MF, ed. *Malariology,* vol. 1. Philadelphia : WB Saunders, 1949 : 698-721.
- Christophers SR, Shortt HE. Malaria in Mesopotamia. *Indian J Med Res* 1921 ; 8 : 508-52.
- Church CJ, Atmosoedjono S, Bangs MJ. A review of Anopheline mosquitoes and Malaria Control strategy in Irian Jaya, Indonesia. *Bull Penelit Kesehat* 1996 ; 23 : 3-17.
- Ciuca M. Le paludisme en Roumanie de 1949 à 1955. *Bull Organ Mond Santé* 1956 ; 15 : 725-51.
- Clarke JL, Pradhan GD, Joshi GP, Fontaine RE. Assessment of the grain store as an unbaited outdoor shelter for mosquitoes of the *Anopheles gambiae* complex and *An. funestus* at Kisumu, Kenya. *J Med Entomol* 1980 ; 17 : 100-2.
- Clarke JK. *A note on blood digestion and egg development in An. merus in the Southern Mozambique.* WHO/MAL/69.686, 1969.
- Clements AN. *The biology of mosquitoes.* London : Chapman & Hall, 1992 : 509 p.
- Clyde DF. Malaria distribution in Tanganyika. Part I. *East Afr Med J* 1962 ; 39 : 528-35.
- Clyde DF. Malaria distribution in Tanganyika. Part VI. Western Tanzania. *East Afr Med J* 1965 ; 42 : 695-707.
- Clyde DF. *Malaria in Tanzania.* London : Oxford University Press, 1967 : 167 p.
- Clyde DF, Msangi AS. Malaria distribution in Tanganyika. Part II. Tanga region. *East Afr Med J* 1963 ; 40 : 71-82.
- Clyde DF, Mzoo FM. Malaria distribution in Tanganyika. Part III. The South-East. *East Afr Med J* 1964 ; 41 : 7-14.
- Clyde DF, Mluba S. Malaria distribution in Tanganyika. Part IV. Central Tanganyika. *East Afr Med J* 1964 ; 41 : 375-85.
- Clyde DF, Elibariki E. Malaria distribution in Tanganyika. Part V. The North. *East Afr Med J* 1965 ; 42 : 438-46.
- Coatney GR, Collins WE, McWarren W, Contacos PG. *The Primate malarias.* Washington : US Government Printing Office, 1971 : 366 p.
- Coene J. Malaria in urban and rural Kinshasa: the entomological input. *Med Vet Entomol* 1993 ; 7 : 127-37.
- Coetzee M, Hunt RH, Braack LE, Davidson G. Distribution of mosquitoes belonging to the *Anopheles gambiae* complex including malaria vectors, South of latitude 15°S. *S Afr J Med Sci* 1993 ; 89 : 227-31.
- Coetzee M, Estrada-Franco JG, Wunderlich CA, Hunt RH. Cytogenetic evidence for a species complex within *Anopheles pseudopunctipennis* Theobald (Diptera: Culicidae). *Am J Trop Med Hyg* 1999 ; 60 (4) : 649-53.
- Coetzee M, Craig M, Le Sueur D. Distribution of African malaria mosquitoes complex belonging to the *Anopheles gambiae* complex. *Parasitol Today* 2000 ; 16 : 74-7.
- Colbourne MJ, Edington GM. Mortality from malaria in Accra. *J Trop Med Hyg* 1954 ; 57 : 203-10.
- Colbourne MJ, Wright FN. Malaria in the Gold Coast. *West Afr J Med* 1955 ; 4 : 3-17 & 161-74.
- Colbourne MJ, Smith SA. *Problems of malaria in the Aden Protectorate.* WHO/MAL/442, 7 april 1964 : 70 p.
- Coleman PG, Goodman CA, Mills A. Rebound mortality and the cost-effectiveness of malaria control: potential impact of increased mortality in late childhood following the introduction of insecticide treated nets. *Trop Med Int Health* 1999 ; 4 : 175-86.
- Collins FH, Porter CH, Cope SE. Comparison of rDNA and mtDNA in the sibling species of *Anopheles freeborni* and *An. hermsi*. *Am J Trop Med Hyg* 1990 ; 42 (5) : 417-23.
- Collins RT, Jung RK, Anoez H, Sutrisno RH, Putut D. *A study on the coastal malaria vectors,* Anopheles sundaicus *and* An. subpictus *in South Sulawesi, Indonesia.* WHO/VBC/79.913, 1979 : 12 p.

Biodiversity of Malaria in the World

- Collins RT, Beljaev AE, Pattanayak S, Agarwala RS. Studies on malaria transmission in Orissa state, India,1981 through 1986. II. Observations on the Anopheles fauna. *J Commun Dis* 1990 ; 22 : 191-204.
- Collins WE, Contracos PG. Immunization of monkeys against *Plasmodium cynomolgi* by X-irradiated sporozoites. *Nat New Biol* 1972 ; 236 : 176-7.
- Coluzzi M. Advances in the study of Afrotropical malaria vectors. *Parassitologia* 1993 ; 35 (suppl.) : 23-9.
- Coluzzi M, Sacca G, Feliciangeli D. Il complesso *A. claviger* nella sottoregione mediterranea. *Cahiers ORSTOM, Entomol Med Parasitol* 1965 : 97-102.
- Coluzzi M, Sabatini A, Petrarca V, Di Deco MA. Chromosomal differentiation and adaptation to human environments in the *Anopheles gambiae* complex. *Trans R Soc Trop Med Hyg* 1979 ; 73 : 483-97.
- Coluzzi M, Petrarca V, Di Deco MA. Chromosomal inversion integration and incipient speciation in *Anopheles gambiae*. *Boll Zool* 1985 ; 52 : 45-63.
- Combemale P, Deruaz D, Villanova D, Guillaumont P. Les insectifuges ou les répellents. *Ann Dermatol Venereol* 1992 ; 119 (5) : 411-34.
- Conlon CP, Berendt AR, Dawson K, Peto TE. Runway malaria. *Lancet* 1990 ; 335 : 472-3.
- Conn J, Puertas YR, Seawright JA. A new cytotype of *Anopheles nuneztovari* from Western Venezuela and Columbia. *J Am Mosq Control Assoc* 1993 ; 9 (3) : 294-301.
- Conn JE, Wilkerson RC, Segura MN, et al. Emergence of a new neotropical malaria vector facilitated by human migration and changes in land use. *Am J Trop Med Hyg* 2002 ; 66 (1) : 18-22.
- Consolim J, Luz E, Pellegrini NJ, Torres PB. The *Anopheles darlingi* Root 1926 and malaria in the Itaipu Lake Parana Brazil, a revision. *Arq Biol Tecnol (Curitiba, Brazil)* 1991 ; 34 (2) : 263-86.
- Coosemans M. Comparaison de l'endémie malarienne dans une zone de riziculture et dans une zone de culture du coton dans la plaine de la Rusizi, Burundi. *Ann Soc Belg Med Trop* 1985 ; 65 (suppl. 2) : 187-200.
- Coosemans M. Recherche épidémiologique dans un foyer de paludisme peu stable en Afrique Centrale. *Mem Acad R Sc OM* 1989 ; 23 (fasc. 3) : 62 p.
- Coosemans M. Développement d'une stratégie de lutte contre le paludisme dans une région rizicole au Burundi. *Bull Mem Acad R Med Belge* 1991 ; 146 (1-2) : 157-65.
- Coosemans M, Wery M, Storme B, Hendrix L, Mfisi B. Épidémiologie du paludisme dans la plaine de la Rusizi, Burundi. *Ann Soc Belg Med Trop* 1984 ; 64 : 135-58.
- Coosemans M, Barutwanayo M. Malaria control by antivectorial measures in a zone of chloroquine-resistant malaria: a successful programme in a rice growing area of the Rusizi Valley, Burundi. *Trans R Soc Trop Med Hyg* 1989 ; 83 (suppl.) : 97-8.
- Coosemans M, Petrarca V, Barutwanayo M, Coluzzi M. Species of the *An. gambiae* complex and chromosomal polymorphism in a rice-growing area of the Rusizi Valley, Burundi. *Parassitologia* 1989 ; 31 : 113-22.
- Coosemans M, Wery M, Mouchet J, Carnevale P. Transmission factors in malaria epidemiology and control in Africa. *Mem Inst Oswaldo Cruz* 1992 ; 87 (suppl. 3) : 385-91.
- Coosemans M, Carnevale P. Malaria vector control: a critical review on chemical methods and insecticides. *Ann Soc Belg Med Trop* 1995 ; 75 (1) : 13-31.
- Coosemans M, Smits A, Roelants P. Intraspecific isozyme polymorphism of *Anopheles gambiae* in relation to environment, behavior and malaria transmission in Southwestern Burkina Faso. *Am J Trop Med Hyg* 1998 ; 58 : 70-4.
- Coosemans M, Guillet P. La protection du voyageur contre les piqûres de moustiques. *Med Mal Infect* 1999 ; 29 (suppl. 3) : 390-6.
- Coppens Y, Picq P. À l'origine de l'humanité. Paris : Fayard, 2001 (2 vol.).
- Corbel V, N'Guessan R, Brengues C, et al. Multiple insecticide resistance mechanisms in *Anopheles gambiae* and *Culex quinquefasciatus* from Benin, West Africa. *Acta Trop* 2007 ; 101(3) : 207-16.
- Cormier-Salem MC. Rivières du Sud. Sociétés et mangroves ouest-africaines. Paris : IRD, 1999 : 416 p.
- Cornevin E. Histoire des peuples de l'Afrique Noire. Paris : Berger Levrault, 1963 : 715 p.
- Cornille-Brogger R, Mathews HM, Storey J, Ashkar TS, Brogger S, Molineaux L. Changing patterns in the humoral immune response to malaria before, during and after the application of control measures: a longitudinal study in the West African savannah. *Bull World Health Organ* 1978 ; 56 : 579-600.
- Correa, Renato R. Da infeção natural, pela Plasmodiose malarica ; do *Anopheles (Kerteszia) cruzi* DK, 1908. *Folia Clin Biol* 1943, 15 : 23.
- Costantini C, Sagnon N, Ilboudo-Sanogo E, Coluzzi M, Boccolini D. Chromosomal and bionomic heterogeneities suggest incipient speciation in *An. funestus* from Burkina Faso. *Parassitologia* 1999 ; 41 : 595-611.
- Cot M, Garde X, Miailhes P, Louis JP, Carnevale P, Louis FJ. Paludisme en zone d'altitude : résultats d'une enquête à Dschang (Ouest Cameroun). *Bull Liaison OCEAC* 1992 ; 100 : 9-13.
- Cot M, Le Hesran JY, Miailhes P, Esveld M, Etya'ale D, Breart G. Increase of birth weight following chloroquine chemoprophylaxis during the first pregnancy. Results of a randomized trial in Cameroon. *Am J Trop Med Hyg* 1995 ; 53 : 581-5.
- Coulibaly CO, Guigemde RT, Lamizana L, Ouedraogo JB, Dabiret E. La part du paludisme dans les affections fébriles en milieu urbain de Ouagadougou, Burkina Faso. *Ann Soc Belg Med Trop* 1991 ; 71 : 5-16.
- Courtois D, Mouchet J. Étude des populations de Culicidés dans le Territoire Français des Afars et des Issas. *Med Trop (Marseille)* 1970 ; 30 : 837-46.
- Coutinho AG. Malaria patterns in North East Swaziland. *S Afr J Epidemiol Infect* 1994 ; 9 : 108-11.
- Coutinho JO, Rachou R, Ferreira M. Considerações em torno de uma inspecção preliminar de malaria em zona de alta endemicidade no Estado de Santa Catarina. *Mem Inst Oswaldo Cruz* 1944 ; 41 : 1.
- Covell G. Notes on the distribution, breeding places, adult habits and relation to malaria of the anopheline mosquitoes of India and the Far East. *J Malaria Inst India* 1944 ; 5 : 399-434.
- Cox FE. Malarial immunity. Indonesian and Sudanese style. *Nature* 1984 ; 309 : 402-3.
- Cox JH, Mouchet J, Bradley DJ. Determinants of malaria in Sub-Saharan Africa. In : Casman E, Dowlatabi H, eds. *The contextual determinants of malaria*. Washingon : Ressources for the Future Press, 2002 : 167-86.
- Coz J. Mission d'études entomologiques dans le sud-ouest de Madagascar. *Arch Serv Anti Palu Madagascar* 1961 ; 15 : 14.
- Coz J. Contribution à l'étude du complexe *An. gambiae*. *Cahiers ORSTOM, Entomol Med Parasitol* 1973a ; 11 : 3-31.
- Coz J. Contribution à la biologie du complexe *An. gambiae* en Afrique Occidentale. *Cahiers ORSTOM, Entomol Med Parasitol* 1973b ; 11 : 33-40.
- Coz J, Hamon J, Sales S, et al. Études entomologiques sur la transmission du paludisme humain dans une zone de forêt humide dense dans la région de Sassandra, Côte d'Ivoire. *Cahiers ORSTOM, Entomol Med Parasitol* 1966, 4 : 13-42.
- Coz J, Picq JJ. Étude en laboratoire de la réceptivité à *Laverania falcipara* d'*An. gambiae* A et d'*An. gambiae* B. *Bull Soc Pathol Exot* 1972 ; 65 : 668-75.
- Crees MJ. Biting activity of mosquitoes and malarial incidences in the South East lowveld of Zimbabwe. *Trans Zimbabwe Sc Assoc* 1996 ; 70 : 21-7.
- Crook S, Cuamba N, Theron D. Inquerito preliminary sobre a distribuicao geograficas da especies do complexo *gambiae* en Moçambique. *Rev Med Moçambique* 1994 ; 5 (suppl. 1) : 5-6.
- Crook SE, Baptista A. The effect of permethrin-impregnated wall-curtain on malaria transmission and morbidity in the suburbs of Maputo, Mozambique. *Trop Geogr Med* 1995 ; 47 (2): 64-7.
- Cross JH, Clarke MD, Irving GS, et al. Intestinal parasites and malaria in Margolembo, Luwu Regency, South Sulawesi, Indonesia. *Southeast Asian J Trop Med Public Health* 1972 ; 3 : 587-93.
- Cross JH, Clarke MD, Carney WP, et al. Parasitology survey in the Palu Valley, Central Sulawesi, Indonesia. *Southeast Asian J Trop Med Public Health* 1975 ; 6 : 366-75.
- Cross JH, Clarke MD, Cole WC, et al. Parasitic infections in humans in West Kalimantan (Borneo). *Trop Geogr Med* 1976 ; 28 : 121-30.
- Crowe S. Malaria outbreak hits refugees in Tanzania. *Lancet* 1997 ; 350 : 41.
- da Cruz Ferreira FS, Pinto AR, Lehmann de Almeida C. Alguns dados sobre a biologia do *An. gambiae* da cidade de Bissau e arredores. *An Inst Med Trop (Lisb)* 1948 ; 5 : 223-50.
- Cuadros J, Calvente MJ, A Benito, et al. Plasmodium ovale malaria acquired in central Spain. *Emerg Infect Dis* 2002 ; 8 : 1506-8.
- Cuamba N, Choi KS, Townson H. Malaria vectors in Angola: distribution of species and molecular forms of the *Anopheles gambiae* complex, their pyrethroid insecticide knockdown resistance (*kdr*) status and *Plasmodium falciparum* sporozoite rates. *Malar J* 2006 ; 5 : 2.
- Curtis CF. Fact and fiction in mosquito attraction and repulsion. *Parasitol Today* 1986 ; 2 : 316-8.
- Curtis CF, White GB. *Plasmodium falciparum* transmission in England: entomological and epidemiological data relative to cases in 1983. *J Trop Med Hyg* 1984 ; 87 : 101-14.

- Curtis CF, et al. *Appropriate technology in vector control*. Boca Raton : CRC Press, 1990 : 45 p.
- Daggy RH. Malaria in Oases of Eastern Saudi Arabia. *Am J Trop Med Hyg* 1959 ; 8 : 223-91.
- D'Alessandro U. Antimalarial drug resistance: surveillance and molecular methods for national malaria control programmes. *Mem Inst Oswaldo Cruz* 1998 ; 93 (5) : 627-30.
- D'Alessandro G, Smiraglia CB, Lavagnino A. *Further studies on the biology of Anopheles labranchiae labranchiae Falleroni in Sicily*. WHO/MAL/71.754, 1971.
- D'Alessandro U, Olaleye BO, McGuire W, et al. Mortality and morbidity from malaria in Gambian children after introduction of an impregnated bednet programme. *Lancet* 1995 ; 345 : 479-83.
- D'Alessandro U, Langerock P, Bennett S, Francis N, Cham K, Greenwood BM. The impact of a national impregnated bed net programme on the outcome of pregnancy in primigravidae in The Gambia. *Trans R Soc Trop Med Hyg* 1996 ; 90 (5) : 487-92.
- D'Alessandro U, Coosemans M. Concerns on long-term efficacy of an insecticide-treated bednet programme on child mortality. *Parasitol Today* 1997 ; 13 : 124-5.
- D'Alessandro U, Buttiëns H. History and importance of antimalarial drug resistance. *Trop Med Int Health* 2001 ; 6 (11) : 845-8.
- Danis M, Mouchet J. *Paludisme*. Paris : Ellipses/AUPELF, 1991 : 240 p.
- Danis M, Mouchet J, Giacomini T, Guillet P, Legros F, Belkaid M. Paludisme autochtone et introduit en Europe. *Med Mal Infect* 1996 ; 26 : 393-6.
- Danis M. Legros F. *Paludisme d'importation. Données épidémiologiques 1999 et 2000*. Paris : Centre national de référence pour les maladies d'importation, 2002.
- Dansgaard W, Tauber H. Glacier oxygen-18 content and Pleistocene ocean temperatures. *Science* 1969 ; 166 : 499-502.
- Dansgaard W, Oeschger H. Past environmental long-term records from the Arctic. In : Oeschger H, Langwau, eds. *The environmental record in glaciers and ice sheets*. New York : John Wiley and Sons, 1989 : 287-318.
- Dansgaard W, Johnsen SJ, Clausen HB, et al. Evidence for general instability of past climate from a 250-kyr ice-core record. *Nature* 1993 ; 364 : 218-20.
- Darriet F, Robert V, Vien NT, Carnevale P. Évaluation de l'efficacité sur les vecteurs du paludisme de la perméthrine en imprégnation sur des moustiquaires intactes et trouées. Doc. mimeo. OMS, WHO/VBC/84. 899 & WHO/MAL/84. 1008, 1984, 20 p.
- Darriet F. Field trial of the efficacy of three pyrethroids in the control of malaria vectors. *Parassitologia* 1991 ; 33 : 111-9.
- Darriet F, Guillet P, Nguessan R, et al. Impact de la résistance d'*Anopheles gambiae s.s.* à la perméthrine et à la deltaméthrine sur l'efficacité des moustiquaires imprégnées. *Med Trop (Marseille)* 1998 ; 58 : 349-54.
- Darsie RF, Cagampang-Ramos A, Kalaw F. The experimental infection of *An. litoralis* from Luzon Island, Philippines, by *P. vivax*. *Southeast Asian J Trop Med Public Health* 1978 ; 9 : 445.
- Darsie RF, Ward RA. Identification and geographical distribution of the mosquitoes of North America, North of Mexico. *Mosq Syst* 1981 ; 1 (suppl.) : 1-313.
- Daruty de Grandpre A, d'Emmery de Charmoy D. *Les moustiques : anatomie, biologie, rôle dans la propagation de la malaria et de la filariose*. Port Louis : The Planters and Commercial Gazette, 1900 : 59 p.
- Das LK, Mohapatra SS, Jambulingam P, Gunasekaran K, Pani SK, Das PK. Malaria and other common ailments among Upper Bonda tribals in Koraput District, Orissa. *Indian J Med Res* 1989 ; 89 : 334-9.
- Das PK, Reuben R, Batra CP. Urban malaria and its vectors in Salem (Tamil Nadu): natural and induced infection with human plasmodia in mosquitoes. *Indian J Med Res* 1979 ; 69 : 403-11.
- Das PK, Das LK, Parida SK, Patra KP, Jambulingam P. Lambdacyhalothrin treated bed nets as an alternative method of malaria control in tribal villages of Koraput District, Orissa State, India. *Southeast Asian J Trop Med Public Health* 1993 ; 24 (3) : 513-21.
- Das SC, Bhuyan M, Baruah I. Active malaria transmission in South Mizoram. *Indian J Malariol* 1990 ; 27 : 111-7.
- Dash AP, Bendle MS, Das AK, Das M, Dwivedi SR. Role of *Anopheles annularis* as a vector in the Inland of Orissa. *J Commun Dis* 1982 ; 14 : 224.
- Daskova NG, Rasnicyn SP. Review of data on susceptibility of mosquitos in USSR to imported strains of malaria parasites. *Bull World Health Organ* 1982 ; 60 (6) : 893-7.
- Davidson G. Further studies of the basic factors concerned in the transmission of malaria. *Trans R Soc Trop Med Hyg* 1955 ; 49 : 339-50.
- Davidson G. *Anopheles gambiae* complex. *Nature* 1962 ; 196 : 907.
- Davidson G. *Likely contacts between insecticides and arthropods of medical importance*. Proceedings of an International Workshop on Resistance to insecticides used in public health and agriculture, Colombo, 26-28 Feb. 1982. Sri Lanka Colombo : National Science Council of Sri Lanka, 1982 : 122-9.
- Davidson G, Draper CC. Field studies of some of the basic factors concerned in the transmission of malaria. *Trans R Soc Trop Med Hyg* 1953 ; 47 : 522-35.
- Davidson G, Sawyer B. Proceedings: Carbamate and organophosphate resistance in *Anopheles albimanus*. *Trans R Soc Trop Med Hyg* 1975 ; 69 (4) : 431.
- Davies CR, Ayres JM, Dyes C, Deane LM. Malaria infection rates of Amazonian primates increase with body weight and group size. *Function Ecol* 1991 ; 5 (5) : 655-62.
- Davis JR, Hall T, Chee EM, Majala A, Minjas J, Shiff CJ. Comparison of sampling anopheline mosquitoes by light-trap and human-bait collections indoors at Bagamoyo, Tanzania. *Med Vet Entomol* 1995 ; 9 : 249-55.
- Deane LM, Deane MP, Ferreira Neto J. Studies on transmission of simian malaria and report of a natural infection of man with *Plasmodium simium* in Brazil. *Bull World Health Organ* 1966 ; 35 : 805-8.
- Deane LM, Ferreira Neto JA, Lima MM. The vertical dispersion of *An. (Kerteszia) cruzi* in a forest in Southern Brazil suggests that human cases of malaria of simian origin might be expected. *Mem Inst Oswaldo Cruz* 1984 ; 79 (4) : 461-3.
- Delacollette C, Van der Stuyft P, Molima K, Delacollette-Lebrun C, Wery M. Étude de la mortalité globale et de la mortalité liée au paludisme dans le Kivu montagneux, Zaïre. *Rev Épidémiol Santé Publique* 1989 ; 37 : 161-6.
- Delacollette C, Van der Stuyft P, Molima K, Hendrix L, Wery M. Indices paludométriques selon l'âge et selon les saisons dans la zone de santé de Katana au Kivu montagneux, Zaïre. *Ann Soc Belg Med Trop* 1990a ; 70 : 263-8.
- Delacollette C, Barutwanayo M, Mpitabakana P. Épidémiologie du paludisme au Burundi. *Med Afr Noire* 1990b ; 37 : 718-21.
- Delacollette C, Taelman H, Wery M. An etiologic study of hemoglobinuria and blackwater fever in the Kivu mountains, Zaire. *Ann Soc Belg Med Trop* 1995 ; 75 : 51-63.
- Delfini LF. *Malaria in Swaziland*. WHO/AFR/MAL/121/2, 2 May 1972 : 24 p.
- Delfini LF. *Report on a visit to Bahrain*, 29 Jan./4 Feb. 1977. WHO/EMRO/1977.
- Delfini LF. *Malaria control in Yemen*, 14 Sept./25 Nov. 1985. WHO/EM/ MAL/212.E 1986.
- Delfini LF. *On a mission to the Sultanate of Oman malaria control Program*, 16 Oct./14 Nov. 1987. WHO/EMRO/1987.
- Delorme DR, Wirtz RA, Loong KP, Lewis GE. Identification of sporozoïtes in *Anopheles maculatus* from Malaysia by enzyme–linked immunosorbent assays. *Trop Biomed* 1989 ; 6 : 21-6.
- Delteil A. Considérations sur le climat et la salubrité à la Réunion. *Arch Med Nav* 1881 ; 36 : 5-45.
- Dempster IE. Notes on the application of the test of organic disease of the spleen as an easy and certain method of detecting malarious localities in hot climate, 1848. Reprinted in *Rec Mal Surv India* 1969.
- Denis MB, Meek SR. Malaria in Cambodia. *Southeast Asian J Trop Med Public Health* 1992 ; 23 (suppl. 4) : 23-8.
- Desfontaine M, Gelas H, Goghomu A, Kouka-Bemba D, Carnevale P. Evaluation of practices and costs of antivectorial control at the family level in central Africa, I. Yaounde City (March 1988). *Bull Soc Pathol Exot Filiales* 1989 ; 82 : 558-65.
- Desfontaine M, Gelas H, Cabon H, et al. Evaluation of practice and costs of vector control on a family level in Central Africa. II. Douala City (Cameroon), July 1988. *Ann Soc Belg Med Trop* 1990 ; 70 : 137-44.
- Desowitz RS, Spark RA. Malaria in the Maprik area of the Sepik region, Papua New Guinea : 1957-1984. *Trans R Soc Trop Med Hyg* 1987 ; 81 : 175-6.
- Detinova TS. Age grouping methods in diptera of medical importance with special reference to some vectors of malaria. *Série des Monographies OMS*, 1962 : n° 47 : 216 p.
- Dev V. *Anopheles minimus*: its bionomics and role in the transmission of malaria in Assam, India. *Bull World Health Organ* 1996 ; 74 : 61-6.
- Develoux M, Chegou A, Prual A, Olivar M. Malaria in the oasis of Bilma, Republic of Niger. *Trans R Soc Trop Med Hyg* 1994 ; 88 : 644.
- Dewit I, Coosemans M, Srikrishnaraj K, Wery M. Population dynamics of anophelines in a malathion treated village in the intermediate zone of Sri Lanka. *Ann Soc Belg Med Trop* 1994 ; 74 : 93-103.

- Dhir SL, Rahim A. Malaria and its control in Afghanistan (1950-54). *Indian J Malariol* 1957, 11 : 73-101.
- Dia A, Lochouarn L, Boccolini D, Costantini C, Fontenille D. Spatial and temporal variations of the chromosomal inversion polymorphism of *Anopheles funestus* in Senegal. *Parasite* 2000 ; 7 : 179-84.
- Diallo DA, Habluetzel A, Cuzin-Ouattara N, *et al*. Widespread distribution of insecticide impregnated curtains reduces child mortality, prevalence and intensity of malaria infection and malaria transmission in rural Burkina Faso. *Parassitologia* 1999 ; 41 : 377-81.
- Diallo S, Ndir O, Faye O, *et al*. Le paludisme dans le district sanitaire Sud de Dakar (Sénégal). 1. Parasitémie et accès paludéens. *Bull Soc Pathol Exot* 1998a ; 91 : 208-13.
- Diallo S, Konate L, Faye O, *et al*. Le paludisme dans le district sanitaire Sud de Dakar (Sénégal). 2. Données entomologiques. *Bull Soc Pathol Exot* 1998b ; 91 : 259-63.
- Diatta M, Spiegel A, Lochouarn L, Fontenille D. Similar feeding preferences of *An. gambiae* and *An. arabiensis* in Senegal. *Trans R Soc Trop Med Hyg* 1998 ; 92 : 270-2.
- Diemkouma. *Prospection au Niger*. Centre Muraz de Bobo-Dioulasso, OCCGE, 1968 : 24 p.
- Diop A, Molez JF, Fontenille D, *et al*. Rôle d'*Anopheles melas* Theobald (1903) dans la transmission du paludisme dans la mangrove du Saloum (Sénégal). *Parasite* 2002 ; 9 : 239-46.
- Dissanaike AS, Nelson P, Garnham PC. *Plasmodium simiovale sp. nov*, a new simian malaria parasite from Ceylon. *Ceylon J Med Sci* 1965 ; 14 : 27-32.
- Dixon KE, Roberts DR, Llewellyn CH. Contribuicao ao estudo epidemiologico da malaria em trecho da Rodovia Transamazonica, Brasil. *Rev Inst Med Trop Sao Paulo* 1979 , 21 : 287-92.
- Djimde A, Doumbo OK, Cortese JF, *et al*. A molecular marker for chloroquine-resistant *falciparum* malaria. *N Engl J Med* 2001 ; 344 : 299-302.
- Doannio JM, Dossou-Yovo J, Diarassouba S, *et al*. La dynamique de la transmission du paludisme à Kafiné, un village rizicole en zone de savane de Côte d'Ivoire. *Bull Soc Pathol Exot* 2002 ; 95 : 11-6.
- Dobson A, Carper R. Biodiversity, health and climatic change. *Lancet* 1993 ; 342 : 1096-9.
- Doby JM, Guigen C. À propos des deux cas "Bretons" de paludisme autochtone, en réalité premiers cas français de paludisme d'aérodrome. *Bull Soc Pathol Exot* 1981 ; 74 : 398-405.
- Dolan G, ter Kuile FO, Jacoutot V, *et al*. Bed nets for the prevention of malaria and anaemia in pregnancy. *Trans R Soc Trop Med Hyg* 1993 ; 87 : 620-6.
- Dong-Xueshu, *et al*. Studies on geographical distribution, ecology and habits, role in malaria transmission and method of control of *Anopheles kunmingensis*. *Zoologic Res* 1990 ; 11 : 317-23.
- Donnelly MJ, Cuamba N, Charlwood JD, Collins FH, Townson H. Population structure in the malaria vector *An. arabiensis* Patton in East Africa. *Heredity* 1999 ; 83 : 408-17.
- Donnelly MJ, Townson H. Evidence for extensive genetic differentiation among populations of the malaria vector *Anopheles arabiensis* in Eastern Africa. *Insect Molec Biol* 2000 ; 9 : 357-67.
- Dossou-Yovo J, Doannio JM, Riviere F, Chauvancy G. Malaria in Côte d'Ivoire wet savannah region: the entomological input. *Trop Med Parasitol* 1995 ; 46 : 263-9.
- Dossou-Yovo J, Doannio JM, Diarrassouba S, Chauvancy G. L'impact de l'aménagement des rizières dans la transmission du paludisme dans la ville de Bouaké (Côte d'Ivoire). *Bull Soc Pathol Exot* 1998a ; 91 : 327-33.
- Dossou-Yovo J, Ouattara A, Doannio JM, Diarrassouba S, Chauvancy G. Enquêtes paludométriques en zone de savane humide de Côte d'Ivoire. *Med Trop (Marseille)* 1998b ; 58 : 51-6.
- Dossou-Yovo J, Diarrassouba S, Doannio J, Darriet F, Carnevale P. Le cycle d'agressivité d'*An. gambiae s.s.* à l'intérieur des maisons et la transmission du paludisme dans la région de Bouaké (Côte d'Ivoire). *Bull Soc Pathol Exot* 1999 ; 92 : 198-200.
- Doumbo O, Sangare O, Toure Y. Le paludisme dans le Sahel : l'exemple du Mali. In : *Maladies tropicales transmissibles*. Paris : John Libbey Eurotext, 1989 : 11-32.
- Doumbo O, Koita O, Traore SF, *et al*. Les aspects parasitologiques de l'épidémiologie du paludisme dans le Sahara malien. *Med Afr Noire* 1999 ; 38 : 103-9.
- Doury P. Le Hoggar, étude médicale. *Arch Inst Pasteur Algérie* 1959 ; 37 : 104-64.
- Dowling MA. *Malaria eradication. Scheme of Mauritius, preliminary report, 21st Dec. 1948*. Port Louis : JE Felix, Acting Government Printer, 1949 : 22 p.
- Dowling MA. Malaria control in Mauritius. *Br Med J* 1952 ; 9 août : 339.
- Dowling MA. Control of malaria in Mauritius. Eradication of *Anopheles funestus* and *Aedes aegypti*. *Trans R Soc Trop Med Hyg* 1953 ; 47 : 177-98.
- Downs WG, Pittendrigh CS. Bromeliad malaria in Trinidad. British West Indies. *Am J Trop Med* 1946 ; 26 : 47-66.
- Downs WG, Pittendrigh CS. Malaria transmitted by Bromeliad-breeding anophelines in Boya. In : Boyd MF, ed. *Malariology*, vol. 1. Philadelphia : WB Saunders, 1949 : 736-48.
- Draper CC, Smith A. Malaria in the Pare Area of North East Tanganyika. Part I. Epidemiology. *Trans R Soc Trop Med Hyg* 1957 ; 51 : 137-51.
- Draper CC, Smith A. Malaria in the Pare Area of North East Tanganyika. Part II. Effects of three years of spraying of huts with dieldrin. *Trans R Soc Trop Med Hyg* 1960 ; 54 : 342-57.
- Draper CC, Lelijveld JL, Matola YG, White GB. Malaria in the Pare area of Tanzania. IV. Malaria in the human population 11 years after the suspension of residual insecticide spraying with special reference to the serological findings. *Trans R Soc Trop Med Hyg* 1972 ; 66 : 905-12.
- Dukeen MY, Omer SM. Ecology of the malaria vector *An. arabiensis* by the Nile in Northern Sudan. *Bull Entomol Res* 1986 ; 76 : 451-67.
- Dupasquier I. *Contribution à l'étude immunopathologique des accès palustres à Plasmodium falciparum*. Thèse Médecine. Paris (Bichat), 1980.
- Duren A. *Essai d'étude d'ensemble du paludisme au Congo Belge*. Mémoires de l'Institut Royal Colonial Belge, Section des Sciences Naturelles et Médicales, 1937 : 86 p.
- Duren AN. Essai d'étude sur l'importance du paludisme dans la mortalité au Congo Belge. *Ann Soc Belg Med Trop* 1951 ; 27 : 129-47.
- Durrheim DN, Braack LE, Waner S, Gammon R. Risk of malaria in visitors to the Kruger National Park, South Africa. *J Travel Med* 1998 ; 5 : 173-7.
- Durrheim DN, Frieremans S, Kruger P, Mabuza A, de Bryun JC. Confidential inquiry into malaria deaths. *Bull World Health Organ* 1999 ; 77 : 263-6.
- Dusfour I, Harbach RE, Manguin S. Bionomics and systematics of the oriental *Anopheles sundaicus* complex in relation to malaria and vector control. *Am J Trop Med Hyg* 2004a ; 71 : 518-24.
- Dusfour I, Linton YM, Cohuet A, *et al*. Molecular evidence of speciation between island and continental populations of *Anopheles (Cellia) sundaicus* Rodenwaldt (Diptera: Culicidae), a principal malaria vector in Southeast Asia. *J Med Entomol* 2004b ; 41 : 287-95.
- Dusfour I, Michaux JR, Harbach RE, Manguin S. Speciation and phylogeography of the Southeast Asian *Anopheles sundaicus* Complex. *Infect Genet Evol* 2007 ; 7(4) : 484-93.
- Dutt AK, Akhtar R, Dutta HM. Malaria in India with particular reference to two West Central States. *Soc Sci Med* 1980 ; 14D (3) : 317-30.
- Dutta HM, Dutt AK, Vishnukumari G. The resurgence of malaria in Tamil Nadu. *Soc Sci Med* 1979 ; 13D (3) : 191-4.
- Dutta P, Baruah .D. Incrimination of *Anopheles minimus* Theobald as a vector of malaria in Arunachal Pradesh. *Indian J Malariol* 1987 ; 24 (2) : 159-62.
- Dutta P, Bhattacharyya DR. Malaria survey in some parts of Namsang Circle of Tirap District, Arunachal Pradesh. *J Commun Dis* 1990 ; 22 : 92-7.
- Dutta P, Bhattacharyya DR, Khan SA, Sharma CK, Mahanta J. Feeding patterns of *Anopheles dirus*, the major vector of forest malaria in North East India. *Southeast Asian J Trop Med Public Health* 1996 ; 27 : 378-81.
- Duverseau YT, Jean-Francois V, Benitez A. *Formation pour la prévention de la malaria : diagnostic de la malaria*. PAHO/HAI/89/023, 1989.

- Edirisinghe JS. Historical references to malaria in Sri Lanka and some notable episodes up to present time. *Ceylon Med J* 1988 ; 33 : 110-7.
- Edrissian GH, Naimi F, Afshar A. Seroepidemiological study of *P. vivax* malaria with suspected long incubation in Iran. *Iranian J Public Health* 1976 ; 5 : 198-206.
- Eisele TP, Lindblade KA, Wannemuehler KA, *et al*. Effect of sustained insecticide-treated bed net use on all-cause child mortality in an area of intense perennial malaria transmission in western Kenya. *Am J Trop Med Hyg* 2005 ; 73 : 149-56.
- Ekanem EE, Asindi AA, Okoi OU. Community-based surveillance of paediatric deaths in Cross River State, Nigeria. *Trop Geogr Med* 1994 ; 46 : 305-8.
- Eldin de Pecoulas P, Basco LK, Wilson CM, Le Bras J, Mazabraud A. Molecular characterisation of airport malaria. *J Travel Med* 1996 ; 3 : 179-81.

- El Gaddal AA, Haridi AA, Hassan FT, Hussein H. Malaria control in Gezira-Managil irrigated scheme of the Sudan. *J Trop Med Hyg* 1985 ; 88 : 153-9.
- El-Hazmi MA, Warsy AS, Al-Swailem AR, Al-Swailem AM, Bahakim HM. Sickle cell gene in the population of Saudi Arabia. *Hemoglobin* 1996 ; 20 : 187-98.
- Elias M. Larval habitat of *Anopheles philippinensis*: a vector of malaria in Bangladesh. *Bull World Health Organ* 1996 ; 74 : 447-50.
- Elias M, Rahman AJ, Begum AJ, Mobarak A, Chowdhury AR. The ecology of malaria carrying mosquito *Anopheles philippinensis* and its relation to malaria in Bangladesh. *Bangladesh Med Res Counc Bull* 1983 ; 13 : 15-28.
- Elissa N, Mouchet J, Rivière F, Meunier JY, Yao K. Resistance of *Anopheles gambiae* to pyrethroids in Ivory Coast. *Ann Soc Belg Med Trop* 1993 ; 73 : 291-4.
- Elissa N, Mouchet J, Rivière F, Meunier JY, Yao K. Sensibilité d'*An. gambiae* aux insecticides en Côte d'Ivoire. *Cahiers Santé* 1994 ; 4 : 95-9.
- Elissa N, Karch S, Bureau P, *et al*. Malaria transmission in a region of savannah-forest mosaic, Haut Ogooue, Gabon. *J Am Mosq Control Assoc* 1999 ; 15 : 15-23.
- Elliott R. The influence of vector behavior on malaria transmission. *Am J Trop Med Hyg* 1972 ; 21 : 755-63.
- El Said S, Beier JC, Kenawy MA, Morsy ZS, Merdan AI. *Anopheles* population dynamics in two malaria endemic villages in Faiyum Governorate, Egypt. *J Am Mosq Control Assoc* 1986 ; 2 : 158-63.
- El Sayed BB, Arnot DE, Mukhtar MM, *et al*. A study of the urban malaria transmission problem in Khartoum. *Acta Tropica* 2000 ; 75 : 163-71.
- Engelbrecht F, Togel E, Beck HP, Enwezor F, Oettli A, Felger I. Analysis of *P. falciparum* infections in a village community in Northern Nigeria: determination of msp2 genotypes and parasite-specific IgG responses. *Acta Tropica* 2000 ; 74 : 63-71.
- Escudié A, Hamon J, Godin J. Le paludisme et l'importance de sa transmission dans la région de Man, République de Côte d'Ivoire. *Riv Malariol* 1962 ; 41 : 9-28.
- Etang J, Manga L, Toto JC, Guillet P, Fondjo E, Chandre F. Spectrum of metabolic-based resistance to DDT and pyrethroids in *Anopheles gambiae s.l.* populations from Cameroon. *J Vector Ecol* 2007 ; 32 : 123-33.
- Etchegorry G, Matthys F, Galinski M, White NJ, Nosten F. Malaria epidemic in Burundi. *Lancet* 2001 ; 357 (9261) : 1046.
- Ettling MB, Shepard DS. Economic cost of malaria in Rwanda. *Trop Med Parasitol* 1991 ; 42 : 214-8.
- Evans AM. Notes on Freetown mosquitoes, with descriptions of new and little-known species. *Am Trop Med Parasitol* 1926 ; 20 : 97-108.
- Eyles DE, Wharton RH, Cheong WH, Warren MW. Studies on malaria and *An. balabacensis* in Cambodia. *Bull World Health Organ* 1964 ; 30 : 7-21.
- Eyraud M, *et al. Rapport sur une mission en Guinée*. Rapport Centre Muraz, OCCGE, Bobo-Dioulasso, 1963.

- Fall M, Sarr M, Ndiaye O, *et al*. Expérience hospitalière du paludisme grave de l'enfant. À propos d'une étude réalisée à l'hôpital d'enfants Albert Royer du CHU de Dakar. *Afrique Méd* 1992 ; 301 : 64-7.
- Fandeur T, Volney B, Peneau C, de Thoisy B. Monkeys of the rainforest in French Guiana are natural reservoirs for *P. brasilianum/P. malariae* malaria. *Parasitology* 2000 ; 120 : 11-21.
- FAO, UNEP, WHO. Disposal of bulk quantities of obsolete pesticides in developing countries. Provisional technical guide. *FAO Pesticide Disposal series (Rome)* 1996 ; 4.
- Faran ME. Mosquito studies (Diptera : Culicidae) XXXIV. A revision of the Albimanus section of the subgenus *Nyssorhynchus* of *Anopheles*. *Contrib Am Entomol Inst* 1980 ; 15 (7) : 215 p.
- Farid MA. Malaria infection in *Anopheles sergenti* in Egypt. *Riv Malariol* 1940 ; 19 : 159-61.
- Farid MA. Ineffectiveness of DDT residual spraying in stopping malaria transmission in the Jordan Valley. *Bull World Health Organ* 1954 ; 11 : 765-83.
- Farid MA. The implications of *Anopheles sergenti* for malaria eradication programmes East of the Mediterranean. *Bull World Health Organ* 1956 ; 15 : 821-8.
- Farid MA. *Assigment report Malaria Eradication Program, Pakistan*. WHOEM/MAL/125, Jul. 1974.
- Farid MA. *Rapport OMS*, 1984.
- Farid MA, Nasir AS, Benthein. *WHO malaria survey team Sultanate of Oman*, 13 April/8 June 1973. WHO/EM/MAL/118, Oct. 1973 ; 57 p.
- Farinaud ME. La lutte contre le paludisme dans les colonies françaises. *Ann Med Pharma Col* 1935 ; 33 : 96.

- Farinaud E, Prost P. Recherches sur les modalités de l'impaludation en milieu Moï et en milieu Annamite. *Bull Soc Pathol Exot* 1939 ; 32 : 762-9.
- Faust EC. Malaria incidence in North America. In : Boyd MF, ed. *Malariology*, vol. 1. Philadelphia : WB Saunders, 1949 : 749-63.
- Favia G, della Torre A, Bagayoko M, *et al*. Molecular identification of sympatric chromosomal forms of *Anopheles gambiae* and further evidence of their reproductive isolation. *Insect Mol Biol* 1997 ; 6 : 377-83.
- Favia G, Lanfrancotti A, Spanos L, Siden-Kiamos I, Louis C. Molecular characterization of ribosomal DNA polymorphisms discriminating chromosomal forms of *Anopheles gambiae s.s. Insect Mol Biol* 2001 ; 10 (1): 19-23.
- Favre VV. *Study of malaria in Russia from the public health angle*. Kharkov, 1903.
- Faye O, Fontenille D, Herve JP, Diack PA, Diallo S, Mouchet J. Le paludisme en zone sahélienne du Sénégal. 1. Données entomologiques sur la transmission. *Ann Soc Belg Med Trop* 1993a ; 73 : 21-30.
- Faye O, Gaye O, Herve JP, Diack PA, Diallo S. Le paludisme en zone sahélienne du Sénégal. *Ann Soc Belg Med Trop* 1993b ; 73 : 31-6.
- Faye O, Gaye O, Faye O, Diallo S. La transmission du paludisme dans des villages proches et éloignés de la mangrove en zone soudanienne, Sénégal. *Bull Soc Pathol Exot* 1994 ; 87 : 157-63.
- Faye O, Gaye O, Fontenille D, *et al*. La sécheresse et la baisse du paludisme dans les Niayes, Sénégal. *Cahiers Santé* 1995a ; 5 : 299-305.
- Faye O, Gaye O, Fontenille D, *et al*. Comparaison de la transmission du paludisme dans deux faciès épidémiologiques au Sénégal : la zone côtière sahélienne et la zone méridionale soudanienne. *Dakar Méd* 1995b ; 40 : 201-7.
- Faye O, Fontenille D, Gaye O, *et al*. Paludisme et riziculture dans le delta du fleuve Sénégal. *Ann Soc Belg Med Trop* 1995c ; 75 : 179-89.
- Faye O, Konate L, Mouchet J, *et al*. Indoor resting by outdoor biting females of *Anopheles gambiae* complex in the Sahel of Northern Senegal. *J Med Entomol* 1997 ; 34 : 285-9.
- Faye O, Gaye O, Fontenille D, *et al*. Aménagements hydro-agricoles et paludisme. In : Brengues J, Hervé JP, eds. *Aménagements hydro-agricoles et santé*. Paris : IRD ORSTOM, 1998 : 103-15.
- Feighner BH, Pak SI, Novakoski WL, Kelsey LL, Strickman D. Re-emergence of *Plasmodium vivax* malaria in the Republic of Korea. *Emerg Infect Dis* 1998 ; 4 : 295-7.
- Fenner F. The effect of changing social organisation on the infectious diseases of man. In : Boyden V, ed. *The impact of civilisation on the biology of man*. Toronto : University of Toronto Press, 1970 : 44-68.
- Fernandes A, Miyar R, Perez O, Shapira A, Lastre M. Relacao entre o diagnostico clinico e laboratorial do malaria. Hospital central de Maputo (HCM 1985). *Rev Med Moçambique* 1994 ; 5 : 37.
- Fernandez-Salas I, Rodriguez MH, Roberts DR, Rodriguez MC, Wirtz RA. Bionomics of adult *An. pseudopunctipennis* in the Tapachula foothills area of Southern Mexico. *J Med Entomol* 1994 ; 31 : 663-70.
- Ferraroni JJ, Hayes J. Aspectos epidemiologicos da malaria no Amazonas. *Acta Amazonica* 1979 (recorded 1981) ; 9 (3) : 471-9.
- Fleming AF, Storey J, Molineaux L, Iroko EA, Attai ED. Abnormal haemoglobins in the Sudan savannah of Nigeria. I. Prevalence of haemoglobins and relationships between sickle cell trait, malaria and survival. *Ann Trop Med Parasitol* 1979 ; 73 : 161-72.
- Floch H, de Lajudie P. Sur les divers indices endémiques du paludisme en Guyane Française. *Bull Soc Pathol Exot* 1946 ; 39 : 440-9.
- Fofana ML, Touré AA. Quelques aspects du changement climatique du Mali. *Assoc Int Climatol* 1994 ; 7 : 318-22.
- Fogg CL, Greenwood B, Gomez-Olive X, Alonso P. The epidemiology of adult malaria infection in a rural area of Mozambique. *Trans R Soc Trop Med Hyg* 2000 ; 94 : 128.
- Foley DH, Paru R, Dagoro H, Bryan JH. Allozyme analysis reveals six species within the *An. punctulatus* complex of mosquitoes in Papua New Guinea. *Med Vet Entomol* 1993 ; 7 : 37-48.
- Foley DH, Meek SR, Bryan JH. The *Anopheles punctulatus* group in the Solomon Island and Vanuatu surveyed by allozyme electrophoresis. *Med Vet Entomol* 1994 ; 8 : 340-50.
- Foley DH, Cooper RD, Bryan JH. A new species of *Anopheles punctulatus* complex in Western Province, Papua New Guinea. *J Am Mosq Control Assoc* 1995 ; 11 : 122-7.
- Foll CV, Pant CP, Lietaert PE. A large-scale field trial with dichlorvos as a residual fumigant insecticide in Northern Nigeria. *Bull World Health Organ* 1965 ; 32 : 531-50.
- Fondjo E, Robert V, Le Goff G, Toto JC, Carnevale P. Le paludisme urbain à Yaoundé, Cameroun. *Bull Soc Pathol Exot* 1992 ; 85 : 57-63.
- Fontaine RE, Najjar AE, Prince JS. The 1958 malaria epidemic in Ethiopia. *Am J Trop Med Hyg* 1961 ; 10 : 795-803.
- Fontaine RE, Pull JH, Payne D, *et al*. Evaluation of fenitrothion for the control of malaria. *Bull World Health Organ* 1978 ; 56 : 445-52.

- Fontaine RE, et al. Report of a mission to Swaziland. WHO/MAL/Geneva, 1987.
- Fontenille D. Hétérogénéité de la transmission des paludismes à Madagascar. *Mem Soc R Belge Entomol* 1992 ; 35 : 129-32.
- Fontenille D, Lepers JP, Campbell GH, Coluzzi M, Rakotoarivony I, Coulanges P. Malaria transmission and vector biology in Manarintsoa, High plateaux of Madagascar. *Am J Trop Med Hyg* 1990 ; 43 : 107-15.
- Fontenille D, Lepers JP, Coluzzi M, Campbell GH, Rakotoarivony I, Coulanges P. Malaria transmission and vector biology on Sainte Marie Island, Madagascar. *J Med Entomol* 1992 ; 29 : 197-202.
- Fontenille D, Campbell GH. Is *Anopheles mascarensis* a new malaria vector in Madagascar? *Am J Trop Med Hyg* 1992 ; 46 : 28-30.
- Fontenille D, Lochouarn L, Diagne N, et al. High annual and seasonal variations in malaria transmission by anophelines and vector species composition in Dielmo, a holoendemic area in Senegal. *Am J Trop Med Hyg* 1997a ; 56 : 247-53.
- Fontenille D, Lochouarn L, Diatta M, et al. Four years on entomological study of the transmission of seasonal malaria in Senegal and the bionomics of *An. gambiae* and *An. arabiensis*. *Trans R Soc Trop Med Hyg* 1997b ; 91 : 647-52.
- Fontenille D, Cohuet A, Awono-Ambene PH, et al. Systématique et biologie des anophèles vecteurs de *Plasmodium* en Afrique : données récentes. *Med Trop (Marseille)* 2003 ; 63 : 247-53.
- Forattini OP. *Entomologia medica. I. Parte Geral, Diptera ; Anophelini*. University of São Paulo, Brazil : Faculdade de Higiene e Saude Publica, 1962 ; vol. 1 : 662 p.
- Forattini OP, Kakitani I, Santos RL, Ueno HM, Kobayashi KM. Role of *An. (Kerteszia) bellator* as malaria vector in Southeastern Brazil. *Mem Inst Oswaldo Cruz* 1999 ; 94 (6) : 715-8.
- Forney JR, Magill AJ, Wongsrichanalai C, et al. Malaria rapid diagnostic devices: performance characteristics of the ParaSight F device determined in a multisite field study. *J Clin Microbiol* 2001 ; 39 (8) : 2884-90.
- Foumane V, Besnard P, LeMire J, Quinda F. *Rapport sur l'Enquête paludométrique menée à Balombo en novembre 2006*. Yaoundé 08 février 2007.
- Freeman T, Bradley M. Temperature is predictive of severe malaria years in Zimbabwe. *Trans R Soc Trop Med Hyg* 1996 ; 90 : 232.
- Frenzel B. Climatic changes in the Atlantic Sub Boreal transition in the Northern Hemisphere. In : *World Climate from 8000 to 0*. London : Royal Meteorological Society, 1991 : 91-123 .
- Fritz GN, Conn J, Cockburn A, Seawright J. Sequence analysis of the ribosomal DNA internal transcribed spacer 2 from populations of *Anopheles nuneztovari*. *Mol Biol Evol* 1994 ; 11 (3) : 406-16.
- Gabaldon A. Malaria control in the neotropical region. In : Boyd MF, ed. *Malariology*, Philadelphia : WB Saunders, 1949 : 1400-15.
- Gabaldon A. El porqué de la persistencia de la transmission de la malaria en Venezuela. *Arch Venezol Puericul Pediatr* 1965 ; 28 : 223-37.
- Gabaldon A. *Anopheles nuneztovari*: an important vector and agent of refractory malaria in Venezuela. *Bol Dir Malariol Saneamiento Ambiental* 1981 ; 21 (1) : 28-38.
- Gabaldon A, Guerrero L, Garcia Martin G. Malaria refractaria en el occidente de Venezuela. *Rev Venezolana Sanid Asist Social* 1963 ; 28 : 513-30.
- Gad AM. Mosquitoes of the oases of the Libyan desert in Egypt. *Bull Soc Entomol Egypte* 1956 ; 40 : 131-6.
- Gaffigan TV, Ward RA. Index to the second supplement to "A catalogue of the mosquitoes of the world" with corrections and additions. *Mosq Syst* 1985 ; 17 : 52-63.
- Gahan JB, Lindquist AW. DDT residual sprays applied in building to control *Anopheles quadrimaculatus*: practical tests. *J Econ Entomol* 1945 ; 38 : 223-35.
- Galloway PR, Lee RD, Hamel EA. In : Montgomery MR, Cohen B, eds. *From death to birth: mortality decline and reproductive change*. Washington : National Academic Press, 1998 : 182-226.
- Gallup JL, Sachs JD. The economic burden of malaria. *Am J Trop Med Hyg* 2001 ; 64 (suppl. 1-2) : 85-96.
- Gamble C, Ekwaru PJ, Garner P, ter Kuile FO. Insecticide-treated nets for the prevention of malaria in pregnancy: a systematic review of randomised controlled trials. *Plos Med* 2007 ; 274(3) : e107
- Ganczakowski M, Town M, Bowden DK, et al. Multiple G6PD deficient variants correlate with malaria endemicity in the Vanuatu archipelago. *Am J Hum Genet* 1995 ; 56 : 294-301.
- Garcia A, Marquet S, Bucheton B, et al. Linkage analysis of blood *P. falciparum* levels: interest of the 5q31-q33 chromosome region. *Am J Trop Med Hyg* 1998 ; 58 : 705-9.
- Gardiner CN, Biggar RJ, Collins WE, Nkrumah FK. Malaria in urban and rural areas of Southern Ghana: a survey of parasitaemia, antibodies and antimalarial practices. *Bull World Health Organ* 1984 ; 62 : 607-13 .
- Garfield R. Malaria control in Nicaragua: social and political influences on disease transmission and control activities. *Lancet* 1999 ; 354 (9176) : 414-8.
- Garfield RM, Frieden T, Vermund SH. Health-related outcomes of war in Nicaragua. *Am J Public Health* 1987 ; 77 (5) : 615-8.
- Garg M, Gopinathan N, Bodhe P, Kshirsagar NA. *Vivax* malaria resistant to chloroquine: case reports from Bombay. *Trans R Soc Trop Med Hyg* 1995 ; 89 : 656-7.
- Garnham PC. Malaria epidemics at exceptionally high altitudes in Kenya. *Br Med J* 1945 ; 14 Juill : 45-7.
- Garnham PC. The incidence of malaria at high altitudes. *J Natl Mal Soc (USA)* 1948 ; 7 : 275-84.
- Garnham PC. Distribution of simian malaria parasites in various hosts. *J Parasitol* 1963 ; 49 : 905-11.
- Garnham PC. *Malaria parasites and other haemosporidia*. Oxford : Blackwell Scientific Publication 1966 : 144 p.
- Garnham PC, Wilson DB, Wilson ME. Malaria in Kigezi, Uganda. *J Trop Med Hyg* 1948 ; 51 : 156-9.
- Garnham PC, Bray RS, Bruce-Chwatt LJ, et al. A strain of *P. vivax* characterised by prolonged incubation. *Bull World Health Organ* 1975 ; 52 : 21-32.
- Garrett-Jones C. Migratory flight in anopheline mosquitoes in the Middle East. *Bull Endem Dis (Baghdad)* 1957 ; 2 : 79-87.
- Garrett-Jones C, Shidrawi GR. Malaria vectorial capacity of a population of *Anopheles gambiae*. *Bull World Health Organ* 1969 ; 40 : 531-45.
- Garros C, Harbach RE, Manguin S. Morphological assessment and molecular phylogenetics of the Funestus and Minimus Groups of *Anopheles* (*Cellia*). *J Med Entomol* 2005 ; 42 : 522-36.
- Garros C, Van Bortel W, Trung HD, Coosemans M, Manguin S. Review of the Minimus Complex of *Anopheles*, main malaria vector in Southeast Asia: from taxonomic issues to vector control strategies. *Trop Med Intern Health* 2006 ; 11 : 102-14.
- Gascon J, Pluymaekaers J, Bada JL. Changing pattern of malaria in Nyarutovu (Rwanda). *Trans R Soc Trop Med Hyg* 1984 ; 78 : 421-2.
- Gautret P, Barreto M, Mendez F, Zorrilla G, Carrasquilla G. High prevalence of malaria in a village of the Colombian Pacific Coast. *Mem Inst Oswaldo Cruz* 1995 ; 90 (5) : 559-60 .
- Gautret P, Coquelin F, Mora-Silvera E, Chabaud AG, Landau I. Chronosexuality of *Plasmodium species* of Central African Muridae. *Parassitologia* 1998 ; 40 : 255-8.
- Gaye O, Diallo S, Faye O, et al. Épidémiologie des endémies parasitaires dans la zone de barrages antisel de Bignona, Sénégal. *Dakar Méd* 1991 ; 36 : 139-44.
- Gazin P, Robert V, Carnevale P. Étude longitudinale des indices paludologiques dans deux villages de la région de Bobo Dioulasso, Burkina Faso. *Ann Soc Belg Med Trop* 1985a ; 65 (suppl. 2) : 181-6.
- Gazin P, Robert V, Akogbeto M, Carnevale P. Réflexions sur les risques d'infection palustre selon la densité et l'infectivité anophéliennes. *Ann Soc Belg Med Trop* 1985b ; 65 : 263-9.
- Gazin P, Robert V, Carnevale P. Le paludisme urbain à Bobo-Dioulasso (Burkina Faso). 2. Les indices paludologiques. *Cahiers ORSTOM, Entomol Med Parasitol* 1987 ; 25 : 27-31.
- Gazin P, Robert V, Cot M, et al. Le paludisme dans l'Oudalan, région sahélienne du Burkina Faso. *Ann Soc Belg Med Trop* 1988a ; 68 : 255-64.
- Gazin P, Cot M, Sana S, et al. La part du paludisme dans les consultations d'un dispensaire sahélien. *Ann Soc Belg Med Trop* 1988b ; 68 : 15-24.
- Gazin P, Robert V, Cot M, Carnevale P. *Plasmodium falciparum* incidence and patency in a high seasonal transmission area of Burkina Faso. *Trans R Soc Trop Med Hyg* 1988c ; 82 : 50-5.
- Gazin P, LeGolf G, Ambassa P, Mulder L, Loué P, Carnevale P. *Étude du paludisme à Edea et Mbébé*. Doc. Tech. OCEAC, 680, SEM, 1989.
- Gbakima AA. Inland valley swamp rice development: malaria, schistosomiasis, onchocerciasis in South Central Sierra Leone. *Public Health* 1994 ; 108 : 149-57.
- Gebreel A. Malaria in Libya. Introduction and historical review. *Garyounis Med J* 1982 ; 5 : 70-1.
- Gebreel AO, Gilles HM, Prescott JE. Studies on the sero-epidemiology of endemic diseases in Libya. IV. Malaria. *Ann Trop Med Parasitol* 1985 ; 79 : 341-7.
- Gebre Mariam M. Malaria. In : Zein AH, Kloss H, eds. *The ecology of health and disease in Ethiopia*. Addis Abeba : Ethiopia's Ministry of Health, 1988 : 136 p.

- Gelfand HM. *Anopheles gambiae* and *An. melas* in a coastal area of Liberia, West Africa. *Trans R Soc Trop Med Hyg* 1955 ; 49 : 508-27.
- Gentile G, Slotman M, Ketmaier V, Powell JR, Caccone A. Attemps to molecularly distinguish cryptic taxa in *Anopheles gambiae s.s. Insect Mol Biol* 2001 ; 10 (1) : 25-32.
- Gentilini M, Danis M, Dallot JY, Richard-Lenoble D, Felix H. Réapparition du paludisme autochtone ? *Ann Med Intern (Paris)* 1978 ; 129 : 405-10.
- Gentilini M, Danis M. Le paludisme autochtone. *Med Mal Infect* 1982 ; 11 : 356-62.
- Genton B, Smith T, Baea K, et al. Malaria: how useful are clinical criteria for improving the diagnosis in a highly endemic area? *Trans R Soc Trop Med Hyg* 1994 ; 88 : 537-41.
- Georghiou GP. Studies on resistance to carbamate and organophosphorus insecticides in *Anopheles albimanus*. *Am J Trop Med Hyg* 1972 ; 21 (5) : 797-806.
- Georghiou GP. *The implication of agricultural insecticides in the development of resistance by mosquitoes with emphasis on control America*. Proceedings International Whorkshop 22-26 Feb 1982. Resistance to insecticides used in Public Health and Agriculture. Colombo : National Science Council of Sri Lanka Publications, 1982 : 95-121.
- Gerry F, Killeen GF, Smith TA, et al. Preventing childhood malaria in Africa by protecting adults from mosquitoes with insecticide-treated nets. *PLoS Med* 2007 ; 4 : e229.
- Gevrey A. *Les Comores*. Pondichéry : Saligny, 1870 : 307 p.
- Ghebreyesus TA, Haile M, Witten KH, et al. Incidence of malaria among children living near dams in Northern Ethiopia: community based incidence survey. *Br Med J* 1999 ; 319 (7211) : 663-6.
- Ghebreyesus TA, Haile M, Witten KH, et al. Household risk factors for malaria among children in Ethiopian highlands. *Trans R Soc Trop Med Hyg* 2000 ; 94 : 17-21.
- Ghosh KK, Chakraborty S, Bhattacharya S, Palit A, Tandon N, Hati AK. *An. annularis* as a vector of malaria in rural West Bengal. *Indian J Malariol* 1985 ; 22 : 65-9.
- Giacomini T, Brumpt LC, Petithory JC. Le paludisme des aéroports. Critères diagnostiques et conséquences médicolégales. *Med Mal Infect* 1984 ; 7/8 : 376-83.
- Giacomini T, Mouchet J, Mathieu P, Petithory JC. Étude de six cas de paludisme contractés près de Roissy-Charles de Gaulle en 1994. Mesures de prévention nécessaires dans les aéroports. *Bull Acad Natl Med* 1995 ; 179 : 335-51.
- Giacomini T, Axler O, Mouchet J, et al. Pitfalls in the diagnosis of airport malaria. Seven cases observed in the Paris area in 1994. *Scand J Infect Dis* 1997 ; 29 : 433-5.
- Giaquinto-Mira M. Notes on the geographical distribution and biology of *Anophelinae* and *Culicinae* in Ethiopia. *Riv Malariol* 1950 ; 29 : 282-313.
- Gibbins EG. Natural malaria infection of house frequenting *Anopheles* mosquitoes in Uganda. *Ann Trop Med Parasitol* 1932 ; 26 : 239-66.
- Giglioli G. Malaria in British Guiana. Part 4. *Agr J Brit Guiana* 1949 ; 10 (1) : 4-12.
- Giglioli G. Eradication of *Anopheles darlingi* from the inhabited areas of British Guiana by DDT residual spraying. *J Natl Mal Soc* 1951 ; 10 : 142-61.
- Giglioli G. Ecological change as a factor in renewed malaria transmission in an eradicated area. A localized outbreak of *Anopheles aquasalis* transmitted malaria on the Demerara River estuary, British Guyana, in the fifteenth years of *An. darlingi* and malaria eradication. *Bull World Health Organ* 1963 ; 29 : 131-45.
- Giglioli ME. Tides, salinity and the breeding of *An. melas* during the dry season in the Gambia. *Riv Malariol* 1964 ; 43 : 245-63.
- Giha HA, Rosthoj S, Dodoo D, et al. The epidemiology of febrile malaria episodes in an area of unstable and seasonal transmission. *Trans R Soc Trop Med Hyg* 2000 ; 94 : 645-51.
- Gilbert SC, Plebanski M, Gupta S, et al. Association of malaria parasite population structure, HLA, and immunological antagonism. *Science* 1998 ; 279 : 1173-7.
- Gil Collado J. *Quelques considérations sur les gîtes larvaires des culicidés espagnols*. Comptes rendus du XIIe Congrès International de Zoologie. Lisbonne, 1935 ; vol. 1 : 2065-78.
- Gil Collado J. La distribucion geografica de las variedades de *Anopheles maculipennis* en España, con breves consideraciones acerca de su biologia. *Riv Malariol* 1937 ; 16 (I) : 276-89.
- Gilles HM, Lawson JB, Sibelas M, Voller A, Allan N. Malaria, anaemia and pregnancy. *Ann Trop Med Parasitol* 1969 ; 63 (2) : 245-63.
- Gillet J. Le paludisme au Congo Belge et au Ruanda-Urundi. *Bull Sc Inst R Colon Belge* 1953 ; 24 : 1342-61.
- Gillies MT. The density of adult *Anopheles* in the neighbourhood of an East African village. *Am J Trop Med Hyg* 1955 ; 4 : 1103-13.
- Gillies MT. The problem of exophily in *An. gambiae*. *Bull World Health Organ* 1956 ; 15 : 437-49.
- Gillies MT. Studies on the dispersion and survival of *An. gambiae* in East Africa by means of marking and release experiments. *Bull Entomol Res* 1961 ; 52 : 99-127.
- Gillies MT. *Assigment report. Lake Nasser development center Asswan. Anopheles gambiae, a potential invader*. Oct./Dec. 1971. WHO/EM/MAC/107, February 1972 : 21 p.
- Gillies MT, Smith A. The effect of a residual house-spraying campaign in East Africa on species balance in the *Anopheles funestus* group. The replacement of *An. funestus* by *An. rivulorum*. *Bull Entomol Res* 1960 ; 51 : 243-53.
- Gillies MT, de Meillon B. *The Anophelinae of Africa south of the Sahara (Ethiopian zoogeographical region)*, 2nd ed. Johannesburg : South African Institute for Medical Research, 1968 ; 54 : 343 p.
- Gillies MT, Coetzee M. *A supplement to the Anophelinae of Africa south of the Sahara (Afrotropical Region)*. Johannesburg : South African Institute for Medical Research, 1987 ; 55 : 141 p.
- Gilroy A. Health in tea gardens of Darjeeling Terai with special reference to malaria. *J Malaria Inst India* 1939 ; 2 : 165-79.
- Giri RS, Roche S, Benthein F, Sarr M. *Report on the malaria situation in Zanzibar Isles*. WHO/ICP/MPD/002 Team, 16 Feb.-19 April 1984.
- Girod R. *La lutte contre la réintroduction du paludisme à la Réunion. Étude entomologique du risque de reprise de la transmission autochtone*. Thèse Doctorat Sciences, Université de la Réunion, 2001.
- Girod R, Salvan M, Denys JC. Lutte contre la réintroduction du paludisme à la Réunion. *Cahiers Santé* 1995 ; 5 : 397-401.
- Girod R, Salvan M, Simard F, Andrianaivolambo L, Fontenille D, Laventure S. Évaluation de la capacité vectorielle d'*An. arabiensis* à l'île de la Réunion : une approche du risque sanitaire lié au paludisme d'importation en zone d'éradication. *Bull Soc Pathol Exot* 1999 ; 92 : 203-9.
- Githeko AK, Brandling-Bennett AD, Beier M, Atieli F, Owaga M, Collins FH. The reservoir of *P. falciparum* malaria in a holoendemic area of Western Kenya. *Trans R Soc Trop Med Hyg* 1992 ; 86 : 355-8.
- Glick JI. Illustrated key to the female *Anopheles* of South-Western Asia and Egypt. *Mosq Syst* 1992 ; 24 :125-53.
- Gogoi SC, Dev V, Phookan S. Morbidity and mortality due to malaria in Tarajulie Tea Estate, Assam, India. *Southeast Asian J Trop Med Public Health* 1996 ; 27 : 526-9.
- Golgi C. Sulla infezione malarica. *G Acad Med Torino* 1885 ; 33 : 734.
- Goma LK. The swamp-breeding mosquitoes of Uganda: records of larvae and their habitats. *Bull Entomol Res* 1960a ; 51 : 77-94.
- Goma LK. Experimental breeding of *Anopheles gambiae* in Papyrus Swamps. *Nature* 1960b ; 187 : 1137-8.
- Goncalves A, Ferrinho P, Dias F. The epidemiology of malaria in Prabis, Guinea-Bissau. *Mem Inst Oswaldo Cruz*, 1996 ; 91 : 11-7.
- Gonzales JM, Olano V, Vergara J, et al. Unstable, low-level transmission of malaria on the Colombian Pacific Coast. *Ann Trop Med Parasitol* 1997 ; 91 (4) : 349-58.
- Gopaul AR, Konfortion P. Roof top breeding of *Anopheles arabiensis* and spread of malaria in Mauritius. *Maurice Inst Bull* 1988 ; 10 : 2-12.
- Gordeev MI, Zvantsov AB, Goriacheva II, Shaikevich EV, Ezhov MN. Description of the new species *Anopheles artemievi* sp.n. (Diptera, Culicidae). *Med Parazitol (Mosk)* 2005 ; 2 : 4-5.
- Gorgas WC. *Sanitation in Panama*. New York : Appleton, 1915.
- Gorham JR, Stojanovich CJ, Scott HG. Illustrated key to the anopheline mosquitoes of Western South America. *Mosq Syst* 1973 ; 5 : 97-156.
- Goswami G, Singh OP, Nanda N, Raghavendra K, Gakhar SK, Subbarao SK. Identification of all members of the *Anopheles culicifacies* complex using allele-specific polymerase chain reaction assays. *Am J Trop Med Hyg* 2006 ; 75 : 454-60.
- Govere J, Durrheim DN, Coetzee M, Hunt R. Malaria in Mpumalanga Province, South Africa, with special reference to the periode 1987-1999. *S Afr J Sci* 2001 ; 97 : 55-8.
- Grab B, Pull JH. Statistical considerations in serological surveys of population with particular reference to malaria. *J Trop Med Hyg* 1974 ; 77 : 222-32.
- Gramiccia G. Endémie palustre au Liban. *Rev Med Moyen Orient* 1953 ; 10 : 293-309.
- Gramiccia G. *Anopheles claviger* in the Middle East. *Bull World Health Organ* 1956 ; 15 : 816-21.
- Gramiccia G, Hempel K. Mortality and morbidity from malaria in countries where malaria eradication is not making satisfactory progress. *J Trop Med Hyg* 1972 ; 75 : 187-92.
- Granja AC, Machungo F, Gomes A, Bergström S, Brabin B. Malaria-related maternal mortality in urban Mozambique. *Ann Trop Med Parasitol* 1998 ; 92 : 257-63.

- Grassi B. *Studi di uno zoologo sulla malaria*. Roma : Reale Academia Lincei, 1900 : 215 p.
- Grassi B, Feletti B. Uber die parasiten der malaria. *Zbl Beskt* 1890 ; 7 : 396-401 et 430-5.
- Grassi B, Bignami A. La malaria propagata per mezzo di peculiari insetti. *Atti Acad Naz Linnei Rc* 1898 ; 7 : 234.
- Grassi B, Bignami A, Bastianelli G. Ciclo evolutivo della semilune nell' *Anopheles claviger*. *Atti Soc Studi Malar* 1899 ; 1 : 14.
- Graves PM, Brabin BJ, Charlwood JD, *et al*. Reduction in incidence and prevalence of *Plasmodium falciparum* in under-5-years-old children by permethrin impregnation of mosquito nets. *Bull World Health Organ* 1987 ; 65 (6) : 869-77.
- Graves P, Gelb and H. *Vaccine for preventing malaria*. Cochrane review, issue n°3 ; update software. Oxford : The Cochrane Library, 2001.
- Green CA, Miles SJ. Chromosomal evidence for sibling species of the malaria vector *Anopheles culicifacies*. *J Trop Med Hyg* 1980 ; 83 : 75-8.
- Green CA, Baimai V, Harrison BA, Andre RG. Cytogenetic evidence for a complex of species within the taxon *Anopheles maculatus*. *Biol J Linnean Soc* 1985 ; 24 : 321-8.
- Green CA, Gass RF, Munstermann LE, Baimai V. Population genetic evidence for two species in *Anopheles minimus* in Thailand. *Med Vet Entomol* 1990 ; 4 : 25-34.
- Green CA, Rattanarithikul R, Pongparit S, Sawadwongporn P, Baimai V. A newly-recognized vector of human malarial parasites in the Oriental Region, *Anopheles pseudowillmori*. *Trans R Soc Trop Med Hyg* 1991 ; 85 : 35-6.
- Green CA, Rattanarithikul R, Charoensub A. Population genetic confirmation of species status of the malaria vectors *Anopheles willmori* and *An. pseudowillmori* in Thailand and chromosome phylogeny of the maculatus group of mosquitoes. *Med Vet Entomol* 1992 ; 6 : 335-41.
- Greenberg AE, Ntumbanzondo M, Ntula N, Mawa L, Howell J, Davachi F. Hospital-based surveillance of malaria-related paediatric morbidity and mortality in Kinshasa, Zaire. *Bull World Health Organ* 1989 ; 67 : 189-96.
- Greenwood BM. Asymptomatic malaria infections. Do they matter? *Parasitol Today* 1987 ; 3 : 206-14.
- Greenwood BM, Bradley AK, Greenwood AM, *et al*. Mortality and morbidity from malaria among children in a rural area of the Gambia, West Africa. *Trans R Soc Trop Med Hyg* 1987a ; 81 : 478-86.
- Greenwood BM, Groenendaal F, Bradley AK, *et al*. Ethnic differences in the prevalence of splenomegaly and malaria in the Gambia. *Ann Trop Med Parasitol* 1987b ; 81 : 345-54.
- Gribbin J. The end of ice ages? *New Scientist* 1989 ; 17 : 48-52.
- Grieco JP, Achee NL, Andre RG, Roberts DR. A comparison study of house entering and exiting behavior of *An. vestitipennis* using experimental huts sprayed with DDT or deltamethrin in the Southern District of Toledo, Belize. *J Vector Ecol* 2000 ; 25 (1) : 62-73.
- Grieco JP, Johnson S, Achee NL, *et al*. Distribution of *Anopheles albimanus*, *Anopheles vestitipennis* and *An. crucians* associated with land use in northern Belize. *J Med Entomol* 2006 ; 43 : 614-22.
- Gringrich JB, Weatherhead A, Sattabongkot J, Pilakasiri C, Wirtz RA. Hyperendemic malaria in a Thai village. Dependence of year-round transmission on focal and seasonally circumscribed mosquito habitats. *J Med Entomol* 1990 ; 27 : 1016-26.
- Grjebine A. Culicidae Anophelinae. Faune de Madagascar, T. XXII. Paris : ORSTOM-CNRS, 1966 : 489 p.
- Grmek MD. La malaria dans la Méditerranée Orientale préhistorique et antique. *Parassitologia* 1994 ; 36 : 1-6.
- Guarda JA, Asayag CR, Witzig R. Malaria reemergence in the Peruvian Amazon Region. *Emerg Infect Dis* 1999 ; 5 (2) : 209-15.
- Guillet P, Germain MC, Giacomini T, *et al*. Origin and prevention of airport malaria in France. *J Trop Med Public Health* 1998 ; 3 : 700-5.
- Guillo du Bodan H. *Contribution à l'étude de la morbidité et de la mortalité des enfants de moins de cinq ans en milieu tropical*. Thèse Médecine, Paris Sud, 1982.
- Guinet F, Diallo DA, Minta D, *et al*. A comparison of the incidence of severe malaria in Malian children with normal and C-trait hemoglobin profiles. *Acta Tropica* 1997 ; 68 : 175-82.
- Gülmezoglu AM, Garner P. *Prevention versus treatment for malaria pregnant women* (Cochrane Review) Issue 1 Update Software. Oxford : The Cochrane Library, 1999.
- Gunasekaran K. Age composition, natural survival and population growth of *Anopheles fluviatilis*, the major malaria vector in the endemic belt of Koraput District, Orissa, India. *Southeast Asian J Trop Med Public Health* 1994 ; 25 : 196-200.
- Gunasekaran K, Sadanandane C, Parida SK, Sahu SS, Patra KP, Jambulingam P. Observations on nocturnal activity and man biting habits of malaria vectors *Anopheles fluviatilis*, *An. annularis*, *An. culicifacies* in the hill tracts of Koraput District, Orissa, India. *Southeast Asian J Trop Med Public Health* 1994 ; 25 : 187-95.
- Gusmao R. The control of malaria in Brazil. In : Casman E, Dowlatabi H, eds. *The contextual determinants of malaria*. Washington : Ressources for the Future Press, 2002 : 59-65.
- Guttoso C. *The Kpain malaria project*. AFR/Mal/61/43. Third African Malaria Conference. WHO CCTA, 30 mai 1962.
- Guy Y. *Les Anophèles du Maroc*. Rabat : Mémoires de la Société des Sciences naturelles et Physiques du Maroc 1959, Série Zoologie : n° 7.
- Guy Y. Bilan épidémiologique du paludisme au Maroc. *Ann Parasitol Hum Comp (Paris)* 1963 ; 38 : 823-57.
- Guy Y, Holstein M. Données récentes sur les anophèles du Maghreb. *Arch Inst Pasteur Algérie* 1968 ; 46 : 142-50.
- Habluetzel AW, Diallo A, Eposito F, *et al*. Do insecticide impregnated curtains reduce all cause of child mortality in Burkina Faso? *Trop Med Int Health* 1997 ; 9 : 855-62.
- Hackett BJ, Gimnig J, Guelbeogo W, *et al*. Ribosomal DNA internal transcribed spacer (ITS2) sequences differentiate *An. funestus* and *An. rivulorum*, and uncover a cryptic taxon. *Insect Mol Biol* 2000 ; 9 : 369-74.
- Hackett LW. The present status of our knowledge of the sub-species of *Anopheles maculipennis*. *Trans R Soc Trop Med Hyg* 1934 ; 28 : 109-40.
- Hackett LW. *Malaria in Europe, an ecological study*. London : Oxford University Press, 1937 : 336 p.
- Hackett LW. Spleen measurements in Malaria. *J Natl Mal Soc* 1944 ; 3 : 121.
- Hackett LW. The malaria of the Andean Region of South America. *Rev Inst Salubr Enferm Trop (Mexico)* 1945 ; 6 (4) : 239-52.
- Hackett LW. Distribution of malaria. In : Boyd MF, ed. *Malariology*, vol. 1. Philadelphia : WB Saunders, 1949 ; vol. 1 : 722-35.
- Hackett LW, Barber MA. Notes on the varieties of *Anopheles maculipennis* in the USSR. *Med Parazitol (Mosk)* 1935 ; 4 : 188-99.
- Hackett LW, Russel PF, Scharff JW, Senior-White R. The present use of naturalistic measures in the control of malaria. *Bull Health Organ League Nations* 1938 ; 7 : 1016-57.
- Haddow AJ, Van Someren EC, Lumsden WH, Harper JO, Gillet JD. The mosquitoes of Bwamba County Uganda. VIII. Records of occurrence, behaviour and habitat. *Bull Entomol Res* 1951 ; 42 : 207-38.
- Haines A, Epstein PR, McMichael AJ. Global health watch: monitoring impacts of environmental changes. *Lancet* 1993 ; 342 : 1464-9.
- Halawani A, Shawarby AA. Malaria in Egypt. *J Egypt Med Assoc* 1957 ; 40 : 753-92.
- Hamon J. Étude biologique et systématique des culicidés de l'Ile de la Réunion. *Mem Inst Sci Madag* 1953 ; 4 : 521-54.
- Hamon J, Dufour G. La lutte antipaludique à la Réunion. *Bull Organ Mond Santé* 1954 ; 11 : 525-56.
- Hamon J, Adam JP, Grjebine A. Observations sur la répartition et le comportement des anophèles de l'Afrique Équatoriale, du Cameroun et de l'Afrique Occidentale. *Bull Organ Mond Santé* 1956a ; 15 : 549-91.
- Hamon J, Rickenbach A, Robert P. Seconde contribution à l'étude des moustiques du Dahomey. *Ann Parasitol Hum Comp* 1956b ; 31 : 619-35.
- Hamon J, Mouchet J. Les vecteurs secondaires du paludisme humain en Afrique. *Med Trop (Marseille)* 1961 ; 21 : 643-60.
- Hamon J, Dedewanou B, Eyraud M. Études entomologiques sur la transmission du paludisme humain dans une zone forestière africaine, la région de Man en République de Côte d'Ivoire. *Bull IFAN* 1962 ; 24 série A : 854-69.
- Hamon J, Maffi M, Ouedraogo CS, Djime D. Note sur les moustiques de la République Islamique de Mauritanie. *Bull Soc Entomol Fr* 1964 ; 69 : 233-53.
- Hamon J, Coz J, Sales S, Ouedraogo C. Études entomologiques sur la transmission du paludisme humain dans une zone de steppe boisée, la région de Dori (République de Haute-Volta). *Bull IFAN* 1965 ; 27 série A (3) : 1115-39.
- Hansford CF. Malaria control in the Northern Transvaal. *S Afr Med J* 1974 ; 48 : 1265-9.
- Harbach RE. Review of the internal classification of the genus *Anopheles* (Diptera: Culicidae): the foundation for comparative systematics and phylogenetic research. *Bull Entomol Res* 1994 ; 84 : 331-42.
- Harbach RE. The classification of genus *Anopheles* (Diptera: Culicidae): a working hypothesis of phylogenetic relationships. *Bull Entomol Res* 2004 ; 94 : 537-53.
- Harbach RE, Baimai V, Sukowati S. Some observations on sympatric populations of the malaria vectors *Anopheles leucosphyrus* and *An. balabacensis* in a village-forest setting in South Kalimantan. *Southeast Asian J Trop Med Public Health* 1987a ; 18 : 241-7.

- Harbach RE, Gingrich JB, Pang LW. Some entomological observations on malaria transmission in a remote village of North-Western Thailand. *J Am Mosq Control Assoc* 1987b ; 3 : 296-301.
- Harbach RE, Roberts DR, Manguin S. Variation in the hindtarsal markings of *Anopheles darlingi* in Belize. *Mosq Syst* 1993 ; 25 (3) : 192-7.
- Harbach RE, Townson H. Mukwaya LG, Adeniran T. Use of rDNA-PCR to investigate the ecological distribution of *Anopheles bwambae* in relation to other members of the *An. gambiae* complex of mosquitoes in Bwamba County, Uganda. *Med Vet Entomol* 1997 ; 11 (4) : 329-34.
- Harbach RE, Kitching IJ. Phylogeny and classification of the Culicidae (Diptera). *System Entomol* 1998 ; 23 : 327-70.
- Hargreaves K, Koekemoer LL, Brooke BD, Hunt RH, Mthembu J, Coetzee M. *An. funestus* resistant to pyrethroid insecticides in South Africa. *Med Vet Entomol* 2000 ; 14 : 181-9.
- Haridi AM. Partial exophily of *Anopheles gambiae* species B in the Khashm Elgirba area in Eastern Sudan. *Bull World Health Organ* 1972 ; 46 : 39-46.
- Harinasuta C, Reynolds DC. *Problems of malaria in the SEAMIC countries*. Proceedings of the 12th SEAMIC Workshop. Bangkok, Thailand, 20-24 August 1984. Tokyo : Southeast Asian Medical Information Center, 1985 : 184 p.
- Harinasuta T, Gilles HM, Sandosham AA. Malaria in Southeast Asia. *Southeast Asian J Trop Med Public Health* 1976 ; 7 (4) : 645-78.
- Harinasuta T. Bunnag D. The clinical features of malaria. In : Wernsdorfer WH, McGregor I, eds. *Malaria principles and practice of malariology*, vol. 1. London : Churchill Livingstone, 1988 ; 709-34.
- Harris AF, Matias-Arnez A, Hill N. Biting time of *Anopheles darlingi* in the Bolivian Amazon and implications for control of malaria. *Trans R Soc Trop Med Hyg* 2006 ; 100 : 45-47.
- Harrison BA. The *Myzomyia* series of *Anopheles* (*Cellia*) in Thailand with emphasis on interspecific variation. Medical entomology studies XIII. *Contrib Am Entomol Inst* 1980 ; 17 : 195 p.
- Harrison BA. Rattanarithikul R, Peyton EL, Mongkolpanya K. Taxonomic changes, revised occurrence records and notes on the *Culicidae* of Thailand and neighbouring countries. *Mosq Syst* 1990 ; 22 : 196-227.
- Harwin RM, Goldsmid JM. Malaria in the Rhodesian highveld. *Rhodesia Sc News* 1972 ; 6 : 167-70.
- Hastenrath S. *The glaciers of equatorial East Africa*. Dordrecht : Reidel Publishing Company, 1984.
- Hasting IM, Watkins WM, White NJ. The evolution of drug-resistant malaria: the role of drug elimination half-life. *Phil Trans R Soc London* 2000 ; B 357 : 505-19.
- Hati AK. Urban malaria vector biology. *Indian J Med Res* 1997 ; 106 : 149-63.
- Haworth J. The global distribution of malaria and the present control effort. In : Wernsdorfer WH, McGregor I, eds. *Malaria*. Edinburgh : Churchill Livingstone, 1988 : 1379 p.
- Hay SI, Snow RW, Rogers DJ. From predicting mosquito habitats to malaria seasons using remotely sensed data: practice, problems and perspectives. *Parasitol Today* 1998 ; 14 : 306-13.
- Hay SI, Rogers DJ, Toomer JF, Snow RW. Annual *Plasmodium falciparum* entomological inoculation rates (EIR) across Africa: literature survey, Internet access and review. *Trans R Soc Trop Med Hyg* 2000 ; 94 : 113-27.
- Hay SI, Rogers DJ, Shanks GD, Myers MF, Snow RW. Malaria early warning in Kenya. *Trends Parasitol* 2001 ; 17 (2) : 95-9.
- Hay SI, Rogers DJ, Randolph SE, *et al*. Hot topic or hot air? Climate change and malaria resurgence in East African highlands. *Trends Parasitol* 2002a ; 18 (12) : 530-4.
- Hay SI, Cox J, Rogers DJ, *et al*. Climate change and the resurgence of malaria in the East African Highlands. *Nature* 2002b ; 415 : 905-9.
- Hayes J, Calderon G, Falcon R, Zambrano V. Newly incriminated anopheline vectors of human malaria parasites in Junin Dpt, Peru. *J Am Mosq Control Assoc* 1987 ; 3 : 418-22.
- Hedman P, Brohult J, Forslund J, Sirleaf V, Bengtsson E. A pocket of controlled malaria in a holoendemic region of West Africa. *Ann Trop Med Parasitol* 1979 ; 73 : 317-25.
- Hehir P. *Malaria in India*. London : Oxford University Press 1927 : 490 p.
- Heinemann SJ, Belkin JN. Collection records of the project "Mosquitoes of Middle America". 8 Central America: Belize (BH), Guatemala (GUA), El Salvador (SAL), Honduras (HON), Nicaragua (NI, NIC). *Mosq Syst* 1977a ; 9 (4) : 403-54.
- Heinemann SJ, Belkin JN. Collection records of the project "Mosquitoes of Middle America". 9 Mexico (MEX, MF, MT, MX). *Mosq Syst* 1977b ; 9 (4) : 483-535.
- Heisch RB. Two years medical work in the Northern frontier District, Kenya Colony. *East Afr Med J* 1947 ; 24 : 3-15.
- Heisch RB, Harper JO. An epidemic of malaria in the Kenya Highlands transmitted by *Anopheles funestus*. *J Trop Med Hyg* 1949 ; 52 : 187-90.
- Hemmer R. Airport malaria in Luxembourg. *Eurosurveillance Weekly* 1999 ; 34.
- Hendrickse RG. The quartan malaria nephrotic syndrome. *Adv Nephrol Necker Hosp* 1976 ; 6 : 229-47.
- Hendrickse RG, Adeniyi A. Quartan malaria nephrotic syndrom in children. *Kidney Int* 1979 ; 16 : 64-74.
- Henry MC, Eggelte TA, Watson P, Van Leeuwen B, Bakker DA, Kluin J. Response of childhood malaria to chloroquine and Fansidar® in an area of intermediate chloroquine resistance in Côte d'Ivoire. *Trop Med Int Health* 1996 ; 1 : 610-5.
- Henry MC, Kone M, Guillet P, Mouchet J. Chloroquino-résistance et lutte antipaludique en Côte d'Ivoire. *Cahiers Santé* 1998 ; 8 : 287-91.
- Henry MC, Rogier C, Nzeyimana I, *et al*. Inland valley rice production systems and malaria infection and disease in the savannah of Côte d'Ivoire. *Trop Med Int Health* 2003 ; 8 : 449-58.
- Henry MC, Assi SB, Rogier C, Dossou-Yovo J, Chandre F, Guillet P, Carnevale P. Protective efficacy of lambda-cyhalothrin treated nets in *Anopheles gambiae* pyrethroid resistance areas of Côte d'Ivoire. *Am J Trop Med Hyg* 2005 ; 73 : 859-64.
- Hernberg CA, Tuomela A. Incubation time of malaria tertiane during an epidemic in Finland in 1945. *Acta Med Scand* 1948 ; 130 (suppl. 206) : 534-6.
- Hervy JP, Le Goff G, Geoffroy B, Hervé JP, Manga L, Brunhes J. *Les anophèles de la région Afrotropicale*. Logiciel d'identification et d'enseignement, CD-ROM. Paris : IRD, 1998.
- Hewitt S, Rowland M, Muhammad N, Kamal M, Kemp E. Pyrethroid-sprayed tents for malaria control: an entomological evaluation in Pakistan. *Med Vet Entomol* 1995 ; 9 (4) : 344-52.
- Highton RB, Van Someren EC. The transportation of mosquitoes between international airports. *Bull World Health Organ* 1970 ; 42 : 334-5.
- Highton RB, Bryan JH, Boreham PF, Chandler JA. Studies on the sibling species of *An. gambiae* and *An. arabiensis* in the Kisumu area, Kenya. *Bull Entomol Res* 1979 ; 69 : 43-53.
- Hightower AW, Ombok M, Otieno R, *et al*. A geographic information system applied to a malaria field study in Western Kenya. *Am J Trop Med Hyg* 1998 ; 58 : 266-72.
- Hii JL, Kan S, Vun YS, *et al*. Transmission dynamics and estimates of malaria vectorial capacity for *Anopheles balabacensis* and *An. flavirostris* on Banggi Island, Sabah, Malaysia. *Ann Trop Med Parasitol* 1988 ; 82 (1) : 91-101.
- Hii JL, Alexander N, Chuan CK, Rahman HA, Safri A, Chan M. Lambdacyalothrin impregnated bednets control malaria in Sabah, Malaysia. *Southeast Asian J Trop Med Public Health* 1995 ; 26 (2) : 371-4.
- Hill AV, Allsopp CE, Kwiatkowski D, *et al*. Common West African HLA antigens are associated with protection from severe malaria. *Nature* 1991 ; 352 : 595-600.
- Hill E, Haydon LG. The epidemic of malaria fever in Natal Province. *S Afr J Hyg* 1905 ; 5 : 467-84.
- Hill RB, Cambournac FJ. Intermittent irrigation in rice cultivation and its effects on yield, water consumption and *Anopheles* production. *Am J Trop Med Hyg* 1941 ; 21 : 123-44.
- Hill WG, Babiker HA. Estimation on numbers of malaria clones on blood samples. *Proc R Soc Lond B Biol Sci* 1995 ; 262 : 249-57.
- *Hippocrates Works* (Trad Jones WHS). London : Loeb Classical Library,1932.
- Hira PR. Koularas A. Studies on malaria in Lusaka. *Med J Zambia* 1974 ; 8 : 32-5.
- Hirsch A. Malaria diseases. In : *Handbook of geographical and historical pathology*. London : Sydenham Society, 1883.
- Ho C. Studies on malaria in new China. *Chin Med J* 1965 ; 84 : 491-7.
- Ho C, Chou TC, Ch'en TH, Hsueh AT. The *Anopheles hyrcanus* group and its relation to malaria in East China. *Chin Med J* 1962 ; 81 : 71-8.
- Hoffman SL, Franke ED, Heligdale, Druilhe In : Hoffman SL, ed. *Malaria vaccine development: a multi-immune response approach*. Washington : American Society for Microbiology, 1996 : 35-75.
- Hogh B, Gamage-Mendis A, Butcher GA, *et al*. The differing impact of choroquine and pyrimethamine/sulfadoxine upon the infectivity of malaria species to the mosquito vector. *Am J Trop Med Hyg* 1998 ; 58 (2) : 176-82.
- Ho Kwei-Ming, Jung K, Ko HL. The physiological age of *Anopheles hyrcanus sinensis* in the Canton area. *Acta Entomol Sinica* 1965 ; 14 : 54-60.

- Holding PA, Stevenson J, Pershu N, Marsh K. Cognitive sequelae of malaria with impaired consciousness. *Trans R Soc Trop Med Hyg* 1999 ; 93 : 529-34.
- Holstein MH. *Biologie d'*Anopheles gambiae*, recherches en Afrique Occidentale Française*. OMS Série des Monographies n°9 ; 1952 : 176 p.
- Holstein M, Le Corroller Y, Addadi K, Guy Y. Contribution à la connaissance des anophèles du Sahara. *Arch Inst Pasteur Algérie* 1970 ; 48 : 7-15.
- Holvoet G, Michielsen P, Vandepitte J. Airport malaria in Belgium. *Lancet* 1982 ; 2 : 881-2.
- Hommel D, Bollandard F, Hullin A. Paludisme grave à *P. falciparum*. Aspects actuels en zone d'endémie guyanaise. *Semaine Hopitaux* 1997 ; 73 : 197-205.
- Hooey DH. Fundamental facts concerning malaria in the North Eastern Transvaal. *S Afr Med J* 1974 ; 48 : 1171-4.
- Houel G, Donadille F. Vingt ans de lutte antipaludique au Maroc. *Bull Inst Hyg Maroc* 1953 ; 13 : 1-51.
- Houghton RA. Effects of land-use change, surface temperature and CO_2 concentration on terrestrial stores of carbon. In : Woodwell GM, Mackensie FT, eds. *Biotic feedbacks in the global climatic system.* New York : Oxford University Press, 1995 : 333-66.
- Hribar LJ. Geographic variation of male genitalia of *Anopheles nuneztovari* (Diptera : Culicidae). *Mosq Syst* 1994 ; 26 : 132-44.
- Htay-Aung, Minn S, Thaung S, *et al*. Well-breeding *Anopheles dirus* and their role in malaria transmission in Myanmar. *Southeast Asian J Trop Med Public Health* 1999 ; 30 : 447-53.
- Hu H, Singhasivanon P, Salazar NP, *et al*. Factors influencing malaria endemicity in Yunnan Province, PR China. *Southeast Asian J Trop Med Public Health* 1998 ; 29 : 191-201.
- Huang SZ. Analysis on epidemic characteristics of *falciparum* malaria in South Henan. *Chin J Parasitol Parasit Dis* 1987 ;5 : 18-20.
- Huang SZ, Lin SX. *Public health in contemporary China*. Beijing : Chinese Social Science Pubication House, 1986 : 248-68.
- Hudleston J. *Programme de prééradication du paludisme, Kaedi, Mauritanie*. WHO/AFR/Mal/74, 1961, 17 p.
- Hudson JE. *Anopheles darlingi* Root (Diptera: Culicidae) in the Suriname rain forest. *Bull Entomol Res* 1984 ; 74 : 129-42.
- Hulme M. Representing twentieth century space-time climate variability. Part I. Development of a 1961-90 mean monthly terrestrial climatology. *Climate* 1999 ; 12 : 829-56.
- Hunt RH, Coetzee M, Fettene M. The *Anopheles gambiae* complex: a new species from Ethiopia. *Trans R Soc Trop Med Hyg* 1998 ; 92 : 231-5.
- Hussain MZ. The vectors of malaria and malaria transmission in Pakistan. *Pakistan J Health* 1951 ; 1 : 69-71.
- Hussain MZ, Talibi SA. Incrimination of the vector of malaria in Federal Karachi area, Pakistan. *Pakistan J Health* 1956 ; 6 : 65-72.
- Hussamedin. *La lutte antipaludique en Turquie*. 2ᵉ Congrès International Paludisme Alger, 19-21 mai 1930 : 60 p.
- Husson AD. Rapport sur la campagne antipaludique de 1908. *Arch Inst Pasteur Tunis* 1909 ; 110-22.
- Hyma S, Ramesh A. The reappearence of malaria in Santhanaur Reservoir and environs: Tamil Nadu, India. *Soc Sci Med* 1980 ; 14D (3) : 337-44.
- Ibadin OM, Airauhi L, Omoigberale AI, Abiodun PO. Association of malarial parasitaemia with dehydrating diarrhoea in Nigerian children. *J Health Popul Nutr* 2000 ; 18 : 115-8.
- IPCC. *Climate change 2001: the scientific basis*. Contribution of Working Group 1 to the Third Assessment Report of the Intergovernmental Panel on Climate Change. Houghton JJ, Ding Y, Griggs DJ, Noguer M, van der Linden PJ, Dai X, Maskell K, Johnson CA, eds. Cambridge, United Kingdom and New York, NY, USA : Cambridge Univesity Press, 2001 : 881 p.
- Isaäcson M. Airport malaria: a review. *Bull World Health Organ* 1989 ; 67 : 737-43.
- Isah HS, Fleming AF, Ujah IA, Ekwenpu CC. Anaemia and iron status of pregnant and non-pregnant women in the Guinea savannah of Nigeria. *Ann Trop Med Parasitol* 1985 ; 79 : 485-93 .
- Ismail IA, Notananda V, Schepens J. Studies on malaria and responses of *Anopheles balabacensis balabacensis* and *An. minimus* to DDT residual spraying in Thailand. Part II. Post-spraying observations. *Acta Tropica* 1975 ; 32 : 206-31.
- Ismail IA, Phinichpongse S, Boonrasri P. Response of *Anopheles minimus* to DDT residual spraying in a cleared forested foothill area in central Thailand. *Acta Tropica* 1978 ; 35 : 69-82.
- Ivorra Cano V. Paludisme. In : Meheus *et al.*, eds. *Santé et maladies au Rwanda*. Bruxelles : AGCD, 1982 : 427-47.

- Iyengar MO. Vectors of malaria in Kabul, Afghanistan. *Trans R Soc Trop Med Hyg* 1954 ; 48 : 319-24.
- Iyengar MO, Mathew MI, Menon MA. Malaria in the Maldive Islands. *Indian J Malariol* 1953 ; 7 : 1-3.
- Jadin JB. Disparition d'*Anopheles funestus* au Rwanda après les traitements insecticides. *Ann Soc Belg Med Trop* 1952 ; 32 : 455-64.
- Jadin JB, Herman F. Paludisme de montagne et action du sulfate de quinine brut sur la malaria. *Ann Soc Belg Med Trop* 1946 ; 26 : 111-6.
- Jadin JB, Fain A. *Anopheles funestus*, transmetteur de paludisme en pays d'altitude (Astrida 1750 m, Ruanda-Urundi). *Ann Soc Belg Med Trop* 1949 ; 29 : 145-50.
- Jadin JB, Fain A. Contribution à l'étude du paludisme en pays d'altitude. *Ann Soc Belg Med Trop* 1951 ; 31 : 353-63.
- Jaenson TG, Gomes MJ, Barreto dos Santos RC, *et al*. Control of endophagic *Anopheles* mosquitoes and human malaria in Guinea Bissau, West Africa by permethrin-treated bed nets. *Trans R Soc Trop Med Hyg* 1994 ; 88 (6) : 620-4.
- Jambou R, Ranaivo L, Raharimalala L, *et al*. Malaria in the highlands of Madagascar after five years of indoor house spraying of DDT. *Trans R Soc Trop Med Hyg* 2001 ; 95 : 14-8.
- James SP, Tate P. New knowledge of the life-cycle of the malaria parasites. *Nature* 1937 ; 139 : 545.
- Janicot S. Impacts régionaux de El Niño : Afrique de l'Ouest. *La lettre de MEDIAS*, numéro spécial El Niño et ses téléconnexions sur l'Afrique et la Méditerranée, Décembre 2000 ; 12 : 34-7.
- Janssens PG, Vincke IH, Bafort J. Le paludisme d'Afrique Centrale. Son influence sur la morbidité et la mortalité des enfants. *Bull Soc Pathol Exot* 1966 ; 59 : 665.
- Janssens PG, Kivits M, Vuylsteke J. *Médecine et hygiène en Afrique Centrale*. Bruxelles : Fondation du roi Baudoin, 1992 : 1632 p.
- Jaujou CM. La lutte antipaludique en Corse. *Bull Organ Mond Santé* 1954 ; 11 : 635-77.
- Jeffrey CM. Epidemiological significance of repeated infections with homologus and heterologus strains and species of *Plasmodium*. *Bull World Health Organ* 1966 ; 35 : 873-82.
- Jelinek T, Loscher T, Nothdurft HD. High prevalence of antibodies against circumsporozoite antigen of *Plasmodium falciparum* without development of symptomatic malaria in travellers returning from Sub-Saharan Africa. *J Infect Dis* 1996 ; 174 : 1376-9.
- Jonchere H, Pfister R. Enquêtes malariologiques en Haute Volta, Côte d'Ivoire et Guinée. *Bull Soc Pathol Exot* 1951 ; 44 : 774-86.
- Joncour G. La lutte contre le paludisme à Madagascar. *Bull Organ Mond Santé* 1956 ; 15 : 711-23.
- Jones TR, Baird JK, Basri H, Purnomo EW, Danu Dirgo EW. Prevalence of malaria in native and transmigrant populations. *Trop Geogr Med* 1991 ; 43 : 1-6.
- Jones WH. Malaria and history. *Ann Trop Med Parasitol* 1908 ; 1 : 529-40.
- Jonkman A, Chibwe RA, Khoromana CO, *et al*. Cost-saving through microscopy-based *versus* presumptive diagnosis of malaria in adult outpatients in Malawi. *Bull World Health Organ* 1995 ; 73 : 223-7.
- Joshi GP, Service MW, Pradhan GD. A survey of species A and B of the *An. gambiae* complex in Kisumu area of Kenya, prior to insecticidal spraying with Fenitrothion. *Ann Trop Med Parasitol* 1975 ; 69 : 91-104.
- Joshi H, Vasantha K, Subbarao SK, Sharma VP. Host feeding patterns of *Anopheles culicifacies* species A and B. *J Am Mosq Control Assoc* 1988 ; 4 : 248-51.
- Joshi H, Subbarao SK, RAghavendra K, Sharma VP. *Plasmodium vivax* enzyme polymorphism in isolates of Indian origin. *Trans R Soc Trop Med Hyg* 1989 ; 83 : 179-81.
- Josse R, Josseran R, Audibert M, *et al*. Paludométrie et variations saisonnières dans la région du projet rizicole de Maga (Nord Cameroun) et dans la région limitrophe. *Cahiers ORSTOM, Entomol Med Parasitol* 1987a ; n° spécial : 63-71.
- Josse R, Merlin M, de Backer L, *et al*. À propos d'une enquête paludométrique menée en saison sèche à Maroua, province de l'extrême Nord, Cameroun. *Bull Liaison OCEAC* 1987b ; 80 : 39-47.
- Josse R, Hengy C, Bailly C, *et al*. Étude épidémiologique du paludisme dans la ville de Nkongsamba, Cameroun. *Med Afr Noire* 1988 ; 35 : 17-24.
- Josse R, Trebucq A, Jaureguiberry G, *et al*. Évaluation des indices paludométriques dans la région forestière de Djoum, Sud Cameroun. *Med Trop (Marseille)* 1990 ; 50 : 47-51.
- Josseran R, Abeso Owono, Foumane V, *et al*. Évaluation des indices paludométriques dans le district de Nsork Région continentale, Guinée Équatoriale. *Bull Liaison OCEAC* 1987 ; fasc. 180 : 49-57.

- Julvez J. *Anthropisation et paludisme. Éco-épidémiologie historique du paludisme dans les archipels du Sud-Ouest de l'Océan Indien.* Thèse Sciences (Ecol hum), Toulouse, 1993 : 350 p.
- Julvez J. Historique du paludisme insulaire dans l'Océan Indien (partie Sud Ouest). Une approche éco-épidémiologique. *Cahiers Santé* 1995 ; 5 : 353-8.
- Julvez J, Isautier H, Pichon G. Aspects épidémiologiques du paludisme dans l'île de la Réunion. Évaluation de certains paramètres constituant le potentiel paludogène. *Cahiers ORSTOM, Entomol Med Parasitol* 1982 ; 20 : 161-7.
- Julvez J, Michault A, Isautier H, Conan H, Galtier J. Études séro-épidémiologiques du paludisme à Mayotte de 1984 à 1986. *Cahiers ORSTOM, Entomol Med Parasitol* 1986 ; 24 : 279-86.
- Julvez J, Galtier J, Ali Halidi MA, Henry M, Mouchet J. Épidémiologie du paludisme et lutte antipaludique à Mayotte, archipel des Comores. *Bull Soc Pathol Exot* 1987 ; 80 : 505-19.
- Julvez J, Mouchet J, Ragavoodoo C. Épidémiologie historique du paludisme dans l'archipel des Mascareignes (Océan Indien). *Ann Soc Belg Med Trop* 1990 ; 70 : 249-61.
- Julvez J, Develoux M, Mounkaila A, Mouchet J. Diversité du paludisme en zone sahélo-saharienne. *Ann Soc Belg Med Trop* 1992 ; 72 : 163-77.
- Julvez J, Mouchet J, Michault A, Fouta A, Hamidine M. Éco-épidémiologie du paludisme à Niamey et dans la vallée du fleuve, République du Niger, 1992-1995. *Bull Soc Pathol Exot* 1997a ; 90 : 94-100.
- Julvez J, Mouchet J, Michault A, Fouta A, Hamidine M. Évolution du paludisme dans l'est sahélien du Niger, une zone écologiquement sinistrée. *Bull Soc Pathol Exot* 1997b ; 90 : 101-4.
- Julvez J, Mouchet J. Anophelism and epidemiological patterns of malaria in the South-West Indian Ocean Archipelagoes. *Res Rev Parasitol* 1998a ; 58 : 161-7.
- Julvez J, Mouchet J. Malaria epidemiology in the Sahel, West Africa. *Res Rev Parasitol* 1998b ; 58 : 181-4.
- Julvez J, Mouchet J, Suzzoni J, Larrouy G, Fouta A, Fontenille D. Les anophèles du Niger. *Bull Soc Pathol Exot* 1998 ; 91 : 321-6.
- Juri MJ, Zaidenberg M, Almiron W. Spatial distribution of *Anopheles pseudopunctipennis* in the Yungas de Salta rainforest, Argentina. *Rev Saude Publica* 2005 ; 39 : 565-70.
- Kachur SP, Elda N, Vely JF, *et al*. Prevalence of malaria parasitemia and accuracy of microscopic diagnosis in Haiti, Oct. 1995. *Rev Panam Salud Publica* 1998 ; 3 (1) : 35-9.
- Kadiki O, Ashraf M. Malaria in Libyan Arab Republic. 1972. Doc Minist of Health. *Trop Dis Bull* 1974 ; 71 : 787-8 .
- Kain KC, Keystone JS, Franke ED, Lanar DE. Global distribution of a variant of the circumsporozoite gene of *Plasmodium vivax*. *J Infect Dis* 1991 ; 164 : 208-10.
- Kaiser PE, Narang SK, Seawright JA, Kline DL. A new member of the *Anopheles quadrimaculatus* complex, species C. *J Am Mosq Control Assoc* 1988 ; 4 : 494-9.
- Kalra NL, Watal BI. A note on *Anopheles leucosphyrus* Doenitz adults in collection of the Malaria Institute of India with distribution records of the *An. b. balabacensis* Baisas and *An. elegans* James in India. *Bull Nat Soc Ind Mal Mosq Dis* 1962 ; 10 : 159-67.
- Kamau L, Lehmann T, Hawley WA, Orago AS, Collins FH. Microgeographic genetic differentiation of *Anopheles gambiae* mosquitoes from Asembo Bay, Western Kenya: a comparison with Kilifi in Coastal Kenya. *Am J Trop Med Hyg* 1998 ; 58 (1) : 64-9.
- Kamau L, Mukabana WR, Hawley WD, *et al*. Analysis of genetic variability in *Anopheles arabiensis* and *Anopheles gambiae* using microsatellite loci. *Insect Mol Biol* 1999 ; 8 : 287-97.
- Kant R, Pandey SD, Sharma RC. Seasonal prevalence and succession of rice field breeding mosquitoes of Central Gujarat. *J Commun Dis* 1992 ; 24 : 164-72.
- Kar I, Subbarao SK, Eapen A, *et al*. Evidence for a new malaria vector species, species E, within *Anopheles culicifacies* complex. *J Med Entomol* 1999 ; 36 : 595-600.
- Kar S, Seth S, Seth PK. Duffy blood groups and malaria in the Ao Nagas in Nagaland, India. *Hum Hered* 1991 ; 41 (4) : 231-5.
- Kar S, Seth S, Seth PK. Prevalence of malaria in Ao Nagas and its association with G6PD and HbE. *Hum Biol* 1992 ; 64 (2) : 187-97.
- Karch S. Breeding of *Anopheles plumbeus* in tyres in France. *J Vector Ecol* 1997 ; 21 : 14.
- Karch S, Mouchet J. *Anopheles paludis* vecteur important du paludisme au Zaïre. *Bull Soc Pathol Exot* 1992 ; 85 : 388-9.
- Karch S, Asidi N, Manzambi ZM, Salaun JJ. La faune anophélienne et la transmission du paludisme humain à Kinshasa, Zaïre. *Bull Soc Pathol Exot* 1992 ; 85 : 304-9.
- Karch S, Garin B, Asidi N, Manzambi Z, Salaun JJ, Mouchet J. Moustiquaires imprégnées contre le paludisme au Zaïre. *Ann Soc Belg Med Trop* 1993 ; 73 (1) : 37-53.
- Karch S, Dellile MF, Guillet P, Mouchet J. African malaria vectors in European aircrafts. *Lancet* 2001 ; 357 (9251) : 235.
- Kariuki SK, Lal AA, Terlouw DJ, *et al*. Effects of permethrin-treated bed nets on immunity to malaria in western Kenya II. Antibody responses in young children in an area of intense malaria transmission. *Am J Trop Med Hyg* 2003 ; 68 : 108-14.
- Kassatsky. Rapport OMS/AFRO, 1994.
- Kengne P, Awono Ambene P, Antonio-Nkondjio C, Simard F, Fontenille D. Molecular identification of *Anopheles nili* group of African malaria vectors. *Med Vet Entomol* 2003 ; 17 : 67-74.
- Kere NK, Parkinson AD, Samrawickerema WA. The effect of permethrin-impregnated bednets on the incidence of *Plasmodium falciparum* in children of North Guadalcanal, Solomon Islands. *Southeast Asian J Trop Med Public Health* 1993 ; 24 (1) : 130-7.
- Ketrangsee S. Status report of malaria in Thailand. *Southeast Asian J Trop Med Public Health* 1992 ; 23 (suppl. 4) : 67-8.
- Keuter M, van Eijk A, Hoogstrate M, *et al*. Comparison of chloroquine, pyrimethamine and sulfadoxine, and chlorproguanil and dapsone as treatment for *falciparum* malaria in pregnant and non-pregnant women, Kakamega district, Kenya. *Br Med J* 1990 ; 301 : 466-70.
- Khan AQ, Talibi SA. Epidemiological assessment of malaria transmission in an endemic area of East Pakistan. *Bull World Health Organ* 1972 ; 46 : 783-92.
- Khin-Maung-Kyi. The anopheline mosquitoes of Burma. *Union Burma J Life Sci* 1971 ; part I to II : 281-493.
- Khin-Maung-Kyi. *Further observations on* Anopheles balabacensis balabacensis *and malaria in Burma*. WHO/MAL/74.838 ; 1974 : 23 p.
- Khin-Maung-Kyi, Winn SM. *Studies on malaria and* Anopheles balabacensis balabacensis *and* An. minimus *in Burma*. WHO/MAL/76.875 ; 1976.
- Kilian AH, Langi P, Talisuna A, Kabagambe G. Rainfall pattern El Niño and malaria in Uganda. *Trans R Soc Trop Med Hyg* 1999 ; 93 : 22-3.
- Killeen GF, Kihonda J, Lyimo E, *et al*. Quantifying behavioural interactions between humans and mosquitoes: evaluating the protective efficacy of insecticidal nets against malaria transmission in rural Tanzania. *BMC Infect Dis* 2006 ; 6 : 161.
- Kirnowardoyo S. Status of *Anopheles* malaria vectors in Indonesia. *Southeast Asian J Trop Med Public Health* 1985 ; 16 (1) : 129-32.
- Kirnowardoyo S, Supalin. Zooprophylaxis as a useful tool for control of *An. aconitus* transmitted malaria in Central Java, Indonesia. *J Commun Dis* 1986 ; 18 (2) : 90-4.
- Kitua AY, Smith T, Alonso PL, *et al*. *Plasmodium falciparum* malaria in the first year of life in an area of intense and perennial transmission. *Trop Med Int Health* 1996 ; 1 : 475-84.
- Kitzmiller JB, Kreutzer RD, Tallaferro E. Chromosomal differences in populations of *Anopheles nuneztovari*. *Bull World Health Organ* 1973 ; 48 (4) : 435-45.
- Kliger IJ. *The epidemiology and control of malaria in Palestine*. Chicago : Chicago University Press, 1930 : 240 p.
- Kloke RG. New distribution of *An. merus* in Zambia. *Afr Entomol* 1997 ; 5 : 361-2.
- Kloos H. Health aspects of resettlement in Ethiopia. *Soc Sci Med* 1990 ; 30 : 643-56.
- Knight KL. Supplement to a catalog of the mosquitoes of the world (Diptera: Culicidae). *Thomas Say Foundation* 1978 ; 6 : 1-107.
- Knight KL, Stones A. *A catalog of the mosquitoes of the world*. Thomas Say Foundation. Entomological Society of America, 1977 : 611 p.
- Kobayashi J, Somboon P, Keomanila H, *et al*. Malaria prevalences and a brief entomological survey in a village surrounded by rice fields in Khammouan province, Lao PDR. *Trop Med Int Health* 2000 ; 5 : 17-21.
- Kochar D, Kumawat BL, Karan S, Kochar SK, Agarwal RP. Severe and complicated malaria in Bikaner, Rajasthan, Western India. *Southeast Asian J Trop Med Public Health* 1997 ; 28 : 259-67.
- Koita O. *Contribution à l'étude épidémiologique du paludisme le long du tronçon malien de la route transsaharienne*. Bamako : Thèse Pharmacie, 1988.
- Konate L. *Épidémiologie du paludisme dans un village de savane soudanienne : Dielmo, Sénégal*. Dakar : Thèse Doct. 3° Cycle, 1991.
- Konate L, Diop A, Sy N, *et al*. Come-back of *An. funestus* in Sahelian Senegal. *Lancet* 2001 ; 358 (9278) : 336.
- Kondrashin AV. Malaria in the WHO South-East Asia Region. *Indian J Malariol* 1992 ; 29 : 129-60.
- Kondrashin AV, Sakya GM. Comparative studies on response to 5 days treatment with primaquine of indigenous and imported cases of *P. vivax* in Nepal in 1974-76. *J Nepal Med Assoc* 1981 ; 19 : 6-15.

- Korenromp EL, Williams BG, Gouws E, Dye C, Snow RW. Measurement of trends in childhood malaria mortality in Africa: an assessment of progress toward targets based on verbal autopsy. *J Infect Dis* 2003 ; 3 (6) : 349-58.
- Kouznetsov RL. *Distribution of anophelines in the Yemen Arab Republic and its relation to malaria.* WHO/MAL/76.879, 1976 : 9 p.
- Kouznetsov RL. Malaria control by application of indoor spraying of residual insecticides in tropical Africa and its impact on community health. *Trop Doct* 1977 ; 7 : 81-91.
- Krafsur ES. *Anopheles nili* as a vector in a lowland region of Ethiopia. *Bull World Health Organ* 1970 ; 42 : 466-71.
- Krafsur ES. Malaria transmission in Gambela, Illubabor Province. *Ethiopian Med J* 1971 ; 9 : 75-94.
- Krafsur ES. The bionomics and relative prevalence of *Anopheles* species with respect to the transmission of *Plasmodium* to man in Western Ethiopia. *J Med Entomol* 1977 ; 14 : 180-94.
- Krafsur ES, Armstrong JC. An integrated view of entomological and parasitological observations on falciparum malaria in Gambela, Western Ethiopian Lowlands. *Trans R Soc Trop Med Hyg* 1978 ; 72 : 348-56.
- Krafsur ES, Armstrong JC. Epidemiology of *P. malariae* infection in Gambela, Ethiopia. *Parassitologia* 1982 ; 24 : 105-20.
- Kroeger A, Mancheno M, Alarcon J, Pesse K. Insecticide-impregnated bed nets for malaria control: varying experiences from Ecuador, Colombia and Peru concerning acceptability and effectiveness. *Am J Trop Med Hyg* 1995 ; 53 : 312-23.
- Krotoski WA, Garnham PC, Bray RS, *et al.* Observations on early and late post-sporozoite tissue stages in primate malaria. I. Discovery of a new latent form of *P. cynomolgi* (the hypnozoite) and failure to detect hepatic forms within the first 24 hours after infection. *Am J Trop Med Hyg* 1982a ; 31 (1) : 24-35.
- Krotoski WA, Bray RS, Garnham PC, *et al.* Observations on early and late post-sporozoite tissue stages in primate malaria. II. The hypnozoite of *P. cynomolgi bastianellii* from 3 to 105 days after infection, and detection of 36 to 40 hours pre-erythrocytic forms. *Am J Trop Med Hyg* 1982b ; 31 (1) : 211-25.
- Kruger A, Rech A, Xin-Zhuan SU, Tannich E. Two cases of autochthonous *Plasmodium falciparum* malaria in Germany with evidence for local transmission by indigenous *Anopheles plumbeus*. *Trop Med Int Health* 2001 ; 6 (12) : 983-5.
- Krzywinski J, Besansky NJ. Molecular systematics of *Anopheles*: from sungenera to Subpopulations. *Annu Rev Entomol* 2003 ; 48 : 111-39
- Kulkarni SM. Detection of sporozoïtes in *An. subpictus* in Bastar District, Madhya Pradesh. *Indian J Malariol* 1983 ; 20 : 159-60.
- Kulkarni SM. Feeding behaviour of anopheline mosquitoes in an area endemic for malaria in Bastar district, Madhya Pradesh. *Indian J Malariol* 1987 ; 24 : 163-71.
- Kulkarni SM, Panda P. Two cases of malaria by split feeding of a naturally infected mosquito. *Indian J Malariol* 1984 ; 21 : 293-4.
- Kumm HW, Bustamante ME, Herrera JR. Report concerning certain anophelines found near the Mexican-Guatemalan frontier. *Am J Trop Med* 1943 ; 23 (3) : 373-6.
- Kuschke WH. The Okawango and its endemic diseases. *Med Proc* 1968 ; 14 : 307-401.
- Kustner HG. Trends in four major communicable diseases. *S Afr Med J* 1979 ; 55 : 460-73.

- Labie D. Aspects génétiques de l'anémie falciforme. *Ann Parasitol Hum Comp* 1992 ; 42 : 1879-84.
- Lacan A. Indices paludométriques et immunité palustre chez l'enfant africain. *Bull Soc Pathol Exot* 1957 ; 50 : 302-8.
- Lacan A. Les anophèles de l'Afrique Équatoriale Française et leur répartition. *Ann Parasitol Hum Comp* 1958 ; 33 : 150-70.
- Lallemant M, Galacteros F, Lallemant-Lecoeur S, *et al.* Haemoglobin abnormalities: an evaluation on new-born infants and their mothers in a maternity unit close to Brazzaville (Congo). *Human Genet* 1986 ; 74 : 54-8.
- Lamb HH. *Climate, history and the modern world.* London : Routledge, 1995.
- Lancien J. Lutte contre la maladie du sommeil dans le Sud-Est Ouganda par piégeage des glossines. *Ann Soc Belg Med Trop* 1991 ; 1 (suppl.) : 35-47.
- Lancisi GM. *De noxiis paludum affluvis corumque remediis.* Roma : Salvieni, 1717.
- Lanckriet C, Bureau JJ, Capdevielle H, Gody JC, Olivier T, Siopathis RM. Morbidité et mortalité dans le service de pédiatrie de Bangui (Centrafrique) au cours de l'année 1990. *Ann Pédiatr (Paris)* 1992 ; 39 : 125-30.
- Langeron M. Anophèles du Grand Atlas et de l'AntiAtlas marocain. *CR Acad Sci* 1938 ; 207 : 260-2.
- Languillon J. Carte épidémiologique du paludisme au Cameroun. *Bull Soc Pathol Exot* 1957 ; 50 : 585-600.
- Languillon J, Mouchet J, Rivola E. Contribution à l'étude du *Plasmodium ovale* dans les territoires français d'Afrique. Sa relative fréquence au Cameroun. *Bull Soc Pathol Exot* 1955 ; 48 : 819-23.
- Languillon J, Mouchet J, Rivola E, Rateau J. Contribution à l'étude de l'épidémiologie du paludisme dans la région forestière du Cameroun. *Med Trop (Marseille)* 1956 ; 16 : 347-78.
- Lantoarilala J, Champetier de Ribes G, Mouchet J. Impact de la lutte antivectorielle sur la morbidité et la mortalité palustres dans un district sanitaire des Hautes Terres de Madagascar. *Bull Soc Pathol Exot* 1998 ; 91 : 87-90.
- Lardeux F, Loayza P, Bouchité B, Chavez T. Host choice and human blood index of *Anopheles pseudopunctipennis* in a village of the Andean valleys of Bolivia. *Malar J* 2007 ; 6 : 8.
- Laserson KF, Wypij D, Petralanda I, Spielman A, Maguire JH. Differential perpetuation of malaria species among Amazonian Yanomami Amerindians. *Am J Trop Med Hyg* 1999a ; 60 (5) : 767-73.
- Laserson KF, Petralanda I, Almera R, *et al.* Genetic characterization of an epidemic of *P. falciparum* malaria among Yanomami Amerindians. *J Infect Dis* 1999b ; 180 : 2081-5.
- de Las Llagas LA. Impact of ecological changes on Anopheles vectors of malaria in some countries of South-East Asia. *Southeast Asian J Trop Med Public Health* 1985 ; 16 : 146-8.
- Latisheve LN. In : Pavlovsky EN. *Epidemic parasitology mission to Iran and parasitological surveys.* Moscow, Leningrad : USSR Academy of Sciences, 1948 : 235-8.
- Laventure S, Rabarison P, Mouchet J, *et al.* Paludisme : perspectives de recherche en entomologie médicale à Madagascar. *Cahiers Santé* 1995 ; 5 : 406-10.
- Laventure S, Mouchet J, Blanchy S, *et al.* Le riz, source de vie et de mort sur les plateaux de Madagascar. *Cahiers Santé* 1996 ; 6 : 79-86.
- Laveran A. Note sur un nouveau parasite trouvé dans le sang de plusieurs malades atteints de fièvre palustre. *Bull Acad Med Paris* 1880 ; 9 : 1235-6.
- Lavoipierre P, Viader F. *A mort les moustiques.* Port Louis : Félix Imp, 1948.
- Layton MC. Malaria in New York City. *Bull New York Acad Med* 1996 ; 73 (2) : 456-8.
- Layton M, Parise ME, Campbell CC, *et al.* Mosquito-transmitted malaria in New York City, 1993. *Lancet* 1995 ; 346 : 729-31.
- Lee VH, Atmosoedjono S, Dennis DT, Suhaepi A, Suwarta A. The anopheline vectors of malaria and bancroftian filariasis in Flores Island, Indonesia. *J Med Entomol* 1983 ; 20 : 577-8.
- Leeson HS. *Anopheline mosquitoes in Southern Rhodesia (1926-1928).* London : London School of Hygiene and Tropical Medicine, 1931 ; 4 : 55 p.
- Lefevre-Witier P. Sur le paludisme en Tassili N'Ajjer (Sahara Central), Algérie. *Bull Soc Pathol Exot* 1968 ; 61 : 596-605.
- Le Gaonach J. Un foyer de paludisme au Hoggar (Tahifet). *Arch Inst Pasteur Algérie* 1939 ; 17 : 438-41.
- Léger M. Quelques documents sur l'indice plasmodial du paludisme en Guadeloupe. *Bull Soc Pathol Exot* 1932 ; 25 : 211-5.
- Le Goff G, Carnevale P, Robert V. Comparaison des captures sur homme et au piège lumineux CDC pour l'échantillonnage des moustiques et l'évaluation de la transmission du paludisme au Sud-Cameroun. *Ann Soc Belg Méd Trop* 1993 ; 73 : 55-60.
- Le Goff G, Toto JC, Nzeyimana I, Guagna LC, Robert V. Les moustiques et la transmission du paludisme dans un village traditionnel du bloc forestier sud-camerounais. *Bull Liaison OCEAC*, Sept 1993 ; 26 (3).
- Le Hesran JY, Fievet N, Deloron P, *et al.* Acquisition de l'immunité antipalustre chez le nourrisson et l'enfant au Cameroun : suivi de deux cohortes. *Med Trop (Marseille)* 1995 ; 55 : 113-4.
- Lehmann T, Besansky NJ, Hawley WA, Fahey TG, Kamau L, Collins FH. Microgeographic structure of *Anopheles gambiae* in Western Kenya based on mtDNA and microsatellite loci. *Mol Ecol* 1997 ; 6 (3) : 243-53.
- Lehmann T, Licht M, Elissa N, *et al.* Population structure of *Anopheles gambiae* in Africa. *J Hered* 2003 ; 94 : 133-47.
- Lemasson JJ, Fontenille D, Lochouarn L, *et al.* Comparison of behaviour and vector efficiency of *Anopheles gambiae* and *Anopheles arabiensis* in Barkedji, a sahelian area of Senegal. *J Med Entomol* 1997 ; 34 : 396-403.
- Lengeler C. *Insecticide treated bednets and curtains for malaria control.* Oxford : Cochrane Review, 1998 : 54 p.
- Lengeler C. Insecticide-treated bed nets and curtains for preventing malaria. *Cochrane Database Syst Rev* 2004 ; 2 : CD000363

- Lengeler C, Cattani J, De Savigny D. *Net gain. A new method for preventing malaria deaths*. International Development Research Center, World Heanth Organization, 1996 : 189 p.
- Lepers JP, Simonneau M, Charmot G. Étude du groupe sanguin Duffy dans la population de Nouakchott, Mauritanie. *Bull Soc Pathol Exot* 1986 ; 79 : 417-20.
- Lepers JP, Deloron P, Rason A, Ramanamirija JA, Coulanges P. Newly transmitted *P. falciparum* malaria in the Central Highland Plateaux of Madagascar: assessment of clinical impact in a rural community. *Bull World Health Organ* 1990a ; 68 : 217-22.
- Lepers JP, Fontenille D, Rason MD, Deloron P, Coulanges P. Facteurs écologiques de la recrudescence du paludisme à Madagascar. *Bull Soc Pathol Exot* 1990b ; 83 : 330-41.
- Lepers JP, Fontenille D, Rason MD, *et al.* Transmission and epidemiology of newly transmitted falciparum malaria in the central highland Plateaux of Madagascar. *Ann Trop Med Parasitol* 1991 ; 85 : 297-304.
- Leroy-Ladurie E. *Histoire du climat depuis l'an 1000.* Paris : Flammarion.
- Le Sueur D, Sharp BL, Appleton CC. Historical perspective of the malaria problem in Natal, with emphasis on the period 1928-1932. *S Afr J Sci* 1993 ; 89 : 232-9.
- Lewis DJ. Observations on *Anopheles gambiae* and other mosquitoes at Wadi Halfa. *Trans R Soc Trop Med Hyg* 1944 ; 38 : 215-29.
- Lewis DJ. The extermination of *An. gambiae* in the Wadi Halfa area. *Trans R Soc Trop Med Hyg* 1949 ; 42 : 393-402.
- Lewis DJ. The anopheline mosquitoes of the Sudan. *Bull Entomol Res* 1956 ; 47 : 475-94.
- Li J, Collins WE, Wirtz RA, Rathore D, Lal A, McCutchan TF. Geographic subdivision of the range of the malaria parasite *Plasmodium vivax. Emerg Infect Dis* 2001 ; 7 (1) : 35-42.
- Li JW. Introduction on malaria history. *J Tradit Chin Med* 1963 ; 8 : 24-6.
- Li ZZ, Zhang M, Li GX. *The study of the control of An. sinensis, An. dirus and malaria prevalence with deltamethrine.* Part III. Field trials of controlling *An. sinensis* group and malaria prevalence by bednets impregnated with deltamethrin. IVe Congrès sur la protection de la Santé humaine et des cultures en milieu tropical, Marseille, 2-4 Juillet 1986. Rapp. et comm. tome II : 6 p.
- Li ZZ, Zhang M, Wu Y, Zhong B, Lin G, Huang H. Trial of deltamethrin impregnated bed nets for the control of malaria transmitted by *Anopheles sinensis* and *Anopheles anthropophagus. Am J Trop Med Hyg* 1989 ; 40 (4) : 356-9.
- Lien JC. Anopheline mosquitoes and malaria parasites in Taiwan. *Kaohsiung J Med Sci* 1991 ; 7 : 207-23.
- Lien JC, Atmosoedjono S, Usfinit AU, Gundelfinger BF. Observations on natural plasmodial infections in mosquitoes and a brief survey of mosquito fauna in Belu Regency, Indonesian Timor. *J Med Entomol* 1975 ; 12 : 333-7.
- Lien JC, Kawegian BA, Partono F, Lami B, Cross JH. A brief survey of the mosquitoes of South Sulawesi, Indonesia, with special reference to the identity of *Anopheles barbirostris* from the Margalembo area. *J Med Entomol* 1977 ; 13 : 719-27.
- Lienhardt C, Ghebray R, Candolfi F, Kien T, Hedlin G. Malaria in refugee camps in Eastern Sudan: a sero-epidemiological approach. *Ann Trop Med Parasitol* 1990 ; 84 : 215-22.
- Lim ES. Current status of malaria in Malaysia. *Southeast Asian J Trop Med Public Health* 1992 ; 23 (suppl. 4) : 43-9.
- Lin CF, Gian HL, Gu ZC, Pang JY, Zheng X. Comparative studies on the role of *Anopheles anthropophagus* and *Anopheles sinensis* in malaria transmission in China. *Chin J Epidemiol* 1990 ; 6 : 360-3.
- Lindberg K. Le paludisme dans l'Iran. *Riv Malariol* 1936 ; 15 : 132-45.
- Lindblade KA, Walker ED, Onapa AW, Katungu J, Wilson ML. Highland malaria in Uganda: prospective analysis of an epidemic associated with El Niño. *Trans R Soc Trop Med Hyg* 1999 ; 93 : 480-7.
- Lindblade KA, Walker ED, Wilson ML. Early warning of malaria epidemics in African highlands using *Anopheles* (Diptera: Culicidae) indoor resting density. *J Med Entomol* 2000 ; 37 (5) : 664-74.
- Lindsay SN, Alonso PL, Armstrong-Schellenberg JR, *et al.* A malaria control using insecticide-treated bednets and targeted prophylaxis in a rural area of the Gambia. *Trans R Soc Trop Med Hyg* 1993 ; 87 (suppl. 2) : 19-28.
- Lindsay SW, Martens WJ. Malaria in the African highlands: past, present and future. *Bull World Health Organ* 1998 ; 76 : 33-45.
- Linley JR, Lounibos LP, Conn J, Duzak D, Nishimura N. A description and morphometric comparison of eggs from eight geographic populations of the South American malaria vector *Anopheles nuneztovari. J Am Mosq Control Assoc* 1966 ; 12 : 275-92.
- Linton YM, Harbach RE, Chang MS, Anthony TG, Matusop A. Morphological and molecular identity of *Anopheles (Cellia) sundaicus* (Diptera: Culicidae), the nominotypical member of a malaria vector species complex in Southeast Asia. *System Entomol* 2001 ; 26 : 357-66.
- Linton YM, Smith L, Harbach RE. Observation on the taxonomic status of *Anopheles subalpinus* Hackett & Lewis and *An. melanoon* Hackett. *Europ Mosq Bull* 2002 ; 13 : 1-7.
- Linton YM, Dusfour I, Howard TM, *et al. Anopheles (Cellia) epiroticus* (Diptera: Culicidae), a new malaria vector species in the Southeast Asian *sundaicus* complex. *Bull Entomol Res* 2005 ; 95 : 329-39.
- Liu C, Qian H, Gu Z, Pan J, Zheng X. Quantitative study on the role of *Anopheles lesteri anthropophagus* in malaria transmission. *Chin J Parasitol Parasit Dis* 1986 ; 4 : 161-4.
- Livadas G. *Is it necessary to continue indefinitely DDT residual spraying programmes? Relevant observations made in Greece.* WHO/MAL/79 ; 1952 : 9 p.
- Livadas G, Belios GD. *Postwar malaria control in Greece.* Proceedings 4th International Congress Tropical Medicine Malaria ; Washington, 1948 ; vol. 2 : 884.
- Livadas GA, Georgiopoulos G. Development of resistance to DDT by *Anopheles sacharovi* in Greece. *Bull World Health Organ* 1953 ; 8 : 497-511.
- Livadas G, Mouchet J, Gariou J, Chastang R. Peut-on envisager l'éradication du paludisme dans la région forestière du Sud Cameroun ? *Riv Malariol* 1958 ; 37 : 229-56.
- Lobel HO, Mathews HM, Kagan IG. Interpretation of IHA titres for the study of malaria epidemiology. *Bull World Health Organ* 1973 ; 49 : 485-92.
- Lobel HO, Najera AJ, Ch'en WI, Monroe P, Mathews HM. *Seroepidemiological investigations of malaria in Guyana.* WHO/MAL/77.884 ; 1977 : 9 p.
- Lochouarn L, Dia I, Boccolini D, Coluzzi M, Fontenille D. Bionomical and cytogenetic heterogeneities of *An. funestus* in Senegal. *Trans R Soc Trop Med Hyg* 1998 ; 92 : 607-12.
- Lockhart JD, Highton RB, McMahon JP. Public health problem arising out of man-made fish ponds in the Western Province of Kenya Fish Culture. *East Afr Med J* 1969 ; 46 : 471-80.
- Lodato G. Campagne antimalaria nel Fezzan : Ubari-Edri. Bonifica del terreno e terapia endovenosa. *Arch Ital Sci Med Trop Parassitol* 1935 ; 16 (1) : 299-310.
- Loevinshon ME. Climatic warming and increased malaria incidence in Rwanda. *Lancet* 1994 ; 343 : 714-8.
- Lo Monaco Croce T. La malaria nella zona di Murzuk. *G Med Militare* 1931 ; 9 : 1.
- Longstreith J, Kondrashin A. Population migration and malaria. In : Casman E, Dowlatabi H, eds. *The contextual determinants of malaria.* Washington : Ressources for the Future Press, 2002 : 270-80.
- Loong KP, Chiang GL, Yap HH. Field studies on the bionomics of *Anopheles maculatus* and its role in malaria transmission in Malaysia. *Southeast Asian J Trop Med Public Health* 1988 ; 19 : 724.
- Lörincz F. Malaria in Hungary. *Riv Malariol* 1937 ; 16(1) : 465-79.
- Loue P, Andela A, Carnevale P. Étude de la morbidité palustre au centre de PMI de l'hôpital Central de Yaoundé, Cameroun. *Ann Soc Belg Med Trop* 1989 ; 69 : 191-208.
- Louis FC. *Rapport Ministère français de la Coopération,* 1999.
- Louis FJ, Foumane V, Bickii J, *et al.* Sensibilité *in vivo* à l'amodiaquine de *P. falciparum* au Cameroun en 1993-94. *Bull Liaison OCEAC* 1994 ; 27 : 119-20.
- Louis JP, Albert JP. Le paludisme en République de Djibouti. *Med Trop (Marseille)* 1988 ; 48 : 127-31.
- Louis JP, Trebucq A, Gelas H, *et al.* Le paludisme-maladie dans la ville de Yaoundé, Cameroun. *Bull Soc Pathol Exot* 1992 ; 85 : 26-30.
- Lourenco de Oliveira R, Guimaraes AE, Arle M, *et al.* Anopheline species, some of their habits and relation to malaria in endemic areas of Rondonia State, Amazon Region of Brazil. *Mem Inst Oswaldo Cruz* 1989 ; 84 (4) : 501-14.
- Lourenco de Oliveira R, Deane LM. Simian malaria at two sites in the Brazilian Amazon. I. The infection rates of *Plasmodium brasilianum* in the non-human primates. *Mem Inst Oswaldo Cruz* 1995 ; 90 (3) : 331-9.
- Lourenco de Oliveira R, Luz SL. Simian malaria at two sites in the Brazilian Amazon. II. Vertical distribution and frequency of anopheline species inside and outside the forest. *Mem Inst Oswaldo Cruz* 1996 ; 91 (6) : 687-94.
- Loyola EG, Arredondo JI, Rodriguez MH, Brown DN, Vaca-Marin MA. *Anopheles vestitipennis,* the probable vector of *P. vivax* in the Lacandon forest of Chiapas, Mexico. *Trans R Soc Trop Med Hyg* 1991 ; 85 (2) : 171-4.

- Lu Bao Lin. The wet irrigation method of mosquito control in rice fields. An experiment of intermittent irrigation in China. Environmental management for vector control in rice fields. FAO. *Irrigation and Drainage* 1984 ; paper 41 : 130-2.
- Lüleyap HU, Alptekin D, Kasap H, Kasap MJ. Detection of knockdown resistance mutations in *Anopheles sacharovi* (Diptera: Culicidae) and genetic distance with *Anopheles gambiae* (Diptera: Culicidae) using cDNA sequencing of the voltage-gated sodium channel gene. *Med Entomol* 2002 ; 39 : 870-4.
- Lumaret R. *Études sur le paludisme à Madagascar*. Doc. ronéo. Antanarivo : SNLP, 1962 : 232 p.
- Lusina D, Legros F, Esteve V, Klerlein M, Giacomini T. Paludisme d'aéroport : quatre nouveaux cas dans la banlieue de Paris durant l'été 1999. *Eurosurveillance Monthly* 2000 ; 5 : 76-80.
- Lutz A. Waldmosquitoes und waldmalaria. *Centralblatt Bakteriol Parasiten Infektionskrank* 1903 ; 33 : 282.
- Lutz W. Impacts of global population trends. In : Casman E, Dowlatabi H, eds. *The contextual determinants of malaria*. Washington : Ressources for the Future Press, 2002 : 239-59.
- Luxemburger C, Perea WA, Delmas G, Pruja C, Pecoul B, Moren A. Permethrin-impregnated bed nets for the prevention of malaria in school children on the Thaï Burmese border. *Trans R Soc Trop Med Hyg* 1994 ; 88 (2) : 155-9.
- Luxemburger C, Thwai KL, White NJ, *et al*. The epidemiology of a Karen population on the Western border of Thailand. *Trans R Soc Trop Med Hyg* 1996 ; 90 : 105-11.
- Luxemburger C, Nosten F, Kyl DE, Kiricharoen L, Chongsuphajaisiddhi T, White NJ. Clinical features cannot predict a diagnosis of malaria or differentiate the infecting species in children living in an area of low transmission. *Trans R Soc Trop Med Hyg* 1998 ; 92 : 45-9.
- Lysenko AJ, Beljaev AE, Rybalka VM. Population studies of *P. vivax*. *Bull World Health Organ* 1977 ; 55 : 541-9.
- Lysenko AJ, Kondrashin AV. *Malariology*. WHO/MAL/99.1089 ; 1999 : 248 p.
- Ma Y, Qu F, Lei X, Dong X. Comparison of rDNA-ITS2 sequences and morphological characters of *Anopheles kunmingensis* and *Anopheles liangshanensis* in China, with discussion on taxonomic status. *Chinese J Parasitol Parasit Dis* 2000 ; 18 : 65-8.
- Macan TT. The anopheline mosquitoes of Iraq and North Persia. In : Anopheles *and malaria in near East*. London : Lewis and Co, London Sch Hyg Trop Med Mem 1950 ; n°7.
- Macdonald G. The analysis of equilibrium in malaria. *Trop Dis Bull* 1952 ; 49 : 813-29.
- Macdonald G. The analysis of malaria epidemics. *Trop Dis Bull* 1953 ; 50 : 871-89.
- Macdonald G. *The epidemiology and control of malaria*. London : Oxford University Press, 1957 : 201 p.
- Machado RL, Povoa MM. Distribution of *Plasmodium vivax* variants (VK210 ; VK247 and *P. vivax*-like) in three endemic areas of the Amazon Region of Brazil and their correlation with chloroquine treatment. *Trans R Soc Trop Med Hyg* 2000 ; 94 : 377-81.
- Madeley J. Le paludisme dans les Iles Salomon. *Santé du Monde* 1988 ; Juin : 14-5.
- Madwar S. A preliminary note on *Anopheles pharoensis* in relation to malaria in Egypt. *J Egypt Med Assoc* 1936 ; 19 : 616-7.
- Maffi M. Contributo alla conoscenza della fauna anofelinica della Somalia. *Riv Malariol* 1958 ; 37 : 73-5.
- Maffi M. La malaria nella regioni del Mudugh e della Migiurtinia, Somalia. *Riv Malariol* 1960 ; 39 : 21-118.
- Maffi M. *Contribution to knowledge of the anopheline fauna of Mauritania*. WHO/MAL/434 ; 1964 : 3 p.
- Magesa SM, Mdira KY, Färnert A, Simonsen PE, Bygbjerg IB, Jakobsen P. Distinguishing *Plasmodium falciparum* treatment failures from re-infections by using polymerase chain reaction genotyping in a holoendemic area in Northeastern Tanzania. *Am J Trop Med Hyg* 2001 ; 65 (5) : 477-83.
- Magnaval JF. *Étude anthropologique d'une population Nigérienne : les Toubous du Nord Est*. Toulouse : Thèse Médecine, 1973 ; 79 : 116 p.
- Maharaj R, Mthembu DJ, Sharp BL. Impact of DDT re-introduction on malaria transmission in KwaZulu-Natal. *S Afr Med J* 2005 ; 95 : 871-4.
- Mahe G, Olivry JC. Changements climatiques et variations des écoulements en Afrique Occidentale et Centrale, du mensuel à l'interannuel. In : van de Ven FHM, Gutknecht D, Loucks DP, Salewicz KA, eds.*Hydrology for the water management of large river basins*. Wallingford : IAHS Publication 1991 ; 201 : 163-72.
- Maheswary NP, Habib MA, Elias M. Incrimination of *Anopheles aconitus* as a vector of epidemic malaria in Bangladesh. *Southeast Asian J Trop Med Public Health* 1992 ; 23 : 798-801.
- Mahmood F, Sakai RK, Akhtar K. Vector incrimination studies and observations on species A and B of the taxon *Anopheles culicifacies* in Pakistan. *Trans R Soc Trop Med Hyg* 1984 ;78 : 607-16.
- Mahmood F, Macdonald M. Ecology of malaria transmission and vectorial capacity of *Anopheles culicifacies sp.* A in rural Punjab, Pakistan. *Pakistan J Med Res* 1985 ; 24 : 95-105.
- Mahon RJ, Miethke PM. *Anopheles farauti* n°3, a hitherto unrecognised biological species of mosquito within the taxon *An. farauti*. *Trans R Soc Trop Med Hyg* 1982 ; 76 : 8-12.
- Maiga MA, Diallo H, Maiga YI. Paludisme en zone irriguée. Enquête épidémiologique dans les villages colons de Kolongotomo (office du Niger, Mali). *Med Afr Noire* 1989a ; 36 : 206-9.
- Maiga MA, Ag Rhaly A, Maiga AS. Évaluation en saison sèche des indices plasmodique et splénique du paludisme dans les campements nomades, sédentaires, du Gourma Malien. *Med Afr Noire* 1989b ; 36 : 240-5.
- Maitland K, Williams TN, Peto TEA, *et al*. Absence of malaria-specific mortality in children in an area of hyperendemic malaria. *Trans R Soc Trop Med Hyg* 1997 ; 91 : 562-6.
- Mak JW, Lim PK, Tan MA, *et al*. Parasitological and serological survey for malaria among the inhabitants of an aborigine village and an adjacent Malay village. *Acta Tropica* 1987 ; 44 : 83-9.
- Mak JW, Jegathesan M, Lim PK, *et al*. Epidemiology and control of malaria in Malaysia. *Southeast Asian J Trop Med Public Health* 1992 ; 23 : 572-7.
- Malakar P, Das S, Saha GK, Dasgupta B, Hati AK. Indoor resting anophelines in North Bengal. *Indian J Malariol* 1995 ; 32 : 24-31.
- Malakooti MA, Biomndo K, Shanks GD. Reemergence of epidemic malaria in the highlands of Western Kenya. *Emerg Infect Dis* 1998 ; 4 : 671-6.
- Maldonado YA, Nahlen BL, Roberto RR, *et al*. Transmission of *Plasmodium vivax* in San Diego County, California, 1986. *Am J Trop Med Hyg* 1990 ; 42 : 3-9.
- Malhotra PR, Sarkar PK, Das NG, Hazarika S, John VM. Mosquito survey in Tirap and Subansiri districts of Arunachal Pradesh. *Indian J Malariol* 1987 ; 24 : 151-8.
- Manga L. La pratique de l'examen parasitologique du paludisme dans les formations sanitaires au Sud Cameroun. *Cahiers Santé* 1994 ; 4 : 119-20.
- Manga L, Traoré O, Cot M, Mooh E, Carnevale P. Le paludisme dans la ville de Yaoundé, Cameroun. 3. Étude parasitologique dans deux quartiers centraux. *Bull Soc Pathol Exot* 1993 ; 86 : 56-61.
- Manga L, Toto JC, Carnevale P. Malaria vectors and transmission in an area deforested for a new international airport in Southern Cameroon. *Ann Soc Belg Med Trop* 1995 ; 75 : 43-9.
- Manga L, Bouchité B, Toto JC, Froment A. La faune anophélienne et la transmission du paludisme dans une zone de transition forêt-savanne au Centre du Cameroun. *Bull Soc Pathol Exot* 1997a ; 90 : 128-30.
- Manga L, Toto JC, Le Goff G, Brunhes J. The bionomics of *An. funestus* and its role in malaria transmission in a forested area of Southern Cameroon. *Trans R Soc Trop Med Hyg* 1997b ; 91 : 387-8.
- Manguin S, Peyton EL, James AC, Roberts DR. Apparent changes in the abundance and distribution of *Anopheles* species on Grenada Island. *J Am Mosq Control Assoc* 1993 ; 9 (4) : 403-7.
- Manguin S, Roberts DR, Peyton EL, *et al*. Biochemical systematics and population genetic structure of *Anopheles pseudopunctipennis*, vector of malaria in Central and South America. *Am J Trop Med Hyg* 1995 ; 53 (4) : 362-77.
- Manguin S, Roberts DR, André RG, Rejmankova E, Hakre S. Characterization of *An. darlingi*, larval habitats in Belize, Central America. *J Med Entomol* 1996a ; 33 (2) : 205-11.
- Manguin S, Roberts DR, Peyton EL, Rejmankova E, Pecor J. Characterization of *Anopheles pseudopunctipennis* larval habitats. *J Am Mosq Control Assoc* 1996b ; 12 (4) : 619-26.
- Manguin S, Wilkerson RC, Conn JE, Rubio-Palis Y, Danoff-Burg JA, Roberts DR. Population structure of the primary malaria vector in South America, *An. darlingi*, using isozyme, random amplified polymorphic DNA, internal transcribed spacer 2 and morphologic markers. *Am J Trop Med Hyg* 1999a ; 60 (3) : 364-76.
- Manguin S, Fontenille D, Chandre F, *et al*. Génétique des populations anophéliennes. *Bull Soc Pathol Exot* 1999b ; 92 (4) : 229-35.
- Mani TR, Tewari SC, Reuben R, Devaputra M. Resting behaviour of anopheline and sporozoïte rates in vectors of malaria along the river Thenpennai (Tamil Nadu). *Indian J Med Res* 1984 ;80 : 11-7.
- Manonmani A, Townson H, Adeniran T, Jambulingam P, Sahu SS, Vijayakumar T. rDNA-ITS2 polymerase chain reaction assay for the sibling species of *Anopheles fluviatilis*. *Acta Trop* 2001 ; 78 : 3-9.

- Manonmani A, Nanda N, Jambulingam P, et al. Comparison of polymerase chain reaction assay and cytotaxonomy for identification of sibling species of *Anopheles fluviatilis* (Diptera: Culicidae). *Bull Entomol Res* 2003 ; 93 : 169-71.
- Manouchehri AV, Ghiasseddin M, Shahgudian ER. *Anopheles dthali* Patton 1905, a new secondary vector in Southern Iran. *Ann Trop Med Parasitol* 1972 ; 66 : 537-8.
- Manouchehri AV, Djanbakhsh B, Eshghi N. The biting cyle of *Anopheles dthali, An. fluviatilis* and *An. stephensi* in Southern Iran. *Trop Geogr Med* 1976 ; 28 : 224-7.
- Manouchehri AV, Zaim M, Emadi AM. A review of malaria in Iran, 1975-90. *J Am Mosq Control Assoc* 1992 ; 8 : 381-5.
- Manson P. Report on haematozoa. *Customs Gaz Med Rep Shangaï* 1877 ; 33 : 13-38.
- Manson P. Experimental proof of the mosquito-malaria theory. *Br Med J* 1900 ; 11 : 949-1266.
- Mara L. Studio sull'epidemiologia malarica del comprensorio agricolo di Tessenei. *Riv Malariol* 1950 ; 29 : 1-49.
- Marbiah NT, Petersen E, David K, Magbity E, Lines J, Bradley DJ. A controlled trial of lambda-cyhalothrin-impregnated bed nets and/or dapsone/pyrimethamine for malaria control in Sierra Leone. *Am J Trop Med Hyg* 1998 ; 58 : 1-6.
- Marchand RP, Quang NT, Hoanh NQ, Vien NT. *The Khanh Phu Malaria Research Project*. Review Meeting 1-2 March 1996. Hanoï : Medical Publishing House 1997 : 168 p.
- Marchiafava E, Celli A. Nuove ricerche sulla infezione malarica. *Arch Sci Med Torino* 1885 ; 9 : 311-30.
- Marchiafava E, Bignami A. *On summer-automnal malaria fevers*. London : The New Sydenham Society, 1894.
- Marchoux E. Le paludisme dans les Dombes et en Camargue. *Bull Acad Med Paris* 1927 ; 97 : 67-89.
- Marneffe H, Sautet J. Infestation sporozoïtique naturelle d'*An. gambiae* au Soudan Français. *Bull Soc Pathol Exot* 1944 ; 37 : 315-6.
- Marques AC. Migrations and the dissemination of malaria in Brazil. International Symposium on Malaria. *Mem Inst Oswaldo Cruz* 1986 ; 81 (suppl. 2) : 17-30 .
- Marques AC. Human migration and the spread of malaria in Brazil. *Parasitol Today* 1987 ; 3 (6) : 166-170.
- Marrama L. *La transmission du paludisme dans une région sub-aride du Sud de Madagascar, l'Androy*. Université Paris IV : Thèse Doctorat, 14 décembre 1999.
- Marrama L, Rajaonarivelo E, Rabarison P, Laventure S. *Anopheles funestus* et la riziculture sur les Plateaux de Madagascar. *Cahiers Santé* 1995 ; 5 : 415-21.
- Marrama L, Laventure S, Rabarison P, Roux J. *Anopheles mascarensis* de Meillon, 1947 : vecteur principal du paludisme dans la région de Fort-Dauphin (Sud-Est de Madagascar). *Bull Soc Pathol Exot* 1999 ; 92 : 136-8.
- Marrelli MT, Branquinho MS, Hoffmann EH, Taipe-Lagos CB, Natal D, Kloetzel JK. Correlation between positive serology for *Plasmodium vivax*-like/*Plasmodium simiovale* malaria parasites in the human and anopheline populations in the State of Acre, Brazil. *Trans R Soc Trop Med Hyg* 1998 ; 92 : 149-51.
- Martet G, Da Conceicao S, Cordoliani G, et al. Le paludisme en République de São Tomé et Principe. *Bull Soc Pathol Exot* 1991 ; 84 : 273-80.
- Martinenko V, Dgedge M, Jarov A, Cuâmba N. Incidencia de malaria na cidade de Maputo. *Rev Med Moçambique* 1994 ; 5 : 37-41.
- Mashaal H. *Assignment report. Malaria control and demonstration project, Saudi Arabia, 1956-1958*. WHO/EM/MAL/37 ; January 1959 : 29 p.
- Mashaal H. Epidemiological assessment of malaria in Sheikhupura and Sialkot districts, West Pakistan during 1961-62. *Paskistan J Health* 1962 ; 12 : 134-41.
- Mason JA. *The ancient civilizations of Peru*. London : Penguin Books, 1961.
- Mason J, Hobbs J. Experimental studies on malaria in a high-incidence zone on the coast of El Salvador. *Bol Oficina Sanit Panam* 1978 ; 84 (1) : 50-64.
- Mastbaum O. Observations of two epidemic malaria seasons (1946 and 1953) before and after malaria control in Swaziland. *Trans R Soc Trop Med Hyg* 1954 ; 48 : 325-31.
- Mastbaum O. Past and present position of malaria in Swaziland. *J Trop Med Hyg* 1957 ; 60 : 119-27.
- Mathew KC, Bradley JT. *Research work on an outbreak of malaria at Assumption and Aldabra Island in 1930*. Victoria : Government Printing Office,1932 : 14 p.
- Mathews HM, Armstrong JC. Duffy blood types and *vivax* malaria in Ethiopia. *Am J Trop Med Hyg* 1981 ; 30 : 299-303.
- Mathis C, Leger M. La faune anophélienne du Tonkin dans ses rapports avec l'endémie palustre. *Publ SMCI* 1911 ; 2 : 83.
- Mathur KK, Harpalani G, Kalra NL, Murthy GG, Narasimham MV. Epidemic of malaria in Barmer district (Thar Desert) of Rajasthan during 1990. *Indian J Malariol* 1992 ; 29 : 1-10.
- Matola YG, White GB, Magayuka SA. The changed pattern of malaria endemicity and transmission at Amani in the Eastern Usambara mountains, North Eastern Tanzania. *J Trop Med Hyg* 1987 ; 90 : 127-34.
- Matson AT. The history of malaria in Nandi. *East Afr Med J* 1957 ; 34 : 431-41.
- Matsumoto WK, Vicente MG, Silva MA, de Castro LL. Comportamento epidemiologico da malaria nos municipios que compoem a Bacia do Alto Paraguai, Mato Grosso do Sul, no periodo de 1990 a 1996. *Cad Saude Publica* 1998 ; 14 (4) : 797-802.
- Mattlet G. Le Kapfura ou Kafindo-findo. *Ann Soc Belg Med Trop* 1935 ; 15 : 521-5.
- Maubert B, Fievet N, Tami G, Boudin C, Deloron P. Cytoadherence of *Plasmodium falciparum* infected erythrocytes in the human placenta. *Parasite Immunol* 2000 ; 22 : 191-9.
- May J, Mockenhaupt FP, Ademowo OG, et al. High rate of mixed and subpatent malaria infections in South West Nigeria. *Am J Trop Med Hyg* 1999 ; 61 : 339-43.
- Mazauric P. *Considérations cliniques sur l'épidémie de Maurice (Océan Indien)*. Montpellier : Thèse Médecine, 1869 : n°79 : 47 p.
- McArthur J. The transmission of malaria in Borneo. *Trans R Soc Trop Med Hyg* 1947 ; 40 : 537-58.
- McCormick MC, Brooks-Gunn J, Workman-Daniels K, Turner J, Peckmah GJ. The health and development station of very low-birth-weight children at school-age. *J Am Med Assoc* 1992 ; 267 : 2204-8.
- McCrae AW. Malaria In : Hatt SA, Langlands BM eds. *Uganda atlas of disease distribution*. Nairobi : East African Publishing House, 1975.
- McGregor IA. Epidemiology, malaria and pregnancy. *Am J Trop Med Hyg* 1984 ; 33 (4) : 517-25.
- McGregor IA, Smith DA. A health, nutrition and parasitological survey in a rural village (Keneba) in West Kiang, Gambia. *Trans R Soc Trop Med Hyg* 1952 ; 46 : 403-27.
- McGreevy PB, Dietze R, Prata A, Hembree SC. Effects of immigration on the prevalence of malaria in rural areas of the Amazon basin of Brazil. *Mem Inst Oswaldo Cruz* 1989 ; 84 : 485-94.
- McGuinness D, Koram K, Bennett S, Wagner G, Nkrumah F, Riley E. Clinical case definitions for malaria: clinical malaria associated with very low parasite densities in African infants. *Trans R Soc Trop Med Hyg* 1998 ; 92 : 527-31.
- Meek SR. Epidemiology of malaria in displaced Khmers on the Thai-Kampuchean border. *Southeast Asian J Trop Med Public Health* 1988 ; 19 : 243-52.
- Meek SR. Vector control in some countries of Southeast Asia: comparing the vectors and the strategies. *Ann Trop Med Parasitol* 1995 ; 89 : 135-47.
- Mehr ZA, Rutledge LC, Morales EL, Meixsell VE, Korte DW. Laboratory evaluation of controlled-released insect repellent formulations. *J Am Mosq Control Assoc* 1985 ; 1 (2) : 143-7.
- de Meillon B. Distribution of *An. gambiae* and *An. funestus*. Malaria research station, Tzaneen Report. *S Afr Inst Med Res* 1933 : 61-5.
- de Meillon B. Observations on *Anopheles funestus* and *Anopheles gambiae* in the Transvaal. *Publ S Afr Inst Med Res* 1934 ; 4 : 195-248.
- de Meillon B. Control of malaria in South Africa by measures directed against the adult mosquitoes in habitations. *Quart Bull Health Org League Nations* 1936 ; 5 : 134-7.
- de Meillon B. Malaria survey in South-West Africa. *Bull Organ Mond Santé* 1951 ; 4 : 333-417.
- de Meillon B. *The anophelini of the Ethiopian geographical region*. Johannesburg : South African Institute for Medical Research, 1957 ; 55 : 272 p.
- de Meillon B, Gear J. Malaria contracted on the Witwaterstrand. *S Afr Med J* 1939 ; 13 : 309-12.
- Mekonnen Y, Beyene P. Urban malaria in Nazareth, Ethiopia: parasitological studies. *Ethiopian Med J* 1996 ; 34 : 83-9.
- Meldrum C. *Weather health and forest: a report of the inequalities of the mortality from malarial fever and other diseases in Mauritius considered in relation to inequalities of temperature, humidity and rainfall*. Port-Louis : Mercantile Rec Cy Print Est, 1881 : 238 p.
- Mendez F, Carrasquilla G, Munoz A. Risk factors associated with malaria infection in an urban setting. *Trans R Soc Trop Med Hyg* 2000 ; 94 : 367-71.
- Mendonca FF, Cerqueira NL. Insects and other arthropods captured by the Brazilian Sanitary Services on landplanes or seaplanes arriving in Brazil between January 1942 and December 1945. *Bol Oficina Sanit Panam* 1947 ; 26 : 22.

- Menelau GJ, Pinheiro EA, Marques AC. Foco de malaria na regiao metropolitana de Recife. *Rev Brasil Malariol D Trop* 1981 ; 33 : 96-108.
- Menon PK, Rajagopalan PK. Seasonal changes in the density and natural mortality of immature stages of the urban malaria vector *Anopheles stephensi* in wells in Pondicherry. *Indian J Med Res* 1979 ; 70 (suppl.) : 123-7.
- Merlin M, Le Hesran JY, Josse R, et al. Évaluation des indices cliniques, parasitologiques et immunologiques du paludisme dans la région de la Baie de Bonny en Afrique Centrale. *Bull Soc Pathol Exot* 1986 ; 79 : 707-20.
- Merlin M, Josse R, Laure JM, et al. Étude épidémiologique du paludisme en saison sèche dans la ville de N'Djamena, République du Tchad. *Bull Liaison OCEAC* 1987 ; 79 : 9-18.
- Merlin M, Dupont A, Josse R, et al. Aspects épidémiologiques du paludisme au Gabon. *Med Trop (Marseille)* 1990 ; 50 : 39-46.
- Mesnil F. *Essai sur la classification et l'origine des sporozoaires.* Paris : Cinquantenaire de la Société de Biologie, 1899 : 258-60.
- de Mesquita B. O impaludismo em Angola. *Bol Geral Med* 1942 ; 2 : 111-120.
- de Mesquita B. Malaria in Angola. *Bol Geral Ultramar* 1952 ; 27 : 3-39.
- Metselaar D. Seven years' malaria research and residual house spraying in Netherlands New Guinea. *Am J Trop Med Hyg* 1961 ; 10 : 327-34.
- Metselaar D, Van Thiel PH. Classification of malaria. *Trop Geogr Med* 1959 ; 11 : 157-61.
- Meunier JY, Safeukui I, Fontenille D, Boudin C. Étude de la transmission du paludisme dans une future zone d'essai vaccinal en forêt équatoriale du Sud Cameroun. *Bull Soc Pathol Exot* 1999 ; 92 : 309-12.
- Meuris S, Piko BB, Eerens P, Vanbellinghen AM, Dramaix M, Hennart P. Gestational malaria: assessment of its consequences on fetal growth. *Am J Trop Med Hyg* 1993 ; 48 (5) : 603-9.
- Meyus H, Lips M, Caubergh H. L'état actuel du paludisme d'altitude au Rwanda-Urundi. *Ann Soc Belg Med Trop* 1962 ; 42 : 771-82.
- Michault A, Isautier H, Julvez J, Blanchy S. *Le paludisme à La Réunion après six années d'éradication : situation, moyens de lutte.* Doc. ronéo. Ministère français de la Recherche, 1985 : 7 p.
- Michel AP, Ingrasci MJ, Schemerhorn BJ, et al. Rangewide population genetic structure of the African malaria vector *Anopheles funestus*. *Mol Ecol* 2005 ; 14 : 4235-48.
- Miles SJ, Green CA, Hunt RH. Genetic observations on the taxon *Anopheles pharoensis* Theobald (Diptera: Culicidae). *J Trop Med Hyg* 1983 ; 86 : 153-7.
- Miller LH, Mason SJ, Dvorak JA, McGuinniss MH, Rothman IK. Erythrocyte receptors for *Plasmodium knowlesi* malaria; the Duffy blood-group determinants. *Science* 1975 ; 189 : 561-3.
- Miller LH, Mason SJ, Clyde DF, McGuinniss MH. The resistance factor to *Plasmodium vivax* in blacks. The Duffy blood-group genotype FyFy. *N Engl J Med* 1976 ; 295 : 302-4.
- Miller LH, McGuinniss MH, Holland PV, Sigmon P. The Duffy blood-group phenotype in American blacks infected with *Plasmodium vivax* in Vietnam. *Am J Trop Med Hyg* 1978 ; 27 : 1069-72.
- Miller MJ. Observations on the natural history of malaria in the semi-resistant West African. *Trans R Soc Trop Med Hyg* 1958 ; 52 : 152-68.
- Miller RI, Ikram S, Armelagos GJ, et al. Diagnosis of *P. falciparum* infections in mummies using the rapid manual ParaSight-F test. *Trans R Soc Trop Med Hyg* 1994 ; 88 : 31-2.
- Misra SP, Nandi J, NArasimham MV, Rajagopal R. Malaria transmission in Nagaland, India. Part 1. Anophelines and their seasonality. *J Commun Dis* 1993 ; 25 : 62-6.
- Missiroli A, Hackett LW, Martini E. Le razze di *Anopheles maculipennis* e la loro importanza nella distribuzione del malaria in alcune regioni d'Europa. *Riv Malariol* 1933 ; 12 : 1-56.
- Miyagi I. Studies on malaria vector in Philippines, especially on *Anopheles balabacensis balabacensis* and monkey malaria in Palawan. *Japan J Trop Med* 1973 ; 1 : 163.
- Miyagi I, Toma T. Studies on the mosquitoes in the Yaeyama Islands. I. Appearances of Anopheline mosquitoes, especially *Anopheles minimus* in Ishigakijima and Iriomotejima. *Japan J Sanit Zool* 1978 ; 29 : 243-50.
- Miyagi I, Toma T. *Anopheles saperoi* Bohart and Ingram, an important vector for malaria epidemic in Okinawajina, Japan, 1948-49. SEAMO workshop on vector borne diseases. *Res Inst Trop Med Manila* 1990 ; 27-29 Nov : 1-7.
- Miyake H, Suwa S, Kimura M, Wataya Y. A variant of *Plasmodium ovale*; analysis of its 18 S ribosomal RNA gene sequence. *Nuc Acids Symp Series* 1997 ; 37 : 293-4.
- Mockenhaupt FP, Falusi AG, May J, et al. The contribution of α thalassaemia to anaemia in a Nigerian population exposed to intense malaria transmission. *Trop Med Int Health* 1999 ; 4 : 302-7.
- Mockenhaupt FP, Rong B, Till H, et al. Submicroscopic *Plasmodium falciparum* infections in pregnancy in Ghana. *Trop Med Int Health* 2000 ; 5 : 167-73.
- Modiano G, Morpugo G, Terrenato L, et al. Protection against malaria morbidity: near-fixation of the alpha-thalassemia gene in a Nepalese population. *Am J Hum Genet* 1991 ; 48 : 390-7.
- Modiano G, Petrarca V, Sirima BS, et al. Different responses to *Plasmodium falciparum* malaria in West African sympatric ethnic groups. *Proc Natl Acad Sci USA* 1996 ; 93 : 13206-11.
- Modiano D, Chiucchiuini A, Petrarca V, et al. Humoral response to *P. falciparum* Pf155/ring-infected erythrocyte surface antigen and Pf332 in three sympatric ethnic groups of Burkina Faso. *Am J Trop Med Hyg* 1998 ; 58 : 220-4.
- Mohammad AM, Ardatl KO, Bajakian KM. Sickle cell disease in Bahrain: coexistence and interaction with glucose-6-phosphate dehydrogenase (G6PD) deficiency. *J Trop Pediatr* 1998 ; 44 : 70-2.
- Molez JF, Desenfant P, Pajot FX, Jacques JR, Duverseau Y, Saint-Jean Y. Le paludisme en Haïti. 2. Présence d'*Anopheles (A.) pseudopunctipennis* Theobald 1901 : première mise en évidence sur l'île d'Hispaniola. *Cahiers ORSTOM, Entomol Med Parasitol* 1987 ; 25 (2) : 75-81.
- Molez JF, Desenfant P, Pajot FX, Jacques JR, Duverseau Y. Le paludisme en Haïti. *Vect Ecol Newslett* 1988 ; 19 : 9.
- Molez JF, Desenfant P, Jacques JR. Bio-écologie en Haïti d'*An. albimanus* Wiedemann,1820. *Bull Soc Pathol Exot* 1998 ; 91 (4) : 334-9.
- Molina R, Benito A, Roche J, et al. Baseline entomological data for a pilot malaria control program in Equatorial Guinea. *J Med Entomol* 1993 ; 30 : 622-4.
- Molina-Cruz A, de Merida AM, Mills K, et al. Gene flow among *Anopheles albimanus* populations in Central America, South America, and the Caribbean assessed by microsatellites and mitochondrial DNA. *Am J Trop Med Hyg* 2004 ; 71 : 350-9.
- Molineaux L. La lutte contre les maladies parasitaires : le problème du paludisme en Afrique. In : Vallin J, Lopez A, eds. *La lutte contre la mort.* INED-UIEGP, Travaux et documents, Cahier n°108. Paris : PUF, 1985 : 1-39.
- Molineaux L. The epidemiology of human malaria as an explanation of its distribution, including some implications for its control. In : Wernsdorfer WH, McGregor I, eds. *Malaria*. Edinburgh : Churchill Livingstone, 1988 : 913-98.
- Molineaux L. Malaria and mortality: some epidemiological considerations. *Ann Trop Med Parasitol* 1997a ; 91 : 811-25.
- Molineaux L. Nature's experiment: what implication for malaria prevention? *Lancet* 1997b ; 349 : 1636-7.
- Molineaux L, Fleming AF, Cornille-Brogger R, Kagan I, Storey J. Abnormal haemoglobin in the Sudan savannah of Nigeria. III. Malaria, immunoglobulins and antimalarial antibodies in sickle cell disease. *Ann Trop Med Parasitol* 1979a ; 73 : 301-10.
- Molineaux L, Shidrawi GR, Clarke JR, Boulzaguet JR, Ashkam TS. Assessment of insecticital impact on the malaria mosquito's vectorial capacity from data on the man-biting rate and age composition. *Bull World Health Organ* 1979b ; 57 : 265-74.
- Molineaux L, Storey J, Cohen JE, Thomas A. A longitudinal study of human malaria in the West African savanna in the absence of control measures: relationships between different *Plasmodium* species, in particular *P. falciparum* and *P. malariae*. *Am J Trop Med Hyg* 1980 ; 29 : 725-37.
- Molineaux L, Gramiccia G. *The Garki Project. Research on epidemiology and control of malaria in a Sudan savanna of West Africa.* Genève : OMS, 1980 : 311 p.
- Monges P, Josse R, Merlin M, et al. Évaluation des indices paludométriques à Bangui. *Bull Liaison OCEAC* 1987 ; 80 : 115-24.
- Montagne L. *Essai de grammaire malgache.* Paris : Société d'Éditions, 1989 : 186 p.
- Montestruc E. Le paludisme à la Martinique. *Bull Soc Pathol Exot* 1936 ; 29 : 193-202.
- Montillier J. Un foyer de paludisme au Gourara : Heiha. *Arch Inst Pasteur Algérie* 1954 ; 32 : 255-65.
- Moorhouse DE, Chooi CK. Notes on the bionomics of *Anopheles campestris* and on its disappearance following house-spraying with residual insecticides. *Med J Malaya* 1964 ; 18 : 184-92.
- Moorthy V, Wilkinson D. Severity of malaria and level of *P. falciparum* transmission. *Lancet* 1997 ; 350 (9074) : 362-3.
- Morillon M, Baudon D, Dai B. Les paludismes au Viêtnam en 1996. Brève synthèse des connaissances épidémiologiques. *Med Trop (Marseille)* 1996 ; 56 : 197-200.
- Morley D, Woodland M, Cuthbertson WF. Controlled trial of pyrimethamine in pregnant women in an African village. *Br Med J* 1964 ; 1 : 667-8.

- Moschkovsky SD, Rashina MG. *Epidemiology and medical parasitology for entomologists*. Moscou : Modgiz, 1951 : 132-7.
- Moscoso Carrasco C. *Bolivia elimina su malaria*. Rapport Ministerio de Salud Publica, 1963 : 108 p.
- Mosha FW, Subra R. *Ecological studies on* Anopheles gambiae *complex sibling species in Kenya. I. Preliminary observations on their geographical distribution and chromosomal polymorphic inversions*. WHO/VBC/82.867 ; 1982 : 9 p.
- Mosha FW, Petrarca V. Ecological studies on *An. gambiae* complex sibling species on the Kenya Coast. *Trans R Soc Trop Med Hyg* 1983 ; 77 : 344-5.
- Motabar M. Malaria and nomadic tribes in Southern Iran. *Cahiers ORSTOM, Entomol Med Parasitol* 1974 ; 12 : 175-8.
- Motabar M, Tabibzadeh I, Manouchehri AV. Malaria and its control in Iran. *Trop Geogr Med* 1975 ; 27 : 71-8.
- Mouchet J. Influence des fleuves sur la biologie d'*An. gambiae* pendant la saison sèche dans le Sud Cameroun. *Bull Soc Pathol Exot* 1962 ; 55 : 1163-71.
- Mouchet J. Prospection sur *Ae. aegypti* et les vecteurs potentiels de fièvre jaune en République Démocratique de Somalie et dans le Territoire français des Afars et des Issas. *Bull Organ Mond Santé* 1971 ; 45 : 383-94.
- Mouchet J. *Mission au Swaziland*. Rapport OMS/AFRO/1987a : 19 p.
- Mouchet J. *Mission au Botswana*. Rapport OMS/AFRO/1987b : 33 p.
- Mouchet J. Agriculture and vector resistance. *Insect Sc Applic (Nairobi)* 1988 ; 9 : 297-307.
- Mouchet J. Malaria in Madagascar. *Res Rev Parasitol* 1998 ; 58 : 185-8.
- Mouchet J, Gariou J. Exophilie et exophagie d'*An. gambiae* Giles 1902 dans le Sud Cameroun. *Bull Soc Pathol Exot* 1957 ; 50 : 446-61.
- Mouchet J, Gariou J. Anophélisme et paludisme dans le département Bamiléké. *Rech Études Camerounaises* 1960 ; 1 : 92-114.
- Mouchet J, Gariou J. Répartition géographique et écologique des anophèles au Cameroun. *Bull Soc Pathol Exot* 1961 ; 54 : 102-18.
- Mouchet J, Cavalié P, Callies JM, Marticou H. L'irritabilité au DDT d'*An. gambiae* et d'*An. funestus* dans le Nord Cameroun. *Riv Malariol* 1961 ; 40 : 191-217.
- Mouchet J, Gariou J. *Anopheles moucheti* au Cameroun. *Cahiers ORSTOM, Entomol Med Parasitol* 1966 ; 4 : 71-81.
- Mouchet J, Carnevale P. Malaria endemicity in the various phytogeographic and climatic areas of Africa, South of Sahara. *Southeast Asian J Trop Med Public Health* 1981 ; 12 : 439-40.
- Mouchet J, Baudon. *Rapport au ministère français de la Coopération*, 1986.
- Mouchet J, Carnevale P. Le paludisme, composante de l'environnement africain. *ORSTOM Actualités* 1988 ; 20 : 1-8.
- Mouchet J, Nadire-Galliot M, Gay F, *et al.* Le paludisme en Guyane : les caractéristiques des différents foyers et la lutte antipaludique. *Bull Soc Pathol Exot* 1989 ; 82 : 393-405.
- Mouchet J, Robert V, Carnevale P, *et al.* Le défi de la lutte contre le paludisme en Afrique tropicale : place et limite de la lutte antivectorielle. *Cahiers Santé* 1991 ; 1 : 277-88.
- Mouchet J, Blanchy S, Rakotonjanabelo A, *et al.* Stratification épidémiologique du paludisme à Madagascar. *Arch Inst Pasteur Madagascar* 1993a ; 60 : 50-9.
- Mouchet J, Carnevale P, Coosemans M, *et al.* Typologie du paludisme en Afrique. *Cahiers Santé* 1993b ; 3 : 220-38.
- Mouchet J, Faye O, Handschumacher P. Les vecteurs de maladies dans les mangroves des rivières du Sud. In : Cormier-Salem MC, ed. *Dynamique et usages de la mangrove dans les pays des rivières du Sud, du Sénégal à la Sierra Leone*. Paris : ORSTOM, 1994 : 117-23.
- Mouchet J, Giacomini T, Julvez J. La diffusion anthropique des arthropodes vecteurs de maladie dans le Monde. *Cahiers Santé* 1995 ; 5(5) : 293-8.
- Mouchet J, Faye O, Julvez J, Manguin S. Drought and malaria retreat in the Sahel, West Africa. *Lancet* 1996 ; 348 (9043) : 1735-6.
- Mouchet J, Laventure S, Blanchy S, *et al.* La reconquête des Hautes Terres de Madagascar par le paludisme. *Bull Soc Pathol Exot* 1997 ; 90 : 162-8.
- Mouchet J, Carnevale P. Entomological biodiversity of malaria in the world. *Res Rev Parasitol* 1998 ; 58 : 189-95.
- Mouchet J, Manguin S, Sircoulon J, *et al.* Evolution of malaria in Africa for the past 40 years: impact of climatic and human factors. *J Am Mosq Control Assoc* 1998 ; 14 : 121-30.
- Mouchet J, Manguin S. Le réchauffement de la planète et l'expansion du paludisme. *Ann Soc Entomol Fr* 1999 ; 35 : 549-55.
- Mount RA. Medical mission to the Yemen, Southwest Arabia, 1951. I. Geomedical observations. *Am J Trop Med Hyg* 1953 ; 2 : 1-12.

- Mpofu SM. Seasonal vector density and disease incidence patterns of malaria in an area of Zimbabwe. *Trans R Soc Trop Med Hyg* 1985 ; 79 : 169-75.
- Muentener P, Schlagenhauf P, Steffen R. Imported malaria (1985-95): trends and perspectives. *Bull World Health Organ* 1999 ; 77 : 560-6.
- Muir DA, Keilany M. *Anopheles claviger* Meigen as a malaria vector in Syria. WHO/MAL/72.757 ; 1972.
- Muirhead-Thomson RC. Studies on the breeding places and control of *Anopheles gambiae* var. *melas* in coastal district of Sierra Leone. *Bull Entomol Res* 1945 ; 36 : 185-252.
- Muirhead-Thomson RC. Recent knowledge about malaria vectors in West Africa and their control. *Trans R Soc Trop Med Hyg* 1947 ; 40 : 512-36.
- Muirhead-Thomson RC. Studies on salt-water and fresh-water *An. gambiae* on the East African Coast. *Bull Entomol Res* 1951 ; 41 : 487-502.
- Muirhead-Thomson RC. Factors determining the true reservoir of infection of *P. falciparum* and *W. bancrofti* in a West African village. *Trans R Soc Trop Med Hyg* 1954 ; 48 : 208-25.
- Muirhead-Thomson RC. The malarial infectivity of an African village population to mosquitoes (*An. gambiae*). *Am J Trop Med Hyg* 1957a ; 6 : 971-9.
- Muirhead-Thomson RC. Notes on the characters of *P. malariae* oocysts of possible value in mixed infections. *Am J Trop Med Hyg* 1957b ; 6 : 980-6.
- Muirhead-Thomson RC. *The winter activities of An. gambiae at high altitudes in Southern Rhodesia*. WHO/MAL/261 ; 1960 : 8 p.
- Muirhead-Thomson RC, Mercier EC. Factors in malaria transmission by *Anopheles albimanus* in Jamaica. Part I. *Ann Trop Med Parasitol* 1952a ; 46 : 103-13.
- Muirhead-Thomson RC, Mercier EC. Factors in malaria transmission by *Anopheles albimanus* in Jamaica. Part II. *Ann Trop Med Parasitol* 1952b ; 46 : 201-13.
- Mukabayire O, Boccolini D, Lochouarn L, Fontenille D, Besansky NJ. Mitochondrial and ribosomal internal transcribed spacer (ITS2) diversity of the African malaria vector, *An. funestus*. *Mol Ecol* 1999 ; 8 : 289-97.
- Mukiama TK, Mwangi RW. Seasonal population changes and malaria transmission potential of *Anopheles pharoensis* and the minor anophelines in Mwea Irrigation Scheme, Kenya. *Acta Tropica* 1989 ; 46 : 181-9.
- Müller P. Uber Zusammenhänge zwischen Konstitution und insectizider Wirkung. *Helvetica Chimica Acta* 1946 ; 29 : 1560-80.
- Müller P. *DDT. Des insektizid dichlorodiphenyltrichlorothan und seine bedentung*. Basel : Birkläuser, 1955.
- Mulligan HW, Baily JD. Malaria in Quetta, Balutchistan. *Rec Mal Surv India* 1938 ; 6 : 289-385.
- Mulumba MP, Wery M, Ngimbi NN, Paluku K, Van der Stuyft P, De Muynck A. Le paludisme de l'enfant à Kinshasa (Zaïre). Influence des saisons, de l'âge, de l'environnement et du standing familial. *Med Trop (Marseille)* 1990 ; 50 : 53-64.
- Mulumba PM, Wery M, Ngimbi NN, Paluku K, De Muynck A, Van der Stuyft P. Relation entre parasitémie à *Plasmodium* et accès fébrile dans différents groupes de population à Kinshasa (Zaïre). *Ann Soc Belg Med Trop* 1994 ; 74 : 275-89.
- Munyantore S. Historique de la lutte antipaludique au Rwanda. *Rev Med Rwandaise* 1989 ; 21 : 14-28.
- Murillo BC, Astaiza VR, Fajardo OP. Biology of *Anopheles (Kerteszia) neivai* H, D, K, 1913 (Diptera: Culicidae) on the Pacific coast of Colombia. III. Light intensity measurements and biting behaviour. *Rev Saude Publica* 1988 ; 22 (2) : 102-12.
- Murphy S, Bremen J. Gaps in the childhood malaria burden in Africa: cerebral malaria, neurological sequelae, anemia, respiratory distress, hypoglycemia and complication of pregnancy. *Am J Trop Med Hyg* 2001 ; 64 : 57-67.
- Mutabingwa TK. Malaria and pregnancy: epidemiology, pathophysiology and control options. *Acta Tropica* 1994 ; 57 (4) : 239-54.
- Mutabingwa TK, Malle LN, de Geus A, Oosting J. Malaria chemosuppression in pregnancy. I. The effect of chemosuppressive drugs on maternal parasitaemia. *Trop Geogr Med* 1993 ; 45 (1) : 6-14.
- Myo Paing, Tun Lin W, Sebastian AA. Behaviour of *Anopheles minimus* in relation to its role as vector of malaria in a forested foothill area of Burma. *Trop Biomed* 1988 ; 5 : 161-6.

- Nagel RL, Fleming AF. Genetic epidemiology of the beta S gene. *Baillieres Clin Haematol* 1992 ; 5 : 331-65.
- Nagpal BN, Sharma VP. Mosquitoes of Andaman Islands. *Indian J Malariol* 1983 ; 20 : 7-13.
- Nagpal BN, Sharma VP. Survey of mosquito fauna of North-Eastern region of India. *Indian J Malariol* 1987 ; 24 : 143-9.
- Nair CP. Malaria in Kashmir province of Jammu and Kashmir State, India. *J Commun Dis* 1973 ; 5 : 22-46.

- Najera JA. A critical review of the field application of a mathematical model of malaria eradication. *Bull World Health Organ* 1974 ; 50 : 449-57.
- Najera JA. Le paludisme et l'action de l'OMS. *Bull Organ Mond Santé* 1989 ; 67 : 347-63 .
- Najera JA. *Malaria control among refugees and displaced populations*. WHO/CTD/MAL/96.6 ; 1996 : 62 p.
- Najera JA. Malaria control: achievements, problems and strategies. *Parassitologia* 2001 ; 43 (1-2) : 1-89.
- Najera JA, Shidrawi GR, Gibson FD, Stafford JS. A large-scale field trial of malathion as an insecticide for antimalarial work in Southern Uganda. *Bull World Health Organ* 1967 ; 36 : 913-35.
- Najera JA, Hempel J. *The burden of malaria*. Genève : OMS, 1996 : 58 p.
- Najera JA, Kouznetsov RL, Delacollette C. *Malaria epidemics: detection and control, forecasting and prevention*. WHO/MAL/98.1084 ; 1998 : 81 p.
- Najera JA, Zaim M. *Malaria vector control: insecticides for indoor residual spraying*. WHO/CDS/WHOPES/2001.3 ; 2001 : 9 p.
- Naji M, Omari M, El Mellouki W, *et al*. Le paludisme d'importation au Maroc. *Rev Int Serv Santé Armées Terre Mer Air* 1985 ; 58 : 241-3.
- Nanda N, Joshi H, Subbarao SK, *et al*. Anopheles fluviatilis complex: host feeding patterns of species S, T and U. *J Am Mosq Control Assoc* 1996 ; 12 : 147-9.
- Nanda N, Das MK, Wattal S, Adak T, Subbarao SK. Cytogenetic characterization of *Anopheles sundaicus* (Diptera: Culicidae) population from Car Nicobar Island, India. *Ann Entomol Soc Am* 2004 ; 97 : 171-6.
- Narang SK, Kaiser PE, Seawright JA. Identification of species D, a new member of the *Anopheles quadrimaculatus* species complex: a biochemical key. *J Am Mosq Control Assoc* 1989 ; 5 : 317-24.
- Nemirovskaia AI, Logvinova ZI, Iasinskii AA. Introduction of malaria into the RSFSR. *Med Parazitol (Mosk)* 1975 ; 44 : 406-11.
- Nethercott AS. Forty years of malaria control in Natal and Zululand. *S Afr Med J* 1974 ; 48 : 1168-70.
- Nevill CG, Some ES, Mung'Ala VO, *et al*. Insecticide-treated bednets reduce mortality and severe morbidity from malaria among children on the Kenya Coast. *Trop Med Int Health* 1996 ; 1 (2) : 139-46.
- Ng'Andu N, Watts TE, Wray JR, Chela C, Zulu B. Some risk factors for transmission of malaria in a population where control measures were applied in Zambia. *East Afr Med J* 1989 ; 66 : 728-37.
- N'Guessan Diplo L, Rey JL, Soro B, Coulibaly A. La mortalité infantile et ses causes dans une sous-préfecture de Côte d'Ivoire. *Med Trop (Marseille)* 1990 ; 50 : 429-32.
- N'Guessan R, Darriet F, Guillet P, *et al*. Resistance to carbosulfan in *Anopheles gambiae* from Ivory Coast, based on reduced sensitivity of acetylcholinesterase. *Med Vet Entomol* 2003 ; 17 : 1-7.
- N'Guessan R, Rowland M, Moumouni TL, Kesse NB, Carnevale P. Evaluation of synthetic repellents on mosquito nets in experimental huts against insecticide-resistant *Anopheles gambiae* and *Culex quinquefasciatus* mosquitoes. *Trans R Soc Trop Med Hyg* 2006 ; 100 : 1091-7.
- Nguyen DM, Tran DH, Harbach RE, Elphick J, Linton YM. A new species of the *Hyrcanus* group of *Anopheles*, a secondary vector of malaria in coastal areas of Southern Vietnam. *J Am Mosq Control Assoc* 2000 ; 16 (3) : 189-98.
- Nguyen Thi Hong. Les lignes biogéographiques Indo-Australiennes. *Ann Biol* 1987 ; 17 : 321-40.
- Nicholson SE. Saharan climates in historic times. In : Williams MAJ, Faure H, eds *The Sahara and the Nile*. Rotterdam : Balkema, 1980 : 173-200.
- Nicholson SE. The historical climatology of Africa. In : Wigley TML, Ingram MJ, Farmer G, eds. *Climate and history*. Cambridge : Cambridge University Press, 1981 : 249-70.
- Nicolescu G, Linton YM, Vladimirescu A, Howard TM, Harbach RE. Mosquitoes of the *Anopheles maculipennis* group (Diptera: Culicidae) in Romania, with the discovery and formal recognition of a new species based on molecular and morphological evidence. *Bull Entomol Res* 2004 ; 94 : 525-35.
- Nigatu W, Abebe M, Dejene A. *Plasmodium vivax* and *P. falciparum* epidemiology in Gambella, South-West Ethiopia. *Trop Med Parasitol* 1992 ; 43 : 181-5.
- Njan Nloga A, Robert V, Toto JC, Carnevale P. *Anopheles moucheti*, vecteur principal du paludisme au Sud Cameroun. *Bull Liaison OCEAC* 1993a ; 26 : 63-7.
- Njan Nloga A, Robert V, Toto JC, Carnevale P. La durée du cycle gonotrophique d'*An. moucheti* varie de trois à quatre jours en fonction de la proximité par rapport aux gîtes de ponte. *Bull Liaison OCEAC* 1993b ; 26 : 69-72.
- Nkhoma WA, Nwanyanwu OC, Kazembe PN, Krogstad D, Wirima JJ, Steketre RW. Cerebral malaria in Malawian children hospitalised with *P. falciparum* infection. *Ann Trop Med Parasitol* 1999 ; 93 : 231-7.
- Nkrumah FK, Perkins IV. Sickle cell trait, hemoglobin C trait and Burkitt's lymphoma. *Am J Trop Med Hyg* 1976 ; 25 : 633-6.
- Nosten F, ter Kuile F, Maelankiri L, *et al*. Mefloquine prophylaxis prevents malaria during pregnancy: a double-blind placebo-controlled study. *J Infect Dis* 1994 ; 169 (3) : 595-603.
- Nosten F, McGready R, Simpson JA, *et al*. Effects of *Plasmodium vivax* malaria in pregnancy. *Lancet* 1999 ; 354 (9178) : 546-9.
- Nosten F, Van Vugt M, Price R, *et al*. Effects of artesunate-mefloquine combination on incidence of *Plasmodium falciparum* malaria and mefloquine resistance in Western Thailand: a prospective study. *Lancet* 2000 ; 356 (9226) : 297-302.
- Nussenzweig RS, Vanderberg J, Most H, Orton C. Protective immunity produced by the injection of X-irradiated sporozoïtes of *Plasmodium berghei*. *Nature* 1967 ; 216 : 160-2.
- Nutsathapana S, Sawasdiwongphorn P, Chitprarop U, Cullen JR. The behaviour of *Anopheles minimus* Theobald subjected to differing levels of DDT selection pressure in Northern Thailand. *Bull Entomol Res* 1986a ; 76 : 303-12.
- Nutsathapana S, Sawasdiwongphorn P, Chitprarop U, Cullen JR, Gass RF, Green CA. A mark-release recapture demonstration of host-preference heterogeneity in *Anopheles minimus* in a Thai village. *Bull Entomol Res* 1986b ; 76 : 313-20.
- Nzeyimana I, Henry MC, Dossou-Yovo J, Doannio JM, Diawara L, Carnevale P. Épidémiologies du paludisme dans le sud-ouest forestier de la Côte d'Ivoire. *Bull Soc Pathol Exot* 2002 ; 95 : 89-94.
- Obsomer V, Defourny P, Coosemans M. The *Anopheles dirus* Complex: spatial distribution and environmental drivers. *Malaria J* 2007 ; 6 : 26 (http://malariajournal.com/contents/6/1/26).
- Ochrymowicz JW, Bakri GE, Hudleston JA. *Rapport sur la prospection faite en vue d'une action antipaludique au Niger*. OMS/AFR/MAL/106. Brazzaville, 1969 : 68 p.
- O'Connor CT. The distribution of anopheline mosquitoes in Ethiopia. *Mosquito News* 1967 ; 27 : 42-54.
- Odetoyinbo JA, Davidson G. *The Anopheles gambiae complex and its role in the malaria transmission in the Islands of Zanzibar and Pemba, Tanzania*. WHO/MAL/68.660 ; 1968 : 5 p.
- Ogata K, Tanaka I, Ito Y, Morii S. Survey of the medically important insects carried by the international aircrafts to Tokyo International Airport. *Japan J Sanit Zool* 1974 ; 25 : 177-84.
- Ogutu BR, Smoak BL, Nduati RW, Mbori-Ngacha DA, Mwathe F, Shanks GD. The efficacy of pyrimethamine-sulfadoxine (Fansidar®) in the treatment of uncomplicated *Plasmodium falciparum* malaria in Kenyan children. *Trans R Soc Trop Med Hyg* 2000 ; 94 (1) : 83-4.
- Olano V, Carrasquilla G, Mendez F. Urban malaria transmission in Buenaventura, Colombia: entomologic aspects. *Rev Panam Salud Publica* 1997 ; 2 (6) : 378-85.
- Olivier M, Develoux M, Chegou A, Loutan L. Presumptive diagnosis of malaria results in a significant risk of mistreatment of children in urban Sahel. *Trans R Soc Trop Med Hyg* 1991 ; 85 : 729-30.
- de Oliveira-Ferreira J, Lourenco de Oliveira R, Teva A, Deane LM, Daniel-Ribeiro CT. Natural malaria infections in anophelines in Rondonia State, Brazilian Amazon. *Am J Trop Med Hyg* 1990 ; 43 (1) : 6-10.
- de Oliveira-Ferreira J, Lourenco de Oliveira R, Deane LM, Daniel-Ribeiro CT. Feeding preference of *Anopheles darlingi* in malaria endemic areas of Rondonia State, Northwestern Brazil. *Mem Inst Oswaldo Cruz* 1992 ; 87 (4) : 601-2.
- Olivier J, Grobler E. Weather malaria incidence relationships in the Nelspruit region. *S Afr J Sc* 1992 ; 88 : 452-3.
- Olivry JC, Chastanet M. Évolution du climat dans le bassin du fleuve Sénégal (Bakel) depuis le milieu du 19e siècle. In : *Changements globaux en Afrique durant le quaternaire*. ORSTOM, Travaux et Documents 1986 ; 197 : 337-43.
- Ollomo B, Karch S, Bureau P, Elissa N, Georges AJ, Millet P. Lack of malaria parasite transmission between apes and humans in Gabon. *Am J Trop Med Hyg* 1997 ; 56 : 440-5.
- Oloo A., Vulule JM, Koech DK. Some emerging issues on the malaria problem in Kenya. *East Afr Med J* 1996 ; 73 : 50-3.
- Olumese PE, Adeyemo AA, Ademowo OG, Gbadegesin RA, Sodeinde O, Walker O. The clinical manifestations of cerebral malaria among Nigerian children with sickle cell trait. *Ann Trop Paediatr* 1997 ; 17 : 141-5.
- Olweny CL, Chauhan SS, Simooya OO, Bulsara MK, Njelesani EK, Van Thuc I. Adult cerebral malaria in Zambia. *J Trop Med Hyg* 1986 ; 89 : 123-9.

- Omer SM, Cloudsley-Thompson JL. Dry season biology of *Anopheles gambiae* in the Sudan. *Nature* 1968 ; 217 : 879-80.
- Omer SM, Cloudsley-Thompson JL. Survival of females *Anopheles gambiae* through a nine month dry season in Sudan. *Bull World Health Organ* 1970 ; 42 : 319-30.
- OMS. Comité d'experts du paludisme, 5e rapport. Genève : OMS, 1954 : Série Rapports Techniques n° 80.
- OMS. Comité d'experts du paludisme, 6e rapport. Genève : OMS, 1957 : Série Rapports Techniques n° 123.
- OMS. *Annual report of the Malaria Eradication Program in Uganda.* 1961.
- OMS. *Terminologie du paludisme et de l'éradication du paludisme.* Genève : OMS, 1964 : 176 p.
- OMS. *Chimiothérapie du paludisme et résistance aux antipaludiques.* Genève, 17-24 Octobre 1972. Genève : OMS, 1973 : Série Rapports Techniques n° 529 : 128 p.
- OMS. Comité d'experts du paludisme, 16e rapport. Genève : OMS, 1974 : Série Rapports Techniques n° 549.
- OMS. Surveillance du paludisme. *Wkly Epidemiol Rec* 1978 ; 53 : 337-8.
- OMS. *Receptivity to malaria and other parasitic diseases.* Reports and studies n°15. Copenhague : Office Régional pour l'Europe, 1979 : 103 p.
- OMS. *Résistance des vecteurs de maladies aux pesticides.* Genève : OMS, 1981a : Série Rapports Techniques n° 655.
- OMS. La situation du paludisme dans le monde en 1979. *Wkly Epidemiol Rec* 1981b ; 56 : 145-9.
- OMS. *Paludisme 1962-1981.* World Health Statist Annual 1983 : 791-5.
- OMS. *Chemistry and specifications for pesticides.* 8th rpt of the WHO Expert Committee on Vector Biology and Control, Geneva ; 8-14 November 1983. Genève : OMS, 1983 : Série Rapports Techniques n° 699 : 46 p.
- OMS. *Résistance aux pesticides des vecteurs et réservoirs de maladies.* Genève : OMS, 1986 : Série Rapports Techniques n° 737 : 94 p.
- OMS. *Report on a technical consultation on research in support of malaria control in the Amazon basin.* TDR/FIELDMAL/SC/AMAZ/88.3 ; 1988 : 25 p.
- OMS. World malaria situation, 1988. *World Health Statist Quart* 1990a ; 43 : 68-79.
- OMS. *Equipment for vector control*, 3e ed. Genève : OMS, 1990b.
- OMS. *A global strategy for malaria control.* Ministerial Conference on Malaria, Amsterdam, 26-27 oct. 1992. Genève : OMS, 1992a : 30 p.
- OMS. *Résistance des vecteurs aux pesticides.* Genève : OMS, 1992b : Série Rapports Techniques n° 818.
- OMS. Flambée de paludisme (Inde). *Wkly Epidemiol Rec* 1994 ; 69 : 321.
- OMS. La situation du paludisme dans le monde en 1993, partie II. *Wkly Epidemiol Rec* 1996a ; 71 : 25-29.
- OMS. *Assessment of therapeutic efficacy of antimalarial drugs for uncomplicated falciparum malaria in areas with intense transmission.* WHO/MAL/96.1077 ; 1996b : 32 p.
- OMS. *Management for poisoning. A handbook for Health Care Workers.* Genève : OMS, 1997 : 314 p.
- OMS. *The WHO recommended classification of pesticides by hazard and guidelines to classification, 1998-1999.* WHO/PCS/98.21, 1998a : 64 p.
- OMS. *The use of artemisinin and its derivatives as antimalarial drugs: report of a joint CTD/DMP/TDR informal consultation, Geneva, 10-12 June 1998.* WHO/MAL/98.1086 ; 1998b : 33 p.
- OMS. Paludisme, 1982-1997. *Wkly Epidemiol Rec* 1999a ; 74 : 265-70.
- OMS. *Strategy to roll back malaria in the WHO European Region.* Copenhague : OMS, 1999b : 16 p.
- OMS. *Maladies transmissibles 2000. Principales activités en 1999 et grands défis pour l'avenir.* WHO/CDS/2000.1, 2000a : 102 p.
- OMS. Severe *falciparum* malaria (Severe and complicated malaria, third edition). *Trans R Soc Trop Med Hyg* 2000b ; 94 (suppl. 1) : 90 p.
- OMS. *Manual for indoor residual spraying: application of residual sprays for vector control.* WHO/CDS/WHOPES/GCDPP/2000.3. Genève : OMS, 2000c : 48 p.
- OMS. *Vade-mecum pour la prise en charge du paludisme grave.* Genève : OMS, 2001a.
- OMS. *Les combinaisons thérapeutiques antipaludiques : rapport d'une consultation technique de l'OMS, 4-5 Avril 2001.* WHO/CDS/RBM/2001.35 ; 2001b : 40 p.
- OMS. *The use of antimalarial drugs.* WHO/CDS/RBM, 2001/33 ; 2001c.
- Omumbo J, Ouma J, Rapuoda B, Craig MH, Le Sueur D, Snow RW. Mapping malaria transmission intensity using geographical information systems (GIS): an example from Kenya. *Ann Trop Med Parasitol* 1998 ; 92 : 7-21.

- Onori E. Differences in *Plasmodium malariae* prevalence in Uganda. *Bull World Health Organ* 1967a ; 37 : 330-1.
- Onori E. Distribution of *Plasmodium ovale* in the Eastern, Western and Northern Regions of Uganda. *Bull World Health Organ* 1967b ; 37 : 665-8.
- Onori E. Malaria in Karamoja District, Uganda. *Parassitologia* 1969 ; 11 : 235-49.
- Onori E. *Report of a mission to Mozambique,* 17 Feb.-13 March 1982. Report to WHO, 1982.
- Onori E, Benthein F. An investigation of the annual cycle of malaria in an area of Uganda. *Parassitologia* 1969 ; 11 : 251-70.
- Onori E, Nushin MK, Cullen JE, Yakubi GH, Mohammed K, Christal FA. An epidemiological assessment of the residual effect of DDT on *Anopheles hyrcanus s.l.* and *An. pulcherrimus* (Theobald) in the North Eastern region of Afghanistan. *Trans R Soc Trop Med Hyg* 1975 ; 69 : 236-42.
- Onori E, Grab B. Indicators for the forecasting of malaria epidemics. *Bull World Health Organ* 1980 ; 58 : 91-8.
- Onyabe DY, Conn JE. Intragenomic heterogeneity of a ribosomal DNA spacer (ITS2) varies regionally in the neotropical malaria vector *Anopheles nuneztovari*. *Insect Mol Biol* 1999 ; 8 (4) : 435-42.
- Orach CG. Morbidity and mortality amongst Southern Sudanese in Koboko refugee camps, Arua District, Uganda. *East Afr Med J* 1999 ; 76 : 195-9.
- Ossi GT. A progress report on malaria eradication in Iraq. *Bull Endem Dis (Baghdad)* 1969 ; 11 : 48-66.
- Ossi GT. Malaria eradication programme in Iraq 1970-1975. *Bull Endem Dis (Baghdad)* 1977 ; 18 : 13-33.
- Ossi GT. Malaria in Iraq for the years 1984 and 1985. *Bull Endem Dis (Baghdad)* 1986 ; 27 : 5-23.
- Oswald G, Lawrence EP. Runway malaria. *Lancet* 1990 ; 335 : 1537.
- Otsuru M, Ohmori Y. Malaria studies in Japan after World War II. Part II. The research of *Anopheles sinensis* sibling species group. *Jpn J Exper Med* 1960 ; 30 : 33-65.
- Ovazza M, Neri P. Vecteurs du paludisme en altitude, région d'Addis Abeba, Ethiopie. *Bull Soc Pathol Exot* 1955 ; 48 : 679-86.

- Packard RM. Agricultural development, migrant labor and the resurgence of malaria in Swaziland. *Soc Sci Med* 1986 ; 22 : 861-7.
- PAHO (Pan American Health Organization). *Status of malaria programs in the Americas.* XLII report, Washington D.C. September 1994. CSP24/INF/2 : 116 p.
- PAHO (Pan American Health Organization). *Status of malaria programs in the Americas.* XLIV report, Washington D.C. September 1996. CD39/INF/2 : 22 p.
- PAHO (Pan American Health Organization). Malaria in the Americas, 1996. *Epidemiol Bull* 1997 ; 18 : 1-8.
- PAHO (Pan American Health Organization). Assessment of the 1980-1998 health situation and trends in the Americas by subregion. *Epidemiol Bull* 1999 ; 20 : 2-10.
- PAHO (Pan American Health Organization). *Report on the status of malaria programs in the Americas (based on 2000 data).* Washington D.C. September 2001. CD43/INF/1 : 23 p.
- PAHO (Pan American Health Organization). Malaria in the Americas: time series, epidemiological data from 1998 to 2004. 2005.
- Paik YH, Ree HI, Shim JC. Malaria in Korea. *Japan J Exper Med* 1988 ; 58 : 55-66.
- Pajot FX. *Rapport sur une mission au Rwanda.* Université de Bordeaux, 1991.
- Pajot FX, Le Pont F, Molez JF, Degallier N. Agressivité d'*Anopheles (Nyssorhynchus) darlingi* Root, 1926 (Diptera : Culicidae) en Guyane Française. *Cahiers ORSTOM, Entomol Med Parasitol* 1977 ; 15 (1) : 15-22.
- Pajot FX, Molez JF, Le Pont F. Anophèles et paludisme sur le Haut-Oyapock (Guyane Française). *Cahiers ORSTOM, Entomol Med Parasitol* 1978 ; 16 (2) : 105-11.
- Pakasa M, Mangani N, Dikassa L. Focal and segmental glomerulosclerosis in nephrotic syndrome: a new profile of adult nephrotic syndrome in Zaire. *Mod Pathol* 1993 ; 6 : 125-8.
- Palmer K. *The papua New Guinea malaria control program.* Meeting of selected malarious countries in Western Pacific and South East Asian Regions, 22 Oct. 1993. WPR/MAL/I/93 Inf. 13.
- Palmer CJ, Makler M, Klaskala WI, Lindo JF, Baum MK, Ager AL. Increased prevalence of *Plasmodium falciparum* malaria in Honduras, Central America. *Rev Panam Salud Publica* 1998 ; 4 (1) : 40-2.
- Pampana EJ. Malaria in Italy and bonifications. *Malayan Med J* 1937 ; 12 : 1-8.
- Pampana EJ. *A textbook of malaria eradication.* London : Oxford University Press, 1969 : 593 p.

- Panday RS. *Anopheles nuneztovari* and malaria transmission in Surinam. *Mosquito News* 1977 ; 37 (4) : 728-37.
- Panday RS. A medical entomological survey in West Surinam. *Surinam Med Bull* 1980 ; 3 : 61-8.
- Panicker KN, Bai MG, Rao B, Viswam K, Murthy US. *Anopheles subpictus*, vector of malaria in coastal villages of South-East India. *Curr Sci* 1981 ; 50 : 694-5.
- Parajuli MB, Shrestha SL, Vaidya RG, White GB. Nation-wide disappearance of *Anopheles minimus* Theobald 1901, previously the principal malaria vector in Nepal. *Trans R Soc Trop Med Hyg* 1981 ; 75 : 603.
- Parent M, Demoulin ML. La faune anophélienne à Yangambi. Biologie d'*An. moucheti* spécialement. *Rec Trav Sci Med Congo Belge* 1943 ; 3 : 159-72.
- Parise ME, Ayisi JG, Nahlen BL, *et al*. Efficacy of sulfadoxine-pyrimethamine for prevention of placental malaria in an area of Kenya with a high prevalence of malaria and human immunodeficiency virus infection. *Am J Trop Med Hyg* 1998 ; 59 (5) : 813-22.
- Park Ross GA. Insecticide as a major measure in control of malaria. *Quart Bull Health Organ League of Nations* 1936 ; 5 : 114-33.
- Parkinson AD. Malaria in Papua New Guinea ; 1973. *Papua New Guinea Med J* 1974 ; 17 : 8-16.
- Partono F, Hudojo, Oemijati S, *et al*. Malayan filariasis in Margolembo, South Sulawesi, Indonesia. *Southeast Asian J Trop Med Public Health* 1972 ; 3 : 537-47.
- Patarroyo ME, Amador R, Clavijo P, *et al*. A synthetic vaccine protects humans against challenge with asexual blood stages of *Plasmodium falciparum* malaria. *Nature* 1988 ; 332 : 158-61.
- Paterson HE. "Saltwater *Anopheles gambiae*" on Mauritius. *Bull World Health Organ* 1964a ; 31 : 635-44.
- Paterson HE. Direct evidence for the specific distinctness of forms A, B and C of the *An. gambiae* complex. *Riv Malariol* 1964b ; 43 : 191-6.
- Paterson HE, Paterson JS, Van Eeden GJ. A new member of the *Anopheles gambiae* complex. A preliminary report. *Med Proc (Med Bydraes)* 1963 ; 9 : 414-8.
- Paterson HE, Paterson JS, Van Eeden GJ. Records of the breeding of saltwater *An. gambiae* at inland localities in Southern Africa. *Nature* 1964 ; 201 : 524-5.
- Pattanayak S, Sharma VP, Kalra NL, Orlov VS, Sharma RS. Malaria paradigms in India and control strategies. *Indian J Malariol* 1994 ; 31 : 141-99.
- Patz JA, Strzepek K, Lele S, *et al*. Predicting key malaria transmission factors, biting and entomological inoculation rates using modelled soil moisture in Kenya. *Trop Med Int Health* 1998 ; 3 : 818-27.
- Paul RE, Hackford I, Brockman A, *et al*. Transmission intensity and *P. falciparum* diversity on the North-Western border of Thailand. *Am J Trop Med Hyg* 1998 ; 58 : 195-203.
- Paz Soldan CE. *La peste verde: instrucciones contra la malaria en la costa de Peru*. Lima : Reforma Medica, 1943.
- Pearson SV. Man and mosquito in Ceylon. *Discovery* 1935 ; 16 : 11-3.
- Pene P, Carrie J. Aspects épidémiologiques du paludisme en zone forestière de Côte d'Ivoire. Abstract 8th International Congress for Tropical Medicine and Malaria. Teheran, 1968 : 1485-6.
- Penilla RP, Rodriguez AD, Hemingway J, Torres JL, Arredondo-Jimenez JI, Rodriguez MH. Resistance management strategies in malaria vector mosquito control. Baseline data for a large-scale field trial against *Anopheles albimanus* in Mexico. *Med Vet Entomol* 1998 ; 12 (3) : 217-33.
- Perez MS. Anemia and malaria in a Yanomami Amerindian population from the Southern Venezuelan Amazon. *Am J Trop Med Hyg* 1998 ; 59 (6) : 998-1001.
- Perez L, Suarez M, Murcia L, *et al*. La malaria en el Amazonas : conocimientos, practicas, prevalencia de parasitemia y evaluacion entomologica en mayo de 1997. *Biomedica* 1999 ; 19 (2) : 93-102.
- Perret JL, Duong TH, Kombila M, Owono M, Nguemby-Mbina C. Résultats d'une recherche systématique d'hématozoaires en médecine interne au Gabon. *Bull Soc Pathol Exot* 1991 ; 84 : 323-9.
- Perry EL. Endemic malaria of the Jeypore Hill Tracts of the Madras Presidency. *Indian J Med Res* 1914 ; 2 : 456-91.
- Petrarca V, Carrara GC, Di Deco MA, Petrangeli G. Osservazioni citogenetiche e biometriche sui membri del complesso *Anopheles gambiae* in Mozambico. *Parassitologia* 1984 ;26 : 247-59.
- Petrarca V, Petrangeli G, Rossi P, Sabatinelli G. Étude chromosomique d'*An. gambiae* et *An. arabiensis* à Ouagadougou (Burkina Faso) et dans quelques villages voisins. *Parassitologia* 1986 ; 28 : 41-61.
- Petrarca V, Sabatinelli G, Di Deco MA, Papakay M. The *Anopheles gambiae* complex in the Federal Islamic Republic of Comores. *Parassitologia* 1990 ; 32 : 371-80.
- Petrarca V, Sabatinelli G, Toure YT, Di Deco MA. Morphometric multivariate analysis of field sample of adult *An. arabiensis* and *An. gambiae s.s. J Med Entomol* 1998 ; 35 : 16-25.
- Petrarca V, Nugud AD, Ahmed MA, Haridi AM, Di Deco MA, Coluzzi M. Cytogenetics of the *An. gambiae* complex in Sudan with special reference to *An. arabiensis*: relationships with East and West African populations. *Med Vet Entomol* 2000 ; 14 : 149-64.
- Peyton EL. A new classification for the *Leucosphyrus* group of Anopheles. *Mosq Syst* 1990 ; 21 : 197-205.
- Peyton EL, Harrison BA. *Anopheles dirus*, a new species of the *Leucosphyrus* group from Thailand. *Mosq Syst* 1979 ; 11 : 40-9.
- Phan Vu Thi. *Épidémiologie du paludisme et lutte antipaludique au Viêtnam*. (Traduit en français par Pham Huy Tien). Hanoï : Med Viêtnam, 1998 : 241 p.
- Phillips-Howard PA, Wood D. The safety of antimalarial drugs in pregnancy. *Drug Safety* 1996 ; 14 : 131-45.
- Pholsena K. The malaria situation and antimalaria program in Laos. *Southeast Asian J Trop Med Public Health* 1992 ; 23 (suppl. 4) : 39-42.
- Pichot J, Deruaz D. Les anophèles du complexe *maculipennis* dans la région lyonnaise. *Lyon Médical* 1981 ; 245 (suppl. 10) : 117-21.
- Picot S, Nkwelle Akeda A, Chaulet JF, *et al*. Chloroquine self-treatment and clinical outcome of cerebral malaria in children. *Clin Exp Immunol* 1997 ; 108 : 279-83.
- Pietra Y, Procacci PG, Sabatinelli G, Kumlien S, Lamizana L, Rotigliano G. Impact de l'utilisation des rideaux imprégnés de perméthrine dans une zone rurale de haute transmission au Burkina Faso. *Bull Soc Pathol Exot* 1991 ; 84 (4) : 375-85.
- Pineli LL, da Araujo ES, de Moraes CA, de Almeida Netto JC. Analise epidemiologica de 266 declaracoes de obito por malaria registradas em Goias, no periodo de 1981 a 1993. *Rev Patol Trop* 1997 ; 26 (2) : 179-84.
- Pithan OA, Confalonieri UE, Morgado AF. A situação de saude dos Indios Yanomami: diagnostico a partir da casa do Indio de Boa Vista, Roraima, 1987-1989. *Cadernos Saude Publica* 1991 ; 7 (4) : 563-80.
- Pitt S, Pearcy BE, Stevens RH, Sharipov A, Satarov K, Banatvala N. War in Tajikistan and re-emergence of *Plasmodium falciparum*. *Lancet* 1998 ; 352 : 1279.
- Pittaluga C. *Investigaciones y estudios sobre el paludisma in España (1901-1903)*. Barcelona, 1903.
- Planton S. Réchauffement global et El Niño : une revue des connaissances actuelles. *Med Mal Infect* 1999 ; 29 : 267-76.
- Pletsch D. Informe sobre una mision efectuada en España en septiembre-noviembre de 1963 destinada a la certificacion de la erradicacion del paludismo. *Rev Sanid Hig Publica (Madr)* 1965 ; 39 : 309-66.
- Plowe CV, Cortese JF, Djimde A, *et al*. Mutations in *Plasmodium falciparum* dihydrofolate reductase and dihydropteroate synthase and epidemiologic patterns of pyrimethamine-sulfadoxine use and resistance. *J Infect Dis* 1997 ; 176 : 1590-6.
- Poirriez J, Landau I, Verhaeghe A, Savage A, Dei-Cas E. Les formes atypiques de *P. vivax*. À propos d'une observation. *Ann Parasitol Hum Comp* 1991 ; 66 : 149-54.
- Polevoy NI, *et al*. Malaria problems and malaria control measures in North Afghanistan. 2. Landscape malariogenic district division of North Afghanistan and reorganisation of malaria control measures system. *Med Parazitol (Mosk)* 1975 ; 44 : 338-44.
- Pope KO, Rejmankova E, Savage HM, Arredondo-Jimenez JI, Rodriguez MH, Roberts DR. Remote sensing of tropical wetlands for malaria control in Chiapas, Mexico. *Ecol Appl* 1994 ; 4 (1) : 81-90.
- Porter CH, Collins FH. Susceptibility of *Anopheles hermsi* to *Plasmodium vivax*. *Am J Trop Med Hyg* 1990 ; 42 (5) : 414-6.
- Porter CH, Collins FH. Phylogeny of nearctic members of the *Anopheles maculipennis* species group derived from the D2 variable region of 28S ribosomal RNA. *Mol Phylogenet Evol* 1996 ; 6 (2) : 178-88.
- Postiglione M. Malaria in Europe. In : *Communicable Diseases (Public Health in Europe n°3)*. Copenhague : Office Régional pour l'Europe de l'OMS, 1974.
- Postiglione M, Venkat Rao V. Malaria in Burma. *Indian J Malariol* 1956 ; 10 : 273-98.
- Postiglione M, Tabanli B, Ramsdale CD. The *Anopheles* of Turkey. *Riv Parassitol* 1973 ; 34 : 127-59.
- Pradhan JN, Shrestha SL, Vaidya RG. Malaria transmission in high mountain valleys of West Nepal, including first record of *Anopheles maculatus willmori* as a third vector of malaria. *J Nepal Med Assoc* 1970 ; 8 : 89-97.
- Prakash A, Mohapatra PK, Bhattacharyya DR, *et al*. Epidemiology of malaria outbreak (April/Mai 1999) in Titabor Primary Health Center, district Jorhat (Assam). *Indian J Med Res* 2000 ; 111 : 121-6.
- Prasittisuk C. Present statut of malaria in Thaïland. *Southeast Asian J Trop Med Public Health* 1985 ; 16 : 141-5.

- Prasittisuk C, Saengchotikrai K, Prasittisuk M, Chaiprasittikul P, Aung-Aung B, Limpaviroj W. *Asymptomatic malaria in highly malarious Provinces in Thailand*. Abstract 4th Conference on Malaria Research. Thailand, 8-10 Feb. 1994 : 31.
- Premji Z, Hamisi Y, Shiff C, Minjas J, Lubega P, Makwaya C. Anaemia and *P. falciparum* infections among young children in an holoendemic area, Bagamoyo, Tanzania. *Acta Tropica* 1995 ; 59 (1) : 55-64.
- Prescott N, Stowers AW, Cheng Q, Bobogare A, Rzepczyk CM, Saul A. *Plasmodium falciparum* genetic diversity can be characterised using the polymorphic merozoïte surface antigen 2(MSA-2) gene as a single locus marker. *Mol Biochem Parasitol* 1994 ; 63 : 203-12.
- Preston-Mafbam K. *Madagascar, a natural history*. Oxford : Facts in File, 1991 : 224 p.
- Price RN, Nosten F, Luxemburger C, *et al*. Effects of Artemisinin derivatives on malaria transmissibility. *Lancet* 1996 ; 347 : 1654-8.
- Pringle G. A summary of malaria and malaria control in Iraq before 1946. *Bull Endem Dis (Baghdad)* 1954 ; 1 : 2-45.
- Pringle G. Experimental malaria infections in "saltwater" and "freshwater" *Anopheles gambiae* from East Africa. *Trans R Soc Trop Med Hyg* 1962 ; 56 (2) : 379-82.
- Pringle G. The effect of social factors in reducing the intensity of malaria transmission in coastal East Africa. *Trans R Soc Trop Med Hyg* 1966a ; 60 : 549-53.
- Pringle GA quantitative study of naturally-acquired malaria infections in *An. gambiae* and *An. funestus* in a highly malarious area of East Africa. *Trans R Soc Trop Med Hyg* 1966b ; 60 : 626-32.
- Pringle G. Experimental malaria control and demography in a rural east African community: a retrospect. *Trans R Soc Trop Med Hyg* 1969 ; 61 : 69-79.
- Pringle G, Avery-Jones S. An assessment of the sporozoite inoculation rate as a measure of malaria transmission in the Ubembe area of North East Tanzania. *J Trop Med Hyg* 1966 ; 69 : 132-9.
- Procacci P.G, Lamizana L, Kumlien S, Habluetzel A, Rotigliano G. Permethrin-impregnated curtains in malaria control. *Trans R Soc Trop Med Hyg* 1991 ; 85 (2) : 181-5.
- Protopopoff P, Van Herp M, Maes P, *et al*. Vector control in a malaria epidemic occurring within a complex emergency situation in Burundi: a case study. *Malar J* 2007 ; 6 : 93.
- Prybylski D, Khaliq A, Fox E, Sarwari AR, Strickland GT. Parasite density and malaria morbidity in the Pakistani Punjab. *Am J Trop Med Hyg* 1999 ; 61 (3): 791-801.

- Qari SH, Ya-Ping Shi, Povoa MM, *et al*. Global occurrence of *Plasmodium vivax*-like human malaria parasite. *J Infect Dis* 1993a ; 168 : 1485-9.
- Qari SH, Ya-Ping Shi, Goldman IF, *et al*. Identification of *Plasmodium vivax-like* human malaria parasite. *Lancet* 1993b ; 341 : 780-3.

- Rabarison P, Ramambanirina L, Rajaonarivelo E, *et al*. Impact de l'utilisation des rideaux imprégnés de deltaméthrine sur la morbidité palustre à Ankazobé sur les Hautes Terres de Madagascar. *Med Trop (Marseille)* 1995 ; 55 (suppl. 4) : 105-8.
- Rabarison P, Rajaonarivelo E, Andrianaivolambo L, Tata E. Éco-éthologie des vecteurs du paludisme dans les deux principales régions rizicoles malgaches : le lac Alaotra et Marovoay. *Arch Inst Pasteur Madagascar* 1999 ; 65 : 48-9.
- Raccurt CP, Bourianne C, Lambert MT, *et al*. Indices paludométriques, écologie larvaire et activités trophiques des anophèles à Djohong, Adamaoua, Cameroun, en saison des pluies. *Med Trop (Marseille)* 1993 ; 53 : 355-62.
- Rachou RG. Algunas manifestações de resistencia de comportamento de insetos aos insecticidas no Brasil. *Rev Brasil Malariol Doencas Trop* 1958 ; 10 : 277-90.
- Rachou RG, Schinazi LA, Moura-Lima M. Preliminary note on the epidemiological studies made in El Salvador to determine the causes of the failure of residual spraying to interrupt the transmission of malaria. *Rev Brasil Malariol Doencas Trop* 1966 ; 18 (3/4) : 763-79.
- Rageau J, Vervent A. *Étude entomologique sur le paludisme aux Nouvelles Hébrides*. Commission du Pacifique Sud, 1959 : doc. 119 : 40 p.
- Raghavendra K, Vasartha K, Subbarao SK, Pillai MK, Sharma VP. Resistance in *Anopheles culicifacies* sibling species B and C to malathion in Andhra Pradesh and Gujarat States, India. *J Am Mosq Control Assoc* 1991 ; 7 (2) : 255-9.
- Rahman KM. Epidemiology of malaria in Malaysia. *Rev Infect Dis* 1982 ; 4 : 985-91.
- Rahman M, Muttalib A. Determination of malaria transmission in Central part of Karachi City and incrimination of *An. stephensi* as the vector. *Pakistan J Health* 1967 ; 17 : 73-84.

- Rahman WA, Abu Hassan A, Adanan CR. Seasonality of *Anopheles aconitus* mosquitoes, a secondary vector of malaria in an endemic village near the Malaysia-Thailand border. *Acta Tropica* 1993 ; 55 : 263-5.
- Rahman WA, Che Rus A, Ahmad AH. Malaria and *Anopheles* mosquitoes in Malaysia. *Southeast Asian J Trop Med Public Health* 1997 ; 28 : 599-605.
- Rahman WA, Adanan CR, Abu Hassan A. A study of some aspects of the epidemiology of malaria in an endemic district in Northern Peninsular Malaysia near Thailand border. *Southeast Asian J Trop Med Public Health* 1998 ; 29 : 537-40.
- Raison JP. *Les Hautes Terres de Madagascar et leurs confins occidentaux*. Paris : ORSTOM/Khartala, 1984, 2 vol.
- Rajagopal R. Studies on persistent transmission of malaria in Burnihat, Meghalaya. *J Commun Dis* 1976 ; 8 : 235-45.
- Rajagopal R. Studies on malaria in Bhutan. *J Commun Dis* 1985 ; 17 : 278-86.
- Rajagopalan PK, Das PK, Pani SP, *et al*. Parasitological aspects of malaria persistence in Koraput district, Orissa, India. *Indian J Med Res* 1990 ; 91 : 44-51.
- Ralisoa Randrianasolo BO, Coluzzi M. Genetical investigations on zoophilic and exophilic *Anopheles arabiensis* from Antananarivo area (Madagascar). *Parassitologia* 1987 ; 29 : 93-7.
- Ramasamy S, Balakrishnan K, Pitchappan RM. Prevalence of sickle cells in Irula, Kurumba, Paniya and Mullukurumba tribes of Nilgiris (Tamil Nadu, India). *Indian J Med Res* 1994 ; 100 : 242-5.
- Rambajan I. Reappearance of *Anopheles darlingi* Root and vivax malaria in a controlled area of Guyana, South America. *Trop Geogr Med* 1984 ; 36 (1) : 61-6.
- Rambajan I. Highly prevalent *falciparum* malaria in North West Guyana: its development history and control problems. *Bull Pan American Health Org (PAHO)* 1994 ; 28 (3) : 193-201.
- Ramsdale CD, Coluzzi M. Studies on the infectivity of tropical African strains of *Plasmodium falciparum* to some Southern European vectors of malaria. *Parassitologia* 1975 ; 17 : 39-48.
- Ramsdale CD, Haas E. Some aspects of epidemiology of resurgent malaria in Turkey. *Trans R Soc Trop Med Hyg* 1978 ; 72 : 570-80.
- Ramsdale CD, Herath PR, Davidson G. Recent developments in insecticide resistance in some Turkish anophelines. *J Trop Med Hyg* 1980 ; 83(1) : 11-9.
- Ramsdale CD, de Zulueta J. Anophelism in the Algerian Sahara and some implications of the construction of a trans-Saharan highway. *J Trop Med Hyg* 1983 ; 86 : 51-8.
- Ramsey JM, Salinas E, Rodriguez MH. Acquired transmission-blocking immunity to *P. vivax* in a population of Southern coastal Mexico. *Am J Trop Med Hyg* 1996 ; 54 (5) : 458-63.
- Ranson H, Jensen B, Vulule JM, Wang X, Hemingway J, Collins FH. Identification of a point mutation in the voltage-gated sodium channel gene of Kenyan *Anopheles gambiae* associated with resistance to DDT and pyrethroids. *Insect Mol Biol* 2000 ; 9(5) : 491-7.
- Rao TR. Malaria control using indoor residual sprays in the Eastern province of Afghanistan. *Bull World Health Organ* 1951 ; 3 : 639-61.
- Rao TR. *The Anophelines of India*. New Delhi : Malaria Research Center, 1984 : 518 p.
- Ratard RC. *Epidemiology of malaria in the New Hebrides*. Thèse MSC, Louisiana State University, 1975 : 57 p.
- Rattanarithikul R, Green CA. Formal recognition of the species of *Anopheles maculatus* group occurring in Thailand, including the description of two new species and a preliminary key to females. *Mosq Syst* 1986 ; 18 : 246-78.
- Rattanarithikul R, Konishi E, Linthicum KJ. Observations on nocturnal biting activity and host preference of anophelines collected in Southern Thailand. *J Am Mosq Control Assoc* 1996a ; 12 : 52-7.
- Rattanarithikul R, Linthicum KJ, Konishi E. Seasonal abundance and parity rates of *Anopheles* species in Southern Thailand. *J Am Mosq Control Assoc* 1996b ; 12 : 75-83.
- Rattanarithikul R, Konishi E, Linthicum KJ. Detection of *Plasmodium vivax* and *P. falciparum* circumsporozoite antigen in anopheline mosquitoes collected in Southern Thailand. *Am J Trop Med Hyg* 1996c ; 54 : 114-21.
- Ragavoodoo C. Situation du paludisme à Maurice. *Cahiers Santé* 1995 ; 5 : 371-5.
- Raynal J. Enquête sanitaire à la Grande Comore en 1925. Observation de paludisme à forme épidémique. *Bull Soc Pathol Exot* 1928 ; 21 : 35-54 & 132-41.
- Redd SC, Kazembe PN, Luby SP, *et al*. Clinical algorithm for treatment of *Plasmodium falciparum* malaria in children. *Lancet* 1996 ; 347 : 223-7.

- Regnaud C, Small J, Naz V. *Rapport sur la fièvre épidémique de l'île Maurice.* Port Louis : Imprimerie du Ceonien, 1868.
- Reid JA. The *Anopheles hyrcanus* group in South-East Asia. *Bull Entomol Res* 1953 ; 44 : 5-76.
- Reinert JF, Kaiser PE, Seawright JA. Analysis of the *Anopheles (Anopheles) quadrimaculatus* complex of sibling species (Diptera: Culicidae) using morphological, cytological, molecular, genetic, biochemical, and ecological techniques in an integrated approach. *J Am Mosq Control Assoc* 1997 ; 13 : 1-102.
- Reisen WK. A quantitative mosquito survey of 7 villages in Punjab Province, Pakistan. *Southeast Asian J Trop Med Public Health* 1978 ; 9 : 587-601.
- Reisen WK, Burns JP, Basio RG. A mosquito survey of Guam, Marianas Islands with notes on the vector borne disease potential. *J Med Entomol* 1972 ; 9 : 319-24.
- Reisen WK, Aslamkhan M. Observations on the swarming and mating behaviour of *Anopheles culicifacies* in nature. *Bull World Health Organ* 1976 ; 54 : 155-8.
- Reisen WK, Mahmood F, Azra K. *Anopheles culicifacies* Giles: adult ecological parameters measured in rural Punjab Province, Pakistan, using capture mark release recapture and dissection methods with comparative observations on *An. stephensi, An. subpictus. Res Popul Ecol* 1981 ; 23 : 39-60.
- Reisen WK, Azra K, Mahmood F. *Anopheles culicifacies*: horizontal and vertical estimates of immature development and survivorship in rural Punjab Province, Pakistan. *J Med Entomol* 1982 ; 19 : 413-22.
- Reisen WK, Milby MM. Population dynamics of some Pakistan mosquitoes: changes of adult relative abundance overtime and space. *Ann Trop Med Parasitol* 1986 ; 80 : 53-68.
- Reisen WK, Pradhan SP, Shrestha JP, Shrestha SL, Vaidya RG, Shrestha JD. Anopheline mosquito ecology in relation to malaria transmission in the Inner and Outer Terai of Nepal, 1987-1989. *J Med Entomol* 1993 ; 30 : 664-82.
- Reiter P. From Shakespeare to Defoe. Malaria in England in the Little Ice Age. *Emerg Infect Dis* 2000 ; 6 : 1-11.
- Rejmankova E, Roberts DR, Harbach RE, et al. Environmental and regional determinants of *Anopheles* larval distribution in Belize, Central America. *Environ Entomol* 1993 ; 22 (5) : 979-92.
- Rejmankova E, Roberts DR, Manguin S, Pope KO, Komarek J, Post RA. *Anopheles albimanus* (Diptera; Culicidae) and cyanobacteria: an example of larval habitat selection. *Environ Entomol* 1996 ; 25 : 1058-67.
- Rejmankova E, Pope KO, Roberts DR, et al. Characterization and detection of *Anopheles vestitipennis* and *Anopheles punctimacula* larval habitats in Belize with field survey and SPOT satellite imagery. *J Vector Ecol* 1998 ; 23 (1) : 74-88.
- Renaudin P, Lombart JP. L'anémie chez les enfants de moins de 1 an à Moundou, Tchad. Prévalence et étiologie. *Med Trop (Marseille)* 1994 ; 54 : 337-42.
- Renjifo S, de Zulueta J. Five years' observations of rural malaria in Eastern Colombia. *Am J Trop Med Hyg* 1952 ; 1 : 598-611.
- Renkonen KO. Uber das Verkommen von malaria in Finnland. *Acta Med Scand* 1944 ; 119 : 261-75.
- Reyes V. *Malaria. Panorama epidemiologico del Ecuador.* Quito : Ministerio de la Salud Publica, 1992 ; 115-23.
- Reyes H. *Lecciones de la erradicacion de la malaria en Chile.* Abstract Congresso Latino-americano de Parasitologia. Santiago, 1999 ; 91.
- Ribeiro H, Casaca VM, Cochofel JA. A malaria survey in the Lobito-Catumbela region, Angola. *An Inst Med Trop (Lisb)* 1964 ; 21 : 337-51.
- Ribeiro H, Carvalho AC. A malaria survey at Luanda, Angola. *An Inst Med Trop (Lisb)* 1964 ; 24 : 181-6.
- Ribeiro H, Ramos HC. *Research on mosquitoes in Angola. IV. The genus Anopheles.* Serie de Zoologia. Lisboa : Garcia de Orta, 1975 ; 4 : 1-40.
- Ribeiro H, da Cunha Ramos H, Pires CA, Capela RA. Research on the mosquitoes of Portugal (Diptera, Culicidae) IV-Two new anopheline records. *Garcia de Orta Ser Zool* 1985 ; 9 : 129-39.
- Ribeiro H, Da Cunha Ramos H, Alves Pires C. *Sobre o vectores dos malaria em Sao Tome e Principe.* Serie de Zoologia. Lisboa : Garcia de Orta, 1983 publ. 1990 ; 15 : 135-52.
- Richard A. *Aspects épidémiologiques et cliniques du paludisme dans les villages de la forêt de Mayombe (RP Congo).* Thèse Médecine, Paris Cochin Port-Royal, 1983.
- Richard A, Zoulani A, Lallemant M, Trape JF, Carnevale P, Mouchet J. Le paludisme dans la région forestière de Mayombe, RP Congo. I. Présentation de la région et données entomologiques. *Ann Soc Belg Med Trop* 1988a , 68 : 293-303.
- Richard A, Lallemant M, Trape JF, Carnevale P, Mouchet J. Le paludisme dans la région forestière de Mayombe, RP Congo. II. Observations parasitologiques. *Ann Soc Belg Med Trop* 1988b , 68 : 305-16.
- Richard A, Lallemant M, Trape JF, Carnevale P, Mouchet J. Le paludisme dans la région forestière de Mayombe, R.P. Congo. III. Place du paludisme dans la morbidité générale. *Ann Soc Belg Med Trop* 1988c ; 68 : 317-29.
- Richard-Lenoble D, Kombila M, Chandenier J, et al. Le paludisme au Gabon. 2. Évaluation des prévalences parasitaires qualitatives et quantitatives sur l'ensemble du pays en milieu scolaire et péri-scolaire. *Bull Soc Pathol Exot* 1987 ; 80 : 532-43.
- Richards FO Jr, Klein RE, Flores RZ, et al. Permethrin-impregnated bed nets for malaria control in Northern Guatemala: epidemiologic impact and community acceptance. *Am J Trop Med Hyg* 1993 ; 49 (4) : 410-8.
- Richie TL, Saul A. Progress and challenges for malaria vaccines. *Nature* 2002 ; 415 : 694-701.
- Rickman LR. *Rapport OMS*, AFR/Mal/89, 6 février 1968.
- Rickman LR, Sawe J, Olando J, Imbwana A. The malaria incidence and species prevalence among the population of the Lambwe Valley, South Nyanza, Kenya. *East Afr Med J* 1972 ; 49 : 739-54.
- Rickman KH, Beaudoin RL, Cassels JS, Sell KW. Use of attenuated sporozoites in immunization of human volunteers against *falciparum* malaria. *Bull World Health Organ* 1979 ; 57 (suppl. 1) : 261-5.
- Rico-Avello C, Rico Y. Aportacion española a la historia del paludismo. *Rev Sanid Hig Publica* 1947 ; 21 : 483-525, 594-625, 691-728.
- Rieckmann KH, Davis DR, Hutton DC. *Plasmodium vivax* resistance to chloroquine? *Lancet* 1989 ; 2 : 1183-4.
- Rihet P, Abel L, Traoré Y, Traoré-Leroux T, Aucan C, Fumoux F. Human malaria: segregation analysis of blood infection levels in a suburban area and a rural area in Burkina Faso. *Genet Epidemiol* 1998 ; 15 : 435-50.
- Riley EM, Wagner GE, Ofori MF, et al. Lack of association between maternal antibody and protection of African infants from malaria infection. *Infect Immun* 2000 ; 68 : 5856-63.
- Ringwald P, Bickii J, Basco LK. Amodiaquine as the first-line treatment of malaria in Yaounde, Cameroon: presumptive evidence from activity *in vitro* and cross-resistance patterns. *Trans R Soc Trop Med Hyg* 1998a ; 92 : 212-3.
- Ringwald P, Bickii J, Basco LK. Efficacy of oral pyronaridine for the treatment of acute uncomplicated *falciparum* malaria in African children. *Clin Infect Dis* 1998b ; 26 : 946-53.
- Rioux JA. Contribution à l'étude des Culicidés (Diptera : Culicidae) du Nord-Tchad. In : Rioux JA, ed. *Mission épidémiologique au Nord-Tchad.* Etampes : Arts et Métiers Graphiques, 1961 : 53-97.
- Rioux JA, Sicart M, Ruffie J. Étude cytogénétique des anophèles du complexe *maculipennis* dans le Sud de la France. *CR Soc Biol Toulouse* 1958 ; 152 : 181-2.
- Rioux JA, Ranque J, Ruffie J. Le problème de l'anophélisme sans paludisme dans les palmeraies de Borkou. In : Rioux JA, ed. *Mission épidémiologique au Nord-Tchad.* Etampes : Arts et Métiers Graphiques, 1961 : 98-104.
- Ripert C, Mannschott C, Malosse D, et al. Étude épidémiologique du paludisme dans la région de Koza, Nord Cameroun. *Med Trop (Marseille)* 1982 ; 42 : 601-9.
- Ripert C, Couprie B, Tribouley J, et al. Vingt enquêtes paludométriques au Cameroun. Corrélations entre indices plasmodiques, spléniques et sérologiques. *Bull Soc Fr Parasitol* 1990 ; 8 : 43-59.
- Ripert C, Same Eboko A, Tribouley J, et al. Étude épidémiologique du paludisme dans la région du futur lac de retenue de la Bini, Adamaoua, Cameroun. *Bull Liaison OCEAC* 1991 ; 97 : 40-4.
- Ripert C, Neves I, Appriou M, et al. Épidémiologie de certaines endémies parasitaires dans la ville de Guadalupe (Rép. De Sao Tomé e Principe). *Bull Soc Pathol Exot* 1996 ; 89 : 259-61.
- Rishikesh N. *Anopheles pulcherrimus* as a probable vector of malaria in Iraq. *Bull Endem Dis (Baghdad)* 1972 ; 13 : 7-13.
- Rishikesh N, Di Deco MA, Petrarca V, Coluzzi M. Seasonal variation in indoor resting *An. gambiae* and *An. arabiensis* in Kaduna. *Acta Tropica* 1985 ; 42 : 165-70.
- Rizzo F, Morandi N, Riccio G, Ghiazza G, Garaveli P. Unusual transmission of *falciparum* malaria in Italy. *Lancet* 1989 ; 1 : 555-6.
- Robert V, Gazin P, Boudin C, Molez JF, Ouedraogo V, Carnevale P. La transmission du paludisme en zone de savane arborée et en zone rizicole des environs de Bobo Dioulasso, Burkina Faso. *Ann Soc Belg Med Trop* 1985 ; 65 (suppl. 2) : 201-14.
- Robert V, Gazin P, Ouedraogo V, Carnevale P. Le paludisme urbain à Bobo Dioulasso, Burkina Faso. 1. Étude entomologique de la transmission. *Cahiers ORSTOM, Entomol Med Parasitol* 1986 ; 24 : 121-8.

- Robert V, Gazin P, Carnevale P. Malaria transmission in three sites surrounding the area of Bobo-Dioulasso, Burkina Faso: the savanna, a rice field and the city. *Bull Soc Vector Ecol* 1987 ; 12 : 541-3.
- Robert V, Carnevale P, Ouedraogo V, Petrarca V, Coluzzi M. La transmission du paludisme humain dans un village de savane du Sud-Ouest du Burkina-Faso. *Ann Soc Belg Med Trop* 1988a ; 68 : 107-21.
- Robert V, Ouari B, Ouedraogo V, Carnevale P. Étude écologique des culicidés adultes et larvaires dans une rizière en vallée du Kou, Burkina Faso. *Acta Tropica* 1988b ; 45 : 351-9.
- Robert V, Petrarca V, Carnevale P, Ovazza L, Coluzzi M. Analyse cytogénétique du complexe *An. gambiae* dans la région de Bobo Dioulasso, Burkina Faso. *Ann Parasitol Hum Comp* 1989 ; 64 : 290-311.
- Robert V, Carnevale P. Influence of deltamethrin treatment of bed nets on malaria transmission in the Kou valley, Burkina Faso. *Bull World Health Organ* 1991 ; 69(6) : 735-40.
- Robert V, Ouedraogo V, Carnevale P. La transmission du paludisme humain dans un village au centre de la rizière de la vallée du Kou, Burkina Faso. *Le paludisme en Afrique de l'Ouest*. Paris : ORSTOM, 1991a : 5-15.
- Robert V, Petrarca V, Coluzzi M, Boudin C, Carnevale P. Étude des taux de parturité et d'infection du complexe *An. gambiae* dans la rizière de la vallée du Kou, Burkina Faso. *Le Paludisme en Afrique de l'Ouest*. Paris : ORSTOM, 1991b : 17-35.
- Robert V, Van den Broek A, Stevens P, et al. Mosquitoes and malaria transmission in irrigated rice-fields in the Benoue Valley of Northern Cameroon. *Acta Tropica* 1992 ; 52 : 201-4.
- Robert V, Le Goff G, Essong J, Tchuinkam T, Faas B, Verhave JP. Detection of *falciparum* malarial forms in naturally infected anophelines in Cameroon using fluorescent anti-25-kD monoclonal antibody. *Am J Trop Med Hyg* 1995 ; 52 : 366-9.
- Robert V, Brey PT. Biting physiology of *Anopheles* affecting *Plasmodium* transmission. *Res Rev Parasitol* 1998 ; 58 : 208.
- Robert V, Awono-Ambene HP, Le Hesran JY, Trape JF. Gametocytemia and infectivity to mosquitoes of patients with uncomplicated *Plasmodium falciparum* malaria attacks treated with chloroquine or sulfadoxine plus pyrimethamine. *Am J Trop Med Hyg* 2000 ; 62 (2) : 210-6.
- Roberts DR, Rodriguez M, Rejmankova E, et al. Overview of field studies for the application of remote sensing to the study of malaria transmission in Tapachula, Mexico. *Prev Vet Med* 1991 ; 11 : 269-75.
- Roberts DR, Chan O, Pecor J, et al. Preliminary observations on the changing roles of malaria vectors in Southern Belize. *J Am Mosq Control Assoc* 1993 ; 9 (4) : 456-9.
- Roberts DR, Laughlin LL, Hsheih P, Legters LJ. DDT, global strategies, and a malaria control crisis in South America. *Emerg Infect Dis* 1997 ; 3 (3) : 295-302.
- Roberts DR, Manguin S, Rejmankova E, et al. Spatial distribution of adult *Anopheles darlingi* and *Anopheles albimanus* in relation to riparian habitats in Belize, CA. *J Vector Ecol* 2002a ; 27(1) : 21-30..
- Roberts DR, Vanzie E, Bangs M, et al. Role of residual spraying for malaria control in Belize. *J Vector Ecol* 2002b ; 27(1): 63-69..
- Roberts DR, Masuoka P, Au AY. Determinants of malaria in the Americas. In : Casman EA, Dowlatabadi H, eds. *The contextual determinants of malaria*. Washington : Resources for the Future Press, 2002c : 35-58.
- Roberts JI. The parasite rate in high altitude malaria. *J Trop Med Hyg* 1949 ; 52 : 160-70, 191-99, 230-7 .
- Roberts JM. The control of epidemic malaria in the Highlands of Western Kenya. 1. Before the campaign. *J Trop Med Hyg* 1964 ; 67 : 161-8.
- Roche J, De Diego JA, Penin P, Santos M, Del Rey J. An epidemiological study of malaria in Bioko and Annobon Islands (Equatorial Guinea). *Ann Trop Med Parasitol* 1991 ; 85 : 477-87.
- Roche J, Benito A, Ayecaba S, Molina R, Alvar J. Le paludisme dans l'île d'Annobon, Guinée Équatoriale, 1991. *Bull Liaison OCEAC* 1992 ; 101 : 23-5.
- Rodenwaldt E, Jusatz H. *World Atlas of epidemic diseases*. Hamburg : Falk Verlag, 1956.
- Rodhain J. Les *Plasmodium* des anthropoïdes de l'Afrique Centrale et leurs relations avec les *Plasmodium* humains. *Bull Acad R Med Belge* 1941 ; 21-6.
- Rodhain F, Boutonnier A, Carteron B, Morvan D. Les Culicidés du Territoire Français des Afars et des Issas. I. Le genre *Anopheles*. *Bull Soc Pathol Exot* 1977 ; 70 : 302-8.
- Rodier GR, Parra JP, Kamil M, Chakib SO, Cope SE. Recurrence and emergence of infectious diseases in Djibouti City. *Bull World Health Organ* 1995 ; 73 : 755-9.
- Rodriguez MH, Gonzalez-Ceron L, Hernandez JE, et al. Different prevalences of *Plasmodium vivax* phenotypes VK210 and VK247 associated with the distribution of *Anopheles albimanus* and *An. pseudopunctipennis* in Mexico. *Am J Trop Med Hyg* 2000 ; 62 (1) : 122-7.
- Rogerson SJ, Chaluluka E, Kanjala M, Mkundika P, Mhango C, Molyneux ME. Intermittent sulfadoxine-pyrimethamine in pregnancy: effectiveness against malaria morbidity in Blantyre, Malawi, in 1997-99. *Trans R Soc Trop Med Hyg* 2000 ; 94 : 549-53.
- Rogier C, Henry MC, Spiegel A. Diagnosis of malaria attacks in endemic areas: theoretical aspects and practical implications. *Med Trop* 2001 ; 61 : 27-46.
- Rognon P. *Biographie d'un désert*. Collection Scientifique Synthèse, Paris : Plon, 1989.
- Romanowsky DL. Zur frage der parasitologie und therapie der malaria. *St Petersburg Medizinische Wochenschrift* 1891 ; 16 : 297-307.
- Romi R, Sabatinelli G, Marjori G. Could malaria reappear in Italy? *Emerg Infect Dis* 2001 ; 7 : 915-9.
- Rongnoparut P, Sirichotpakorn N, Rattanarithikul R, Yaicharoen S, Linthicum KJ. Estimates of gene flow among *Anopheles maculatus* populations in Thailand using microsattelite analysis. *Am J Trop Med Hyg* 1999 ; 60 : 508-15.
- Rooth I, Björkman A. Fever episodes in a holoendemic malaria area of Tanzania. *Trans R Soc Trop Med Hyg* 1992 ; 86 : 479-82.
- Ropelewski C. The great El Niño of 1997 and 1998: impact on precipitation and temperature. *Consequences* 1999 ; 5 (2) : 17-25.
- Ropelewski C, Halpert M. Global and regional scale precipitation pattern associated with the El Niño-Southern oscillation. *Month Weather Rev* 1987 ;115 : 1606-26.
- Roper C, Elhassan IM, Hviid L, et al. Detection of very low level *P. falciparum* infections using the nested polymerase chain reaction and a reassessment of the epidemiology of unstable malaria in Sudan. *Am J Trop Med Hyg* 1996 ; 54 : 325-31.
- Roper MH, Torres RS, Goicochea CG, et al. The epidemiology of malaria in an epidemic area in the Peruvian Amazon. *Am J Trop Med Hyg* 2000 ; 62 (2) : 247-56.
- Rosa-Freitas MG. *Anopheles* (*Nyssorhynchus*) *deaneorum*: a new species in the *albitarsis* complex. *Mem Inst Oswaldo Cruz* 1989 ; 84 (4) : 535-43.
- Rosa-Freitas MG. Deane LM, Momen H. A morphological, isoenzymatic and behavioural study of ten populations of *Anopheles (Nyssorhynchus) albitarsis* Lynch-Arribalzaga, 1878, including from the type-locality, Baradero, Argentina. *Mem Inst Oswaldo Cruz* 1990 ; 85 (3) : 275-89.
- Rosenberg R, Maheswary NP. Forest malaria in Bangladesh. I. Parasitology. II. Transmission by *An. dirus*. III. Breeding habits of *An. dirus*. *Am J Trop Med Hyg* 1982 ; 31 : 175-82, 183-91,192-201.
- Rosenberg R, Wirtz RA, Lanar DE, et al. Circumsporozoïte protein heterogeneity in the human malaria parasite *Plasmodium vivax*. *Science* 1989 ; 245 : 973-6.
- Rosenberg R, Andre RG, Somchit L. Highly efficient dry season transmission of malaria in Thailand. *Trans R Soc Trop Med Hyg* 1990 ; 84 : 22-8 .
- Ross R. Malaria in Greece. *J Trop Med* 1906 ; 9 : 341-7.
- Ross R. *The prevention of malaria*. London : John Murray, 1911 : 23 p.
- Ross R. *Researches on Blackwater fever in Southern Rhodesia*. Mems London Sch Hyg Trop Med 1932 ; 6 : 262 p.
- Ross R. *The prevention of malaria*. (2nd ed.) London : John Murray, 1941 : 573 p.
- Ross R, Annett HE, Austen EE. *Report to the malaria expedition of the Liverpool School of Tropical Medicine and Medical Parasitology*. Memoir II, 1900.
- Rossi P, Belli A, Mancini L, Sabatinelli G. Enquête entomologique longitudinale sur la transmission du paludisme à Ouagadougou, Burkina Faso. *Parassitologia* 1986 ; 28 : 1-15.
- Roubaud E. Recherches sur la transmission du paludisme par les anophèles français de régions non palustres. *Ann Inst Pasteur* 1918 ; 32 (9) : 430-62.
- Roubaud E. Les conditions de nutrition des anophèles en France (*Anopheles maculipennis*) et le rôle du bétail dans la prophylaxie du paludisme. *Ann Inst Pasteur* 1920 ; 34 : 181-228.
- Roubaud E. Les raisons de l'absence en Europe septentrionale de l'endémie palustre estivo-automnale. *Bull Soc Pathol Exot* 1925 ; 18 : 279-87.
- Roubaud E. Principes et possibilités de la prophylaxie animale du paludisme. *Arch Inst Pasteur Tunis* 1937 ; 26 : 625-64.
- Rougemont A, Breslow N, Brenner E, et al. Epidemiological basis for clinical diagnosis of childhood malaria in endemic zone in West Africa. *Lancet* 1991 ; 338 : 1292-5.

- Rowland M, Hewitt S, Durrani N, Bano N, Wirtz R. Transmission and control of *vivax* malaria in Afghan refugee settlements in Pakistan. *Trans R Soc Trop Med Hyg* 1997 ; 91 : 252-5.
- Rowland M, Durrani N, Hewitt S, *et al*. Permethrin-treated chaddars and top-sheets: appropriate technology for protection against malaria in Afghanistan and other complex emergencies. *Trans R Soc Trop Med Hyg* 1999 ; 93 : 465-72.
- Roy RG, Moorthy BS, Franco S, Balasubramaniam V. Malaria in Minicoy Island, India. *J Commun Dis* 1974 ; 6 : 265-9.
- Rozeboom LE, Laird RL. *Anopheles (Kerteszia) bellator* as a vector of malaria in Trinidad, BWI. *Am J Trop Med* 1942 ; 22 : 83.
- Rozendaal JA. Observations on the biology and behavior of Anophelines in Suriname rainforest with special reference to *An. darlingi* Root. *Cahiers ORSTOM, Entomol Med Parasitol* 1987 ; 25 (1) : 33-43.
- Rozendaal JA *Epidemiology and control of malaria in Suriname with special reference to* An. darlingi. Thèse doctorat, Rijksuniversiteit te Leiden, 1990 171 p.
- Rozendaal JA. Relations between *An. darlingi* breeding habitats, rainfall, river level and malaria transmission rates in the rain forest of Suriname. *Med Vet Entomol* 1992 ; 6 : 16-22.
- Rozendaal JA. *Vector control*. Genève : OMS, 1997 : 412 p.
- Rubio JM, Benito A, Roche J, *et al*. Semi-nested multiplex polymerase chain reaction for detection of human malaria parasites and evidence of *P. vivax* infection in Equatorial Guinea. *Am J Trop Med Hyg* 1999 ; 60 : 183-7.
- Rubio-Palis Y, Wirtz RA, Curtis CF. Malaria entomological inoculation rates in Western Venezuela. *Acta Tropica* 1992 ; 52 : 167-74.
- Rubio-Palis Y, Zimmerman RH. Ecoregional classification of malaria vectors in the neotropics. *J Med Entomol* 1997 ; 34 (5) : 499-510.
- Ruebush TK. Zeissig R, Koplan JP, Klein RE, Godoy HA. Community participation in malaria surveillance and treatment. III. An evaluation of modifications in the volunteer collaborator network of Guatemala. *Am J Trop Med Hyg* 1994 ; 50 (1) : 85-98.
- Russel PF, Jacob VP. On the epidemiology of malaria in the Nilgiris District, Madras Presidency. *J Malaria Inst India* 1942 ; 4 : 349-92.
- Russel PF, West LS, Manwell RD, Macdonald G. *Practical malariology*. London : Oxford University Press 1963 : 750 p.
- Sabatinelli G. Determinants of malaria in the WHO European Region. In : Casman E, Dowlatabadi H, eds. *The contextual determinants of malaria*. Washington : Resources for the Future Press, 2002 : 66-92.
- Sabatinelli G, Bosman A, Lamizana L, Rossi P. Prévalence du paludisme à Ouagadougou et dans le milieu rural limitrophe en période de transmission maximale. *Parassitologia* 1986a ; 28 : 17-31.
- Sabatinelli G, Rossi P, Belli A. Étude sur la dispersion d'*An. gambiae* dans une zone urbaine à Ouagadougou, Burkina Faso. *Parassitologia* 1986b ; 28 33-9.
- Sabatinelli G, Petrarca V, Petrangeli G. Données préliminaires sur le complexe An. gambiae dans la RFI des Comores. *Parassitologia* 1988 ; 30 (suppl.) : 178-9.
- Sabatinelli G, Blanchy S, Majori G, Papakay M. Utilisation du poisson larvivore *Poecilia reticulata* sur la transmission du paludisme en RFI des Comores. *Ann Parasitol Hum Comp* 1991 ; 66 : 84-8.
- Sabatinelli G, Gokcinar T, Serttas S, Ejov M. The malaria epidemiological situation in Turkey. *Parassitologia* 2000 ; 42 (suppl. 1) : 150.
- Sabesan S, Jambulingam P, Krishnamoorthy K, *et al*. Natural infection and vectorial capacity of *Anopheles culicifacies* Giles in Rameswaram Island (Tamil Nadu). *Indian J Med Res* 1984 ; 80 : 43-6.
- Sachs J, Malaney P. The economic and social burden of malaria. *Nature* 2002 ; 415 : 680-5.
- Sakya GM. Present status of malaria in Nepal. *J Nepal Med Assoc* 1981 ; 19 21-8.
- Salazar NP, Miranda ME, Santos MN, de Las Llagas LA. The malaria situation in the Philippines with special reference to mosquito vectors. *Southeast Asian J Trop Med Public Health* 1988 ; 19 : 709-12.
- Saliou P, Vergeau B, Alandry G, *et al*. Deux nouveaux cas de paludisme autochtones en région Parisienne illustrant deux modes de contamination différents. *Bull Soc Pathol Exot* 1978 ; 71 : 342-7.
- Saliternik Z. An outbreak of malaria along the Israeli waistline in 1955. *Briut Hazbur (Public Health) Jerusalem* 1960 ; 3 : 217.
- Saliternik Z. Field investigations on the bionomics of *An. sergenti* in Israël during the years 1961-1965. *Isr J Entomol* 1967 ; 2 : 145-62.
- Saliternik Z. Reminiscences of the history of malaria eradication in Palestine and Israël. *Isr J Med Sci* 1978 ; 14 : 518-20.
- Sallum MA, Wilkerson RC, Forattini OP. Taxonomic study of species formely identified as *Anopheles mediopunctatus* and resurrection of *An. costai* (Diptera: Culicidae). *J Med Entomol* 1999 ; 36 (3) : 282-300.

- Sallum MA, Peyton EL, Wilkerson RC. Six new species of the *Anopheles leucosphyrus* group, reinterpretation of *An. elegans* and vector implications. *Med Vet Entomol* 2005 ; 1 : 158-99.
- Samarawickrema WA, Parkinson AD, Kere N, Galo O. Seasonal abundance and biting behaviour of *An. punctulatus* and *An. koliensis* in Malaita Province, Solomon Islands, and a trial of permethrin impregnated bednets against malaria transmission. *Med Vet Entomol* 1992 ; 6 : 371-8.
- Samba EM. The burden of malaria in Africa. *Afr Health* 1997 ; 19(2) : 17.
- Same-Eboko A, Lohoue J, Essono E, Ravinet L, Ducret JP. Résolution rapide des accès palustres à *P. ovale* par l'artesunate (Arsumax®). *Med Trop (Marseille)* 1999 ; 59 : 43-5.
- Sampaio MR, Turcotte S, Martins VF, Cardoso EM, Burattini MN. Malaria in the Indian reservation of "Vale do Javari", Brazil. *Rev Inst Med Trop S Paulo* 1996 ; 38 (1) : 59-60.
- Sandosham AA. Malaria in rural Malaya. *Med J Malaya* 1970 ; 24 : 221-6.
- Sandoval JJ, Saraiva MG, Amorin RD, *et al*. Malaria na cidade de Manaus : vulnerabilidade e receptividade. *Rev Soc Bras Med Trop* 2000 ; 30 (suppl. 1) : 67.
- Saugrain J, Taufflieb R. Anophélisme sans paludisme au Nord Tchad. *Bull Soc Pathol Exot* 1960 ; 53 (2) : 150-2.
- Sautet J. Quelques détails sur l'anophélisme au Soudan Français. *Med Trop (Marseille)* 1942 ; 2 : 21-27.
- Sautet J. État actuel du paludisme et de l'anophélisme dans la région méditerranéenne. *Rech Trav Hist Nat Inf* 1944 ; 1 : 176-96.
- Sautet J, Ranque J, Vuillet F, Vuillet J. Quelques notes parasitologiques sur le paludisme et l'anophélisme en Mauritanie. *Med Trop (Marseille)* 1948 ; 8 : 32-9.
- Sautet J, Quilici M. À propos de quelques cas de paludisme autochtone. *Presse Med* 1971 ; 79 : 542.
- Savage HM, Rejmankova E, Arredondo-Jimenez JI, Roberts DR, Rodriguez MH. Limnological and botanical characterization of larval habitats for two primary malarial vectors, *Anopheles albimanus* and *Anopheles pseudopunctipennis*, in coastal areas of Chiapas state, Mexico. *J Am Mosq Control Assoc* 1990 ; 6 (4) : 612-20.
- Sawabe K, Takagi M, Tsudo Y, *et al*. Genetic differentiation among three populations of *Anopheles minimus* of Guangxi and Yunnan Provinces in the People's Republic of China. *Southeast Asian J Trop Med Public Health* 1997 ; 28 : 440-9.
- Sawada P. Malaria after the war. *Nippon Naikagaku-Zasshi* 1949 ; 31 : 1-8.
- Sawadipanich Y, Baimai V, Harrison BA. *Anopheles dirus* species E: chromosomal and crossing evidence for another member of the *dirus* complex. *J Am Mosq Control Assoc* 1990 ; 6 : 477-81.
- Scanlon JE, Sandhinand U. The distribution and biology of *Anopheles balabacensis* in Thailand. *J Med Entomol* 1965 ; 2 : 61-9.
- Scarpassa VM, Tadei WP, Suarez MF. Population structure and genetic divergence in *Anopheles nuneztovari* from Brazil and Columbia. *Am J Trop Med Hyg* 1999 ; 60 (6) : 1010-8.
- Scarpassa VM, Tadei WP. Enzymatic analysis in *Anopheles nuneztovari*. *Braz J Biol* 2000 ; 60 (4) : 539-50.
- Schapira A. Determinants of malaria in Oceania and East Asia. In : Casman E, Dowlatabadi H, eds. *The contextual determinants of malaria*. Washington : Resources for the Future Press, 2002 : 93-109.
- Schapira A, Ravaonjanahary C. *Rapport sur une mission au Rwanda*. OMS/AFRO/Genève, 3 au 14 juin 1993.
- Schaudinn F. Untersuchungen uber den generationswechsel bei Coccidien. *Zoologische Jahrbucher* 1899 ; 13 : 197-292.
- Schenone H, Olea A, Rojas A, Garcia N. Malaria in Chile: 1913-2001. *Rev Med Chil* 2002 ; 130 : 1170-6.
- Schreck CE, Kline D, Smith N. Protection afforded by the insect repellent jacket against four species of bitting midges (*Dipt. culicoides*). *Mosquito News* 1979 ; 39 : 739-42.
- Schuffner WA. Two subjects from the epidemiology of malaria. *Mededell vd Burg Geneesk n Nederl Infië* 1919 : 9.
- Schultz LJ, Steketee RW, Macheso A, Kazembe P, Chitsulo L, Wirima JJ. The efficacy of antimalarial regimens containing sulphadoxine-pyrimethamine and/or chloroquine in preventing peripheral and placental *Plasmodium falciparum* infection among pregnant women in Malawi. *Am J Trop Med Hyg* 1994 ; 51 (5) : 515-22.
- Schuurkamp GI. *The epidemiology of malaria and filariasis in the OK Tedi Region of Western Province, Papua New Guinea*. PhD Thesis, University of Papua New Guinea, 1992.
- Schwetz J. Sur une épidémie mystérieuse, suspecte et soupçonnée de paludisme constatée dans une agglomération indigène d'un très haut plateau du Ruanda. *Ann Soc Belg Med Trop* 1941 ; 21 : 37-61.

- Schwetz J. Recherches sur la limite altimétrique du paludisme dans le Congo Oriental et sur la cause de cette limite. *Ann Soc Belg Med Trop* 1942 ; 22 : 183-208.
- Schwetz J, Baumann H, Peel E, Belhommet. Contribution à l'étude de l'infection malarienne chez les Pygmées de la forêt de l'Ituri, Congo Belge. *Bull Soc Pathol Exot* 1934 ; 27 : 199-208.
- Schwetz J, Bauman H. *Recherche sur le paludisme dans les villages et camps des mines d'or de Kilo (Congo Belge).* Mémoires de l'Institut Royal Colonial Belge, Section des Sciences Naturelles et Médicales, 1941 ; 11 : 75 p.
- Scorza JV, Tallaferro E, Rubiano H. Comportamiento y susceptibilidad de *Anopheles nuneztovari* Gabaldon, 1940 a la infeccion con *P. falciparum* y *P. vivax*. *Bol Dir Malario Saneamiento Ambiental* 1976 ; 16 (2) : 129-36.
- Scott JA, Brogdon WG, Collins FH. Identification of single specimens of *Anopheles gambiae* complex by the polymerase chain reaction. *Am J Trop Med Hyg* 1993 ; 49 (4) : 520-9.
- Seboxa T, Snow RW. Epidemiological features of severe paediatric malaria in North Western Ethiopia. *East Afr Med J* 1997 ; 74 : 780-3.
- Sedaghat MM, Linton YM, Oshaghi MA, Vatandoost H, Harbach RE. The *Anopheles maculipennis* complex (Diptera: Culicidae) in Iran: molecular characterization and recognition of a new species. *Bull Entomol Res* 2003 ; 93 : 527-35.
- Sen AK, John VM, Krishnan KS, Rajagopal R. Studies on malaria transmission in the Tirap District, Arunachal Pradesh. *J Commun Dis* 1973 ; 5 : 98-110.
- Senevet G, Andarelli L. *Les anophèles de l'Afrique du Nord et du Bassin Méditerranéen*. Paris : Lechevallier, 1956.
- Sergent ED. Définition de l'immunité et de la prémunition. *Arch Inst Pasteur Algérie* 1950 ; 28 : 429-40.
- Sergent ED, Sergent ET, Parrot L, Donatien A. Le paludisme en Corse. Étude épidémiologique. *Bull Soc Pathol Exot* 1921 ; 14 : 685-710.
- Sergent ED, Sergent ET. *L'armée d'Orient délivrée du paludisme*. Paris : Masson, 1932.
- Sergent ET. Les épidémies de paludisme et la météorologie en Algérie. *Bull Soc Pathol Exot* 1932 ; 25 : 133-6.
- Sergiev VP, Baranova AM, Orlov VS, *et al. Importation of malaria into the USSR from Afghanistan, 1981-89*. WHO/MAL/92.1064 ; 1992 : 6 p.
- Service MW. The ecology of the mosquitoes of the Northern Guinea savannah of Nigeria. *Bull Entomol Res* 1963 ; 54 : 601-32.
- Service MW. Some basic entomological factors concerned with the transmission and control of malaria in Northern Nigeria. *Trans R Soc Trop Med Hyg* 1965 ; 59 : 291-6.
- Service MW. Contribution to the knowledge of the mosquitoes of Gabon. *Cahiers ORSTOM, Entomol Med Parasitol* 1976 ; 14 : 259-63.
- Service MW. Mortalities of the immature stages of species B of the *Anopheles gambiae* complex in Kenya. Comparison between rice fields and temporary pools, identification of predators and effects of insecticidal spraying. *J Med Entomol* 1977 ; 13 : 535-45.
- Service MW, Joshi GP, Pradhan GD. A survey of *An. arabiensis* and *An. gambiae* in the Kisumu area of Kenya following insecticidal spraying with Fenitrothion. *Ann Trop Med Parasitol* 1978 ; 72 : 377-86.
- Shalaby AM. Survey of the mosquito fauna of Fezzan, South Western Lybia. *Bull Soc Entomol Egypte* 1972 ; 56 : 301-11.
- Shanks GD, Karwacki JJ, Singharaj P. Malaria in displaced persons along the Thai Burmese border. *Southeast Asian J Trop Med Public Health* 1990 ; 21 : 39-43.
- Shanks GD, Biomndo K, Hay SI, Snow RW. Changing patterns of clinical malaria since 1965 among a tea estate population located in the Kenya highlands. *Trans R Soc Trop Med Hyg* 2000 ; 94 : 253-5.
- Sharma RC, Gautam AS, Orlov V, Sharma VP. Relapse pattern of *Plasmodium vivax* in Kheda district, Gujarat. *Indian J Malariol* 1990 ; 27 : 95-9.
- Sharma RS. Urban malaria and its vectors *Anopheles stephensi* and *An. culicifacies* in Gurgaon, India. *Southeast Asian J Trop Med Public Health* 1995 ; 26 : 172-6.
- Sharma SK, Nanda N, Dutta VK, *et al.* Studies on the bionomics of *Anopheles fluviatilis* s.l. and the sibling species composition in the foothills of Shiwalik Range, India. *Southeast Asian J Trop Med Public Health* 1995 ; 26 : 566.
- Sharma VP. Re-emergence of malaria in India. *Indian J Med Res* 1996 ; 103 : 26-45.
- Sharma VP. Determinants of malaria in Southeast Asia. In : Casman E, Dowlatabadi H, eds. *The contextual determinants of malaria*. Washington : Resources for the Future Press, 2002 : 110-32.
- Sharma VP, Uprety HC. Preliminary studies on irrigation malaria. *Indian J Malariol* 1982 ; 19 : 139-42.
- Sharma VP, Mehrotra KN. Final words on malaria's return. *Nature* 1983 ; 302 : 372.
- Sharma VP, Sharma RC. Bioenvironmental control of malaria in Nadiad, Kheda district, Gujarat, India. *Indian J Malariol* 1987 ; 23 : 95-118.
- Sharp BL, Le Sueur D. Malaria in South Africa. The past, the present and selected implications for the future. *S Afr Med J* 1996 ; 86 : 83-9.
- Shawarby AA, Mahdi AH, Shenouda ME, *et al.* Further trials for entomological and parasitological evaluation of some insecticides against *An. pharoensis* in UAR, 1965. *J Egypt Public Health Assoc* 1967a ; 42 : 159-70.
- Shawarby AA, Mahdi AH, Kolta S. Prospective measures against *An. gambiae* invasion to UAR. *J Egypt Public Health Assoc* 1967b ; 42 : 194-9.
- Shears P, Berry AM, Murphy R, Nabil MA. Epidemiological assessment of the health and nutrition of Ethiopian refugees in emergency camps in Sudan, 1985. *Br Med J* 1987 ; 295 : 314-8 .
- Shelley AJ. Observations on the behaviour of *An. gambiae* sp. B in Kambole village in the Zambesi Valley, Zambia. *Ann Trop Med Parasitol* 1973 ; 67 : 237-47.
- Shidrawi GR, Gillies MT. *Anopheles paltrinieri* n.sp. from the Sultanate of Oman. *Mosq Syst* 1987 ; 19 : 201-11.
- Shihab KI, Ali NA, Dorky KA, Jawad AH, Abdul Latif YA, Habeen RN. Immunological and parasitological survey in areas of Iraq where malaria transmission has been interrupted since several years. *Bull Endem Dis (Baghdad)* 1987 ; 28 : 17-28.
- Shilulu JI, Maier WA, Seitz HM, Orago AS. Seasonal density, sporozoite rates and entomological inoculation rates of *An. gambiae* and *An. funestus* in a high-altitude sugarcane growing zone in Western Kenya. *Trop Med Int Health* 1998 ; 3 : 706-10.
- Shousha AT. Destruction de *Anopheles gambiae* en Haute Égypte, 1942-45. *Bull Organ Mond Santé* 1948 ; 1 : 343-86.
- Shrestha SL. Anophelines of Nepal and their relation to malaria eradication. *J Nepal Med Assoc* 1966 ; 4 : 148-54.
- Shrestha SL. Dynamics of malaria transmission with reference to development projects in Nepal. *J Commun Dis* 1985 ; 17 : 287-92.
- Shrestha SL, Parajuli MB. Reappearance of malaria in Terai area of Nepal and incrimination of *An. annularis* Van der Wulp. *J Nepal Med Assoc* 1980 ; 18 : 11-8.
- Shukla RP, Pandey AC, Mathur A. Investigation of malaria outbreak in Rajasthan. *Indian J Malariol* 1995 ; 32 : 119-28.
- Shukla RP, Nanda N, Pandey AC, Kohli VK, Joshi H, Subbarao SK. Studies on the bionomics of *Anopheles fluviatilis* and its sibling species in Nainital district UP. *Indian J Malariol* 1998 ; 35 : 41-7.
- Shulman CE, Dorman EK, Talisuna AO, *et al.* A community randomized controlled trial of insecticide-treated bednets for the prevention of malaria and anaemia among primigravid women on the Kenyan coast. *Trop Med Int Health* 1998 ; 3 (3) : 197-204.
- Shulman CE, Dorman EK, Cutts F, *et al.* Intermittent sulfadoxine-pyrimethamine to prevent severe anaemia secondary to malaria in pregnancy: a randomised placebo-controlled trial. *Lancet* 1999 ; 353 (9153) : 632-6.
- Shute PG, Lupascu GH, Branzei P, *et al.* A strain of *P. vivax* characterised by prolonged incubation. *Trans R Soc Trop Med Hyg* 1977 ; 70 : 474-81.
- Sidhu AB, Verdier-Pinard D, Fidock DA. Chloroquine resistance in *Plasmodium falciparum* malaria parasites conferred by *pfcrt* mutations. *Science* 2002 ; 298 : 210-3.
- Silva-Vasconcelos AA, Kato MY, Mourao EN, *et al.* Biting indices, host-seeking activity and natural infection rates of Anopheline species in Boa Vista, Roraima, Brazil from 1996 to 1998. *Mem Inst Oswaldo Cruz* 2002 ; 97 (2) : 151-61.
- Silvain JF. *Étude de l'écologie d'Anopheles (Nyssorhynchus) aquasalis Curry, 1932 en relation avec l'épidémiologie du paludisme en Guyane Française*. Paris : ORSTOM, 1979 : 122 p.
- Silvain JF, Pajot FX. Écologie d'*An. (Nyssorhynchus) aquasalis* Curry, 1932 en Guyane Française. 1. Dynamique des populations imaginales, caractérisation des gîtes larvaires. *Cahiers ORSTOM, Entomol Med Parasitol* 1981 ; 19 (1) : 11-21.
- Simard F, Fontenille D, Lehmann T, *et al.* High amounts of genetic differentiation between populations of the malaria vector, *An. arabiensis* from West Africa and Eastern outer islands. *Am J Trop Med Hyg* 1999 ; 60 : 1000-9.
- Simard F, Lehmann T, Lemasson JJ, Diatta M, Fontenille D. Persistance of *Anopheles arabiensis* during the severe dry season conditions in Senegal: an indirect approach using microsatellite loci. *Insect Mol Biol* 2000 ; 9 : 467-79.
- Simic C. Le paludisme en Yougoslavie. *Bull Organ Mond Santé* 1956 ; 15 : 753-66.

- Singh GP, Chitkara S, Kalra NL, Makepur KB, Narasimham MV. Development of a methodology for malariogenic stratification as a tool for malaria control. *J Commun Dis* 1990 ; 22 : 1-11.
- Singh N, Singh OP, Sharma VP. Dynamics of malaria transmission in forested and deforested regions of Mandla District, Central India (Madhya Pradesh). *J Am Mosq Control Assoc* 1996 ; 12 : 225-34.
- Singh N, Saxena A, Chand SK, Valecha N, Sharma VP. Studies on malaria during pregnancy in a tribal area of Central India, Madhya Pradesh. *Southeast Asian J Trop Med Public Health* 1998 ; 29 : 10-7.
- Singh N, Mishra AK, Chand SK, Sharma VP. Population dynamics of *Anopheles culicifacies* and malaria in the tribal area of Central India. *J Am Mosq Control Assoc* 1999 ; 15 : 283-90.
- Singh OP, Chandra D, Nanda N, Sharma SK, Htun PT, Adak T, Subbarao SK, Dash AP. On the conspecificity of *Anopheles fluviatilis* species S with *Anopheles minimus* species C. *J Biosci* 2006 ; 31 : 671-7.
- Singhanetra-Renard A. Population movement. Socio-economic behavior and the transmission of malaria in Northern Thailand. *Southeast Asian J Trop Med Public Health* 1986 ; 17 : 396-405.
- Singhasivanon P, Thimasarn K, Yimsamran S, *et al.* Malaria in tree crop plantations in South-Eastern and Western provinces of Thailand. *Southeast Asian J Trop Med Public Health* 1999 ; 30 : 399-404.
- Sinton JA, Singh HJ. The numerical prevalence of parasites in relation to fever in chronic benign tertian malaria. *Indian J Med Res* 1931 ; 18 : 871-9.
- Siziya S, Watts TE, Mason PR. Malaria in Zimbabwe. *Central Afr J Med* 1997 ; 43 : 251-4.
- Slooff R. Field observations on the biting activity of *An. koliensis* Owen. *Trop Geogr Med* 1961 ; 13 : 67-76.
- Slooff R. *Observations on the effect of residual DDT spraying on behavior and mortality in species of Anopheles punctulatus group*. Leiden : Sythoff Editions, 1964 : 144 p.
- Sloof R. *Visit to malaria control project unit, Male, Maldives*. Travel report to WHO Dir., June 1988.
- Slooff R, Verdrager J. Anopheles balabacensis balabacensis *Baisas 1936 and malaria transmission in the South-Eastern areas of Asia*. WHO/VBC/72.765 ; 1972 : 25 p.
- Slutsker L, Khoremana CO, Hightower AW, *et al.* Malaria infection in infancy in rural Malawi. *Am J Trop Med Hyg* 1996a ; 55 (suppl. 1) : 71-6.
- Slutsker L, Bloland P, Steketee RW, Wirima JJ, Heymann DL, Breman JG. Infant and second year mortality in rural Malawi: causes and descriptive epidemiology. *Am J Trop Med Hyg* 1996b ; 55 (suppl. 1) : 77-81.
- Smalley ME, Sinden RE. *Plasmodium falciparum* gametocytes. Their longevity and infectivity. *Parasitology* 1977 ; 74 : 1-8.
- Smalley ME, Brown J. *Plasmodium falciparum* gametocytogenesis stimulated by lymphocytes and serum from infected Gambian children. *Trans R Soc Trop Med Hyg* 1981 ; 75 : 316-7.
- Smeaton MJ, Slater PJ, Robson P. Malaria from a "commuter" mosquito. *Lancet* 1984 ;1 : 845-6.
- Smith A. Resting habits of *An. gambiae* and *An. pharoensis* in salt bush and in crevices in the ground. *Nature* 1961 ; 190 : 1220-1.
- Smith A. Malaria in the Taveta area of Kenya and Tanganyika. III. Entomological findings three years after the spraying period. *East Afr Med J* 1962 ; 39 : 553-64.
- Smith A. Studies on *An. gambiae* and malaria transmission in the Umbugwe area of Tanganyika. *Bull Entomol Res* 1964 ; 55 : 125-37.
- Smith A. Malaria in the Taveta area of Kenya and Tanzania. IV. Entomological findings six years after the spraying period. *East Afr Med J* 1966 ; 43 : 7-18.
- Smith A, Draper CC. Malaria in the Taveta area of Kenya and Tanganyika. I. Epidemiology. *East Afr Med J* 1959a ; 36 : 99-113.
- Smith A, Draper CC. Malaria in the Taveta area of Kenya and Tanganyika. II. Results after three and a half years treatment of huts with dieldrin. *East Afr Med J* 1959b ; 36 : 629-43.
- Smith A, Pringle G. Malaria in the Taveta area of Kenya and Tanzania. V. Transmission eight years after the spraying period. *East Afr Med J* 1967 ; 44 : 469-74.
- Smith A, Hansford CF, Thompson JF. Malaria along the Southernmost fringe of its distribution in Africa: epidemiology and control. *Bull World Health Organ* 1977 ; 55 : 95-103.
- Smith EC. Child mortality in Lagos, Nigeria. *Trans R Soc Trop Med Hyg* 1943 ; 36 : 287-303.
- Smith T, Genton B, Baea K, *et al.* Relationships between *Plasmodium falciparum* infection and morbidity in a highly endemic area. *Parasitology* 1994 ; 109 : 539-49.
- Smith T, Charlwood JD, Kitua AY, *et al.* Relationships of malaria morbidity with exposure to *P. falciparum* in young children in a highly endemic area. *Am J Trop Med Hyg* 1998 ; 59 : 252-7.
- Smith T, Felger I, Tanner M, Beck HP. The epidemiology of multiple *P. falciparum* infections. Premunition in *P. falciparum* infection: insights from the epidemiology of multiple infections. *Trans R Soc Trop Med Hyg* 1999 ; 93 : 59-64.
- Smith T, Leuenbergen R, Lengeler C. Child mortality and malaria transmission intensity in Africa. *Trends Parasitol* 2001 ; 17 (3) : 145-9.
- Smits A, Roelants P, Van Bortel W, Coosemans M. Enzyme polymorphisms in the *Anopheles gambiae* complex related to feeding and resting behavior in the Imbo Valley, Burundi. *J Med Entomol* 1996 ; 33 : 545-53.
- Smrkovski LL, Escamilla J, Wooster MT, Rivera DG. A preliminary survey of malaria in Occidental Mindoro, Philippines. *Southeast Asian J Trop Med Public Health* 1982 ; 13 : 181-5.
- Snounou G, Pinheiro L, Goncalves A, *et al.* The importance of sensitive detection of malaria parasites in the human and insect hosts in epidemiological studies as shown by the analysis of field samples from Guinea Bissau. *Trans R Soc Trop Med Hyg* 1993 ; 87 : 649-53.
- Snow RW, Rowan K, Lindsay S, Greenwood B. A trial of bed nets as a malaria control strategy in a rural area of the Gambia, West African. *Trans R Soc Trop Med Hyg* 1988 ; 82 : 212-5.
- Snow RW, Armstrong-Schellenberg JR, Peshu N, *et al.* Periodicity and space-time clustering of severe childhood malaria on the Kenyan Coast. *Trans R Soc Trop Med Hyg* 1993 ; 87 : 386-90.
- Snow RW, Bastos de Azevedo I, Lowe BS, *et al.* Severe childhood malaria in two areas of markedly different *falciparum* transmission in East Africa. *Acta Tropica* 1994 ; 57 : 289-300.
- Snow RW, Marsh K. Will reducing *P. falciparum* transmission alter malaria mortality among African children? *Parasitol Today* 1995 ; 11 : 188-90.
- Snow RW, Omumbo JA, Lowe B, *et al.* Relation between severe malaria morbidity in children and level of *P. falciparum* transmission in Africa. *Lancet* 1997 ; 349 : 1650-4.
- Snow RW, Peshu N, Forster D, *et al.* Environmental and entomological risk factors for the development of clinical malaria among children on the Kenyan Coast. *Trans R Soc Trop Med Hyg* 1998a ; 92 : 381-5.
- Snow RW, Gouws E, Omumbo J, *et al.* Models to predict the intensity of *Plasmodium falciparum* transmission: applications to the burden of disease in Kenya. *Trans R Soc Trop Med Hyg* 1998b ; 92 : 601-6.
- Snow RW, Craig M, Deichmann V, Marsh K. Estimating mortality, morbidity and disability due to malaria among Africa's non pregnant population. *Bull World Health Organ* 1999 ; 77 : 620-40.
- Sodeinde O, Gbadegesin RA, Ademowo OG, Adeyemo AA. Lack of association between *falciparum* malaria and acute diarrhea in Nigerian children. *Am J Trop Med Hyg* 1997 ; 57 : 702-5.
- Soeiro A. Malaria em Moçambique. *An Inst Med Trop (Lisb)* 1956 ; 13 : 615-34.
- Soeiro A, Morais T. de Subsidios para o estudo da endemia de malaria no distrito do Niassa. *An Inst Med Trop (Lisb)* 1959 ; 16 : 169-78.
- Soekirno M, Bang YH, Sudomo M, Pemayun TP, Fleming CA. *Bionomics of Anopheles sundaicus and other anophelines associated with malaria in coastal areas of Bali, Indonesia*. WHO/VBC/83.885 ; 1983 : 13 p.
- Somboon P, Suwonkerd W, Lines JD. Susceptibility of Thai zoophilic Anophelines and suspected malaria vectors to local strains of human malaria parasites. *Southeast Asian J Trop Med Public Health* 1994 ; 24 : 766-70.
- Somboon P, Aramrattana A, Lines J, Webber R. Entomological and epidemiological investigations of malaria transmission in relation to population movements in forest areas of North-West Thailand. *Southeast Asian J Trop Med Public Health* 1998 ; 29 : 3-9.
- Somboon P, Walton C, Sharpe RG, *et al.* Evidence for a new sibling species of *Anopheles minimus* from the Ryukyu Archipelago, Japan. *J Am Mosq Control Assoc* 2001 ; 17 : 98-113.
- Somboon P, Thongwat D, Choochote W, Walton C, Takagi M. Crossing experiments of *Anopheles minimus* species C and putative species E. *J Am Mosq Control Assoc* 2005 ; 21 : 5-9.
- Some ES. Effects and control of Highland malaria epidemic in Uasin Gishu District, Kenya. *East Afr Med J* 1994 ; 71 : 2-8.
- Somo-Moyou R, Mittelholzer ML, Sorenson F, Haller L, Sturchler D. Efficacy of Ro 42-1611 (arteflene) in the treatment of patients with mild malaria: a clinical trial in Cameroon. *Trop Med Parasitol* 1994 ; 45 : 288-91.
- Sony PN, Sharp BL. Severity of malaria and level of *P. falciparum* transmission. *Lancet* 1997 ; 350 : 363.
- Soper FL, Wilson DB. *Anopheles gambiae in Brazil, 1930 to 1940*. New York : The Rockefeller Foundation, 1943 : 262 p.
- Sorre M. *Les fondements biologiques de la géographie humaine*. Paris : Librairie Colin, 1943.

- Sousa CA, Pinto J, Almeida AP, Ferreira C, do Rosario VE, Charlwood JD. Dogs as a favoured host choice of *An. gambiae s.s.* of Sao Tome, West Africa. *J Med Entomol* 2001 ; 38 : 122-5.
- Southammavong M. *Lieux de contamination des cas de paludisme hospitalisés dans la ville de Vientiane (Laos) en 1996.* Mémoire de DEA. Paris : Université Pierre et Marie Curie, 1997 : 40 p.
- de Souza SL, Noronha CV, Dourado MI. Migration and malaria: a controlled study in the urban area of Camacari, Bahia, Brazil. *Ciencia e Cultura* 1988 ; 40 (5) : 490-4.
- Spencer T, Spencer M, Venters D. Malaria vectors in Papua New Guinea. *Papua New Guinea Med J* 1974 ; 17 : 22-30.
- Stafford Smith DM. Mosquito records from the Republic of Niger, with reference to the construction of the new "Trans-Sahara highway". *J Trop Med Hyg* 1981 ; 84 : 95-100.
- Steffan WA. A check list and review of the mosquitoes of the Papuan subregion. *J Med Entomol* 1966 ; 3 : 179-237.
- Storey J, Fleming AF, Cornille-Brogger R, Molineaux L, Matsushima T, Kagan I. Abnormal haemoglobins in the Sudan savannah of Nigeria. IV. Malaria immunoglobulins and antimalaria antibodies in haemoglobin AC individuals. *Ann Trop Med Parasitol* 1979 ; 73 : 311-5.
- Stowers AW, Miller LH. Are trials in new world monkeys on the critical path for blood-stage malaria vaccine development? *Trends Parasitol* 2001 ; 17 (9) : 415-9.
- Strickland GT, Zafar-Latif A, Fox E, Khaliq AA, Chowdhry MA. Endemic malaria in four villages of the Pakistani province of Punjab. *Trans R Soc Trop Med Hyg* 1987 ; 81 : 36-41.
- Strickland GT, Fox E, Hadi H. Malaria and splenomegaly in the Punjab. *Trans R Soc Trop Med Hyg* 1988 ; 82 : 667-70.
- Suarez MF, Quinones ML, Palacios JD, Carrillo A. First record of DDT resistance in *Anopheles darlingi*. *J Am Mosq Control Assoc* 1990 ; 6 (1) : 72-4.
- Subbarao SK. The *Anopheles culicifacies* complex and control of malaria. *Parasitol Today* 1988 ; 4 : 72-5.
- Subbarao SK, Vasantha K, Raghavendra K, Sharma VP, Sharma GK. *Anopheles culicifacies*: sibling species composition and its relationship to malaria incidence. *J Am Mosq Control Assoc* 1988 ; 4 : 29-33.
- Subbarao SK, Vasantha K, Joshi K, *et al.* Role of *Anopheles culicifacies* sibling species in malaria transmission in Madhya Pradesh State, India. *Trans R Soc Trop Med Hyg* 1992 ; 86 (6) : 613-4.
- Subbarao SK, Nanda N, Vasantha K, *et al.* Cytogenetic evidence for three sibling species in *Anopheles fluviatilis*. *Ann Entomol Soc Am* 1994 ; 87 : 116-21.
- Subbarao SK, Sharma VP. *Anopheles species* complexes and malaria control. *Indian J Med Res* 1997 ; 106 : 164-73
- Sucharit S, Komalamisra N, Leemingsawat S, Apiwathnasorn C, Thongrungkiat S. Population genetic studies on the *Anopheles minimus* complex in Thailand. *Southeast Asian J Trop Med Public Health* 1988 ; 19 : 717-23.
- Suguna SG, Rathinam KG, Rajavel AR, Dhanda V. Morphological and chromosomal descriptions of new species in the *Anopheles subpictus* complex. *Med Vet Entomol* 1994 ; 8 : 88-94.
- Sukowati S, Baimai V, Harun S, Dasuki Y, Andris H, Efriwati M. Isoenzyme evidence for three sibling species in the *Anopheles sundaicus* complex from Indonesia. *Med Vet Entomol* 1999 ; 13 : 408-14.
- Suleman M. Malaria in Afghan refugees in Pakistan. *Trans R Soc Trop Med Hyg* 1988 ; 82 : 44-7.
- Sulzer AJ, Cantella R, Colichon A, Gleason NN, Walls KW. A focus of hyperendemic *P. malariae*-*P. vivax* with no *P. falciparum* in a primitive population in the Peruvian Amazon jungle. *Bull World Health Organ* 1975 ; 52 : 273-8.
- Sundararaman S. The behaviour of *An. sundaicus* Rodenwaldt in relation to the application of residual insecticides in Tjilatjap, Indonesia. *Indian J Malariol* 1958 ; 12 : 129-56.
- Sundararaman S, Soeroto RM, Siran M. Vectors of malaria in Mid-Java. *Indian J Malariol* 1957 ; 11 : 321-38.
- Surtees G. Large-scale irrigation and arbovirus epidemiology, Kano Plain, Kenya. I. Description of the area and preliminary studies on the mosquitoes. *J Med Entomol* 1970 ; 7 : 509-17.
- Sweeney AW. *Anopheles farauti* n°2 as a possible vector of malaria in Australia. *Trans R Soc Trop Med Hyg* 1980 ; 74 : 830-1.
- Sweeney AW. A review of chemical control of malaria vectors in the South West Pacific Region. In : Laird M, Miles JW, eds. *Integrated mosquito control methodologies: biocontrol and other innovative components, and future directions*. London : Academic Press, 1983 : 143-58.
- Sweeney AW. Larval salinity tolerances of the sibling species of *Anopheles farauti*. *J Am Mosq Control Assoc* 1987 ; 3 : 589-92.
- Swellengrebel NH. The malaria epidemic of 1943-46 in the province of North Holland. *Trans R Soc Trop Med Hyg* 1950 ; 43 : 445-76.
- Swellengrebel NH, Anneke S, de Meillon B. Malaria investigation in Transvaal and Zululand. *Publ S Afr Inst Med Res* 1931 ; XXVIII : 245-76.
- Swellengrebel NH, Schoute E, Kraan H. Investigations on the transmission of malaria in some villages North of Amsterdam. *Bull Health Organ League Nations* 1936 ; 5 : 295-352.
- Swellengrebel NH, de Buck A. *Malaria in the Netherlands.* Amsterdam : Schetelma & Holkema, 1938 : 267 p.
- Swellengrebel NH, Van der Kuyp RG. Health of white settlers in Suriname. *Royal Col Inst Amsterdam, Dep Trop Hyg* 1940 ; 16.
- Symes CB. Insects in aeroplanes. *Rec Med Res Lab Nairobi* 1935 ; 6 : 16 p.
- Symes CB. Present state of malaria in Nairobi. *East Afr Med J* 1940 ; 17 : 339-55.
- Tadei WP, Dutary Thatcher B, *et al.* Ecologic observations on anopheline vectors of malaria in the Brazilian Amazon. *Am J Trop Med Hyg* 1998 ; 59 (2) : 325-35.
- Tadei WP, Dutary Thatcher B. Malaria vectors in the Brazilian Amazon: *Anopheles* of the subgenus *Nyssorhynchus*. *Rev Inst Med Trop São Paulo* 2000 ; 42 (2) : 87-94.
- Taha TT, Broadhead RL. A comparative epidemiological study of malaria between children of Northern and Southern Sudan. *J Trop Pediatr* 1986 ; 32 : 117-9.
- Takken W, Snellen WB, Verhave JP, Knols BG, Atmosoedjono S. *Environmental measures for malaria control in Indonesia and historical review on species sanitation.* Wageningen Agricultural University Papers, 1990 : 167 p.
- Tami A, Mubyazi G, Talbert A, Mshinda H, Duchon S, Lengeler C. Evaluation of Olyset insecticide-treated nets distributed seven years previously in Tanzania. *Malar J* 2004 ; 3 : 19.
- Tang Am Nguyen, Anh Hao Luong, Thi Huyen Vu. Utilisation d'insecticide dans la lutte contre le paludisme au Sud du Viêtnam. *Cahiers Santé* 1991 ; 1 (3) : 215-20.
- Tang Am Nguyen, Le Quy Riec, Vu Thi Huyen, Nguyen Bieh Lan. Études entomo-épidémiologiques du paludisme dans la zone côtière d'Ho Chi Minh Ville, 1990-1992. *Cahiers Santé* 1993 ; 3 : 464-73.
- Tang Lin-Hua, Qian Hui-Lin, Xu Shu-Hui. Malaria and its control in the People's Republic of China. *Southeast Asian J Trop Med Public Health* 1991 ; 22 : 467-76.
- Tanner M, Beck HP, Felger I, Smith T. The epidemiology of multiple *P. falciparum* infections. *Trans R Soc Trop Med Hyg* 1999 ; 93 (suppl. 1) : 1-2.
- Tatem AJ, Rogers DJ, Hay SI. Estimating the malaria risk of African mosquito movement by air travel. *Malar J* 2006 ; 5 : 57. http://www.malariajournal.com/content/5/1/57
- Tauil PL. Comments on the epidemiology and control of malaria in Brazil. *Mem Inst Oswaldo Cruz* 1986 ; 81 (suppl. 2) : 39-41.
- Taylor B. Changes in the feeding behaviour of a malaria vector *An. farauti* following the use of DDT as a residual spraying in houses in British Solomon Islands. *Trans R Entomol Soc London* 1975 ; 127 : 277-92.
- Taylor CE, Toure YT, Coluzzi M, Petrarca V. Effective population size and persistence of *Anopheles arabiensis* during the dry season in West Africa. *Med Vet Entomol* 1993 ; 7 : 351-7.
- Taylor C, Toure YT, Carnahan J, *et al.* Gene flow among populations of the malaria vector, *Anopheles gambiae*, in Mali, West Africa. *Genetics* 2001 ; 157 : 743-50.
- Taylor KA, Koros JK, Nduati J, *et al. Plasmodium falciparum* infection rates in *An. gambiae*, *An. arabiensis* and *An. funestus* in Western Kenya. *Am J Trop Med Hyg* 1990 ; 43 : 124-9.
- Taylor P. The malaria problem in Zimbabwe. Epidemiology. *Central Afr J Med* 1985 ; 31 : 163-5.
- Taylor P, Mutambu SL. A review of the malaria situation in Zimbabwe with special reference to the period 1972-1981. *Trans R Soc Trop Med Hyg* 1986 ; 80 : 12-9.
- Teklehaimanot A. *Report on a mission to Ethiopia, 4 August-13 September 1991.* WHO/Geneva, 1991.
- Temu EA, Minjas JN, Coetzee M, Hunt RH, Shiff CJ. The role of four anopheline species in malaria transmission in coastal Tanzania. *Trans R Soc Trop Med Hyg* 1998 ; 92 : 152-8.
- Terrenato L, Shrestha S, Luzatto G, *et al.* Decreased malaria morbidity in the Tharu people compared to sympatric populations in Nepal. *Ann Trop Med Parasitol* 1988 ; 82 : 1-11.
- Testa J, Baquillon G, Delmont J, Kamata G, Ngama G. Gestation et indices parasitaires de *P. falciparum* dans une étude à Bangui, République Centrafrique. *Med Trop (Marseille)* 1987 ; 47 : 339-43.
- Tewari SC, Appavoo NC, Mani TR, Reuben R, Ramadas V, Hiriyan J. Epidemiological aspects of persistent malaria along the River Thenpennaï (Tamil Nadu). *Indian J Med Res* 1984 ; 80 : 1-10.

- Tewari SC, Hiriyan J, Reuben R. Survey of the anopheline fauna of the Western Ghats in Tamil Nadu, India. *Indian J Malariol* 1987 ; 24 : 21-8.
- Thaithong S. *Genetic diversity of Plasmodium falciparum in Thailand*. Abstract 4th Conference on Malaria Research Thailand, 8-10 Feb. 1994 : 7.
- Theander TG. Unstable malaria in Sudan: influence of the dry season. Malaria in areas of unstable and seasonal transmission. Lessons from Daraweesh. *Trans R Soc Trop Med Hyg* 1998 ; 92 : 589-92.
- Theobald FV. *A monograph of the Culicidae or Mosquitoes*, vol. 2. London : British Museum, 1901 : 305-6.
- Thevasagayam ES, Yap S, Chooi CK. *Deterioration of thatch roofs after house spraying with DDT in a malaria eradication programme in Peninsular Malaysia and the prevention of such deterioration by the use of malathion*. WHO/MAL/78.899 ; 1978 : 9 p.
- Tho Vien N, Dinh Bai B, Van Son M, Van Thong T, Tuyen Quang N, Tan N. Évaluation des mesures antivectorielles contre le paludisme dans le centre du Viêtnam (1976-1991). *Cahiers Santé* 1996 ; 6 : 97-101.
- Thompson R, Hogh B. Malaria in a densely populated suburban area of Maputo, Mozambique. *Rev Med Moçambique* 1994 ; 5 (suppl. 1) : 47.
- Thompson R, Begtrup K, Cuamba N, et al. The Matola malaria project: a temporal and spatial study of malaria transmission and disease in a suburban area of Maputo, Mozambique. *Am J Trop Med Hyg* 1997 ; 57 : 550-9.
- Thuriaux MC. Notes on the epidemiology of malaria in the Yemen Arab Republic. *Ann Soc Belg Med Trop* 1971 ; 51 : 229-37.
- Tia E, Akogbeto M, Koffi A, et al. Pyrethroid and DDT resistance of *Anopheles gambiae* s.s. (Diptera: Culicidae) in five agricultural ecosystems from Côte d'Ivoire. *Bull Soc Pathol Exot* 2006 ; 99(4) : 278-82.
- Tin F. Malaria control in Myanmar. *Southeast Asian J Trop Med Public Health* 1992 ; 23 (suppl. 4) : 51-4.
- Todd JE, de Francisco A, O'Dempsey TJ, Greenwood BM. The limitation of verbal autopsy in a malaria endemic region. *Ann Trop Paediatr* 1994 ; 14 : 31-6.
- Tomaszunas S. Malaria in sea farers. 1. The magnitude of the problem and the strategy of its control. *Bull Inst Marit Trop Med Gdynia* 1998 ; 49 : 53-61.
- Toole MJ, Waldman RJ. Prevention of excess mortality in refugee and displaced populations in developing countries. *JAMA* 1990 ; 263 : 3296-302.
- Toole MJ, Waldman RJ. The public health aspects of complex emergencies and refugee situations. *Ann Rev Public Health* 1997 ; 18 : 283-312.
- della Torre A, Fanello C, Akogbeto M, et al. Molecular evidence of incipient speciation within *Anopheles gambiae* s.s. in Western Africa. *Insect Mol Biol* 2001 ; 10 (1) : 9-18.
- Torres JR, Magris M, Villegas L, Torres VM, Dominguez G. Spur cell anaemia and acute haemolysis in patients with hyperreactive malarious splenomegaly. Experience in an isolated Yanomami population of Venezuela *Acta Tropica* 2000 ; 77 (3) : 257-62.
- Toumanoff C. *L'anophélisme en Extrême Orient*. Paris : Masson, 1936 : 429 p.
- Toumanoff C, Simon M. Quelques observations sur la faune culicidienne de la Basse-Guinée (Conakry et Presqu'île de Kaloum). *Bull Soc Pathol Exot* 1956 ; 49 : 667-74.
- Touré YT, Petrarca V, Coluzzi M. Comparaison des taux d'infection par des sporozoïtes et des filaires dans les diverses formes du complexe *An. gambiae* dans un village du Mali. *Ann Ist Super Sanita (Rome)* 1986 ; 22 : 215-7.
- Touré YT, Petrarca V, Traoré SF, et al. The distribution and inversion polymorphism of chromosomally recognized taxa of the *Anopheles gambiae* complex in Mali, West Africa. *Parassitologia* 1998 ; 40 : 477-511.
- Traoré O, Le Goff G, Doumde N, et al. Évaluation *in vivo* de la chimiosensibilité de *P. falciparum* à la chloroquine dans la région de Moundou. *Bull Liaison OCEAC* 1992 ; 101 : 26-7.
- Traoré Y, Rinet P, Traoré-Leroux T, et al. Analyse des facteurs génétiques contrôlant l'infection palustre chez l'homme. *Cahiers Santé* 1999 ; 9 : 5-9.
- Trape JF. Malaria and urbanization in Central Africa: the example of Brazzaville. IV. Parasitological and serological surveys in urban and surrounding rural areas. *Trans R Soc Trop Med Hyg* 1987a ; 81 (suppl. 2) : 26-33.
- Trape JF. Étude sur le paludisme dans une zone de mosaïque forêt-savane d'Afrique Centrale, la region de Brazzaville. II. Densités parasitaires. *Bull Soc Pathol Exot* 1987b ; 80 : 520-31.
- Trape JF, Peelman P, Morault-Peelman B. Criteria for diagnosing clinical malaria among a semi-immune population exposed to intense and perennial transmission. *Bull Soc Pathol Exot* 1985 ; 79 : 435-42.
- Trape JF, Zoulani A. Études sur le paludisme dans une zone de mosaïque forêt-savane d'Afrique Centrale, la région de Brazzaville. I. Résultats des enquêtes entomologiques. *Trans R Soc Trop Med Hyg* 1987a ; 81 (suppl. 2) : 84-99.
- Trape JF, Zoulani A. Malaria and urbanisation in Central Africa. Part II. Results of entomological surveys and epidemiological analysis. *Trans R Soc Trop Med Hyg* 1987b ; 81 (suppl. 2) : 10-8.
- Trape JF, Zoulani A. Malaria and urbanisation in Central Africa: the example of Brazzaville. Part III. Relationships between urbanisation and the intensity of malaria transmission. *Trans R Soc Trop Med Hyg* 1987c, 81 (suppl. 2) : 19-25.
- Trape JF, Quinet MC, Nzingoula S, et al. Malaria and urbanization in Central Africa: the example of Brazzaville. V. Pernicious attacks and mortality. *Trans R Soc Trop Med Hyg* 1987a ; 81 (suppl. 2) : 34-42.
- Trape JF, Zoulani A, Quinet .C. Assessment of the incidence and prevalence of clinical malaria in semi-immune children exposed to intense and perennial transmission. *Am J Epidemiol* 1987b ; 126 : 193-201.
- Trape JF, Lefebvre-Zante E, Legros F, et al. Vector density gradients and the epidemiology of urban malaria in Dakar, Senegal. *Am J Trop Med Hyg* 1992 ; 47 : 181-9.
- Trape JF, Rogier C, Konate L, et al. The Dielmo project, a longitudinal study of natural malaria infection and the mechanisms of protective immunity in a community living in a holoendemic area of Senegal. *Am J Trop Med Hyg* 1994 ; 51 : 123-37.
- Trape JF, Rogier C. Combating malaria mortality and morbidity by reducing transmission. *Parasitol Today* 1996 ; 12 : 236-40.
- Trape JF, Pison G, Preziosi MP, et al. Impact de la résistance à la chloroquine sur la morbidité palustre. *CR Acad Sci Paris, Sciences de la Vie/Life Sciences*, 1998 ; 321(série 3) : 689-97.
- Trung HD, Van Bortel W, Sochantha T, et al. Malaria transmission and major malaria vectors in different geographical areas of Southeast Asia. *Trop Med Intern Health* 2004 ; 9 : 230-7.
- Trzaska S. Impacts régionaux de El Niño : Afrique Australe. *La lettre de MEDIAS*, numéro spécial El Niño et ses téléconnexions sur l'Afrique et la Méditerranée, Décembre 2000 ; 12 : 30-3.
- Tsuda Y, Takagi M, Toma T, Sugiyama A, Miyagi I. Mark-release-recapture experiment with adult *Anopheles minimus* on Ishigaki Island, Ryukyu Archipelago, Japon. *J Med Entomol* 1999 ; 36 : 601-4.
- Tula AN. Malaria transmission in the highlands of Ethiopia. *Trans R Soc Trop Med Hyg* 1993 ; 87 : 347.
- Tulu AN, Abose T, Balcha F, Degu G. Early results of an epidemiological study of malaria in the lower Arbaminch Valley, Southern Ethiopia. *Trans R Soc Trop Med Hyg* 1993 ; 87 : 347-8.
- Tun-Lin W, Htay-Aung, Moe-Moe, et al. Some environmental factors influencing the breeding of *An. balabacensis* complex in domestic wells in Burma. *J Commun Dis* 1987 ;19 : 291-9.
- Turley J, Orellana E, Hunt S, et al. *P. vivax* malaria, San Diego County, California, 1986. *MMWR Morbid Mortal Wkly Rep* 1986 ; 35 : 679-81.

- Udhayakumar V, Qari SH, Patterson P, Collins WE, Lal AA. Monoclonal antibodies to the circumsporozoite protein repeats of a *Plasmodium vivax-like* human malaria parasite and *Plasmodium simiovale*. *Infect Immun* 1994 ; 62 (5) : 2098-100.
- Ulloa A, Rodriguez MH, Arredondo-Jimenez JI, Fernandez-Salas I. Biological variation in two *Anopheles vestitipennis* populations with different feeding preferences in southern Mexico. *J Am Mosq Control Assoc* 2005 ; 21 : 350-4.
- Upatham ES, Prasittisuk C, Ratanatham S, et al. Bionomics of *An. maculatus* complex and their role in malaria transmission in Thailand. *Southeast Asian J Trop Med Public Health* 1988 ; 19 : 259-69.

- Vaid BK, Nagendra S, Paithane PK. Spring transmission of malaria due to *An. culicifacies* in North Western Madhya Pradesh. *J Commun Dis* 1974 ; 6 : 270.
- Vaisse D, Michel R, Carnevale P, et al. Le paludisme à *P. falciparum* et le gène de la drépanocytose en RP Congo. II. Manifestations cliniques du paludisme selon la parasitémie et le génotype hémoglobinique. *Med Trop (Marseille)* 1981 ; 41 : 413-23.
- Van Bortel W, Delacollette C, Barutwanayo M, Coosemans M. Deltamethrin-impregnated bednets as an operational tool for malaria control in an hyperendemic region of Burundi: impact on vector population and malaria morbidity. *Trop Med Int Health* 1996 ; 1 (6) : 826-35.

- Van Bortel W, Trung HD, Manh ND, Roelants P, Verle R, Coosemans M. Identification of two species within the *Anopheles minimus* complex in Northern Viêtnam and their behavioural divergences. *Trop Med Int Health* 1999 ; 4 : 257-65.
- Van den Ende J, Lynen L, Elsen P, *et al.* A cluster of airport malaria in Belgium in 1995. *Acta Clin Belg* 1998 ; 53 : 259-63.
- Van der Stuyft P, Manirankunda L, Delacollette C. L'approche du risque dans le diagnostic du paludisme-maladie en région d'altitude. *Ann Soc Belg Med Trop* 1993 ; 73 : 81-9.
- Veeken H. Malaria and gold fever. *Br Med J* 1993 ; 307 : 433-4.
- Velema JP, Alihonou EM, Chippaux JP, Van Boxel Y, Gbedji E, Adegbini R. Malaria morbidity and mortality in children under three years of age on the coast of Benin, West Africa. *Trans R Soc Trop Med Hyg* 1991 ; 85 : 430-5.
- Venkat Rao V. Malaria in Orissa. *Indian J Malariol* 1949 ; 3 : 159.
- Venkat Rao V, Ramakrishna V. Fresh-water form of *An. sundaicus*. *Indian J Malariol* 1950 ; 4 : 235.
- Vercruysse J. Étude entomologique sur la transmission du paludisme humain dans le bassin du fleuve Sénégal (Sénégal). *Ann Soc Belg Med Trop* 1985 ; 65 (suppl. 2) : 171-9.
- Vercruysse J, Jancloes M. Étude entomologique sur la transmission du paludisme humain dans la zone de Pikine (Sénégal). *Cahiers ORSTOM, Entomol Med Parasitol* 1981 ; 19 : 165-78.
- Vercruysse J, Jancloes M, Van den Velden L. Epidemiology of seasonal *falciparum* malaria in an urban area of Senegal. *Bull World Health Organ* 1983 ; 61 : 821-31.
- Verdrager J. Angkor, le mystère de la ville morte et *An. dirus*. *Med Trop (Marseille)* 1992 ; 52 : 377-84.
- Verdrager J. Localized permanent epidemics: the genesis of chloroquine resistance in *Plasmodium falciparum*. *Southeast Asian J Trop Med Public Health* 1995 ; 26 : 23-8.
- Verhoeff FH, Brabin BJ, Chimsuku L, Kazembe P, Russell WB, Broadhead RL. An evaluation of the effects of intermittent sulfadoxine-pyrimethamine treatment in pregnancy on parasite clearance and risk of low birthweight in rural Malawi. *Ann Trop Med Parasitol* 1998 ; 92 (2) : 141-50.
- Verhoeff FH, Brabin BJ, Hart CA, Chimsuku L, Kazembe P, Broadhead RL. Increased prevalence of malaria in HIV-infected pregnant women and its implications for malaria control. *Trop Med Int Health* 1999 ; 4 (1) : 5-12.
- Verle P, Binh LN, Lieu TT, Yen PT, Coosemans M. ParaSight,-F test to diagnose malaria in hypo-endemic and epidemic prone regions of Vietnam. *Trop Med Int Health* 1996 ; 1 (6) : 794-6.
- Verle P, Tuy TQ, Lieu TT, Kongs A, Coosemans M. New challenges for malaria control in Northern Vietnam. *Res Rev Parasitol* 1998 ; 58 (3-4) : 169-74.
- Verle P, Nhan DH, Uyen TT, *et al.* Glucose-6-phosphate dehydrogenase deficiency in Northern Vietnam. *Trop Med Int Health* 2000 ; 5 : 203-6.
- Vermeil C. Contribution à l'étude des Culicidés du Fezzan (Libye) : présence d'*An. broussesi* à El Barka (Territoire de Rhat). *Bull Soc Pathol Exot* 1953 ; 46 : 445-54.
- Vermylen M. Répartition des anophèles de la République du Rwanda et de la République du Burundi. *Riv Malariol* 1967 ; 46 : 13-22.
- Vien NT, Tan HX, Manh ND, *et al.* Étude du paludisme transmis par *An. minimus* à Gia Lam, Hanoï. *Bull Information LCPMP* 1992 ; 2 : 28-34.
- Villalobos CE. *Malaria y sembradios de arroz en el valle de Camana*. Lima : Directoria General Sanidad, 1942.
- Vincke IH, Jadin JB. Contribution à l'étude de l'anophélisme en pays d'altitude. *Ann Soc Belg Med Trop* 1946 ; 26 : 483-500.
- Vincke IH, Lips M. Un nouveau *Plasmodium* d'un rongeur sauvage du Congo, *Plasmodium berghei* n.sp. *Ann Soc Belg Med Trop* 1948 ; 28 : 97-104.
- Vinetz JM, Li J, McCutchan TF, Kaslow DC. *Plasmodium malariae* infection in an asymptomatic 74-years-old Greek woman with splenomegaly. *N Engl J Med* 1998 ; 338 : 367-71.
- Viriyakosol S, Siripoon N, Petcharapirat C, *et al.* Genotyping of *P. falciparum* isolates by the polymerase chain reaction and potential uses in epidemiological studies. *Bull World Health Organ* 1995 ; 73 : 85-95.
- Viswanathan DK. The seasonal prevalence of malaria transmitted by *An. fluviatilis* in different regions of Bombay Presidency. *J Malaria Inst India* 1945 ; 6 : 253-7.
- Viswanathan DK. A review of immunity and endemicity in malaria and a discussion on their relationship with malaria control. *Indian J Malariol* 1951 ; 5 : 251-69.
- Viswanathan DK, Rao TR. The behaviour of *Anopheles fluviatilis* James as regards the time of entry into houses and of feeding. *J Malaria Inst India* 1943 ; 5 : 255-60.
- Vittor AY, Gilman RH, Tielsch J, *et al.* The effect of deforestation on the human-biting rate of *Anopheles darlingi*, the primary vector of *falciparum* malaria in the Peruvian Amazon. *Am J Trop Med Hyg* 2006 ; 74 : 3-11.
- Voelckel J, Mouchet J. Quelques aspects et résultats de la désinsectisation systématique en milieu urbain tropical. *Med Trop (Marseille)* 1959 ; 19 : 266-93.
- Voituriez B, Jacques G. *El Niño. Réalité et fiction*. Paris : UNESCO, Collection COI Forum Océans, 1999.
- Voller A, Bray RS. Fluorescent antibody staining as a measure of malaria antibody. *Proc Soc Exper Biol Med* 1962 ; 110 : 907-10.
- Von Seidlein L, Milligan P, Pinder M, *et al.* Efficacy of artesunate plus pyrimethamine-sulfadoxine for uncomplicated malaria in Gambian children: a double-blind randomised controlled trial. *Lancet* 2000 ; 355 (9220) : 2080.
- Vyslouzil J. Does malaria exist in Assab at the present time? *Ethiopian Med J* 1971 ; 9 : 153-4.
- Vythinlingam I, Phetsouvanh R, Keokenchanh K, *et al.* The prevalence of *Anopheles* (Diptera: Culicidae) mosquitoes in Sekong Province, Lao PDR in relation to malaria transmission. *Trop Med Intern Health* 2003 ; 8 : 525-35.

- Walker J. Malaria in a changing world: an Australian perspective. *Int J Parasitol* 1988 ; 28 : 947-53.
- Walliker D. *Cloning of malaria parasites*. WHO/MAL/81.939 ; 1981 : 7 p.
- Walter P, Garin FJ, Blot P, Philippe E. Placenta et paludisme. *J Gynecol Obstet Biol Reprod (Paris)* 1981 ; 10 : 535-42.
- Walton GA. On the control of malaria in Freetown, Sierra Leone. I. *P. falciparum* and *An. gambiae* in relation to malaria occurring in infants. *Ann Trop Med Parasitol* 1947 ; 41 : 380-407.
- Walton C, Somboon P, O'Loughlin SM, *et al.* Genetic diversity and molecular identification of mosquito species in the *Anopheles maculatus* group using the ITS2 region of rDNA. *Infect Genet Evol* 2007 ; 7 : 93-102.
- Wanderley DM, da Silva RA, Andrade JC. de Aspectos epidemiologicos da malaria no Estado de Sao Paulo, Brasil, 1983 a 1992. *Rev Saude Publica* 1994 ; 28 (3) : 192-7.
- Wang KA, Qian HL. The review of epidemic situation of malaria from 1977 to 1986. *Chin Dis Surv* 1988 ; 8 : 5-8.
- Wanson M, Berteaux M. Note sur l'infectivité de l'*Anopheles brunnipes*. *East Afr Med J* 1944 ; 21 : 272-3.
- Ward RA. Medical entomology, Dipt. : Culic. In : Buck AA, *et al.* eds. *Health and diseases in rural Afghanistan*. Baltimore : York Press, 1972a.
- Ward RA. Mosquitoes of Afghanistan. An annoted checklist. *Mosq Syst* 1972b ; 4 : 93-7.
- Ward RA. *Recent changes in the epidemiology of malaria relating to human ecology*. Washington : Proceedings 15th International Congress Entomology 1977.
- Ward RA. Second supplement to "A catalog of the mosquitoes of the world". *Mosq Syst* 1984 ; 16 : 227-70.
- Ward RA. Third supplement to "A catalog of the mosquitoes of the world". *Mosq Syst* 1992 ; 24 : 177-230.
- Ward RA, Jordan B, Gillogly AR, Harrison FJ. *Anopheles litoralis* and *Anopheles barbirostris* group on the Island of Guam. *Mosquito News* 1976 ; 36 : 99-100.
- Ward RA, Jordan B. *Anopheles barbirostris*, confirmation of introduction on Island of Guam. *Mosquito News* 1979 ; 39 : 802-3.
- Warren M, Cheong WH, Fredericks HK, Coatney GR. Cycles of jungle malaria in West Malaysia. *Am J Trop Med Hyg* 1970 ; 19 : 383-93.
- Warren M, Collins WE, Jeffery GM, Skinner JC. The seroepidemiology of malaria in Middle America. II. Studies on the Pacific Coast of Costa Rica. *Am J Trop Med Hyg* 1975 ; 24 (5) : 749-54.
- Watkins WM, Mosobo M. Treatment of *Plasmodium falciparum* malaria with pyrimethamine-sulfadoxine: selective pressure for resistance is a function of long elimination half-life. *Trans R Soc Trop Med Hyg* 1993 ; 87 : 75-8.
- Watson M. Twenty five years malaria control. *Malayan Med J* 1928 ; 3 : 710.
- Weill M, Lutfalla G, Mogensen K, *et al.* Comparative genomics: insecticide resistance in mosquito vectors. *Nature* 2003 ; 423(6936) : 136-7.
- Weir WR, Hodges JM, Wright JF, Higgins AF, Corringham RE. Atypical *falciparum* malaria: case report. *Br Med J* 1984 ; 289 : 178.

- Wenlock RW. The incidence of *Plasmodium* parasites in rural Zambia. *East Afr Med J* 1978 ; 55 : 268-76.
- Wenlock RW. The epidemiology of tropical parasitic diseases in rural Zambia and the consequences for public Health. *J Trop Med Hyg* 1979 ; 82 : 90-8.
- Wernsdorfer W. *Report on mission to the Sudan*. WHO/Mal/77, 1977.
- Wernsdorfer W. *Report on a visit to Gezira Province, DR of the Sudan.7-14 and 16-17 August 1977*. WHO/Mal/Geneva, 1977.
- Wernsdorfer G, Wernsdorfer W. Malaria in the middle Nile basin and its bordering regions. *Z Tropenmed Parasitol* 1967 ; 18 : 17-44.
- Wernsdorfer WH, McGregor I. *Malaria principles and practice of malariology*. Edinburgh : Churchill Livingstone, 1988, 2 vol. : 1818 p.
- Wery M. *Stratification of malarious areas in Africa. A few examples*. WHO/MAL/86.1033 ; 1986 : 18 p.
- Wery M, Coosemans M. La résistance médicamenteuse dans le paludisme. *Ann Soc Belg Med Trop* 1980 ; 60 (2) : 137-62.
- Wesenberg-Lund C. Sur les causes du changement intervenu dans le mode de nourriture d'*Anopheles maculipennis*. *CR Séances Soc Biol* 1921 ; 85 : 383-6.
- Weyer F. Beobachtungen an Hausanophelen in zusammenhang mit der rassenfrage bei *An. maculipennis*. *Z Parasitol* 1933 ; 6 : 288-334.
- Whang CH. Hibernation of mosquitoes in Korea. *Mosquito News* 1961 ; 21 : 17-20.
- Wharton RH. The habit of adult mosquitoes in Malaya. III. Feeding preferences of anophelines. *Ann Trop Med Parasitol* 1953 ; 47 : 272-84.
- Wharton RH, Eyles DE, Warren M, Moorhouse DE, Sandosham AA. Investigations leading to the identification of members of the *Anopheles umbrosus* group as the probable vectors of mouse deer malaria. *Bull World Health Organ* 1963 ; 29 : 357-74.
- Whitbourne D. Notes on the infantile mortality of the colony of Lagos, Nigeria. *West Afr J Med* 1930 ; 4 (2) : 39-45.
- White GB. The *Anopheles gambiae* complex and malaria transmission around Kisumu, Kenya. *Trans R Soc Trop Med Hyg* 1972 ; 66 : 572-81.
- White GB. Biological effects of intraspecific chromosomal polymorphism in malaria vector populations. *Bull World Health Organ* 1974 ; 50 : 299-306.
- White GB. Systematic reappraisal of the *Anopheles maculipennis* complex. *Mosq Syst* 1978 ; 10 : 13-44.
- White GB. *Anopheles bwambae n. sp*, a malaria vector in the Semliki Valley, Uganda, and its relationships with other sibling species of the *An. gambiae* complex. *Syst Entomol* 1985 ; 10 : 501-22.
- White GB, Magayuka SA, Boreham PF. Comparative studies on sibling species of the *An. gambiae* complex: bionomics and vectorial activity of species A and B at Segera, Tanzania. *Bull Entomol Res* 1972 ; 62 : 295-317.
- White GB, Rosen P. Comparative studies on sibling species of the *Anopheles gambiae* Giles complex. II. Ecology of species A and B in savannah around Kaduna, Nigeria, during transition from wet to dry season. *Bull Entomol Res* 1973 ; 62 : 613-25.
- White GB, Tessfaye F, Boreham PF, Lemma G. Malaria vector capacity of *An. arabiensis* and *An. quadriannulatus* in Ethiopia: chromosomal interpretation after six years storage of field preparations. *Trans R Soc Trop Med Hyg* 1980 ; 74 : 683-4.
- White IM, Harbach RE, Sandlant GR. *Fauna malesiana: interactive key for mosquito vectors of human disease (Diptera: Culicidae)*. CD-ROM. Biodiversity Centre of ETI, Associated Party Software. Paris : UNESCO-Publishing, 2004.
- WHO. Pesticides and their application for the vectors and pests of public health importance. WHO/CDS/WHOPES/GCDPP/2006.1.
- WHO. World malaria report. 2005. http://www.rbm.who.int/wmr2005/html/1-1.htm
- Wijesundera MS. Malaria outbreaks in new foci in Sri Lanka. *Parasitol Today* 1988 ; 4 : 147-50.
- Wildling E, Winkler S, Kremsner PG, Brandts C, Jenne L, Wernsdorfer WH. Malaria epidemiology in the province of Moyen Ogoov, Gabon. *Trop Med Parasitol* 1995 ; 46 : 77-82.
- Wilkerson RC. Redescription of *Anopheles punctimacula* and *An. malefactor* (Diptera: Culicidae). *J Med Entomol* 1990 ; 27 (2) : 225-47.
- Wilkerson RC. *Anopheles calderoni n. sp*, a malarial vector of the Arribalzagia series from Peru, (Diptera: Culicidae). *Mosq Syst* 1991 ; 23 (1) : 25-38.
- Wilkerson RC, Sallum MA. *Anopheles forattinii*: a new species in series Arribalzagia (Diptera: Culicidae). *J Med Entomol* 1999 ; 36 (3) : 345-54.
- Wilkerson RC, Li C, Rueda LM, *et al*. Molecular confirmation of *Anopheles (Anopheles) lesteri* from the Republic of South Korea and its genetic identity with *An. (Ano.) anthropophagus* from China (Diptera: Culicidae). *Zootaxa* 2003 ; 378, 1-14.
- Wilkes TG, Matola YG, Charlwood JD. *Anopheles rivulorum*, a vector of human malaria in Africa. *Med Vet Entomol* 1996 ; 10 : 108-10.
- Willcox MC, Beckman L. Haemoglobin variants, α-thalassaemia and G6PD types in Liberia. *Hum Hered* 1981 ; 31 : 339-47.
- Willcox MC, Bjorkman A, Brohult J. *Falciparum* malaria and α-thalassemia trait in Northern Liberia. *Ann Trop Med Parasitol* 1983 ; 77 : 335-47.
- Willcox MC, Bjorkman A, Brohult J. The effect of persistent malarial infections on haemoglobin A2 levels in Liberian children. *Trans R Soc Trop Med Hyg* 1985 ; 79 : 242-4.
- Williams N. Malaria strains appear to gang up against immune defenses. *Science* 1998 ; 279 : 1136.
- Williamson WA, Gilles HM. Malumfashi endemic disease research project. II. Malariometry in Malumfashi, Northern Nigeria. *Ann Trop Med Parasitol* 1978 ; 72 : 323-8.
- Wilson DB. Malaria in Madagascar. *East Afr Med J* 1947 ; 24 : 171-8.
- Wilson DB. Malaria in British Somaliland. *East Afr Med J* 1949 ; 26 : 283-91.
- Wilson DB, Garnham PC, Swellengrebel NH. A review of hyperendemic malaria. *Trop Dis Bull* 1950 ; 47 : 677-98.
- Wilson DB, Wilson ME. Rural hyperendemic malaria in Tanganyika territory. Part II. *Trans R Soc Trop Med Hyg* 1962 ; 56 : 287-93.
- WMO. *WMO statement on the status of the global climate in 1997*. Geneva : WMO, 1998 : 877.
- WMO. *WMO statement on the status of the global climate in 1998*. Geneva : WMO, 1999 : 896.
- Wolfe HL. Epidemiological data concerning one year of a malaria surveillance pilot project in Southern Rhodesia. *Bull World Health Organ* 1964 ; 31 : 707-20.
- Wolfe HL. *Plasmodium ovale* in Zambia. *Bull World Health Organ* 1968 ; 39 : 947-8.
- Woodruff AW, Adamson EA, El Suni A, Maughan TS, Karu M, Bundru N. Infants in Juba, Southern Sudan: the first six months of life. *Lancet* 1983 ; 30 : 262-4.
- Xu JJ, Feng LC. Studies on *Anopheles hyrcanus* group of mosquitoes in China. *Acta Entomol Sinica* 1975 ; 18 : 77-104.
- Xu J, Liu H. Border malaria in Yunnan, China. *Southeast Asian J Trop Med Public Health* 1997 ; 28 : 456-9.
- Yacob M, Swaroop S. The forecasting of epidemic malaria in the Punjab. *J Malaria Inst India* 1944 ; 5 : 319-35.
- Yacob M, Swaroop S. Investigation of long-term periodicity in the incidence of epidemic malaria in the Punjab. *J Malaria Inst India* 1945 ; 6 : 39-51.
- Yadav RS, Sharma VP, Ghosh SK, Kumar A. Quartan malaria: an investigation on the incidence of *Plasmodium malariae* in Bisra PHC, district Sundargarh, Orissa. *Indian J Malariol* 1990 ; 27 : 85-94.
- Yadava RL, Sharma RS. Malaria problem and its control in North-Eastern states of India. *J Commun Dis*,1995 ; 27 : 262-6.
- Yang B. Studies on some biological characteristics of *Plasmodium vivax* isolated from tropical and temperate zones of China. *Chin Med J* 1996 ; 109 : 266-71.
- Yao WL, Shen JH, Zhang ML, Wang YL, Zhang HP, Wang QD. Studies on antimalarials. VII Synthesis of alpha-(alkylaminomethyl)-2-phenyl-4-quinazoline-methanols. *Acta Pharma Sinica* 1984 ;19 (1) : 76-8.
- Yap HH. Effectiveness of soap formulations containing deet and permethrin as personal protection against outdoor mosquitoes in Malaysia. *J Am Mosq Control Assoc* 1986 ; 2 (1) : 63-7.
- Young MD, Eyles DE, Burgess RW, Jeffery GM. Experimental testing of the immunity of Negroes to *Plasmodium vivax*. *J Parasitol* 1955 ; 41 : 315-8.
- Yuan YU Studies on two forms of *Anopheles minimus* in China. *Mosq Syst* 1987 ;19 : 143-5.
- Zahar AR. Review of the ecology of malaria vectors in the WHO Eastern Mediterranean Region. *Bull World Health Organ* 1974 ; 50 : 427-40.
- Zahar AR. *Vector bionomics in the epidemiology and control of malaria*. Part I. The WHO African region and the WHO Eastern Mediterranean region. A. West Africa. VBC/85.1, 1985a. B. Equatorial Africa, C. Southern Africa. VBC/85.2, 1985b. D. East Africa, E. Eastern Outer Islands, F. Southwestern Arabia. VBC/85.3, 1985c.
- Zahar AR. *Vector bionomics in the epidemiology and control of malaria*. Part II. The WHO European region and the WHO Eastern Mediterranean region. 1990, VBC/90.1, VBC/90.2. et VBC/90.3.

- Zahar AR. *Vector bionomics in the epidemiology and control of malaria.* Part III. The WHO South East Asia Region and the WHO Western Pacific Region. 1996, CTD/MAL/96.1 et 1994, CTD/MAL/94.1.
- Zahar AR, Dabbagh HS. Malaria survey in North Western part of Saudi Arabia. *Bull Endem Dis (Baghdad)* 1959 ; 3 : 111-28.
- Zahar AR, et al. *Epidemiological evaluation of DDT spraying with studies on behaviour of* Anopheles pharoensis *in Egypt, United Arab Republic.* WHO/MAL/66.566 ; 1966 : 34 p.
- Zaim M. Malaria control in Iran. *J Am Mosq Control Assoc* 1987 ; 3 : 392-6.
- Zaim M, Javaherian Z. Occurrence of *Anopheles culicifacies* species A in Iran. *J Am Mosq Control Assoc* 1991 ; 7 : 324-6.
- Zavortink TJ, Poinar GO. *Anopheles* (*Nyssorhynchus*) *dominicanus* sp. n. (Diptera: Culicidae) from Dominican Amber. *Ann Entomol Soc Am* 2000 ; 93(6) : 1230-5.
- Zeidler O. Verbindungen von chloral mit brom und chlorbensol. *Berchte Deutschen Chemis Gesellschaft* 1874 ; 7 : 1180-1.
- Zhang ZX. An outbreak of *vivax* malaria in the final stage of malaria eradication in Haifeng, Guangdong Province. *Chin J Parasitol Parasit Dis* 1986 ; 4 : 228.
- Zhang BX, Sheng BL, Zhang HJ, *et al.* Malaria. In : Zheng G, ed. *Historical experience on preventive medicine in new China.* Beijing : People's Health Publishing House, 1998 : 286-307.
- Zhou Zu-Jie. The malaria situation in the People's Republic of China. *Bull World Health Organ* 1981 ; 59 : 931-6.
- Zhou Zu-Jie. Curent status of malaria in China. *Proc Asian Pac Conf Malaria* 1985 : 31-9.
- Zimmerman RH. Ecology of malaria vectors in the Americas and future direction. *Mem Inst Oswaldo Cruz* 1992 ; 87 (suppl. 3) : 371-83.
- Zimmerman RH, Galardo AK, Lounibos LP. Arruda M, Wirtz R. Bloodmeal hosts of *Anopheles* species (Diptera: Culicidae) in a malaria-endemic area of the Brazilian Amazon. *J Med Entomol* 2006 ; 43 : 947-56.
- Zucker JR. Changing patterns of autochthonous malaria transmission in the United States: a review of recent outbreaks. *Emerg Infect Dis* 1996 ; 2 (1) : 37-43.
- de Zulueta J. Insecticide resistance in *Anopheles sacharovi*. *Bull World Health Organ* 1959 ; 20 : 797-822.
- de Zulueta J. Changes in the geographical distribution of malaria throughout history. *Parassitologia* 1987 ;29 : 193-205.
- de Zulueta J. Forty years of malaria eradication in Sardinia. A new appraisal of a great enterprise. *Parassitologia* 1990 ; 32 : 231-6.
- de Zulueta J, Kafuko GW, Cullen JR, Pedersen CK. The results of the first year of a malaria eradication pilot project in Northern Kigezi, Uganda. *East Afr Med J* 1961 ; 38 : 1-26.
- de Zulueta J, Kafuko GW, Cullen JR. An investigation of the annual cycle of malaria in Masaka District, Uganda. *East Afr Med J* 1963 ; 40 : 469-88.
- de Zulueta J, Kafuko GW, McCrae AW, Cullen JR, Pedersen CK, Wasswa DF. A malaria eradication experiment in the Highlands of Kigezi, Uganda. *East Afr Med J* 1964 ; 41 : 102-20.
- de Zulueta J, Garrett-Jones C. An investigation on the persistence of malaria transmission in Mexico. *Am J Trop Med Hyg* 1965 ; 14 : 63-77.
- de Zulueta J, Chang TH. *Report for certification of malaria eradication in the Republic of Cyprus.* Doc. OMS non publié, 1967.
- de Zulueta J, Ramsdale CD, Coluzzi M. Receptivity to malaria in Europe. *Bull World Health Organ* 1975 ; 52 : 109-11.
- de Zulueta J, Ramsdale CD, Cianchi R, Bullini L, Coluzzi M. On the taxonomic status of *Anopheles sicaulti*. *Parassitologia* 1983 ; 25 : 73-92.

Species Index

Abbreviations used throughout the index

Afr: Afrotropical Region
Amer: American Regions
Aust: Australasian Region
Or: Oriental Region
Pal: Palaearctic Region
Ubi: ubiquitous

An: *Anopheles*
Alg: algae
Bact: entomopathogenic bacteria
Fung: entomopathogenic fungus
Haemopar: haemoparasite

P: *Plasmodium*
Pha: phanerogam
Par: parasite
Syn: synonymy with

Plants (including bacteria)

Acacia xantholacca (Afr, Pha): 165, 320
Artemisia annua (Or, Pha): 4, 6, 10, 352
Avicennnia sp. (Ubi, Pha): 71, 91, 94, 104
Azolla (Alg): 376
Bacillus thuringiensis (Bact): 252, 367, 376, 377

Ceratophyllus sp.: 202
Cinchona (Amer, Pha): 4, 9, 266, 288, 302, 339, 345, 357
Cinchona ledgeriana (Amer, Pha): 4
Eleocharis: 277
Naja: 202

Nosema algerae (Fung): 221
Paspalum (Pha): 91, 94, 104, 152, 156
Rhizophora sp. (Ubi, Pha): 72, 91, 94, 104
Spirogyra (Ubi, Alg): 279

Protozoa (and hosts)

Adeleidae (Par, insects): 12, 13
Coccidiomorpha (sporozoan): 12
Eimeriidae (Par, vertebrates digestive tract): 12, 13
Haemoproteus (Haemopar, vertebrates): 12, 13
Haemosporidae (Haemopar, vertebrates): 12, 13
Hepatocystis (Haemopar, vertebrates): 12, 13, 15
Laverania (Afr, humans, apes): 13, 14
Leucocytozoonidae (birds): 13
Oscillarium malariae: 4
Plasmodidae (Haemopar): 12, 13
P. s.g. Carinia (lizards): 13
P. s.g. Giovannolaia (birds): 13

P. s.g. Haemamoeba (birds): 13
P. s.g. Huufia (birds): 13
P. s.g. Laverania (humans, apes): 13, 14
P. s.g. Novyella (birds): 13
P. s.g. Ophidellia (snakes): 13
P. s.g. Plasmodium (mammals): 13, 14
P. s.g. Sauromoeba (lizards): 13
P. s.g. Vinckeia (rodents): 13
P. agamae (Afr, saurians): 94
P. bastianelli (Or, primates): 15
P. berghei (Afr, rodents): 124, 126
P. brasilianum (= *P. malariae*) (Amer, primates): 13, 14, 37, 265, 280, 289, 293, 294
P. cynomolgi (Or, monkeys): 5, 14, 15, 209
P. cynomolgi bastianelli (Or, primates): 195
P. eylesi (Or, gibbons): 15

P. falciparum (Ubi, humans): 3-6, 10, 11, 13-17, 23-26, 28, 29, 31, 33, 34, 37-39, 40-43, 49-53, 55, 63, 76, 78, 80, 86, 90, 92, 94, 95, 97, 102-107, 109, 111, 116-122, 127, 131, 133, 135-138, 140, 143, 144, 149, 153-156, 158, 159, 161, 162, 167, 170-172, 176, 178, 183, 184, 186, 187, 195, 202, 206, 207, 210-220, 223-225, 228-231, 235, 237-239, 241-243, 245, 247-251, 254, 255, 257-262, 265-270, 272, 274-276, 278-294, 296-298, 301-303, 305-307, 316, 319, 325, 328, 331-336, 342, 346, 347, 353, 354, 355, 357, 359, 372, 374, 375, 382-385
P. giganteum (Afr, lizards) : 94
P. hylobati (Or, gibbons): 15
P. inui (Or, monkeys): 13, 15
P. jeffreyei (Or, orang-utans): 15

P. knowlesi (Or, monkeys): 14, 15
P. malariae (= *P. brasilianum*) (Ubi, primates): 3-6, 13, 14, 23, 25, 33, 37, 39, 40, 49, 63, 76, 90, 94, 95, 97, 102, 104-106, 109, 110, 120, 121, 124, 126, 128, 133, 137, 138, 144, 148, 149, 158, 159, 162, 176, 183, 184, 194, 214, 218, 219, 229, 230, 238, 242, 243, 245, 248-250, 254, 257, 258, 261, 265-270, 272, 274, 278-282, 285-290, 292-294, 296, 302, 305, 306, 325, 334, 347
P. mexicanum (Amer, lizards): 13
P. ovale (humans): 4-6, 10, 13, 14, 23-26, 38-40, 76, 94, 95, 97, 104, 110, 116, 118, 121, 124, 133, 137, 144, 148, 158, 162, 176, 184, 194, 229, 239, 347
P. pitheci (Or, orang-utans): 15
P. reichenowi (Afr, chimpanzees): 13, 14, 126
P. rodhaini (= *P. malariae*) (Afr, chimpanzees): 14, 126
P. schwetzi (Afr, chimpanzees, gorillas): 13, 14, 126
P. simiovale (= *P. vivax-like*) (Amer, Or, primates): 13, 14, 25, 195, 280, 296
P. simium (Amer, primates): 13, 14, 25, 37, 265, 280, 294, 295
P. vinckei (Afr, rodents): 117, 124
P. vivax (Ubi, humans): 3-6, 10, 13-15, 23-25, 27, 28, 33, 34, 37-41, 49, 50, 52, 53, 59, 63, 64, 76, 86, 97, 104, 107, 112, 118, 119, 124, 132, 133, 136-140, 143, 144, 155, 158, 164, 170-172, 176, 178, 182-184, 187, 194, 195, 203, 206-220, 223-225, 228-230, 235-240, 242, 243, 245, 247-251, 254, 256, 258-263, 265-272, 274-294, 296-298, 302, 303, 305-307, 313, 316, 325, 328, 329, 331, 334, 335, 347, 350,-353, 355, 359, 373, 374, 382, 383
P. vivax collinsi (Ubi, humans): 25, 280
P. vivax hibernans (Pal, humans): 25, 38, 230, 243, 263
P. vivax-like (= *P. simiovale*) (Amer, Or, primates): 13, 14, 25, 195, 272, 280, 296
P. yangi (Or, gibbons): 15
P. yoeli (Afr, rodents): 118

Arthropods

Aedes sp.: 13, 17, 66, 97
Aedes s.g. *Diceromyia*: 66
Aedes s.g. *Stegomyia*: 66, 367
Aedes aegypti 5, 97, 340, 367
Aedes simpsoni: 97
Anophelinae: 12, 13, 15, 37
Anopheles: 15
An. s.g. *Anopheles*: 15, 189, 195, 275, 276
An. s.g. *Cellia*: 15, 189, 195, 231
An. s.g. *Kerteszia*: 15, 20, 274-276, 280, 288, 295, 298
An. s.g. *Lophopodomyia*: 15
An. s.g. *Nyssorhynchus*: 12, 15, 275, 276, 280, 294
An. s.g. *Stethomyia*: 15
An. aconitus (Or): 18, 189, 202, 203, 207, 210, 211, 215-217, 315, 316
An. adenensis (Afr): 75, 140
An. albimanus (Amer): 18, 20, 25, 63, 266-269, 271-277, 282-289
An. albitarsis (Amer): 270, 273, 276, 280, 296, 297
An. alexandroeschingarevi (Pal): 231
An. allopha (Amer): 18, 276, 280, 296, 297
An. annularis (Or): 18, 189, 207-211, 215, 220
An. annulipes (Aust): 182
An. anthropophagus (Pal, Or): 18, 62, 195, 207, 214, 236, 237, 261, 316, 374, 375
An. aquasalis (Amer): 18, 20, 268-270, 273, 275, 276, 277, 278, 285-287, 291-293, 317, 322
An. arabiensis (Afr): 7, 15, 16, 18, 20, 27, 37, 45, 60, 66-72, 79-84, 86-93, 97-100, 104, 105, 107-112, 114-117, 125, 130, 132, 135, 137-143, 145, 146, 148, 152, 156, 158, 159, 161-167, 170-174, 178, 179, 188, 231, 238, 249, 254, 307, 314, 315, 317-319, 321, 322, 329, 332, 333, 367, 368, 375, 377-379
An. aruni (Afr): 72, 152, 166, 167
An. atroparvus (Pal): 7, 15, 17, 18, 19, 62, 230, 231, 233-235, 238, 239, 242, 243, 317, 333
An. aztecus (Amer): 266, 2734, 280, 282
An. balabacensis (Or): 16, 18, 20, 189, 190, 194, 198-200, 203, 215-218
An. bambusicolus (Amer): 280
An. bancrofti (Aust): 182
An. barbirostris (Or): 18, 189, 203, 215, 217
An. barbumbrosus (Or): 181, 182
An. basilii (Pal): 231
An. beklemishevi (Pal): 15, 231, 234, 235, 243, 263
An. bellator (Amer): 18, 268, 270, 272, 274, 276, 280, 285, 292, 298
An. benarrochi (Amer): 289
An. boliviensis (Amer): 280
An. braziliensis (Amer): 18, 273, 276, 280, 296
An. brucei (Afr): 72, 167
An. brunnipes (Afr): 18, 67, 75, 92, 114, 125, 126
An. bwambae (Afr): 16, 67, 72, 148
An. calderoni: 273
An. cambournaci: 231
An. campestris (Or): 18, 189, 203, 215, 216
An. candidiensis (Or), variant of *An. jeyporiensis*: 261
An. carnevalei (Afr): 74, 97, 116
An. chrystii (Afr): 75, 314
An. cinereus (Afr): 124, 247, 314
An. claviger (Pal): 5, 18, 237, 247, 248, 250, 260
An. clowi (Aust): 182
An. confusus (Afr): 72, 152, 153, 167
An. costai (Afr): 295
An. costalis: 148, 178
An. coustani (Afr): 18, 75, 177, 178
An. cruzii (Amer): 270, 273, 274, 276, 280, 294, 298
An. culicifacies (Or, Pal): 7, 16, 20, 62, 67, 138, 140, 188, 190, 204-2076, 209, 219-221, 223-226, 238, 254-257, 316, 322, 376, 377, 379
An. culicifacies A (Or, Pal): 18, 75, 189, 223, 238, 255, 257, 315-317
An. culicifacies B (Or): 189, 205, 225, 316
An. culicifacies C (Or): 18, 189
An. culicifacies D (Or): 18, 189
An. culicifacies E (Or): 18, 189, 205, 206, 220, 225, 311
An. darlingi (Amer): 7, 16, 18, 20, 21, 63, 266-270, 273-278, 282-284, 286-298, 314, 316-318, 322, 323, 367
An. deaneorum (Amer): 18, 276, 280, 296
An. dirus (Or): 9, 16, 20, 21, 23, 52, 62, 188-190, 192-194, 198-202, 208, 210-213, 261, 313-316, 318, 3201, 323, 328, 367, 375
An. dirus A (= *An. dirus*) (Or): 18, 21, 189, 198, 211, 213, 214, 261
An. dirus B (= *An. cracens*) (Or): 18, 189, 198, 215, 216
An. dirus C (= *An. scanloni*) (Or): 18, 189, 198

Species Index

An. dirus D (= *An. baimaii*) (Or): 18, 21, 189, 198, 210, 214, 220, 365

An. dirus E (Or) (= *An. elegans*): 189

An. dispar: 200, 201

An. donaldi (Or): 18, 189, 203, 215, 216

An. dravidicus (Or): 200, 201

An. dthali (Afr, Pal): 18, 67, 76, 87, 112, 135, 138, 140, 141, 238, 254

An. elegans (Or): 198

An. elutris: 231

An. elutus (Or): 231

An. epiroticus (Or): 201, 202, 209, 211, 214, 216

An. fallax: 231

An. farauti (Aust): 7, 16, 181-184, 186, 187, 365, 373, 375

An. farauti n°1 (Aust): 18, 180-182, 186, 187

An. farauti n°2 (Aust): 181, 182, 187

An. farauti n°3 (Aust): 181, 182

An. farauti n°4 (Aust): 182

An. farauti n°5 (Aust): 182

An. farauti n°6 (Aust): 182

An. farauti n°7 (Aust): 182

An. flavicosta (Afr): 75, 104, 105, 166

An. flavirostris (Or): 189, 202, 203, 215-217, 316

An. fluminensis (Or): 289

An. fluviatilis (Or, Pal): 9, 16, 18, 52, 62, 75, 188-190, 194, 197, 202, 204, 205, 209, 210, 219-221, 223, 224, 226, 238, 257-260, 313, 375

An. forattinii (Amer): 280, 295

An. freeborni (Amer): 18, 266, 273, 275, 279, 282

An. funestus (Afr): 16, 18, 20, 25, 37, 44, 45, 60, 66, 67, 72, 73, 76, 78-83, 86-95, 97-102, 104, 105, 107-120, 123, 124, 126-128, 137-143, 145, 146, 148, 149, 152-154, 158, 159, 161, 162, 164-167, 169-179, 301, 304, 307, 314-318, 321, 322, 332, 333, 368, 374, 377, 379, 383

An. fuscivenosus (Afr): 72, 167

An. galvaoi (Amer): 276, 280

An. gambiae (Afr): 7, 11, 15-17, 20, 23, 25, 27, 60, 66, 67-73, 78, 79, 82-84, 86, 89, 91, 93-95, 97, 98, 100-106, 108-111, 113, 115-119, 122, 124, 125, 127, 135, 138, 143, 145-148, 150-154, 156, 162-165, 167, 170, 173-176, 178, 179, 247-249, 270, 287, 301, 304, 315, 317, 318, 322, 323, 331-333, 335, 336, 340, 341, 378, 379, 383

An. gambiae s.s. (Afr): 16, 18, 21, 26, 37, 45, 66-71, 73, 75, 77, 79, 81-84, 88-95, 97, 100, 102-105, 107-111, 114-120, 122, 123, 125, 130-132, 135, 137, 142, 143, 145, 146, 148-152, 156, 158, 161-165, 167, 170-178, 313-319, 322, 332, 367, 374-379

An. greeni (Or): 200, 201

An. hanckoki (Afr): 95

An. hargreavesi (Afr): 18, 67, 76, 100-102, 104, 119

An. hectoris (Amer): 266

An. hermsi (Amer): 18, 273, 275, 276, 279, 282, 329

An. hispaniola (Pal): 112, 247, 248

An. homunculus (Amer): 273, 274, 276, 280

An. hyrcanus (Pal): 18, 189, 207, 236, 251, 259, 260, 316-318

An. introlatus (Or): 198

An. jeyporiensis (Or): 189, 207, 213, 214

An. karwari (Aust): 181, 182

An. koliensis (Aust): 18, 181-184, 186, 187

An. kunmingensis (Or) (Syn *An. liangshanensis*): 207, 214, 236, 237

An. labranchiae (Pal): 3, 5, 15, 17, 18, 62, 229-235, 238, 239, 241, 246-249, 306, 315, 332

An. laneanus (Amer): 280

An. leesoni (Afr): 72, 152, 167, 202

An. lesteri (Or): 189, 207, 214, 236, 237, 261, 263, 316, 373, 374

An. lesteri anthropophagus (Or): 237

An. letifer (Or): 18, 189, 204, 215, 216

An. leucosphyrus (Or): 7, 16, 18, 198, 200, 202, 215

An. leucosphyrus A (= *An. latens*) (Or): 189, 216, 217

An. leucosphyrus B (= *An. leucosphyrus*) (Or): 189, 200

An. lewisi (Pal): 231

An. litoralis (Or): 18, 189, 203 ,215, 218

An. ludlowi (Or): 215

An. maculatus (Or): 18, 189, 193, 200-202, 208-211, 214-216, 314

An. maculipennis (Pal): 7, 15, 18, 62, 63, 188, 230-235, 238, 242, 243, 245, 246, 251, 256, 257, 260, 275, 319, 329

An. maculipennis s.l. (Pal): 5, 15

An. mangyanus (Or): 18, 189, 203, 215

An. marajoara (Amer): 18, 276, 280, 297

An. marshalli (Afr): 124, 126, 167, 314

An. martinius (Pal): 15, 231, 232, 260

An. mascarensis (Afr): 18, 60, 67, 75, 170, 171, 173, 177, 178

An. mediopunctatus (Amer): 280, 295

An. melanoon (Pal): 18, 231, 232, 234, 235, 251

An. melas (Afr): 15, 16, 18, 20, 67, 71, 72, 83, 90, 91-95, 97-99, 102-104, 114, 116, 118, 119, 123, 125, 155, 156, 340, 375

An. merus (Afr): 15, 16, 18, 20, 67, 71, 141, 142, 145, 151, 152, 158, 161, 163, 164, 167, 173, 176-178

An. messeae (Pal): 5, 7, 15, 18, 19, 62, 230, 231-235, 238, 239, 242, 243, 245, 260, 261, 263, 319

An. minimus (Or): 16, 20, 23, 52, 62, 74, 188, 190, 193-199, 202, 204, 208-211, 213, 214, 220, 260, 261, 311, 313, 315, 316, 318, 320, 323, 328, 367, 375

An. minimus A (= *An. minimus*) (Or): 18, 21, 189, 197, 198, 211, 213, 214, 260, 378

An. minimus C (= *An. harrisoni*) (Or): 18, 72, 189, 197, 198, 204, 211, 214, 260, 378

An. minimus E (Or): 197, 214, 263

An. moucheti (Afr): 17, 18, 20, 67, 74, 75, 78, 83, 93, 96, 114-120, 122, 123, 126, 128, 135, 142, 148

An. moucheti bervoesti (Afr): 75

An. moucheti nigeriensis (Afr): 104

An. multicolor (Pal): 112, 238, 249, 315

An. neivai (Amer): 273, 274, 276, 280, 287, 288, 293

An. nemophilous (Or): 198

An. nili (Afr): 16, 20, 67, 74, 78, 79, 83, 92-94, 97, 100-102, 104, 105, 107, 113-117, 119, 120, 123, 125, 126, 128, 135, 137-139, 141, 142, 156, 161

An. nili s.l. (Afr): 18, 74

An. nimpe (Or): 189, 202, 207, 236

An. nivipes (Or): 18, 189, 203, 207-211, 213, 315, 316

An. notanandai (Or): 200, 201

An. nuneztovari (Amer): 9, 18, 273-276, 278, 286, 287, 289-292, 294, 297, 316

An. obscurus (Afr): 17, 104

An. oswaldoi (Amer): 273, 276, 280, 286, 289, 292, 294, 296, 297

An. ovengensis (Afr): 74, 116

An. paltrinieri (Pal): 238, 255

An. paludis (Afr): 17, 18, 67, 75, 114, 116, 117, 119, 126

An. parensis (Afr): 72, 152

An. pattoni (Pal): 238

An. petragnani (Pal): 237

An. pharoensis (Afr, Pal): 18, 20, 67, 75, 88, 89, 102, 114, 116, 130, 135, 137-140, 142, 145, 146, 148, 153, 156, 161, 164, 317

An. philippinensis (Or): 16, 18, 189, 203, 207, 209-211, 220

An. plumbeus (Pal): 18, 238

An. pseudopunctipennis (Amer): 16, 20, 63, 264, 266-269, 273-275, 278, 279, 282-290, 373, 377

An. pseudowillmori (Or): 18, 189, 193, 200, 201, 211, 214, 314

An. pulcherrimus (Or, Pal): 18, 188, 189, 195, 207, 223, 236, 237, 259, 260, 316
An. punctimacula (Amer): 273, 280
An. punctulatus (Aust): 18, 61, 180-187
An. quadriannulatus (Afr): 15, 16, 67, 72, 125, 138, 152, 158, 160, 162-164, 167, 378
An. quadrimaculatus (Amer): 18, 234, 266, 273, 275, 276, 279, 281, 329, 334
An. rangeli (Amer): 273, 280, 289, 290
An. rennelensis (Or): 182
An. rivulorum (Afr): 18, 72, 111, 142, 152, 167
An. rivulorum-like (Afr): 72
An. rufipes (Afr): 21, 104, 112
An. sacharovi (Pal): 3, 5, 8, 15, 17, 18, 62, 188, 226, 229-235, 238, 239, 241-244, 246, 250, 251, 256-258, 260, 306, 316, 317, 379
An. saperoi (Pal): 208, 215, 263
An. sawadwongporni (Or): 18, 189, 193, 200, 201, 209, 211, 314
An. selengensis (Pal): 231
An. sergentii (Pal): 18, 62, 75, 112, 188, 207, 230, 231, 235, 246-250, 254, 255, 367, 377
An. shannoni (Amer): 295
An. sicaulti (Pal) (Syn *An. labranchiae*): 15, 18, 230-233, 247, 248
An. sinensis (Or, Pal): 18, 62, 189, 195, 207, 214, 215, 230, 236, 237, 243, 260, 261, 263, 316, 373-375, 379
An. somalicus (Afr): 74, 116
An. splendidus (Or): 214
An. stephensi (Or, Pal): 7, 16, 18, 62, 75, 188, 189, 206, 207, 210, 221, 223, 224, 226, 238, 253-259, 315, 321, 322, 367, 377
An. strodei (Amer): 276, 280, 290, 296
An. subalpinus (Pal) (Syn *An. melanoon*): 231, 232, 235, 251
An. subpictus (Or): 18, 181, 182, 189, 202, 207-209, 214, 215, 217, 221, 225, 226, 315, 316, 321, 322, 332, 377
An. sundaicus (Or): 16, 18, 20, 62, 189, 194, 200-202, 209-211, 213-217, 316, 340
An. sundaicus D (Or): 201, 209, 210
An. sundaicus E (Or): 201, 216, 217
An. superpictus (Or, Pal): 18, 62, 188, 189, 195, 207, 223, 224, 230, 231, 236, 241, 242, 245, 246,250, 251, 254, 256-260
An. takasagoensis (Or): 16, 198
An. tessellatus (Or): 18, 189, 208, 214, 215, 225, 316
An. triannulatus (Amer): 18, 276, 280, 289, 294, 296, 297
An. trinkae (Amer): 273, 276, 280, 289
An. umbrosus (Or): 203
An. vagus (Or): 18, 189, 208, 215, 322
An. vaneedeni (Afr): 72, 167
An. varuna (Or): 18, 189, 203, 208
An. vestitipennis (Amer): 18, 267, 273, 275, 279, 280, 283, 284
An. willmori (Or): 18, 189, 200, 201, 208-210
An. wellcomei (Afr): 119, 139
An. ziemanni (Afr): 119, 130, 138
Bironella (Aust, anophelinae): 15
Chagasia (Amer, anophelinae): 15, 37
Chrysops dimidiata (Afr, tabanidae): 96
Chrysops silacea (Afr, tabanidae): 96
Culex sp.: 5, 13, 17, 66, 363, 365, 377, 379
Culex quinquefasciatus (Ubi, culicinae): 6, 175, 177, 332, 364, 366, 376, 377, 379
Culicinae: 12, 13
Culicoides sp. (ceratopogidae): 12
Glossina tachinoides (Afr, muscidae): 83, 114
Herculia migrivitta (Aust, lepidopteran): 216
Hippoboscidae: 12
Ornithodoros moubata (Afr, mite): 164
Phlebotomus argentipes (Or, psycodidae): 222
Simulim damnosum s.l. (Afr, simulidae): 71
Stomoxys sp. (Ubi, muscidae): 12

Vertebrates

Mammals

Aotus trivirgatus (Amer): 14
Alouatta fusca (Amer): 294
Alouatta seniculus (Amer): 293
Ateles paniscus (Amer): 293, 294
Callicebus personatus (Amer): 294
Callithris anita (Amer): 294
Cebus apella (Amer): 294
Homo erectus (Afr, Or, Pal): 132, 304, 324

Homo ergaster (Afr): 132, 304
Homo habilis (Afr): 132, 304
Homo sapiens sapiens (Ubi): 132, 301 304, 312, 324
Pithecia pithecia (Amer): 293
Saguinus midas (Amer): 293
Saimiri sciureus (Amer): 15
Saimiri ustus (Amer): 294
Thamnomys surdaster (Afr): 117, 124, 126

Reptiles and fish

Aphanius dispar (Afr, Pal): 140, 256, 377
Bothriospondylus madagascariensis (Afr): 64
Gambusia affinis (Amer, Ubi): 169, 235, 248, 252, 340, 377
Oreochromis spilurus (Afr): 141, 377

Achevé d'imprimer par Corlet, Imprimeur, S.A. - 14110 Condé-sur-Noireau
N° d'Imprimeur : 109451 - Dépôt légal : janvier 2008 - *Imprimé en France*